PRINCIPLES OF HEALTH CARE ETHICS

Second Edition

PRINCIPLES OF HEALTH CARE ETHICS

Second Edition

Edited by

Richard E. Ashcroft

Queen Mary, University of London, Barts and the London Medical School,
Institute of Health Sciences Education, London, UK

Angus Dawson

Centre for Professional Ethics, School of Law, Keele University, Staffordshire, UK

Heather Draper

Centre for Biomedical Ethics, University of Birmingham, Birmingham, UK

John R. McMillan

Philosophy Department, The University of Hull, Hull, UK

John Wiley & Sons, Ltd

Other Wiley Editorial Offices

John Wiley & Sons Inc., 111 River Street, Hoboken, NJ 07030, USA

Jossey-Bass, 989 Market Street, San Francisco, CA 94103-1741, USA

Wiley-VCH Verlag GmbH, Boschstr. 12, D-69469 Weinheim, Germany

John Wiley & Sons Australia Ltd, 42 McDougall Street, Milton, Queensland 4064, Australia

John Wiley & Sons (Asia) Pte Ltd, 2 Clementi Loop #02-01, Jin Xing Distripark, Singapore 129809

John Wiley & Sons Canada Ltd, 6045 Freemont Blvd, Mississauga, Ontario, L5R 4J3, Canada

Wiley also publishes its books in a variety of electronic formats. Some content that appears in print may not be available in electronic books.

Anniversary Logo Design: Richard J. Pacifico

Library of Congress Cataloging-in-Publication Data

Principles of health care ethics. – 2nd ed. / edited by Richard E.
Ashcroft... [et al.].
          p.; cm.
  Includes bibliographical references and index.
ISBN-13: 978-0-470-02713-4
    1. Medical ethics. I. Ashcroft, Richard E.
[DNLM: 1. Ethics, Clinical. 2. Bioethical Issues. 3. Biomedical
Technology–ethics. 4. Delivery of Health Care–ethics.
5. Professional-Patient Relations–ethics. 6. Social Medicine. WB 60 P957 2007]
R724.P69 2007
174.2–dc22   2006038748

British Library Cataloguing in Publication Data

A catalogue record for this book is available from the British Library

ISBN 978-0-470-02713-4

Typeset in 9/11pt Times by Thomson Digital
Printed and bound in Great Britain by Antony Rowe Ltd, Chippenham, Wiltshire
This book is printed on acid-free paper responsibly manufactured from sustainable forestry
in which at least two trees are planted for each one used for paper production.

Contents

Contributors

TINEKE A. ABMA Professor, Department of Health Ethics and Philosophy, PO Box 616, Faculty of Health Sciences, Universiteit Maastricht, 6200 MD Maastricht, The Netherlands. Email: t.abma@zw.unimaas.nl

PASCALE ALLOTEY Chair in Race and Diversity, School of Health Sciences and Social Care, and, Centre for Public Health Research, Brunel University, Uxbridge UB8 3PH, UK. Email: Pascale.Allotey@brunel.ac.uk

DAVID W. ARCHARD Director, Institute for Philosophy & Public Policy (IPPP), Furness College, Lancaster University, Lancaster LA1 4YG, UK. Email: d.archard@lancaster.ac.uk

ADRIENNE ASCH Edward and Robin Milstein Professor of Bioethics, Wurzweiler School of Social Work, Albert Einstein College of Medicine, Yeshiva University, 2495 Amsterdam Avenue, New York, NY 10033, USA. Email: asch@yu.edu

RICHARD E. ASHCROFT Professor of Biomedical Ethics, Queen Mary University of London, Barts and the London Medical School, Institute of Health Sciences Education, 38–40 New Road, London E1 2AX, UK. Email: r.ashcroft@qmul.ac.uk

NAFSIKA ATHANASSOULIS Lecturer in Ethics, Centre for Professional Ethics, School of Law, Keele University, Staffordshire, ST5 5BG, UK. Email: n.athanassoulis@peak.keele.ac.uk

MARGARET P. BATTIN Distinguished University Professor, Division of Medical Ethics, 260 Central Campus Drive, Room 341, University of Utah, Salt Lake City, UT 84112-9156, USA. Email: battin@utah.edu

TOM L. BEAUCHAMP Professor of Philosophy, Department of Philosophy, Georgetown University, New North 215–37th and O Streets, NW Washington, DC 20057, USA. Email: beauchat@georgetown.edu

GRAHAM M. BEHR Consultant Psychiatrist and Honorary Senior Lecturer in Psychiatry, South Paddington Team, Central and North West London Mental Health NHS Trust, 7A Woodfield Road, London, W9 2NW, UK. Email: graham.behr@nhs.net

SOLOMON R. BENATAR Professor of Medicine, Director Bioethics Centre, Department of Medicine, University of Cape Town, J Floor Old Main Building, Groote Schuur Hospital, Observatory 7925, Western Cape, South Africa. Email: sbenatar@uctgsh1.uct.ac.za or solly.benatar@utoronto.ca

PIERS BENN Lecturer, Division of Epidemiology, Public Health and Primary Care, Imperial College London, Reynolds Building, St Dunstan's Road, London W6 8RP, UK. Email: p.benn@imperial.ac.uk

REBECCA BENNETT Senior Lecturer in Bioethics, The Centre for Social Ethics and Policy, School of Law, University of Manchester, Williamson Building, Oxford Road, Manchester M13 9PL, UK. Email: rebecca.bennett@manchester.ac.uk

TIM BOND Reader in Counselling and Professional Ethics, Graduate School of Education, University of Bristol, 35 Berkeley Square, Bristol, BS8 1JA. Email: Tim.Bond@bristol.ac.uk

ANNETTEE J. BRAUNACK-MAYER Associate Professor, Discipline of Public Health, The University of Adelaide, Mail Drop 207, Adelaide SA 5005, Australia. Email: annette.braunackmayer@adelaide.edu.au

DAN W. BROCK Frances Glessner Lee Professor of Medical Ethics at Harvard Medical School and Chair of the Division of Medical Ethics, Harvard Program in Ethics and Health, Harvard Medical School, 641 Huntington Avenue, 4th Floor, Boston, MA 02115, USA. Email: dan_brock@hms.harvard.edu

HOWARD BRODY University Distinguished Professor, Family Practice, Philosophy, and Centre for Ethics and Humanities in the Life Sciences, B100 Clinical Center, Michigan State University, East Lansing, MI 48824, USA. Email: Howard.Brody@ht.msu.edu

LINDA S. CARR-LEE Research Associate/Course Coordinator, Division of Medical Ethics, LDS Hospital, 8th Ave and C Street, Salt Lake City, UT 84143, USA. Email: Linda.Carr-Lee@intermountainmail.org

ADRIAN CARTER Office of Public Policy and Ethics, Institute for Molecular Bioscience, and The Queensland Brain Institute, University of Queensland, Ritchie Building (64A) (C Wing), St Lucia, QLD, 4072, Australia. Email: adrian.carter@uq.edu.au

RUTH CHADWICK Professor, CESAGen: ESRC Centre for Economic and Social Aspects of Genomics: a Lancaster-Cardiff collaboration, Cardiff Law School, Cardiff University, Museum Avenue, Cardiff CF10 3XJ, UK. Email: chadwickr1@cardiff.ac.uk

IAIN CHALMERS Editor, James Lind Library, The James Lind Initiative, Summertown Pavillion, Middle Way, Oxford OX2 7LG, UK. Email: Ichalmers@jameslindlibrary.org

JAMES F. CHILDRESS Hollingsworth Professor, Institute for Practical Ethics and Public Life, University of Virginia, PO Box 400800, Charlottesville, VA 22904, USA. Email: jfc7c@virginia.edu

ANGUS CLARKE Department of Medical Genetics, University Hospital of Wales, Health Park, Cardiff CF14 4XN, UK. Email: clarkeaj@cardiff.ac.uk

MIKE CLARKE Professor, Director, UK Cochrane Centre, NHS R&D Programme, Summertown Pavillion, Middle Way, Oxford OX2 7LG, UK. Email: mclarke@cochrane.co.uk, mike.clarke@ctsu.ox.ac.uk

STEVEN S. COUGHLIN Epidemiology and Applied Research Branch, Division of Cancer Prevention and Control, National Center for Chronic Disease Prevention and Health Promotion, Centers for Disease Control and Prevention, 4770 Buford Highway, NE (K-55), Atlanta, GA 30341, USA. Email: sic9@cdc.gov

HAROLD COWARD Director, Centre for Studies in Religion and Society, University of Victoria, PO Box 3045, Victoria, BC V8W 3P4 Canada. Email: csrs@uvvm.uvic.ca

ALAN CRIBB Professor of Bioethics and Education, Centre for Public Policy Research, King's College London, Strand, London WC2R 2LS, UK. Email: alan.cribb@kcl.ac.uk

GARRETT CULLITY Associate Professor, Department of Philosophy, The University of Adelaide, Adelaide SA 5005, Australia. Email: garrett.cullity@adelaide.edu.au

ANTHONY J. CULYER Chief Scientist, Institute for Work & Health, 481 University Avenue, Toronto, ON, M5G 2E9, Canada. Email: aculyer@iwh.on.ca

DANIELA CUTAŞ Research Fellow, CSEP/IMLAB, School of Law, University of Manchester, Williamson Building, Oxford Road, M13 9PL, UK. Email: Daniela.Cutas@manchester.ac.uk

MARION DANIS Head, Section on Ethics and Health Policy, Department of Clinical Bioethics, Warren G. Magnuson Clinical Center, Building 10 Room 1C118, National Institutes of Health, Bethesda, MD 20892-1156, USA. Email: mdanis@nih.gov

ANGUS DAWSON Senior Lecturer in Ethics and Philosophy, Centre for Professional Ethics, School of Law, Keele University, Staffordshire, ST5 5BG, UK. Email: a.j.dawson@keele.ac.uk

DAVID DEGRAZIA Professor of Philosophy, Department of Philosophy, George Washington University, Phillips 525, Washington DC 20052, USA. Email: ddd@gwu.edu

JACK DOWIE Emeritus Professor of Health Impact Analysis, Public Health and Policy Dept, London School of Hygiene and Tropical Medicine, Keppel Street, London WC1E 7HT, UK. Email: Jack.Dowie@lshtm.ac.uk

HEATHER DRAPER Reader in Biomedical Ethics, Centre for Biomedical Ethics, Department of General Practice and Primary Care, Primary Care Clinical Sciences Building, University of Birmingham, Edgbaston, Birmingham B15 2TT, UK. Email: h.draper@bham.ac.uk

REBECCA S. DRESSER Daniel Noyes Kirby Professor of Law and Professor of Ethics in Medicine, School of Law and School of Medicine, Washington University in St Louis, Law School-Box 1120, One Brookings Drive, St Louis, MO 63130, USA. Email: dresser@wulaw.wustl.edu

STEVEN D. EDWARDS Centre for Philosophy, Humanities and Law in Healthcare, School of Health Science, University of Wales, 7th Floor Vivian Building, Swansea SA2 8PP, UK. Email: s.d.edwards@swansea.ac.uk

EZEKIEL EMANUEL Chair, Department of Clinical Bioethics at the Warren G. Magnuson Clinical Center, National Institutes of Health, 10 Center Drive, Building 10, Room 1C118, Bethesda, MD 20892-1156, USA. Email: eemanuel@nih.gov

J.S. EMMANUEL Consultant Psychiatrist and Honorary Senior Lecturer in Psychiatry, Central and North West London Mental Health NHS Trust, 7A Woodfield Road, London, W9 2NW, UK.

VERONICA ENGLISH Deputy Head of Medical Ethics Department, British Medical Association, BMA House, Tavistock Square, London WC1H 9JP, UK. Email: venglish@bma.org.uk

MARTYN EVANS Professor of Humanities in Medicine, Centre for Arts and Humanities in Health and Medicine, University of Durham, Dawson Building, Science Site, South Road, Durham DH1 3HP, UK. Email: h.m.evans@durham.ac.uk

JAMES FLORY MD Student, School of Medicine, University of Pennsylvania, 295 John Morgan Building, 3620 Hamilton Walk, Philadelphia, PA 19104-6055, USA.

BENNETT FODDY Research Student, Centre for Applied Philosophy and Public Ethics, University of Melbourne, Victoria 3010, Australia; and Australian Stem Cell Centre, Monash University, Victoria 3800, Australia. Email: bennett@foddy.net

NORMAN MICHAEL FORD Director, Caroline Chisholm Centre for Health Ethics, East Melbourne; Senior Honorary Research Fellow, Bioethics, Monash University, Melbourne; Lecturer in Bioethics, Melbourne College of Divinity, Australia. Email: nford@mercy.com.au

LESLIE P. FRANCIS Alfred C. Emery Professor of Law, S.J. Quinney College of Law, University of Utah, 332 South 1400 East, Salt Lake City, UT 84112-0730, USA. Email: Francisl@law.utah.edu

JIM GALLAGHER Centre for Ethics in Public Policy and Corporate Governance, Glasgow Caledonian University, 70 Cowcaddens Road, Glasgow G4 0BA, UK. Email: Jim.Gallagher@scotland.gsi.gov.uk

KERRY A. GALVIN Junior Research Fellow, Department of Anatomy and Structural Biology, University of Otago, PO Box 913, Dunedin, New Zealand.

GRANT GILLETT Neurosurgeon and Professor of Medical Ethics, Dunedin Hospital and Otago Bioethics Centre, University of Otago Medical School, Dunedin PO Box 913, New Zealand. Email: grant.gillett@stonebow.otago.ac.nz

SIMONA GIORDANO Lecturer, The Centre for Social Ethics and Policy, School of Law, University of Manchester, Williamson Building, Oxford Road, Manchester M13 9PL, UK. Email: simona.giordano@manchester.ac.uk

ROBERT E. GOODIN Research School of Social Sciences, Building 09, Australian National University, Canberra ACT 0200, Australia. Email: goodinb@coombs.anu.edu.au

HANNAH GRANKVIST Tema Health and Society, The Department of Health and Society – IHS, Linköping University, SE-581 83 Linköping, Sweden. Email: hannah.grankvist@ihs.liu.se

WAYNE HALL Director, Office of Public Policy and Ethics, Institute for Molecular Bioscience, and School of Population Health, University of Queensland, St Lucia QLD 4072, Australia. Email: w.hall@imb.uq.edu.au

JOHN HARRIS Sir David Alliance Professor of Bioethics, The Centre for Social Ethics and Policy, School of Law, University of Manchester, Williamson Building, Oxford Road, Manchester M13 9PL, UK. Email: John.harris@manchester.ac.uk

ANDREAS HASMAN Research Associate, PPIP Profect Manager for Technology Appraisals, National Institute for Health and Clinical Excellence, MidCity Place, 71 High Holborn, London WC1V 6NA, UK. Email: Andreas.Hasman@nice.org.uk

MATTI HÄYRY Professor of Bioethics and Philosophy of Law, Centre for Social Ethics and Policy, The University of Manchester, Williamson Building, Oxford Road, Manchester M13 9PL, UK. Email: matti.hayry@manchester.ac.uk

ADAM HEDGECOE Senior Lecturer, Department of Sociology, School of Social Sciences, University of Sussex, Falmer, Brighton BN1 9QN, UK. Email: a.m.hedgecoe@sussex.ac.uk

ROGER HIGGS Professor of General Practice and Primary Care, Population Sciences & Health Care Research, Guy's, King's & St Thomas' School of Medicine, 5 Lambeth Walk, London SE11 6SP, UK. Email: roger.higgs@kcl.ac.uk

SØREN HOLM rofessorial Fellow in Bioethics, Cardiff Law School, Cardiff University, Law Building, Museum Avenue, Cardiff CF10 3AX, UK. Email: holms@cardiff.ac.uk

JAMES HUGHES Public Policy Studies, Trinity College, 300 Summit Street, Hartford, CT 06106, USA. Email: james.hughes@trincoll.edu

JONATHAN HUGHES Director, Centre for Professional Ethics, School of Law, Keele University, Staffordshire ST5 5BG, UK. Email: j.a.hughes@peak.keele.ac.uk

JULIAN C. HUGHES Honorary Clinical Senior Lecturer, Psychiatry of Old Age Service, North Tyneside General Hospital, Rake Lane, North Shields NE29 8NH, UK. Email: julian.hughes@nhct.nhs.uk or j.c.hughes@ncl.ac.uk

RICHARD HUXTABLE Senior Lecturer in Medical Law and Ethics/Deputy Director, Centre for Ethics in Medicine, University of Bristol, 73 St Michael's Hill, Bristol BS2 8BH, UK. Email: R.Huxtable@bristol.ac.uk

JENNIFER JACKSON Park House, Leathley, Nr Otley, North Yorkshire LS21 2JU, UK. Email: J.C.Jackson@leeds.ac.uk

JAY A. JACOBSON Professor of Internal Medicine, Chief of the Division of Medical Ethics, LDS Hospital, 8th Ave and C Street, Salt Lake City, UT 84143, USA. Email: jay.jacobson@intermountainmail.org

BRUCE JENNINGS Director, Center for Humans and Nature, 109 West 77th Street, Suite 2, New York, NY 10024, USA. Email: brucejennings@humansandnature.org

STEPHEN D. JOHN Lecturer, Department of History and Philosophy of Science, University of Cambridge, Free School Lane, Cambridge, CB2 3RH, UK. Email: sdj22@cam.ac.uk

VANESSA JOHNSTON School of Population Health, Faculty of Medicine Dentistry and Health Sciences, University of Melbourne, Parkville, Victoria 3010, Australia. Email: v.johnston2@pgrad.unimelb.edu.au

MONIQUE F. JONAS Centre for Professional Ethics, School of Law, Keele University, Staffs ST5 5BG, UK. Email: m.jonas@peak.keele.ac.uk

D. GARETH JONES Professor and Head of Department of Anatomy and Structural Biology, University of Otago, PO Box 913, Dunedin, New Zealand. Email: gareth.jones@stonebow.otago.ac.nz

ALBERT R. JONSEN 1333 Jones St., Apt. 502, San Francisco, CA 94109, USA. Email: ARJONSEN@aol.com

ERIC T. JUENGST Director, Center for Genetic Research Ethics and Law, Department of Bioethics, School of Medicine, Tower Annex 211, Case Western Reserve University, 10900 Euclid Avenue, Cleveland, OH 44106-4976, USA. Email: etj2@case.edu

NIKLAS JUTH Lecturer, Department of Philosophy, Göteborg University, Box 200, SE-40530 Göteborg, Sweden. Email: Niklas.Juth@filosofi.gu.se

JACOB E. KURLANDER Medical Student, School of Medicine, University of Michigan, 1500 E. Medical Center Drive Ann Arbor, MI 48109, USA. Email: jkurland@umich.edu

DAVID LAMB 294 Leigh Road, Chandlers Ford, SO5 3AU, UK. Email: davidlamb884@btinternet.com

LAURENS LANDEWEERD PhD Student, Department of Health Ethics and Philosophy, Faculty of Health and Science, University of Maastricht, PO Box 616, 6200 MD, Maastricht, The Netherlands. Email: l.landeweerd@zw.unimaas.nl

REIDAR K. LIE Senior Investigator, Department of Clinical Bioethics, National Institutes of Health, Building 10, Room 1C118, Bethesda, MD 20892, USA. Email: rlie@well.com

HILDE LINDEMANN Associate Professor, Philosophy Department, Michigan State University, 503 South Kedzie Hall, East Lansing, MI 48824, USA. Email: hlinde@msu.edu

PEKKA LOUHIALA Director of Research, Department of Public Health, Faculty of Medicine, University of Helsinki, PO Box 41 (Mannerheimintie 172), FIN-00014, Finland. Email: pekka.louhiala@helsinki.fi

NEIL C. MANSON Lecturer, Institute for Philosophy & Public Policy (IPPP), Furness College, Lancaster University, Lancaster LA1 4YG, UK. Email: n.manson@lancaster.ac.uk

SARAH MARCHAND Independent Scholar. Email: sarahmmarchand@gmail.com

MATT MATRAVERS Head, Department of Politics, University of York, Room: D/D205, York YO10 5DD, UK. Email: matt@matravers.demon.co.uk

JOHN MCKIE Research Fellow, Centre for Health Economics, Faculty of Business and Economics, Monash University, Victoria 3800, Australia. Email: john.mckie@buseco.monash.edu.au

SHEILA A.M. MCLEAN Director, Institute of Law and Ethics in Medicine, The School of Law, Stair Building, 5–8 The Square, University of Glasgow, Glasgow G12 8QQ, UK. Email: S.A.M.McLean@law.gla.ac.uk

JOHN R. MCMILLAN Senior Lecturer, Philosophy Department, The University of Hull, Room: L173 (Larkin Building - West), Hull HU6 7RX, UK. Email: John.McMillan@hyms.ac.uk

DAVID A. MCNAUGHTON Department of Philosophy, Florida State University, Tallahassee, FL 32306-1500, USA. Email: dmcnaugh@mailer.fsu.edu

PAUL B. MILLER Department of Philosophy, University of Toronto, 215 Huron Street, 9th Floor Toronto, Ontario M5S 1A2, Canada. Email: paul.miller@utoronto.ca

CHRISTIAN MUNTHE Head of Department of Philosophy, Göteborg University, Box 200, SE-40530 Göteborg, Sweden. Email: christian.munthe@phil.gu.se

THOMAS H. MURRAY   President, The Hastings Center, 21 Malcolm Gordon Road, Garrison, NY 10524-5555, USA. Email: murrayt@thehastingscenter.org

AINSLEY J. NEWSON   Lecturer in Biomedical Ethics, Centre for Ethics in Medicine, University of Bristol, 3rd Floor, Hampton House, Cotham Hill, Bristol BS6 6AU, UK. Email: ainsley.newson@bristol.ac.uk

JING-BAO NIE   PhD Lecturer, Otago Bioethics Centre, University of Otago Medical School, PO Box 913, Dunedin, New Zealand. Email: jing-bao.nie@stonebow. otago.ac.nz

LISBETH NIELSEN   EU ENHANCE Project Manager, Centre for Ethics in Medicine, University of Bristol, Hampton House, Cotham Hill, Bristol BS6 6AU, UK. Email: Lisbeth.Nielsen@bristol.ac.uk

LENNART Y. NORDENFELT   Professor, Department of Health and Society, Linköping University, 58183 Linköping, Sweden. Email: lenno@ihs.liu.se

JUSTIN OAKLEY   Director, Centre for Human Bioethics, School of Philosophy and Bioethics, Monash University, Victoria 3800, Australia. Email: justin.oakley@arts. monash.edu.au

ONORA O'NEILL   Principal, Newnham College, Sidgwick Avenue, Cambridge, CB3 9DF, UK. Email: oon20@ cam.ac.uk

MICHAEL PARKER   Professor of Bioethics and Director, The Ethox Centre, Department of Public Health and Primary Health Care, University of Oxford, Gibson Building/Block 21, Radcliffe Infirmary, Woodstock Road, Oxford OX3 6HE, UK. Email: michael.parker@ethics-and-communication-in-health.oxford.ac.uk

ROBERT A. PEARLMAN   Chief, Ethics Evaluation Service, Veterans Administration Puget Sound Health Care System, 1660 S. Columbian Way, Seattle, WA 98108, USA. Email: robert.pearlman@med.va.gov

GUIDO PENNINGS   Department of Philosophy and Moral Science, Ghent University, Blandijnberg 2, B-9000 Gent, Belgium. Email: Guido.Pennings@Ugent.be

HILARY PICKLES   Director of Public Health and Medical Director, Hillingdon Primary Care Trust, Kirk House, 97-109 High Street, Yiewsley, West Drayton, Middlesex UB7 7HJ,UK. Email: Hilary.Pickles@hillingdon. nhs.uk

THOMAS W. POGGE   Professorial Research Fellow, Centre for Applied Philosophy and Public Ethics, The Australian National University, LPO Box 8260, Canberra, ACT 2601, Australia. Email: tp6@columbia.edu

DAVID P.T. PRICE   Professor of Medical Law, De Montfort Univesity, The Gateway, Leicester, LE1 9BH, UK. Email: dpp@dmu.ac.uk

J. PIERS RAWLING   Department of Philosophy, Florida State University, Tallahassee, FL 32306-1500, USA. Email: prawling@mailer.fsu.edu

JEFF RICHARDSON   Professor and Foundation Director, Centre for Health Economics, Faculty of Business and Economics, Monash University, Victoria 3800, Australia. Email: Jeffrey.Richardson@BusEco.monash. edu.au

WENDY ROGERS   Associate Professor Medical Ethics & Health Law, Department of Medical Education, Flinders University, GPO Box 2100, Adelaide 5001, South Australia. Email: wendy.rogers@flinders.edu.au

FRED ROSNER   Attending Physician, Mount Sinai Services at Elmhurst Hospital Center, Elmhurst, New York and Professor of Medicine, Mount Sinai School of Medicine, New York; 750 Elvira Avenue, Far Rockaway, NY 11691, USA. Email: fsrosner@att.com

J. P. RUDDOCK   Crisis Resolution Service Manager, Central and North West London Mental Health NHS Trust, 7A Woodfield Road, London, W9 2NW, UK.

ABDULAZIZ SACHEDINA   Frances Myers Ball Professor of Religious Studies, Department of Religious Studies, University of Virginia, PO Box 400126, Charlottesville, VA 22904-4126, USA. Email: aas@virginia.edu

JULIAN SAVULESCU   Director, Oxford Uehiro Centre for Practical Ethics, University of Oxford, Littlegate House, St Ebbes Street, Oxford OX1 1PT, UK. Email: julian.savulescu@philosophy.ox.ac.uk

DORIS SCHROEDER   Acting Head of Centre, Centre for Professional Ethics, University of Central Lancashire, Preston PR1 2HE, UK. Email: dschroeder@uclan.ac.uk

UDO SCHUKLENK   Head of Centre for Ethics in Public Policy and Corporate Governance, Glasgow Caledonian University, 70 Cowcaddens Road, Glasgow G4 0BA, UK. Email: Udo.Schuklenk@gcal.ac.uk

ROSAMUND SCOTT   Reader in Law, Centre of Medical Law and Ethics, King's College London, The Strand, London, WC2R 2LS, UK. Email: rosamund.scott@kcl. ac.uk

MICHAEL J. SELGELID   Centre for Applied Philosophy and Public Ethics (CAPPE), and Menzies Centre for Health Policy, LPO Box 8260, The Australian National University, Canberra ACT 2601, Australia. Email: Michael. Selgelid@anu.edu.au

TOM SHAKESPEARE Research Fellow, Policy, Ethics and Life Sciences Research Centre (PEALS), University of Newcastle upon Tyne, Bioscience Centre, Times Square, Newcastle NE1 4EP, UK. Email: t.w.shakespeare@ncl.ac.uk

MARK SHEEHAN Research Fellow, Program on Ethics and the New Biosciences, Suite 7, Littlegate House, 16/17 St. Ebbes Street, Oxford OX1 1PT, UK. Email: mark.sheehan@philosophy.ox.ac.uk

SUSAN SHERWIN University Research Professor, Department of Philosophy, Dalhousie University, Halifax, NS B3H 4P9, Canada. Email: susan.sherwin@dal.ca

ANNE SLOWTHER Medical Education, Warwick Medical School, Medical Teaching Centre, Gibett Hill Campus, Room 103B, Coventry CV4 7AL, UK. Email: a-m.slowther@warwick.ac.uk

CHARLES B. SMITH 159 W Broadway #411, Salt Lake City, Utah 84101-1926, USA.

RICHARD SMITH Co-founder, Committee on Publication Ethics, 35 Orlando Road, London SW4 0LD, UK. Email: richardswsmith@yahoo.co.uk

ANN SOMMERVILLE Head of Medical Ethics Department, British Medical Association, BMA House, Tavistock Square, London WC1H 9JP, UK. Email: asommerville@bma.org.uk

TOM SORELL John Ferguson Professor of Global Ethics, Director of the Centre for the Study of Global Ethics, Department of Philosophy, School of Social Sciences, The University of Birmingham, Edgbaston, Birmingham B15 2TT, UK. Email: t.sorell@bham.ac.uk

NATALIE STOLJAR Department of Philosophy, Leacock Building, McGill University, 855 Sherbrooke Street West, Montreal, Quebec H3A 2T7, Canada. Email: natalie.stoljar@mcgill.ca

JEREMY SUGARMAN Phoebe R. Berman Bioethics Institute, Johns Hopkins University, Hampton House 351, 624 N. Broadway, Baltimore, MD 21205, USA. Email: jsugarm1@jhmi.edu

TUIJA TAKALA Lecturer in Bioethics and Moral Philosophy, School of Law, The University of Manchester, Oxford Road, Manchester, M13 9PL, UK; and Department of Social and Moral Philosophy, University of Helsinki, Finland. Email: Tuija.Takala@manchester.ac.uk,

TESSA TAN TORRES Coordinator, Global Programme on Evidence for Health Policy, World Health Organization, Avenue Appia 20, 1211 Geneva 27, Switzerland. Email: tantorrest@who.int

HOLLY TAYLOR Health Policy and Management, Faculty Research, Johns Hopkins Bloomberg School of Public Health, Hampton House 353, 624 N. Broadway, Room 493 Baltimore, MD 21205, USA. Email: htaylor@jhsph.edu

RUUD H.J. TER MEULEN Chair/Director, Centre for Ethics in Medicine, University of Bristol, Hampton House, Cotham Hill, Bristol BS6 6AU, UK. Email: r.terMeulen@bristol.ac.uk

COLIN TYLER Senior Lecturer in Political Theory, Department of Politics and International Studies, University of Hull, Cottingham Road, Hull HU6 7RX, UK. Email: C.Tyler@hull.ac.uk

SUZANNE UNIACKE Reader in Applied Ethics, Philosophy, Room L171, Larken Building – West, University of Hull, Hull HU6 7RX, UK. Email: s.m.uniacke@hull.ac.uk

THEO VAN WILLIGENBURG Kant Academy, Oudegracht 291, 3511 PA Utrecht, The Netherlands. Email: vanwilligenburg@kantacademy.nl

ROBERT M. VEATCH Kennedy Institute of Ethics, Georgetown University, Washington, DC 20057, USA. Email: veatchr@georgetown.edu

MARCEL VERWEIJ Senior Researcher and Lecturer, Ethics Institute, Utrecht University, Postbus 80.103, 3508 TC Utrecht, The Netherlands. Email: m.f.verweij@ethics.uu.nl

ADRIAN WALSH Acting Head of School and Senior Lecturer, School of Social Science, The University of New England, Armidale, NSW 2351, Australia. Email: awalsh@pobox.une.edu.au

CHARLES WEIJER Canada Research Chair (Tier I), Associate Professor of Philosophy and Medicine, Department of Philosophy, Talbot College, University of Western Ontario, London, Ontario N6A 3K7, Canada. Email: cweijer@uwo.ca

DAVID WENDLER Head of the Unit on Vulnerable Populations, Department of Clinical Bioethics, National Institutes of Health, 10 Center Drive Building 10, Room 1C118, Bethesda MD 20892-1156, USA. Email: Dwendler@cc.nih.gov

ALAN P. WERTHEIMER Senior Research Fellow, Clinical Bioethics Department, National Institutes of Health (NIH), Building 10 – Magnuson CC, Room 1C118, 10 Center Drive, Bethesda, MD 20892-1156, USA. Email: aw355w@nih.gov

GUY A.M. WIDDERSHOVEN Professor, Department of Health Ethics and Philosophy, PO Box 616, Faculty of Health Sciences, Universiteit Maastricht, 6200 MD Maastricht, The Netherlands. Email: G.Widdershoven@ZW.unimaas.nl

HEATHER WIDDOWS   Senior Lecturer in Global Ethics, Centre for the Study of Global Ethics, University of Birmingham, Edgbaston Park Road, Edgbaston, Birmingham B15 2TT, UK. Email: H.Widdows@bham.ac.uk

DANIEL WIKLER   Mary B. Saltonstall Professor of Ethics and Population Health, Department of Population & International Health, Harvard School of Public Health (Bldg 1, Room 1210), 665 Huntington Avenue, Boston, MA 02115, USA. Email: wikler@hsph.harvard.edu

STEPHEN WILKINSON   Professor of Bioethics, Centre for Professional Ethics, School of Law, Keele University, Staffordshire ST5 5BG, UK. Email: s.wilkinson@peak.keele.ac.uk

TIMOTHY M. WILKINSON   Senior Lecturer, Faculty of Medical and Health Sciences, School of Population Health, University of Auckland, Private Bag 92019, Auckland, New Zealand. Email: m.wilkinson@auckland.ac.nz

JAMES G.S. WILSON   Centre for Professional Ethics, School of Law, Keele University, Keele, Staffs ST5 5BG, UK. Email: j.g.wilson@peak.keele.ac.uk

SIMON WOODS   Director of Learning, Policy Ethics and Life Sciences Research Institute, University of Newcastle, Bioscience Centre, Times Square, Newcastle upon Tyne, NE1 4EP, UK. Email: Simon.Woods@newcastle.ac.uk

Foreword: Raanan E. Gillon

It is such a delight to welcome this second and new edition of Principles of Health Care Ethics. While my own energy was inadequate to accepting the task of once again editing a hundred-author textbook, it was clear that a new edition was due and this new collection, brought together and edited by my excellent erstwhile colleague Richard Ashcroft and his associates, is in my view superb. The first edition of this book was born, in the early 1990s, of two intentions. One was to create a textbook covering most of the substantive issues in medical ethics written by a wider, more international, range of authors than the mainly American collections that already existed. The second intention was that the hundred or so authors would in their chapters all to some extent use, and or reflect upon, the Beauchamp and Childress four principles approach to medical ethics. The authors of the first edition fulfilled both intentions handsomely.

In this second edition the first intention is maintained and extended. The writers are cosmopolitan not only geographically but also in terms of perspectives and disciplines, and while the main issues of health care ethics represented in the first edition are all covered there are some fascinating additions within the new edition's four main areas of concern.

Thus in the context of methodologies in health care ethics (HCE) there are new chapters on virtue theory, universalism and relativism, liberalism and communitarianism, deliberative bioethics, hermeneutics, empirical approaches to bioethics, the relationship of medical humanities to HCE, and a fascinating chapter on reflective equilibrium as a method in HCE. In the context of particular HCE issues there are welcome new chapters on ethics in primary care, conflicts between practitioners' personal beliefs and their care of patients, the role of conscience in health care practice, responses to violent and abusive patients, ethical issues in relation to performance enhancement in sport, ethical challenges created by contemporary emphasis on patient choice, ethical issues in relation to disability, and ethical aspects of 'medical tourism'. In the section on 'medicine in

society' consideration of ethical issues in health promotion, public health and epidemiology is expanded and new chapters on ethical issues of bioterrorism, disaster relief, care of refugees and asylum seekers, and a chapter on doctors and human rights are timely additions. In the last section, on ethical issues in research and new technologies, health care research and genetics get a more intensive and contemporary treatment than in the first edition, including chapters on human cloning and stem cell research. There are also new chapters addressing xenotransplantation, vaccination to prevent addiction, psychosurgery and neuroimplantation, along with a final trio considering obligations of the pharmaceutical industry, obligations of patients, and reflections on ethics consultations and ethics committees in health care institutions.

As for my second intention in the first edition- that authors should in presenting their subjects also reflect (whether positively or negatively) on the four principles approach- this, as indicated above, has been replaced by a wide range of alternative methodological approaches, and no special emphasis on the four principles. In this context let me simply state that the four principles approach got a very good airing in the first edition and in this edition their use is lucidly explained and stoutly if synoptically defended by one of their originators, Tom Beauchamp. I won't repeat my responses to objections to the approach that I offered in the first edition. Suffice it to assert that I stand by those responses and to add that during the more than twenty five years that I have supported the use of these universalisable prima facie principles in health care ethics I have not encountered either plausible objections to any one of them, nor plausible candidates for necessary additional principles that can not themselves be encompassed by one, or by some combination, of the four principles. Even the proposed additional principle of preserving and not taking human life is quite capable of justification by means of a combination of the four principles. I would suggest to readers of the new edition that they might usefully ask themselves whether any one of the individual chapters is incompatible with the four principles approach.

For my own part I continue to value the four principles approach as a way of bringing people of different faiths, different cultures, different moral and political perspectives, together in a common if basic set of prima facie moral commitments and of providing them with a common if basic moral language and a common if basic moral analytic framework. If the widespread 'grass roots' acceptance of these principles in international health care ethics is anything to go by they will eventually be recognised to be of international relevance and acceptability not just in health care ethics but in ethics more generally. When (yes, and if) this prediction becomes a reality I hope that Tom Beauchamp and Jim Childress will get the Nobel Peace Prize that they'll deserve!

In pursuit of an increase in world harmony it would be a great development, in my opinion, for medical ethicists to come together to promote the enormous potential moral acceptability of the four principles across all moral cultures, (including the considerable variety of moral cultures represented in this book) and then to concentrate on remaining problems. These can be (admittedly over-simply) categorised in terms of interpretation of the principles; further investigation of their scope of application (to whom or to what do we owe these four prima facie obligations?); and most difficult of all, how should we deal with conflicts between the principles when these arise, as in practice they so often do? In this last context especially, judgement plays an obviously crucial role. But just what is judgement, how is it done, how should it be done? Kant pointed out that there could be no rules for judgement between conflicting rules, on pain of an infinite regress. What then? Maybe it is in the context of judgement between conflicting moral rules, principles and values that intuition, emotion, a sense of fit, perhaps even aesthetic sensibility, do or should play an important role? Judgement, especially moral judgement, is a theme that I hope will get a thorough airing in the third edition of Principles of Health Care Ethics. Meanwhile I heartily commend the second.

Raanan E. Gillon MB BS FRCP(LOND)
BA(Philosophy) HonRCM Hon DSc(OXON)
Emeritus Professor of Medical Ethics,
Imperial College London

Foreword: Tony Hope

In his famous essay on Tolstoy Isaiah Berlin divided thinkers into foxes and hedgehogs. The fox knows many things; the hedgehog knows one big thing. Those who are driven to find unifying principles and ideas, like Plato, were classified by Berlin as hedgehogs. Those who, like Aristotle, prefer a less systematic approach, and like to consider each issue in its own terms, are the foxes.

The first edition of this book was a fox in hedgehog's clothing. It presented itself as unified under the 'four principles of biomedical ethics'. The editors of this second edition have thrown off the prickly outer garments and relished its foxiness. This is a book of byzantine proportions: a treasure trove for anyone with even the slightest initial interest in biomedical ethics. Indeed this book demonstrates that biomedical ethics is a microcosm of culture broadly conceived.

Principles of Health Care Ethics is unique. There is no other source-book that provides such diversity within the field. Here you can explore Eastern as well as Western approaches; examine the value of scientific studies in ethics, or of bizarre thought experiments. You can read about specific issues arising in clinical care, or gaze into a future when drugs might be widely used not only to treat disease but also to enhance health and abilities. There are twenty chapters on political and social issues and almost as many on the ethics of medical research and new technologies.

The first edition of *Principles of Health Care Ethics* was a constant companion for me, although one that was rather too frequently 'borrowed'. This second edition is even more exciting. A book of reference; and also a book to explore.

Tony Hope
Professor of Medical Ethics
University of Oxford

Preface

Ranaan Gillon's first edition of Principles of Health Care Ethics was published in 1994, and quickly became established as the leading single volume companion to the ethical issues in modern health care. In his Preface to that first edition, he defined it as having two principal purposes:

> [...] to provide a collection of papers accessible to English-speaking health care workers internationally, introducing the wide range of issues that comprise health care ethics from a wide variety of perspectives – a variety that was more international, multidisciplinary and less predominantly American bioethical, than earlier collections. The second motive was a desire to invite each writer at least to consider in his or her contribution a common moral theme – notably that of the four prima facie principles of health care ethics and their scope of application... (Gillon (1994): xxi)

This second edition retains the first objective, but does not retain the second. Since 1994, there has been an enormous expansion in the range of topics covered in modern health care and biomedical ethics, but there has also been a shift in the philosophical centre of gravity of the field. In this preface we describe how we decided to reshape the volume in the light of current priorities in health care and biomedical ethics.

A great strength of the first edition of this volume was its commitment to a single analytical and moral framework – the so-called "Four Principles" approach created by Thomas Beauchamp and James Childress's Principles of Biomedical Ethics, now in its fifth edition, and popularised and extended by a number of authors, most notably Raanan Gillon himself. The first edition devoted almost a third of its contents to chapters examining different philosophical, political and religious frameworks from the point of view of their convergence or divergence from the Four Principles framework. Many of these chapters retain their value as

independent contributions to the scholarly and professional literature. As Raanan Gillon argues in his foreword to this second edition, the Four Principles approach could serve both as the core common ground which might serve as what Rawls termed an overlapping consensus between those who share quite different substantive moral and metaphysical views of the world, and as a process or mechanism for creating agreement among such people. Several of the chapters in the present volume develop this idea, notably the opening chapter by Thomas Beauchamp. Nevertheless we felt that the state of scholarly debate no longer supported taking this approach to organising what we intended as an overview of the field for both new students and established workers in the field.[1] This volume is therefore *Principles of Health Care Ethics* in a different sense of the word "principles": the fundamental topics and issues covered in a way which will allow people new to the field, or to specific topics within it, to grasp the essential issues.

Methodologically, health care and biomedical ethics is far more diverse now than in 1994. We have seen the rapid growth of both empirical studies which have attended more to the differences between specific moral perspectives than to what they may have in common, and of different philosophical methodologies for analysing cases and for interpreting the ethical, legal, and social challenges posed by new health technologies and by tough decisions in health policy. We do not think that the field is in a phase of synthesis in which extracting common principles is either easy or intellectually helpful. Instead, we felt that it was important to give a sense of the diversity of intellectual approaches to ethical problems in health care. So, we chose authors for each essay who were recognised authorities on the topics they were discussing, and gave them considerable freedom as to the approach they took to presenting the topic. We

---

[1]For a discussion of the current state of play regarding the Four Principles approach in health care ethics, see the special issue of the Journal of Medical Ethics published in honour of Raanan Gillon on his retirement: Journal of Medical Ethics 2003; 29(5): 265-312, and more recently Dawson and Garrard (2006)

encouraged them to write as for a readership of intelligent, but not yet well informed, readers, such as we meet in our upper level undergraduate or Master's courses. We asked each author to write new, state of the art articles, so as to give a picture of the latest thinking on each topic. In most cases, authors have set out specific arguments, taking into account contrary views, but giving their own analysis. In some cases, the articles have more of a survey article character, especially where the topic is more empirical in nature or where controversy is widespread. The editors are all philosophers, and we have favoured philosophical over legal or social science approaches to our chosen topics, but in many cases the articles do present empirical as well as theoretical, and positive as well as normative material, and some articles present a legal analysis of the topic. This diversity reflects the multidisciplinary nature of modern scholarship and research in health care ethics.

Each section opens with a brief overview of its contents by the section editor responsible for it. The first section introduces the main methodological and intellectual approaches to health care and biomedical ethics in general. This section will be of particular help to the reader who needs an orientation to the different philosophical methods in modern English-speaking philosophical health care ethics. The second section introduces the main ethical challenges in health care practice. This book is principally concerned with health care ethics, rather than biomedical ethics. Health care ethics is the study of ethical challenges in the delivery of health care. It is wider than medical ethics, which is concerned with the ethical challenges of medical care and the profession of medicine. Biomedical ethics is principally concerned with the ethical challenges of modern high technology applied to health care, rather than with the challenges of professional care. Naturally the three areas – health care ethics, medical ethics, biomedical ethics – overlap, but our emphasis is mainly on health care practice rather than policy. That noted, major growth areas in health care and biomedical ethics over the past ten years

are public health ethics (concerned both with the ethics of protecting and promoting public health, and with the ethics of allocation of care between different competing needs and people) and the ethics of new technologies in health care. Section three gives an overview of public health ethics, and section four gives an overview of research ethics and ethics of new technologies in health care.

Preparing this volume for the press has been a challenge, but almost always an enjoyable one. We first invited chapters from May 2005, and received the last chapter complete from its authors in October 2006. By the time you read this, some issues may have moved on, but we hope they won't have moved on too much! From the very beginning we have had warm encouragement both from Raanan Gillon and from Lucy Sayer, our editor at John Wiley. We have had excellent practical support throughout from Lucy and from her colleague Juliet Booker. Most of all we thank our contributing authors, who have produced what we think are outstanding chapters with efficiency and grace. Time will tell whether there is a third edition, and, if so, whether it will have a more unified intellectual structure as the first edition did. Our challenge to you, as readers, is to advance the topics we have covered, and – if you find the task to your taste, to produce an intellectual synthesis. Raanan strongly believes that this is possible – we are more sceptical. But over to you!

REFERENCES

Dawson AJ, Garrard E (2006) In defence of moral imperialism: four equal and universal prima facie principles. Journal of Medical Ethics 32: 200–204

Gillon R (1994) Preface: Medical ethics and the four principles. In Gillon R (ed.) Principles of Health Care Ethics Chichester: John Wiley (first edition): xxi–xxxi

Richard E. Ashcroft, Angus Dawson,
Heather Draper and John R. McMillan

PART I

METHODOLOGY AND PERSPECTIVES

SECTION ONE: MORAL THEORY AND HEALTH CARE ETHICS

One of the guiding thoughts for the second edition of *Principles* was to commission a collection of high quality chapters that could not only serve as a general introduction to health care ethics but also provide a resource that is sufficiently detailed for postgraduate students. Given that this section discusses the major methodologies and perspectives that are relevant to health care ethics, many of the chapters introduce moral theory at a fairly advanced level.

The first edition of *Principles* demonstrated the utility and applicability of the four principles approach for a broad array of issues in health care ethics. While the second edition does not attempt to do this, it does begin with and include a number of chapters discussing this approach. Beauchamp and Childress developed and refined their four principles approach in the years following the first edition of *Principles* and the first chapter of the second edition begins with an account of the mature theory by Beauchamp.

The next four chapters present important interpretations and theories of each of the principles. Stoljar and Cullity consider different theoretical accounts of autonomy and beneficence, respectively. Interest in justice theory has moved beyond simply discussing distributional justice within a nation state, and attention has turned to more international issues. Pogge's *Responsibilities for poverty-related ill health* presents his influential account

of global justice. Tyler explains the relevance of the liberalism/communitarianism debate for health care ethics.

Veatch played an important role in the principles debate, and in *How many principles?*, he considers the merits of other principle-based approaches to health care ethics that use fewer or more than four principles. One important question about the application of principles to biomedical ethics is: what role do they play in practical moral reason? In Chapter 7, Jonsen gives an account of practical casuistry and how it interfaces with the use of principles in moral reason.

The next eight chapters show how a number of normative moral theories can be applied to health care ethics. Rather than simply giving an account of the different versions of utilitarianism, Häyry gives an interesting account of the way the utilitarian arguments function in bioethics. There is a tendency for introductions to ethics to mention only Kant when introducing deontology, with the consequence that some students assume that deontology implies Kantianism or absolutism. McNaughton and Rawling give an exceptionally clear account of what deontology is and contrast Kant's version with Ross's. O'Neill gives a concise account of Kantian ethics and its origins in Kant's moral philosophy. Sherwin outlines a very useful taxonomy of the four major approaches to feminist bioethics. In Chapter 12, Oakley explains the nature, application and problems of virtue theory. Sheehan describes the important differences between the descriptive and metaethical versions of moral relativism.

SECTION TWO: THEOLOGICAL APPROACHES TO HEALTH CARE ETHICS

One of the most popular features of the first edition of *Principles* was the way it considered religious approaches to health care ethics, and this edition includes a section on 'theological approaches to health care ethics'. Inevitably, it was not possible to discuss every religion that says something important about health care ethics, or even to have a chapter on each of the major religions. Nonetheless, readers who want an introduction to some of the fundamental articles of various faiths that enter into debates about health care ethics will find these chapters of value. Widdows, Rosner, Sachedina, Hughes and Coward explain what is distinctive about Christian, Jewish, Islamic, Buddhist and South Asian approaches to health care ethics (respectively). Nie offers a useful critique of the idea that there is something distinctive about Asian Bioethics.

SECTION THREE: METHODOLOGY AND HEALTH CARE ETHICS

One of the most important aspects of the development of bioethics since the first edition of *Principles* is the proliferation of methodological approaches to health care ethics. Brody offers an illuminating account of narrative ethics, and this chapter is followed by a description of the ways in which empirical methods can be incorporated into health care ethics by Sugarman, Pearlman and Taylor. Hedgcoe questions whether the emergence of empirical methods in health care ethics is merely reinventing medical sociology. Thought experiments are pervasive in philosophy and are an important rhetorical strategy in health care ethics too. Walsh gives an especially useful description of the ways in which thought experiments can contribute to argument in health care ethics.

Parker's chapter begins with the recognition that the debate about health care ethics has a political dimension and proceeds to give a typology of the deliberative democratic approaches that can be employed. Just as ethics is intertwined with politics, it is in a complicated relationship with the law, and McLean illustrates some of the ways in which law and ethics are interdependent.

Evans explains what is distinctive about the Medical Humanities, while van Willigenburg shows how Rawls's concept of Reflective Equilibrium can be applied as a method in health care ethics. Widdershoven and Abma's chapter is similar in that they also show how a philosophical concept, hermeneutics, can be employed as a method in health care ethics.

The last 10 chapters in Part one are similar in that they all explain moral concepts, distinctions or doctrines that are central to health care ethics. Chapter 29 is by Childress, and he makes a number of very useful distinctions between the different forms of paternalism. The concept of a 'medical need' can play an important role in prioritisation, and Culyer distinguishes and evaluates the theoretical possibilities. Rights theory is important and often not explained with the clarity with which Wilson has written Chapter 31. 'Exploitation' has always been an important moral concept for health care ethics, but now that it is becoming accepted as a key principle for research ethics, a clear understanding of it is essential. Chapter 32 is by Wertheimer and shows how his theory of exploitation (arguably the most influential and successful account developed thus far) can be applied to health care ethics. The remaining chapters explain important concepts such as Competence to Consent (Jonas), The Doctrine of Double Effect (Uniacke), Ordinary and Extraordinary Means (John), Acts and Omissions (Takala), Personhood and Moral Status (Newson), and Commodification (Wilkinson).

John R. McMillan

1

The 'Four Principles' Approach to Health Care Ethics

TOM L. BEAUCHAMP

My objective is to explain the so-called four principles approach and to explain the philosophical and practical roles these principles play. I start with a brief history and then turn to the four principles framework, its practicality, and philosophical problems of making the framework specific.

THE ORIGINS OF PRINCIPLES IN HEALTH CARE ETHICS

Prior to the early 1970s, there was no firm ground in which a commitment to principles or even ethical theory could take root in biomedical ethics. This is not to say that physicians and researchers had no principled commitments to patients and research subjects. They did, but moral principles, practices and virtues were rarely discussed. The health care ethics outlook in Europe and America was largely that of maximizing medical benefits and minimizing risks of harm and disease. The Hippocratic tradition had neglected many problems of truthfulness, privacy, justice, communal responsibility, the vulnerability of research subjects and the like (Jonsen, 1998; Pellegrino & Thomasma, 1993). Views about ethics had been largely confined to the perspectives of those in the professions of medicine, public health and nursing. No sustained work combined concerns in ethical theory and the health care fields.

Principles that could be understood with relative ease by the members of various disciplines figured prominently in the development of biomedical ethics during the 1970s and early 1980s. Principles were used primarily to present frameworks of evaluative assumptions so that they could be used, and readily understood, by people with many different forms of professional training. The distilled morality found in principles gave people a shared and serviceable group of general norms for analysing many types of moral problems. In some respects, it could even be claimed that principles gave the embryonic field of bioethics a shared 'method' for attacking its problems, and this gave some minimal coherence and uniformity to bioethics.

There were two primary sources of the early interest in principles in biomedical ethics. The first was the *Belmont Report* (and related documents) of the National Commission for the Protection of Human Subjects (Childress et al., 2005; National Commission for the Protection of Human Subjects of Biomedical and Behavioral Research, 1978), and the second was the book entitled *Principles of Biomedical Ethics*, which I co-authored with James F. Childress. I here confine discussion to the latter.

Childress and I began our search for the principles of biomedical ethics in 1975. In early 1976 we drafted the main ideas for the book, although only later would the title *Principles of Biomedical Ethics* be placed on it (Beauchamp & Childress, 1979). Our goal was to develop a set of principles suitable for biomedical ethics. Substantively, our proposal was that traditional preoccupation of health care with a beneficence-based model of health care ethics be shifted in the direction of an autonomy model, while also incorporating a wider set of social concerns, particularly those focused on social justice. The principles are understood as the standards of conduct on which many other moral claims and judgements depend. A principle, then, is an essential norm in a system of moral thought, forming the basis of moral reasoning. More specific rules for health care ethics can be formulated *by reference to* these four principles, but neither rules nor practical judgements can be straightforwardly *deduced* from the principles.

Principles of Health Care Ethics, Second Edition   Edited by R.E. Ashcroft, A. Dawson, H. Draper and J.R. McMillan

THE FRAMEWORK OF PRINCIPLES

The principles in our framework have always been grouped under four general categories: (1) respect for autonomy (a principle requiring respect for the decision-making capacities of autonomous persons); (2) nonmaleficence (a principle requiring not causing harm to others); (3) beneficence (a group of principles requiring that we prevent harm, provide benefits and balance benefits against risks and costs); (4) justice (a group of principles requiring appropriate distribution of benefits, risks and costs fairly). I will concentrate now on an explication of each of the principles and how they are to be understood collectively as a framework of principles.

RESPECT FOR AUTONOMY

Respect for autonomy is rooted in the liberal moral and political tradition of the importance of individual freedom and choice. In moral philosophy personal autonomy refers to personal self-governance: personal rule of the self by adequate understanding while remaining free from controlling interferences by others and from personal limitations that prevent choice. 'Autonomy' means freedom from external constraint and the presence of critical mental capacities such as understanding, intending and voluntary decision-making capacity (Childress, 1990; Engelherdt, 1996; Katz, 1984; Kukla, 2005). The autonomous individual acts freely in accordance with a self-chosen plan, analogous to the way an independent government manages its territories and sets its policies. A person of diminished autonomy, by contrast, is in some respect controlled by others or incapable of deliberating or acting on the basis of his or her desires and plans.

To respect an autonomous agent is to recognize with due appreciation that person's capacities and perspectives, including his or her right to hold certain views, to make certain choices, and to take certain actions based on personal values and beliefs. The moral demand that we respect the autonomy of persons can be expressed as a *principle* of respect for autonomy, which should be stated as involving both a negative obligation and a positive obligation. As a negative obligation, autonomous actions should not be subjected to controlling constraints by others. As a positive obligation, this principle requires both respectful treatment in disclosing information and actions that foster autonomous decision making.

Many autonomous actions could not occur without others' material cooperation in making options available. Respect for autonomy obligates professionals in health care and research involving human subjects to disclose information, to probe for and ensure understanding and voluntariness, and to foster adequate decision making. True respect requires more than mere noninterference in others' personal affairs. It includes,

at least in some contexts, building up or maintaining others' capacities for autonomous choice while helping to allay fears and other conditions that destroy or disrupt their autonomous actions. Respect, on this account, involves acknowledging the value and decision-making rights of persons and enabling them to act autonomously, whereas disrespect for autonomy involves attitudes and actions that ignore, insult, demean or are inattentive to others' rights of autonomy.

Many issues in professional ethics concern failures to respect a person's autonomy, ranging from manipulative underdisclosure of pertinent information to nonrecognition of a refusal of medical interventions. For example, in the debate over whether autonomous, informed patients have the right to refuse medical interventions, the principle of respect for autonomy suggests that an autonomous decision to refuse interventions must be respected. Although it was not until the late 1970s that serious attention was given to rights to refuse for patients, this is no reason for thinking that respect for autonomy as now understood is a newly added principle in our moral perspective. It simply means that the implications of this principle were not widely appreciated until recently (Faden & Beauchamp, 1986).

Controversial problems with the principle of respect for autonomy, as with all moral principles, arise when we must interpret its significance for particular contexts and determine precise limits on its application and how to handle situations when it conflicts with other moral principles. Many controversies involve questions about the conditions under which a person's right to autonomous expression demands actions by others, and also questions about the restrictions society may rightfully place on choices by patients or subjects when these choices conflict with other values. If restriction of the patient's autonomy is in order, the justification will always rest on some competing moral principles such as beneficence or justice.

NONMALEFICENCE

Physicians have long avowed that they are obligated to avoid doing harm to their patients. Among the most quoted principles in the history of codes of health care ethics is the maxim *primum non nocere*: 'Above all, do no harm'. British physician Thomas Percival furnished the first developed modern account of health care ethics, in which he maintained that a principle of nonmaleficence fixes the physician's primary obligations and triumphs even over the principle of respect for the patient's autonomy in a circumstance of potential harm to patients:

> To a patient…who makes inquiries which, if faithfully answered, might prove fatal to him, it would be a gross and unfeeling wrong to reveal the truth. His right to it is suspended, and even annihilated; because…it would be deeply injurious to himself, to his family, and to the public. And he has the strongest

claim, from the trust reposed in his physician, as well as from the common principles of humanity, to be guarded against whatever would be detrimental to him (Percival, 1847).

Many basic rules in the common morality are the requirements to avoid causing a harm. They include rules such as do not kill, do not cause pain, do not disable, do not deprive of pleasure, do not cheat and do not break promises (Gert, 2005). Similar, but more specific prohibitions are found across the literature of biomedical ethics, each grounded in the principle that intentionally or negligently caused harm is a fundamental moral wrong.

Numerous problems of nonmaleficence are found in health care ethics today – some involving blatant abuses of persons and others involving subtle and unresolved questions. Blatant examples of failures to act nonmaleficently are found in the use of physicians to classify political dissidents as mentally ill, thereafter treating them with harmful drugs and incarcerating them with insane and violent persons (Bloch & Reddaway, 1984). More subtle examples are found in the use of medications for the treatment of aggressive and destructive patients. These common treatment modalities are helpful to many patients, but they can be harmful to others.

A provocative question about nonmaleficence and physician ethics has been raised by Paul S. Appelbaum in an investigation of 'the problem of doing harm' through testimony in criminal contexts and civil litigation – for example, by omitting information in the context of a trial, after which a more severe punishment is delivered to the person than likely would have been delivered. Appelbaum presents the generic problem as one of nonmaleficence:

If physicians are committed to doing good and avoiding harm, how can they participate in legal proceedings from which harm may result? If, on the other hand, physicians in court abandon medicine's traditional ethical principles, how do they justify that deviation? And if the obligations to do good and avoid harm no longer govern physicians in the legal setting, what alternative principles come into play? . . . Are physicians in general bound by the principles of beneficence and nonmaleficence? (Appelbaum, 1990)

BENEFICENCE

The physician who professes to 'do no harm' is not usually interpreted as pledging never to cause harm, but rather to strive to create a positive balance of goods over inflicted harms. Those engaged in medical practice, research and public health know that risks of harm presented by interventions must often be weighed against possible benefits for patients, subjects and the public. Here we see the importance of beneficence as a principle beyond the scope of nonmaleficence.

In ordinary English the term *beneficence* connotes acts of mercy, kindness, charity, love and humanity. In its most general meaning, it includes all forms of action intended to benefit other persons. In health care ethics beneficence commonly refers to an action done to benefit others, whereas benevolence refers to the character trait or virtue of being disposed to act for the benefit of others. The principle of beneficence refers to a moral obligation to act for the benefit of others. No demand is more important when taking care of patients: the welfare of patients is medicine's context and justification. 'Beneficence' has long been treated as a foundational value – and sometimes as the foundational value (Pellegrino, 1994; Pellegrino & Thomasma, 1988) – in health care ethics.

The principle of beneficence requires us to help others further their important and legitimate interests, often by preventing or removing possible harms. This principle includes rules such as 'maximize possible benefits and minimize possible harms' and 'balance benefits against risks'. Many duties in medicine, nursing, public health and research are expressed in terms of a positive obligation to come to the assistance of those in need of treatment or in danger of injury. The harms to be prevented, removed or minimized are the pain, suffering and disability of injury and disease. The range of benefits that might be considered relevant is broad. It could even include helping patients find appropriate forms of financial assistance and helping them gain access to health care or research protocols. Sometimes the benefit is for the patient, at other times for society.

Some writers in health care ethics suggest that certain duties such as not to injure others are more compelling than duties to benefit them. They point out that we do not consider it justifiable to kill a dying patient in order to use the patient's organs to save two others, even though benefits would be maximized, all things considered. The obligation not to injure a patient by abandonment has been said to be stronger than the obligation to prevent injury to a patient who has been abandoned by another (under the assumption that both are moral duties). Despite the attractiveness of these notions that there is a hierarchical ordering rule, Childress and I reject such hierarchies on grounds that obligations of beneficence do, under many circumstances, outweigh those of nonmaleficence. A harm inflicted by not avoiding causing it may be negligible or trivial, whereas the harm that beneficence requires we prevent may be substantial. For example, saving a person's life by a blood transfusion clearly justifies the inflicted harm of venipuncture on the blood donor. One of the motivations for separating nonmaleficence from beneficence is that these principles themselves come into conflict. As the weights of the two principles can vary, there can be no mechanical decision rule asserting that one obligation must always outweigh the other.

Perhaps the major theoretical problem about beneficence is whether the principle generates general moral duties that are incumbent on *everyone* – not because of a professional role, but because morality itself makes a general demand of benefi-cence. Many analyses of beneficence in ethical theory (most notably utilitarianism, Kagan, 1989; Miller, 2004; Singer, 1993; 1999) seem to demand severe sacrifice and extreme generosity in the moral life – for example, giving a kidney for transplantation or donating bone marrow to a stranger. Consequently, some moral philosophers have argued that such beneficent action is virtuous and a moral ideal, but not an ob-ligation, and therefore that there is no principle of beneficence of the sort proclaimed in the four principles approach.

I agree, of course, that the line between what is required and what is not required by the principle is difficult to draw, and that drawing a precise line independent of context is impossible. I do not agree, however, with the radical view that there are no obligations of beneficence – neither general nor specific obligations. I return to this problem of weighing, judging and specifying below in a discussion of the notion of *prima facie* duties.

JUSTICE

Every civilized society is a cooperative venture structured by moral, legal and cultural principles of justice that define the terms of cooperation. A person in any such society has been treated justly if treated according to what is fair, due or owed. For example, if equal political rights are due all citizens, then justice is done when those rights are accorded. The more re-stricted notion of *distributive justice* refers to fair, equitable and appropriate distribution in society. Usually this term re-fers to the distribution of primary social goods such as eco-nomic goods and fundamental political rights, but burdens are also within its scope. Paying for forms of national health insurance is a distributed burden; medical-welfare checks and grants to do research are distributed benefits.

There is no single principle of justice in the four princi-ples approach. Somewhat like principles under the heading of beneficence, there are several principles, each requiring specification in particular contexts. But common to almost all theories of justice – and accepted in the four principles approach – is the minimal (formal) principle that like cases should be treated alike, or, to use the language of equality, equals ought to be treated equally and unequals unequally. This elementary principle, or formal principle of justice, states no particular respects in which people ought to be treated. It merely asserts that whatever respects are relevant, if persons are equal in those respects, they should be treated alike. Thus, the formal principle of justice does not tell us how to determine equality or proportion in these matters, and it lacks substance as a specific guide to conduct.

Many controversies about justice arise over what should be considered the relevant characteristics for equal treat-ment. Principles that specify these relevant characteristics are often said to be 'material' because they identify relevant properties for distribution. Childress and I take account of the fact that philosophers have also developed diverse theo-ries of justice that provide sometimes conflicting material principles. We try to show that there are some merits in egalitarian theories, libertarian theories and utilitarian theories, and we defend a mixed use of principles in these theories. We think that these three theories of justice all capture some of our intuitive convictions about justice and that they can all be tapped as resources that will help to produce a coherent conception of justice.

However, many issues of justice in health care ethics are not easily framed in the context of traditional principles and abstract moral theories (Buchanan, 1997; Buchanan et al., 2000; Daniels, 1985; 2006; Powers & Faden, 2006). For example, some basic issues in health care ethics in the last three decades centre on special levels of protection and aid for vulnerable and disadvantaged parties in health care sys-tems. These issues cut across clinical ethics, public health ethics and research ethics. The four principles approach tries to deal with several of these issues, without producing a grand theory for resolving all issues of justice. For example, we address issues in research ethics about whether research is permissible with groups who have been repeatedly used as research subjects, though the advantages of research are calculated to benefit all in society. We argue that as medical research is a social enterprise for the public good, it must be accomplished in a broadly inclusive and participatory way, and we try to specify the commitments of such generaliza-tions. Thus, we incorporate principles of justice but do not produce a general theory of justice.

THE FRAMEWORK OF FOUR PRINCIPLES AND THE EVOLUTION OF THE THEORY

The choice of our four types of moral principle as the frame-work for moral decision-making in bioethics derives in part from professional roles and traditions. As noted earlier, health professionals' obligations and virtues have for centu-ries (as found in codes and learned writings on ethics) been framed by professional commitments to provide medical care and to protect patients from disease, injury and system failure. Our principles build on this tradition, but they also significantly depart from it by including parts of morality that traditionally have been neglected in health care ethics, especially through the principles of respect for autonomy and justice. All four types of principles are needed to pro-vide a comprehensive framework for biomedical ethics, but this general framework is abstract and spare until it has been further specified – that is, interpreted and adapted for particular circumstances.

Principles of Biomedical Ethics has evolved appreciably since the first edition in its understanding of abstractness and the demands of particular circumstances. This is not because the principles have changed, but because over the years Childress and I have altered some of our views about the grounding of the principles and about their practical significance. Two major changes deserve special attention. The first is our development of the idea that the four principles are already embedded in public morality – a universal common morality – and are presupposed in the formulation of public and institutional policies. The second is our adoption of Henry Richardson's account of the specification of moral norms. These changes of theory and their significance will be discussed in the next two sections.

THE CENTRALITY OF THE COMMON MORALITY

The source of the four principles is what we, Childress and I, call *the common morality* (a view only incorporated at the point of the third edition of *Principles*, following the language of Alan Donagan). The common morality is applicable to all persons in all places, and all human conduct is rightly judged by its standards. The following are examples of *standards of action* (rules of obligation) in the common morality: (1) 'do not kill'; (2) 'do not cause pain or suffering to others'; (3) 'prevent evil or harm from occurring'; (4) 'rescue persons in danger'; (5) 'tell the truth'; (6) 'nurture the young and dependent'; (7) 'keep your promises'; (8) 'do not steal'; (9) 'do not punish the innocent'; (10) 'treat all persons with equal moral consideration'.

Why have such norms become parts of a common morality, whereas other norms have not? To answer this question, I start with an assumption about the primary goal – that is, objective – of the social institution of morality. This objective is to promote human flourishing by counteracting conditions that cause the quality of people's lives to worsen. The goal is to prevent or limit problems of indifference, conflict, suffering, hostility, scarce resources, limited information, and the like. Centuries of experience have demonstrated that the human condition tends to deteriorate into misery, confusion, violence and distrust unless norms of the sort just listed (1–10) – the norms of the common morality – are observed. When complied with, these norms lessen human misery and preventable death. It is an overstatement to maintain that all of these norms are necessary for the *survival* of a society (as some philosophers and social scientists have maintained (Bok, 1995), but it is not too much to claim that these norms are necessary to *ameliorate or counteract the tendency for the quality of people's lives to worsen or for social relationships to disintegrate* (Mackie, 1977; Warnock, 1971).

These norms are what they are, and not some other set of norms, because they have proven over time that their observance is essential to realize the objectives of morality. What justifies them is that they achieve the objectives of morality, not the fact that they are universally shared across cultures. It is conceivable, of course, that the set of norms that is shared universally is not the same set of norms as the set pragmatically justified by their conformity to the objectives of morality. I agree that if another set of norms would better serve the objectives of morality, then that set of norms ought to displace the norms currently in place. However, I believe that there are no good candidates as alternatives to these norms.

What Childress and I call 'principles' simply are the most general and basic norms of the common morality. In *Principles of Biomedical Ethics*, we devote an entire chapter to each principle in the attempt to explain its nature, content, specification and the like. The assumption behind the argument in each chapter is that our framework of four principles should incorporate and articulate the most general values of the common morality.

Our framework encompasses several types of moral norms, including not only principles, but also rules, rights and moral ideals. We treat principles as the most general and comprehensive norms, but we make only a loose distinction between rules and principles. Rules, we argue, are more precise and practical guides to action that depend on the more general principles for their justification. We defend several types of rules, all of which should be viewed as specifications of principles. These include substantive rules (e.g. truth telling, confidentiality and privacy rules), authority rules (e.g. rules of surrogate authority and rules of professional authority) and procedural rules (e.g. rules for determining eligibility for organ transplantation and rules for reporting grievances to higher authorities).

THE *PRIMA FACIE* CHARACTER OF PRINCIPLES AND RULES

These principles and rules (or other norms in the common morality) can in some circumstances be justifiably overridden by other moral norms with which they conflict. For example, we might justifiably not tell the truth in order to prevent someone from killing another person, and we might justifiably disclose confidential information about a person in order to protect the rights of another person. Principles, duties and rights are not *absolute* (or unconditional) merely because they are *universal*. There are exceptions to all principles, each of which is merely presumptive in force.

Oxford philosopher W. D. Ross developed a theory that has been part of *Principles* since the first edition. Ross's theory is intended to assist in resolving problems of conflict between principles. His views are based on an account of *prima facie* duties, which he contrasts with actual duties. A *prima facie* duty is one that is always to be acted upon unless it conflicts on a particular occasion with another duty. One's *actual* duty, by contrast, is determined by an examination of the respective weights of competing *prima facie* duties in particular situations. When principles contingently conflict, no supreme principle is available – in the four principles approach – to determine an overriding obligation. Therefore, discretionary judgement becomes an inescapable part of moral thinking that relies on principles.

Here is an example. A physician has confidential information about a patient who is also an employee in the hospital where the physician practises. The employee is seeking advancement in a stress-filled position, but the physician has good reason to believe this advancement would be devastating for both the employee and the hospital. The physician has duties of confidentiality, nonmaleficence and beneficence in these circumstances. Should the physician break confidence? Could the matter be handled by making thin disclosures only to the hospital administrator and not to the personnel office? Can such disclosures be made consistent with one's general commitments to confidentiality? Addressing these questions through a process of moral justification is required to establish one's actual duty in the face of these conflicts of *prima facie* duties. I will discuss how this is to be done in the section below on specification.

Once we acknowledge that all general principles have exceptions, we are free to view every moral conclusion that is supported by a principle and every principle itself as subject to modification or reformulation. Change of this sort is to be accomplished through specification, the means by which principles come to have real practical value.

THE SPECIFICATION OF PRINCIPLES AND RULES

To say that principles have their origins in and find support in the common morality and in traditions of health care is not to say that their appearance in a developed system of biomedical ethics is identical to their appearance in the traditions from which they spring. Many authors have correctly pointed out that *prima facie* principles underdetermine moral judgements because there is too little content in such abstract principles to determine concrete outcomes. Every norm and theory contains regions of indeterminacy that need reduction through further development of their commitments in the system, augmenting them with a more specific moral content. I turn, then, to these questions: 'How does the *prima facie* conception of principles work in practical bioethics?'; 'How are general principles to reach down to concrete policies?'; 'How does one fill the gap between abstract principles and concrete judgements?'

The answer is that principles must be specified to suit the needs and demands of particular contexts, thus enabling principles to overcome their lack of content and to handle moral conflict. Specification is a process of reducing the indeterminateness of abstract norms and providing them with specific action-guiding content (Degrazia & Beauchamp, 2001; DeGrazia, 1992; Richardson, 1990; 2000). For example, without further specification, 'do no harm' is too abstract to help in thinking through problems such as whether physicians may justifiably hasten the death of patients. The general norm has to be specified for this particular context.

Specification is not a process of *producing* or *defending* general norms such as those in the common morality; it assumes that they are available. Specifying the norms with which one starts (whether those in the common morality or norms that were previously specified) is accomplished by *narrowing the scope* of the norms, not by explaining what the general norms *mean*. The scope is narrowed, as Henry Richardson puts it, by 'spelling out where, when, why, how, by what means, to whom, or by whom the action is to be done or avoided' (Richardson, 2000). For example, the norm that we are obligated to 'respect the autonomy of persons' cannot, unless specified, handle complicated problems of what to disclose or demand in clinical medicine and research involving human subjects. A definition of 'respect for autonomy' (as, say, 'allowing competent persons to exercise their liberty rights') might clarify one's meaning in using the norm, but would not narrow the general norm or render it more specific.

Specification adds content to general norms. For example, one possible specification of 'respect the autonomy of persons' is 'respect the autonomy of competent patients when they become incompetent by following their advance directives'. This specification will work well in some medical contexts, but will not be adequate in others, thus necessitating additional specification. Progressive specification can continue indefinitely, gradually reducing the conflicts that abstract principles themselves cannot resolve. However, to qualify all along the way as a specification, some transparent connection must always be maintained to the initial norm that gives moral authority to the resulting string of norms.

Now we come to a critical matter about particular moralities, by contrast to the common morality. There is always the possibility of developing more than one line of specification of a norm when confronting practical problems and moral disagreements. It is simply part of the moral life that different persons and groups will offer different (sometimes conflicting) specifications, potentially creating multiple particular moralities. On any problematic issue (such as abortion, animal research, aid in disaster relief, health inequities, euthanasia, etc.) competing specifications are likely to be offered by reasonable and fair-minded parties, all of whom are committed to the common morality. We cannot hold persons to a higher standard than to make judgements conscientiously in light of the relevant basic and specified norms, while attending to the available factual evidence. Conscientious and reasonable moral agents will understandably disagree with equally conscientious persons over moral weights and priorities in circumstances of a contingent conflict of norms.

Nothing in the model of specification suggests that we can always eliminate circumstances of intractable conflicting judgements. However, we should always try to do so by justifying whatever specification we put forward. This suggests that specification as a method needs to be connected to a model of justification that will support some specifications and not others. Only brief attention can be paid here to this difficult philosophical problem.

JUSTIFYING SPECIFICATIONS USING THE METHOD OF COHERENCE

A specification is justified, in the four principles approach, if and only if it maximizes the coherence of the overall set of relevant, justified beliefs. These beliefs could include empirically justified beliefs, justified basic moral beliefs and previously justified specifications. This is a version of so-called wide reflective equilibrium (Daniels, 1979; 1996). No matter how wide the pool of beliefs, there is no reason to expect that the process of rendering norms coherent by specification will come to an end or be perfected. Particular moralities are, from this perspective, continuous works in progress – a process rather than a finished product. There is no reason to think that morality can be rendered coherent in only one way through the process of specification. Many particular moralities present coherent ways to specify the common morality. Normatively, we can demand no more than that agents faithfully specify the norms of the common morality with an attentive eye to overall coherence.

The following are some of the criteria for a coherent (and therefore, according to this model, justified) set of ethical beliefs: consistency (the avoidance of contradiction); argumentative support (explicit support for a position with reasons); intuitive plausibility (the feature of a norm or judgement being secure in its own right); compatibility or coherence with reasonable nonmoral beliefs (in particular, coherence with available empirical evidence); comprehensiveness (the feature of covering the entire moral domain or as much of it as possible); simplicity (reducing the number of moral considerations to the minimum possible without sacrifice in terms of the other criteria) (DeGrazia, 2003; DeGrazia & Beauchamp, 2001).

CONCLUSION

I have explained, and argued in defence of, what has often been called the four principles approach to biomedical ethics, and now increasingly called *principlism* (Arras, 1994;

Gert et al., 1997; Evans, 2000; Strong, 2000; Winkler, 1996). The four clusters of principles derive from both considered judgements in the common morality and enduring and valuable parts of traditions of health care. Health care ethics has often been said to be an 'applied ethics', but this metaphor may be more misleading than helpful. It is rarely the case that we simply apply a principle to resolve a tough problem. We will almost always, I have argued, be engaged in collecting evidence, reasoning and specifying general principles. This is how problems should be treated and how progress can be made in health care ethics. From this perspective, the four principles form only a starting point – the point where the practical work begins.

REFERENCES

Appelbaum PS. The parable of the forensic physician: ethics and the problem of doing harm. *Int J Law Psychiatry* 1990; **13**: 249–59.

Arras JD. Principles and particularity: the roles of cases in bioethics. *Indiana Law J* 1994; **69**: 983–1014.

Beauchamp TL, Childress JF. *Principles of Biomedical Ethics.* New York: Oxford University Press, 1979.

Bloch S, Reddaway R. *Soviet Psychiatric Abuse: The Shadow Over World Psychiatry.* Boulder, CO: Westview Press, 1984; Chapter 1.

Bok S. *Common Values.* Columbia, MO: University of Missouri Press, 1995; pp. 13–23, 50–9.

Buchanan A. Health-care delivery and resource allocation. In: Veatch R, ed. *Medical Ethics*, 2nd edition. Boston: Jones and Bartlett Publishers, 1997.

Buchanan A, Brock D, Daniels N, Wikler D. *From Chance to Choice: Genetics and Justice.* New York: Cambridge University Press, 2000.

Childress JF. The place of autonomy in bioethics. *Hastings Center Report* 20, 1990; pp. 12–16.

Childress JF, Meslin EM, Shapiro HT, eds. *Belmont Revisited: Ethical Principles for Research with Human Subjects.* Washington, DC: Georgetown University Press, 2005.

Daniels N. Wide reflective equilibrium and theory acceptance in ethics. *J Philos* 1979; **76**: 256–82.

Daniels N. *Just Health Care.* New York: Cambridge University Press, 1985.

Daniels N. Wide reflective equilibrium in practice. In: Sumner LW, Boyle J, eds. *Philosophical Perspectives on Bioethics.* Toronto: University of Toronto Press, 1996.

Daniels N. *Just Health.* New York: Cambridge University Press, 2006.

DeGrazia D. Moving forward in bioethical theory: theories, cases, and specified principlism. *J Med Philos* 1992; **17**: 511–39.

DeGrazia D. Common morality, coherence, and the principles of biomedical ethics, *Kennedy Inst Ethics J* 2003; **13**: 219–30.

DeGrazia D, Beauchamp TL. Philosophical foundations and philosophical methods. In: Sulmasy D, Sugarman J, eds. *Methods of Bioethics.* Washington, DC: Georgetown University Press, 2001; pp. 33–6.

Engelhardt HT Jr. *The Foundations of Bioethics*, 2nd edition. New York: Oxford University Press, 1996.

Evans JH. A sociological account of the growth of principlism. *Hastings Center Report* 30, 2000; pp. 31–8.

Faden RR, Beauchamp TL. *A History and Theory of Informed Consent*. New York: Oxford University Press, 1986.

Gert B. *Morality*. New York: Oxford University Press, 2005.

Gert B, Culver CM, Clouser KD. *Bioethics: A Return to Fundamentals*. New York: Oxford University Press, 1997; Chapter 4.

Jonsen AR. *The Birth of Bioethics*. New York: Oxford University Press, 1998; p. 3ff.

Kagan S. *The Limits of Morality*. Oxford: Clarendon Press, 1989.

Katz J. *The Silent World of Doctor and Patient*. New York: The Free Press, 1984.

Kukla R. Conscientious autonomy: displacing decisions in health care. *Hastings Center Report*, 2005; pp. 34–44.

Mackie J. *Ethics: Inventing Right and Wrong*. London: Penguin, 1977; p. 107ff.

Miller RW. Beneficence, duty, and distance. *Philos Public Aff* 2004; **32**: 357–83.

National Commission for the Protection of Human Subjects of Biomedical and Behavioral Research. *The Belmont Report: Ethical Principles and Guidelines for the Protection of Human Subjects of Research*. Washington, DC: DHEW Publication OS 78–0012 1978.

Pellegrino E. The four principles and the doctor–patient relationship: the need for a better linkage. In: Gillon R, ed. *Principles of Health Care Ethics*. Chichester: John Wiley & Sons, Ltd, 1994.

Pellegrino E, Thomasma D. *For the Patient's Good: The Restoration of Beneficence in Health Care*. New York: Oxford University Press, 1988.

Pellegrino ED, Thomasma DC. *The Virtues in Medical Practice*. New York: Oxford University Press, 1993; pp. 184–9.

Percival T. *Medical Ethics; or a Code of Institutes and Precepts, Adapted to the Professional Conduct of Physicians and Surgeons*. Manchester: S. Russell, 1803; pp. 165–6. Percival's work was the pattern for the American Medical Association's (AMA) first code of ethics in 1847.

Powers M, Faden R. *Social Justice: The Moral Foundations of Public Health and Health Policy*. New York: Oxford University Press, 2006.

Richardson HS. Specifying norms as a way to resolve concrete ethical problems. *Philos Public Aff* 1990; **19**: 279–310.

Richardson HS. Specifying, balancing, and interpreting bioethical principles. *J Med Philos* 2000; **25**: 285–307.

Singer P. *Practical Ethics*, 2nd edition. Cambridge: Cambridge University Press, 1993.

Singer P. Living high and letting die. *Philos Phenomenol Res* 1999; **59**: 183–7.

Strong C. Specified principlism. *J Med Philos* 2000; **25**: 285–307.

Warnock GJ. *The Object of Morality*. London: Methuen & Co., 1971; pp. 15–26.

Winkler E. Moral philosophy and bioethics: contextualism versus the paradigm theory. In: Sumner LW, Boyle J, eds. *Philosophical Perspectives on Bioethics*. Toronto: University of Toronto Press, 1996.

2

Theories of Autonomy[1]

NATALIE STOLJAR

The philosophical notion of personal autonomy (or free agency) has been characterized in different ways: as a fundamental right which justifies further rights such as those of abortion or free speech; as a basic political good of liberal political theory; as a character ideal on a par with courage or integrity; and as a necessary state or capacity of full moral agents. Although there are many conceptions of autonomy, there is a common theme. Being autonomous is usually taken to mean being self-governing in one way or another; an autonomous state is one in which one's will is genuinely *one's own*.

In health care ethics, the requirement to respect autonomy has usually been conceived as the requirement to secure a patient's voluntary and informed consent to a medical procedure or treatment. This notion of consent has placed the emphasis on the actions of the health care provider (see Dodds, 2000). The provider is required to provide accessible, relevant and complete information and to refrain from interference in the patient's decision-making processes. In brief, the *absence* of certain autonomy-undermining conditions – in particular those of coercion and ignorance – is sufficient to secure a patient's autonomy.

Contemporary theories of autonomy challenge this minimalist notion, however, and suggest that agents' (and therefore patients') decision-making processes must satisfy some extra *positive* conditions to secure autonomy. Consider, for example, two typical failures of personal autonomy: first, an agent who habitually and uncritically adopts others' social preferences and values as his own; second, an agent who has so internalized the outlooks and mores of the family in which she grew up that these are treated as authoritative without critical reflection (Feinberg, 1986, p. 32). Although in neither case is there any overt interference or coercion, both agents lack autonomy because both fail to exhibit a characteristic necessary for autonomy, for example a capacity of 'subjecting these governing ideals to rational criticism and then modifying them when necessary' (Feinberg, 1986, p. 32). I propose at the end of this chapter that health care ethics should adopt a richer conception of the requirement of patient autonomy and shift its focus from the actions of the health care provider to the situation of the patient, in particular to the social context that affects the patient's preference formation and decision-making processes.

Conceptions of autonomy in the contemporary literature have been divided into two rough classes: Kantian conceptions and non-Kantian – or procedural – conceptions. Broadly speaking, each reflects a different approach to the following question: How can agents be genuinely self-governing in the face of the physical and social forces in which they are embedded and which appear to determine their states and capacities? Traditional Kantian conceptions endorse a version of *incompatibilism*, namely the thesis that genuine free agency cannot be reconciled with socialization or physical determinism. They characterize autonomy by introducing either idealized conditions of free agency or metaphysical conceptions of the autonomous self.

Non-Kantian conceptions are *compatibilist*, and they attempt to explicate autonomy within the network of physical and social forces in which agents operate. The key task of these conceptions is to distinguish the conditions in which socialization is autonomy undermining from the conditions in which it is not.

This chapter traces the main theories of autonomy in the current philosophical literature. (It does not attempt to survey discussions of autonomy within the literature on health care ethics specifically.) The first section outlines the traditional Kantian account which conceives of moral autonomy as an ability of rational agents to formulate universal moral

---

[1] This chapter is an updated and somewhat revised version of my entry on the philosophy of autonomy in the *Elsevier Encyclopedia of the Social and Behavioral Sciences* (2001).

Principles of Health Care Ethics, Second Edition   Edited by R.E. Ashcroft, A. Dawson, H. Draper and J.R. McMillan

principles. These moral principles are said to originate in the will of the agent and to be, in this sense, the agent's 'own'. The second section turns to three illustrations of procedural accounts of autonomy: *endorsement*, *historical* and *self-knowledge* accounts.[2] Each proposes a condition on critical reflection that distinguishes autonomous from nonautonomous preference formation. The third section describes neo-Kantian responses to procedural analyses. These propose that autonomy requires a kind of normative competence, namely an ability to identify norms, for example, moral norms or norms that are 'correct' for an agent to endorse. The fourth section outlines two further approaches – *psychological* and *self-realization* – both of which focus on the relationship between conceptions of autonomy and the nature of the autonomous agent. In the final section, I briefly discuss the consequences for health care ethics.

THE KANTIAN CONCEPTION OF AUTONOMY

A major strand in theories of autonomy is derived from the philosophy of Immanuel Kant. For Kant, autonomy has a special meaning: 'Autonomy of the will is the property the will has of being a law unto itself (independently of every property belonging to the objects of volition)' (Kant, 1785, 1948, p. 108). Rational beings make the moral law for themselves and can regard themselves as authors of the law. Thus, autonomy is manifested when rational agents 'will' the moral law. An important feature of the moral law is that it is a categorical, not a hypothetical, imperative. When an agent formulates a categorical imperative, he formulates a maxim of the form 'I ought to do this', not of the form 'I ought to do this if I desire that'. For example, an agent formulates the moral law when she wills 'I ought not to lie' but formulates a hypothetical imperative when she wills 'I ought not to lie if I desire not to be punished for lying'. The act of formulating the moral law is an act of a pure autonomous will: It is untainted by the influence of the desires and interests that an agent may have relative to a particular situation. The pure autonomous will amounts to a metaphysical conception of the self, to be distinguished from empirical conceptions of the self. The metaphysical self is unconstrained by desires, interests and social forces. Thus, Kant's conception of freedom is incompatibilist.

A contemporary parallel of Kant's conception of autonomy is John Rawls' influential notion of free and rational agents formulating principles of justice in the 'original position' (Rawls, 1971). Rawls argues that rational agents formulate principles of justice from behind a 'veil of ignorance', namely from a position in which they are making decisions about how a society will function before they know who in this society they will turn out to be. In the original position, they

have abstracted away from a particular location in the society to which the principles of justice apply. This means that such agents, like Kantian agents, are uninfluenced by the particular desires and preferences arising from being embedded in an actual situation. Because of this, their formulation of the principles of justice is genuinely *self*-originating.

The Kantian conception of autonomy has two aspects. First, the categorical imperative provides a standard according to which we can judge whether a particular example of moral reasoning is autonomous. If the moral reasoning issues in the categorical imperative, then it is autonomous. Otherwise, it is not. Second, autonomy is a function of a metaphysical conception of the self, because autonomy manifests itself when the Kantian 'true' self is expressed through the formulation of the moral law. Both aspects of the Kantian view are contentious. Critics challenge the notion of a universally valid moral law as well as the concept of a pure autonomous will, which is said to be implausibly metaphysical. In addition, Rawls' account of the agent operating in the original position has been criticized as unfaithful to empirical reality. Feminists and communitarians have argued that this agent is 'atomistic'; that is, existing in a vacuum divorced from the social relations in which actual agents are embedded (e.g. Sandel, 1982). No such agent exists because agents are always the product of family influences, socialization and so on. Moreover, an agent stripped of desires, interests and preferences cannot engage in the imaginative moral reasoning required to formulate principles of justice. A further difficulty is that the Kantian conception is said to lead to an impoverished account of the *value* of autonomy. It is associated with the claim that autonomous agents are, and ought to be, self-sufficient, which in turn is associated with the character ideal of the 'self-made man'. Critics – especially feminists – have challenged this character ideal and questioned whether self-sufficiency, or 'substantive independence', is really a value that a theory of autonomy, or normative theories in general, should promote. They have argued that a conception of autonomy should not exclude the possibility of agents having significant relationships of interdependency such as those obtaining with family members (see Friedman, 1997).

PROCEDURAL THEORIES OF AUTONOMY

Since the 1970s, *procedural* theories have been dominant. On procedural theories, it is enough that agents' reasoning processes satisfy certain formal and procedural conditions for the outcomes of those processes (decisions, preferences and desires) to count as autonomous. Procedural accounts are 'content neutral'. There are no specific beliefs, goals

---

[2]See Stacey (2005a) for additional illustrations of procedural theories of autonomy.

or values that the autonomous agent must adopt. Nor are there any standards or conditions external to the agent that operate as touchstones of autonomous reasoning or place constraints on the contents of agents' preferences and desires. Procedural theories, therefore, are congenial to the concerns of critics of the Kantian conception.

AUTONOMY AS ENDORSEMENT

Perhaps the most prominent procedural approaches are those of Gerald Dworkin and Harry Frankfurt (Dworkin, 1970, 1988; Frankfurt, 1971). Both argue that what distinguishes autonomous from nonautonomous critical reflection is *endorsement* – an agent's sense of engagement or identification with his preferences or desires. In Frankfurt's terms, an autonomous will is *the will the agent wants*. Consider the difference between a willing and an unwilling drug addict. Frankfurt argues that although both are addicted, only the unwilling addict is nonautonomous. He is a 'passive bystander' with respect to the desire to use drugs, whereas the willing addict engages and identifies with that desire, and hence endorses it. In Frankfurt's account, the idea of endorsement is spelt out using a hierarchical distinction between different levels of desire. First-order desires – such as a desire to inject heroin – are autonomous just in case they are endorsed by second-order desires – such as a desire to desire to inject heroin (Frankfurt, 1971).[3]

Important objections have been raised to endorsement accounts. The first focuses on their hierarchical nature. Even if first-order desires can be characterized as endorsed with respect to second-order desires, this is not sufficient to ensure autonomy unless the second-order desires themselves are endorsed. The problem results in a regress unless we introduce a qualitative distinction among levels, for example, between higher-order *values* and first-order *desires* (Watson, 1975). However, the regress objection can be generalized to many hierarchical accounts, because whatever the nature of the higher-order level, one can always question whether it truly represents free agency. The second-order level itself will always be the outcome of the social forces influencing the agent. A second objection is that the endorsement condition is too stringent. Suppose out of habit an agent chooses to go on vacation to the same destination every year. The fact that the agent fails to attend critically to the desire and does not endorse it each time should not rule out its being autonomous. Third, it has been suggested that the endorsement condition is too weak. The endorsement account relies on the idea that although the unwilling addict intentionally injects himself with heroin, he prefers not to. As he prefers not to inject himself, he does not endorse the desire to inject himself. It has been argued that (all things considered) intending to do something

and preferring to do something are indistinguishable, and thus if an agent intends to so something, he also prefers to do it and endorses it. Therefore, in so far as the unwilling addict intends to inject himself with the drug, he also endorses it. The objection claims that endorsement merely distinguishes intentional from nonintentional agency, not autonomous from nonautonomous agency. The apparent lack of autonomy of the unwilling addict is not due therefore to a lack of endorsement (Buss, 1994).

AUTONOMY AS HISTORICAL CRITICAL REFLECTION

Most hierarchical approaches to autonomy are *structural* or *ahistorical*. They propose conditions that an agent's *existing* motivational state must satisfy. An important difficulty for structural variants of the hierarchical approach is the 'problem of manipulation' (see e.g. Stacey, 2005b). Suppose a hypnotist inserts into the agent a hierarchy of desires that satisfies Frankfurt's conditions. Because Frankfurt's analysis is ahistorical, this motivational state counts as autonomous when it appears not to be. A possible solution is to introduce conditions that allow reflection on the historical processes of development of the motivational state. For example, Gerald Dworkin analyses autonomy as 'a second-order capacity of persons to reflect critically on their first-order preferences, desires, wishes and so forth and the capacity to accept or attempt to change these in the light of higher-order preferences and values' (Dworkin, 1988, p. 20). A capacity allows reflection on the processes by means of which an agent acquires desires and preferences. It also distinguishes between an agent's autonomy on the one hand and a particular exercise of autonomy on the other hand. A related approach *requires* reflection on the processes of development of desires. The *historical criterion of autonomy* proposes that an agent is autonomous with respect to a certain preference or desire only if she does not resist its development when attending to the process of its development or would not have resisted had she attended to the process (Christman, 1990, 1991). Notice that this criterion can account for preferences formed out of habit because, although in most cases of habit agents do not attend each time to the process of development of their preferences, it is true that they *would not* have resisted the process *had* they attended to it.

The historical criterion is difficult to maintain in the face of apparent counterexamples. Consider agents who have internalized an oppressive ideology, for example a young student who is so influenced by the norms of the fashion industry that she devotes an excessive amount of time and energy to her appearance. Such agents are usually

---

[3]For a more precise summary of Frankfurt's position and objections to it, see Stacey (2005b). For essays on Frankfurt's theory, see Buss & Overton (2005).

characterized as nonautonomous with respect to the norms of the ideology, yet the historical condition cannot adequately explain why. Even had the student reflected on the fashion norms that she has internalized, as well as the processes of development of her preferences and its relationship to the norms, she probably would not have resisted the norms or the development of her preferences. The very fact that the ideology is effectively internalized makes it unlikely that an agent would resist the development of preferences based on the ideology (Benson, 1990). The historical condition therefore does not account for cases that are thought to be paradigms of nonautonomous preference-formation.

AUTONOMY AS SELF-KNOWLEDGE

Another set of procedural conceptions proposes that *authenticity* is the key factor in explicating autonomy. Having one's own will is having the will one *really* wants. One important approach characterizes authenticity in terms of self-knowledge. For example, Diana Tietjens Meyers argues that self-discovery is a necessary capacity for achieving autonomy (e.g. Meyers, 1989, 2005). Suppose an agent – Martin – has 'always been groomed to follow in his father's footsteps [and] his parents have taught him to feel deeply guilty whenever he disappoints their expectations' (Meyers, 1989, p. 46). He dutifully completes medical school and ends up as a successful surgeon. Although there are opportunities along the way for Martin to 'probe' his feelings and reconsider his career path, it does not occur to him to do so. Meyers suggests that Martin's 'insensitivity to his own responses' and 'blindered approach to life' indicate that whereas 'He may be doing what he wants, . . . there is no reason to suppose that he is doing what he really wants' (Meyers, 1989, p. 47). The distinction between doing what one wants and doing what one really wants is important for a range of cases in which authenticity is questionable. For instance, conventional gender roles can shape values and desires through being omnipresent in culture or instilled since birth by family socialization. Meyers points out that the enforcement of gender roles can interfere with a person's ability to distinguish between apparent and authentic desires.

The challenge for this conception of autonomy is to give a plausible account of the difference between 'real' and 'apparent' desires as well as to identify how self-knowledge fails in cases of failures of autonomy. One possibility is to argue that agents lack self-knowledge by having inaccurate beliefs about themselves, specifically about the desires and motivations in question. Perhaps Martin's 'real' wishes are being covered up by his failure to scrutinize. The desires to be a doctor operate on the surface, but his deep, 'true' desires are to follow some other career path. As his beliefs that he wants to be a doctor are based on apparent desires, they are

false beliefs about himself, and he lacks self-knowledge. A difficulty for this characterization, however, is that it may seem to employ a metaphysical notion of the self as the bearer of real desires. Even if it does not, it must rely on the agent experiencing internal conflict among desires, and failing to probe or scrutinize in response to such experiences. The apparent desires are the unscrutinized ones, and the real desires are the ones that would have emerged had the agent scrutinized her apparent desires. Often, however, there is no experienced dissonance among desires, and no opportunity for 'real' desires to emerge. How should we characterize the notion of an authentic self in these cases?

NEO-KANTIAN THEORIES

The many objections to procedural conceptions of autonomy have given rise to a new category of approaches, namely 'substantive' approaches. These have begun to achieve prominence and to challenge the dominance of procedural conceptions. The new substantive accounts introduce *external* and relational conditions on agents' preferences and desires. On procedural accounts, the internal processes necessary for autonomous reasoning are both necessary and sufficient for autonomy. On substantive accounts, procedural criteria may be necessary for autonomy; however, they are not sufficient. Broadly speaking, there are two versions of substantive account: neo-Kantian accounts which characterize autonomy as having 'normative substance' (Richardson, 2002), and non-normative versions which characterize the external conditions of autonomy as social or psychological in some way. I sketch neo-Kantian accounts in this section and non-normative substantive accounts in the next section.

Some neo-Kantian accounts place direct normative restrictions on the content of agents' preferences.[4] For example, suppose an agent's preference is analysed as autonomy undermining when it interferes with the agent's normal functioning (Buss, 1994, p. 106). 'Normal functioning' is spelt out using a normative notion – that of well-being, or human flourishing – and thus the agent's reasoning processes are subject to a normative constraint. However, theories that place direct normative constraints on the contents of agents' preferences risk collapsing the notion of autonomy – that of *self*-government or *self*-rule – into another notion entirely, that of *right*-rule (Benson, 2005, p. 132). Instead, proponents of neo-Kantian approaches have introduced the notion of *normative competence*: the failure of autonomy corresponds to a failure of competence or a capacity to identify norms and apply them to one's own decision-making processes. Consider JoJo, the son of an evil and sadistic tyrant. JoJo

---

[4]Benson (2005) contains a helpful discussion of the different substantive theories of autonomy and a comprehensive list of the authors identified with different versions (see especially footnotes 5, 40 and 41).

is raised to respect his father's values and emulate his desires, so that he thoroughly internalizes his father's evil and sadistic world view. Let us suppose that on procedural theories JoJo is counted as autonomous because he identifies with his first-order desires in the appropriate ways, has the desires he *really* wants, and so on. It has been proposed that he is neither free nor morally responsible because his upbringing has blocked his capacity to distinguish right from wrong (Wolf, 1987). Similarly, the young student who has internalized the ideology of the fashion industry can be characterized as having internalized certain *false* norms such as that most women's natural physical appearance is deficient. The internalization of the norm blocks her capacity to effectively criticize this 'false construal of [her] personal value', and hence her ability to distinguish correct from incorrect norms – her normative competence – is flawed (Benson, 1991). It is the failure of normative competence that explains the failure of autonomy. Normative competence approaches do not collapse autonomy into the notion of right-rule because 'normatively competent persons can choose what is unreasonable or wrong or value what is bad because competence lies some distance short of perfect evaluative perception or responsiveness' (Benson, 2005, pp. 133–4).

One controversial issue raised by normative competence accounts is that of the status of the moral and other norms that autonomous agents identify. For example, it has been argued that moral norms are objective because they derive from the requirements of objective reason (Wolf, 1990). If this is right, the capacity required for autonomy is a capacity to 'track' objective features of the world. The idea that morality is objective – moral realism – is controversial despite being a well-known and widely supported position. Moreover, realism about nonmoral norms is often thought to be less plausible than moral realism. An additional difficulty for normative competence accounts is the charge that they conflate autonomy with moral responsibility. In the case of JoJo, for example, it may be that the comprehensiveness of his socialization absolves him from full moral responsibility for his acts, but does it follow that the acts are not the product of his own agency? The wish to maintain a conceptual distinction between responsibility and autonomy has led to a revision of the normative competence approach (Benson, 1994).

PSYCHOLOGICAL APPROACHES

Neither procedural nor neo-Kantian conceptions of autonomy give much emphasis to the social context of the autonomous agent, and how psychological and other features of the agent may be necessary for producing and maintaining autonomy. Several recent theories developed by feminists and others ad-dress this aspect of the problem, focusing particularly on the putative incompatibility between autonomy and oppression. On *psychological approaches*, certain kinds of psychological impairment, such as impairments of self-confidence and self-esteem, are construed as autonomy undermining. Moreover, these impairments are the products of social and relational features of agents, not of their internal psychological states considered in isolation. Consider a person who is believed (erroneously) by her family and the medical establishment to be mentally unstable because she is passionate, excitable and 'prone to emotional outbursts in public' (Benson, 1994). Because she trusts these external judgements of her character and behaviour, she becomes disoriented and loses her self-confidence and self-esteem. Her will is still intact because she can still put her preferences and desires into effect. But due to her lack of a sense of self-worth, she also lacks certain important attitudes to her own decisions that seem to be necessary for those decisions to be autonomous. She is not 'behind' her decisions and does not treat them as authoritative. Such failures of a sense of assurance in one's own capacity to form preferences and make decisions (for example, failures of self-confidence, self-trust or a sense of self-worth) can be caused by a variety of psychological states, including many arising from oppression.[5]

Psychological accounts have several advantages. First, they do not rely on metaphysical conceptions of the self, but rather situate agents within the network of social relations that affect them. As a result, they take an important step towards understanding the effects of oppression and how oppression is incompatible with autonomy. Second, these accounts do not require that autonomous agents have preferences and desires with specific contents, and nor do they appeal to objective conceptions of value. They do, however, place weaker external constraints on desires and preferences, and hence they are not purely procedural or content neutral.

Nevertheless, there are questions to be raised. For example, how exactly is the psychological impairment (that is the lack of self-esteem, self-trust or self-confidence) tied to the failure of autonomy? One suggestion is that the absence of self-worth erodes agents' sense of themselves as competent 'to answer for one's conduct in light of normative demands that, from one's point of view, others might appropriately apply to one's actions' (Benson, 1994, p. 660). Agents therefore are not autonomous because they do not see themselves as authoritative with respect to the normative demands that the community places on them. However, in certain typical cases of nonautonomous decision making, this link between the lack of a sense of self-worth and the lack of normative competence does not seem to be present. In the case of the young student who has internalized fashion ideology, one may suppose that

---

[5]For discussions of self-trust in the context of health care ethics see, for example, McLeod (2002) and McLeod & Sherwin (2000).

a low sense of self-worth accompanies her commitment to these norms. Yet it is not clear that her lack of self-esteem interferes with her sense of herself as normatively competent to answer the fashion world's expectations. Indeed, she seems to wish to increase her sense of self-worth by living up to these norms, which she takes as applicable to her. In this sense, she is very much 'behind' her commitment to these norms. A second issue is whether the psychological impairment itself is constitutive of the lack of autonomy, or rather it causes the breakdown of some other constitutive process. Psychological conceptions claim that the reasoning capacities of agents are fully intact despite the psychological impairment, and hence that the failure of autonomy is due to the absence of a necessary psychological or emotional state such as that of sense of self-worth. A proponent of a procedural conception may respond that an agent's lack of a sense of self-worth makes it impossible for her critical reflection to operate appropriately. Hence the lack of self-worth may lead to a *procedural* failing that is responsible for the agent's lack of autonomy.

THE IMPLICATIONS FOR HEALTH CARE ETHICS

Current theories of autonomy recommend a shift away from autonomy conceived as voluntary and informed consent to a richer, more complex account of autonomy in which the social context of the patient plays an important role. For example, 'the decision about whether or not to use hormone replacement therapy at menopause is complicated by factors other than inadequate and inconsistent evidence' (McLeod & Sherwin 2000, p. 269). A decision to use hormone replacement therapy may be influenced not only by medical considerations (for example that it is likely to reduce the risk of heart disease) but also by the cultural situations of the particular agent and that of women as a group. A patient's 'normative competence' – that is, her ability to evaluate cultural norms which she takes as applicable to her and to reject them if they are inapplicable – may be diminished; and her self-confidence and self-trust in her own decision making may be reduced. McLeod and Sherwin comment that a cultural norm that is oppressive to women, such as that looking young is attractive and valued whereas looking old is unattractive and devalued, may influence a decision about whether to take hormone replacement therapy. Self-trust may be difficult to achieve when the agent is aware of the influence of oppressive cultural norms on her own thinking (McLeod & Sherwin 2000, p. 269).

Thus, it is not enough to secure the autonomy of a patient in health care contexts to ensure only the *absence* of interference or ignorance. In addition health care providers must attempt to enhance certain positive conditions that are likely to generate autonomous, or *more* autonomous,

reasoning. Certain specific recommendations may be deduced from the theories above. First, the health care provider must be informed about the social situation (including family and other social relationships) of patients because the social situation will have affected the development of capacities necessary for autonomy or the exercise of autonomous reasoning in this particular case. Second, providers must recognize that different individuals have different capacities for autonomous reasoning and that even the same individual will exercise these capacities to different degrees at different times. Third, whether a patient is in an oppressed group – in short, a patient's race, class or gender – is likely to affect their ability to engage in autonomous reasoning either in general or about certain specific cases. For example, certain kinds oppression may impede the development of the capacity of critical reflection that is required for autonomy. Alternatively, norms and values implicit in ideologies of oppression may be taken (incorrectly) by the agent to be applicable to her. In such cases, the provider should encourage imaginative rejection of the oppressive norms and consideration of other options. Finally, providers must be aware of potential psychological impediments to autonomous reasoning deriving from the social and family situation of the patient but also from the relationship with the health care provider. A patient's relationship with a provider will have the potential to either enhance or undermine a patient's sense of self-worth and self-confidence and therefore her ability to make autonomous decisions.

REFERENCES

Benson P. Freedom and value. *J Philos* 1987; **84**: 465–86.

Benson P. Autonomy and oppressive socialization. *Soc Theory Pract* 1991; 17: 385–408.

Benson P. Free agency and self-worth. *J Philos* 1994; **91**: 650–68.

Benson P. Feminist intuitions and the normative substance of autonomy. In: Taylor JS, ed. *Personal Autonomy: New Essays on Personal Autonomy and Its Role in Contemporary Moral Philosophy.* Cambridge: Cambridge University Press, 2005.

Buss S, Overton L, eds. *The Contours of Agency.* Cambridge, MA: MIT Press, 2005.

Buss S. Autonomy reconsidered. In: French PA, Uehling TA, Wettstein HK, eds. *Midwest Studies in Philosophy* XIX. Minneapolis, MN: University of Minnesota Press, 1994.

Christman J, ed. *The Inner Citadel: Essays on Individual Autonomy.* New York: Oxford University Press, 1989.

Christman J. Autonomy and personal history. *Can J Philos* 1990; **20**: 1–24.

Christman J. Liberalism and individual positive freedom. *Ethics* 1991; **101**: 343–59.

Christman J, Anderson J, eds. *Autonomy and the Challenges of Liberalism: New Essays.* Cambridge: Cambridge University Press, 2005.

Dodds S. Choice and control in feminist bioethics. In: Mackenzie C, Stoljar N, eds. *Relational Autonomy. Feminist Essays on Autonomy, Agency and the Social Self*. New York: Oxford University Press, 2000; p. 214.

Dworkin G. Acting freely. *Nous* 1970; **3**: 367–83.

Dworkin G. *The Theory and Practice of Autonomy*. New York: Cambridge University Press, 1988.

Feinberg J. Autonomy. *Harm To Self*. Oxford: Oxford University Press, 1986. Reprinted: *The Inner Citadel*, 1986 (page references are to the latter).

Frankfurt H. Freedom of the will and the concept of a person. J Philos 1971; **68**: 5–20. Reprinted in *The Inner Citadel*.

Frankfurt H. *The Importance of What We Care About*. Cambridge: Cambridge University Press, 1988.

Friedman M. Autonomy and social relationships: rethinking the feminist critique. In: Meyers DT, ed. *Feminists Rethink the Self*. Boulder, CO: Westview Press, 1997.

Hill TE Jr. The Kantian conception of autonomy. In: Christman J, ed. *The Inner Citadel: Essays on Individual Autonomy*. New York: Oxford University Press, 1989.

Kant I. *Groundwork of the Metaphysic of Morals* (Translated and analysed by Paton HJ). New York: Harper & Row, 1785, 1948.

Mackenzie C, Stoljar N, eds. *Relational Autonomy. Feminist Essays on Autonomy, Agency and the Social Self*. New York: Oxford University Press, 2000a.

Mackenzie C, Stoljar N. Introduction: autonomy refigured. In: Mackenzie C, Stoljar N, eds. *Relational Autonomy. Feminist Essays on Autonomy, Agency and the Social Self*. New York: Oxford University Press, 2000b.

McLeod C. *Self-Trust and Reproductive Autonomy*. Cambridge, MA: MIT Press, 2002.

McLeod C, Sherwin S. Relational autonomy, self-trust and health care for patients who are oppressed. In: Mackenzie C, Stoljar N, eds. *Relational Autonomy. Feminist Essays on Autonomy, Agency and the Social Self*. New York: Oxford University Press, 2000.

Meyers DT. *Self, Society and Personal Choice*. New York: Columbia University Press, 1989.

Meyers DT. Decentralizing autonomy. Five faces of selfhood. In: Christman J, Anderson J, eds. *Autonomy and the Challenges of Liberalism: New Essays*. Cambridge: Cambridge University Press, 2005.

Rawls J. *A Theory of Justice*. Oxford: Oxford University Press, 1971.

Rawls J. Kantian constructivism in moral theory: the Dewey lectures. *J Philos* 1980; **77**: 515–72.

Reath A. Ethical autonomy. In: Craig E, ed. *Routledge Encyclopedia of Philosophy*. Oxford: Routledge, 1998; vol. 1.

Sandel M. *Liberalism and the Limits of Justice*. Cambridge: Cambridge University Press, 1982.

Taylor JS, ed. Introduction. In: *Personal Autonomy: New Essays on Personal Autonomy and Its Role in Contemporary Moral Philosophy*. Cambridge: Cambridge University Press, 2005a.

Taylor JS, ed. *Personal Autonomy: New Essays on Personal Autonomy and Its Role in Contemporary Moral Philosophy*. Cambridge: Cambridge University Press, 2005b.

Watson G. Free agency. *J Philos* 1975; **72**: 205–20.

Wolf S. *Freedom Within Reason*. New York: Oxford University Press, 1990.

Wolf S. Sanity and the metaphysics of responsibility. In: Schoeman F, ed. *Responsibility, Character and the Emotions*. New York: Cambridge University Press, 1987.

3

Beneficence

GARRETT CULLITY

Since the point of health care is to benefit the person to whom it is provided, all questions in health care ethics are in one way or another about beneficence: its scope, limits and proper expression. This chapter provides a general introduction to beneficence and its treatment within moral philosophy, and then discusses its application to a number of important issues in the ethics of health care.

'Beneficence' is now an uncommon word in ordinary English discourse. Since it was first coined,[1] it has been used with different meanings, broader and narrower. At its broadest, it has been used to refer to *doing good* generally – as its etymology would suggest (Frankena, 1987). According to some writers, it now has a much narrower meaning in ordinary English: it 'connotes acts of mercy, kindness, and charity': (Beauchamp & Childress, 2001). In the study of ethics, however, it has come to be used with a meaning intermediate between these two. On this usage, beneficence is appropriately furthering the welfare of others, from that motive.

This is not as broad as the first usage, since it excludes doing good accidentally or in ways other than by promoting others' welfare. On the other hand, it is not as narrow as the second. Saving your life, for example, need not be an act of mercy; but it would also be odd to describe it as kind or charitable. It is simply the minimally decent thing to do. However, as long as it is motivated by the recognition of your interests in receiving help, it counts as beneficent, on the usage now prevailing in ethical theory.

So understood, beneficence has a strong claim to be *the* characteristic attitude of the moral point of view. When we contrast self-interest with morality, the distinction being drawn is between seeking only to further one's own welfare and seeking also to further the welfare of others. This is at the core of all cultures' conception of morality. It is therefore not surprising to find that there have been prominent attempts to construct theories that seek to derive the whole

of morality from a foundation of beneficence. These will be discussed further below.

Some ways of furthering other people's welfare are naive, foolish or even pernicious. If beneficence is something there is reason to admire, recommend and practise, it must amount to *appropriately* furthering others' welfare (from that motive). Notice that this covers two points. Beneficence furthers those forms of welfare that it is appropriate for us to further, and it does so in the right way.

Obviously, then, a central question in interpreting the moral requirements of beneficence is what distinguishes appropriate from inappropriate ways of furthering welfare. Examining that question is a major focus of this chapter. Other questions I shall discuss along the way include: What is meant by talking about 'requirements' of beneficence, and how far do such requirements extend? How are such requirements justified? What is welfare? What are the sub-varieties of beneficence? What is its relationship to other moral requirements, and what determines which of them prevails in particular cases? The latter part of the chapter will demonstrate the relevance of answers to these questions to some prominent issues in health care ethics.

SPECIAL AND GENERAL REQUIREMENTS OF BENEFICENCE AND THEIR LIMITS

An influential idea, endorsed by both Kant (1996) and Mill (1998), is that beneficence is an 'imperfect duty'. I have a duty to treat others beneficently, but have discretion over when and towards whom I perform beneficent actions: I need not be doing so all the time. This attractive idea needs interpretation and defence, however. It is not plausible that the exercise of beneficence is always

---

[1]*OED* gives 1531 for its first appearance in English, though of course it comes from much older Latin antecedents.

Principles of Health Care Ethics, Second Edition   Edited by R.E. Ashcroft, A. Dawson, H. Draper and J.R. McMillan
© 2007 John Wiley & Sons, Ltd

morally discretionary. If I could easily save your life, it is not morally discretionary whether I do so, and if I am a nurse, it is not morally discretionary which of my patients I choose to look after. Beneficent actions like these are 'morally required' – not performing them is morally wrong. Kant and Mill ought to be read in a way that allows them to agree with this point.

Some beneficent actions appear to be morally required and others morally discretionary. It makes sense, then, to ask how we are to identify the boundary between the two. It is clear enough how to answer this for those requirements of beneficence that derive from relationships of special responsibility (such as the relationship between nurse and patient): here, we should refer to the responsibility-creating role and the expectations it is reasonable to attach to it. However, identifying the boundary between required and discretionary beneficence is a more difficult problem when it comes to our general relationship towards other needy people. At any one time, the world contains a vast number of people in desperate need of help, and aid organizations stand ready to receive my contributions towards helping them. If it is a requirement of beneficence that I give desperately needed help to another person when the cost to me of helping that person is insignificant, why does this requirement not apply to me in respect of each of those needy people? For a clear statement of this problem, see Fishkin (1982).

Moral philosophers have offered diverging responses to this problem. Arguably closest to moral 'common sense' is the view that the general requirements of beneficence are limited by considerations of the overall cost to an agent of helping others. Helping others is morally required when, overall, it does not significantly impinge on my own welfare; once it does that, it becomes discretionary. However, the recommendation of moral 'common sense' is not by itself a strong defence of a moral judgement. What is required is a fuller explanation (which moral philosophers have attempted in several different forms) of *why* general requirements of beneficence cannot impinge significantly on my own welfare. My own attempt to explain this is set out in Cullity (2004).

THE JUSTIFICATION OF BENEFICENCE

How do we justify judgements about the requirements of beneficence? We want to be able to do so for two reasons. First, we ought to be able to say something in defence of the idea that beneficence *is* morally important. But secondly, we also want guidance about how to prioritize it in relation to the other things that seem morally important: the protection of rights, justice, fidelity to commitments, open dealing with others, and so on.

One popular answer to this question treats beneficence itself as the foundation for the whole of morality. Theories in the 'welfarist' tradition do this: they claim that moral rightness is determined by the production of the greatest overall welfare. Utilitarianism is the most famous theory of this kind: it adds the further claim that welfare consists entirely in happiness. Utilitarianism in effect explains the moral importance of beneficence by saying that morality *is* impartial beneficence (Foot, 1988, p. 236; Warnock, 1971). Anything else that has moral importance derives that importance from its effects on welfare; and that tells us how to prioritize different moral considerations when they conflict. We ought to protect others' rights, keep our commitments to them and so on, insofar as doing so best promotes welfare, but no further.

In opposition to this are those views which claim that the moral importance of beneficence is to be derived from something else more fundamental. Historically, the three most influential such views have emphasized contractualist, Kantian and Aristotelian ideas, respectively.

Contractualists see the whole of morality as arising from the norms we have reason to agree on to regulate our interaction with each other: plausibly, a graduated set of norms for beneficence will be included. An idea advocated in different forms by different thinkers is a 'mutual insurance' argument for a requirement of mutual aid. This appeals to the reasons we have to agree to assist each other by offering mutual assurances of protection against calamities. We have reason to agree to require from each other limited forms of assistance in protection of our most important interests, but not to impose such onerous requirements of beneficence that we impair our ability to live independently fulfilling lives (Scanlon, 1998).

While this contractualist approach appears to have had an important influence on Kant's thinking about beneficence (Herman, 1984), contemporary Kantians emphasize also a second, potentially independent line of thought. This treats respect for autonomy as the foundation from which beneficence should be derived. On this view, morality is the set of practical requirements that governs our recognition of each other as autonomous equals. Our most fundamental interests – the ones calling for protection by moral requirements – are interests in autonomous agency. These are the interests which ground requirements of beneficence, but which also must be protected by limiting those requirements. For accounts of this Kantian argument, see Herman (2002), Hill (1993) and Buchanan (1982, pp. 41–3). Caution is needed in understanding the role which autonomy plays in Kant's own thought about the foundation of morality: on this, see O'Neill (2003).

A third approach is inspired by Aristotle's discussion of friendship in the *Nicomachean Ethics*. This emphasizes the way in which beneficence creates relationships of friendship and community between those who have a concern for each other's welfare. It thus create goods the possession of which is at the heart of a flourishing human life (Wallace, 1978), (Blum, 1980). This view again suggests a way of thinking about how beneficence is limited by our other moral priorities: the task for moral thought is to combine these priorities in the way that best conduces to a flourishing life.

So, we might treat beneficence as morally fundamental and seek to derive the rest of morality from it, or we might treat something else as morally fundamental and derive from it the importance of beneficence. There is a further possibility. This is that there are several fundamental, mutually irreducible sources of moral requirements, and beneficence is one of them. This kind of 'pluralistic' view seems to offer a close fit with ordinary moral thought and has become influential in thinking about health care ethics. The four-principle approach (Beauchamp and Childress, 2001) is a prominent example. For a survey of others, see Veatch (in press). When we ought to promote others' welfare, it does not seem that this is because doing so will help us achieve something else more fundamental. So beneficence does seem to be a basic source of moral requirements. But there are other moral requirements that do not seem readily reducible to a concern for welfare. I ought to respect people's entitlements to decline needed help, to pursue projects that are misguided or involve personal sacrifice, and to refuse to be used in the service of others' welfare; and I also ought to contribute to general schemes of cooperation even when they are large enough to mean that my joining in confers no perceptible benefit on anyone.

BENEFICENCE AND WELFARE

Beneficent action seeks to promote others' welfare – or to put it another way (as I have been doing already) to promote their interests, do what is good for them or benefit them. For guidance on what beneficence requires from us, then, it is natural to look for an account spelling out what human welfare consists in.[2] There are three main possibilities.[3]

One kind of account – with a long pedigree, dating back to the ancient Epicureans – tries to locate this in the nature of our experience. For example, hedonistic theories hold that welfare consists in pleasure: the best state for a person at any time, and the best life for a person overall, is the most

pleasant. Accounts of this kind confront the serious problem of pleasant experiences based on false beliefs. If I live under the happy illusion that my children are flourishing and my work is seriously regarded, then that does not make me well-off. On the contrary, I am badly off in two different respects: first, my children are languishing and my work is ignored, and, secondly, I am unaware of this.

The second and most popular kind of theory of welfare – a desire- or preference-based theory – can be formulated in a way that avoids this objection. If we say that a person's welfare consists in the satisfaction of those desires that are not based on ignorance, then we avoid the problem just mentioned, while preserving the attractive feature that a person's welfare will depend on what she takes an interest in. However, there remain two significant problems. One is that it seems we can have desires for objects unconnected with our own welfare, the satisfaction of which makes us no better off. The other, deeper problem is that it seems to get the explanatory relationship between welfare and desires the wrong way around. Usually, we desire things because we recognize their goodness: it is not our happening to desire them that makes them good. If I suffered a bizarre psychological change which made me prefer that my children languish and my work is ignored, that would not make these things good for me: it would itself be bad for me.

The alternative to these accounts is a view on which things are beneficial and harmful to us independently of whether we succeed in appreciating this. Philosophers have proposed different candidate lists of goods that are intrinsic contributors to welfare. Four kinds of goods that appear on most such lists are, first, goods of fellowship, a broad category comprising personal relationships of friendship and love as well as participation in communities; secondly, experiences of enjoyment and pleasure; thirdly, achievements in the course of worthwhile projects; and fourthly, knowledge that is worth having about oneself and the world – See for example Griffin (1986, p. 67). I shall mention a fifth below.

Clearly, there is scope for debate about the exact extension of any such list and about how exactly the content of any such list is derived. However, one thing that seems clear without having to tackle those questions is that certain other goods will be instrumental to the intrinsic goods on any plausible list. Money is one of these; another is health. Having money or good health but not using them to attain anything else that is good would not give you a good life. They are not good in themselves. But lacking these things can significantly

[2]This is not the only possible approach. An alternative is to try to give an independent psychological characterization of the attitude of caring for a person, and then to use this to derive an account of the appropriate objects of this attitude. This seeks to derive the content of welfare from that of beneficence, rather than the other way around. For this approach, see Darwall (2002).

[3]For further discussion, see Griffin (1986), which remains the best introduction to this topic.

impair your ability to attain the things that *are* good in themselves.

The primary reason of beneficence governing the provision of health care is therefore to supply an important instrumental good – health – to those who need it. However, an important secondary reason should not be overlooked. If goods of fellowship feature amongst the core components of human welfare, then the expression of solidarity and support for the needy is itself an important benefit we can, and should, confer upon them.

THE VIRTUES OF BENEFICENCE

Like many moral qualities, beneficence can be attributed both to particular actions and to people who characteristically perform them. Used in the latter way, it names a virtue – or rather, a family of overlapping virtues.[4] A list of these would include at least the following: kindness, generosity, compassion, sympathy, considerateness, sensitivity, loyalty, friendliness and affectionateness, as well as what I called above decency, meaning by that a readiness to render effective help to others in an emergency. These qualities differ from each other in various ways. They differ in their degree of emotional involvement (sympathy involves being upset by others' distress, decency need not), their characteristic expression (considerateness anticipates others' needs, compassion responds to them once they arise) and their scope (loyalty arises within preexisting relationships, kindness can be either selective or general). Given these differences, people can possess some of these virtues without others – or can possess these virtues in their relationships to some people but not to others. What unifies them is that they are ways of treating others' welfare as a reason for helping them.

Listing the virtues associated with beneficence reminds us of the way in which some expectations of beneficence attach with special relationships which one bears towards some but not all other people. There are two broad classes of such relationships to consider. One concerns those personal relationships of friendship, family relationship and communal association that give us reasons for special concern for others' welfare. But the other concerns those professional relationships that are understood to be directed towards aspects of a person's welfare. It is the job of financial advisors to promote the financial interests of their clients, the job of lawyers to promote their clients' legal interests and the job of social workers to help their clients to avoid social deprivation. In presenting yourself to others as a practitioner of one of these professions, you present yourself as offering to serve these aspects of their welfare, and this gives them an entitlement to expect that you will do so conscientiously.

BENEFICENCE AND HEALTH CARE

The professional field that is most obviously governed in this way by expectations of beneficence is of course health care. The relationship between health care professionals and their patients is governed by a mutual understanding that the role of the former is to use their medical expertise for the benefit of the latter. The expectations and entitlements thus created provide the core of health care ethics. Accordingly, the most prominent issues in health care ethics are all issues about the proper exercise of beneficence. The main ones concern its scope, its proper expression, its relationship with other ethical priorities, and the exercise of authority in making judgements about it. The remainder of the chapter offers a brisk treatment of each of these topics, drawing attention to the ways in which the general points made above can help us to think about them.

SCOPE

Two groups of problems in health care ethics are problems about the scope of beneficence. First, there is the problem of demarcating those to whom it applies. Familiar issues about the beginning and end of life arise here. Thinking of the core responsibilities of health care professionals as responsibilities of beneficence does not make the resolution of these issues automatic, but it does at least tell us how to think about them. The primary questions to ask are which human beings have a welfare, and which kinds of action have an impact on that welfare. It will obviously matter whether we accept or reject an experiential account of welfare. Rejecting it means that we cannot take sentience to be the key moral question about the beginning or end of life. On the other hand, what is relevant to beneficence is the impact a death will have on actual, and not merely potential, welfare. This is the primary question to ask; it is not the only one, however. Beneficence is the *appropriate* furthering of others' welfare. The important secondary question, then, is whether the promotion of welfare for those who have it is being achieved by morally objectionable means (and if so, in what ways are those means objectionable).

The other important question about scope concerns which aspects of patients' welfare are the responsibility of health care workers. If we understand the primary application of beneficence to health care as deriving from the special relationship of trust that is created between professionals and their patients, this suggests a simple answer. The professional

---

[4]For an objection to thinking of beneficence itself as a virtue, see Frankena (1982, pp. 66–8).

responsibility of health care workers is to further the medical interests of their patients. A corresponding restriction applies to the other professions that generate special requirements of beneficence. My financial advisor should apply her professional expertise to telling me what is in my financial interests: her job is not to tell me how to live. In the same way, it might be argued that any views that health care professionals may have about the nonmedical aspects of my welfare are irrelevant to doing their job. A minister of religion (or a philosopher?) might claim professional expertise in giving general advice on the best way for a person to live. But this is not the role of a medical professional.

It has seemed equally obvious to some writers how this answer should be applied to some practical controversies. For example, an orthodox view about euthanasia is this. It may be best, overall, for a person's life to end. However, it is not the business of medical staff to make an overall judgement about what is best, overall, for a patient (any more than a lawyer or financial advisor should be guided by such judgements in their dealings with clients). The job of medical staff is to tend to the medical interests of their patients, and these can never be served by killing them. Actively killing a patient can never have a *medical* justification (Callahan, 1992).

However, on reflection, this approach proves to be too simple. To see this, consider the widely held view that it can at least sometimes be right not to seek to prolong a life through medical intervention. This seems to be part of a sensible and humane attitude towards palliative care for the dying (Weir, 1989). It raises the following important point. If we conceive of 'medical interests' in a way which means that it can be bad for me overall – detrimental to my overall welfare – to have my medical interests furthered, then there will sometimes be no good reason to further my medical interests. More broadly, there will only be good reason for medical staff to serve a patient's medical interests to the extent that this furthers his overall welfare. And this in turn means that we collectively have a good reason not to confer on medical staff the responsibility of furthering the medical interests of their patients when this is detrimental to their overall welfare.

It is sometimes argued on these grounds that doctors' responsibilities extend to promoting the overall welfare of their patients (Pellegrino & Thomasma, 1988). However, this overlooks a more plausible intermediate position. The proper aim of medical staff treating me is to further my medical interests, *insofar as this is in my overall interests*. This is consistent with the source of special requirements of beneficence in relation to medicine, which is that medical staff offer to use their expertise for their patients' benefit. We can say this without ceding authority to medical staff to act on judgements about their patients' overall interests. It is a patient's prerogative to do that. But medical professionals

may have special expertise about the extent to which different forms of medical treatment will contribute towards or detract from their patients' overall well-being. And this expertise is something that it is their role to exercise for the benefit of their patients.

PROPER EXPRESSION

A question often discussed in textbooks of professional ethics is how to find a 'balance' between professionalism and personal concern. This is a question about the proper expression of beneficence in professional contexts. The discussion so far suggests that, in the health care context, we should think about it as follows.

As my doctor, your professional responsibility is not to be my friend, but to provide me with competent medical treatment.[5] However, for any given course of medical treatment, there will be more and less considerate ways of delivering it. And reasons of considerateness should govern your choice between them: there is the same case for thinking this as for accepting that such reasons should govern your dealings with other people generally. Being treated considerately is itself an important benefit.

Notice, moreover, that it is not just that nonprofessional reasons of considerateness provide a way of breaking a tie between ways of delivering medical treatment that are of equal professional merit. That this is wrong is suggested by our discussion of the scope of beneficence in health care. It is the responsibility of health care professionals to provide me with the health care that it is in my interests to receive. Given two forms of treatment that are equally effective in medical terms, it is better for me to receive the one that treats me with more consideration. Therefore, it is the responsibility of health care professionals to provide it to me.

RELATIONSHIP TO OTHER ETHICAL PRIORITIES

Broadly speaking, there are two ways in which ethical theories can tell us to think about our competing ethical priorities. As we saw earlier, some theories offer us one fundamental ethical value or principle by reference to which all of our ethical priorities are to be ordered; others give us a plurality of fundamental ethical principles, the importance of which is not to be derived from a single master-principle. Views of the latter kind are attractive in making room for different ethical principles that do not seem readily reducible to each other, but face the objection that they are of little help in dealing with cases in which those principles conflict. Proponents of such views often resort to the metaphor of 'balancing' competing principles against each other. This has the merit of encouraging us

---

[5]For arguments to the contrary, see Pellegrino and Thomasma (1981) and Englehardt (1996).

to respect experienced and reflective opinion about cases of moral conflict, rather than to search for a simple algorithm for moral decision-making. However, talk of 'balancing' is rarely a helpful way of thinking about the relationship between beneficence and other important ethical considerations. I shall briefly illustrate this with reference to Beauchamp and Childress's influential version of pluralism, which sees beneficence as one of four fundamental principles of health care ethics, alongside the respect for autonomy, justice and nonmaleficence.

A clear view of the relationship between beneficence and respect for autonomy requires an awareness of two different points. First, autonomy is a constituent of welfare. Earlier, I mentioned four intrinsic contributors to welfare: autonomy is a fifth (see Griffin, 1986, p. 67). A life containing friendships, achievements, enjoyments and knowledge which you have chosen for yourself is better for you, in virtue of this self-authorship, than one in which the same goods have been dictated for you. When we think, as adults, that it is bad for us to be treated like children, we are endorsing this idea. Secondly, however, autonomy seems important independently of its contribution to welfare. It seems sometimes to be the case that I ought to respect your autonomous decisions even though it would be better for you to be forced to act differently, all things (including the impact on your autonomy) considered.

These two ideas are consistent with each other. It makes sense to think that autonomy is important as a contributor to well-being, and also important independently of its contribution to well-being. Having noticed this, we find that both ideas have straightforward applications to health care ethics.

First, most cases in which good medical practice requires respect for autonomy are cases in which it is *bad* for us not to have our autonomy respected. It is bad for us to be lied to, to have our privacy invaded, to be subjected to medical procedures without our consent. It is therefore seriously misleading to think of these as cases in which respect for autonomy outweighs beneficence. They are cases in which beneficence – a proper concern for welfare – dictates respect for autonomy.

However, there are also cases in which a proper respect for autonomy extends beyond a beneficent concern for welfare. This follows from our treatment of the scope of beneficence in health care. There is an important distinction to be observed between the decisions about my medical welfare that fall within the professional expertise of medical

staff and those broader decisions about my overall welfare that do not. This means two things: my doctor should leave nonmedical decision-making to me, but should not use this as an excuse for abdicating responsibility for medical decisions. Where my personal, nonmedical priorities are affected by a choice between two medically equivalent procedures, giving the decision to me could be an appropriate way of respecting my autonomy. But it is a mistake to think that my autonomy is being respected by failing to take responsibility for decisions that fall within the field of medical expertise forming the basis of the professional relationship.

Saying this does not involve 'balancing' beneficence against respect for autonomy: rather, it involves being clear about the scope of beneficence in health care and the way in which it restricts the appropriate field for medical judgements about patients' welfare. Moreover, it also seems wrong to think that respect for autonomy is acting as a 'side-constraint' on beneficence – a prohibition on taking certain illicit means to pursue beneficent ends.[6] Here, respect for autonomy does not provide an independent constraint on the practice of medical beneficence; rather, the proper scope of medical beneficence dictates certain forms of respect for autonomy.[7]

Turn next to the issues often described as conflicts between beneficence and justice. These prominently include the allocation of health care resources. Should public funds be used to pay for procedures that will improve the health of many people by a modest amount, or for more expensive procedures that may yield bigger improvements for a few badly-off people? Principled ways can be found for making quantitative comparisons of this kind – for example, in terms of 'quality-adjusted life years' (Nord, 1999). And they can seem to give rise to conflicts between beneficence and justice. Overall welfare might be maximized by benefiting the many, but justice may seem to dictate helping the badly off rather than those who are already significantly better - off (Lockwood, 1988).[8]

However, it is again unhelpful to think of this as a conflict between beneficence and something else. Rather, it is better characterized as a problem concerning the application of beneficence. Should medical beneficence treat welfare aggregatively? A case against doing so might be developed along the following lines. The primary relationship governing the ethics of health care is that between an individual patient and individual health professional. As my doctor, your treatment of me should be based exclusively on a concern for *my* welfare. What you do to

---

[6] Here I am disagreeing with (Englehardt 1996, p. 70).

[7] I am not arguing that respect for autonomy *never* provides a 'side-constraint' on beneficence; only that it is not doing so here.

[8] For further discussion of the issues surrounding the justification for giving priority to the worst off, and how the worst off are to be defined, see Brock (2002). The question I raise in the text is only one of many that bear on the ethics of health care resource allocation: others include the desert of the recipients, and how to prioritize treating current needs in competition with preventing future ones.

me should not be guided by what is best for others. However, the same applies to your relationship to each of your other patients. This means that you can face the problem of how to allocate scarce resources in doing what is best for each of them. In resolving this problem, it is clear that you can justify not giving them to me if there is someone else who needs them more. (For any complaint I can make about not getting those resources, the other patient would have a stronger ground for complaint if you gave them to me instead of her.)[9] It is harder to see how you can justify leaving my needs unmet in order to help several less needy patients. When you examine the responsibilities created by your relationships to each of your patients, it can make sense to make a series of pairwise comparisons of benefits and costs to the different individuals involved, but what is harder to see is how it can be relevant to cite the aggregate benefit to a group in justification of your treatment of any individual. And arguably, if the ethics of health care is grounded in the individual relationships of professionals to patients, this tells against the systematic allocation of health care resources to maximize aggregate benefits, rather than to help the neediest. When medical administrators allocate medical resources, they are resourcing individual relationships of professional beneficence between doctors and patients. The strongest reasons of beneficence are generated by the greatest needs. Therefore, these generate the strongest claims on resources.

This is a sketch of an argument needing fuller development. However, it does already suggest that the issue here is not a matter of 'balancing' beneficence against justice. Rather, the issue is whether beneficence, as the *appropriate* furthering of others' welfare, tells us to approach the needs of different individuals by giving priority to those with the greatest needs or by the aggregation of overall welfare.[10]

More briefly, let me note the application of the same point to the issues often presented as conflicts between beneficence and nonmaleficence. When we are dealing with a single individual, there is no need to invoke a principle of nonmaleficence to guide our treatment of her in addition to a principle of beneficence. Promoting her welfare implies not inflicting a net harm on her. However, it can seem that we do need to invoke two separate principles in order to explain some judgements about choices between different people – for example, the judgement that it is wrong to harm some subjects in the course of a medical research project in order to benefit others later. This can seem to require us to say that nonmaleficence has priority over beneficence. But once more, this is questionable. If the ethical norms governing the practice of medicine derive from the individual relationships between doctor and patient, that is enough to explain why imposing a net harm on one of them cannot be justified by greater benefits to others. Imposing a net harm on a person is always incompatible with the requirement of beneficence that properly governs the relationship of a medical professional to a patient.

AUTHORITY IN MAKING JUDGEMENTS

The foregoing discussion has some clear implications for the question where authority should lie in exercising judgements about a person's welfare. We have seen the need to distinguish between those parts of a person's welfare which call for judgements of medical expertise and those which do not. In the treatment of competent adult patients, the latter judgements should not be arrogated by medical staff, nor the former avoided. This leaves open the question of where decision-making authority should lie in the treatment of children and incompetent adults. Decisions about the medical aspects of their welfare are rightly taken by medical professionals. How about decisions concerning those nonmedical aspects of a person's welfare – including what priority to give to good health in relation to other goods – that can have a bearing on choices between different forms of medical treatment? Our discussion suggests three things. First, when an adult has clearly expressed views about his overall welfare, the fact that he is now incompetent does not justify disregarding them. Secondly, the ideal way in treating incompetent patients who have expressed no such views is an open discussion between medical staff and near relatives, generating a consensual decision about what is best overall for the patient. When the patient's views about his welfare cannot be established, others with relevant knowledge and a concern for his welfare will have to think about that directly.[11] And thirdly, when such a consensus cannot be reached, what beneficence will recommend is that there should be an institutional and legal structure in place which is likeliest to result in patients' interests receiving the best protection. Identifying the best such structure remains beyond the scope of this chapter.

---

[9] Compare (Scanlon, 1998), Chapter 5, Section 9.

[10] For the view that benevolence is unable to give us guidance in choosing between the good of different individuals, and needs to be supplemented by justice, see Rawls (1971, Section 30).

[11] Thinking about what a patient's own preferences would have been can be relevant to answering that question; but the question to answer in this case is the direct one: what *is* best for the patient; not how the patient would have answered that question. On this issue, see Dresser and Robertson (1989).

REFERENCES

Beauchamp TL, Childress JF. *Principles of Biomedical Ethics.* New York: Oxford University Press, 2001; p. 166.

Blum L. *Friendship, Altruism and Morality.* London: Routledge & Kegan Paul, 1980.

Brock DW. Health resource allocation for vulnerable populations. In: Danis M, Clancy C, Churchill LR, eds. *Ethical Dimensions of Health Policy.* New York: Oxford University Press, 2002; pp. 283–309.

Buchanan AE. Philosophical foundations of beneficence. In: Shelp E, ed. *Beneficence and Health Care.* Dordrecht: D. Reidel, 1982; pp. 33–62.

Callahan D. When self-determination runs amok. *Hastings Cent Rep* 1992; **22**: 52–5.

Cullity G. *The Moral Demands of Affluence.* Oxford: Clarendon Press, 2004

Darwall S. *Welfare and Rational Care,* Princeton: Princeton University Press, 2002.

Dresser RA, Robertson JA. Quality of life and non-treatment decisions for incompetent patients. *Law Med Health Care* 1989; **17**: 234–44.

Englehardt HT. *The Foundations of Bioethics.* New York: Oxford University Press, 1996; pp. 296–9.

Fishkin JS. *The Limits of Obligation.* New Haven: Yale University Press, 1982; pp. 3–7

Foot P. Utilitarianism and the virtues. In: Scheffler S, ed. *Consequentialism and Its Critics.* Oxford: Oxford University Press, 1988; pp. 224–42.

Frankena WK. Beneficence in an ethics of virtue. In: Shelp EE, ed. *Beneficence and Health Care.* D. Reidel: Dordrecht, 1982; pp. 63–81.

Frankena WK. Beneficence/benevolence. *Soc Philos Policy* 1987; **4**: 1–20.

Griffin J. *Well-Being: Its Meaning, Measurement and Moral Importance.* Oxford: Clarendon Press, 1986.

Herman B. Mutual aid and respect for persons. *Ethics,* 1984; **94**: 577–602.

Herman B. The scope of moral requirement. *Philos Public Aff* 2002; **30**: 227–56.

Hill TE. Beneficence and self-love: a Kantian perspective. *Soc Philos Policy* 1993; **10**: 1–23.

Kant I. *The Metaphysics of Morals.* Cambridge: Cambridge University Press, 1996; **6**: 390–91.

Lockwood M. Quality of life and resource allocation. In: Bell JM, Mendus S, eds. *Philosophy and Medical Welfare.* Cambridge: Cambridge University Press, 1988; pp. 35–55.

Mill, JS. *Utilitarianism.* Oxford: Oxford University Press, 1998; Ch. 15, para 15.

Nord E. *Cost-Value Analysis in Health Care: Making Sense Out of QALYs.* Cambridge: Cambridge University Press, 1999.

O'Neill O. Autonomy: The emperor's new clothes. *Proc Aristotelian Soc* 2003; **77**(Suppl.): 1–21.

Pellegrino ED, Thomasma DC. *A Philosophical Basis of Medical Practice.* New York: Oxford University Press, 1981; pp. 64–6.

Pellegrino ED, Thomasma DC. *For the Patient's Good: The Restoration of Beneficence in Health Care.* New York: Oxford University Press, 1988.

Rawls J. *A Theory of Justice,* Cambridge: Harvard University Press, 1971.

Scanlon TM *What We Owe to Each Other.* Cambridge MA: Harvard University Press 1998; pp. 223–9.

Veatch, RM. How many principles for bioethics? In: McMillan J, ed. *Principles of Health Care Ethics.* London: Wiley (in press).

Wallace JD. *Virtues and Vices.* Ithaca: Cornell University Press, 1978; Ch. 5.

Warnock GJ. *The Object of Morality.* London: Methuen, 1971; pp. 29–30.

Weir RF. *Abating Treatment with Critically Ill Patients.* Oxford: Oxford University Press, 1989.

4

Responsibilities
for Poverty-Related Ill Health

THOMAS POGGE[1]

My view on justice in regard to health is distinctive in two ways. First, I hold that the strength of our moral reasons to prevent or to mitigate particular medical conditions does not depend only on what one might call distributional factors, such as how badly off the people affected by these conditions are in absolute and relative terms, how costly prevention or treatment would be and how much patients would benefit from given treatment. Rather, it depends also on relational factors, that is, on how we are related to the medical conditions they suffer. This point is widely accepted in regard to conduct. You have, for instance, stronger moral reason to make sure that people are not harmed through your own activities than you have to ensure that they are not harmed through other causes (others' negligence or their own, say, or bad weather). And your moral reason to help an accident victim is stronger if you were materially involved in causing her accident.

I assert an analogous point also in regard to any social institutions that agents are materially involved in upholding: in shaping an institutional order, we should be more concerned, morally, that it not contribute substantially to the incidence of medical conditions than we should be that it prevent medical conditions caused by other factors. Thus, we should design any institutional order so that it prioritizes the alleviation of those medical conditions it substantially contributes to. In institutional contexts as well, what is important to moral assessment is not merely the distribution of health outcomes as such, but also whether and how social factors contribute to their incidence. The latter consideration is needed to distinguish different degrees of responsibility for medical conditions and for their prevention and mitigation.

My second thesis builds on the first. It is generally believed that one's moral reason to help prevent and mitigate others' medical conditions is stronger when these others are compatriots than when they are foreigners. I reject this belief in regard to medical conditions in whose incidence one is materially involved. People can be so involved through their ordinary conduct or through their role in upholding an institutional order. In the case of ordinary interpersonal relations, for example, one's moral reasons to drive carefully and to assist victims of any accident one has caused do not weaken when one is travelling abroad and among foreigners. And in institutional contexts, we ought especially to ensure that any institutional order we help impose avoids causing health problems and prioritizes the alleviation of any health problems it does cause. Here my second thesis holds that this responsibility is not sensitive to whether the medical conditions at stake are suffered by foreigners or by compatriots.

Combining both theses, I hold then that foreigners' medical conditions in whose incidence we are materially involved have greater moral weight for us than compatriots' medical conditions in whose incidence we are not materially involved.

In interpersonal contexts, this combined thesis is not likely to be very controversial. Suppose, two children have been injured by speeding drivers and money is needed to pay for an expensive medical treatment necessary to restore their health and appearance completely. In one case, the child is a foreigner and you were the driver. In the other case, the child is a compatriot and someone else was the driver. My view entails that in a situation like this you have

[1] This paper is reprinted, with some updates and revisions, from *Ethics & International Affairs* 2002; 16/2: 71–79. A longer version, "Relational Conceptions of Justice: Responsibilities for Health Outcomes,' appeared in Sudhir Anand, Fabienne Peter, and Amartya Sen, eds., *Public Health, Ethics, and Equity* (Oxford: Clarendon Press, 2004). I am grateful to the editors for permission to reuse this material here.

(other things being equal) stronger moral reason to buy the expensive treatment for the foreign child; and most would probably agree.

In institutional contexts, by contrast, my view is likely to be quite controversial. It might be stated as follows: Foreigners' medical conditions, if social institutions we are materially involved in upholding substantially contribute to their incidence, have greater moral weight for us than compatriots' medical conditions in whose causation we are not materially involved. This combined thesis is radical if social institutions we are materially involved in upholding do substantially contribute to the incidence of medical conditions abroad. Is this the case?

SOCIAL INSTITUTIONS, POVERTY AND HEALTH

Many kinds of social institutions can substantially contribute to the incidence of medical conditions. Of these, economic institutions – the basic rules governing ownership, production, use, and exchange of natural resources, goods, and services – have the greatest impact on health. This impact is mediated, for the most part, through poverty. By avoidably engendering severe poverty, economic institutions substantially contribute to the incidence of many medical conditions. And persons materially involved in upholding such economic institutions are then materially involved in the causation of such medical conditions.

In our world, poverty is highly relevant to human health. In fact, poverty is far and away the most important factor in explaining existing health deficits. Because they are poor, 850 million people are malnourished and 2600 million lack access to basic sanitation (UNDP, 2005, p. 24), 1197 million lack access to safe water (UNDP, 2004, pp. 129–30), 2200 million lack access to essential drugs (www.fic.nih.gov/about/summary.html), 1000 million have no adequate shelter and 2000 million have no electricity (UNDP, 1998, p. 49). Poverty-related causes account for about one third of all human deaths, some 18 million every year (WHO, 2004, p. 120–5) including 10.6 million children under age 5 (UNICEF 2005, inside front cover).

This massive poverty is not due to overall scarcity. The '$2/day' poverty line corresponds today to the purchasing power of annually ca. $1100 in the US and about $250 in a typical poor country. Living on average 42% below this

line, the 2735 million people who are poor by this standard thus have aggregate annual income of roughly $400 billion. By contrast, the aggregate gross national incomes of the 24 'high-income OECD countries' (Organisation for Economic Co-operation and Development) with 919 million citizens amount to over $30,760 billion (World Bank, 2005). However daunting the figure of 2735 million poor people may sound, global inequality is now so enormous that plausible reforms doubling or even tripling the income of the poor solely at the expense of the high-income countries would barely be felt in the latter.[2]

It cannot be denied that the distribution of income and wealth is heavily influenced by economic institutions, which regulate the distribution of a jointly generated social product. What can be said, and is said quite often, is that the economic institutions that substantially contribute to severe poverty in the developing world are *local* economic institutions in whose imposition we, citizens of the developed countries, are not materially involved. Economists tirelessly celebrate the success stories of the Asian tigers or of Kerala (a state in India), leading us to believe that those who remain hungry have only their own institutions and governments (and hence themselves and their own compatriots) to blame. Even the philosopher Rawls feels called upon to reiterate that poverty has local explanations: 'The causes of the wealth of a people and the forms it takes lie in their political culture and in the religious, philosophical, and moral traditions that support the basic structure, as well as in the industriousness and cooperative talents of its members, all supported by their political virtues. . . . Crucial also is the country's population policy' (Rawls, 1999b, p. 108).

It is quite true, of course, that local economic institutions, and local factors more generally, play an important role in the reproduction of extreme poverty in the developing world. But this fact does not show that the social institutions we are materially involved in upholding play no substantial role. That the effects of flawed domestic institutions are as bad as they are is often due to global institutions – to the institution of the territorial state, for instance, which allows affluent populations to prevent the poor from migrating to where their work could earn a decent living (see Carens, 1987). Global institutions also have a profound impact on the indigenous institutional schemes of developing countries. By assigning those who can gain effective power in a developing country the authority to borrow in the name of its

[2]It is claimed that the world's richest individuals could comfortably solve much of the problem out of their income from safe investments: 'The additional cost of achieving and maintaining universal access to basic education for all, basic health care for all, reproductive health care for all women, adequate food for all and safe water and sanitation for all is … less than 4% of the combined wealth of the 225 richest people in the world' (UNDP, 1998, p. 30). The WHO Commission on Macroeconomics and Health (chaired by Jeffrey Sachs) has sketched how deaths from poverty-related causes could be reduced by 8 million annually at a cost of $62 billion/year (*The Economist*, 22 December 2001, pp. 82–3).

people and to confer legal ownership rights in the country's resources, our global institutional order greatly encourages the undemocratic acquisition and exercise of political power in especially the resource-rich developing countries.[3]

The national institutional schemes of developed countries, too, can have a profound influence on the national institutional schemes of developing countries. An obvious example is that, until quite recently, most developed countries (though not, after 1977, the United States) have allowed their firms to pay bribes to officials of developing countries and even to deduct such bribes from their taxable revenues.[4] Such authorization and moral support for bribery have greatly contributed to the now deeply entrenched culture of corruption in many developing countries.

If the social institutions of the developed countries and the global institutional order these countries uphold contribute substantially to the reproduction of poverty, then it is hard to deny that we citizens of developed countries are therefore materially involved in it as well. It is true, of course, that these institutions are shaped by our politicians. But we live in reasonably democratic states where we can choose politicians and political programmes from a wide range of alternatives, where we can participate in shaping political programmes and debates, and where politicians and political parties must cater to the popular will if they are to be elected and re-elected. If we really wanted our domestic and international institutions to be shaped so as to avoid reproducing extreme poverty, politicians committed to that goal would emerge and be successful. But the vast majority of citizens of the developed countries want national and global institutions to be shaped in the service of their own interests and therefore support politicians willing so to shape them. At least the citizens in this large majority can then be said to be materially involved in the reproduction of poverty and the associated health deficits. And they, at least, have then stronger moral reason to discontinue their support, and to help the foreign victims of current institutions, than to help fund most services provided under ordinary health programmes (such as Medicare) for the benefit of their compatriots – or so the view I have outlined would suggest.

Superficially similar conclusions are sometimes defended on cost/benefit grounds, by reference to how thousands of children in the developing countries can be saved from their trivial diseases at the cost of terminal care for a single person in a developed country.[5] My view, by contrast,

turns on the different ways in which we are related to the medical conditions of others and thus may tell us to favour foreigners even if costs and benefits are equal.

This summary of my larger view on health equity was meant to be introductory, not conclusive. Seeing what is at stake, I would expect even the most commonsensical of my remarks about the explanation of global poverty to be vigorously disputed; and I certainly do not believe that this brief outline can lay such controversies to rest.

TREATING RECIPIENTS JUSTLY VERSUS PROMOTING A JUST DISTRIBUTION

The justice of judicanda – conduct, persons and social institutions – is often thought to depend solely on the distribution of relevant goods and ills that they bring about. On such a view, alternative arrangements of a health care system, for instance, are assessed solely on the basis of the distribution of health outcomes each would tend to produce. By focusing exclusive moral attention on those affected, such a view deploys what one might call a passive concept of justice.

An important alternative to this passive concept adds an essential place for (what I call) the *agents* of justice, for those who have or share moral responsibility for a judicandum. I call it the active concept of justice, because it diverts some attention from those affected by a judicandum to those who shape it. This modification is significant in several ways: for something to be unjust, there must be some identifiable agent or agents responsible for its injustice or for making it (more) just. Some agents may have responsibilities with respect to some injustice while others do not – unlike you, I may have no moral reason to seek to prevent or to remedy a minor injustice in your spouse's conduct towards your children. There may also be gradations, as when moral responsibility with regard to the injustice of some institutional order varies from agent to agent within its scope; being privileged or influential may strengthen moral responsibilities, being poor or burdened by many other responsibilities may weaken them. Furthermore, as this last thought suggests, there may be competing claims – one may have responsibilities with regard to several injustices and may then have to decide how much of an effort one ought to make with regard to each. These issues concerning responsibilities and their prioritization are crucial for giving justice a determinate role in the

---

[3] See Lam and Wantchekon (1999), Wantchekon (1999), and Pogge (2002) chapters 4 and 6.

[4] Only in 1997 did the developed states sign a *Convention on Combating Bribery of Foreign Public Officials in International Business Transactions* (www.oecd.org/dataoecd/4/18/38028044.pdf), which requires them to enact laws against the bribery of foreign officials. "But big multinationals continue to sidestep them with ease" (*The Economist*, 2 March 2002, pp. 63–65).

[5] Representative examples of such lines of argument are Singer 1972, Rachels 1979, Kagan 1989 and Unger 1996.

real world. And they tend to be overlooked from the start, or grossly oversimplified, when the topic is approached in terms of the passive concept of justice.[6]

Associated with these contrasting concepts of justice are two fundamentally different ways of understanding contemporary egalitarian liberalism. One variant sees its core in the idea that no citizen ought to be worse off on account of unchosen inequalities. This idea, duly specified, defines an ideal society in which no person is worse off than others except only as a consequence of free and informed choices this person has made. In such a society, social institutions and perhaps all other humanly controllable factors as well, are then to be aimed at promoting such a solely choice-sensitive overall distribution of quality of life.[7] The other variant sees the core of egalitarian liberalism in the idea that a liberal society, or state, ought to treat all its citizens equally in terms of helps and hindrances. Such *equal* treatment need not be *equality-promoting* treatment. Pre-existing inequalities in, for example, genetic potentials and liabilities–however unchosen by their bearers–are not society's responsibility and not to be corrected or compensated at the expense of those favoured by these inequalities.

The health equity theme provokes the most forceful clash of these two variants of egalitarian liberalism. One side seems committed to the indefinite expansion of the health-care system by using it to neutralize (through medical research, treatment, alleviation and compensation) all handicaps, disabilities and other medical conditions from which persons may suffer through no fault of their own. The other side seems committed to the callous (if not cruel) view that we, as a society, need to do no more for persons whose health is poor through no fault of ours than for persons in good health.[8] Most contemporary theorists of justice take the purely recipient-oriented approach, though they do not explicitly consider and reject the relational alternative I propose. Much of the current debate is focused on the question of how we are to judge the justice of overall distributions or states of affairs in a comparative way.[9]

But *should* we judge the justice of conduct, people and/or social rules solely by their impact on the quality of such overall distributions? With respect to conduct, most would reject this purely recipient-oriented mode of assessment. Abstractly considered, a situation in which everyone has at least one eye and one kidney is surely morally better than (an otherwise similar) one in which some, through no fault of their own, have no functioning eye or kidney while many others have two. But actions and persons promoting such an abstractly better distribution are nevertheless judged gravely unjust.

Cases of this kind may be used to draw the conclusion that we ought to distinguish between *treating recipients justly* and *promoting a good distribution among recipients*. With respect to social rules, a similar distinction would seem to be called for and for similar reasons. Just social rules for the allocation of donated kidneys favour those who, through no fault of their own, have no functioning kidney over those who have one; such rules thereby promote a better distribution of kidneys over recipients. Just social rules do not, however, mandate the forced redistribution of kidneys from those who have two to those who have none, even though doing so would likewise promote a better distribution of kidneys over recipients. Nor are just rules ones that produce a better distribution of kidneys by engendering severe poverty that compels some people to sell one of their kidneys so as to obtain basic necessities for themselves and their families.

Medical conditions that are intrinsically identical need not then be morally on a par. The moral weight of renal failures to which an institutional order avoidably gives rise depends on how patients came to be dependent on a single kidney. Was the other one forcibly taken from them through a legally authorized medical procedure (forced redistribution)? Were they obliged to sell it to obtain food? Or did it atrophy on account of a genetic defect? How important the avoidance, prevention and mitigation of renal failures are for the justice of an institutional order depends on which of these scenarios it would exemplify. Once again,

---

[6]Witness Rawls's generic natural duty to promote just institutions, which leaves all such more specific questions of responsibility out of account (Rawls 1999a, pp. 99, 216, 293–4).

[7]The main champion of the view that all such factors — social institutions and practices, conventions, ethi, and personal conduct — should be pressed in the service of promoting a just distribution so understood is Cohen (1989, 1992, 1997, 2000). For a detailed critique of this view, see Pogge (2000).

[8]Advocates of the first view could also be accused of callousness in that the huge demands they make in behalf of persons whose health is poor through no fault of their own will, in the real world, shrink the domain of recipients, typically in line with national borders. The billions of dollars required for providing our compatriots with all the 'services needed to maintain, restore, or compensate for normal species-typical functioning' (Daniels 1985, p. 79) would suffice to save countless millions who now die from poverty-related causes, such as malnutrition, measles, diarrhoea, malaria, tuberculosis, pneumonia, and other cheaply curable but all-too-often fatal diseases. On the view I have sketched, citizens in affluent countries have stronger moral reason to prevent and mitigate most of the latter medical conditions suffered by foreigners than most of the former medical conditions suffered by compatriots.

[9]Some main contributors are Sen (1982, 1992), Dworkin (1981a, 1981b, revised and expanded in 2000), Rawls (1982), Cohen (1989), and Arneson (1989). See also Galston (1980), Griffin (1986), Elster and Roemer (1991), and Pogge (1995).

treating recipients justly does not boil down to promoting the best distribution among them – what matters is how social rules *treat*, not how they *affect*, the set of recipients.

This simple thought has been remarkably neglected in contemporary work on social justice. It is not surprising, of course, that it plays no role in consequentialist theorizing. Consequentialists, after all, hold that social rules (as well as persons and their conduct) should be judged by their impact on the overall outcome, irrespective of how they produce these effects. Consequentialists hold, that is, that the justice of social rules is determined exclusively by the quality of the overall distribution (of goods and ills, or quality of life) produced by these rules.

But it *is* remarkable that supposedly deontological approaches, such as that developed by Rawls and his followers, likewise make the justice of social rules depend exclusively on the overall distribution these rules produce. As the thought experiment of the original position makes vivid, Rawls agrees with consequentialists that the moral assessment of a social order should be based solely on what overall distribution of goods and ills it, in comparison to its feasible alternatives, tends to produce among its recipients. By judging any social order in this purely recipient-oriented way, Rawls ensures from the start that it is judged exclusively by its 'output' in terms of what overall distribution of quality of life it produces among its participants – without regard to the diverse *ways* in which it affects the quality of life of these persons.[10]

RELATIONAL RESPONSIBILITIES

The most plausible alternative structure for a conception of social justice would involve weighting the impact that social institutions have on relevant quality of life according to how they have this impact. Let me illustrate this structure by distinguishing, in a preliminary fashion, six basic ways in which a social order may have an impact on the medical conditions that persons suffer. This illustration distinguishes scenarios in which some particular medical condition suffered by certain innocent persons can be traced to the fact that they, due to the arrangement of social institutions, avoidably lack some vital nutrients V (the vitamins contained in fresh fruit, perhaps, which are essential to good health). The six scenarios are arranged in order of their moral weight, according to my intuitive, pre-reflective judgment[11]:

- In scenario 1, the nutritional deficit is *officially mandated*, paradigmatically by the law: legal restrictions bar certain persons from buying foodstuffs containing V.
- In scenario 2, the nutritional deficit results from *legally authorized* conduct of private persons: sellers of foodstuffs containing V lawfully refuse to sell to certain persons.
- In scenario 3, social institutions *foreseeably and avoidably engender* (but do not specifically require or authorize) the nutritional deficit through conduct they stimulate: certain persons, suffering severe poverty within an ill-conceived economic order, cannot afford to buy foodstuffs containing V.
- In scenario 4, the nutritional deficit arises from private conduct that is *legally prohibited but barely deterred*: sellers of foodstuffs containing V illegally refuse to sell to certain persons, but enforcement is lax and penalties are mild.
- In scenario 5, the nutritional deficit arises from social institutions *avoidably leaving unmitigated the effects of a natural defect*: certain persons are unable to metabolize V due to a treatable genetic defect, but they avoidably lack access to the treatment that would correct their handicap.
- In scenario 6, finally, the nutritional deficit arises from social institutions *avoidably leaving unmitigated the effects of a self-caused defect*: certain persons are unable to metabolize V due to a treatable self-caused disease – brought on, perhaps, by their maintaining a long-term smoking habit in full knowledge of the medical dangers associated with it – and avoidably lack access to the treatment that would correct their ailment.

This differentiation of six ways in which social institutions may be related to the goods and ills persons encounter is

---

[10] The full story about Rawls's theory is somewhat more complicated in that he is actually offering two distinct criteria of justice. One is the public criterion by reference to which citizens are to assess and reform the basic structure of their society. For this role, Rawls proposes his two principles conjoined with the two priority rules. In justifying this proposal, Rawls appeals to the original position in which rational deliberators, each representing the higher-order interests of one citizen with unknown characteristics, are to agree on one public criterion of justice from a list of candidates. One can thus think of the original position as a meta-criterion for ranking candidate public criteria of justice. Clearly, this meta-criterion is purely recipient-oriented, attending only to information about how citizens would fare (in terms of their stipulated three higher-order interests) with various public criteria and the basic structure designs each might justify under various given conditions. And this fact biases the parties' deliberations in favour of a purely recipient-oriented public criterion, which attends only to information about how citizens would fare in terms of social primary goods.

[11] Other things must be presumed to be equal here. The moral weight of the health impact declines as we go through the list. But a morally less weighty such impact may nevertheless outweigh a weightier one if the former is more severe or affects more persons or is more cheaply avoidable than the latter. In this way, an advantage in reducing scenario-4 type deficits may outweigh a much smaller disadvantage in engendering scenario-3 type deficits, for example.

preliminary in that it fails to isolate the morally significant factors that account for the descending moral weight of the relevant medical conditions. Lacking the space to do this here, let me merely venture the hypothesis that what matters is not merely the *causal* role of social institutions, how they figure in a complete causal explanation of the nutritional deficit in question, but also (what one might call) the implicit *attitude* of social institutions towards this deficit.[12]

My preliminary classification is surely still too simple. In some cases one will have to take account of other, perhaps underlying causes; and one may also need to recognize interdependencies among causal influences and fluid transitions between the classes.[13] Bypassing these complications here, let me emphasize once more the decisive point missed by the usual accounts of justice: to be morally plausible, a criterion of social justice must take account of – and its application thus requires information about – the particular relation between social institutions and human quality of life, which may determine whether some institutionally avoidable deficit is an injustice at all and, if so, how great an injustice it is. Such a criterion must take into account, that is, not merely the comparative impact a social order has on the distribution of quality of life, but also *how* it exerts this influence. If this is right, then it is no truer of social rules than of persons and conduct that they are just if and insofar as they promote a good overall distribution. Appraising overall distributions of goods and ills (or of quality of life) may be an engaging academic and theological pastime, but it fails to give plausible moral guidance where guidance is needed: for the assessment and reform of social rules as well as of persons and their conduct.

CONCLUSION

An institutional order can be said to contribute substantially to medical conditions if and only if it contributes to their genesis through scenarios 1, 2 and 3. Supposing that at least the more privileged adult citizens of affluent and reasonably democratic countries are materially involved in upholding not only the economic order of their own society but also the global economic order, we can say two things about such citizens: pursuant to my second thesis, they have equally strong moral reason to prevent and mitigate *compatriots'* medical conditions due to avoidable poverty engendered by *domestic* economic institutions as they have to prevent and mitigate *foreigners'* medical conditions

due to avoidable poverty engendered by *global* economic institutions. And pursuant to my combined thesis, they have stronger moral reason to prevent and mitigate foreigners' medical conditions due to avoidable poverty engendered by global economic institutions than to prevent and mitigate compatriots' medical conditions that are not due to mandated, authorized or engendered deficits.

In the United States, some 40 million mostly poor citizens avoidably lack adequate medical insurance. Due to their lack of coverage, many of these people, at any given time, suffer medical conditions that could be cured or mitigated by treatment not in fact accessible to them. This situation is often criticized as manifesting an injustice in the country's social order. Now imagine that the poverty of the 40 million were so severe that it not only rendered them unable to gain access to the medical care they need (scenarios 5 and 6), but also exposed them to various medical conditions owing specifically to poverty-related causes (scenario 3). This additional feature, which does play a substantial role for some fraction of the 40 million, considerably aggravates the injustice, and it is central to the plight of the world's poorest populations. The global poor generally lack access to adequate care for the medical conditions they suffer, of course. But the main effect of an extra $50 or $100 of annual income for them would not be more medical care, but much less need for such care. If they were not so severely impoverished, they would not suffer in the first place most of the medical conditions for which, as things are, they also cannot obtain adequate treatment.

I have tried to lend some initial plausibility to the view that such poverty-induced medical conditions among the global poor are, for us, morally on a par with poverty-induced medical conditions among the domestic poor and of greater moral weight than not-socially-induced medical conditions among poor compatriots. In the first two cases, but not in the third, we are materially involved in upholding social institutions that contribute substantially to the incidence of medical conditions and of the countless premature deaths resulting from them.

REFERENCES

Arneson R. Equality and equality of opportunity for welfare. *Philos Stud* 1989; **56**: 77–93.

Carens J. Aliens and citizens: the case for open borders. *Rev Polit* 1987; **49**: 251–73.

---

[12] This implicit attitude of social institutions is independent of the attitudes or intentions of the persons shaping and upholding these institutions. Only the former makes a difference to how just the institutions are – the latter only make a difference to how blameworthy persons are for their role in imposing them.

[13] The case of smoking, for instance, may exemplify a fluid transition between scenarios 2 and 6 insofar as private agents (cigarette companies) are legally permitted to try to render persons addicted to nicotine.

Cohen GA. On the currency of egalitarian justice. *Ethics* 1989; **99**: 906–44.

Cohen GA. Incentives, inequality, and community. In: Peterson G, ed. *The Tanner Lectures on Human Values XIII*. Salt Lake City: University of Utah Press, 1992

Cohen GA. Where the action is: on the site of distributive justice. *Philos Public Aff* 1997; **26**: 3–30.

Cohen GA. *If You're an Egalitarian, How Come You're so Rich?* Cambridge, MA: Harvard University Press, 2000.

Daniels N. *Just Health Care*. Cambridge: Cambridge University Press, 1985.

Dworkin R. What is equality? Part 1: Equality of welfare. *Philos Public Aff* 1981a; **10**: 185–246.

Dworkin R. What is equality? Part 2: Equality of resources. *Philos Public Aff* 1981b; **10**: 283–345.

Dworkin R. *Sovereign Virtue*. Cambridge, MA: Harvard University Press, 2000.

Elster J, Roemer J, eds. *Interpersonal Comparisons of Well-Being*. Cambridge: Cambridge University Press, 1991.

Galston W. *Justice and the Human Good*. Chicago: University of Chicago Press, 1980.

Griffin J. *Well-Being*. Oxford: Clarendon Press, 1986.

Kagan S. *The Limits of Morality*. Oxford: Oxford University Press, 1989.

Lam R, Wantchekon L. Dictatorships as a political Dutch disease, Working paper 795. Yale University, 1999. Also at www.library.yale.edu/socsci/egcdp795.pdf.

Pogge, T. Three problems with contractarian–consequentialist ways of assessing social institutions. *Soc Philos Policy* 1995; **12**: 241–66.

Pogge T. On the site of distributive justice: reflections on Cohen and Murphy. *Philos Public Aff* 2000; 29: 137–69.

Pogge. T. *World Poverty and Human Rights*. Cambridge: Polity Press, 2002.

Rachels J. Killing and starving to death. *Philosophy* 1979; **54**: 159–71.

Rawls, J. Social unity and primary goods. In: Sen A, Williams B, eds. *Utilitarianism and Beyond*. Cambridge: Cambridge University Press, 1982.

Rawls, J. *A Theory of Justice*. Cambridge, MA: Harvard University Press 1999a [1971].

Rawls J. *The Law of Peoples*. Cambridge, MA: Harvard University Press, 1999b.

Sen, A. Equality of what? In: *Choice, Welfare and Measurement*. Cambridge: Cambridge University Press, 1982.

Sen A. *Inequality Reexamined*. Cambridge, MA: Harvard University Press, 1992.

Singer P. "Famine, affluence and morality. *Philos Public Aff* 1972; **1**: 229–43.

UNDP (United Nations Development Program). *Human Development Report 1998*. New York: Oxford University Press, 1998. Also at hdr.undp.org/reports/global/1998/en.

UNDP (United Nations Development Program). *Human Development Report 2004*. New York: UNDP, 2004. Also at hdr.undp.org/reports/global/2004.

UNDP (United Nations Development Program). *Human Development Report 2005*. New York: UNDP. Also at hdr.undp.org/reports/global/2005.

Unger P. *Living High and Letting Die: Our Illusion of Innocence*. Oxford: Oxford University Press, 1996.

UNICEF (United Nations Children's Fund). *The State of the World's Children 2005*. New York: UNICEF, 2005 (also at www.unicef.org/sowc05/english).

Wantchekon L. Why do Resource Dependent Countries Have Authoritarian Governments? Working Paper, Yale University, 1999. Also at www.yale.edu/leitner/pdf/1999-11.pdf.

WHO (World Health Organisation). *The World Health Report 2004*. Geneva: WHO Publications, 2004. Also at www.who.int/whr/2004.

World Bank. *World Development Report 2006*. New York: Oxford University Press, 2005.

5

Liberalism and Communitarianism

COLIN TYLER

Contemporary liberal philosophy came to prominence in the West in the early 1970s as a reaction against utilitarianism. Those philosophers whom some opponents have called (rather problematically) 'communitarian' arose in the late 1970s and early 1980s as a reaction to liberalism's new direction, especially as that was expressed in the writings of John Rawls and his followers. Consequently, in order to understand the liberal and communitarian perspectives on health care ethics, one must first understand the utilitarian theories against which they still contend.

Utilitarianism has always aspired to be a practical philosophy, and utilitarians such as Peter Singer have paid particular attention to medical questions (for example, Singer, 1995). In fact, it has exerted a major influence in medical ethics and public policy, standing as it does at the root of health economics. Philosophically, the doctrine's key claim is that an action is good to the extent that it helps to maximize aggregate utility experienced within the community. (An agent is good to the extent that she seeks to maximise aggregate utility.) At the most fundamental level, 'utility' equates to individual feelings of pleasure and 'disutility' equates to individual feelings of pain. (Frequently, scholars hesitate to use the term 'happiness,' which refers to a state of character in the Aristotelian tradition.) In that utilitarianism judges the value of an action by assessing its results, it is a form of 'consequentialism'. As it is concerned with the individual's feelings (as opposed to, say, the enlargement of freedom or the enforcement of personal rights), it is a form of 'welfarism'. In public policy discussions, the 'community' to which utilitarians refer is usually taken to be the inhabitants of a politically defined territory, such as the state or health authority.

It is commonly claimed that not only do utilitarians lack a convincing method for making interpersonal comparisons of utility, but that they lack a practicable understanding of 'pleasure' and 'pain'. Some utilitarians have used the satisfaction of the expressed preferences of individuals as their metric of pleasure and pain. Yet, few wish to give significant weight to poorly thought-out preferences, particularly in medical decisions where frequently a solid grasp of complex technical knowledge is required in order to make competent assessments of the available options for intervention. The situation is complicated further by the fact that health is only one of the things for which people have preferences. How is a utilitarian to judge authoritatively between preferences for, say, a healthy lifestyle and much stronger and definite preferences for smoking or eating enjoyable but high-fat food? As Henry Sidgwick observed optimistically, 'men seem to attach great value to the ample gratification of bodily appetites and needs: . . . and though they do not often deliberately sacrifice health to this gratification . . . still one may say that they are habitually courageous in pressing forward to the very verge of this imprudence, (Sidgwick, 1907, p. 154).

It has been noted that the methods of conventional health economics are founded on forms of utilitarianism, predominantly through analyses of cost-effectiveness, cost-benefit and cost-utility (Zweifel & Breyer, 1997, ch. 2). Each of these approaches attempts to weigh human lives and health states on a common scale as a proxy for calculations of pleasure and pain (for example, by ascribing monetary values to alternative health outcomes and the costs of securing those outcomes or by attempting to measure 'quality-adjusted life years' (QALYs)) (Williams, 1995, p. 221). Often, such approaches attempt to ascribe cardinal values to the alternatives. The advantages to these approaches are clear. For example, they allow managers to claim that scientific calculation justifies providing treatment for the young at the expense of treatment for the elderly. Furthermore, they allow the government to cap health spending on the grounds that the health budget is now being used more effectively.

Principles of Health Care Ethics, Second Edition   Edited by R.E. Ashcroft, A. Dawson, H. Draper and J.R. McMillan
© 2007 John Wiley & Sons, Ltd

From a liberal point of view, however, utilitarianism faces a number of other serious problems. Firstly, it seems facile to attempt to reduce the various dimensions and complexities of alternative health outcomes to a single measure (utility), particularly when money is used as a proxy for utility. Secondly, to the extent that these measures refer to individuals' revealed preferences, they fall foul of the problem, mentioned above, of evaluating the quality of reasoning that gave rise to those preferences (Burchardt, 2005). For many contemporary liberals, however, utilitarianism's most significant problem is its failure to respect individuals as free and equal persons. Instead, utilitarianism values individuals only to the extent that they experience the pleasures and pains (or, say, QALYs) that are aggregated to produce the greatest social good. It accords no intrinsic value to the fair distribution of health care. As John Rawls puts it, 'Utilitarianism does not take seriously the distinction between persons, (Rawls, 1972, p. 24). Sir Bernard Williams, a moral philosopher and chair of many government committees on the ethics of public policy, concluded that 'utilitarianism, both in theory and practice, is alarmingly good at combining technical complexity with simple-mindedness . . .. Simple-mindedness consists in having too few thoughts and feelings to match the world as it really is . . .. [T]he simple-mindedness of utilitarianism disqualifies it totally [as a method of making social choices], (Williams, 1973, pp. 149–50, 135–50).

In contrast to utilitarianism's pursuit of aggregate pleasure, the dominant liberal position is that the institutions and rules on which a social system is based are legitimate only to the extent that, when taken together and over the long term, they respect all citizens as free and equal persons. The classic defence of such a position is found in the moral and political philosophy of Immanuel Kant, for whom it has been written, 'one should act in such a way that, in a community whose members all acted that way, one would order one's life according to reason and the lives of all would be enhanced' (Campbell et al, 2005, p. 4) The primary objective for Kant was to be a rational moral agent: someone who deliberated on the actions and forms of life open to them in order to act consistently towards every person. In that sense, Kant valued the quality of one's will above all else: 'Power, riches, honor, even health and that complete well-being and satisfaction with one's condition called *happiness*, produce boldness and thereby often arrogance as well unless a good will is present which corrects the influence of these on the mind' (Kant, 1996, p. 49).

Over the years, Kant's ideal has been variously reinterpreted. Some liberals have argued that the individual's actions should be structured by a system of inalienable property rights found in the world (these rights should function as moral and legal boundaries or 'side-constraints' on what the individual may legitimately do). In a very influential right libertarian book *Anarchy, State and Utopia* (1974), Robert Nozick attacked Williams' claim that 'Leaving aside preventive medicine, the proper ground of distribution of medical care is ill health: this is a necessary truth' (Williams, 1962, p. 121); quoted in (Nozick, 1974, p. 233). To Nozick's mind, Williams approaches the issue from a totally wrong angle. Rather than health care being provided according to the patients' needs for treatment, it should be made available according to the price that doctors and hospitals can charge given current effective demand: 'why must the internal goal of the activity take precedence over, for example, the person's particular purpose in performing the activity? . . . just because [the doctor] has this [medical] skill, why should *he* bear the costs of the desired allocation, why is he less entitled to pursue his own goals, within the special circumstances of practicing medicine, than everyone else?' (Nozick, 1974, p. 234). Medical care should be distributed on the grounds of the effective demand of the ill person, that is, according to her personal desire and ability to pay.

Nozick's view is somewhat in the minority among mainstream academic liberals, with the latter being primarily concerned with social justice, see Rice (2001). Ronald Dworkin, for example, bases his theory of social justice in health care (the 'prudent insurance' ideal, Dworkin, 2000, p. 311) on what he describes as 'an extremely appealing assumption: a just distribution [of health resources] is one that well-informed people create for themselves by individual choices, provided that the economic system and the distribution of wealth in the community in which these choices are made are themselves just' (Dworkin, 2000, p. 313). Achieving these background conditions of justice requires three very demanding things (Dworkin, 2000, pp. 311–2). First, that income and wealth are distributed as fairly as possible, with 'fairness' entailing at least a reduction in the extremes of wealth and poverty of the type found in contemporary America. Second, that 'everything . . . that good doctors know . . . is generally known by the public at large as well'. Third, that no one is able to predict who will be ill or injured in the future. Once these three conditions have been satisfied, Dworkin believes individuals should be left free to purchase whatever medical care they require 'in as free a market as we can imagine' (Dworkin, 2000, p. 312). Individuals may choose to form health insurance cooperatives among themselves or to devise other schemes to provide for their predicted future medical needs. Whatever happens, Dworkin holds that the subsequent level of medical expenditure 'is the morally appropriate amount for [the community] to spend', and that concerns of justice require no further redistribution of health expenses by the state. He then uses this prudent insurance ideal to justify a limited national health service for 'our own, imperfect, and unjust community' (Dworkin, 2001, pp. 313, 313–9). Other contemporary liberals also hold that the primary aim of public policy, state action and civic life should be to facilitate and respect the autonomous lives of each of its individual citizens. The late John Rawls' treatment – which he called 'justice as fairness' – is the most influential contemporary liberal theory of social justice. He begins by attempting to isolate those qualities and capacities that make individual human beings subjects of justice. In other words, he asks what is it about a human being that makes it plausible to say that she has acted unfairly, and what makes it problematic to say the same thing about building, plants or 'lower' non-human animals?

Rawls holds that in the long run we seek a good life. What this good life consists in – what each of us has to do in order to feel that we live such a life – is shaped partly by our humanity. We would not lead a good life were we to face starvation say, or death by exposure, involuntarily. Yet, on their own, our capacities for physical suffering cannot make us subjects of justice because justice presupposes responsibility and responsibility presupposes self-conscious agency. The first quality is self-consciousness: we are aware of ourselves as beings with desires and reason, living in a world with other such beings and other objects. Secondly, we are conscious of ourselves as living in a world which changes over time, and thirdly and importantly, which we can choose to change in accordance with our desires and plans over time. This third quality is rational agency or autonomy. The majority of the complexities of the individual's good life are unique to her as a particular autonomous being, and precisely which sort of life the individual values depends on her particular character and circumstances. In Rawls' terms, each of us shares a 'thin theory of the good' (to lead an autonomous life) but not a 'thick theory of the good' (we do not all want to live the same life). Rawls bases his liberalism on the thin good of the autonomous life.

The most obvious and significant ways in which concerns about autonomy inform the ethics of current medical practice are through the notions of 'competence' and 'consent'. As Margaret Brazier has observed, from the perspective of modern medical law '[t]he right of the patient, who is sufficiently rational and mature to understand what is entailed in treatment, to decide for herself whether to agree to that treatment is a basic human right' (Brazier, 2003, p. 91, Chapters 4 and 5). There are obvious problems in realizing this ideal of patient autonomy. First, difficult decisions remain even when one appeals to the single criterion of respecting personal autonomy. The patient's request for an abortion clashes with doctors' religious prohibition against taking (what they judge to be) life. Both concerns are given force through an appeal to autonomy. The clash is irresolvable within this framework, reflecting the unavoidable tragedies that punctuate a normal human life, where right conflicts with right, rather than right

with wrong (Bradley, 1965, pp. 71, 85–92).Second, can someone truly consent to a particular course of medical treatment if they cannot understand or evaluate it to any significant degree (if they lack the requisite mental abilities)? This same problem is encountered in any area where decisions rely on professional expertise or complex technical knowledge. In what senses, if any, do we consent to the laws when we treat the judgements of civil servants and politicians as proxies for our own, or do we act when we follow the advice of solicitors and barristers? Even if consent is weak in health care, autonomy requires openness and honesty from the medical professional. In part, this is because in doctor–patient relations as with politicians and solicitors, 'If truth is the first casualty, trust must be the second' (Higgs, 1985, p. 188). In part also, however, it is because autonomy requires independence not manipulation no matter how well intentioned the latter may be. Being truthful and open with a patient may cause them a great deal of pain, even depression, but it does at least show them respect as an autonomous being. This is one substantive point at which, all other things being equal, liberalism and utilitarianism diverge. Honesty may lead to a decrease in aggregate utility, but it does respect the fundamental moral equality of the patient and the doctor, and can form a significant basis of the patient's feeling of self-respect and control.

Personal autonomy requires more than simply a diversity of attractive options. The autonomous individual must have the resources to be able to use these options. This is a decisive factor when designing a fair health service in that it determines the nature and value of the resources that facilitate living a healthy life. In many cases, these resources are primarily financial. Yet, as Rawls has pointed out, frequently many other types of resources are also needed:

> suppose that the basic structure of society distributes certain primary goods, that is, things that every rational man is presumed to want. These goods normally have a use whatever a person's rational plan of life. For simplicity, assume that the chief primary goods at the disposition of society are rights and liberties, powers and opportunities, and income and wealth. (Later on . . . the primary good of self-respect has a central place.) These are the social primary goods. Other primary goods such as health and vigor, intelligence and imagination, are natural goods; although their possession is influenced by the basic structure, they are not so directly under its control (Rawls, 1972, p. 53).

For Rawls, social primary goods should be used as components of indices of the expectations which it is reasonable for members of society to have when pursuing their chosen plans of life over a long term (Rawls, 1972, section 15). The government should use these indices to determine the fairest distribution of resources throughout the society. A society is fair to the extent that it is organized so as to distribute resources in accordance with two abstract principles of justice. The first is that 'Every person is to have an equal right to the most extensive total system of equal basic liberties compatible with a similar system of liberty for all' (Rawls, 1972, p. 302). The second principle requires that 'Social and economic inequalities are to be arranged so that they are both:

(a) to the greatest benefit of the least advantaged, consistent with the just savings principle, and
(b) attached to offices and positions open to all under conditions of fair equality of opportunity' (Rawls, 1972, p. 302).

The technicalities of these very influential principles need not detain us beyond noting that the first has absolute (or 'lexical') priority over the first part of the second principle ('the difference principle') (you cannot give up your basic rights in order to gain more social and economic resources), and that the difference principle has lexical priority over the second part of the second principle.

For Rawls, in practice the government needs to be concerned only with the expectations of those persons who are least advantaged by the scheme of social cooperation in which they participate. In other words, institutions, norms, laws and policies should seek to raise to the highest possible level the expectations of the worst-off section in society (worst-off in terms of access to primary goods). The particular expectations of all other sections of society can be left to the vagaries of the system of social cooperation. Individuals, he writes, 'share in primary goods on the principle that some can have more if they are acquired in ways which improve the situation of those who have less' (Rawls, 1972, p. 94). (The pivotal belief here is that in a free society inequalities provide incentives for hard work, the benefits of which 'trickle down' to less advantaged sectors.) One of the great strengths of this approach, to Rawls' mind, is that it requires an ordinal measure of (dis)advantage rather than cardinal one: the government needs only to determine that group x gains the least from living in a society, not that group x is half as advantaged as the next least advantaged group or a tenth as advantaged as the most advantaged group.

Rawls is emphatic, however, that he is not concerned with how well individuals use their primary goods: 'Justice as fairness . . . does not look behind the use which persons make of the rights and opportunities available to them in order to measure, much less to maximize, the satisfaction they achieve. Nor does it try to evaluate the relative merits of different [thick] conceptions of the good' (Rawls, 1972, p. 94). Rawls sees this agnosticism as a necessary implication of the requirement that a free society treat its members as free and equal beings. (For a very interesting extended discussion of the implications of Rawls' theory for health care ethics, see Daniels (1985)).

Rawls' later writings stress the political justification of primary goods, arguing that they are significant because they enable individuals to function as citizens within a stable and fair scheme of social cooperation (Rawls, 1993, pp. 178–90). More specifically, they enable individuals to develop and exercise 'two moral powers'. The first 'is the capacity for a sense of justice: it is the capacity to understand, to apply, and to act from (and not merely in accordance with) the principles of justice that specify the fair terms of social cooperation . . . The other moral power is a capacity for a conception of the good: it is the capacity to have, to revise, and rationally to pursue a conception of the good' (Rawls, 2001, pp. 18–9). The second moral power is important because a just society must be founded upon the 'thin' conception of the good understood as an autonomous life. Thick conceptions are relevant to justice only to the extent and because they are endorsed critically and self-consciously by autonomous agents.

The political turn in Rawls' later liberalism has profound implications for his understanding of a fair health care system. Towards the end of the book *Justice as Fairness. A Restatement*, he argues carefully that schemes of educational and health resources should be designed and delivered in the manner that is most likely to 'enable' individuals 'to be normal and fully cooperating members of society over a complete life and to maintain their status as free and equal citizens' (Rawls, 2001, p. 169). Specifically, he sketches what justice requires society to provide for citizens when they are either 'seriously ill or suffer from severe accidents from time to time' (Rawls, 2001, pp. 172, 171–6). He highlights three key points. First, the particular set of primary social goods is not determined universally via an abstract form of philosophical reflection, but for each particular society at 'the constitutional, legislative, and judicial stages as more information is made available, and particular social conditions can be taken into account' (Rawls, 2001, p. 172). Second, as citizens we have legitimate claims on government and its agencies to provide us with resources from the collective stock, including both 'personal goods and services, . . . as in the case of health care' and 'public goods (in the economist's sense), as in the case of measures ensuring public health (clean air and unpolluted water, and the like)' (Rawls, 2001, p. 172). Third, to be legitimate the index of primary social goods must be able to respond effectively to 'the various contingencies' citizens face over 'the normal course of a complete life', including 'the illnesses and accidents that befall them' (Rawls, 2001, pp. 172–3). In this sense, 'the expectation' of an assured provision of health care at a certain level (calculated by estimated cost) is included as part of . . . [the social] minimum [or welfare net]' (Rawls, 2001, p. 173). Our claims for medical treatment that will enable us to participate as citizens in our society are legitimate and must be weighed in calculations regarding the use of scarce resources to meet the normal functions of the state (welfare provision, defence and so on). Treatment that is unlikely to serve that end has no legitimate claim on public resources: 'cosmetic medicine, say, is not offhand a need at all' (Rawls, 2001, p. 174). (Presumably, Rawls is referring merely to cosmetic treatment on the basis of vanity rather than real disfigurement).

Amartya Sen has objected that Rawls' theory neglects 'the *actual living* that people manage to achieve' with resources, '(or going beyond that, on the *freedom* to achieve actual livings that one can have reason to value)' (Sen, 1999, p. 73). Sen's alternative – 'the capabilities approach' – tries to remedy this alleged deficiency. On the basis of this view, the government should be concerned with the individual's 'capability', understood as 'the alternative combinations of functionings that are feasible for her to achieve (or, less formally put, the freedom to achieve various lifestyles)' (Sen, 1999, p. 75). The functionings referred to here are:

> the various things a person may value doing or being. The valued functionings may vary from elementary ones, such as being adequately nourished and being free from avoidable disease, to very complex activities or personal states, such as being able to take part in the life of the community and having self-respect (Sen, 1999, pp. 75, 309n 40).

Sen argues that precisely which resources are required, how many are required and their relative importance for an individual to realise her capabilities, will depend on her particular society and circumstances to a far greater degree than is allowed for by Rawls' primary goods approach. Sen believes that defining poverty in terms of 'capabilities deprivation' has a number of strengths: 'the approach concentrates on deprivations that are *intrinsically* important (unlike low income, which is only *instrumentally* significant)': it highlights causes of poverty other than low income, such as restricted access to health care; it shows that 'the impact of income on capabilities is contingent and conditional' (Sen, 1999, pp. 88–9). That capabilities that are possessed by individuals rather than Rawlsian groups is especially significant as it allows for a more nuanced conception of need and deprivation, in which those who have greater natural health requirements, such as the disabled, children and, relative to men, women, tend to have a greater claim on the pool of available resources even if they fall within the same income group, class or even family. Moreover, he claims that his capabilities approach is better able to accommodate cultural variations. Rawls held that neither of these criticisms was significant, as the particular components of the set of primary goods to be delivered in a community and their relative weights are to be determined at the legislative level, in the light of local circumstances.

The dispute between Sen and Rawls is one for the reader to pursue (in the first instances, see Sen (1980, 1992)). A more radical critique of primary goods has been launched by so-called 'communitarian' philosophers. To the extent that 'communitarianism' is anything more than a term of abuse, it is characterized by the (rather vague) contention that the practices that can give meaning and structure to an individual's existence, together with the virtues associated with those practices, are inherently socially derived and situated. On the basis of this view, the appropriate activities of a profession tend to change as its social context changes, as do the resources required to participate in those activities. Michael Walzer's critique of Rawlsian primary good starts with the claim that goods are embodied meanings. They are constituted by the ways they are understood in society and by the purposes that society understands them to properly serve: 'They are not and they cannot be idiosyncratically valued' (Walzer, 1983, p. 7). Consequently, '[fair] distributions are patterned in accordance with shared conceptions of what the goods are and what they are for' (Walzer, 1983, p. 7). Walzer denies the very possibility of there being then, except in the most abstract terms, a 'single set of primary or basic goods conceivable across all moral and material worlds': as societies vary so must goods, and as a particular society changes so do the meanings (and nature) of its goods (Walzer, 1983, p. 8).

Walzer develops and defends this framework in many areas, including social membership, paid employment, the duties of professional offices, education and familial relations. He also focuses on 'Security and welfare,' under which heading he includes health care in modern industrialized countries and especially the United States. His discussion of social justice in the distribution of health care in modern societies is founded upon three principles: 'that every political community must attend to the needs of its members as they collectively understand those needs; that the goods that are distributed must be distributed in proportion to need; and that the distribution must recognize and uphold the underlying equality of membership' (Walzer, 1983, p. 84). Nowadays, there is, he claims, a 'common appreciation' that public investment in such a fundamental good as health care (whether 'to finance research, build hospitals, and pay the fees of doctors in private practice') means that when push comes to shove, 'the services that these expenditures underwrite must be equally available to all citizens' (Walzer, 1983, p. 90). His interesting argument has radical implications for the organization of medical services.

Alasdair MacIntyre (another 'communitarian') holds, in Janet Coleman's words, that 'practices [such as 'being a doctor *qua* doctor'] never have a goal or goals fixed for all time but goals themselves are transmuted by the history of the activity so that every practice (read virtue) has its own history' (Coleman, 1994, pp. 82–3). MacIntyre provides a detailed and subtle underpinning for this historical understanding of practices and virtues. He characterizes a 'practice' as 'any coherent and complex form of socially es-tablished cooperative human activity through which goods internal to that form of activity are realized in the course of trying to achieve those standards of excellence which are appropriate to, and partially definitive of, that form of activity, with the result that human powers to achieve excellence, and human conceptions of the ends and goods involved, are systematically extended' (MacIntyre, 1985, p. 187).

The good internal to the practice of medicine is not simply what individual doctors, the medical community or the health authority decides medical treatment should achieve. Instead, it is the purpose that gives medicine its value in the wider community. It is the reason why medicine is valued in the particular culture where the particular doctors practise (Miller, 1994, pp. 250–1, 255–6). MacIntyre is appealing to the values that structure the wider community rather than the wishes or plans of current formal post-holders. In spite of its appeal to convention then, his 'communitarianism' provides a critical standard against which the actions and especially the goals of office-holders should be judged. The relationships between clinicians, managers, governments, patients and the wider community should take the form of on-going dialogues: '. . . no practices can survive for any length of time unsustained by institutions . . . . [Yet, w]ithout [virtues], without justice, courage and truthfulness, practices could not resist the corrupting power of institutions' (MacIntyre, 1985, p. 194). The necessary interrelation of practices, virtues and institutions has special significance in the context of the influence of economic utilitarianism on the medical profession. If it is the case that the United Kingdom's National Health Service is increasingly structured by concerns arising from cost-based analyses of the types outlined above, then the tendency will be, as the nineteenth century social theorist Thomas Carlyle noted in more general context, for 'Cash Payment . . . [to grow] to be the universal sole nexus of man to man' (Carlyle, 1971, p. 193). This would be (is already?) one effect of what Williams called utilitarianism's simple-mindedness: namely, 'having too few thoughts and feelings to match the world as it really is' (Williams, 1973, pp. 149–50). The sense of professionalism and care that informed medical practice in the National Health Service, and which finds canonical (if in practice qualified) expression in the Hippocratic oath, is in danger of being eroded by the commercial consciousness of contemporary institutionalized medicine.

Some political theorists have attempted to reconcile and extend the theories of goods that underpin Rawlz and Walzer's theories of social justice in health care (Tyler, in press). This entry will conclude by highlighting a problem that is faced by liberals and 'communitarians' alike. It might be asked, are both approaches simple-minded when they take persons to be the subjects of their respective theories? Social primary goods, functionings and capabilities and goods as embodied meanings, as well as virtues and traditions, can be used only by persons. Non-persons are akin to Joseph Raz's 'the Man in the Pit'.

> A person falls down a pit and remains there for the rest of his life, unable to climb out or to summon help. There is just enough ready food to keep him alive without (after he gets used to it) any suffering. He can do nothing much, not even move much. His choices are confined to whether to eat now or a little later, whether to sleep now or a little later, whether to scratch his left ear or not . . . . His options are all short term and negligible in their significance and effects (Raz, 1986, p. 373–4).

Yet, clearly not all beings that have interests (beings for whom life can go better or worse) are persons. If my cat is a person then she is so in only a very limited way. Nevertheless, her capacity to feel pleasure and especially pain mean that she is worthy of moral concern. Newborn children and severely mentally disabled humans lack the capacities for personhood in the same way that most non-human animals do (the higher-order primates seem to have a good claim to personhood). Nevertheless, the sentience of these 'non-persons' makes them legitimate objects of moral concern. There are some things that is deplorable to to them. Indeed, the wrongness of certain treatment is compounded greatly by the vulnerability that necessarily attends their lack of personhood. These facts create real problems for liberals and communitarians writing about health care ethics. At one point, Rawls acknowledged that he has 'put aside the more extreme cases of persons with such grave disabilities that they can never be normal contributing members of social cooperation' (Rawls, 2001, p. 170). Given the centrality of personhood (the capacity for autonomous agency) in his theory, this seems more than a device to simplify his argument. He cannot accommodate non-persons within his theory, simply because they cannot be subjects of justice or citizens. The same holds true for any theory that relies on notions of personhood or justice in any of its many forms. Just how much headway liberals and 'communitarians' have made in addressing the uncomfortable implications of their shared commitments remains a matter of dispute (Dworkin, 1993: chapters 1, 3 and 8; Guest, 2002).

REFERENCES

Bradley AC. Hegel's theory of tragedy. In: *Oxford Lectures on Poetry*, London: MacMillan, 1965; pp. 67–95.

Brazier M. *Medicine, Patients and the Law,* 3rd edition. Harmondsworth: Penguin, 2003.

Burchardt T. Just happiness? Subjective wellbeing and social policy. In: Pearce N, Paxton W, eds. *Social Justice. Building a Fairer Britain.* London: Politico's, 2005; pp. 240–60.

Campbell, A., Gillett, G., and Jones, G. *Medical Ethics.* Fourth edition. Oxford: Oxford University Press, 2005.

Carlyle T. 'Chartism.' In: Shelston A, ed. *Thomas Caryle: Selected Writings*, Harmondsworth: Penguin, 1971; pp. 149–232.

Coleman J. MacIntyre and Aquinas. In: Horton J, Mendus S, eds. *After MacIntyre. Critical perspectives on the work of Alasdair MacIntyre*. Notre Dame, Indiana: University of Notre Dame Press, 1994; pp. 65–90.

Daniels N. *Just Health Care*. Cambridge: Cambridge University Press, 1985.

Dworkin R. *Life's Dominion: An Argument about Abortion and Euthanasia*, London: HarperCollins, 1993.

Dworkin R. *Sovereign Virtue: The Theory and Practice of Equality.* Cambridge, MA: Harvard University Press, 2000.

Guest S. The value of art. *Art Antiquity Law* 2002; **7**: 305.

Higgs R. On telling patients the truth. In: Lockwood M, ed. *Moral Dilemmas in Modern Medicine*. Oxford: Oxford University Press, 1985; pp. 187–202.

Kant I. Groundwork of the metaphysic of morals. In: Gregor MJ, ed. and translator. *Practical Philosophy*. Cambridge: Cambridge University Press, 1996; pp. 37–108.

MacIntyre A. *After Virtue: A Study in Moral Theory.* 2nd edition. London: Duckworth, 1985.

Miller D. Virtues, practices and justice. In: Horton J, Mendus S, eds. *After MacIntyre. Critical Perspectives on the Work of Alasdair MacIntyre*. Notre Dame, Indiana: University of Notre Dame Press, 1994; pp. 245–64.

Nozick R. *Anarchy State and Utopia*. Oxford: Blackwell, 1974.

Rawls J. *A Theory of Justice*. Oxford: Oxford University Press, 1972.

Rawls J. *Political Liberalism*. New York: New York: Columbia University Press, 1993.

Rawls J. In: Erin K, ed. *Justice as Fairness: A Restatement*. Cambridge, MA: Belknapp Harvard, 2001.

Raz J. *The Morality of Freedom*. Oxford: Clarendon Press, 1986.

Rice T. Individual autonomy and state involvement in health care. *J Med Ethics* 2001; **27**: 240–4.

Sen A. Equality of what? In: McMurrin SM, ed. *Tanner Lectures on Human Values,* Vol. 1. Salt Lake City: University of Utah Press, 1980

Sen A. *Inequality re-examined*. Cambridge, MA: Harvard University Press, 1992.

Sen A. *Development as Freedom*. Oxford: Oxford University Press, 1999.

Sidgwick H. *Methods of Ethics*. Seventh Edition. London: MacMillan, 1907.

Singer P. *Rethinking Life and Death: The Collapse of Our Traditional Ethics*. Oxford: Oxford University Press, 1995.

Tyler C. Human well-being and the future of the WTO. In: Lee SD, McBride S, eds. *Neo-liberalism, State Power and Global Governance*, London: Springer-Kluwer (in press).

Walzer M. *Spheres of Justice. A Defence of Pluralism and Equality.* Oxford: Basil Blackwell, 1983

Williams A. Economics, QALYs and medical ethics – a health economist's perspective. *Health Care Anal* 1995; **3**: 221–6.

Williams B A. critique of utilitarianism. In: Smart JJC, Williams B, eds. *Utilitarianism For and Against*. Cambridge: Cambridge University Press, 1973; pp.75–155.

Williams B. The idea of equality. In: Laslett P, Runciman WG, eds. *Philosophy, Politics, and Society.* 2nd series. Blackwell: Oxford, 1962; pp. 110–31.

Zweifel P, Breyer F. *Health Economics*. Oxford: Oxford University Press, 1997.

6

How Many Principles for Bioethics?

ROBERT M. VEATCH

It is common in bioethics literature, to see references to 'the four principles', often without bothering to name them. It is common, but by no means universal. Some bioethics theories are not based on principles at all: virtue theories, casuistry, human rights approaches and codes that appear in certain health professional and religious groups. Principle-based theories are those that articulate a small set of general, abstract, right-making characteristics of action – most famously beneficence, nonmaleficence, autonomy and justice. Other theories do not use the language of principles, but nevertheless present short general lists of normative moral criteria for morally right action calling them duties (sometimes *prima facie* duties), rules or 'appeals'. This chapter explores these theories that put forward lists of principles or functionally similar considerations.

In order to compare different principle-based approaches, we need to define the limits of what we will include. As I use the term, principle-based approaches are a branch of normative theory of right action. Thus, virtue-based approaches and axiological theories (value theories) are excluded. For example, care theory – insofar as care is presented as a virtue, a trait of good character – is not included (Veatch, 1998). Likewise, casuistry (Jonsen, 1988) and collections of rules or rights will not be included. The American Hospital Association's 'Patient's Bill of Rights' (American Hospital Association, 1992) and the American Nurses Association's 'Codes of Ethics for Nurses,' (American Nurses Association, 2001) are both essentially examples of compendia of moral insights that are open-ended lists (even though the ANA Code has buried in some of its statements what a philosopher could identify as principles – such as autonomy or self-determination and beneficence).

Some restrict principle-based ethics even further. They would limit their attention to principled approaches that do not provide anything more than an intuitive balancing of conflicting appeals based on the judgement of the decision-maker. Sometimes referred to as 'principlism', these theories based on nonordered lists surely make up a major set of principle-based approaches, but that restriction seems too confining (Clouser and Gert, 1994). I will include any theory in biomedical ethics that includes a list of principles or their close equivalent regardless of how potential conflicts among principles are to be resolved.

One common view today, presented in the critically important *Principles of Biomedical Ethics* by Tom Beauchamp and James Childress as well as elsewhere, is that moral theory has its grounding in a set of pre-theoretical insights that are shared by all humans or at least by all reasonable humans (Beauchamp and Childress, 2001, pp. 2–5). Often referred to as the 'common morality', this set of pre-theoretical insights gets shaped by different cultural groups into normative theories. Names are given to common moral norms that, through the influences of the culture's language and concepts, eventually emerge as principles or their equivalent. As such it is plausible that somewhat different names get used. A somewhat different scope or range of behaviours is defined as right-making. What one theorist calls beneficence might be subdivided into two principles called beneficence and nonmaleficence – principles that affirm that actions are right insofar as they produce benefit and avoid harm, respectively. To make matters more complex, the more inclusive meaning of beneficence – the meaning that covers both positive and negative aspects of producing good consequences – might be given a different name. Hence, many theories call the broader norm 'utility', while the American Belmont Report from the National Commission for the Protection of Subjects of Biomedical and Behavioral Research persists in calling the principle 'beneficence' even though it makes clear that it includes both aspects – what Beauchamp and Childress would call beneficence and nonmaleficence.

Principles of Health Care Ethics, Second Edition   Edited by R.E. Ashcroft, A. Dawson, H. Draper and J.R. McMillan

ALTERNATIVE LISTS OF PRINCIPLES

Looking at ethics this way, it is apparent that many different normative theories rely on principle lists when presenting their formulation of morally right action. It is worth compiling a working list of the alternatives. In this section of the chapter, I set out several examples of lists of principles that appear in principle-based theories. In the following section, I examine the question of the significance of the differences among the lists.

SINGLE-PRINCIPLE THEORIES

Utilitarianism

That utility is an example of a principle makes clear that some principle-based normative theories can incorporate only a single principle. Utilitarianism has only one principle (although that principle is interpreted so as to cover what some theorists would express as two separate principles: beneficence and nonmaleficence). The single principle of utility, as classically formulated, strives to maximize aggregate net utility by taking into account the amount and probability of benefits and harms, combining the possible net benefits for each individual affected by alternative courses of action.

There are problems with single-principle theories even though they have attracted many adherents. Beauchamp and Childress have insisted that beneficence and nonmaleficence must be kept distinct. As we shall discuss later, lumping both production of benefit and the avoidance of harm into a single principle makes it more difficult to address some questions about the relation between benefit and harm.

Hippocratism

In traditional medical ethics a similar consequence-maximizing principle also prevails, but, following the Hippocratic Oath, the goal is to maximize benefit for the individual patient and to protect the patient from harm. No introduction of benefits and harms to others is permitted as it is in classical utilitarianism. Nevertheless, the standard Hippocratic ethic is usually treated as a single-principle theory – one that strives to maximize net utility for the patient. A modern version of Hippocratism is seen in the medical ethical theory of Edmund Pellegrino and David Thomasma in which they claim all medical ethics can be subsumed under their principle of 'beneficence in trust' (Pellegrino & Thomasma, 1988). With sophistication lacking in traditional Hippocratic theory, they attempt to account for a wide range of moral insights – including respect for patient autonomy – within this single principle. I know of no other comparable moral theory in any branch of ethics

other than Hippocratic ethics that relies on a single principle of utilitarian character but systematically excludes all consequences not accruing to a single person such as the patient.

Libertarianism

Another single-principle approach is libertarianism. Here the core principle is not utility, but liberty or autonomy: that action is morally right that respects the autonomy of the person by not interfering with actions derived from substantially autonomously chosen life plans. The critical problem for autonomy as a single-principle theory is whether it can adequately account for our moral insights if left standing as our only moral principle. Although most (but not all) moral theories include autonomy, almost all see fit to include something else – either principles that promote maximizing consequences (beneficence and nonmaleficence) or those that require other behaviours (such as a principle of justice that requires distributing goods according to some end-state pattern considered to be morally correct).

A strong case is made that normative ethics cannot be reduced to either utility-maximization or liberty-preservation. Hence, multiple-principle approaches to bioethics have become common.

MULTIPLE-PRINCIPLE THEORIES

The four-principle theory introduced by Tom Beauchamp and James Childress that became the core approach in the first edition of *The Principle of Health Care Ethics* is one example of a multiple-principle theory, but other examples exist as well. Theories with lists ranging from two to ten principles (or their close equivalents) have emerged. This section catalogues those theories.

Two-Principle Approaches

Beneficence and Nonmaleficence

A utilitarian who takes the Beauchamp/Childress claim seriously that nonmaleficence needs to be kept conceptually distinct from beneficence, might be said to have a two-principle theory of biomedical ethics. Insisting on two separate principles related to maximizing consequences has distinct advantages over merely endorsing utility as the sole principle of an ethic. Maintaining two distinct principles provides the conceptual and linguistic means for addressing the question of how avoiding harm should be related to production of benefit.

Many classic utilitarians follow Bentham in assuming that considerations of benefit and harm get integrated into a single measure of utility by combining them arithmetically. The benefits are taken as positive units, whereas the harms are taken as negative ones. All the benefits can be added while the harms are subtracted.

While the standard Benthamite calculus worked arithmetically, many people in health care intuitively integrate benefits and harms a different way. They calculate the ratio. They conclude that a course that produces the largest possible benefit–harm ratio is moral. This is common, for example, in cost–benefit analysis as well as in bedside clinical ethics.

The approach is sometimes referred to as the 'geometric method' of comparing benefits and harms (Veatch, 2003). This is the most plausible way of justifying randomized clinical trials in which one wants to compare a standard treatment that offers small benefits and small risks of harm with an experimental treatment that offers proportionally larger amounts of each. When the ratios are the same, one is said to be in 'equipoise', and when researchers as a community are more or less in equipoise randomization is said to be justified (Freedman, 1987; Veatch, 2002). As arithmetic comparison would not support equipoise in these cases, it is apparent that standard Benthamite calculation is not favoured. (When ratios are the same, the difference between a large expected benefit and a large expected harm of the experimental treatment will be greater than the difference between the smaller expected benefit and the smaller expected harm of the standard treatment.)

At the very least, such an example illustrates that using the geometric and arithmetic methods will sometimes – in fact usually – produce different answers. One of the objections to collapsing consequences into a single principle of utility (or beneficence in the broader sense) is that it masks the interesting controversies between alternative ways of processing considerations of benefit and harm.

Even more troublesome is the possibility that a normative theory might want to consider whether benefits and harms have different standing or priority in morality. Some theories hold that avoiding harm is a weightier or a prior moral duty. One should first make sure that no harm is done by one's actions and only then set out to see if one can do good. That is the most plausible meaning of the medical ethical slogan *primum non nocere* if it means something other than maximizing utility (Jonsen, 1977). A number of moral theories including those of W. D. Ross (Ross, 1930) and Bernard Gert (Gert et al., 1997 p. 9) attempt to treat a duty to avoid harm differently from a duty to produce good. Holding on to two different principles – beneficence and nonmaleficence – makes all the analysis of mechanisms for combining benefit and harm considerations easier. For a single-principle theorist who puts forward utility as his or her only principle, all of these issues must be buried as ways of operationalizing one's single principle rather than leaving these controversies out in the open, which is more likely if two separate principles are maintained.

Engelhardt's Principles of Permission and Beneficence

A theory that distinguishes beneficence and nonmaleficence as separate principles is not the only two-principle approach. The philosopher-physician H. Tristram Engelhardt has adopted two principles in his *Foundations of Bioethics*: permission and beneficence (Engelhardt, 1996, p. 103). In his first edition, he used the terms 'autonomy' and 'beneficence' (Engelhardt, 1986, p. 66), but in either case his is a theory relying on two principles – one commanding the first priority that strives to protect the freedom of individuals to live their lives as they see fit as long as they do not interfere with similar rights of others, and another that holds that good ought to be done by one's actions. For Engelhardt the principle of permission is more basic. '[o]ne can have the possibility of coherent resolution of moral disputes by agreement without granting the principle of beneficence' (Engelhardt, 1996, p. 105).

Engelhardt's theory does not insist on the separation of beneficence and nonmaleficence into separate principles. Beneficence presumably can come in both positive and negative forms (although harming others would not be permitted without satisfying the prior principle of permission). Moreover, Engelhardt does not include a separate and free-standing principle of justice. For him, 'Most appeals to the principle of justice can be understood as being at root a concern with beneficence' (Engelhardt, 1996, p. 121). Thus, he does not recognize a separate moral requirement based on the patterning of the distribution of the good. He follows Mill and the utilitarians in holding that the needy deserve special priority in the distribution of the good only because that tends to be beneficence maximizing.

The Belmont Report: A Three-Principle Approach

In the United States, research with human subjects is governed by the Belmont Report, the first official government-mandated study of ethical principles (National Commission for the Protection of Human Subjects of Biomedical and Behavioral Research, 1978). The National Commission for the Protection of Human Subjects of Biomedical and Behavioral Research worked with its staff, which included philosophers, to produce an ethical document that provided the moral foundation for its recommendations. Three principles were articulated: respect for persons, beneficence and justice. These, of course, have a striking similarity to the four principles of Beauchamp and Childress that constitute the primary list used in *The Principles of Health Care Ethics* as well as much of the popular literature in contemporary medical ethics.

The listing is similar, but not identical. Most strikingly in the Belmont Report, beneficence functions in the broader sense that includes what we normally refer to as nonmaleficence. It works in the Belmont Report much like a principle of utility with positive and negative consequences incorporated into a single metric. 'Beneficence thus requires that we protect against risk of harm to subjects . . .' (National Commission, 1978, p. 16). Respect for persons functions in many ways as does Beauchamp and Childress's respect for autonomy. It provides the intellectual home for informed consent and other moral requirements to show respect for the autonomy of subjects. Added to the account of respect for persons, however, are anomalous paragraphs that handle the protection of persons who are not capable of self-determination. 'Respect for the immature and the incapacitated may require protecting them as they mature or while they are incapacitated' (National Commission, 1978, p. 5). Thus, the protection of nonautonomous persons is placed by the Commission under the general principle of respect for persons rather than beneficence.

The similarities between the three Belmont principles and Beauchamp and Childress's four is not accidental. Although the three Belmont principles had apparently already been conceptualized prior to his appearance, Tom Beauchamp became part of the staff of the Commission and was responsible for preparing much of the Belmont Report draft (Beauchamp, 2003b, pp. 17–46). He has noted the differences between his own principles and those generated by the group effort of the Commission) (Beauchamp, 2003b, p. 23).

Beauchamp and Childress: The Four-Principle Approach

The well-known four-principle approach thus had its origins in the work that was going on simultaneously with the preparation of the three-principled Belmont Report, although certain differences are apparent. The four principles themselves have shown signs of evolution. The first edition in 1979 speaks merely of the 'principle of autonomy', although that edition already made clear that it was respect for the autonomy of others that was critical (Beauchamp and Childress, 1979, p. 58). It is not until the third edition that they formally shift to calling the principle 'respect for autonomy' (Beauchamp and Childress, 1989, p. 67). Moreover, already in that first edition the authors were linking respect for autonomy with respect for persons. Referring to the work of Immanuel Kant and his notion that we ought to respect others as persons, they say, 'This aspect of the principle of autonomy is often referred to as the principle of respect for persons, because it demands respect not for a utilitarian or any other reason expect that another is a person and therefore rightfully a rational determiner of his or

her own destiny' (Beauchamp and Childress, 1979, p. 59). Of course, highlighting that the element of persons that grounds respect is that persons are rightfully rational determiners of their own destiny makes clear the incompatibility of this notion of respect for persons and that of Belmont, which wants respect for persons to do the work of protecting those who are not rational determiners of their destiny.

Beauchamp and Childress include a second moral characteristic that goes beyond maximizing consequences. Justice is an independent moral notion – one that places inherent moral weight in the way that goods are distributed. The pattern of the good as well as the amount counts morally.

Baruch Brody: A Five-Appeals Approach

In moving to an example of a five-principle approach we need to confront the theoretical question of whether principles must always be called *principles*. The best known proponent of a bioethical theory that contains five elements is Baruch Brody in his 1988 volume, *Life and Death Decision Making* (Brody, 1988). In that volume, before turning to three chapters of analysis of cases involving life and death issues, he presents a theoretical framework for practising biomedical ethics that involves what he calls 'conflicting appeals'. In the second chapter he presents five appeals that have many of the qualities of principles (at least in most cases).

This raises the question of whether it is legitimate to include in our discussion of lists of principles those ethical theorists whose approaches do not explicitly refer to *principles*. If we characterize ethical principles as abstract right-making characteristics of actions or rules, then Brody's 'appeals' surely qualify at least in some cases. In this discussion of the general problem of how many principles there are in bioethical theory, I take lists of appeals to qualify regardless of whether the authors formally use the term *principle*. Furthermore, Brody's theory of resolution of conflict among his appeals uses a 'balancing' or 'judgment' approach in much the same way that many principlists do (Brody, 1988, pp. 75, 77). He thus meets even the narrower definition of principle-based approaches that limits principlism to theories that intuitively balance competing claims.

Two of Brody's appeals are direct analogues of what we have seen as principles. One of his appeals is to 'respect for persons'. Another is to the 'consequences of our actions,' which I take to be similar in all relevant respects to the principle of utility or the combined consideration of beneficence and nonmaleficence (Brody, 1988, pp. 32, 17). It is easiest to make the case that Brody's appeals are functional principles in these two examples. A third appeal is to the 'rights' (Brody, 1988, p. 22). Although expressed in the language of rights rather than principles, Brody's examples make clear that he is talking precisely about the moral right-making characteristics that other theorists express in the language of duty or principle.

It is with the fourth and fifth appeals of Brody that the story gets more complicated. One of these he calls the 'appeal to cost-effectiveness and justice' (Brody, 1988, p. 42). Although the justice component of this appeal closely parallels the Belmont and Beauchamp/Childress principles, the 'cost-effectiveness' element does not seem to fit. Cost-effectiveness is usually accounted for as a moral requirement of beneficence or utility. If the principle calls for maximizing of net good consequences, then getting as much good as possible per unit of resources is necessary. Hence, rather than listing cost-effectiveness as a separate principle or appeal, most theorists would assume it is already accounted for under the rubric of an appeal to consequences. Moreover, most theorists who have moved beyond the two-principle approach of Engelhardt would insist that the right-making characteristic of action that is singled out in the principle of justice is conceptually distinct from that in utility maximizing. Thus, a case can be made that Brody's appeal to cost-effectiveness is redundant with his appeal to consequences while both are included in the same appeal as justice conflates two different moral notions.

Finally, among his five appeals Brody lists an appeal to the virtues. Here he clearly moves beyond what would normally be included among the principles since virtue theory identifies persistent dispositions of character that make persons praiseworthy rather than characteristics of actions or rules that make behaviours morally right conduct.

Thus there is some slippage in cataloguing Brody's five appeals as a theory that contains five 'principles'. One could at least argue that an appeal to the virtues is out of place since virtues are not right-making characteristics of action at all. Nevertheless, Brody's list has many elements that suggest it could count as an alternative list of principles.

W.D. Ross: Six *Prima Facie* Duties

If it is legitimate to include in our lists of principles some work of theorists who use some alternative term, then surely W.D. Ross deserves consideration. He is the intellectual grandfather of principlists often acknowledged by them as their predecessor. Beauchamp and Childress in their first edition not only acknowledge him, but also use the term 'principle' to refer to his *prima facie* duties (Beauchamp and Childress 1979, p. 39). I will take it that there is no significant difference except one of terminology.

Ross's famous list of *prima facie* duties can be numbered in several different ways, but I will count the list as containing six items – mainly because that is the way he numbers it. His list includes some items that we have encountered regularly, such as beneficence and nonmaleficence ('not injuring others') (Ross, 1930). Idiosyncratically, he includes

as a separate item, the duty of self-improvement – reserving beneficence to actions that benefit others. A fourth consideration is justice.

Ross classifies two other items on the basis of whether the duty rests on previous acts of one's own or previous acts of others. Duties resting on previous acts of one's own are divided into those that rest on a promise (including the duty not to tell lies) and those that result from previous wrongful acts one has committed, which generate a duty of reparation. Duties resting on previous acts of others can generate duty of gratitude. It is apparent that this list could be re-grouped to generate some number other than six duties. Promise keeping, truth telling and reparation could easily be seen as separate principles. That suggests the list could be crafted as eight duties (or principles). On the contrary, if the duty of self-improvement were collapsed into beneficence, the number could be seven. Most strikingly, Ross, in spite of his intellectual link to Kant, includes no duty of respect for autonomy in his list.

Seven-Principle Approaches

Next we might consider principle lists that include seven items. My own principle list in *A Theory of Medical Ethics* (Veatch, 1981) would be an example. Influenced by W. D. Ross as well as William Frankena and my colleagues Tom Beauchamp and James Childress, my principle-based theory has, over the past decades, contained seven items. I include beneficence and nonmaleficence as well as justice, but do not handle the remaining areas exactly the way either Ross or Beauchamp and Childress do.

I often distinguish between consequence maximizing of the classical social utilitarian type and that of the more individualistic Hippocratic type. Moreover, I sometimes combine beneficence and nonmaleficence, using the short-hand term of utility. Hence, I can speak of Hippocratic and social utility as two separate principles – noting that both kinds of utility maximizing must deal with the problem of how beneficence and nonmaleficence get incorporated. In biomedical ethics it is often as important at least to differentiate utility considerations that are limited to the welfare of the patient from those that take into account the welfare of other parties as it is important to distinguish positive elements of welfare from negative ones.

It is, however, in the realm of Ross's duties resulting from previous acts of oneself and others that I most sharply differ from Beauchamp and Childress (although the differences in the end are not great). I was uncomfortable with the Beauchamp/Childress handling of autonomy (or respect for autonomy). Primarily, I was concerned that autonomy or respect for autonomy failed to give attention to duties of respect that we owe to those who are not substantially autonomous agents. I believe that there are duties of respect owed to children, babies and the senile that bear no direct relation to whether they are, ever were, or ever will be autonomous agents.

From Ross I note that we owe *prima facie* fidelity to promises and truthfulness even to those who are not autonomous agents. I thus include in my normative theory of right action a principle of fidelity that holds that there are duties of fidelity to commitments (including promises made). I also include a principle of veracity that holds that there are *prima facie* duties to avoid lying. (I generally understand the limited duty to tell the truth to be derived from the relationships one has with others. Hence, a physician has a duty to tell the truth – not merely avoid lying – because of implied promises made in the establishment of the doctor–patient relationship). In contrast to Ross, I would also include the principle of respecting autonomy (which I usually have referred to simply as the principle of autonomy although I certainly agree that the principle merely requires respecting autonomy, not actually requiring autonomous actions). I take all three of these elements (fidelity, veracity and autonomy) to be aspects of respect for humans. I do not limit the requirement of respect merely to autonomous humans. I do not even limit it to humans who are 'persons' – a distinction I shall take up in the final section of this chapter.

I am not convinced that these three elements, which I have usually treated as independent moral principles, exhaust the moral requirements of respect. In particular, I have been concerned that many moral theories hold that there is something intrinsically immoral about killing a human being. Often, in both religious and secular moral theories, this is seen as a morally wrong-making characteristic independent of whether the killing actually harms the one who is killed.

By contrast Beauchamp and Childress handle the moral prohibition on killing as part of the principle of nonmaleficence. The implication is that there is nothing intrinsically immoral about killing a human unless that action also does harm to the human's interest. This would cover many garden-variety murders, but interestingly does not normally include merciful killings such as the Dutch euthanasia or physician-assisted suicides on the request of competent persons who believe they would be better off dead. Thus, Beauchamp and Childress seem to be locked into the position that there is nothing wrong with merciful killing except when it does harm.

By contrast, I think it is important to include in one's catalogue of moral principles at least the possibility that killing of a human is a wrong-making characteristic of actions. I see it as part of a Kantian lack of respect for the intrinsic worth of humans (leaving open the possibility that a similar conclusion might be reached for certain nonhuman animals as well). Thus, I have usually grouped avoidance of killing of humans along with the principles of fidelity, veracity and autonomy as aspects of respect that we owe to one another, recognizing, of course, that these principles may have to be overridden by competing principles in certain cases. Thus, I have generally put forward a list of seven principles: beneficence, nonmaleficence, fidelity, veracity, autonomy, avoidance of killing and justice. I have often, however, added Ross's gratitude and reparation to the list, which would make my position a nine-principle theory. I have no principled reason to exclude them, although they do not often arise as critical in medical ethical deliberations.

Bernard Gert: A Ten-Rule Approach

One other prominent list in bioethical theory deserves consideration: Dartmouth philosopher Bernard Gert with his colleagues, Charles Culver and K. Danner Clouser, has developed a list of ten general moral rules (Gert et al. 1997). Their approach must be added to this discussion with care since they insist on limiting principlism to those principle-based theories that intuitively balance competing moral claims. Moreover, they explicitly reject the language of principles in favour of what they call 'moral rules'.

In spite of these claims, I believe that, assuming principle-based theories cover more than those theories that intuitively balance competing claims, the Gert/Culver/Clouser approach functions much the same way as principle-based theories do. Their list puts forward general right-making considerations hierarchically related to more specific moral rules and rights statements as well as moral judgements in specific cases.

There is another complexity with their theory. Gert and his colleagues claim all their rules are based on an overarching principle of not harming. 'The purpose of morality is to minimize the amount of evil or harm suffered by those protected by morality' (Gert et al. 1997, p. 7). Their moral rules simply detail the list of behaviours required to avoid causing harm. Hence, one could classify their theory as a one-principle theory based on nonmaleficence with ten specifications of rules to be followed to achieve what that principle requires.

One can also, however, fruitfully view their theory as a ten-rule (or ten-principle) theory. Their ten rules dovetail well with other principle lists we have examined. Listed together with the analogous principles, they include the following: 'do not deprive of freedom' (autonomy), 'do not deceive' (veracity), 'do not kill' (avoidance of killing) and 'do not cheat', as well as 'obey the law' (both of which are plausibly manifestations of the principle of fidelity). They also include the notion of 'do your duty' by which they mean do the duties associated with one's role, another manifestation of fidelity. Another group of their rules is a more direct derivation from nonmaleficence: 'do not cause pain', 'do not disable' and 'do not deprive of pleasure'. In short each of their rules can be linked to one of the principles we have already considered, and the only principles that are not somehow represented in the moral rules are the principles of beneficence and justice. They explicitly claim (however implausibly) that justice is subsumed under the notion of lessening of harm (Gert et al. 1997, p. 25). Beneficence, they claim is not a moral rule, but rather related to the 'moral rules', what is encouraged but not required (Gert et al. 1997, pp. 77, 80).

WHAT IS THE RIGHT NUMBER OF PRINCIPLES?

It is apparent that many formulations of lists of principles are possible. Although four is a convenient number lodged about midway between the single-principle theories and those that produce longer lists, there is no theoretical or 'principled' reason why the number should be four. The existence of multiple lists is also something of a problem for Beauchamp/Childress and Gert/Culver/Clouser because their efforts include two of the most forceful defences to the claim that normative ethics derives in some way from a 'common morality' (Beauchamp and Childress, 2001, pp. 2–5; Beauchamp, 2003; Gert et al. 2000). Each of them, therefore, seems committed to the view that there is some common moral grounding underlying normative ethical theory. One might think that this view should commit them (and all the other theorists we have considered) to coming up with the same list of moral principles (*prima facie* duties or moral rules).

That is not the case, however. Common morality theory holds that all humans share some common set of pre-theoretical moral insights (or would share them if they were stripped of biases and cultural distortions, and linguistic conventions could be reconciled). Thus, disproving the common morality thesis is difficult because one can claim that differences that do occur can be explained by biases or cultural distortions or are merely linguistic variations. Hence, a principle list that omits justice could be the result of a theorist overly exposed to libertarian ideas that attribute concerns about unfairness to psychological confusion. One such as Ross's, that omits autonomy, might be attributed to a theorist with inadequate appreciation of the requirements of respect for persons.

More obviously, some differences among the lists we have considered can be attributed to linguistic convention. What some call principles others call *prima facie* duties or rules. What some call respect for persons others call respect for autonomy and still others simply shorten it to a principle of autonomy. No doubt real substantive differences remain among these lists. Respecting autonomy does not cover all that is implied by respecting persons. In particular it does not seem to command respect for nonautonomous persons (or at least those who will never be autonomous). Even 'respect

for persons' seems to beg the question of whether we owe respect to humans who are not and never will be persons according to various theories of personhood. It seems fair to conclude, however, that much of the difference seen among these lists is to be explained by linguistic and social conventions that even the theorists would concede amount to cultural accretion. For example, I am more and more inclined to treat four of my principles (fidelity, veracity, autonomy and avoidance of killing) as four aspects or specifications of an overarching principle of respect for humans. In the end, it probably does not matter whether my position is described in this regard as including seven principles (including these four along with beneficence, nonmaleficence and justice) or merely four principles (beneficence, nonmaleficence, justice and respect for humans, the last of which in turn contains four more specific manifestations).

The movement from a set of pre-theoretical moral insights that are widely if not universally shared to specific normative theories which surely will reflect linguistic and cultural conventions is a major step. This surely explains much of the variation among principle lists. No doubt, there are also real substantive differences among these lists. Some of the substantive differences may show up in the number of principles on the various lists. In the end, however, the number of principles explicated in the various theories may have more to do with the linguistic and cultural conventions than with the substantive differences. The number of principles on one's list will no doubt depend on both the conventions and the substance.

REFERENCES

American Hospital Association. *A Patient's Bill of Rights*. Chicago: American Hospital Association, 1992.

American Nurses Association. *Code of Ethics for Nurses with Interpretive Statements*, Washington, DC: American Nurses Association, 2001.

Beauchamp TL, Childress JF, eds. *Principles of Biomedical Ethics*, 1st edition. New York: Oxford University Press, 1979.

Beauchamp TL, Childress JF, eds. *Principles of Biomedical Ethics*, 3rd edition. New York: Oxford University Press, 1989.

Beauchamp TL, Childress JF. *Principles of Biomedical Ethics*, 5th edition. New York: Oxford University Press, 2001.

Beauchamp TL. A defense of the common morality. *Kennedy Institute of Ethics Journal* 2003a; **13**: 259–74.

Beauchamp TL. The origins, goals, and core commitments of the Belmont Report and the Principles of Biomedical Ethics. In: Walter JK, Klein EP, eds. *The Story of Bioethics: From Seminal Works to Contemporary Explorations*. Washington, DC: Georgetown University Press, 2003b.

Brody B. *Life and Death Decision Making*. New York: Oxford University Press, 1988.

Clouser KD, Gert B. Morality vs. principlism. In: Gillon R, ed. *Principles of Health Care Ethics*. New York: John Wiley & Sons, Inc., 1994.

Engelhardt HT. *The Foundations of Bioethics*. New York: Oxford University Press, 1986.

Engelhardt HT. *The Foundations of Bioethics*. 2nd edition. New York: Oxford University Press, 1996.

Freedman B. Equipoise and the ethics of clinical research. *N Engl J Med* 1987; **317**: 141–5

Gert B, Culver CM, Clouser KD. *Bioethics: A Return to Fundamentals*. New York: Oxford University Press, 1997.

Gert B, Culver CM, Clouser KD. A common morality versus specified principlism: reply to Richardson. *J Med Philos* 2000; **25**(3): 308–22.

Jonsen AR. Do no harm: axiom of medical ethics. In: Spicker SF, Engelhardt, HT Jr., eds. *Philosophical Medical Ethics: Its Nature and Significance*. Boston: D. Reidel Publishing Co., 1977; pp. 27–41.

Jonsen AR, Toulmin S. *The Abuse of Casuistry: A History of Moral Reasoning*. Berkeley: University of California Press, 1988.

National Commission for the Protection of Human Subjects of Biomedical and Behavioral Research. *The Belmont Report: Ethical Principles and Guidelines for the Protection of Human Subjects of Research*. Washington, D.C.: US Government Printing Office, 1978.

Pellegrino ED, Thomasma DC. *For the Patient's Good: The Restoration of Beneficence in Health Care*. New York: Oxford University Press, 1988.

Ross WD. *The Right and the Good*. Oxford: Oxford University Press, 1930; p. 21.

Veatch RM. *A Theory of Medical Ethics*. New York: Basic Books, 1981.

Veatch RM. The place of care in ethical theory. *J Med Philos* 1998; **23**: 210–24.

Veatch RM. Indifference of subjects: an alternative to equipoise in randomized clinical trials. *Social Philosophy & Policy* 2002; **19**(2): 295–323.

Veatch RM. *The Basics of Bioethics*, 2nd edition. Upper Saddle River, NJ: Prentice-Hall, 2003; pp. 55–7.

7

Casuistical Reasoning In Medical Ethics

ALBERT R. JONSEN

The field of bioethics was created when philosophers and theologians began to notice the troubling questions that physicians and scientists were asking themselves about the effects of emerging technology on the moral dimensions of their work. In the decades after World War II, medical science leaped ahead and medical practice changed dramatically. A cascade of new drugs wiped out ancient diseases and supported patients through chronic diseases that were once fatal. Technological devices such as pacemakers and ventilators sustained failing organs and transplantation replaced them. Diagnostic tests revealed many conditions in time for treatment or beyond treatment. Even the secrets of reproduction were opened to manipulation. Scientists in the laboratory provided physicians in the clinic a panoply of possibilities that had never been within their range. The media rang with announcements of medical miracles from heart transplant to *in vitro* fertilization.

By the 1960s, these new methods, miraculous as they were, began to show their problematic side. Critical moments of illness, once surely fatal, could be overcome but with what promise for the future? Chronic diseases could be managed, but their deteriorating effect on the body continued. A transplanted kidney or heart was a gift of hope that often failed. Scientists and practitioners who saw these effects were forced to ask whether the benefits of the new medicine were worth the costs, pain and disappointment. Of course, this question made little sense if asked in general: saving life and restoring health are goods to be desired and fostered. But if asked about particular cases, where benefits and costs could be assessed in the circumstances, it was open to answers.

In the late 1960s, persons trained in the disciplines of moral philosophy and moral theology began to participate in the conversation with health professionals, scientists

and legal scholars about moral questions in medicine and science. Philosophers and theologians traditionally reflect on general problems, abstract issues, theoretical formulations and logical reasoning. Indeed, the early discussions in the biomedical world were at the level of generalization: should we proceed with genetic engineering? Should heart transplants be done? Should patients be allowed to die by 'pulling the plug'? However, clinicians are not accustomed to such generalized discussions: they focus on cases. So the philosophers and theologians who entered the conversation with doctors and scientists quickly learnt that in medical care the moral questions are stimulated by cases, particular instances in which actual persons are being treated in specific ways in definite circumstances. These novice bioethicists might have recalled the words of Aristotle, 'agents are compelled at every step to think out for themselves what the circumstances demand, just as happens in the arts of medicine and navigation. Prudence is not concerned with universals only; it must also take cognisance of particulars...because it is concerned with conduct, and conduct has its sphere in particular circumstances' (Aristotle, 1976).

This intense concentration on the particulars of medical cases presented a problem for those trained in moral philosophy. That discipline had, for many years, cultivated an approach to ethics that turned away from cases and towards theory. One of the seminal books in English modern moral philosophy, G. E. Moore's *Principia Ethica* (1903), opened with the assertion that there is 'a study different from Ethics and one much less respectable, the study of Casuistry... (although Ethics cannot be complete without it)'. He goes on, 'The defects of Casuistry are not defects of principle; no objection can be taken to its aim and object. It has failed because... the casuist had been unable to distinguish, in the cases which he treats, those elements upon which their value

Principles of Health Care Ethics, Second Edition   Edited by R.E. Ashcroft, A. Dawson, H. Draper and J.R. McMillan
© 2007 John Wiley & Sons, Ltd

depends'. Moore's predecessors in Continental and British moral philosophy had, since the late Renaissance and Enlightenment, reflected on the psychological and logical foundations of moral reasoning and constructed theories to ground morality in rationality. After Moore, most moral philosophers in the English tradition and those affected by the Vienna Circle turned their attention to the meaning of the vocabulary of moral discourse: what did words such as 'right' and 'good' mean, since they do not appear to refer to the objects of empirical perception. Casuistry, a 'less respectable branch of moral philosophy' in Moore's words, was hardly noticed. Philosophers neither analysed cases nor did they reflect, in anything but a cursory way, on the theoretical conditions under which universal principles could be brought to bear on particular circumstances (Moore, 1998).

In one corner of the scholarly world of ethics, a tradition of case analysis had survived. Roman Catholic moral theology had developed Casuistry, called 'Cases of Conscience', to a high art in the 17th century and, although that art had been severely ridiculed and had eventually deteriorated into a tired and rather shabby technique, it retained an important place. That place was guaranteed by the Roman Catholic practice of private confession of sins to a priest for absolution. Priests were required to judge the seriousness of sins confessed and impose proportionate penance. Thus, the exact circumstances of an action, the relevance of excuses and the persuasiveness of justifications entered into their judgement. Thus, casuistry remained an integral part of Roman Catholic (and Anglican) moral theology. It also remained vigorous within Orthodox Judaism.

Some scholars, familiar with historical casuistry (and often disdainful of the debilitated casuistry of latter day moral theology), became active participants in the conversation about medical ethics. Recognizing the interest in medical cases as an analogue to their own concern about judgement in particular moral cases, they saw possibilities for a contribution to the methodology of the new medical ethics. In 1988, Stephen Toulmin and I published a study of historical casuistry, suggesting that its methods could be rehabilitated and re-invigorated for use in modern ethical discourse. 'Casuistry', once a word of ridicule in common discourse, began to regain its righteous place as a method of moral reasoning in the Aristotelian tradition. Toulmin and I attempted to revive Casuistry by revealing its method or its underlying form of reasoning. It was our intention in *The Abuse of Casuistry* to revise the classical casuistical methodology for use in contemporary moral argumentation.

Casuistry always begins with a case. What is a case? The English word, 'case', has two distinct meanings. It means 'the instance of a thing occurring, an actual state of affairs'. A totally different meaning is 'that which encloses or contains something, as box, bookcase, briefcase'. The first meaning derives from the Latin, *casus*, an event,

from *cadere*, to happen; the second derives from the Latin, *capsa*, from *capere*, to hold, which comes into the Romance languages as '*cassa*'. These are very different meanings and derivations, yet for the purpose of explaining 'case method' they are illuminating. The most colloquial use of the first meaning, for example, 'well, it was the case that...' is made into technical jargon in medicine and in law, for example, 'this is a case of pneumonia', or 'this is a case of treason', meaning this is a particular instance of the general condition called pneumonia or the crime called treason. This use of jargon can remind us of the second meaning of 'case'. A complex human event, filled with behaviours, beliefs, motivations, emotions, must be enclosed or 'boxed'. Its components that are so tumbled together in life are sorted out into compartments so that they can be seen more distinctly.

It is important, at the beginning of a discussion of casuistry, to distinguish two rather distinct ways of being a casuist. The first way is the way of metaethical casuistry. Some scholars maintain that cases are the sum and substance of ethics. All ethical principles are abstracted from cases; ethical theory is, in some fashion, derived from them. Any ethical property merely reflects multitudes of cases. A second way of casuistry is practical casuistry. The practical casuist does not make metaethical claims about the primacy of cases. Principles and theories stand on their own rational grounds. However, the practical casuist maintains that, when decisions and actions are under consideration, principles and theories must be seen in the light of the circumstances in which those decisions and actions are undertaken. Some might say that principles and theories are 'applied', suggesting that these elements of ethics have sufficient substance and clarity that, when imposed on a case, a solution appears. Others prefer to say that principles and theories are 'interpreted' in the setting of the case. The present author has been accused of being a metaethical casuist: he thinks of himself as a practical casuist: he also thinks that his practice of casuistry interprets principles and theory rather than applies them to the case. In the rest of this essay, he will suggest how this interpretation is performed.

FIRST STEP IN CASUISTICAL REASONING: DETERMINATION OF TOPICS

This sorting out or boxing is, in part, what the classical rhetoricians called the elucidation of topics. A topic (*topos* in Greek means 'place') designates a standard 'place in the mind' which stores certain common and invariant lines of reasoning, either about some general feature of existence such as causality, proportion, sequence or about some particular form of existence, such as the human institutions of marriage, education, warfare, administration of justice and so forth. The classical rhetoricians suggested that, whenever, for instance, one was making an argument about causality, one would have to refer to the contiguity of cause and effect, the temporal priority of one over the other, the sufficient and necessary relationship of both. This form of argument penetrated all cases in which causality was in question. The special topics designate those features that define certain forms of human life and activity. Marriage, for example, (in its traditional form) will consist of two persons of opposite gender, joined by agreement or contract in a lasting union involving co-habitation and mutual sexual activity for the procreation and education of children. Arguments about the advisability and value of marriage and about responsibilities within it will dwell within this general pattern; arguments against traditional marriage must contest the same set of topics. The point of the ancient rhetorician-casuists in proposing the relevance of topics is to place the particular and variable circumstances of any instance of marriage, or warfare, or any other human activity, within a general framework that distinguishes that activity from others. This situates or places the argument so that particular assertions can be associated with familiar features, and persons can be helped to appreciate the issues that are at stake.

In my book, *Clinical Ethics,* I and my colleagues, Drs Mark Siegler and William Winslade, suggest that the complex practice of providing medical care to a patient can be seen to consist of at least four morally relevant topics. These are the 'boxes' into which all particular cases of clinical care can be sorted. The first topic is about medical indications, the physical signs and symptoms that suggest to persons that they seek the aid of health professionals, and that health professionals recognize as reasons to respond to requests and as starting points for employment of their skills of diagnosis and therapy. The second topic is about patient preferences, the perceptions, assessments and choices that lead people to seek help, direct its progress and seek its results. The third topic is about the qualify of life, the physical, intellectual, affective and social states that persons wish to attain by means of health interventions and the objective ability of those interventions to contribute to such states. The fourth topic is about contextual features, the social, organizational, administrative, financial and legal structures within which health interventions take place and which enhance or limit their efficacy. Any particular instance of the medical relationship takes place within these four topics: every case has these four dimensions.

Take a particular case: a man who is bleeding severely is brought to an emergency department . The doctors and nurses recognize that he needs a blood transfusion. He refuses to be transfused, saying he is a follower of the Jehovah's Witness faith, which considers transfusion a sin. What should the doctors and nurses do? 'Bleeding' and 'needs a transfusion' are medical indications. 'Says he is Jehovah's Witness and refuses the transfusion' are patient preferences. The providers know the patient's quality of life will be nil, as he will be dead; the patient believes his qualify of life will be in the splendour of salvation, if he dies faithful to God's command. The fact that the patient is father of several young children, the mission of the hospital and its emergency department, the extant law, the possibility for malpractice claims, the distress of the hospital staff, the doctrine of the Jehovah's Witness faith and the rallying of the local congregation to support their brother are contextual features (Jonsen et al., 1998). This is, then, a 'case of refusal of medical care'.

Although it is easy to recognize it as such, it is not easy to analyse the particular case at hand. A general philosophical response to the case might be, 'The principle of respect for autonomy dictates that the patient's refusal be respected' and the philosopher might go on to provide strong arguments to justify the principle of respect for autonomy. On the contrary, another might say, 'The medical maxim, "do no harm" requires that the transfusion be given, regardless of the patient's objection'. However, those faced with the question, 'what shall I do' (which includes the patient, his family and fellow believers, as well as the doctors, nurses, administrators and legal counsel) cannot be satisfied with these responses. It is generally accepted, in ethics and in law, that competent patients may refuse medical care, but in this case, can that general principle be implemented?

This question can be answered only when we examine in detail the actual features of this case. We need quite specific information about this patient's medical condition, its causes, his past medical history, and his physical and psychological status at admission. We need to know just how urgent is the need for transfusion and whether there are alternatives. We have to be better informed about his personal beliefs and the tenets of his faith, as well as about the relevant policies and legal provisions that might apply. In other words, each of the four topics must be filled with information specific to this case. When this is done, it might be seen that, given the blood loss, the need for blood transfusion is not urgent or, conversely, that even a transfusion might be useless. We might learn that he himself is not expressing this preference but someone who brings him or that he expresses it only vaguely in his confusion. We might find that, although we believed that he would be expelled from his congregation if we administered blood against his will, he would, however, be received with love as one who had been wronged. We might be astonished to learn from legal counsel that the hospital policy and the state law acknowledge the right of Jehovah's Witnesses to refuse transfusions even at risk to life. These particular features of this specific case are crucially important: they allow us to move towards an ethical resolution. Thus, the first act of casuistical reasoning is to determine the topics of relevance to the general enterprise within which the case arises and then to sort out the details of the specific case into the appropriate topics. In summary, topics are, to use a term from computer sciences, a platform on which to build an application, namely, the analysis of the specific circumstances of the case.

THE SECOND ACT OF CASUISTICAL REASONING: INTERPRETATION OF PRINCIPLES AND MAXIMS

Specific cases are, in reality, always a riot of detail and it is the details that attract attention. Casuistical reasoning begins by sorting those details in an orderly way. The development of topics is the method for doing such sorting. However, the conjunction of the topics and the factual details reveals not merely an empirical state of affairs, but begins, as well, to disclose the moral dimensions of the case. Human practices have embedded in them a host of normative features that say not only how persons engaged in that practice do behave but also how they ought to behave. Morality is not in itself an institution or practice; it is a particular way of acting within a variety of institutions and practices, and the particular way is dictated by what are generally called moral principles, rules, norms or values.

Almost as soon as bioethics appeared, its scholars attempted to articulate principles that would serve to guide moral thinking through the complexity of new problems and cases. The National Commission for Protection of Human Subjects of Biomedical and Behavioral Research was mandated by the US Congress 'to conduct a comprehensive investigation and study to identify the basic ethical principles that should underlie the conduct of biomedical and behavioural research involving human subjects' (National Research Act, 1974). Philosopher Tom Beauchamp and theologian James Childress produced a book that has given theoretical shape to the field of bioethics; they entitled it *The Principles of Biomedical Ethics* (Beauchamp and Childress, 1979). They identified the principles as respect for autonomy, beneficence, nonmaleficence and justice. The term 'principle' has always been part of the English vernacular of ethics. However, despite its common use, its meaning has neither been consistent nor clear. Since the 18th century, authors used it to refer to a variety of elements of ethics: the foundation for moral sentiment, the work of reason, virtues, motives and norms. It is now common for ethicists to simply identify it, as do Beauchamp and Childress, as an 'action guide'. Apart from this variety of usage, serious metaethical problems surround the notion of principle: in what sense is a principle obligatory, not merely action guiding but action obliging? How do principles and exceptions fit? Can there be a true conflict of moral principles? These myriad questions about the existence, nature and function of principles have not deterred bioethicists from 'identifying' those that seem

most appropriate to bioethics and employing them to illuminate and elucidate problems. The first edition of this volume, edited by Raanan Gillon, was an impressive example of this adoption of a principled approach to bioethical questions (Gillon, 1994).

The word 'principle' was well known to the classical rhetorician-casuists. Thomas Aquinas had opened his treatise on ethics by stating that the *prima et communissima principia* of the natural law were self-preservation, preservation of the species and preservation of social life (Aquinas). However, the casuists rarely use the term. Rather, they prefer to use a word no longer found in ethical writing, namely, 'maxims'. These were the '*maxima sententia*' or 'significant opinions' that expressed in pithy ways the standards of behaviour that any rational person who understood the practice would see as obligatory or prudently wise. Maxims served as the fulcrum of any persuasive argument. They were statements that the hearers would acknowledge at face value, needing no proof in themselves but giving the colour of truth to the conclusions drawn about the case. Maxims fit the work of casuistry because they come from common discourse about moral matters rather than from abstract theorizing. They are, almost in their very formulation, open to exceptions, contrasts and comparisons. Yet, like principles, they have the ring of truth to them.

There are multitudes of moral maxims, invoked in all sorts of cases. Some maxims are framed as common sense advice, such as 'honesty is the best policy' or 'the truth will out'. Other maxims take a more lofty tone, such as 'truthfulness is the essential ingredient in trust' or 'thou shalt not bear false witness'. Moral arguments pivot on these maxims. Thus, someone might say, 'The President was wrong to deceive the American people, because he forfeits their trust: after all, truth is the essential ingredient in trust'. The argument may then go on to show that trust is the basis for political authority and effectiveness, using other maxims to make that point. Maxims go by very fast in moral discourse, since it is seldom necessary to stop and demonstrate, explain or justify the maxims invoked. However, maxims themselves might be challenged, and then the argument moves to another plane where the relatively unreflective maxims must be transmuted into principles.

Principles are stated in a more general fashion, as 'universal', and are related to more general theories of moral justification. Contemporary moral philosophy has concentrated intently on the problem of giving theoretical explanations for the origin and certainty of moral principles. So much intellectual effort was expended on this search that the more humble maxims of classical rhetoric-casuistry have been forgotten. Instead of the multitude of maxims that inhabit common moral discourse, modern moral philosophy attempts to identify one or several very general principles that encompass a wide swath of moral issues. Modern bioethics, for example, commonly refers to four fundamental principles, respect for autonomy, nonmaleficence, beneficence and justice. The challenge to moral discourse consists in relating the very specific details of particular cases to the sweeping range of an abstractly defined moral principle. How does the principle of autonomy resolve the case of this Jehovah's Witness believer arriving at this clinic at this time? It should be clear that, in addition to the principle of autonomy, many other moral maxims are at play in the case – how can this patient be helped and not harmed? Are we somehow bound by a belief that we do not understand and share? Is it right to let a person die because of a belief that is not rationally justifiable? Is it right to allow this person, who is the father of a family, to leave his wife and children fatherless? Would it not be better to force a transfusion on him and let him be welcomed back to family and congregation not as a sinner but as one whom we have sinned against? These and other maxims provide the moral ambiance of the case. Still, how do we find the route to travel between these moral maxims and the facts of the case, so that we might arrive at a resolution useful to those who must make a decision?

At the most abstract level, two principles, beneficence and respect for autonomy, strive for attention in the case of the Jehovah's Witness believer. These principles are apparently conflicting. As the factual details of the case emerge, however, these abstract principles begin to take on (or lose) importance. If the details show that the patient had in fact reached critically low haemoglobin levels to sustain organic perfusion and life and also reveal that he is a truly committed believer and is (or was at the moment of admission to the hospital) clear and competent in expressing his beliefs, the two competing principles remain in balance. This patient can be benefited by transfusion; he competently rejects transfusion. However, as more detail about the nature of his beliefs and the doctrines of his church appear and as possible medical alternatives are considered, weight may begin to shift. Without pursuing the case in detail, the accumulation of details may finally weigh down the principle of autonomy to the point where its importance becomes manifest: it may become clear that the beneficence that sustains organic life by blood transfusion is not, for this patient, a benefit. It will give him not the gift of life but a burden of guilt, perhaps not even his own but, in his belief, a sin he has occasioned for others. Even his continued fatherly presence may be less a benefit than an example of infidelity to divine commands. The abstract principles of beneficence and autonomy take on their respective weight as the factual details relative to the topics and maxims are filled out and amplified. This is the second essential act of casuistical reasoning.

However, even though circumstances exert a powerful pull on the abstract principles, the casuist must appreciate that principles and maxims, abstract though they may be, carry some weight in themselves. Failure to appreciate the weight of principles allows good casuistry to collapse into situationism: the ethical doctrine that circumstances alone determine the moral quality of decision and action (Jonsen, 1993). A proper philosophical consideration of the source, meaning and importance of principles of morality is a necessary prelude to Casuistry. Unfortunately, the scope of this chapter makes such an examination impossible.

THE THIRD STEP IN CASUISTICAL REASONING: ARGUMENT BY ANALOGY

A final step in casuistical reasoning must be noted. Where does the casuist find the grounds for testing his conclusions in the particular case? The casuist seeks those grounds in other cases. The conclusions in a contested case are compared to conclusions in similar cases in which the relation between principles, maxims and the circumstances suggest an obvious resolution. The casuist reflects on the similarities and differences between the contested case and the uncontested cases – similarities and differences that are manifested in the actual circumstances of each case. In the uncontested case, the maxim and the circumstances are such that no other maxim has the weight to challenge or to uphold an exception to the rule. The casuist notes, 'this case is very like or somewhat like, the previous case of X', and then asks what it is about the instant case that might call for a different judgement than did the prior case. For example, the maxim that parents should determine what is best for their children is, in the usual circumstances of familial life, an uncontested maxim, even though many parents may make ill-considered judgements. However, given the circumstance that the parents are devoted believers in a sect that forbids medical care for children, another maxim, the protection of a vulnerable human being, grows strong enough to challenge the first maxim. Cases can then be lined up in which the uncontested case stands as a paradigm and other cases stand at various distant removes: at the first remove, the parents' faith does not forbid medical care but rather recommends that prayer be the first recourse; at the second remove the belief forbids all but emergency treatment; at the third remove, it forbids all medical attention without exception. At each remove, the danger to the child increases and the moral challenge to parental authority grows stronger. This simple example (which in reality might be very complex) shows how the circumstances change the case, modify the moral judgement about it and justify different practical responses to it. The contested case is an analogy, a similar yet relevantly different instance in a series of cases in which the paradigm case is the most clear and compelling.

The casuist needs a relatively clear test of right and wrong. These are found in cases rather than in principles or theories. The judgement in one case, with its pattern of circumstances and maxims, is clearly and incontestably right and so becomes the paradigm against which other similar cases, with diverging patterns of circumstances and maxims, can be tested. In classical casuistry, for example, a 'just war' was a military action that was launched after timely declaration, justified by a clearly just reason, carried out with due proportion between aggression and the goal and providing for protection of innocent noncombatants. The just war casuists were not so foolish as to believe that such a war had ever been fought or would be ever fought. Rather, they were proposing maxims that conscientious rulers or generals could attempt to realize in the circumstances of their political and military manoeuvring. These maxims found their way into international rules of war and, while certainly never perfectly realized, went far to keep warfare within humane limits. Certain actual wars attain paradigmatic status in some respects: the Allies fought World War II for a just cause, the obliteration of Nazi aggression. In other respects, clear departures from the paradigm can be properly condemned: saturation bombing by the Allies in World War II violated the maxim of noncombatant immunity.

These are central activities of casuistry: the designation of topics, the interpretation of maxims and principles in the light of circumstances and the use of analogical reasoning...They are open to abuse as the description of topics, the choice of appropriate analogies and the description of circumstances may be subjective and coloured by cultural bias. The casuist may check his subjectivity by placing himself within the long conversation of his casuistic colleagues, but only up to the point where he must choose the appropriate analogy and weigh the current circumstances. Here the 'prudence' or 'practical wisdom' of the casuist, his ability to consider fairly and comprehensively the circumstances of this case, in the light of relevant principles, becomes central. It is a virtue or talent of the experienced casuist. Casuistry, then, is both conservative and creative: It places cases within a tradition and then moves the tradition ahead by the decision in the present case. The primary check on unfettered ingenuity now becomes the response of the contemporary casuistic community and the broader community to the new resolution of the new case. That response is usually not slow in coming, if the case is a notable one that addresses a current and widely felt moral problem. In Roman Catholicism, the response of the casuistic community is supplemented by hierarchical authority, which is granted the right to determine doctrinal truth about morality and may, on occasion, contradict the consensus of casuists. In Judaism and in Islam, respected scholars and scholarly councils are sometimes granted a similar but far less absolute authority in matters of morality and religious law. In the secular world of bioethics, a vigorous community of casuists has come into existence (many bioethicists would repudiate the title but utilize the technique). They are ready to argue through the topics, maxims and principle and analogies and give critical support to the proposed resolutions of cases. It is this modern Casuistry that allows persons faced with critical decisions in the care of patients to reach reasonable, if not final solutions and to move ahead with the confidence that they have given full, reasonable consideration to the ethical aspects of the case. Casuistry is, then, not moral philosophy as such but is, as G.E. Moore suggested, necessary to moral philosophy as it approaches real decisions and actions.

REFERENCES

Aquinas. *Summa Theologiae* I–II, 94.2.

Aristotle. *The Ethics of Aristotle.* Thomson JAK, Tredennick H, eds and trans. London: Penguin Books, 1976; II, ii, 1104; vi, vii, 1141, pp. 93, 213.

Beauchamp T, Childress J. *Principles of Biomedical Ethics.* New York: Oxford University Press, 1979.

Gillon R, *Principles of Health Care Ethics.* Chicester, UK: John Wiley & Sons, 1994.

Jonsen AR, Siegler M, Winslade W. *Clinical Ethics.* New York: McGraw-Hill, 1998; pp. 1–12, 74–6.

Jonsen AR. Casuistry, situationism and laxity. In: Vaux K, ed. *Joseph Fletcher: Memoir of an Ex-Radical. Reminiscence and Reappraisal.* Louisville, KY: John Knox Press, 1993.

Moore GE. *Principia Ethica.* Cambridge: Cambridge University Press, 1903; pp. 4–5. For a more detailed and referenced history of philosophy's turn from cases to theory, see Jonsen AR. *The Birth of Bioethics.* New York: Oxford University Press, 1998; Chapter 3.

NATIONAL RESEARCH ACT 1974, Public Law 93–348.

8

Utilitarianism and Bioethics

MATTI HÄYRY

INTRODUCTION

Three notable approaches to philosophical bioethics are based on the three main normative theories in European moral thinking. These are the Aristotelian view, which stresses the role of social relationships and good character traits; the Kantian teaching, which emphasizes respect for human beings as rational agents with duties and rights; and the utilitarian doctrine, which focuses on happiness, well-being, and the material outcomes of our actions.

This chapter outlines utilitarianism as a moral theory, describes some of its applications to bioethics and explores the objections that can be raised against the theory and its applications. I will first portray what the basic elements of any type of utilitarianism are and then go on to list the main variations to these central themes. I will then review the possible and actual uses of the theory in medical and health care settings and conclude by taking stock of the criticisms that have been levelled at the most prevalent version of the view both by ethicists from other camps and by utilitarians themselves.

THE BASIC ELEMENTS OF UTILITARIANISM

Utilitarianism comes in many forms, but most of them lay weight on *consequences* rather than rules or character traits, place the concepts of *good and bad* before the ideas of right and wrong, advocate *impartiality* instead of any kind of favouritism and concentrate on the *maximization* of quantitative factors sooner than engage in analyses of qualitative distinctions (Häyry, 1994).

The starting point of the theory is that our actions, inactions, choices and policies (hereinafter 'actions' for short)

have consequences for ourselves and for other entities. According to this view, all these can matter morally, but nothing else can. Actions can be described as vicious, or they can be said to violate rights, but if they have no adverse outcomes, utilitarians standardly refuse to condemn them. This means that when we want to know what the moral status of actions is, we must study their consequences to the exclusion of everything else.

Consequences matter morally insofar as they are or promote 'good' or 'bad' – categories that are defined either explicitly or implicitly, by every utilitarian theory. Outcomes that *are* good or bad tend to make actions *intrinsically* right or wrong, outcomes that *promote* good or bad tend to make them *instrumentally* right or wrong. In the end, there is no rigid distinction between the two because all the effects of what we do, or fail to do, should be a part of the analysis.

In the assessment of the goodness and badness of consequences, all entities that matter in the moral sense must be taken equally and impartially into account. Consequences to entities that do not matter, on the other hand, are not directly considered. Because the good or bad that befalls them can have an impact on entities that do matter, they can form an indirect part of the calculations.

Maximization normally lies at the core of utilitarian ethics. The better the consequences cumulatively are, the more morally valuable the actions are. Good net outcomes are better than bad, very good net outcomes are superior to the not-so-good and the lesser of two evils is to be preferred. Action alternatives with the best consequences are right and we should perform (any) one of them. An action alternative which alone has the indisputably best consequences is our moral duty and we ought to perform it (Moore, 1912).

A statistically probable form of utilitarianism could state the following. The moral rightness of our actions depends

Principles of Health Care Ethics, Second Edition   Edited by R.E. Ashcroft, A. Dawson, H. Draper and J.R. McMillan
© 2007 John Wiley & Sons, Ltd

ultimately on the goodness of their consequences, not on their conformity to rules or on their being virtuous. Physical health and psychological well being are good, whereas illness and suffering are bad. All and only beings that are capable of well-being and suffering are to be taken equally into account. Their well-being should be maximized and their illness and suffering should be minimized.

Actual forms of utilitarianism vary according to what sorts of consequences are accounted for, what is considered to be good or bad, what the range of impartiality is and what is maximized and how.

VARIETIES OF UTILITARIANISM

TYPES OF CONSEQUENCES

The consequences accounted for in utilitarian theories can be *actual*, *probable*, *possible* or *morally expected*.

Actual consequences are the states of affairs that eventually come about as a result of our actions. It is impossible for us to know what all these are because every little thing that we do changes in subtle ways the rest of world history. What we do has an effect on what we and other people do in the future, and in the end the stroke of the butterfly's wing in England can become a factor in the outbreak of a tropical storm in Brazil. This is why a distinction must be drawn in this model between a 'criterion of morality' and 'action-guiding principles'. The former, in this case the actual consequences of our activities, tells us what the right action was, but only when history has come to its end. Any discussion of the ultimate morality of our behaviour needs to involve a fictional judge, who by definition knows everything that goes on in the world (Hare, 1981). As we are not such omniscient observers, we need to figure out what to do on other grounds, for instance, by acting according to some specified set of rules of thumb or by considering the most probable outcomes of what we do.

Probable consequences are the states of affairs that are most likely to come about as a result of our actions. Here the criterion of morality is the same as the best action-guiding principle. As we almost always know more about the immediate impact of our choices than about the ensuing future events, it is natural that temporal proximity will direct our choices to some degree, although no theoretical priority needs to be given to the most instant prospects. More remote outcomes will, of necessity, be assessed in the light of our personal or cultural expectations and attitudes – with optimism or pessimism and with or without taking risks.

Possible consequences are the states of affairs that *can* come about as a consequence of our actions. Strong pessimism or optimism and extreme risk-aversion or risk-taking can lead to the choice of this option. Taken to its limit, however, this line ceases to be a form of utilitarianism – decisions will be based purely on precaution or hope (Häyry, 2005). With extremely bad or good consequences these considerations may serve as an auxiliary decision-making principle.

Morally expected consequences are the states of affairs that come about only if everybody acts in a prescribed manner. A focus on them makes more sense in policy decisions, in the context of which sanctions can be installed, than elsewhere. It requires in many cases a prior value judgement which has no utilitarian justification. For instance, both restrictive and liberal sex education in schools could, in principle, work if only adolescents followed them.

DEFINITIONS OF GOOD AND BAD

Good and bad can in utilitarian theories be defined in terms of *pleasure and pain* (or otherwise 'naturally'), *ideal elements of a good life* ('intuitively'), *nonfanatical preferences* or *rational desires* and *interests*, *well-being* or *needs* ('objectively').

Jeremy Bentham (1789), the founder of classical utilitarianism, defined good and bad as pleasure and pain and contended that qualitative differences among them are not morally significant. The joy a person gets by playing a children's game is as important as the elevation another person achieves by reading poetry. Pleasure and pain are in Bentham's model subjectively felt yet objective and commensurable entities. John Stuart Mill (1861), Bentham's follower, argued in his turn that 'higher' pleasures should be given more weight in the utility calculations than 'lower' ones. According to him, these more advanced enjoyments involve complex mental functions and would be preferred by a person who has experienced both.

G. E. Moore (1903) criticized all theories of value which equate 'the good' with natural properties. He rejected those forms of utilitarianism which commit the 'naturalistic fallacy'. By this he meant views which claim that the word 'good' simply means, say, 'pleasure'. Everything that is good can, he said, give us pleasure, but the questions 'Is this pleasurable?' and 'Is this good?' still refer to different categories in our minds. Moore's own intuition was that the best things in life have to do with aesthetic enjoyment and social experiences like art and friendship. Longer lists of similar ideal goods have been presented by others, although the comparison of vastly diverse values is difficult when we try to calculate which action alternatives have the best consequences.

R. M. Hare (1981) advocated a model in which the good is defined as that which a person prefers. Because people sometimes seem to prefer immoral things (such as racism), preferences which are 'fanatical' are excluded from this model. Hare argued that people can think in seriously dangerous ways only if their attitudes or stupidity prevent them from grasping what morality is actually about. This is why fanatical preferences can be excluded as erroneous. R. B. Brandt (1979) promoted a similar idea by defining 'good' as the satisfaction of rational desires. These are desires that survive a scrutiny he called 'cognitive psychotherapy'. The basic idea is that if we think through the consequences of our actions to ourselves and others, we cannot rationally try to fulfil desires which have reckless or harmful connotations.

In theory, the good in utilitarianism can be defined in any nonmoral way. Objectively or intersubjectively determined interests, well-being, and needs are viable options. If they can be described well, they give a good basis for inter-personal comparisons (and sometimes even wider comparisons between persons and other beings). Unless a 'felt', subjective element is added, however, they can be criticized for ignoring individuals and their lives. Harsh forms of paternalism can ensue, if we conclude that other people are always better judges of our good than we ourselves are.

Good and bad cannot be defined in moral terms within utilitarianism. Since the goodness and badness of consequences are the only basis of morality, it would be circular to claim that morality is the basis of the goodness and badness of the consequences.

ENTITIES THAT MERIT IMPARTIAL CONSIDERATION

The entities accounted for impartially in utilitarian theories can be *people, sentient beings, living beings or species,* or *persons defined in nonmoral ways.*

In legal, policy and professional decision-making, the people to be taken into account can be citizens, patients or clients. Human beings as members of the species *Homo sapiens* are also an alternative, although this option has not been too popular lately. Yet another alternative would be to include all and only rational beings in the Enlightenment spirit which lies at the core of utilitarian thinking. And it would be possible to include all social, communicative or reciprocal beings.

The rational and social nature of beings has not often been favoured in this school of thought as the fundamental criterion of equal consideration. Sentience, or the ability to experience pleasure and pain, has been a more popular option, at least in principle. Bentham (1789) gave expression to this idea when he wrote: '[T]he question is not, Can they *reason*? nor, Can they *talk*? but, Can they *suffer*?' Sentience, taken seriously, extends the sphere of morality to many non-human animals. On the contrary, human beings who are not sentient such as embryos, early foetuses, and the irreversibly comatose are excluded. The meaning of 'impartial consideration' is, however, often unclear even if sentience is emphasized. Few utilitarian theorists have argued that pain in animals should be avoided with the same intensity as should pain in humans.

Theoretically speaking, the demand for impartiality could be extended to all living individuals. This could form the basis of an 'environmental utilitarianism', although this variation has never been fully developed. Even beyond individuals, the survival and well being of species or ecosystems could be considered – a line that was partly explored by Herbert Spencer (1879–93). An anthropocentric reading of this can easily lead to social Darwinism and to attempts to design the best possible human race.

Persons defined in nonmoral ways are currently the most prevalent contenders for utilitarian consideration. Individuals capable of directing their actions according to their own preferences or interests can fall within this category, although a set of rational faculties is usually required, too. Continued self-awareness as a subject of mental states seems to be a minimum requirement (Singer, 1979), and some call for an ability to value one's own life (Harris, 1985). Views based on nonmoral personhood sometimes struggle to explain how to treat future, potential, prospective, and currently dormant persons. These groups include unborn and newly born human beings, possible children people think about having, and individuals who are asleep, unconscious, or severely demented or intellectually disabled.

FORMS OF MAXIMIZATION

Maximization in utilitarianism can be understood in terms of *good consequences, bad consequences or both; acts or rules; mental states or individuals;* and *individuals or societies.*

One way to optimize the moral value of actions is to maximize their net good consequences. This 'positive' type of balancing is how maximization is in most cases understood in utilitarian thinking. An alternative would be to concentrate on the minimization of bad consequences like suffering. Practical decision-making often has this 'negative' element, because suffering has a certain urgency that we feel should be addressed. A theoretical difficulty for the latter route is that pain and discomfort could best be eliminated by the removal of all sentient beings, including the entire humanity, and ethicists usually shy away from this solution.

The traditional idea in utilitarianism is to assess the consequences of individual acts. But it has also been suggested that behaviour is good when it conforms to rules whose existence is thought to have the best consequences, regardless of the impact of the behaviour in and by itself. The 'rule' version may, strictly speaking, collapse either into the 'act' variant of the theory, or fail to be utilitarian at all (Lyons, 1965). A combination of the two ideas can be found in R. M. Hare's (1981) 'two-tier' view, in which we should normally act 'intuitively', that is, by the rules of thumb that prevail in our societies, but in difficult cases rise to a 'critical' level where the consequences of individual acts are made the ultimate standard of morality.

Bentham (1789) contended in his famous dictum that we should aim at 'the greatest happiness of the greatest number'. This can be interpreted as saying that people as such do not matter, only the pleasure and absence of pain 'in them' (Rawls, 1972). If individuals are seen as containers of good physical and mental states rather than separate individuals, many kinds of paradoxical situations can arise. One of these is described by Derek Parfit (1986) in his 'repugnant conclusion' argument, which shows that a miserable huge population would be, in utilitarian terms, better than a happy smaller one. This conclusion, and others like it, can probably be avoided by concentrating on individuals more than on happiness, but the utilitarian character of the ensuing view can become problematic in the process (Häyry, 1994).

As pleasure and pain are only felt by individuals, utilitarians often lean, in practice, towards liberal democracy. It is possible, in theory, to conceive of a strictly paternalistic society based on the theory (Stephen, 1873), and if straightforward maximization is taken seriously, it cannot matter how the greatest aggregate well-being is achieved. Some of the most renowned utilitarians have argued, however, that the demands of human nature make individual liberty crucial for the promotion of the greatest happiness (Mill, 1859).

BIOUTILITARIANISM

UTILITARIANISM IN HEALTH CARE ETHICS

Some elements of utilitarianism are taken for granted in today's health policies and medical ethics. Health and well-being are promoted, illness and suffering are removed, risks of harm are eliminated and reduced, and people are treated, in theory at least, without undue favouritism. But views on utilitarianism are not necessarily associated with these elements of health policy and medical ethics. They are linked with a specific form of the creed which has attracted the epithet 'bioutilitarian' (Silvers, 2000).

Health policies in most affluent societies reflect the ideal of the greatest happiness of the greatest number. Publicly financed health services promote the impartial maximization of well-being. Public health activities aim to decrease morbidity and mortality in entire populations. Quality-of-life assessments define values which can then be promoted in clinical and policy practice. And health economists make their calculations with an eye on efficiency – the optimization of good over bad.

Medical ethics in liberal political environments echoes utilitarian credos on freedom and democracy. Patients can in many parts of the world refuse treatments that they see as useless. Lifestyle choices are in most cases left to individuals unless harm to others ensues. Reproductive choices are respected on the grounds that restrictions would be detrimental to people's well-being. Bioscientific research is by and large allowed, provided that consent procedures are in place and the safety of the researchers and the general public are secured. Other liberal theories can make similar claims to these ideals, but they are in no way alien to the basic tenets of utilitarianism, either.

The main current perception of the theory is, however, centred on 'bioutilitarianism', which is one of the main Anglo-Australian branches of philosophical bioethics. The main originators and advocates of this view have included R. M. Hare (1975), Jonathan Glover (1977), Peter Singer (1979), John Harris (1985) and Julian Savulescu (2001).

SOME BIOUTILITARIAN VIEWS

In the early 1990s, 'bioethics' was widely considered synonymous with utilitarian medical ethics, and the whole discipline was criticized for the controversial views presented mainly by Singer and Harris.

Singer's contributions include views on our treatment of seriously ill babies (Kuhse and Singer, 1985) and on our use of animals in research and food production (Singer, 1975). According to him, the lives of newborn infants may be actively taken when their existence would otherwise be short and miserable due to their health condition. He has also argued that the birth of children with disabilities may be prevented by terminations of pregnancy, especially if they are replaced by nondisabled ones. And he has contended that 'higher' non-human animals like chimpanzees, gorillas and orang-utans should not be used as experimental subjects in situations in which we feel that the use of intellectually disabled humans would be inappropriate.

The views held by Harris (1985; 1998) on the lives of unborn and newly born human beings are similar to those nurtured by Singer. In addition, he has presented some striking ideas about resource allocation, organ retention and bioscientific research. One of his arguments is that it would be rational and hence morally right to take the lives of innocent people and use their vital organs for transplantation on those who need them to survive (Harris, 1975; 1980). More recently, he has argued that it would be right to buy vital organs from willing individuals and to sell them to those who need them (Erin and Harris, 2003). He also advocates the view that we have a shared duty to conduct bioscientific research, to allow it and to act as experimental subjects in trials that advance science and technology (Harris, 2005).

Savulescu has during recent years confirmed his position as the most unswerving acolyte of the bioutilitarian cause as pioneered by Singer and Harris. In a widely commented article (Savulescu, 2001), he argues that *in vitro* fertilization, prenatal genetic diagnosis and embryo selection should be employed to produce the best children possible, both in terms of health and in terms of non-health-related traits and qualities, including intelligence. A keen champion of biomedical research, he has also maintained (Savulescu, 2002) that far from being contrary to human dignity, as some have claimed, human embryonic stem cell research, properly understood, is one of the best ways to respect and to promote it.

WHITHER BIOUTILITARIANISM?

Although bioutilitarian views form, by and large, a unified whole and have remained basically the same during the last three decades, the theoretical emphasis of the doctrine seems to be shifting, and in some cases oscillating, between *immediate* and *morally expected* consequences; *actual* and *rational* preference satisfaction; *sentient beings* and *persons*; and the *reduction of individual suffering* and the *exclusion of individuals who could suffer*.

Singer's (1979) views on infanticide originally centred on alleviating and eliminating the pain and suffering of hopelessly ill newborns. This was a concrete consideration of the immediate consequences of the actions and inactions of medical professionals in neonatal units. Harris (1975; 1980) in his 'survival lottery' organ retention model studied the impact of a rational and, to him, morally sensible system. This is a more theoretical construction which gives much less weight to the instant consequences of implementing the suggested plan. Harris and Savulescu's current advocacy of advanced bioscience, in its turn, is based on an optimistic reading of the future. As all pessimistic and precautionary prospects are rejected as irrational, it seems that here a moral choice of how the world should be shaped precedes any genuine calculations of actual or expected utility.

There is a similar shift from simple, empirically observable pleasures and pains to more fictional, rational preference satisfaction. Suffering infants show distress, and so do primates experimented on and people dying of organ failure. Their inclinations and aversions can be deduced in a relatively straightforward manner. But when it comes to neonatal screening and abortions based on reduced physical and mental capacities, the situation is different. People with disabilities do not necessarily suffer in any way. To reach the bioutilitarian conclusions on their fate, their real-life experiences must be replaced by their 'rational preferences', which are construed by thought experiments on the kind of life that 'any reasonable person' would like to have (Harris, 2000). The thought experiment model has been extended to the fictional choices of future generations and embryos, as well (Harris, 2002; Savulescu, 2002).

Another shift, or perhaps fluctuation, in bioutilitarian premises occurs between sentient beings and persons as entities that matter morally. According to the applications of the theory, beings who are aware of their own continued existence and who can value it should be respected as 'persons'. These beings ought not to be killed against their wishes, although their lives may be ended at their own considered request. One oversight in these deliberations concerns the fact that late foetuses and terminal, unconscious patients can be sentient. Their suffering could be assessed by others, but normally this consideration does not enter the bioutilitarian evaluation. The lack of personhood seems to cancel out reflections on pain in the case of foetuses, and a person's prior request is usually seen to trump any further reflections in end-of-life decisions.

An interesting tension appears at the interface of the minimization of individual suffering and the exclusion of individuals whose lives would be less than perfect. Bioutilitarian arguments often evoke images of people who suffer and whose suffering should be eased by the isolated choices we make. In many cases, however, repeated and socially sanctioned choices form patterns, which can become coercive without anybody intending to make them so. Prenatal genetic screening for undesirable traits is quite possibly a case in point. Initially solitary decisions to exclude individuals with disabilities can surreptitiously become policies, and these can have social consequences which are mostly ignored in bioutilitarian argumentation.

BIOUTILITARIAN CONCLUSIONS AND PREMISES

Proponents of the bioutilitarian view condone many medical practices that are condemned or disapproved of by others. Among these are abortions wanted by the pregnant woman, even extremely late ones, because persons are not directly affected and because appeals to principles like the sanctity of life or the dignity of human beings can be ignored as irrational. All requests for voluntary euthanasia, the active killing of patients included, should be granted because competent persons should be assisted to die as they wish. Infanticide is acceptable, if the child's condition is hopeless or its quality of life would be very low, provided that this is what the parents wish and no one else can take custody. This is because persons are not killed, emotional arguments are inadmissible and references to the wrongness of murder are irrelevant in this context. Apart from permitting life taking in many traditional medical settings, bioutilitarians advocate technological advances which have been objected to on grounds of justice, equality and precaution. According to them, we should sanction regulated voluntary organ sales, because they respect everybody's autonomy and because the possible injustice surrounding the arrangement is not created by it. We should authorize genetic selection requested by parents, as this respects their liberty and no persons are harmed. Scientists ought to be allowed to conduct human embryonic stem cell research, as persons are not harmed and symbolic concerns are irrelevant. Human reproductive cloning can be condoned if issues of safety can be resolved. And all genuine medical and genetic enhancements of our offspring must be permitted, lest we produce future human beings who are not as healthy or intelligent as they could have been.

The views and normative conclusions presented so far make it possible to extrapolate some likely bioutilitarian tenets on consequences, values, impartiality and optimization. The moral rightness of our actions depends on the goodness of their immediate or morally expected, rather than their probable or possible, consequences. What rational or reasonable persons, as defined by bioutilitarians, prefer is good; what they disfavour is bad. All beings that are or will actually be capable of valuing their lives are to be equally accounted for and so can some other sentient beings be, but potential persons do not count as such. The rational preference satisfaction of present and future persons should be maximized, by technological means where feasible.

EXTERNAL CRITICISMS OF BIOUTILITARIANISM

PRACTICAL OBJECTIONS

External criticisms of bioutilitarianism (that is, objections launched by people who do not buy into its credos) are often based on practical moral disagreements, and their logic is simple. Late abortions, active euthanasia, infanticide, organ sales, genetic selection, and human embryonic stem cell research are wrong; the bioutilitarian doctrine condones them; therefore, the doctrine must be mistaken. Or, human reproductive cloning and all future genetic enhancement technologies would be wrong; bioutilitarians would condone some of these; therefore, they are wrong. The gist here is that certain popular intuitions concerning disputed practices can be used to establish the immorality of views that would allow them.

THEORETICAL OBJECTIONS

On a more theoretical level, bioutilitarians have been externally accused of going against the *sanctity* and *dignity* of human life; of promoting the *commodification* and *exploitation* of human beings and of using them as a *mere means*; of ignoring *social consequences*, *structural injustice* and the slide towards a *consumerist society*; and

of *missing the point* of morality by making analyses and calculations the core of moral considerations.

As for violations of sanctity and dignity, many theorists believe that human life has intrinsic value which makes it wrong to end lives actively. Some of them maintain that this worth is bestowed upon humans by God or Nature, while others argue that it is based on our standing as free and rational agents, or on our genetic constitution (Häyry, 2004a). If these theorists are right, bioutilitarians can be rightfully accused of advocating practices that go against humanity.

Some argue that organ sales, however carefully they are regulated, will inevitably turn human beings into commodities, and this is bound to reduce our mutual respect. As the poor would probably be inclined to sell and the rich to buy, exploitation and economic injustice would also be issues. An independent argument, or another way of formulating the same idea, is that in organ sales and other potentially demeaning activities people would be used as a mere means to the ends of others, which is deeply immoral (Green, 2001). If any of this is true, bioutilitarianism encourages wickedness by condoning organ sales and other commodifying practices.

Others have raised objections based on social consequences, structural injustice and impending consumerism (Levitt and Häyry, 2005). Bioutilitarians usually defend free individual choices on abortion, euthanasia, organ sales, genetic tests, medical treatments and other things related to health care and bioscience. One problem with this is that the choices of individuals can converge and become coercive societal norms. If genetic tests are available for congenital diseases and disabilities, parents often feel forced to authorize them. When norms like this emerge in coercive circumstances, say, in conditions where people with disabilities are discriminated against, the new norms can reinforce existing unjust structures (Koch, 2005). And the stress on individual choices in a market society can lead to consumerism in health care, which in its turn can be seen to erode the ethical solidity of the system.

Ethicists from diverse backgrounds have thought that, in one way or another, all forms of utilitarian thinking completely miss the point of morality (Foot, 1988; Jackson, 2006; Maclean, 1993; Rawls, 1972). By insisting that only consequences count, utilitarians ignore moral rights, duties and virtues. By stressing rational preferences as the only source of value, they dismiss the ethical significance of life, culture and tradition. By focusing on individuals, they deny the importance of family ties, friendship, community and society. And by overlooking the ordinary use of moral language, they sanction practices that normally repel decent people, such as baby killing and murder.

THE VALIDITY AND SOUNDNESS OF THE EXTERNAL OBJECTIONS

Can the external objections against bioutilitarianism be regarded as *valid* and *sound*?

In the assessment of moral theories, criticisms can be said to be valid if they correctly identify a feature of the assessed view and present a clear alternative to it. All the points presented in the above against bioutilitarianism meet both criteria. Some of them identify practical implications of the doctrine and offer opposite norms as the alternative. Others identify theoretical elements of the creed and suggest competing theories as viable options.

What about soundness? Ethical objections can be seen as sound if the alternatives they present are correct, or at least more correct than the assessed view. The correctness of moral views, again, can be evaluated by coherence, consistency and intuitive acceptability. Some of the critical views and observations have these features for some people. But bioutilitarianism can also be coherent, consistent and intuitively acceptable to its proponents, so the question turns out to be, whose views are more correct? In theory, the correctness of moral doctrines can be assessed by the method of 'reflective equilibrium' (Daniels, 1979). Views reach this balance when their practical conclusions and theoretical underpinnings are, put together, at their most acceptable. The difficulty is that both bioutilitarians and their critics can believe themselves to have reached this state, despite minor residual hiccups which presumably feature in any theory that claims wide coverage in moral matters. This is why external critics, in essence, end up saying, 'You're wrong because you don't agree with me'. And while saying this they are right from their own viewpoint, there are no guarantees that their objections reach the ones they aim to criticize.

INTERNAL CRITICISMS OF BIOUTILITARIANISM

The same conclusion can hold true of internal (intra-utilitarian) criticism – in the end, theorists within the school of thought just disagree as to which contested points can be accepted. Internal objections can, however, be slightly more focused than external ones because there is also accord, and this can make the precise points of dispute more visible. Utilitarians can agree that consequences go before rules and virtues, good precedes right, impartiality is paramount and maximization is an ideal, yet disagree on the finer points of all these tenets (Takala, 2003).

Some critical questions that can be posed by utilitarians are as follows. Why should ethicists concentrate on the immediate or morally expected consequences, when *probable* consequences arguably offer the most neutral alternative? Why should they focus on the preferences of fictional ('rational' or 'reasonable') persons, when *actual* persons are the ones performing and affected by the actions assessed? Why should our attention be focused on the beginning and end of life, when everything that matters is experienced *during* it? And why should maximization automatically be attempted by technological means even when *social* and *political* solutions are available?

In many cases bioutilitarians focus on the immediate consequences of actions. Choice is paramount, and if people are denied what they have decided to go for, the first consequence is that their freedom is limited. In the light of this, other considerations are easily dismissed – including arguments from indirect and cumulative impacts, 'slippery slopes' and 'precaution'. If future outcomes enter the calculation at all, they do so in the form of 'morally expected' consequences. This means that in claims made for the proposed solution its potential benefits are evaluated expecting that everyone will act in a bioutilitarian manner. Both restrictions ignore many actual and probable consequences, the former mainly in the name of convenience or economy of argumentation and the latter on ideological grounds.

People's actual concerns are often overlooked by bioutilitarians on the basis that they are irrational. Irrational concerns, according to them, include those inspired by religion, tradition, sentiments, and deontological and teleological moralities. But if the point of the exercise is to maximize people's preference satisfaction, it is difficult to see what could justify the replacement of their actual desires with fictional, 'rational' ones.

Bioutilitarians have manifestly concentrated on issues involving the beginning and end of life, first on the selection of the best individuals and then on extending and finally ending their lives as they wish. This reverence for 'perfect lives' brings the view much closer to Kantian reflections on 'humanity' and Aristotelian contemplations on 'flourishing' than is customary in other forms of utilitarian thinking. Since preferences are satisfied during one's lifetime, whatever its length and regardless of its level of perfection, the limitation seems unwarranted.

One typical bioutilitarian way to seek perfection is the selection of the 'best babies' by prenatal or preimplantation genetic diagnosis or testing. This has been objected to by noting that the problems remain for the 'imperfect', and that the issue could be handled better by social inclusion and tolerance (Häyry, 2004b). Whatever the merits of this case, insofar as bioutilitarians calculate consequences and assess options selectively, they stray from their original creeds.

Utilitarianism in bioethics, as opposed to current forms of bioutilitarianism, could concentrate on the probable consequences of actions, an exercise which would ideally involve empirical studies as well as thought experiment; focus on people's actual preferences, bearing in mind that some of them may clash with those of others; widen the scope of inquiries to the lives and experiences of 'imperfect' as well as 'perfect' individuals; and explore all solutions, including social and political arrangements, to maximise the good and minimize the bad impacts of what we do and fail to do.

ACKNOWLEDGEMENTS

This chapter was produced as a part of the projects *Public Policies, Law and Bioethics: A Framework for Producing Public Health Policy Across the European Union by Examining Concepts of European and Universal Ethical Standards* (EuroPHEN), financed between 2003 and 2006 by the European Community (QLRT-2001-02320); and *Ethical and Social Aspects of Bioinformatics* (ESABI), financed between 2004 and 2007 by the Academy of Finland (SA 105139). My thanks are due to these institutions for their support, and to Peter Herissone-Kelly for checking my English.

REFERENCES

Bentham J. *An Introduction to the Principles of Morals and Legislation.* London: Methuen, 1789/1970.

Brandt RB. *A Theory of the Good and the Right.* Oxford: Clarendon Press, 1979.

Daniels N. Wide reflective equilibrium and theory acceptance in ethics. *J Philos* 1979; **76**: 256–82.

Erin CA, Harris J. An ethical market in human organs. *J Med Ethics* 2003; **29**: 137–8.

Foot P. Utilitarianism and the virtues. In: Scheffler S, ed. *Consequentialism and Its Critics.* New York: Oxford University Press, 1988.

Glover J. *Causing Death and Saving Lives.* Harmondsworth: Penguin Books, 1977.

Green RM. What does it mean to use someone 'as a means only'? Rereading Kant. *Kennedy Inst Ethics J* 2001; **11**: 247–61.

Hare RM. Abortion and the golden rule. *Philos Public Aff* 1975; **4**: 201–22.

Hare RM *Moral Thinking: Its Levels, Method and Point.* Oxford: Clarendon Press, 1981.

Harris J Scientific research is a moral duty. *J Med Ethics* 2005; **31**: 242–8.

Harris J. *Clones, Genes, and Immortality: Ethics and the Genetic Revolution.* Oxford: Oxford University Press, 1998.

Harris J. *The Value of Life.* London: Routledge & Kegan Paul, 1985.

Harris J. *Violence and Responsibility.* London: Routledge & Kegan Paul, 1980.

Harris J. Intimations of immortality: the ethics and justice of life-extending therapies. In: Freeman MDA, ed. *Current Legal Problems.* Vol. 55. Oxford: Oxford University Press, 2002; pp. 65–95.

Harris J. Is there a coherent social conception of disability? *J Med Ethics* 2000; **26**: 95–100.

Harris J. The survival lottery. *Philosophy* 1975; **50**: 81–7.

Häyry M. *Liberal Utilitarianism and Applied Ethics.* London: Routledge, 1994.

Häyry M. Another look at dignity. *Camb Q Healthc Ethics* 2004a; **13**: 7–14.

Häyry M. If you must make babies, then at least make the best babies you can? *Hum Fertil* 2004b; **7**: 105–12.

Häyry M. Precaution and solidarity. *Camb Q Healthc Ethics* 2005, **14**: 199–206.

Jackson J. *Ethics in Medicine.* Cambridge: Polity, 2006.

Koch T. The ideology of normalcy – the ethics of difference. *J Disabil Policy Stud* 2005; **16**: 123–9.

Kuhse H, Singer P. *Should the Baby Live? The Problem of Handicapped Infants.* Oxford: Oxford University Press, 1985.

Levitt M, Häyry M. Overcritical, overfriendly. A dialogue between a sociologist and a philosopher on genetic technology and its applications. *Med, Health Care Philos* 2005; **8**: 377–83.

Lyons D. *Forms and Limits of Utilitarianism.* Oxford: Clarendon Press, 1965.

Maclean A. *The Elimination of Morality: Reflections on Utilitarianism and Bioethics.* London: Routledge, 1993.

Mill JS. *On Liberty.* Reprinted in Mill JS *On Liberty and The Subjection of Women.* Wordsworth: Ware, Hertfordshire, 1859/1996; pp. 1–114.

Mill JS. *Utilitarianism.* Indianapolis: Hackett Publishing Company, 1861/1979.

Moore GE. *Principia Ethica.* Cambridge: Cambridge University Press, 1903.

Moore GE. *Ethics.* Oxford: Oxford University Press, 1912.

Parfit D. *Reasons and Persons.* Oxford and New York: Oxford University Press, 1986.

Rawls J. *A Theory of Justice.* Oxford: Oxford University Press, 1972.

Savulescu J. Procreative beneficence: why we should select the best children. *Bioethics* 2001; **15**: 413–26.

Savulescu J. The embryonic stem cell lottery and the cannibalization of human beings. *Bioethics* 2002; **16**: 508–29.

Silvers A. Super villainous or mild mannered? Does Singer's position threaten real people or only philosophically constructed ones? *APA Newsletter* 2000; **99**(2): available on the World Wide Web: http://www.apa.udel.edu/apa/publications/newsletters/v99n2/medicine/article-silvers.asp (accessed 15 May 2006).

Singer P. *Animal Liberation.* New York: The New York Review of Books, 1975.

Singer P. *Practical Ethics.* Cambridge: Cambridge University Press, 1979.

Spencer H. *Principles of Ethics* I-II. Indianapolis: Liberty Classics, 1879–93/1978.

Stephen JF. *Liberty, Equality, Fraternity.* Cambridge: Cambridge University Press, 1873/1967.

Takala T. Utilitarianism shot down by its own men? *Camb Q* 2003; **13**: 170–8.

9

Deontology[1]

DAVID A. MCNAUGHTON AND J. PIERS RAWLING

INTRODUCTION

Which actions does morality require of us? What does it forbid and what does it permit? In trying to find some general answers to these questions, moral theorists typically start from commonsense morality, from what ordinary people think about moral issues. In deciding how to act, people often think about the consequences of their actions: they try to find the action that leads to the best overall outcome. One moral theory, act-consequentialism, claims that this is the *only* consideration that is relevant to moral choice. The right action – the one we are required to do – is the one that produces the most good; it is wrong to do less good than we could.

Act-consequentialism seems, however, to conflict with commonsense morality. Although we should be concerned to make things go as well as possible for everyone, most people do not think that this exhausts morality, or even identifies some of its most crucial elements. Are we not, for instance, sometimes required to aid our loved ones, even if we do not thereby produce the best overall? And are there no limits on what we may do to produce good, or limits on what we must do to produce it? Deontology contrasts with consequentialism in its answers to these questions, and is, in one of its versions, the theory we favour.

COMMON SENSE MORALITY

Here are three areas of ordinary moral thought in which considerations other than the amount of good our actions would produce are normally taken to be relevant to what we morally ought to do.

OPTIONS

Act-consequentialism appears very demanding. Given the amount of poverty in the world, maximizing the good would require the better off to make enormous sacrifices to help the very poor. Most people believe that, though they should do something to help those less fortunate, there is nothing wrong with devoting a lot of time, effort and money to one's own happiness and the happiness of those one cares about. There is some point, perhaps hard to determine, at which someone has done all that they are *required* to do by way of helping strangers. At that point they are morally permitted, or have an *option*, not to do more. We admire those who make the extra sacrifice, but it is supererogatory – more than morality requires. Act-consequentialism, however, seems to leave no room for supererogation.

Deontologists do not deny that morality can be very demanding. We may be obliged to make significant sacrifices – even of our lives – rather than breach a serious constraint (see below) or betray a friend. But we are not constantly required to be promoting the general good.

DUTIES OF SPECIAL RELATIONSHIP (OR SPECIAL OBLIGATIONS)

Many people believe that not only are we *permitted* to do more for those close to us, but we are often *required* to put their interests first. We *owe* things to those with whom we have special relationships – such as our friends, colleagues and family members – that we do not owe to strangers. Our own children, for example, have a claim on our attention and resources that other people's children do not. It follows that it would be wrong to neglect our own children, even if we could thereby do slightly more good for other children.

[1]Some of this material is taken from our contribution to 'Deontology' in *Ethics in Practice*, 3rd edition, LaFollette H, ed. Oxford: Blackwell (2007) pp. 31–44. We are grateful to Blackwell for permission to reproduce this material.

Principles of Health Care Ethics, Second Edition   Edited by R.E. Ashcroft, A. Dawson, H. Draper and J.R. McMillan

CONSTRAINTS

In addition to our special obligations, many people believe that we have a duty to avoid seriously harming *anyone* unless, perhaps, they are a threat or deserve punishment. We should not lie, kill innocent people or torture. These prohibitions *constrain* us in what we may do to *any* person (not just those close to us), even in pursuit of good ends. People differ in how stringent these constraints are. Some think them as absolute or exceptionless. Roman Catholic moral theology has traditionally held that one may never intentionally kill an innocent person, even to prevent, say, two other innocents from being intentionally killed. Kant infamously argued that it would be wrong to lie, even to prevent murder. Others hold that, though constraints are always a significant consideration, they may be overridden, especially to avoid catastrophe. Either way, such constraints would sometimes *require* us not to maximize the good.

DISTINGUISHING DEONTOLOGY FROM ACT-CONSEQUENTIALISM

How does consequentialism differ from deontology? A traditional answer points to their contrasting accounts of the relation between the right and the good. Act-consequentialism holds that the good wholly determines the right – which act is right depends solely on the amount of good it produces. Deontologists maintain, by contrast, that other considerations, of the kind discussed in previous sections, are also relevant and that consequentialism fails to take them into account. How might an act-consequentialist respond to this charge?

She might plead guilty, but claim that ordinary moral thinking is confused and unreliable as a guide to moral thinking. Since consequentialism is the correct theory, we should eliminate elements in our moral thinking that do not conform to it. Let us call this the defiant strategy.

Alternatively, she might deny that her theory puts her at odds with common sense morality. Consider special obligations: there might be good consequentialist reasons for encouraging people to do more for those close to them than for strangers. We are in a better position to benefit our nearest and dearest since we know their needs and we are more motivated to help them. So we will do more good by focusing much of our attention on them. Or consider constraints. It is not very often that killing an innocent will have the best results, so we may want to discourage the thought that it could ever be permissible. If our valuable reluctance to kill the innocent were weakened then

people might be tempted to kill when doing so would not produce the best results. In short, from a consequentialist perspective, things might go better if people were guided by common sense morality, rather than directly making decisions using consequentialist criteria. Let us call this the conformist strategy.

We do not have space here to consider whether the conformist strategy is defensible. Even if it were, act-consequentialism would still differ from deontology concerning what makes acts right. The conformist strategy points out that in less than perfect conditions – imperfect knowledge and imperfect motivation to be moral – we may well do better to act in accordance with the dictates of ordinary morality than to try to produce the best results and thereby inadvertently make things worse. But, for the act-consequentialist, the right act remains the one that maximizes value. Under ideal conditions of knowledge and motivation, therefore, the virtuous agent should never produce less good than she could. The deontologist disagrees: she believes that, even under these conditions, we are sometimes permitted, and even required, to do just that.

The three elements of common sense morality to which we have drawn attention are distinct, so that it would be possible, for example, to believe (like Ross) that there are special obligations and constraints, but no options. Or (as we are inclined to do) one might accept that there are special obligations and options, but deny that there are constraints. Or (like some Kantians) one might accept constraints and (perhaps) options, while leaving less room for special obligations. Or (like Scheffler) one might accept only options. Which elements must one accept in order to qualify as a deontologist? A key feature of deontology is the claim that we are sometimes *required* not to maximize the good. So a deontological theory must include this claim. Options only give us *permission* not to maximize the good, but duties of special relationship and constraints can require us not to do so. Thus one or both of these features will typically be part of any deontology.

Can we say more about what characterizes deontology? We could supply a list of the various duties of special obligation and constraints. But is there a unifying theme to such a list? Ross, for example, gives a list that includes – in addition to beneficence (producing good results) – fidelity (to promises and commitments), gratitude, reparation and avoiding harming others. These considerations, he plausibly maintained, were distinct, and none is reducible to any of the others.[2] However, it has been suggested (originally by Nagel 1986) that the considerations that fall under our

---

[2]For a discussion of whether Ross's theory exhibits sufficient unity see McNaughton (1996).

three headings do at least share a common *form*: they are all *agent-relative*.

AGENT-RELATIVITY AND AGENT-NEUTRALITY

The distinction between the agent-neutral and the agent-relative may be introduced by reference to reasons for acting[3]. Roughly, someone's reason is agent-relative if, at base, there is reference within it to her. For example, rational egoism is an agent-relative theory – it holds that each agent has reason to promote only *her own* good, whereas act-consequentialism is an agent-neutral theory – it holds that each of us has reason to promote *everyone's* good. Another way of making this point (which we owe to Parfit (1987) is that consequentialism gives us the *common* aim of promoting the general or impersonal good, whereas according to egoism each of us has the *distinct* aim of promoting his personal good: I have reason to pursue my good, you yours. In contrast to act-consequentialism, deontology is an agent-relative theory: at its base, there are agent-relative as well as agent-neutral moral reasons. Each of the three elements in deontology incorporates agent-relativity.

Special obligations are obviously agent-relative. I am required to care for *my* family, you for *yours*: we have distinct aims. Act-consequentialism might allow that parental care giving is valuable, but on this view we would have the common aim of promoting parental care-giving in general. That would require that I neglect my own children if I can thereby increase the total amount of parental care giving – a claim that deontology denies.

Constraints are also agent-relative. Suppose I can only prevent you from killing two innocents by killing one myself. If there are constraints, then each of us has strong (or even overriding) moral reason not to kill anyone ourselves. Constraints give each of us distinct aims: I have reason not to kill anyone *myself*; you have reason not to kill anyone *yourself*. Thus although you will do wrong in killing the two, I should not kill the one in order to prevent you. Consequentialism, by contrast, holds that everything else equal, it is right to kill an innocent myself to save two: killing innocents is bad, so I have an agent-neutral moral reason to contribute to the common aim of minimizing such killing.

Options need not be agent-relative in their formulation. They simply permit us not to maximize the good. But the standard rationale for admitting options into a moral theory is agent-relative. Each of us is morally permitted to give special weight to *our own* interests, just because they are ours.

RULE-CONSEQUENTIALISM: A DEONTOLOGY IN DISGUISE?

Act-consequentialism is not the only version of consequentialism. Perhaps its most popular rival is rule-consequentialism, which offers a 'two-stage' account of justification. Rule-consequentialism assesses acts, not in terms of their contribution to the good, but by whether they conform to the best set of rules governing human conduct. Rules, however, are assessed by their contribution to the good. The best set of rules is the one whose general acceptance would produce most good. Thus, according to rule-consequentialism, 'an act is wrong if and only if it is forbidden by the code of rules whose internalization by the overwhelming majority . . . has maximum expected value' (Hooker, 2000, p. 32). Which rules are best is determined, in part, by the psychological make-up of human beings. They must, for example, be simple enough for ordinary people to learn and sufficiently appealing that the majority of people can be persuaded to follow them. Given these restrictions, acceptable rules will probably be close to the rules of common sense morality. In particular, rule-consequentialism is likely to include constraints, options and special obligations. There will, for example, be a fairly simple rule against killing the innocent, since having a more complicated rule that allowed killing whenever it would do most good might be disastrous. Given our natural concern for our nearest and dearest and the need for companionship and security, there will also be rules permitting, and even requiring, us to give priority to the claims of friends and family.

How are we to classify rule-consequentialism? Despite its name, it might seem to have more in common with deontology. It agrees with deontology that it is often wrong to do the act that will produce the most good and that some of the moral rules we should follow are agent-relative in form. However, we follow Hooker, a leading rule-consequentialist, in classifying this theory as fundamentally agent-neutral and thus consequentialist. Each form of consequentialism assesses something, at its base, in terms of impersonal or agent-neutral value. But what they assess varies: act-consequentialism assesses acts, while rule-consequentialism assesses rules. As Hooker notes, this makes 'the agent-relativity in rule-consequentialism . . . derivative. Agent-relative rules are justified by their role in promoting agent-neutral value' (Hooker, 2000, p. 110). Deontology, by contrast, holds that some agent-relative considerations are *underivatively* relevant. They have weight in their own right, not merely in virtue of their serving some further purpose.

---

[3]But see McNaughton and Rawling (1991) for discussion of some problems for this approach.

VARIETIES OF DEONTOLOGY

KANT

Kant's moral theory is the best known example of a deontology. As it is discussed in chapter 10 we only mention points that are relevant to our discussion. First, Kant strongly rejects the whole consequentialist approach to moral theory. He denies that the value of its consequences is relevant to the rightness of an act, and he claims that there are kinds of action, such as lying, which are *always* wrong. Second, he gives structure to his theory by offering us the categorical imperative test to determine whether an act is required, permissible or forbidden. Finally, failure to act in accordance with the results of that test is to be, in some strong sense, irrational. Famous though it is, Kant's is not the only nor, in our view, the most plausible deontological theory.

ROSSIAN DEONTOLOGY

How can we find out which moral considerations are fundamentally relevant to how we ought to act? Ross's answer is that we do this by reflecting on our intuitions about contrasting cases. (Ross 1930, chapter 2) Does, for example, having made a promise make a difference? Ross claims that no one would deny that, if we could give an equal amount of help to two people, the fact that I had made a promise to one of them would make it right to help that one. Such reflection, he claims, eventually reveals a number of basic moral considerations, which he formulates as a list of moral principles or duties. As we have seen, his suggested list includes agent-relative duties of promise keeping, gratitude, reparation and not harming others,[4] as well as an agent-neutral requirement to promote the good. These duties are, he says, only *prima facie* (or, as we prefer, *pro tanto*) since, though each is relevant to determining what is right, no duty automatically trumps any of the others in cases where they conflict. Indeed, there is no general method for resolving such conflicts: which duty is the weightier depends on the complexities of the particular circumstance. Where keeping a promise will harm someone, for example, what we ought to do will depend on how serious the promise is, to whom it was made, how much harm we would do in keeping it and so on. To weigh all these factors correctly requires discernment and judgement.

The items on Ross's list are intended to be basic in two ways. First, they are *underivative*, in that they are not instances of some more general principle. So, for example, the duty to pay one's debts is derivative because it is an instance of the more general duty to keep promises. But the latter duty is underivative because it is not itself an instance of some yet more general duty. Second, they are basic in the sense that they are *self-evident* and need no justification. We can see their truth directly, without reasoning from further premises. Indeed, Ross strongly implies that they not only require no further justification but that none is available. He thus rejects the Kantian claim that such basic principles rest on a common foundation. For Ross there is no test that principles must pass to earn their place on the list.

Of the two deontological theories we have looked at so far, Kant's and Ross's, which is the more attractive? This depends, in part, on what one is looking for in a moral theory. Kant's programme is remarkably ambitious; Ross's is very modest. Kant seeks a *grounding* for common-sense morality, whereas Ross holds that none is available and none is needed. Kant supposes that, at bottom, there is something that morality is about; Ross makes no such assumption. Kant offers a test that purports to show that acting immorally is indisputably *irrational*, rather in the way that it is irrational to contradict oneself. Ross holds that there are moral reasons, but failure to appreciate them would be a sign of moral insensitivity or immaturity, rather than a gross failure of reasoning. Kant maintains that certain kinds of action, such as lying, are morally unacceptable in all cases; Ross rules nothing out in advance – it all depends on the facts of the particular case. Ambitious theories may be exciting and stimulating in a way that modest ones are not, but that does not make them correct. Not only may they fail to realize their ambitions, but those ambitions may themselves be misguided. It may, for example, be an error to suppose that our moral thought stands in need of special justification, or that a successful moral theory should provide unequivocal guidance in perplexing cases. In our view, the modesty of Ross's account is a strength, not a weakness.

PARTICULARIST DEONTOLOGY

To what extent can morality be codified into a set of rules or principles? Some moral theorists think that there are *strong* moral principles that tell us that we are always forbidden (or required) to act in certain ways. Thus Kant claimed that lying is always wrong. Others, such as Ross, think there are only *weak* principles that tell us that certain features always matter, morally speaking The features on Ross's list of *prima facie* duties are supposed always to count for (or against) the rightness of an act. Particularists, however, doubt the existence of even weak principles and deny that we need them to engage in moral thinking. On their view,

---

[4]This last is, we think, agent-relative for Ross: he does not appear to countenance doing harm oneself in order to minimize the total amount of harm.

almost any feature can be morally relevant and none need always be relevant – it all depends on the context. So, for example, the fact that an act brings pleasure often counts in its favour, but not, perhaps, when the pleasure is sadistic. That it would bring sadistic pleasure is *no* reason to perform an act.

Who is right – Ross or the particularist? The matter is hotly disputed. Ross seems to be mistaken about one member of his list – promise-keeping. In normal circumstances the fact that I would be breaking a promise does indeed count against acting in that way. But promises extracted by fraud or force are null and void, as are promises to do something immoral. Suppose I promise to perform a contract killing. It is implausible to hold that, though, all things considered, I ought not to do it, yet the fact that I promised gives me *some* moral reason to do it. However, other considerations on Ross's list seem more plausible candidates. How could an act's being just, for example, not count in its favour?

DEFENDING DEONTOLOGY

There is nothing puzzling about the consequentialist claim that the amount of (agent-neutral) good we could do is morally relevant. Deontology, however, claims that there is also an *underivative* agent-relative component to morality, and this does seem puzzling. How can the *mere* fact that some act will be good or bad for *me*, or for *my* nearest and dearest, itself make a moral difference? Or how can the *mere* fact that *I*, rather than someone else, will kill an innocent be morally relevant? In what follows we try to meet this challenge in the case of special relationships and options, while conceding that it is harder to meet it in the case of constraints.

SPECIAL RELATIONSHIPS AND THE TIES THAT BIND

On our view, we have underivative, agent-relative, moral ties to certain people in virtue of our relationships with them. Consider the tie of friendship. Such ties are agent-relative: part of my reason for helping Eve rather than Adam is that Eve is *my* friend. These ties are underivative because such reasons do not depend wholly on considerations about the general value of friendship. Friendship is valuable, but that fact does not explain *my* tie to Eve. Finally, the ties of friendship have a moral component. It is not just that friends like and support each other. In addition, your friend has the *right* to expect *your* loyalty and support because she is *your* friend. If you betray her, she has a moral complaint against you that no one else has. The (tacit) acknowledgement of a moral tie between friends appears essential to friendship.

Friends come through for one another; someone who did not even recognize this would not be loyal and so would not be a friend.

Act-consequentialism does get something right: we only have reason to act when it will do some good. But how much good I can do is not the only factor. Who will receive the good also matters. Friends have stronger claims than others to my good offices. Which act would be right depends on two factors: the good I can do someone and the strength of the claim she has on me.

If this is right, then consequentialism has a serious strike against it. Loyalty is essential to friendship. Loyalty involves the recognition of an underivative agent-relative obligation to one's friends. Consequentialism has no place for underivative agent-relative obligations; thus it has no room for friendship. But friendship, as is generally acknowledged by consequentialists, is an important intrinsic good. Consequentialism holds that the good is to be promoted; but here is a good that it apparently cannot accommodate.

How might the consequentialist respond? Act-consequentialists, as we saw, may opt for a strategy of defiance or conformity. Those who favour defiance may deny that the moral point of view has room for friendship. Morality, on this approach, requires giving equal weight to everyone's interests. Since we are not even permitted, still less required, to favour any group of people, the consistent act-consequentialist cannot have friends.

Unsurprisingly, most act-consequentialists reject this stark approach and opt for the conformist strategy. We saw earlier (see Section Distinguishing Deontology From Act-Consequentialism) that an agent might do better in achieving consequentialist goals if she did not think about which act is right on each occasion, but instead had dispositions to favour friends and family. Pursuing this line, the act-consequentialist might concede that friendship requires loyalty, but then maintain that loyalty does not require that there actually be moral ties, only that people *believe* there to be such ties. So act-consequentialism might encourage people falsely to believe that they have special obligations.

A serious objection to this strategy, however, is that it pictures the ideal moral agent as someone who is fundamentally mistaken about what makes acts right or wrong. In effect, such a consequentialist is saying: consequentialism is the theory you have most reason to believe, but it would be better, from the consequentialist perspective, if no one believed it. If not actually incoherent, this position is certainly uncomfortable. Simpler and better to accept that special obligations exist, unless there are compelling reasons to believe that they do not. But no such reasons have been offered.

Rule-consequentialism does rather better. Unlike act-consequentialism, it acknowledges that one can be acting rightly in favouring friends, but it fails to capture friendship because it maintains that preferential treatment of friends can be justified only by appeal to the general good:

> Moral requirements of loyalty are . . . needed . . . when affection isn't up to the job. . .. [S]pecial moral obligations towards family and friends can then be justified on the ground that internalization of these obligations gives people some assurance that some others will consistently take a special interest in them. Such assurance answers a powerful psychological need (Hooker, 2000, p. 141).

This does not yield genuine loyalty. Friends have moral reason not to let us down, and assurance is engendered in part by a belief that they will respond to this reason. (This is not to say that the only reasons here are moral.) But for rule-consequentialism, the *moral* reason for John not to let Mary down is the general assurance that results from the internalization of a rule requiring the special treatment of 'friends', not anything special about his relationship with Mary.

A final objection to our account. Morality requires us to be impartial, but do not duties of special relationship require us to be *partial* to our friends, and so on? No. In our view, we show partiality in allocating goods only if we give the claims of one person or group more weight than we are *warranted* in doing. To favour those who have a claim on us is not to show an unacceptable favouritism. We do that only when we give *undue* or *inappropriate* weight to the interests of our nearest and dearest.

OPTIONS

Each of us has special personal reason to pursue our own benefit, just by virtue of it being ours. I have personal reason to care about my pain that I cannot have to care about yours, namely that it is mine. This does not mean that I have no reason to care about your pain, nor does it commit me to denying that pain is equally bad whoever has it. But each agent has moral permission not to maximize the good when the cost to *her* would be significant.[5] An agent is allowed, in determining what she is morally required to do, to accord greater weight to the cost borne by her than to the cost borne by others. The act-consequentialist denies this: whether an act is morally permitted, on her view, depends solely on the amount of impersonal value it would produce. She might try to soften that view by arguing that if too much is required of agents they will become disillusioned or exhausted and so do less good than if they had more modest targets. But that strategy allows us to favour

ourselves merely as a concession to our weakness, not as an acknowledgment of a right.

In our view there has to be some balance between the demands that the needs of others put on us and our right to live our own lives. Determining where that balance lies is notoriously difficult. But this does not entail that there is no balance to be struck.

Moreover, the act-consequentialist denies room for supererogation (acting beyond the call of duty): she maintains that the person who bears great personal cost in maximizing the good, although admirable in the extreme, would be doing something morally wrong if she did otherwise.

Rule-consequentialism appears to do better. An agent who follows the rules does not act wrongly: she does enough good – to do more would be meritorious but is not required. The presence of this personal space, however, stems from impersonal costs: we are psychologically resistant to making significant sacrifices, and this makes it too expensive to inculcate a more demanding rule. But this resistance is understood as a regrettable flaw, not a mark of personal reasons. Rule-consequentialism denies the *moral* significance of personal reasons at the fundamental level. They matter only because of the cost of training people to ignore them.

CONSTRAINTS

Constraints, though often regarded as the most distinctive feature of deontology, seem harder to justify than options or duties of special relationship. Consider an absolute constraint against (intentionally) killing an innocent person. Suppose Anne and several other innocents are about to be shot by Bert, but he agrees to let the others go if you shoot Anne. The constraint forbids you to do it. Yet, as Scheffler (1994) points out, this appears inexplicable: Anne is going to be shot, but at least you can prevent the other shootings.

Some advocates of constraints might concede that you should shoot Anne in this case, but they would object to your shooting some unthreatened innocent in order to save Bert's intended victims. But even this weaker position does not, in the end, evade the standard 'irrationality objection' to constraints: that they forbid their own violation *even to minimize such violation*.

An important feature of constraints, as understood by traditional deontology, is that they are underivative. Rule-consequentialism incorporates prohibitions against, say, killing the innocent, but these are *derivatively* 'justified by their role in promoting agent-neutral value' (Hooker, 2000, p. 110). In that sense, rule-consequentialism does not include constraints.

We have defended special obligations and options by contending that, in addition to the amount of good we do,

---

[5]For an extended defence of this approach, see Scheffler (1994), *passim*.

what we might call positional facts – that the good would accrue to *my* friends or to *me* – are also morally relevant. Constraints, however, cannot be similarly defended. Constraints, unlike duties of special relationship, single out no group on the basis of my relationship to its members, thus they cannot rest on my being more closely related to some than others. Could they be justified on the grounds that my violating a constraint, even to prevent worse actions by others, is bad *for me*, and so something I have personal reason to avoid? After all, many of us have an understandable reluctance to get our hands dirty. But that thought, at best, *might* ground a *permission* not to violate the constraint. It cannot ground a *requirement* not to do so.

Constraints, then, embody as fundamental the fact of your agency. It is the bare fact that you would be doing the killing that rules out your killing an innocent as a means to preventing other innocents suffering a like fate. Since constraints are fundamental, we should not expect to find a deeper justification for them. Their being fundamental does not, however, preclude our defending constraints, as we did with special obligations and options, by explicating their nature in ways that make their force clearer. The problem is that we can find no explication of constraints that dispels their air of irrationality.

Given that air of irrationality, it is unsurprising that many deontologists have nevertheless attempted to find a deeper justification, but such attempts to explain why agency matters seem to presuppose the very point at issue (see Scheffler, 1994, ch. 4). Thus it is said (in a Kantian vein) that persons deserve respect in view of their unique importance as rational moral agents. But why does such respect forbid you to harm others rather than requiring you to minimize harm? It may be said that just as we owe particular duties to others in view of our special relationships with them, so we owe to everyone else a duty not to harm them because of our general relationship with them. But what is that relationship? Perhaps that of being fellow humans or fellow persons. Whatever the answer, the problem remains: why does our standing in that relationship ground a *constraint* against harming as opposed to a duty to minimize harm?

Some defenders of constraints[6] have complained that in seeing constraints as *agent*-relative, recent attempts to ground constraints have wrongly focused on agency. Rather, they claim, we should focus on a *patient*-centred justification – on what it is about innocents that entails the existence of constraints against harming them. But this does not seem to help. Innocents do not deserve to be harmed; ideally, then, we should not harm them. But what are we to do in our non-ideal world in which innocents are under threat?

If we deny there are constraints, however, would not we have to abandon the many intuitions that seem to support their existence? Not necessarily. Many intuitions that appear to be support constraints may actually rest on other features. We may, for example, think it wrong to take $10 from one person in order to enrich another by $20. But our grounds for that (depending on the circumstances) might be that the harm of taking $10 *honestly possessed* outweighs the benefit of bestowing $20 *unearned*. Second, we may think it wrong to do considerable harm to one person in order to prevent small harms to a large number. But that may have nothing to do with agency but be explained by the fact that no number of small harms to different people, when added together, is as bad as a serious harm to one person.

We are tentatively proposing, then, a morality devoid of constraints (as traditionally understood) but incorporating underivative duties of special obligation and options. Is such a theory worthy of the name of deontology? Yes. Ours is a theory that acknowledges underivative agent-relative requirements not to maximize the good.

REFERENCES

Brook R. Agency and morality. *J Philos* 1991, **88**: 190–212

Hooker B. *Ideal Code, Real World.* Oxford: Clarendon Press, 2000.

Kamm F. Nonconsequentialism. In: LaFollette H, ed. *The Blackwell Guide to Ethical Theory.* Oxford: Blackwell, 2000; pp. 205–26.

McNaughton D, Rawling P. Agent-relativity and the doing-happening distinction. *Philos Stud* 1991; **63**: 167–85.

McNaughton D, Rawling P. Deontology and agency. *Monist* 1993; **76**: 81–100.

McNaughton D. An unconnected heap of duties? *Philos Q* 1996; **46**: 433–47.

Nagel T. *The View from Nowhere.* Oxford: Oxford University Press, 1986; ch. 9.

Parfit D. *Reasons and Persons*, revised edition. Oxford; Clarendon Press, 1987; p. 27.

Ross WD. *The Right and the Good.* Oxford: Clarendon Press, 1930.

Scheffler S. *The Rejection of Consequentialism*, revised edition. Oxford: Clarendon Press, 1994.

---

[6]See for instance Brook (1991), Kamm (2000). For discussion see McNaughton and Rawling (1993).

10

Kantian Ethics[1]

ONORA O'NEILL

Kantian ethics originates in the ethical writings of Immanuel Kant (1724–1804). These writings remain the most influential attempt to vindicate universal ethical principles that respect the dignity and equality of human beings without presupposing theological claims or a metaphysical conception of the good. Kant's systematic, critical philosophy centres on an account of reasoning about action, which he uses to justify principles of duty and virtue, a liberal and republican conception of justice with cosmopolitan scope and an account of the relationship between morality and hope.

Numerous contemporary writers also advance views of ethics which they, and their critics, think of as Kantian. However, some contemporary work is remote from Kant's philosophy on fundamental matters such as human freedom and reasoning about action. It converges with Kant's ethics in claiming that we lack a substantive account of the Good (so that teleological or consequentialist ethics are impossible), in taking a strong view of the equality of moral agents and the importance of universal principles of duty which spell out what it is to respect them, and in stressing an account of justice and rights with cosmopolitan scope.

Both Kant's ethics and contemporary Kantian ethics have been widely criticized for preoccupation with rules and duties and for lack of concern with virtues, happiness or personal relationships. A number of these criticisms apply more accurately to recent Kantian ethics than to Kant's ethics.

KANT'S ETHICS

Kant's main writing on ethics and politics can be found in *The Groundwork of The Metaphysic of Morals* (1785), *The Critique of Practical Reason* (1788), *The Metaphysics*

of Morals (1797) and in numerous sections of other works and freestanding essays. Throughout these writings he insists that we cannot derive ethical conclusions from metaphysical or theological knowledge of the Good (which we lack) or from a claim that human happiness is the sole good (which we cannot establish). We lack the basis for a teleological or consequentialist account of ethical reasoning, which therefore cannot be simply a matter of means-ends reasoning towards some fixed and knowable good.

Yet if reasoning about action, that is practical reasoning, is not means-end reasoning, what can it be? Kant's alternative account proposes simply that reasons for action must be reasons for all. He insists that we can have reasons for recommending as moral requirements only those principles of action which could be adopted by all concerned, whatever their particular desires, social identities, roles or relationships. Correspondingly, practical reasoning must reject any principles that cannot be principles for all concerned, which Kant characterizes as non-universalizable principles.

Kant gives this rather limited, modal conception of practical reasoning some grand names. He calls it the 'supreme principle of morality' and the 'Categorical Imperative'. He formulates this fundamental principle of ethics in various ways. The formulation most discussed in the philosophical literature runs, 'Act only on that maxim [principle] through which you can at the same time will that it become a universal law' (Kant, 1785, p. 421). The formulation that has had and still has the greatest cultural resonance requires us to treat others with impartial respect. It runs 'treat humanity... never simply as a means, but always at the same time as an end' (Kant, 1785, p. 429). The equivalence of these two formulations of the Categorical Imperative is

---

[1] Adapted from the Routledge Encyclopedia. Reproduced by permission of Taylor and Francis Group Ltd.

Principles of Health Care Ethics, Second Edition   Edited by R.E. Ashcroft, A. Dawson, H. Draper and J.R. McMillan
© 2007 John Wiley & Sons, Ltd

far from obvious. One way of glimpsing why Kant thought they were equivalent is to note that if we treat others as persons rather than as things then we must not destroy or impair their abilities to act. Indeed we must leave it open to them to act on the same principles that we act on; hence, we must act on universalizable principles. On Kant's view, one of the worst features of consequentialist ethics is that it not merely permits but requires that persons be used as mere means if this will produce better results than other available acts.

Kant claims that the Categorical Imperative can be used to justify the underlying principles of human duties. For example, we can show by a *reductio ad absurdum* argument that promising falsely is not universalizable. Suppose that everyone was to adopt the principle of promising falsely: since then there would be much false promising, trust would be destroyed and many would find that they could not get their false promises accepted, contrary to the hypothesis of universal adoption of the principle of false promising. A maxim of promising falsely is not universalizable, so the Categorical Imperative requires us to reject it. Parallel arguments can be used to show that principles such as those of coercing or doing violence are not universalizable, and so it is a duty to reject these principles.

Kant calls duties such as these perfect (i.e. complete) duties. These are duties which can observed by each towards all others. He also provides arguments to establish the principles of certain imperfect (i.e. incomplete) duties, such as those of helping others in need or developing one's own talents. One way in which imperfect duties are unavoidably incomplete is that they cannot be observed towards all others: nobody can help all others in need, or develop all possible talents. Kant calls these imperfect duties as 'duties of virtue'.

The derivation of principles of duty from his conception of practical reason is the core of Kant's ethics, and it provides the context for his discussion of many other themes. These include the difference between internalizing principles and merely conforming to them in outward respects ('acting out of duty' versus 'acting according to duty'); the place of happiness in a good life; the need for judgement in moving from principle to act; the justification of state power, despite the fact that it coerces; and the justification of a cosmopolitan account of justice. He also develops the connections between his distinctive conceptions of practical reason and of freedom, and his equally distinctive view of religion, which he sees as a matter not of knowledge but of reasoned hope for a future in which morality can be fully realized. In some works Kant articulates reasoned hope in religious terms; in others he articulates it in political and historical terms as a hope for a better future for us worldly humans.

CONTEMPORARY KANTIAN ETHICS

Much contemporary work on ethics is commonly labelled Kantian, in the main because it does not derive an account of right action from one of good results, but rather sees the right as prior to the Good. In contemporary Kantian work obligations and rights are the fundamental ethical notions. Such work is often called deontological ethics (the term derives from the Greek word for ought). Deontological ethical theories are contrasted with teleological or consequentialist theories, which treat the good as prior to the right. Deontological theories are concerned with ethically required action, hence with principles, rules or norms, with obligations, prohibitions and permissions, and with justice and injustice, but not with virtues, good lives, moral ideals and personal relationships (see Fried, 1978 and Gewirth, 1978).

Deontological ethics has many distinct forms. Many versions endorse one or another interpretation of the Kantian demand to respect persons, and hold that moral principles should be universal in the sense that they are formulated as principles that hold for all; few mention Kant's minimalist strategy for justifying specific universally binding principles as those we must live by if we reject non-universalizable principles. Indeed, many deontological ethical theories rely on conceptions of freedom, reason and action which are unlike Kant's, and often on theories that resemble those typically used by consequentialists.

One prominent range of contemporary 'Kantian' positions seeks to justify principles of justice by showing that they *would* be agreed to by all concerned under certain hypothetical conditions. They draw on the thought that agreements and contracts are good reasons for action, and suggest that all ethical claims are to be justified by showing that they are based, if not on actual then on hypothetical agreements or contracts. These sorts of theories are often called contractarian or contractualist; they are contemporary versions of social contract theories.

Some contractualists take a Hobbesian rather than a Kantian approach (for example, Alan Gewirth). They argue that principles of justice are those on which instrumentally rational persons, guided by their individual preferences, would agree. Other contractualists take a more Kantian approach. They argue that principles of justice are those which would be accepted or agreed to by persons who are not merely instrumentally rational but use certain other reasonable procedures.

The best known exponent of Kantian contractualism is John Rawls, whose *A Theory of Justice* (1971) identifies principles of justice as those that would be agreed by rational and self-interested beings in circumstances which ensure that their choosing will be reasonable as well as rational. He argues that principles of justice would emerge if they were chosen by all concerned in a hypothetical situation devised to ensure impartiality and hence agreement. Rawls calls this hypothetical situation 'the original position' and represents it as one in which persons are ignorant of their own social position and personal attributes, hence of their own advantage; thus, they cannot but be impartial.

He claims that rational persons in this hypothetical situation would choose principles of justice that prescribe equal rights for all and the highest attainable level of well-being for the worst off. Since everything that differentiates individuals (and so could provide a basis for disagreement, bargaining or a need to seek agreement) is carefully excluded from the original position, it is not obvious why principles chosen in it should be thought of as matters of agreement, or why the parties to the original position should be thought of as contracting with one another. Nor is it clear why the fact that certain principles would be agreed to under these conditions justifies those principles to those in other situations. Why are principles that would be agreed to under conditions that do not obtain binding under conditions that actually obtain?

In *A Theory of Justice,* Rawls (1971) argued that principles that would be so agreed are binding in other situations because they cohere, or form a 'reflective equilibrium' with our 'considered moral judgements'. Principles are justified not merely because the instrumental reasoning of the hypothetically ignorant would select them, but because we would reasonably judge them as congruent with our most carefully considered moral views. In his later book *Political Liberalism*, Rawls depicts these principles as the outcome not of hypothetical agreement in an original position, but as the hypothetical agreement of persons who are not only rational but reasonable, in the sense that they are willing to abide by principles given the assurance that others will do so too. (Rawls, 1993, p. 49). Principles and institutions are just if they are the focus of reasonable agreement by all concerned.

Jürgen Habermas (1993) has also advocated versions of Kantian ethics that stress agreement between agents. In his earlier work he argued that the test of justification or legitimation is that a proposal would be agreed in a hypothetical 'ideal speech situation', in which communication was undistorted. In a more recent work, he has argued that legitimation of norms is achieved through processes of public discourse to which each can contribute and in which all can agree.

INDIVIDUAL AUTONOMY AND PRINCIPLED AUTONOMY

Both Kant and contemporary exponents of Kantian ethics stress the importance of *autonomy* for morality. But here too there is much more divergence than is commonly appreciated, because the conceptions of autonomy invoked are quite different. The conceptions of *individual autonomy* and of *rational individual autonomy* that have played a large part in the late twentieth century moral and political philosophy, and in areas such as bioethics, view it as a property that individuals manifest in choosing freely, or in choosing freely and rationally. It is difficult to see how individual autonomy could be enough for morality, although plausible to think that it may be necessary for morality.

By contrast, Kant advances a conception of *principled autonomy* that he thinks of as basic to morality. He construes autonomy not as a property of individuals, but as a property of certain principles that individuals may adopt or reject. On the basis of Kant's account, *autonomous principles* are those principles that could be willed for all: they have both law-like form and universal scope. They could be proposed to and justified to anybody. By contrast, heteronomous principles are principles that indeed have law-like form, but lack universal scope, so could not be adopted by or justified to all others. Heteronomous principles are not principles of morality, although action on them is often compatible with moral requirements (we may do the right thing for the wrong reason). Heteronomous action may be individually autonomous, but they violate the demand for principled autonomy that is one of the hallmarks of Kant's account of morality.

CRITICISM OF KANTIAN ETHICS

Both Kant's ethics and contemporary Kantian ethics have been criticized from many quarters. The critics evidently include those who advocate one or another form of teleological or consequentialist theory, who believe that it is possible to establish an account of the Good, from which a convincing account of the right, and specifically of justice, can be derived. However, they also include a variety of writers who reject consequentialist thinking, including communitarians, virtue ethicists, Wittgensteinians and feminist thinkers.

The most common and general criticisms are that, because they concentrate on principles or rules of right conduct and justice, both Kant's ethics and Kantian ethics are doomed to be either empty and formalistic or rigidly uniform in their prescriptions (both the complaints cannot be true). The charge of empty formalism is based on the correct observation that principles underdetermine action; it is usually countered with the equally correct observation that quite indeterminate principles (e.g. 'Stay within the budget' or 'All religions are to be tolerated') can set significant constraints on action, so they are not empty. The charge of rigidly uniform prescriptivity is based on the thought that rules prescribe, so must regiment. It is usually countered by the reminder that because rules can be indeterminate, they need not be regiment: universal principles need not be uniformly prescriptive. An ethical theory that applies to principles can be more than empty and less than rigid.

Other critics object that because Kantian ethics focuses on obligations and rights, and in good measure on justice, it either must or does neglect other ethical categories, and in particular the virtues, good character or good lives. Some critics go further in claiming that 'Natural and human rights... are fictions', and, by implication, that both Kant's ethics and Kantian ethics are based on fictitious claims (MacIntyre, 1981). Others have argued that different obligations inevitably conflict in some cases, and that this renders all deontological ethics incoherent. Yet others have laid particular stress on the point that by requiring impartial respect for all, Kantian ethics wholly ignores the place of happiness, emotions, personal integrity and above all personal relationships in the good life. They have claimed that we must choose between an ethic of justice and one of care; between an ethic of rules and one of relationships; between an ethic of duty and one of virtue; and that the latter term of each pair is to be preferred.

BACK TO KANT?

Some of these criticisms are accurately aimed at significant features of various forms of contemporary Kantian writing in ethics; many of them are less apt as criticisms of Kant's ethics. Several recent writers have suggested that Kant's ethics is the most convincing form of Kantian ethics, and that its distinctive features are strengths rather than weaknesses: they may be thought of as reviving the neo-Kantian slogan 'back to Kant'. Many of these writers accept much of the critique of deontological ethics, but think that not all the criticisms apply to Kant's ethics, of which they offer detailed interpretations. Part of their effort has gone into works on Kant's conceptions of action, reason and freedom, and part into works on his ethics. They have pointed out that Kant's account of practical reason and of its vindication does not assume either that all reasoning about action is instrumentally-rational pursuit of preferred ends, or that ethical vindication is located in hypothetical agreements or contracts reached by reasonable procedures. They have stressed that Kant's conception of practical reason is based on universalizability rather than impartiality or reciprocity, and that he views obligations rather than rights as basic to ethics. They have insisted that impartial respect for persons and a cosmopolitan approach to justice are not morally negligible matters,

and have criticized communitarians, virtue ethicists and some feminist thinkers for not taking justice seriously. They have also pointed out that Kant offers accounts of the virtues, the role of happiness in the good life, and judgement, and argued that his position is not damagingly individualistic and that he acknowledges the importance of institutions and of social and personal relationships in human life (see Hill (1992), Korsgaard (1996), Herman (1993) and O'Neill (1989)).

REFERENCES

Fried C. *Right and Wrong.* Cambridge, MA: Harvard University Press, 1978. (Forthright defence of deontological ethics).

Gewirth, A. *Reason and Morality.* Chicago: University of Chicago Press, 1978. (Rational justification of deontological ethics).

Habermas J. *Between Facts and Norms: Contributions to a Discourse Theory of Law and Democracy,* William R, translator. Cambridge: Polity Press, 1993. (Habermas's most recent extended discussion of questions of normative justification).

Herman B. *The Practice of Moral Judgement.* Cambridge, MA: Harvard University Press, 1993. (Essays on the use of Kantian ethical reasoning; argues that it can be sensitive to context).

Hill TE Jr. *Dignity and Practical Reason in Kant's Moral Theory.* Ithaca NY: Cornell University Press, 1992. (Essays on Kant's ethics, and especially on respect for persons.)

Kant I. *Groundwork of the Metaphysic of Morals* (1785) (Groundwork) (Paton HJ, translator). London: Hutcheson, 1949; New York: Harper and Row, 1964. Page numbers are those of the Prussian Academy edition, given in the margins of this and most editions. (Kant's classic, short, if difficult introduction to his ethics)

Kant I. *The Critique of Practical Reason* (1788) (Becktrans LW, translator). New York: Library of Liberal Arts, Macmillan Publishing, 1993. (Kant's most abstract account of his ethics; particular stress on reason and the highest good).

Kant I. *The Metaphysics of Morals* (1797) (Gregor M, translator). Cambridge: Cambridge University Press, 1991. (Kant's accounts of justice and of the virtues.)

Korsgaard CM. *Creating the Kingdom of Ends.* Cambridge: Cambridge University Press, 1996. (Essays on the Categorical Imperative and its implications.)

MacIntyre A. *After Virtue: A Study in Moral Theory.* London: Duckworth, 1981, p. 67. (Vigorous criticism of Kantian ethics from a distinctive neo-Aristotelian viewpoint).

O'Neill O. *Constructions of Reason: Explorations of Kant's Practical Philosophy.* Cambridge: Cambridge University Press, 1989. (Essays on Kant's vindication of reason and its implications for ethics).

O'Neill O. Kant's virtues. In: Crisp R, ed. *How Should One Live: Essays on the Virtues?* Oxford: Oxford University Press, 1996; pp. 77–97. (Critical account of Kant on virtue.)

O'Neill O. Autonomy: The Emperor's New Clothes, The Inaugural Address. *Proc Aristotelian Soc* 2003; **LXXVII**: 1–21.

Pasternak L, ed. *Immanuel Kant: Groundwork of the Metaphysic of Morals.* Routledge, 2002 (useful recent selection of articles).

Rawls J. *A Theory of Justice.* Cambridge MA: Harvard University Press, 1971. (Very influential work on liberal political philosophy; many Kantian aspects).

Rawls J. Kantian Constructivism in Moral Theory: The Dewey Lectures. *J Philos* 1980; **77**: 515–72. (Rawls's reconsideration of his theory of justice, discusses the importance of pluralism and the impossibility of justifying a conception of the good to all).

Rawls J. *Political Liberalism.* New York: Columbia University Press, 1993 (Reworks Rawls's theory of justice, grounding it in a distinctive conception of public reason).

Stratton-Lake P. *Kant, Duty and Moral Worth*, London: Routledge, 2000. (Discussion of central themes of Kant's ethics.)

Williams B. *Ethics and the Limits of Philosophy.* London: Fontana, 1985. (Varied and thoughtful criticism of Kantian ethics).

Wood A. *Kant's Ethical Thought.* Cambridge: Cambridge University Press, 1999 (Reliable and recent commentary on Kant's ethics).

11

Feminist Approaches to Health Care Ethics

SUSAN SHERWIN

INTRODUCTION

Feminist approaches to health care ethics are rooted in feminist practice and feminist theory. Feminist practice is a broad and diverse collection of activities occurring around the globe aimed at promoting women's equality through identifying and challenging practices that support inequality. Feminist theory, for its part, is a rich, complex, diverse conversation that embraces a multitude of views and perspectives. The unifying theme that distinguishes activities and theories as feminist is that they recognize gender as an important, if problematic, category of analysis.[1] Specifically, feminists tend to share the three part view that gender inequality exists, it is unjust, and social and political actions can help to correct existing inequities. It is important to keep in mind, however, that feminists differ in their views as to how to characterize the normative ideal of gender equality and also as to how best to go about achieving that goal. Most believe that we must attend to the complex ways in which gender interacts with other aspects of social injustice – particularly those based on race, sexual orientation, age, socioeconomic class and disability – and that we must work to promote social equality in all areas.

Because feminists view gender and other forms of inequality as moral as well as political problems, the work of feminism is, in a fundamental sense, a moral quest. Feminist ethics is, at its core, an approach to ethics that places a very high priority on exploring and addressing questions of social justice, particularly gender justice. It requires us to explore why gender and other forms of injustice have remained largely invisible in the work of mainstream ethical theorists and to find ways of correcting this oversight. These questions are particularly urgent within the realm of bioethics since gender, along with other forms of embodiment which constitute the basis of discriminatory practices, seems often to be a factor in the ways in which health and health care are conceptualized and delivered.

For many engaged in feminist bioethics, a principal task is to correct distortions within mainstream bioethics that occur when insufficient attention is paid to the role of gender in the analyses offered. It is important to stress, however, that feminist bioethics goes beyond modifications of non-feminist work: often, it involves expanding the scope of bioethics by identifying new sets of moral issues that must be explored, alternative concepts that must be considered and distinct ways of framing problems under discussion.

Although theorists working in feminist ethics and feminist bioethics naturally concentrate on theoretical questions in their disciplines, there are many feminist activists engaged in related activities with regard to practices that disadvantage women. Women's health care has long been a primary site for feminist political activism and analysis and feminist bioethics can trace its lineage to the activities of those in the women's health movement (Norsigian et al. 1999). In addition, feminist bioethical theorists have been inspired by the multiple feminist critiques within the academy, particularly those directed at the primary disciplines that constitute bioethics (i.e., philosophy, religious studies, anthropology, literature, history as well as medicine, nursing and social work). Within the feminist work concerning health, there is no linear relation from

---

[1] Many feminists have found it useful to distinguish gender (the social norms regarding behavioural expectations of women and men) from sex (the physiological basis of distinguishing females from males) even though these categories tend to be complicated, overlapping and problematic.

Principles of Health Care Ethics, Second Edition   Edited by R.E. Ashcroft, A. Dawson, H. Draper and J.R. McMillan
© 2007 John Wiley & Sons, Ltd

theory to practice (or from practice to theory, for that matter) but rather an on-going multi-level exploration by those seeking to improve the health and status of women and members of other socially disadvantaged groups.

In the remainder of this chapter, I shall unpack this brief overview by examining some of the major feminist approaches to ethics and bioethics and looking more closely at how these approaches play out within contexts of health care ethics. Although there are many ways to organize the work of feminist bioethics (e.g. historically, according to the kinds of problems addressed, or according to disciplines it is rooted in), I shall adopt an approach that reflects on some key distinctions among approaches to feminist theorizing.[2]

FEMINIST APPROACHES

As a response to the existing patterns of gender inequality, feminism generally begins with a critique of the practices that sustain such patterns and then undertakes the challenging work of imagining positive alternatives. Many of these critiques explore the ways gender is conceptualized and deployed. Assumptions about gender are pervasive throughout the history of Western thought. For centuries, most people believed that there are many important differences between men and women that extend far beyond the anatomical. They generally concurred with Aristotle that women are physically inferior to men and, hence, are destined to fulfil different (and inferior) social roles. The dominant view was androcentrism, that is the belief that the male sets the norm for the species both in the sense of defining what is normal and also serving as the ideal against which all others are to be measured. This ideological position has had a profound impact on scientific, philosophical and political thought. The species is referred to as 'mankind' and 'woman' is constructed always as 'other' – as atypical, problematic and different.

Feminists have revealed multiple ways in which assumptions about gender pervade thought and distort people's understanding of the world. By dividing the human world into two distinct, dichotomous categories, it becomes easy to assume that many other distinctions map tidily onto these two groups. Thus, characteristics commonly associated with men (or at least with ideal men) – rationality, strength, impartiality – are reflected in opposing traits that are generally

associated with women – emotionality, weakness, partiality. The fact that gender is a socially constructed phenomenon that captures norms a society deems appropriate for each sex (masculinity and femininity) does little to undermine the deeply entrenched hold such expectations have on people. Nor does it seem to matter that even the supposedly clear underlying biology that determines who is physically male and who is physically female is ambiguous and problematic.[3] There are many counter-examples to the prevailing gender norms (women who display rationality and men who display 'feminine' emotions). As well, gender norms are complicated by norms associated with other forms of difference that are salient in a society, such as those associated with race, ethnicity, socio-economic class, age, (dis)ability status and sexuality: the stereotypes assigned to a poor black man in the West are quite different from those attached to an affluent white one. Even though gender is a situated concept that varies according to many complicating social conditions, traditional gender expectations are resilient to all confounding evidence and continue to structure the ways in which humans treat one another and also the ways academics theorize. Feminism's project of naming and troubling gender assumptions (e.g. Little, 1996) has a valuable role to play within bioethics.

The pattern of neglecting or misrepresenting women has been pervasive in ethics as in other areas of inquiry. Within ethics, feminists have offered several inter-related critiques of traditional approaches to ethics. These critiques object to the fact that traditional ethics focuses on questions and methods that are of particular concern to men (interactions that occur among strangers within the public sphere) and it neglects or trivializes questions and methods that are typically associated with women (relations within the private sphere such as families and communities). Historically, ethical theorists commonly refused to recognize women as full moral agents and developed theoretical approaches to ethics that seemed designed to enforce this exclusion. Currently, no major ethical theorist explicitly denies moral agency to women, but many offer theories that have the implication that women do not fully measure up to their purported norms (Okin, 1989).

There are four main feminist responses to the exclusionary assumptions of traditional ethics. For convenience, I have assigned each a generic label, but it is important to note that these are neither discrete nor exhaustive categories; many feminists draw on more than one type of theory in particular aspects of their work and others do not fit eas-

---

[2]Other overviews of feminist bioethics, organized by different principles have been provided by Susan M. Wolf (1996) in her Introduction to Feminism & Bioethics, Rosemarie Tong (1997) and Anne Donchin (2004, 2006).

[3]Physical sex can be determined by genitalia, by chromosomes or by gonads, hormones or genes. Although in the majority of cases, these all cohere, in a significant minority of cases, there can be discrepancies among these different measures or ambiguity within one (notably genitalia). Such people are categorized as intersexed; others prefer to describe themselves as transsexuals when they feel their gender identity does not reflect their anatomical sex, or transgendered when they wish to claim an alternative gender for themselves.

ily within this taxonomy.[4] The four positions are: (1) liberal theorists whose central aim is to emphasize the facts about women's equal capabilities (relative to men's) to act as moral agents and, on this basis, to demand explicit inclusion and attention to gender equality; (2) care theorists whose followers believe that women approach ethics differently from men and insist on equal recognition for women's distinctive approach; (3) oppression theorists whose proponents focus on the political injustice of oppression and look for ways to modify the concepts and applications of traditional ethics to ensure recognition of this problem and redress for inequalities; and (4) continental and postmodern theorists whose proponents challenge both the underlying conceptual scheme of gender that rigidly dichotomizes the world into two categories and the effort to identify universal moral values, demanding more local, situated approaches to ethical problems. Each of these strategies has its counterpart within feminist approaches to bioethics.

LIBERAL FEMINISM

The earliest and still most popular efforts to correct ethical and political theories and practices that exclude women are ones that seek to have women recognized as morally equal to men and, therefore, entitled to equal consideration. In 1792, Mary Wollstonecraft published *A Vindication of the Rights of Women*, in which she accepted the Enlightenment view that moral status rests on the capacity of moral agents to reflect rationally and impartially and argued that women as well as men have this capacity. She espoused an egalitarian social philosophy that would guarantee the same rights and opportunities to women as to men, including the right to education. Wollstonecraft reasoned that if women were not hobbled by ignorance they would be able to demonstrate their equal moral and political worth and take their rightful place in a society that respected the individual rights of all its citizens. This theme was picked up by John Stuart Mill and Harriet Taylor Mill in Mill's 1869 book *On the Subjection of Women* and it has become so widely accepted in many parts of the world as to become mainstream thought. Gender equality is guaranteed under the constitution of many nations and is expressly supported by the United Nations Universal Declaration of Human Rights. The core idea of liberal feminism is that women and men are the same with respect to morally relevant characteristics, particularly reason. Whatever differences exist between the sexes have no moral significance and cannot serve as the basis for differential political, legal, or social rights.

Within ethics, the liberal defence of fundamental equality requires us to treat women and men as equally qualified moral agents entitled to comparable rights and responsibilities. It is reflected in the effort to use gender inclusive language ('he or she' rather than simply a supposedly generic 'he') and by demands for political equality. Within bioethics, it takes the form of efforts to avoid gender stereotypes in the construction of cases and to find ways of ensuring that medical interventions do not actively discriminate against women (e.g. through the widespread use of selective abortion to terminate the lives of female foetuses).

Issues of particular relevance to women, such as those concerning reproduction and, especially, abortion, are addressed through a lens that tries to remove the gender disadvantage attached to mandatory pregnancy. Women's health activists generally rely on a liberal framework when they invoke freedom of choice in the campaign for access to safe, legal abortion services. For example, although Judith Jarvis Thomson's (1971) classic essay, 'A Defense of Abortion' did not use the term 'feminist', it made a powerful case for respecting women's property rights in their own bodies, showing that a state imposed duty to carry an unwanted pregnancy to term could only be defended if the state made comparable demands on all citizens to act to preserve human lives whenever they had the opportunity. While previously most authors treated pregnancy and hence abortion as unique phenomena, unlike any other human experience and, hence, subject to distinctive rules, Thomson's implicit commitment to gender equality allowed her to demonstrate that what is really at issue is the unacceptable role of the state in coercing one person to support the life of another.

Liberal feminist arguments are often found in other areas of reproductive ethics. For example, Bonnie Steinbock (1992, 2002) defends individual women's right to be free of legal prosecution for endangering their foetuses even through illegal drug use and the right of individual women to choose abortion even for the purposes of sex selection. Laura Purdy (1996) argues vigorously for women's right to choose in all aspects of reproduction, including participation in commercial surrogacy arrangements provided efforts are made to avoid exploitative contracts that undervalue the actual labour involved. Mary Mahowald (1992) seeks to improve equality in health care for women and children, though she often has to move beyond liberalism and into Marxist theory to make her case.

The arguments for equal worth and equal treatment have proven very powerful in the struggle for equal rights in health care as in other spheres. For example, the perspective of liberal feminism has allowed women to

---

[4]These are my own efforts at assigning labels, not the theorists' own description of their work; some would surely resist the reductionist implications of the labels I have assigned their work.

lobby effectively for equal access to medical training for women and other social minorities and to demand better representation among senior administrators, educators and funding agencies (Sherwin, 1992). Others have an impact on research practices by virtue of their objections to the under-representation of women in clinical research trials and the subsequent absence of data needed to properly manage women's health care (Dresser, 1992; Faden et al. 1996; Merton, 1996). Unfortunately the impact of equality arguments has proven limited, for there remain many significant aspects of inequality that continue to occur in health contexts despite widespread acceptance of the equality principle at the heart of liberal approaches.

ETHICS OF CARE

Some feminists actively resist the liberal move to understand gender equality as gender sameness. They believe that there are important differences between women and men that must be addressed. On this view, the difficulty with traditional approaches to ethics is not a failure to recognize that women can behave the same as men, but rather a failure to appreciate qualities that are particularly associated with women. These feminists seek to restore value to the traits and activities that are commonly found among women. They see the effort to stress sameness as requiring women to develop the skills and dispositions of men while devaluing their traditional roles. So, for example, sameness efforts typically minimize the importance of domestic sphere skills in favour of encouraging women to participate fully within the public sphere of work, politics, business, and so on. In contrast, difference theorists emphasize the value of abilities and activities traditionally assigned to women in connection with their responsibilities in the home. In particular, they urge celebration and appreciation of women's inclination towards nurturing behaviours. In the context of ethics, this takes the form of validating women's particular approach to moral reasoning – an approach that is identified by the label 'ethics of care'.

Although there are various ways of approaching an ethic of care, there are some features common to most versions, including the following beliefs: that women are more inclined to adopt such an approach than men; that we should abandon the project of reducing all of ethics to abstract, universal principles and make room for values such as love, trust, care, responsibility; that we need to attend to particular contextual details in our ethical reasoning; that ethics must account for the question of responsibilities to those who are dependent on others; and that there is moral importance in preserving relationships.

Although Carol Gilligan (1982) is a moral psychologist, not an ethicist, she is undoubtedly the most influential figure in the area of ethics of care. In her landmark 1982 book, *In a Different Voice: Psychological Theory and Women's Moral Development*, Gilligan put forward evidence that many women approach moral problems in a distinctly different way than men do. Where all the male subjects in her studies sought to resolve moral problems – both actual and hypothetical – through appeal to general, abstract rules (what she labelled 'an ethics of justice'), many of the female subjects focused on contextual details of the dilemmas they were asked to resolve. Frequently, the girls and women sought ways to modify the situation to preserve relationships and attend to the needs of all participants. Gilligan dubbed this alternative, feminine approach to moral reasoning, 'an ethics of care', though she also refers to it as an 'ethics of responsibility' since the problem of balancing responsibilities to self and others is often at the core of concerns she recorded. Gilligan argued that a competent moral agent should be skilled in both approaches and able to switch between an ethics of justice and one of care according to the circumstances occasioning moral deliberation. Other care theorists (e.g. Nel Noddings, 1984) have proposed that care ethics is superior to traditional ethics and ought to supplant it as the primary mode of moral reasoning. Some theorists have proposed that we go further in promoting a female-inspired ethics and make maternal–child relationships a moral paradigm instead of the mainstream orientation to basing ethics on interactions among strangers (e.g. Held, 1993; Ruddick, 1989).

Joan Tronto (1993) has proposed an important variation on the ethics of care, arguing that questions concerning the responsibility for attending to the human needs among us should be placed at the centre of our moral and political thinking rather than relegated to some other discipline or left at the margins of ethics. She proposes that we identify four distinct phases of caring: caring about (recognizing that someone is in need of care), taking care of (assuming responsibility for delivering needed care), care-giving (doing the hands-on labour of providing care) and care-receiving (acknowledging that care has been received and giving feedback as to whether it is adequate to the need). To be effective and morally sound, these four phases must all be valued (although at present, the latter two are devalued) and integrated. Although Tronto offers a promising picture for a practical feminist bioethics, no one has yet worked out how to operationalize her theory within the context of health care.

The value of some version or other of an ethics of care has been particularly welcomed by those working in traditionally female fields such as nursing (Nelson, 1992; Noddings, 1992). Its focus on contextual details with particular attention to the needs of participants has also been seen as especially valuable in the context of clinical bioethics, where the task is to determine the right way to proceed with specific patients rather than to determine general policies to be applied universally. Many feminists find that it captures more accurately the complexities of women's deliberations regarding matters of procreation than does an ethics of justice, since women often feel the multiple layers of responsibility facing them in deciding if they can support a (nother) child or one with special needs. (Interestingly, much of Gilligan's original research involved interviews with pregnant women contemplating abortion.)

The attention to care for people who are dependent in some ways has led to important feminist work on caring for people with particular needs. For example, Jennifer Parks (2003) explores ethical issues in home care. Other theorists take on questions concerning our treatment of people with disabilities and the ways in which medicine and philosophy presuppose that everyone prefers to live independently (e.g. Parens and Asch, 2000; Silvers et al. 1999).

Attention to relationships requires us to pay attention to the importance of trust. Annette Baier (1986) first put these concepts on the map of feminist ethics in her important paper titled 'Trust and Anti-Trust'. Some feminist bioethicists (e.g. C. McLeod, 2002) have taken up the issue in exploring the role of trust and self-trust in interactions between patients and their doctors.

Finally, a number of feminist theorists have adopted aspects of care ethics, including its commitment to attending to relationships, in efforts to reinterpret key ethical concepts, especially personhood and autonomy in relational ways rather than purely abstract ways. See, for example, Donchin (1995), Dodds (2000), Mackenzie & Stoljar (2000) and Sherwin (2003).

OPPRESSION THEORISTS

Although all feminists share liberal feminists' goal for equality between men and women, and most share care theorists' appreciation of the limits of relying on a purely abstract ethics of justice approach to moral deliberation, some believe that it is a mistake to focus primarily on the situation of individuals and to rely on an ethics that valorizes women's socialization to nurturing behaviour as a response to systemic inequality. Many feminists understand inequality to be a problem between social groups, not just the individual members of each group. They see systematic patterns of discrimination affecting many different dimensions of society – from the private, domestic sphere to the economic sphere, the world of law and politics, religion and even academic research. Sexism, or male domination, involves greater power attached to males than to females in multiple areas of life, just as racism involves differential access to power and privilege based on racial categorization, ablism reflects the systemic disadvantage experienced by people with disabilities, and heterosexism captures the privilege available to those who identify and live as heterosexuals. These power differentials can only be appreciated if we

see them as affecting social groups, not just the individual members who make up a social group. For any particular woman, it is usually possible to find a man who is more disadvantaged than she – in most cases, because he belongs to another disadvantaged social group (e.g. a racial minority). What is problematic is how women (racial minorities, people with disabilities, non-heterosexuals) generally are likely to be disadvantaged relative to comparable men (or members of relevant privileged groups).

Such systematic bias is commonly referred to as 'oppression'. Iris Marion Young (1990) has explicated this concept by identifying five different varieties ('faces') of harm that oppression might take: exploitation, marginalization, cultural imperialism, violence and powerlessness. Indeed, some of these harms can only be calculated at the level of groups. For example, under cultural imperialism the dominant group controls key tools of culture formation and the experiences of oppressed minorities are either ignored or misleadingly represented through pejorative stereotypes. This phenomenon does not make sense at the level of the individual: it refers to ways in which one group represents another *as a group* – individuals are affected only when assumptions are made about their character or abilities based on stereotypical norms for the group. Cultural imperialism is problematic because it shapes false cultural beliefs about the character, activities and value of members of both groups.

Other types of group harms such as violence, exploitation or powerlessness, can be understood when they apply to individuals, but they assume a different meaning when they occur in the context of group oppression. For example, gender is a causal factor in many attacks against women (especially, but not solely, sexual assaults), as race often is in attacks against blacks, and sexuality is in attacks against gay men. If we look only at the particular harms of a series of attacks on individuals, we may record the suffering of the victims and their loved ones, but we will not see how each one connects with other gender or race or sexuality-based violence to diminish the opportunities and social status of women, racial minorities and homosexuals. That is why hate crimes are particularly insidious even though the impact on the individual victims may be quite analogous to the impact of a comparable attack precipitated by 'personal' reasons.

Feminists who focus on patterns of oppression do not believe that these systematic forms of group-based practices can be fully appreciated or corrected by insisting on the equality of all individuals without attending to harms that operate on the level of groups. Thus, they find the strategies of liberal feminism insufficient to capture their concerns. They also worry that the approach of care ethics may serve to reinforce the social conditioning of women that seems to support their continued participation in oppressive social practices. Insofar as Tronto's political version of care ethics promises to illuminate systemic patterns of discrimination, it seems to fit more closely within the category of oppression oriented feminism.

Feminists such as Morgan (1991) and Sherwin (1992, 1998) who seek to place oppression (or group-based power differentials) firmly on the agenda of ethics propose that we expand our list of ethical concerns to ensure that we always interrogate practices or policies to determine how each contributes to existing patterns of oppression, especially as they affect women: does it worsen or exacerbate current inequalities? Is it likely to improve the situation? Or is it neutral with respect to social group differences? As well, we need to ask whether there are alternative practices or policies we might adopt that would make a larger contribution to reducing social inequalities. Some feminists direct us to look at particular groups of women who are vulnerable to specific types of oppression. For example, Abby Wilkerson (1998) focuses on health experiences of lesbians, Dorothy Roberts (1996) addresses the lives of women of colour, Christine Overall (2003) explores attitudes about ageing women and Shelley Tremain (1999) examines the situation of women with disabilities.

In the context of bioethics, this approach leads to several important innovations. It directs us to rethink the traditional subject matter of bioethics and explore the role that gender (and/or race, class, disability, etc.) might play in our analysis. For example, when reflecting on moral questions regarding reproduction, we need to consider how different policies might affect the status of oppressed social groups. If we consider the impact of various approaches to assisted human reproduction on women and children, we have reason to be concerned about the ways in which increased effort to ensure the birth of children with a genetic connection to their social parents reinforces social norms about the importance of biological reproduction in every woman's life. Feminists also question the implication that different values are attached to different lives under a social policy that encourages some couples to spend huge sums of money to produce a child when so many children lack provision for even their basic needs. On a related front, where other bioethicists worry about the moral legitimacy of embryonic stem cell research because such research results in the death of the embryo, feminist theorists are concerned that the embryos in question can only be produced in the first place through eggs collected from women in risky procedures and often under conditions of duress. Feminists also note that other forms of embryo research are aimed at finding ways of manipulating the genetic material to facilitate enhancement of desired traits and avoidance of 'undesired' traits, particularly those experienced by people with disabilities.

Oppression-based theorists have also sought to expand the scope of bioethics. They have insisted that the domain of research ethics move beyond questions of informed consent and protection of human subjects to include discussion of the ethics of the systematic exclusion of women from many clinical trials, and to moral evaluation of the research agenda itself (Baylis et al. 1998). Some feminists have challenged the role of medicine in setting norms for sexual behaviours and turning some sexual activities into pathologies (Wilkerson, 1998). They note that medicine's efforts to treat homosexuality as a disease in need of cure is a way of regulating sexual conduct and reinforcing heterosexual norms, along with the gender stereotypes they support. Others have challenged mainstream bioethics approaches to questions of resource allocation in health care, objecting that a focus on distributive justice without attending to matters of social justice simply repeats existing patterns of inequity (Nelson and Nelson, 1996).

CONTINENTAL AND POSTMODERN FEMINISMS

Some feminists are sceptical of all of the approaches reviewed above. Some, such as Mary Rawlinson (2001), situate their work in the Continental tradition of philosophy and adapt insights from such influential theorists as Foucault, Derrida or Irigrary, focusing on the masculinist bias within language itself and the influence it has on medical thinking. Others, such as Janet Farrell Smith (1996), are inspired by Jurgen Habermas's communicative ethics and its explanatory power for feminist bioethics.

Margrit Shildrick (1997) represents the approach of theorists who adopt a postmodern orientation that objects to all efforts that directly or implicitly accept gender as a clearly defined, universal boundary. Because gender falsely divides humanity into two distinct groups, we should not strive for gender equality; rather we need to emphasize the distortions inherent in all concepts that refer to politically salient categories of human difference. Shildrick argues that theories that ignore important bodily differences assume the traditional paradigm (male, white, free of disability) as the norm, or ideal, and implicitly treat all bodily differences from that norm as inferior. To uncover the inherent sexism and other biases within bioethics (and, more deeply, within ethics, political theory and epistemology), it is essential to deconstruct common assumptions and to resist efforts to make de-contextualized universal claims. Universalizing theories are inevitably exclusionary of some and unstable; as such, they are misguided. In their place, she proposes 'an ethic in which differences are acknowledged, respected and allowed to flourish as the very basis of moral discourse' (Shildrick, 1997, p. 6). In other words, bioethics must begin with the embodied experiences of patients so that it can explore the social and ethical meaning of their needs for health care. Like theorists from all traditions, postmodern feminists seek to build a feminist bioethics that is inclusive rather than exclusionary and is able to value women without making essentialist assumptions.

CONCLUSION

Rough and imprecise as they are, these four major categories of feminist approaches to bioethics provide a framework for seeing how different insights guide feminist work in bioethics. Although they do not divide the world of feminist bioethicists neatly or accurately – many (perhaps most) feminist theorists and activists draw on more than one conception in different aspects of their work – they allow us to see some of the major themes played out in the work of feminist bioethicists to date. Other taxonomies would allow us to see how different feminist theorists approach specific topics in bioethics such as euthanasia, competency, allocation of resources, reproduction and so on. I suggest that what can be seen as common among all feminist contributions to bioethics is an appreciation of the fact that no matter what the topic, it is always worth asking the core feminist question: what does this question/practice/policy mean for women and for other minorities?

REFERENCES

Baier AC. Trust and antitrust. *Ethics* 1986; **96**: 231–60.

Baylis F, Downie J, Sherwin S. Reframing Research Involving Humans. *The Politics of Women's Health*, 1998.

Dodds S. Choice and control in feminist bioethics. In: Mackenzie C, Stoljar N, eds. *Relational Autonomy*, 2000.

Donchin A. Reworking autonomy: toward a feminist perspective. *Camb Q Health Care Ethics* 1995; **4**(1): 44–55.

Donchin A. Feminist bioethics. In: Zalta EN, ed. *The Stanford Encyclopedia of Philosophy*, 2006 edition, 2004 (URL: http://plato.stanford.edu/entries/feminist-bioethics/).

Dresser R. Wanted: single, white male for medical research. *Hastings Center Rep* 1992; **22**(1): 24–9.

Faden R, Kass N, McGraw D. Women as vessels and vectors: lessons from the HIV epidemic. In: Wolf SM, ed. *Feminism & Bioethics: Beyond Reproduction*. Oxford: Oxford University Press, 1996.

Gilligan C. *In a Different Voice: Psychological Theory and Women's Moral Development*. Cambridge MA: Harvard University Press, 1982.

Held V. *Feminist Morality: Transforming Culture, Society, and Politics*. Chicago: University of Chicago Press, 1993.

Little MO. Why a feminist approach to bioethics? *Kennedy Inst Ethics J* 1996; **6**(1): 1–18.

Mackenzie C, Stoljar N, eds. *Relational Autonomy: Feminist Perspectives on Autonomy, Agency, and the Social Self*. Oxford: Oxford University Press, 2000.

Mahowald M. *Women and Children in Health Care: An Unequal Majority*. Oxford: Oxford University Press, 1992.

McLeod C. *Self-Trust and Reproductive Autonomy*. Cambridge, MA: MIT Press, 2002.

Merton V. Ethical obstacles to women in biomedical research. In: Wolf SM, ed. *Feminism & Bioethics*, 1996.

Morgan KP. Women and the knife: cosmetic surgery and the colonization of women's bodies. *Hypatia* 1991; **6**(3): 25–53.

Nelson HL. Against caring. *J Clin Ethics* 1992; **3**(1): 8–15.

Nelson HL, Nelson JL. Justice in the allocation of health care resources: a feminist account. In: Wolf S, ed. *Feminism & Bioethics*, 1996.

Noddings N. *Caring: A Feminine Approach to Ethics and Moral Education*. Berkeley: University of California Press, 1984.

Noddings N. In defense of caring. *J Clin Ethics* 1992; **3**(1): 15–8.

Norsigian J, Diskin V, Doress-Worters P, Pincus J, Sunford W, Suenson N. The Boston women's health group collective and *our bodies, ourselves*: a brief history and reflection, *JAMWA* 1999; **54**(1): 35–9.

Okin SM. *Gender, Justice and the Family*. New York: Basic Books 1989.

Overall C. *Aging, Death, and Human Longevity: A Philosophical Inquiry*, Berkeley: University of California Press, 2003.

Parens E, Asch A, eds. *Prenatal Testing and Disability Rights*. Washington D.C.: Georgetown University Press, 2000.

Parks JA. *No Place Like Home: Feminist Ethics and Home Health Care*. Bloomington: Indiana University Press, 2003.

Purdy LM. *Reproducing Persons: Issues in Feminist Bioethics*. Ithaca, NY: Cornell University Press, 1996.

Rawlinson M. The concept of a feminist bioethics. *J Med Philos* 2001; **26**(4): 405–16.

Roberts DE. Reconstructing the patient: starting with women of color. In: Wolf S, ed. *Feminism & Bioethics*, 1996.

Ruddick S. *Maternal Thinking: Toward a Politics of Peace*. Boston: Beacon Press, 1989.

Sherwin S. *No Longer Patient: Feminist Ethics and Health Care*. Philadelphia, PA: Temple University Press, 1992.

Sherwin S. Coordinator, Canadian Health Care Ethics Research Network. *The Politics of Women's Health: Exploring Agency and Autonomy*. Philadelphia PA: Temple University Press, 1998.

Sherwin S. The importance of ontology for feminist policy-making in the realm of reproductive technology. *Can J Philos* 2003; **26**: 273–95.

Shildrick M. *Leaky Bodies and Boundaries: Feminism, Postmodernism and (Bio)ethics*. London: Routledge, 1997.

Silvers A, Wasserman D, Mahowald MB. In: *Difference, Discrimination: Perspectives on Justice in Bioethics and Public Policy*. Lanham, MD: Rowman & Littlefield, 1999.

Smith JF. Communicative ethics in medicine: the physician-patient relationship. In S Wolf, ed. *Feminism & Bioethics*, 1996.

Steinbock B. The relevance of illegality. *Hastings Center Rep* 1992; **2**(1): 19–22.

Steinbock B. Sex selection: not obviously wrong. *Hastings Center Rep* 2002; **32**(1): 23–28.

Thomson JJ. A Defense of abortion. *Philos Public Aff* 1971; **1** (1): 47–66.

Tong R. *Feminist Approaches to Bioethics: Theoretical Reflections and Practical Applications*. Boulder, CO: Westview Press, 1997.

Tremain S, ed. *Bodies of Knowledge: Critical Perspectives on Disablement and Disabled Women*. Toronto: Women's Press, 1999.

Tronto J. *Moral Boundaries: A Political Argument for and Ethic of Care*. New York: Routledge, 1993.

Wilkerson AL. *Diagnosis Difference: The Moral Authority of Medicine*. Ithaca NY: Cornell University Press, 1998.

Wolf SM, ed. *Feminism & Bioethics: Beyond Reproduction*. Oxford: Oxford University Press, 1996.

Young IM. *Justice and the Politics of Difference*. Princeton: Princeton University Press, 1990.

12

Virtue Theory

JUSTIN OAKLEY

A perfectly natural way of expressing our admiration or condemnation for what someone did is by asking, 'What sort of person would do a thing like that?' Going out of one's way to help a needy stranger can be regarded not simply as providing help but as acting generously, and overcoming fearsome obstacles to attain an important goal can be seen not just as displaying strength of will but as acting courageously. Similarly, adverse judgements of how someone acted can express a kind of bewilderment not only at harm done or at any rights that may have been violated, but also at the sort of person who would do such a thing. For example, inflicting suffering upon someone in certain circumstances can be regarded as malevolent or malicious, in addition to being harmful or disrespectful. An important feature of act evaluations like generous, courageous, malevolent and malicious is that they necessarily make reference to the character or dispositions that determines the person's action. Virtue Theory – or Virtue Ethics, as it is more often called – is an approach to ethics that picks up on these common ways of judging actions. It holds that actions cannot be properly judged as right or wrong without reference to the character of an agent.

Virtue ethics draws inspiration from the ideas of ancient Greek philosophers such as Aristotle, who regarded ethics as essentially about what is a good life for human beings, and what sort of person one needs to become to live such a life. Many of these ideas had an enduring impact on the Western philosophical tradition, but they fell from favour in the late eighteenth and early nineteenth centuries due to the growing influence of both rights-based and utilitarian approaches to ethics, among other things. However, dissatisfaction with those approaches in the closing decades of the twentieth century has prompted a reconsideration of virtue-based perspectives on ethics, and there is currently much exciting work being done in developing virtue ethics and its applications to a variety of practical questions.

THE NATURE OF VIRTUE ETHICS

Virtue ethics can be used to evaluate actions, emotions, and persons and their lives. Much contemporary discussion of virtue ethics focuses on its approach to the evaluation of *actions*. The virtue ethics criterion of right action can be stated broadly as follows:

> **V**: An action is right if and only if it is what an agent with a virtuous character would do in the circumstances.

Because virtue ethics regards a right action as one that a virtuous person would do in certain circumstances; it makes reference to character essential in the justification of right action (Hursthouse, 1999, pp. 28–31; Oakley and Cocking, 2001, pp. 9–15). For example, it is right to save a wounded stranger by the roadside (whether or not he has a right to your help), because that is what a person with the virtue of benevolence would do. And it is ordinarily right to keep a promise made to someone on their deathbed, even though living people would benefit from its being broken, because that is what a person with the virtue of justice would do (Hursthouse, 1999, p. 36; 1996, p. 25; Foot 1977, p. 106). Of course, the formulation of the virtue ethics criterion of right action in **V** above is very general, and if the approach is to be used to guide and justify actions, this criterion clearly needs to be supplemented by an account of *which* character-traits are virtues. Nevertheless, this bare formulation already reveals a key difference between virtue ethics and standard forms of Kantian and Utilitarian approaches to ethics, whereby the rightness of an act is determined by whether the act is in accordance with certain rules or by whether it maximizes expected utility. Neither of these approaches, as standardly defined, makes reference to character essential to the justification of right action.

Principles of Health Care Ethics, Second Edition   Edited by R.E. Ashcroft, A. Dawson, H. Draper and J.R. McMillan
© 2007 John Wiley & Sons, Ltd

Before explaining in more detail the sort of character that a virtuous agent in **V** would have, we need to clarify how the virtue ethics criterion of right action is to be used in evaluating actions. For as it stands, **V** could be interpreted as stating a purely *external* criterion of right action, which could be met whatever one's motives or dispositions, so long as one has a good idea of what a virtuous agent would do in particular circumstances. Or **V** could be taken as incorporating certain *internal* requirements, whereby one acts rightly only if one acts from the kinds of motives and dispositions that a virtuous agent would act from in the circumstances. What the examples mentioned so far may not make sufficiently apparent is that the virtue ethics criterion of right action is to be interpreted in the second of these ways – that is, doing what the virtuous agent would do involves not merely the performance of certain acts, but acting from certain dispositions and (in many cases) certain motives. For example, acting as someone with the virtue of benevolence would act not only involves providing assistance to another but also includes having and acting from a genuine concern for the well-being of that person and a disposition to have and act from that concern in particular kinds of situations. As Aristotle (1980, VI, 13, 1144b26–6) put it, 'It is not merely the state in accordance with the right rule, but the state that implies the *presence* of the right rule, that is virtue'. Acting as the virtuous agent would act typically involves acting from certain motives, though with the virtue of justice one can act justly from a variety of motives, so long as one acts from a *disposition* that incorporates an appropriate sense of justice. Indeed, every virtue embodies what might be called a *regulative ideal*, involving the internalization of a certain conception of excellence such that one is able to adjust one's motivation and conduct so that they conform to that standard. Thus, while most but not all virtues are motive-dependent, all virtues involve regulative ideals and so include internal requirements of some kind.

Indeed, a striking difference between virtue ethics and standard Utilitarian and Kantian ethical theories is the close connection made by virtue ethics between motive and rightness. Most forms of Utilitarianism and Kantianism which go beyond mere theoretical possibilities hold that, generally speaking, one can act rightly whatever one's motivation – so long as one maximizes expected utility or acts in accordance with duty, one has done the right thing, whether one's motives were praiseworthy, reprehensible or neutral. As we have seen, however, virtue ethics holds that acting rightly, in many situations, requires acting from a particular sort of motivation because this is part of what is involved in doing what a virtuous person would do in the circumstances. Apart from its historical links with Aristotle's ethics, this strong connection between motive and rightness has considerable intuitive plausibility. Many people believe, for example, that the rightness of giving a gift to a friend depends partly on whether one acts from motives appropriate to the occasion, like affection and friendly feeling – giving out of a sense of duty may not actually be the right thing to do here. This is not to say that virtue ethics takes the rightness of an act to depend *entirely* on its motivation (though some philosophers [e.g. Slote, 2001] have recently argued that the approach is most plausibly developed along such lines). For most virtue ethicists would regard an act that is well-motivated but fails to uphold the regulative ideal relevant to a particular virtue as an act that does not meet the criterion of right action stated in **V**.

Another key difference between virtue ethics and classical forms of Utilitarianism is that many contemporary exponents of virtue ethics argue that virtues are intrinsic goods which are plural, and so the goodness of the virtues cannot be reduced to a single underlying value, such as utility (see Oakley 1996). The goodness of integrity, for example, does not consist simply in the utility (e.g. pleasure) that the agent or others gain from this. (This irreducible plurality of the virtues is not incompatible with the notion of an underlying unity of the virtues, a concept held by many ancient Greek philosophers; however, many modern virtue ethicists reject suggestions of a unity between the different virtues.) This commitment to evaluative pluralism can in certain circumstances make it difficult to determine what ought to be done. What if, for instance, the honest thing to do seems to conflict with the kind thing to do, as when a friend asks you whether his wife is having an affair, and you happen to know that she is? Hursthouse (1991, p. 231) argues that 'someone hesitating over whether to reveal a hurtful truth..., thinking it would be kind but dishonest or unjust to lie, may need to realize, with respect to these particular circumstances, not that kindness is more (or is less) important than honesty or justice, and not that honesty or justice sometimes requires one to act unkindly or cruelly, but that one does people no kindness by concealing this sort of truth from them, hurtful though it may be'. Further, in cases of genuine conflict between two virtues where, for instance, kindness does seem to demand dishonesty or where honesty would be unkind, virtue ethics can allow that acting in accordance with either of these virtues may be right. For it recognizes that there can be circumstances where not all virtuous people (acting in character) would necessarily act in the same way. The evaluative pluralism of contemporary virtue ethics acknowledges that determining what is right can involve taking account of competing ethical considerations, and looking towards what a moral exemplar would do can be particularly instructive here, for an exemplar has taken account of the competing considerations and reached an all things considered judgement about what is to be done.

Thus, the appeal to what a virtuous agent would do not only emphasizes the importance of motivation in right action, but also acknowledges how exemplars can point the way to sound ethical judgement in circumstances where the plural values that are the virtues conflict.

However, it should be acknowledged that some contemporary variants of Kantian and Utilitarian approaches have suggested that reference to character could play an essential role in justifying actions. For example, Barbara Herman (1993) has argued that the rightness of an act could be determined by reference to whether a good Kantian agent, whose character is regulated by a commitment to not acting impermissibly, would have performed such an act. And some utilitarians have argued that to act rightly is to act as the good Utilitarian agent would, where such an agent is disposed to follow rules or to have aversions or inclinations towards act-types that – when followed or had by people generally – maximize expected utility (see e.g. Brandt, 1989). Sometimes these suggestions are put simply as theoretical possibilities, rather than fully worked out ethical theories, with their implications for practice traced out. Nevertheless, distinguishing virtue ethics from these contemporary versions of Kantian and Utilitarian views requires filling in the details about what character-traits count as virtues. So, just as Kantians and Utilitarians need to detail their general criteria of rightness by specifying what rules we are to act in accordance with, or what expected utility consists in, virtue ethicists must likewise provide details about what the virtues are. For virtue ethics to be capable of guiding action, the criterion of right action in **V** needs to be completed with an account of the virtues.

Broadly speaking, virtue ethicists take one of the following two approaches to specifying and grounding the character-traits that a virtuous agent would have. The majority of virtue ethicists take the Aristotelian view that the virtues are character-traits that we need to have in order to live flourishing human lives (see Foot, 1978; Hursthouse, 1999). Character-traits such as benevolence, courage and justice count as virtues on this approach because an individual cannot flourish as a human being without having such traits. According to Aristotle, what counts as a good human life is determined by what sort of creatures we are, by what it is in our nature to be and to do. Aristotle believes that the characteristic activity of human beings is the exercise of our rational capacity, and he argues that only by living virtuously is our rational capacity to guide our lives expressed in an excellent way. There is a sense, then, in which someone lacking the virtues would not be living a *human* life. So, virtuous character-traits form part of an interlocking web of intrinsic goods, which includes other goods such as friendship and knowledge, and these intrinsic goods when governed by the central virtue of practical wisdom (or *phronesis*) are

together constitutive of *eudaimonia*, a happy or flourishing life for human beings. Thus, for example, friendship is a necessary part of *eudaimonia* because humans are naturally social creatures, and because without friendship it is difficult, if not impossible, to have adequate knowledge of oneself (see Aristole, 1980, XI 9)). Other Aristotelian virtues include integrity, temperance, pride and magnanimity.

However, some virtue ethicists reject the Aristotelian claim that the virtues are given by what humans need in order to flourish. For example, Michael Slote (1992) has argued that the virtues are to be derived from common-sense views about what character-traits we typically find admirable – as exemplified in the lives of figures such as Albert Einstein and Mother Teresa – whether or not those traits help the individual who has them to flourish in Aristotle's sense. And, drawing on Nietzsche and other philosophers, Christine Swanton (2003) argues that virtues are dispositions to respond to morally significant features of objects in an excellent way, whether or not such dispositions are good *for* the person who has them. For example, a great artist's creative drive can be a virtue, Swanton (2003, p. 82–3) argues, even if this drive leads the artist to suffer bipolar disorder – such an artist's creative drive need not bring about a flourishing life, but it is nevertheless an excellent way of responding to value, and can certainly result in a life that is justifiably regarded as successful in some sense (even if only posthumously).

APPLICATIONS OF VIRTUE ETHICS

One area where Aristotelian virtue ethics has a natural application is in professional roles. In ordinary life the character-traits that qualify as virtues are given by their connections with *eudaimonia*, the overarching goal of a good human life. The virtues in various professional contexts can be derived through a similar teleological structure. For example, *health* is clearly a central goal of medicine, and which of a doctor's character-traits count as professional virtues are those which help the doctor serve the goal of patient health. For example, medical beneficence would qualify as a virtue, as it focuses doctors on patients' own interests and curbs a tendency towards the unnecessary interventions in defensive medicine. Similarly, trustworthiness helps with effective diagnosis and treatment by helping patients feel comfortable about revealing intimate details about themselves, and medical courage helps doctors work towards healing patients by facing risks of infection when necessary (Oakley & Cocking, 2001, p. 93).

Likewise, an account of the virtues in legal practice can be given by considering which character-traits help lawyers serve the central legal goal of justice (of some kind). On this approach, traits which are vices in ordinary life, such as callousness and moral indifference to others' shortcomings, could be regarded as virtues in, say, a criminal defence lawyer working within an adversarial system. In highlighting the links between virtuous character-traits and the proper goal(s) of the profession in question, virtue ethics also takes seriously the notion of professional integrity. That is, where a patient autonomously requests a doctor to perform a procedure that is irreconcilable with the medical goal of serving patient health, a virtuous doctor can justifiably refuse to comply with this request. A doctor in this situation could legitimately tell the patient 'I cannot with my doctor's hat on do this for you'. This sort of refusal is distinct from a refusal based on conscientious objection, which makes no necessary reference to the proper goals of the profession. The moral relevance of the goals of a profession to evaluating the conduct of individual professionals is also apparent when those goals are contravened. So, for example, one acts wrongly in torturing another, but it is even worse for a *doctor* to torture another person – doctors profess to be healers, and torturing is the opposite of healing.

Professional roles also provide an interesting context in which to study the implications for virtue ethics of research in social psychology suggesting that the variations in behaviour displayed by different individuals in a given context may be better explained by minor situational variations, than by the assumptions we commonly make about differences in character-traits between those individuals (see Doris, 1998; 2002). For despite the role that situational factors may play in explaining why some individuals and not others act corruptly in certain professional contexts, the actions of whistleblowers suggests that the character of at least some professionals can be a powerful determinant of beneficent actions and leads them to persist in the face of significant situational obstacles and personal risks. So while research into situational influences on helping actions and other behaviour might indicate that truly virtuous actions are less common than we might like to think, acting from appropriate professional virtues may not be an unattainable ideal.

Virtue ethics has also been applied in illuminating ways in analysing the morality of abortion and euthanasia. Philippa Foot (1977) argues that death is a good to the person who dies, not merely when they want to die, but when their life lacks a minimum of basic human goods, such as autonomy, friendship and moral support. Foot then argues that where a competent individual in such circumstances requests assistance in dying, fulfilling this request is consistent with the virtues of both justice and charity. A virtue ethics approach to euthanasia would also emphasize the importance of a sympathetic and supportive doctor–patient relationship, which many patients requesting euthanasia (in countries where this practice is legally available) say they value highly (see van der Maas et al. 1991, p. 673).

Rosalind Hursthouse's virtue ethics analysis of the morality of abortion also sheds new light on the issues there. Hursthouse (1987; 1991) argues that the morality of abortion is fundamentally a matter of the motivation and character expressed by the woman seeking abortion, rather than about the competing rights of the mother and her foetus. Noticing that people can exercise their rights virtuously or viciously, Hursthouse argues that an adolescent girl requesting an abortion may be showing an appropriate humility about her current level of development, whereas a woman seeking a late abortion on frivolous grounds may show herself as self-centred and callous (see Oakley 1998).

Virtue ethics could also provide an interesting perspective on various issues in research ethics. For example, an important current concern in the ethical oversight of research on humans is the problem of researcher conflict of interest. Some medical researchers have ties to the pharmaceutical companies that often sponsor such research, and questions sometimes arise about whether decisions made by researchers with such links might compromise the protection of research subjects. Although there may be no rights violated or harm done to subjects, conflicts of interest are nevertheless ethically problematic because they involve researchers being guided by values that are inappropriate to their role. A virtue-based approach to research ethics could bring out the wrongness of conflicts of interest by providing an account of the proper goals of research as an activity and of what character-traits in researchers enable them to serve those goals.

OBJECTIONS TO VIRTUE ETHICS

Some object to virtue ethics on the grounds that it is too vague to guide action or that virtuous agents can sometimes do terrible things. The vagueness worry seems to be raised less often now, in light of the detail that virtue ethicists often provide about what the virtues are and how they would apply in a given situation. It is interesting to consider whether truly virtuous agents really can act wrongly. Sometimes the examples used in support of this claim involve agents who act wrongly precisely because they are deficient in the relevant virtue, or they lack another virtue which the situation warrants. Alternatively, the actions of virtuous agents can indeed bring about bad consequences, but where this is due to such agents having nonculpably false beliefs, it is far from clear that the agent acted wrongly here. Few ethical theories would charge an agent with having acted wrongly in circumstances where a well-motivated action results in bad consequences which were unforeseeable at the time the agent acted.

A more recent objection to virtue ethics is the worry that it rests on a questionable kind of subjectivism about value. That is, the virtue ethics criterion of right action in V could be taken as suggesting that value cannot be specified independently of the virtuous agent. Virtue ethics seems to imply that something *becomes* valuable because it is what the virtuous agent would do, whereas it seems more plausible to regard agents as virtuous because they are people who are appropriately responsive to what is independently valuable (see Baron et al. 1997, p. 139; Hurka, 2001; Darwall, 2005). However, this objection seems to arise from a misunderstanding of Aristotelian virtue ethics. The character-traits that count as virtues, on this approach, are those that enable us to live a humanly flourishing life. It is this latter notion that confers value on some character-traits over others. We cannot live a flourishing life without the virtues, but the notion of a flourishing life is the basis of the virtues. In this respect, virtue ethics has an analogous justificatory structure to rule-utilitarianism. Virtues justify actions in the same way that the rules of rule-utilitarianism justify actions. But in neither case is this some sort of ethical primitive, without a further justificatory basis. Yet while there is a further justificatory basis, in neither rule-utilitarianism nor virtue ethics is it possible to connect the underlying justificatory basis (maximizing utility; or human flourishing) directly with right action – the connection is given through the rules (in rule-utilitarianism) and the virtues (in virtue ethics).

CONCLUSION

Although some theorists have responded to recent objections by suggesting certain modifications to the virtue ethics criterion of right action, there is considerable consensus among contemporary virtue ethicists that **V**, or something very similar, can provide a distinctive and compelling standard for evaluating how we act, and offers an illuminating alternative to Kantian and Utilitarian theories. It has been customary to introduce virtue ethics by saying that it has revived an ancient approach to ethics. But if recent and ongoing work on this approach is anything to go by, virtue ethics is not only alive and well but has a very bright future.

REFERENCES

Aristotle. *The Nicomachean Ethics* (Ross WD, translator). Oxford: Oxford University Press, 1980.

Baron M, Pettit P, Slote M. *Three Methods of Ethics: A Debate.* Oxford: Blackwell, 1997.

Brandt R. Morality and its critics. *Am Philos Q* 1989; 26.

Darwall S. Critical notice of virtue ethics: a pluralistic view (by Christine Swanton), *Australas J Philos* 2005; **83**: 589–97.

Doris JM. *Lack of Character: Personality and Moral Behaviour.* New York: Cambridge University Press, 2002.

Doris, John M. Persons, situations, and virtue ethics. *Nous* 1998; **32**: 504–30.

Foot P. Euthanasia. *Philos Public Aff* 1977; **6**: 85–112.

Foot P. *Virtues and Vices.* Berkeley: University of California Press, 1978.

Herman B. *The Practice of Moral Judgment,* Cambridge, MA: Harvard University Press, 1993.

Hurka T. *Virtue, Vice, and Value.* Oxford: Oxford University Press, 2001.

Hursthouse R. *Beginning Lives.* Oxford: Blackwell, 1987.

Hursthouse R. Normative virtue ethics. In: Crisp R, ed. How Should One Live? *Essays on the Virtues.* Oxford: Clarendon Press, 1996.

Hursthouse R. *On Virtue Ethics,* Oxford: Oxford University Press, 1999.

Hursthouse R. Virtue theory and abortion. *Philos Public Aff* 1991; **20**: 223–46.

Oakley J, Cocking D. *Virtue Ethics and Professional Roles.* Cambridge: Cambridge University Press, 2001.

Oakley J. A virtue ethics approach. In: Kuhse H, Singer P, eds. *A Companion to Bioethics.* Oxford: Blackwell, 1998.

Oakley J. Varieties of virtue ethics. *Ratio* 1996; **9**: 128–52.

Slote M. *From Morality to Virtue.* New York: Oxford University Press, 1992.

Slote M. *Morals from Motives.* Oxford: Oxford University Press, 2001.

Swanton C. *Virtue Ethics, A Pluralistic View.* Oxford: Oxford University Press, 2003.

van der Maas PI, van Delden JJ, Pijnenborg L, Looman, CW (1991) Euthanasia and other medical decisions concerning the end of life. *Lancet* 1991; **338**: 669–74.

13

Moral Relativism

MARK SHEEHAN

People do things differently: they live their lives differently, they care about different things and most importantly they differ about what things count as right and wrong, permissible and impermissible. Moral relativists think that we observe something important about the nature of morality when we see these differences and the disagreement they often precipitate. Most commonly moral relativists think that there really is no right answer to moral questions because morality is relative to culture or society. The particular moral values that people hold depend on the culture in which they live or were raised.

The initial attractiveness of moral relativism can be characterized in various different ways. One way is through the 'anti-imperialist' thought, 'Who are we to judge?' – Why think we know better what is right and wrong than some other culture? Why think that we can say of them that they have it wrong? – This is a concern about moral authority:

> 'If we want to oppose cruelty, or defend free speech, or outlaw child sex, we need the conviction that it is not 'just us', voicing a contingent or accidental aspect of how we feel. We want to hold that truth is on our side ...'(Blackburn, 2001, p. 38)

But when we look around and reflect on the status of our own deeply held views when contrasted with those with whom we differ, it seems that there is very little to separate our views from those with whom we disagree. These thoughts might have two effects on us. They might make us feel uneasy about our moral convictions – why are we so committed to them when there is no obvious reason that they are better than anyone else's? Moreover, we might, on these grounds, think that we should not judge those with whom we differ. After all, their moral values are as good as ours.

One way of trying to get clear about these issues is to examine other kinds of disagreement compared to moral disagreement. Disagreement about facts often looks to be resolvable by appeal to evidence or argument. If someone is not willing to accept the evidence we tend to look for alternative, perhaps psychological explanations of the refusal. Disagreement about taste looks very different. If I like coffee with milk and you do not, there is no way to resolve the disagreement – *de gustibus non disputandum*. At the cultural level, we can see the same kinds of differences – the French way is to have cheese before dessert, the English way is the reverse. The relativist will think that moral disagreement is more like disagreements of taste than disagreements about facts. Those who oppose relativism think the reverse.

Before looking at these issues, some distinctions are useful. There are two more obvious kinds of moral relativism that are often distinguished in the literature: descriptive moral relativism and metaethical moral relativism. Descriptive moral relativism is a view about the actual variation of moral views across societies and cultures. It holds that, as a matter of fact, there is widespread divergence in moral values and judgements between the peoples of the world both currently and across time. Metaethical moral relativism is a view about the nature of morality and most often involves the nature of moral truth and justification. The metaethical moral relativist thinks that there is no absolute moral truth; there are only different views about what is right and wrong.

One final distinction: the opponents of relativism come in many shapes and sizes but they all do think that moral judgement is not relative. So someone opposing descriptive moral relativism will think that there is some moral agreement across cultures and someone opposing metaethical relativism will think that there are some moral truths. In what follows I will refer to opponents of relativism as objectivists. Following Wiggins, a subject matter is objective if and only if there are questions about it that admit of answers that are simply and plainly true (Wiggins, 1995, p. 243).

In the third and fourth sections below we will consider both of these positions in some detail. However first, it is instructive to examine the relation between moral relativ-

Principles of Health Care Ethics, Second Edition   Edited by R.E. Ashcroft, A. Dawson, H. Draper and J.R. McMillan
© 2007 John Wiley & Sons, Ltd

ism and tolerance or, more generally, the normative consequences of moral relativism of either stripe.

TOLERANCE

Our obligation to be tolerant of those whose views, ways and customs are not like ours is often taken to be an important feature of moral relativism. Indeed for many it is the crucial, defining element of the position. If our moral judgements cannot be privileged over others – our judgements and values are no more right than others – then it would seem that we have no grounds on which to judge those whose moral views are different from ours.

Given this, it is natural to think that we ought always to be tolerant of others. But this looks to involve the relativist in a contradiction. Understood in this strong way, the relativist seems to be making an absolute moral claim of precisely the kind that is supposed not to exist. The moral relativist cannot both require that we are always tolerant and claim that there are no absolute moral truths.

David Wong (1984; 1993) suggests that relativists need not be committed to such a strong tolerance claim. He argues that tolerance is only a requirement of our particular (i.e. western liberal) morality and is to be thought of as a feature of our own culturally influenced moral values. So the requirement that we ought be tolerant is not an absolute one that applies to all but, as a key part of our own cultural viewpoint, is one that applies specifically to us. Though tolerance is required of us, we cannot impose it on others. This move gets the relativist out of the contradiction by restricting the tolerance claim to 'us'.

Another way in which we might weaken the tolerance claim is by allowing exceptions to the rule. Generally, we might think, we should be tolerant of moral differences but there will be some cases where the disagreement is too great. Again, the justification for this comes from our own morality. Being tolerant is an important value but there are some things that are sometimes more important. When these more important things are under threat, our obligation to be tolerant is overridden. Genocide and slavery are good examples of this. In both of these cases our obligation to be tolerant is outweighed by the violations to individual freedoms and liberties that genocide and slavery involve. We think that protecting these freedoms and liberties is more important than being tolerant.

The important move in both of these ways of weakening the tolerance claim is to recognize that our culture's morality will make claims on us that, consistent with the relativist position, will not be applicable to others. So some acts performed by an 'outsider' will be objectionable enough to us to warrant intolerance and some will not – we may be prepared to tolerate very mild forms of circumcision but we will not tolerate genocide.

Importantly, the lesson here is that the relativist and the objectivist need not differ substantially on the tolerance issue – or at least on the tolerance issue as it applies to 'us'. The cost of this lesson for the relativist is the loss of the strong tolerance claim. The moral relativist need not be committed to a prohibition on judging others because we can weaken the tolerance claim to allow exceptions. The requirement to tolerate the views of others can consistently be understood to be a product of one's own moral system.

DESCRIPTIVE (MORAL) RELATIVISM

As we saw above, descriptive moral relativism is an empirical thesis about the variation in moral systems across societies and cultures. A cursory glance at the various moral systems is enough to suggest that there is indeed significant variation. In this section we examine the plausibility of this claim.

APPARENT MORAL DIFFERENCES

On reflection some of the observed differences can be explained in terms other than moral disagreement. Consider the well-worked examples of the Inuit and the Callatians (Levy, 2002; Rachels, 1999; Wiggins, 2006). The traditional practice of the Inuit tribes was to abandon their elderly in the snow. On the face of it this practice looks to be wrong according to us. However, in a context where resources are extremely scarce such decisions look difficult to avoid. It is easy to see how such resource allocation decisions become an entrenched part of the culture and the moral system of the Inuit tribes. In this case the apparent difference in moral judgement is explained by a closer examination of the context of the judgement. We cannot conclude from this that the Inuit have (radically) different values to us, instead the situations in which they find themselves have led to systematically different judgements.

Not all divergence can be explained by a straightforward appeal to context. According to Herodotus, the Callatians had the practice of eating their dead fathers. Herodotus' Greeks thought this practice barbaric. We might suppose that the Callatians believed that a person's soul remained in their body after death and that by consuming the dead, the soul of the deceased would be transferred to the living. By eating their fathers, the Callatians ensured that they retained an all-important connection with them. The substance of these beliefs is not that important, rather what matters is the fact that they are beliefs about the workings of the world. The Callatians and the Greeks differ not in the value of respect and honour to be accorded to the dead but in the nature and workings of the soul. If we believed as we have supposed the Callatians might have, then eating the deceased may be morally required for us also.

Finally, some disagreement between cultures might be understood in terms of a natural variation between people rather than as a fundamental difference at the cultural level. There are some moral issues – we might call them 'essentially contestable' – about which we can expect disagreement. How to distribute resources is one example. Faced with a decision about how to divide up the pot of health care resources, for example, it is reasonable for people who are well disposed to find a fair solution to differ (Daniels & Sabin, 2002). At the cultural level, a marker for these kinds of issues might come from within our own culture. So, for instance, we might think that some variation is to be expected about when and to what extent abortion is permissible – and this is in the nature of the case; the particular clash of values involved can be resolved, reasonably, in a number of ways.

These explanations should not however lead us to think that all variation can be handled in this way. We can find examples of cultural practices for which the above explanations do not work. Two well known ones come from Spartan Greece and medieval Japan. Connected to their warrior culture, the Spartans had the practice of leaving sick or weak infants in the hills to die. In medieval Japan the Samurai had the practice of *tsujigiri* – trying out a new sword on a random passer-by – in order to avoid the dishonour of a sword not working properly in battle (Midgely, 1981). In both cases the explanations above do not provide a satisfactory answer (Levy 2002, pp. 101, 110). They are both importantly connected to fundamental differences in moral values between their culture and ours.

Where does this leave us with respect to descriptive moral relativism? In the end I think it will depend on how we understand the nature of morality. Both sides of the debate must agree that there is difference at some level but its significance will depend on the level at which the basic moral principles are described. For instance James Rachels concludes that 'there are some moral rules that all societies will have in common, because those rules are necessary for society to exist' (Rachels, 1999, p. 30). (It is interesting to compare this view to Wong's, discussed in next section.) Without a thoroughly worked-out account of these necessary rules it is hard to see how this could be true. If the rules are specified too closely then there is a danger that there will be or have been a culture that failed to have one of them – for example the Spartans falsify the rule that all cultures must value the lives of children. If the rules are specified too broadly then it might look platitudinous that all cultures agree; for example, all cul-tures must have rules relating to a concept of respect or its equivalents.

'CULTURE' AS A VAGUE CONCEPT

In all of this we have been speaking of cultural variation as though cultures were fixed, discrete entities. The reality of course is that cultures and, more particularly, cultural values are fluid and amorphous. Moreover the variation that we seem to see across cultures is very often mirrored within them. One way to see these problems is to consider how we can individuate the relevant cultural groups. When are we to think of British, English, Catholic, African, urban, working class, liberal or male as the relevant grouping? The problem for the relativist of course is that if 'culture' or 'cultural values' are too vague or changeable, we will lose the sense of what it means for some moral judgement to be 'true in that culture' or for the judgements that any individual makes to reflect the culture's values.

Neil Levy (2002) provides a response to these problems by drawing an analogy with language. Like cultures, he suggests, languages are similarly difficult to define and yet we have no difficulty understanding the properties of languages and the differences between them. There is a good deal of mingling between languages at their edges and there is a good deal of variation within languages. It is easy to see the mingling; there are many French words that have been adopted by and assimilated into English and vice versa. Among others, Levy cites 'gourmet', 'garage', and 'chauffeur' as examples of French words that are now 'entirely naturalized' (Levy, 2002, pp. 106–7). The variation within languages is clearly illustrated by dialects and other regional variations – it is easy to find examples of regional divergence: Cockney-rhyming slang for example. In spite of these differences we are still able to talk coherently about the English language. We are able to make judgements about grammar, semantics and vocabulary all relativized to English.

And so it is with culture. The ways in which cultures and cultural values vary looks very similar to the variation between and within language. By analogy then it makes sense to make judgements about the moral values of a culture or sub-culture being careful that they are properly relativized and based on sufficiently robust common features of the culture in question.

There is a further, related problem here for the relativist – how are we to determine what counts as the moral values of a culture? (See Levy, 2002; Moody Adams, 1997) We can illustrate the issue here by reflecting on the idea of 'western liberal' culture mentioned earlier. The idea that freedom and liberty are very highly valued in western liberal society certainly rings true – indeed it seems to be a very good example of how well the analogy with language works. But how do we know this is true or how would we go about finding out what else is true of western liberal society? A vast empirical study might yield some interesting results, but it would hardly be definitive. What for instance would we say if the majority of people surveyed did not value liberty and freedom highly at all? We might also try to find a particularly representative individual, but this too runs into trouble. We might pick a particular person for reasons that end up presupposing the values for which we are looking – a US democrat, for example, might give us the kind of story we would expect. Alternatively we might pick someone who fits better into a sub-culture, say from a particular socio-economic class or ethnic group. Finally, we might look at official documents – laws, policies, institutional regulations and the like – in an effort to extract the key moral tenets of a culture. The problem in this case will be change and representation. Why think that the policies of a particular government, for instance, accurately capture the moral values of the culture?

Where are we to this point? This last point is a significant one but it is not one that is devastating for the descriptive moral relativist. There does need to be some way of determining what the moral values of a culture are but this is a project, for philosophers and social scientists, on which progress could be made. The analogy with language gives us reason to be confident.

METAETHICAL RELATIVISM

In this section we focus on the metaethical relativist's position and its relationship to other 'nearby' positions. In particular we will look, in a little more detail, at David Wong's 'moderate' relativist position as well as an attempt to soften the objectivist position to accommodate some of the lessons of the preceding discussions.

As we saw at the outset, the metaethical relativist thinks that there is no absolute moral truth; there are only different views about what is right and wrong. More substantively the moral relativist often has a story to tell about how we come to think that there are things that are 'really' right or wrong. For the relativists that we have been considering (i.e. cultural relativists), this story suggests that what we think is right and wrong is importantly connected to or determined by the culture to which we belong or in which we were raised. Other kinds of metaethical relativists also think that there is no absolute moral truth but might differ in their account of how we come to have the moral views that we do. So, subjectivists typically would count as relativists; they hold that there is no (absolute) moral truth because moral judgements are not the kind of things that are capable of being true or false. Simon Blackburn's view

is of note here (see Blackburn, 1998; 2001). Blackburn's view, quasi-realism, is to be counted as relativist only on this broad, non-normative account of relativism – that is as comprising the claim that there is no absolute moral truth. Instead, moral values are an extension of attitudes and desires. In this case morality is not relative to culture but to each individual subject (though of course an individual is likely to be influenced by their culture amongst other things).

On the opposite side of the fence, objectivists typically believe (unsurprisingly) that there are moral truths and that these truths give us the appropriate authority or justification to be confident of judgements in accord with their favoured account of these truths. Part of what is at issue here connects with our initial way of capturing the moral relativist's impulse – what gives us the special status or privileged position to judge the values and practices of others – who are we to judge? One way to understand much of the history of moral philosophy is as an attempt to come up with a satisfactory answer to this question. In each case the quest is to find the standpoint from which to judge.

Understood in this way, these objectivist attempts are responses to the relativist's position – if we can come up with a satisfactory answer to the 'who are we to judge?' question then we seem to be in a better (or at least more justified) position in cases of conflict. This is not the place to discuss these various attempts as many will be discussed in other chapters of this volume. The important point here is that the relativist cannot object to the objectivist by repeating the 'who are we to judge?' claim. Criticisms of these approaches instead need to be of the theories themselves as adequate accounts of morality and, in particular, by undermining the ability of the theory to achieve the required 'authority'.

MODERATE RELATIVISM

An important feature of David Wong's work on relativism is his insistence that the relativist's position is typically characterised too harshly. One reason for this is the assumption that

> 'one's moral confidence, one's commitment to act on one's values, is somehow dependent on maintaining the belief that one's morality is the only true or the most justified one (Wong, 1984, p. 449)'.

This assumption suggests a tight connection between the metaethical claim concerning the truth or justifiability of moral claims and our confidence in the normative judgements that we are prepared to endorse. It certainly seems correct that if I did believe that my morality was true or the most justified then I would have confidence in my own moral judgements. It is less clear that such a belief is the only source of 'moral confidence'.

In arguing for his position, Wong urges that the relativist can hold a moderate position – that is, a position which sticks to the metaethical claim that there is no one true morality but makes fewer claims about tolerance and perhaps some claims of correctness. He suggests that morality has the function of regulating two types of conflict of interest: inter-personal and intra-personal. Inter-personal conflicts of interest are those where two people, say, want the same thing. Intra-personal conflicts occur when two impulses within an individual pull in opposite directions. In each culture and society the ways in which the particular moral system fulfils this function is likely to be different with no one way being the best.

'Moralities, on this picture, are social creations that evolve to meet certain needs. The needs place conditions on what could be an adequate morality ... the complexity of our nature makes it possible for us to prize a variety of goods and to order them in different ways, and this opens the door for a substantial relativism to be true (Wong, 1984, p. 446.)

The contextual and historical details of a culture will thus ensure difference between the moral systems that grow up in different places. All of these systems however are supposed to function in the same way – to regulate the two types of conflict. There may be some moralities that fail to perform this regulatory function. Thus while this position insists that there is no single true morality it leaves open the possibility that some might be false.

MODERATE OBJECTIVISM

David Wiggins has developed an objectivist position that is similarly 'softened' by the concerns raised by the relativist. There are two main strands to Wiggins' position that are relevant here: (1) the way in which the position is softened towards some of the relativist's points and (2) the way in which the position is to be understood as objectivist. We will deal with each of these in order.

Perhaps the key point of softening in Wiggins' approach involves the idea of authority. As we saw initially one way of understanding the challenge of relativism is through the challenge that it seems to pose to the authority of our own moral convictions. In order to secure this authority the objectivist seems to be required to show that we can have the authority that absolute truth would bring. Alternatively put, in order to avoid the conclusion that moral judgements are like judgements of taste, the objectivist seems to have to demonstrate that moral judgements are very much like the paradigm cases of judgements of fact. We are tempted to think that what is required to regain the authority of our

convictions is the ability to convince everyone – faced with stark cultural disagreement between us and them about what ought to be done, the only things that seem good enough are reasons that will convince them.

Wiggins argues that this expectation is an unreasonable one (Wiggins, 1993, p. 307). Instead he suggests three options: incommensurability, perseverance and underdetermination. First it may be that 'us' and 'them' come from such different 'forms of life' (civilizations or cultures) that 'any semblance of agreement on the question what one ought to do or what is good is only a semblance' (Wiggins, 1990, p. 75). Here the respective understanding on either side is so different that there is not enough common ground or common language on which to build any progress.

Second, there may be a genuine question that we share and where our disagreement is non-trivial. Here Wiggins urges perseverance. The thought is that by uncovering the 'deep' differences of perspective, both conceptual and responsive, one or both sides can come to see or understand the other's standpoint. This seems reasonably common – one finds oneself (suddenly) seeing or feeling what it is like from the 'other side'. The idea here is that perseverance would or could achieve agreement or a resolution of the dispute. Whether such a strategy works or not is more a matter of the individuals concerned and the circumstances of their involvement. In the enterprise of trying to understand one another egos, temperament, claims of authority and attitudes of superiority can get in the way. Finally, there may be situations where, although there is a real issue, a real question of what ought to be done, it is not clear that any of the parties is in a position to decide and to be justified – 'there is no manifest possibility of any winning set of considerations ever being mustered' (Wiggins, 1990, p. 76).

On this picture of moral disagreement only the second option offers any prospect of resolution. The only authority that the objectivist can claim, then, is as a result of the process of perseverance and this only after hindrances like egos and temperament have been put aside. It is in this context that possibility of moral truth arises and for Wiggins this happens when we arrive at the point where 'there is nothing else to think'. A particular moral claim, 'X is wrong', is true when, after bringing to bear the full argumentative, conceptual and emotional resources, we realise that there is nothing else to think but that X is wrong.

Wiggins uses the example of slavery. Here there is a wealth of considerations that can be produced to show that slavery is unjust and insupportable and these considerations are such as to show that there is nothing else to think but that slavery is unjust and insupportable (Wiggins, 1990, p. 71). Raimond Gaita discusses this issue in a way that well illustrates the point here. He writes:

The slave owner denies that the slave has his kind (the slave owner's kind) of individuality: the kind of individuality that shows itself in our revulsion in being numbered rather than being called by name; the kind of individuality that gives human beings the power to haunt those who have wronged them, in remorse. If the slave owner could be haunted by the slave girl he raped, then her days as a slave would be numbered (Gaita, 1991, p. 159).

What this passage and the rest of Gaita's discussion brings out is how the concepts of 'individuality', 'human being' and 'person' themselves are invested with an emotional and responsive power that cannot be disentangled from them. These kinds of emotions and responses are caught up with the idea of taking someone seriously as an individual. They illustrate the full force, not of what it is to *treat* someone as a human being, but of conceiving of them as 'other to my one' (Gaita, 1991, p. 159). This kind of investigation of, as we might say, the psychology of the slave owners shows how their understanding of those who were their slaves failed to approach their conception of those who were 'fully human'. It trades on an understanding of the full range of our evaluative and emotional resources and seeks to show how these resources cohere. In the face of this understanding and in the face of this diagnosis of the slave owner we are to see that there is nothing else to think.

Importantly, what is shown by these kinds of considerations is not that there is nothing else *for us* to think but that there is nothing else to think, simpliciter. The thought is that the arguments, etc. are mounted from the level of a perspective that is not particular, that aims at an abstraction from the 'for us' to one involving simply one person to another. What is shown, then, by these arguments is that the price of not thinking that slavery is unjust and insupportable is that one opts out of the point of view that is common between people and which is aimed at by the considerations and arguments brought forward. This common point of view is not culturally or socially specific even though particular ways of expressing it might be.

As I have described it here, Wiggins' position first adjusts the aims of the objectivist enterprise by allowing that there are significant limits to the kind of success that can be hoped for. In cases where perseverance is called for, we can come to some moral truths when the wealth of considerations in our moral repertoire lead us to the view that there is nothing else to think.

What are we to say more generally about the prospects for the moderate positions surrounding metaethical relativism? I have not in the above been critical of either of the moderate positions partly because my aim has been to begin to show that the issues with which this debate is concerned are deep and subtle. Wong's position makes use of the range of resources available to the objectivist whereas Wiggins' view draws heavily on the tradition of subjectivism.

Wong is right that relativism is often depicted in a poor and extreme light – and by those who ought to know better. However, the kinds of relativistic claims that are made on the margins of moral philosophy and in the broad sweeping statements of the more popular press are often the best examples of crude, unthinking relativism at its worst. Both, clearly, are to be avoided.

REFERENCES

Blackburn S Relativism. In: Hugh L, ed. *The Blackwell Guide to Ethical Theory*. Oxford: Blackwell, 2001; pp. 38–52.

Blackburn S. *Ruling Passions*, Oxford: Clarendon Press, 1998.

Daniels N, Sabin J. *Setting Limits Fairly*. New York: Oxford University Press, 2002.

Gaita R. *Good and Evil: An Absolute Conception*. London: Macmillan, 1991.

Levy N. *Moral Relativism: A Short Introduction*. Oxford: Oneworld Publications, 2002.

Midgely M. On trying out one's new sword. In: *Heart and Mind: The Varieties of Moral Experience*, New York: Harvester Press, 1981.

Moody-Adams MM. *Fieldwork in Familiar Places: Morality, Culture, and Philosophy*. Cambridge, MA: Harvard University Press, 1997.

Rachels J. *The Elements of Moral Philosophy*, 3rd edition. New York: McGraw-Hill, 1999.

Wiggins D. *Ethics: Twelve Lectures on the Philosophy of Morality*. London: Penguin Books, 2006.

Wiggins D. Cognitivism, naturalism, and normativity: a reply to Peter Railton. In: Haldane J, Wright C, eds. *Reality, Representation and Projection*. Oxford; Oxford University Press, 1993.

Wiggins D. Moral cognitivism, moral relativism and motivating moral beliefs. *Proc Aristotelian Soc* 1990; **91**: 61–85.

Wiggins D. Objective and subjective in ethics, with two postscripts about truth. *Ratio (New Series)* 1995; **8**: 243–58.

Wong DB. *Moral Relativity*. Berkeley CA: University of California Press, 1984.

Wong DB. Relativism. In: Peter S. ed. *A Companion to Ethics*. Oxford: Blackwell, 1993; pp. 442–50.

14

Christian Approaches to Bioethics

HEATHER WIDDOWS

In attempting to describe what is 'Christian Bioethics', the key question is 'What is 'Christian' about Christian bioethics?'. In other words, what is it that makes 'Christian' bioethics different from 'secular' bioethics? In order to answer this question and to provide an outline of Christian bioethics, or Christian approaches to bioethics, this chapter will begin by exploring Christian ethics. It will examine the range of Christian ethics and, to illustrate the breadth of this range, it will consider two very different forms of Christian ethics: that of divine command ethics and Gustafson's 'theocentric ethics'. The chapter will then proceed to examine how these differences in Christian ethics play out in bioethics. To do this most effectively a test case will be used to provide a central focus, that of the status of the embryo, as it appears in discussion about the ethics of abortion, reproductive technologies and genetic and stem cell research. The chapter will conclude with an attempt to find some shared characteristics or tendencies in different versions of Christian bioethics in order to see if any meaningful distinction can be made between Christian and secular bioethics.

WHY STUDY CHRISTIAN BIOETHICS

Before moving on to address these issues of Christian ethics and bioethics, it is pertinent to ask why we are still interested in Christian approaches to bioethics in the current context of 'Western bioethics'. Western bioethics is predominantly secular and tends to assume, at least implicitly, a secular liberal worldview that is endorsed by bioethicists and their audiences. Religious reasoning is not explicitly included in most secular accounts of bioethical reasoning. Indeed, the very fact that there is a separate chapter on 'Christian bioethics' suggests that Christian bioethics is something distinct from the topic addressed in the rest of the volume, that of mainstream bioethics.

(Reflect on how often religious concerns are presented as core considerations for ethical decision-making rather than as 'alternative perspectives' in this, and any other mainstream, volume on bioethics.)

However, although 'religious views' are largely excluded from Western, and particularly Anglo-American bioethics, religious concerns continue to be important in bioethics for two reasons. First, bioethics derived from the moral concerns of a Christian context and the Christian heritage of many of the key concerns of bioethics are still detectable, although this is increasingly less true and the Christian preoccupations out of which bioethics grew are less dominant than they once were. Second, even as evidence of religious concerns in bioethics recede, religious belief remains a primary factor, indeed for many people the most important factor, in moral reasoning. This is not just true in the loosely termed 'non-Western' world, but also in parts of the West; particularly the United States which, despite its huge Christian population, continues to produce 'secular' bioethics which largely ignores the views of these prominent religious groups. Thus, one could argue that understanding Christian bioethics is important not only for believers, but also for all bioethicists, if they are to engage adequately with ethical issues in the contemporary climate. Non-religious secular practitioners and scholars must have some understanding of Christian bioethics, and faith bioethics in general, if they are to communicate with and understand the reasons for the ethical decisions of their patients and audiences.

CHRISTIAN ETHICS

Having provided some rationale as to the importance of understanding faith based ethics, the chapter will now turn to the task of outlining Christian bioethics. To address only Christian bioethics is to fail to address the bioethics

Principles of Health Care Ethics, Second Edition   Edited by R.E. Ashcroft, A. Dawson, H. Draper and J.R. McMillan
© 2007 John Wiley & Sons, Ltd

arising from other faiths, and the points of similarity and dissimilarity between Christian bioethics and the bioethics of other faiths and their relationship with secular liberal frameworks. However, the remit of this chapter, as will become abundantly clear, is already broad, and thus, while recognizing that some understanding of faith-based bioethics would be valuable, the discussion will be limited to the Christian faith.

In order to describe Christian bioethics, we will begin by attempting to understand 'Christian ethics'. The first important fact to recognize when considering Christian ethics is the complexity of the field; defining 'Christian ethics' is no easy task. There is no one source of Christian ethics, despite the shared sacred text and belief in one God, no one set of moral rules or principles, and no single attitude or particular perspective that all Christians, or even most Christians, could be said to agree on or to share. In addition, the positions that Christians are likely to take on any given subject are not necessarily predictable by the outsider. There is no direct relationship which allows one to predict accurately a person's moral convictions on the basis of knowing whether and which faith community they belong to. For example, it is not uncommon for Christians to agree with secular ethicists at the expense of their fellow Christians. For instance, in an example we shall return to, and contrary to assumptions which are often made about what Christians believe, Christians are divided on the 'status of the embryo', and some Christian thinkers would 'morally justify an abortion' (Gustafson, 1985, p. 495). It is not to say that their faith does not influence Christian perspectives on such issues – it does and profoundly does so – but how individuals, groups and denominations interpret their faith and attempt to live out their beliefs differs from group to group and even from one individual believer to another.

However, all Christians will consider acts from the perspective of a believer, assessing right and wrong in the context of their faith. Thus, with regard to the example of the status of the embryo all Christians are likely to include in their reasoning a concern for the sacredness of life (an issue which is less important in secular bioethicists – although this too is a generalization). Consequently, even Christians who endorse abortion will not do so lightly. It is perhaps the element of sacredness which sets ethical decisions in the context of the whole of life and within a spiritual framework which may prove to be the only common element in Christian ethical decision-making. Although a spiritual perspective is not necessarily exclusive to Christians or to people of faith, more emphasis is placed on such awareness in Christian ethics than in secular ethics. Whether this emphasis and context is the closest we can come to finding common ground between Christians is a question we will return to in the final section of the chapter. However, even if a recognition of the sacred and an awareness of the spiritual could be said

to be held by all Christians, it would still be unclear whether such a commonality between Christians would be primary and more important than other shared perspectives, for example between liberals and conservatives. If we return to the example of the status of the embryo, the Christian who accepts abortion and believes that while regrettable it is compatible with the Christian life is arguably far closer to the liberal secular bioethicist in terms of shared values than to other Christians and other people of faith.

From the outset then it is important to recognize that there are many 'Christian ethics', which derive from many diverse individuals, groups and denominations. Moreover, views about what constitutes Christian ethics and how Christian ethics relate to non-Christian ethics are strongly held and fiercely defended. On the one hand some Christian thinkers, such as the famous Karl Barth, deny all continuation between Christian and non-Christian ethics (Fairweather and McDonald, 1984, p. 127; Gustafson, 1975, p. 149). From such perspectives the only valid form of ethics is Christian ethics, as correct ethical thinking comes from divine revelation alone. For Barth all other sources of ethical knowledge are flawed as human reason is fundamentally and irredeemably corrupt and 'fallen'; thus 'general ethical discussion is a work of human pride and presumption... Such ethics is not genuine but illegitimate' (Fairweather and McDonald, 1984, p. 127). On the other hand, other Christians believe that secular and Christian thinking is similar and draws on similar sources and addresses similar concerns. In essence, for such thinkers, the moral reasoning process is the same; what is different is that Christians have additional sources of moral knowledge to draw on and additional considerations derived from their faith to take into account. Such a model dramatically reduces the significance of the difference between Christians and non-Christians, as non-Christians too bring convictions and concerns from their own value-frameworks which bear on their moral judgements: for example, political, cultural and ethnic preoccupations and perspectives.

Thus, Christian ethics is regarded by some as distinctive and exclusive with no continuity within the moral framework and reasoning processes of non-Christians. Conversely, Christian ethics can also denote an ethics similar in form and content to so-called secular ethics – similar in sources and methodology but informed and enriched by the Christian's belief system and faith perspective. Between these two extremes a myriad of possible Christian ethical approaches abound, all of them vigorously asserted and defended by their proponents.

TYPES OF CHRISTIAN ETHICS

In order to clarify further the varieties of Christian ethics and to illustrate the types of moral reasoning that

Christians employ when approaching ethical issues, we will consider two types of Christian ethical approach: that of divine command ethics, and the 'theocentric' approach of Gustafson. Gustafson asserts a distinctively Christian element to ethics but suggests that Christian and secular ethics are largely coextensive – and it is this similarity, rather than his distinctive theological ethics, which is relevant to the discussion of this chapter.

First we will consider divine command types of Christian ethics which are probably closest to the picture non-believers tend to have of what constitutes Christian ethics. Certainly, it is a common assumption made by non-religious persons that morality for believers consists in following the 'rules' or laws of God. This rule following is precisely the divine command model, for acts are right or wrong depending on whether or not they accord with the commands of God. Accordingly, divine command theories are 'formulated using only three basic concepts; they are notions of ethical requirement, ethical permission and ethical prohibition' (Quinn, 1978, p.26). In other words acts are required if, and only if, God commands them, forbidden if, and only if, God forbids them, and permitted if, and only if, God does not forbid them. Such an understanding of the nature of moral value one might imagine provides a simple and relatively workable moral framework. And one would expect to find in Christian communities where 'divine choice is the defining condition of moral reality' (Johnson, 1994, p. 42) a clear, well-defined set of moral rules which simply require adherence. However, despite the simplicity which divine command theories appear to promise, this model is not as unproblematic as it might appear. There are many difficulties which beset divine command theories and which have been the source of debate in theological and philosophical circles since the beginnings of theorising about morality. These roughly fall into two groups of issues: the first concerns theoretical contradictions and the second the practical implications of endorsing such a position.

Debates regarding the theoretical flaws in the divine command theory have a long history which can be traced back to the very beginnings of Western Philosophy and to Plato's *Euthyphro* dialogue (Euthyphro, Plato, 1989). The question raised in the *Euthyphro* is whether actions are 'good' because God (or in Plato's case the gods) wills them so or whether God wills good actions because they are good. There are problems with both of these answers.

In the first instance we have no 'moral' standard as such, but only the commands of God; thus a 'right' action could become a 'wrong' action if God so commanded. In such a scenario, moral goodness is a moveable feast, for example 'if God were to command that Smith tortures children then it would be required that Smith tortures children' (Quinn, 1978, p. 31). If the second is true, then it cannot be the case that good actions are such simply because of the commands

of God. For many Christians this is an unacceptable position as not only does it mean that morality is arbitrary and open to change as God wills, but it also prevents the believer from asserting that God is good or loving or as having any moral attributes. For if morality is what God deems it to be, then it is meaningless to say that 'God is good', as we must know what goodness is independently of God's commands if we are to deem God to be good; 'for clearly we could not judge anything to be *perfectly* good unless we could judge that it was good, and... our criterion must be at least logically independent of God' (Nielsen, 1982, p. 340). To adopt this alternative would imply that morality is an independent standard to which even God must defer. This conclusion limits the omnipotence of God, again something that many Christians cannot accept.

Which side of the debate to come down on remains a problem for believers and, despite the longevity of this debate, no conclusion has yet been reached and it seems set to continue. Defenders of the theory have been unconvinced by the theoretical criticisms from Plato onwards, and contemporary proponents are defiant, asserting that 'philosophers have not succeeded in refuting certain divine command theories, and, therefore, are not justified in rejecting them' (Quinn, 1978, p. 23).

The second difficulty with divine command theories is practical and twofold, related first to discovering and interpreting divine commands and second to the implications of the theory for non-Christians. First then, even if one believes that moral values derive from the commands of God, there are still difficulties about how such values are to be discovered and how they should be interpreted in context. For example, Christians who believe that God's commands are revealed in Scripture have to negotiate conflicting passages and different interpretations. Moreover, knowing the commands of God is complicated when tradition, denomination and personal religious experience are added to the picture. Not only is the task of deciphering the commands of God in general a difficulty, but also God can override His general commands with specific commands to individuals (for example, as in various Biblical stories, such as that of Abraham and Isaac, where Abraham is commanded to sacrifice his son). In such situations one only has the individual's testimony that they have been commanded in a certain way; the dangers of such claims are abundantly clear. Any act could be deemed moral (however immoral it would normally be judged to be) if it is claimed to be a command of God. Thus, determining morality according to divine command theories is not as simple and automatic as one might imagine.

Second, if one follows the logic of divine command theories then 'nothing is morally good or bad if there is no God' (Westmoreland, 1996, p. 17), because if morality is following the commands of God, there is no moral framework outside of the religious framework. The divine command theory is exclusive – unless one recognizes and adheres to the commands of God one cannot be moral – and, accordingly, the non-believer has no source of moral knowledge. Such a conclusion many Christians have found unpalatable and in conflict with their experience, for 'we seem capable of knowing that various actions are right or wrong without knowing what (or whether) God commands' (Westmoreland, 1996, p. 19). The wish to assert some shared moral framework has led theologians to attempt to escape this implication; for example, Adams puts forward a '*modified* divine command theory' (Adams, 1981, p. 83). In his modified theory Adams asserts that 'in some ordinary (and ... imprecise) sense of "mean", what believers and non-believers mean by "wrong" in ethical contexts may well be partly the same and partly different' (Adams, 1981, p. 103). However, even though Adams wishes to assert some continuity between the moral world of the Christian and the non-Christian, the grounds by which he can do this in a divine command theory, however modified, are unclear. Moral values either derive from the will of God or they do not, and if they do then it would seem that moral understanding is exclusively the preserve of the believer.

As a result of these theoretical and practical difficulties many Christian ethicists have sought alternative moral frameworks. For the purpose of showing the range of Christian ethics, we will consider an alternative view in which Christian and non-Christian moral frameworks are, for the most part, the same. This position is set out by James Gustafson who frames his book on this subject, *Can Ethics be Christian?*, on a case study of a 'moral action' by a non-Christian colleague. The colleague's action he judges to be morally exemplary and argues that the colleague's 'dispositions and the actions that followed could have been judged to be exemplary of the Christian moral life' (Gustafson, 1975, p. 147). However, despite judging his colleague's action as a moral one and suggesting that Christians and non-Christians largely share the same moral sensibility, Gustafson still wishes to say that being a Christian provides a crucial dimension to moral decision-making processes, without denying the moral sensibilities of non-believers. Such a position is hard to maintain; something which Gustafson recognizes, and thus he asks 'is it conceivable that members of the Christian community would act under any circumstances in a way that could not be justified by principles on which presumably all rational persons could agree? Is it conceivable that a "moral" act by a Christian can be justified by only a "religious" reason?' (Gustafson, 1975, p. 166). For him the answer to this question is that such circumstances would be extremely rare, but possible, for example, when a person's only reason for action is 'their commitment and loyalty to Jesus Christ, and to the Christian "way of life"' (Gustafson, 1975,

p. 167). Therefore, for Gustafson, ethics is enriched for the believer as Christians can make moral decisions from their faith perspectives because of their obedience to God and ideals of the Christian way of life which a non-believer could not make. Indeed such decisions may be difficult for a non-believer to understand as 'such obedience is not easily justified on the basis of rational self-interest, or even on a proper balance of self-regard and other-regard' (Gustafson, 1975, p. 168). However, these cases are not common and, for Gustafson, there is much that is similar in Christian and non-Christian moral decision-making.

In this theory of Christian ethics then the Christian and the non-Christian share the same moral world, which is not the case if one adopts a divine command model. Thus for Gustafson there are not 'a whole unique set of moral values and principles for Christians' (Gustafson, 1975, p. 168). Rather, for all human beings, 'moral activity comes into being within relationships between persons and others' (Gustafson, 1975, p. 13) and it is from these relations of 'mutuality that moral obligations and claims emerge' (Gustafson, 1975, p. 13). Accordingly, and because of the nature of moral demands arising from relationships, Christians and non-Christians all have reasons to be moral and inhabit moral frameworks according to which right actions are determined. Thus he asserts, 'that morality can be interpreted to have other ultimate grounds than Christian theological grounds cannot be gainsaid... That persons and communities can have reasons for being moral other than those of the Christian faith and tradition is equally uncontradictable' (Gustafson, 1975, p. 173). Moreover, the moral framework for the Christian and the non-Christian is shared and mutually comprehensible for most moral acts. Thus, for the majority of occasions believers and non-believers can agree on what the correct, or best, moral action is in a certain instance, and both can deem a particular disposition or act 'good'.

For Gustafson then, acts are moral acts for Christians for all of the same reasons they are moral for non-Christians; however, for the Christian they also have religious significance. Moral striving and action, for the believer, takes on additional significance and is regarded by the believer as a manifestation of his or her faith. According to Gustafson for the 'serious Christian (and I believe also the devout Jew and Moslem), every moral act is a religiously significant act' (Gustafson, 1975, p. 174). However, despite the differences in how the religious person understands his or her moral action, for Gustafson there is no difference between the moral worlds of the Christian and the non-Christian, only between how the moral acts are interpreted in terms of faith commitment. Gustafson then is at the other end of the spectrum from the divine command ethicists. He presents us with a moral framework within which the moral worlds of the Christian and the non-Christian are coextensive.

Our consideration of but two instances of Christian ethics, albeit from opposite ends of the spectrum, has shown how difficult it is to characterize Christian ethics, which is the first stage in our attempt to outline a Christian approach to bioethics. What is now abundantly clear is that to speak of *a* Christian ethics is misleading and ignorant of the diverse nature of Christian approaches to ethics. The spectrum of Christian ethics stretches, as we have seen, from those who regard Christian ethics as exclusive and who struggle to account for the moral convictions of non-Christians to Christian ethicists like Gustafson who believe that in nearly every case a non-Christian and a Christian act for the same moral reasons.

CHRISTIAN BIOETHICS

Given the difficulties in establishing a single Christian approach to ethics and having illustrated the great difference between those who term themselves Christian ethicists, it will come as no surprise that 'Christian Bioethics' is similarly difficult to define and that Christian approaches to bioethics are similarly numerous and divergent in their assertions. At one end of the Christian bioethics spectrum, like the Christian ethics spectrum, are those who assert that Christian and non-Christian bioethics are separate and in conflict and at the other end there are those who assert that Christian and non-Christian bioethics overlap to the point of convergence.

In parallel with Christian ethics there are Christian bioethicists who endorse a distinctively Christian approach to ethics, such as H Tristham Englehardt, Jr. who asserts the values of what he terms 'traditional Christianity' (which draws predominantly on the Church Fathers and he describes as the 'Christianity of the first millennium' (Englehardt, 2000)). Englehardt finds relatively little overlap between Christian and non-Christian moral decision-making, and he judges his form of traditional Christianity to be in conflict with contemporary 'liberal cosmopolitanism' (Englehardt, 2000). In a similar vein, Corinna Delkeskamp-Hayes suspects that Christian authors who wish to make their faith-based thinking applicable in the secular world run the risk of perverting their specifically Christian insight (Delkeskamp Hayes, 2002). At the other end of the Christian bioethics spectrum, again in parallel with Christian ethics, there are thinkers who claim Christian and non-Christian bioethics inhabit the same world and draw on the same values and use similar processes of moral reasoning, for there are 'not two ethics systems... one for Christians and another for the public world' (Seifert, 2002, p. 97).

In order to explore some of these issues and consider how they are worked out in practical decision-making, we will introduce and explore the test case of abortion and the related but wider issue of the status of the embryo. We will

focus on abortion for a number of reasons: first because abortion remains a core issue in bioethics; second, the issue of abortion is one which is often assumed to be a fault-line dividing religious persons from non-religious persons; and third, the abortion debate and particularly how one considers the status of the embryo, has profound implications for other cutting edge issues, such as reproductive technologies, genetic therapy and manipulation and the more controversial issues of stem cells and cloning.

The issue of the status of the embryo, for our purposes the 'test case' to explore Christian approaches to bioethics, reveals that when it comes to determining the rights and wrongs of practice, there is no more unity in Christian bioethics than there is in the theory of Christian ethics. Christian bioethicists endorse conflicting positions and can be found in both 'pro-life' and 'pro-choice' camps (the 'pro-life' and 'pro-choice' terms have been used for ease of comprehension, but the emotive and contested assumptions and implications of these terms should be borne in mind whenever one considers the topic of abortion).

If we consider the Christian bioethicists who are 'pro-life' and anti-abortion we find thinkers like Englehardt. Englehardt considers both contraception and abortion to be forbidden; indeed he would deem abortion to be murder: one should consider 'any action taken to expel an embryo from the womb, as equivalent to murder' (Englehardt, 2000, p. 281) – a relatively common view amongst Christians who assert that the foetus is a person from conception. Also in this camp are most self-defined 'Evangelical Christians' (although in theological terms, all Christians are strictly speaking 'evangelical'). Evangelical Christians, along with certain Roman Catholic groups, have been most the most vocal in putting forward a 'pro-life' Christian position on abortion in the popular debate. They argue that abortion is immoral on the grounds that the 'Bible teaches: (1) that the foetus is a person, and (2) that abortion is murder' (Simmons, 2001, p. 207). In support of this view biblical quotes are used (for example, Exodus 20:13; Psalms 139; Genesis 9:6), all of which are believed to support the view that 'fetuses, embryos, and unwanted pregnancies all fall into the same category – human beings who are precious and highly valued in the sight of God' (Leber, 2001, p. 197). Such positions are often couched in very emotional terms and there are many organizations and groups who, from their belief perspective, actively oppose abortion. One such organization is 'Operation Rescue' which is dedicated to 'saving *in utero* babies who are about to be killed by an abortionist' (Leber, 2001, p. 195).

On this key issue in bioethics then there are believers who assert a very clear and absolute stance, derived from knowing the will of God and from biblical authority, that abortion is wrong. This, these thinkers and activists would assert, is *the* Christian approach to abortion, and they would deny the validity, and indeed the Christianity, of any other approach to abortion. However, to assert that the foetus is a person and that abortion is murder and therefore against the will of God is not the end of the story, and other, also Christian, thinkers have drawn other conclusions and have argued, for example, that 'there are logical, moral, and biblical-theological reasons for not accepting the easy equation of conceptus with person' (Simmons, 2001, p. 207). Such critics of the anti-abortion view dispute the scriptural evidence, the biblical interpretation and the theological framework of such positions (Simmons, 2001) and moreover suggest that a hard-line anti-abortion stance conflicts with other central Christian beliefs (Shoenig, 2001).

Thus, and contrary to the way the 'Christian' position is often portrayed, even in this supposedly defining bioethical issue a single Christian position or approach cannot be identified. Even to make broad generalizations about the position of 'the majority of Christians', if such a thing could be discovered, or to state the position of believers of different denominations would be misleading. For example, the Roman Catholic Church condemns contraception and abortion; however, clearly there are many Roman Catholic women who do not heed these prescriptions but who continue to consider themselves Catholic. Moreover, there are Catholic theologians and ethicists who question the anti-abortion stance of the Roman Catholic Church; for example, Maguire writes after a visit to an abortion clinic that 'I have held babies in my hands and now I held this embryo. I know the difference' (Maguire, 2001, p. 205). Accordingly, he does not call for the prohibition of abortions but rather asserts that 'there are no moral grounds for political consensus against this freedom on an issue where good experts and good people disagree' (Maguire, 2001, p. 205). Therefore our exploration of our test case, that of abortion, has served to reinforce the breadth of Christian ethics, and our supposition that to say there is a Christian approach to bioethics would be misleading. If we expand this test case into some of the issues we identified as being linked to abortion by virtue of also being concerned with the status of the embryo, we can see that the difficulty in asserting a single Christian position on these key bioethical issues is reinforced.

Englehardt takes a conservative position which forbids prenatal testing and states that 'any action against a zygote or embryo at any stage must be forbidden' (Englehardt, 2000, p. 281). He also takes a firm line on reproductive technology, forbidding all third-party reproductive technology; the only artificial reproductive technology he permits is donor insemination by husband (DIH) and in this case the couple should 'seek spiritual guidance so that their struggle to have a child does not distract from their pursuit of the Kingdom of God, does not cause them great spiritual harm' (Englehardt, 2000, p. 254). For many

Christians, as for Englehardt, the issues raised by reproductive technologies and other uses of embryos, such as for stem cell research, are the same as abortion, and if abortion should be condemned so should these other technologies. For example, Samuel B Casey has described the destruction of so-called spare embryos, created for the *in vitro* fertilization (IVF) process, in the following way: the 'remaining "potential infants" – in a chilling reminder of another Holocaust involving persons considered by their Nazi executioners to be "sub-human" – were thawed out, destroyed with saline solution, and incinerated with other biological waste' (Casey, 2000, p. 154).

However, as we would expect, such positions are contested by other Christians. For example, Maura Ryan, from the Roman Catholic tradition, uses Roman Catholic social thought to justify certain forms of assisted reproduction, particularly IVF which is her primary concern. Like Englehardt, she too rejects third party forms of assisted reproduction on the ground that 'we are adopting forms of symbolic understandings of reproduction that undermine our personal and social capacities to appreciate and embody these core reproductive and marital values' (Ryan, 2001, pp. 55–56). However, she does not share his rejection of non-third party forms of assisted reproduction. From her perspective, by prioritizing relationships over acts and psychospiritual and social dimensions of parenthood over biological and genetic dimensions, some forms of assisted reproduction can be deemed acceptable to the Christian. From the tenets of Roman Catholic social teaching, Ryan argues that viewing reproduction in a social, relational context includes respecting 'the natural *telos* of the sexual act, its proper setting in marriage, and its intrinsic reproductive finality' (Ryan, 2001, p. 113). Accordingly, she asserts the limited acceptance of assisted reproduction, which she believes acknowledges the 'importance of the capacity to reproduce as a dimension of human flourishing without ignoring the social effects of reproductive choices' (Ryan, 2001, p. 115). Thus, even Christians who come from similar traditions and share similar convictions and use similar sources can make different decisions about the rightness and wrongness of particular interventions and procedures.

Likewise, when we move from reproductive technologies to issues of research and the use of embryos we again find very different views. Not surprisingly, there are those who regard any such research as unacceptable to the Christian and who deem such research as prohibited and even dangerous. Leber comments that the use of '"tissue" from abortion to help treat Parkinson's and other diseases... may sound very appealing at first, but such thinking has already opened the door to barbaric practices that are making their appearance slowly and discreetly as they did in Nazi Germany' (Leber, 2001, p. 197). Groups have mobilized because of their beliefs that such practices are fundamentally anti-Christian.

For example, the Center for Bioethics and Human Dignity (IL, US) promotes Biblical and Christian values and published a statement opposing such research and launched a coalition: *On Human Embryos and Stem Cell Research: The Founding Statement of the 'Do No Harm: The Coalition of Americans for Research Ethics* (CARE) (http://www.stemcellresearch.org/statement/statement.htm). The coalition works to oppose all such research and use of embryos, and its objectives are: 'To advance the development of medial treatments and therapies that do not require the destruction of human life, including the human embryo…[and]… to support continuation of the federal law prohibiting the federal funding of research that would require the destruction of human life, including human embryos' (Casey, 2000, p. 166). However, and again not surprisingly, this position is not the only available one and is challenged by other Christian groups, such as the *Religious Coalition for Reproductive Choice*, which defends pro-choice positions from a believer's perspective (http://www.rcrc.org/about/index.htm). Likewise, Christians write in favour of genetic research; for example, Francis Collins, who though not unconcerned about the ethical issues involved, states that 'the promise of this research is so great that the most unethical thing we can do is to slow it down' (Collins, 2002, p. 3).

Not only are there different positions from different perspectives, but all Christians do not even agree on which ethical issues are most important and should be focused upon. For example, as discussed above, for Englehardt the debates about abortion, reproductive technologies and stem cell and other research are the same ethical debate concerned with the status of the embryo. However, others believe the issues are different and argue that 'responses to the question whether it would be right to engage in abortion will not necessarily apply to the question whether it would be right to use preimplantation genetic diagnosis (PGD) or germline interventions on early embryos' (Cohen, 2003, p. 105). Moreover, a number of prominent 'contemporary Anglican thinkers have taken the development of the primitive streak at approximately fourteen days after conception as the time after which early embryos are owed moral consideration' (Cohen, 2003, p. 122). For these theologians then reproductive techniques like IVF and PGD and research on embryos raise different and separate questions from those of the abortion debate. The different focus of Christian thinkers was illustrated further in our discussion when we considered the perspective of Ryan, whose focus when discussing the ethics of reproductive technology was not on the status of the embryo but on the importance of fulfilling the ideals of the family as part of the Christian life. Thus, once again we are left with a confusing array of vastly divergent perspectives. Christians disagree not only in their conclusions about what are right and wrong perspectives and practices but also in their methodologies and reasoning, and even with regard to what are the most pertinent issues from the Christian perspective.

A CHRISTIAN APPROACH TO BIOETHICS?

The vast differences in Christian ethics and Christian bioethics are now abundantly clear. Yet, having stated that it is not possible to define a single Christian approach to ethics and bioethics, nor even a group of Christian approaches to ethics and bioethics, this final section of the paper will seek commonalities within this complex field. However, though such an attempt will be made the insights of the previous discussion will be borne in mind, in particular, the recognition that a so-called Christian view may in fact be more similar to a secular position than to other Christian views. Thus even if a common theme is found in Christian bioethics, it must be recognized that Christian element of any position may not be the most important or the most distinctive factor in any perspective. To try to find commonality after this discussion, which has illustrated beyond doubt the varieties of Christian ethics, may seem contradictory. However, simply because one recognizes that there is no single Christian approach to bioethics, it does not mean that we should not consider the question of whether there are any shared perspectives or shared tendencies which may characterize the Christian element in these diverse positions.

At the end of this chapter we return to the suggestion of the first section that despite the disagreements about the Christian framework, sources of authority and processes of moral reasoning, there may still be a shared Christian element. The claim is that perhaps, after all, some difference may be traced, however tentatively, between secular ethicists and Christian ethicists as a whole. Namely, for the Christian, there is a real sense that what one decides truly matters (and matters eternally). For the Christian, there are right and wrong, or at least better and worse, answers to these bioethical questions; they are not matters of opinion or preference. Therefore, ethically speaking, Christian bioethicists, unlike many Anglo-American bioethicists – to use crude caricatures – are very unlikely to be utilitarians. In addition, the background against which the Christian bioethicist makes these decisions is a spiritual one where health and happiness in this life is not the only concern. If we return to the test case of this chapter, that of the status of the embryo (from abortion to stem cell therapy), what all the Christian thinkers have in common is a recognition of the importance – or, in religious language, of the sacredness – of life and a belief that moral decisions are symbolic of their religious convictions. Accordingly, none of the Christian thinkers who accept abortion and research on embryos think that there is no moral issue to be addressed.

For all these thinkers and despite their disagreements the status of the embryo is a moral issue, and an issue which does have a correct answer.

Objections might be raised to suggesting that only Christians (or religious persons) have a belief in the special importance of life which is akin to the religious concept of sacredness. And indeed such an understanding still continues in secular bioethics; however, it would be fair to say that it is no longer the case that this is always true. Therefore, and as the Christian heritage which informed the secular tradition recedes, it may be that a divide between Christian and non-Christian bioethicsits will increasingly emerge around the issue of the intrinsic value of human life. At this point a distinctively Christian view of bioethics may appear which, though covering a wide variety of positions, is characterized by a shared sense of sacredness and a spiritual framework which confers fundamental value to human life.

The beginnings of such a divergence between how Christians frame their debates is perhaps already evident in debates about how life is valued, for example, in the death and dying debate. When considering end of life decisions it is likely that prolonging life will be of less importance to the believer than to the non-believer (although again this is an over-generalization), and all Christians would agree that 'pursuing health and the means to stay alive should not be of ultimate human value' (Boyle, 2002, p. 79). Some Christians would assert that the difference between the way that believers and non-believers conceive of and value human life is profound: For example, Seifert describes the secular attitudes he believes are embodied in Western, and predominantly secular, health care as a 'horrible reversal of the true hierarchy of values when health is placed above life' (Seifert, 2002, p. 113) and Schotsmans berates the 'idolatrous ideology of health' (Schotsmans, 2002, p. 131). However although Christians have criticized dominant contemporary values which promote the extension of life over the living of a good life, it is not only Christian writers who bemoan the 'medicalisation of death' (Taboada, 2002, p. 65; Khushf, 2002, p. 172). Non-Christian ethicists also worry about this issue and there is much discussion about what constitutes a 'good death' in the West (Dickenson, 2000). However, although there are non-Christians who are critical of the tendency of Western medicine to focus on prolonging life, all Christians are likely to share this opinion and to recognize the 'finitude of human life' and 'the importance of proper preparation for death' (Englehardt and Cherry, eds, 2002, p.36). Thus, perhaps what we can say about a Christian approach to bioethics is that Christian approaches of all types embody a respect for the sacredness of life and they make decisions within a spiritual framework.

CONCLUSION

In summary, then, our attempt to outline a Christian bioethics or a Christian approach to bioethics has shown that such an attempt is flawed as there is no single Christian approach to bioethics. This was true at the theoretical and methodological level when we considered Christian ethics, from which Christian bioethics is derived, and at a practical level when we turned to bioethics and our test case of the status of the embryo – in the issues of abortion, reproductive technologies and research. Having illustrated the impossibility of outlining a Christian approach to bioethics, in the final section we explored whether any generalizations, however broad, could be made about Christian approaches to bioethical issues. It was suggested, very tentatively, that a distinction, however minor, between Christian and non-Christian bioethics could be found in Christian understandings of sacredness and the belief that ethical decisions have spiritual significance and should be considered against a wider spiritual background.

If we now attempted to answer the question set out at the beginning of the chapter of 'what is Christian about Christian bioethics?', we would have to conclude that the answer could be 'very much' or 'very little', depending on the type of Christian bioethics we are discussing. However, in the shared sense of the sacredness of human life considered in a spiritual context, a distinction between secular and Christian bioethics may perhaps, and very cautiously, be drawn. Moreover, if secular bioethics continues to move away from the Christian values from which it was derived this distinction may increase, enabling a clearer answer to the question of this chapter. However, such a divide may not be desirable, as the values of sacredness and spirituality are potentially of value to the secular bioethicist (as the non-Christian thinkers argued in relation to a good death). Therefore, perhaps we should not be focusing on the difference between Christian bioethics and secular bioethics, but asking why these values are less evident in contemporary secular bioethics than they once were and whether in losing these perspectives valuable insights have been lost.

BIBLIOGRAPHY

Adams R. A modified divine command theory of ethical wrongness. In: Helm P, ed. *Divine Commands and Morality.* Oxford: Oxford University Press, 1981; pp 83–108.

Boyle J. Limiting access to health care: a traditional Roman Catholic analysis. In: Engelhardt HT Jr, Cherry MJ, eds. *Allocating Scare Medical Resources: Roman Catholic Perspectives.* Washington: Georgetown University Press, 2002; pp. 77–95.

Casey SB. How the law will shape our life and death decisions In: Cameron NMdeS, Daniels SE, Barbara JW, eds. *BioEngagement: Making a Christian Difference Through Bioethics Today.* 2000; pp. 143–66.

Cohen CB. The moral status of early embryos and new Genetic Interventions. In: Smith DH, Cohen CB, eds. *A Christian Response to the New Genetics: Religious, Ethical and Social Issues.* New York: Rowman and Litterfield Publishers, 2003; pp 105–30.

Collins FS. Human genetics. In: Kilner JF, Hook CC, Uustal DB, eds. *Cutting Edge Bioethics: A Christian Exploration of Technologies and Trends.* Cambridge: WM B Eerdmans Publishing Co, 2002.

Delkeskamp-Hayes C. Between secular reason and the spirit of christianity. In: Engelhardt HT Jr, Cherry JM, eds. *Allocating Scare Medical Resources: Roman Catholic Perspectives.* Washington: Georgetown University Press, 2002; pp. 275–96.

Dickenson D, Johnson M, Katz JS, eds. In: *Death, Dying and Bereavement.* London: Sage Publications, 2000.

Englehardt HT. *The Foundations of a Christian Bioethics.* Lisse: Swets and Zeitlinger Publishers, 2000.

Englehardt HT Jr, Cherry MJ, eds. *Allocating Scarce Medical Resources: Roman Catholic Perspectives.* Georgetown University Press, 2002.

Fairweather ICM, McDonald JIH. *The Quest for Christian Ethics: An Inquiry into Ethics and Christian Ethics.* Edinburgh: The Handsel Press, 1984.107

Gustafson JM. *Can Ethics be Christian?* Chicago: The University of Chicago Press, 1975.

Gustafson JM. Abortion – a reformed perspective. In: Gill R, ed. *A Textbook of Christian Ethics.* Edinburgh: T&T Clark, 1985; pp. 488–99.

Johnson JL. Procedure, substance and the divine command theory. *Philos Religion* 1994; **35:** 39–55.

Kaveny, Cathleen, M. Developing the Doctrine of Distributive Justice: Methods of distribution, redistribution and the role of time in allocation of intensive care resources. In: Engelhardt HT Jr, Cherry MJ, eds. *Allocating Scare Medical Resources: Roman Catholic Perspectives.* Washington: Georgetown University Press, 2002; pp. 177–99.

Khushf G. Beyond the question of limits: Institutional guidelines for the appropriate use of critical care. In: Engelhardt HT Jr, Cherry MJ, eds. *Allocating Scare Medical Resources: Roman Catholic Perspectives.* Washington: Georgetown University Press, 2002; pp. 157–76.

Leber G. We must rescue them. In: Baird RM, Rosenbaum SE, eds. *The Ethics of Abortion.* New York: Prometheus Books, 2001; pp. 195–8.

Maguire DC. A Catholic theologian at an abortion clinic. In: Baird RM, Rosenbaum SE, eds. *The Ethics of Abortion.* New York: Prometheus Books, 2001; pp. 199–206.

Nielsen Kai. God and the Basis of Morality. *J Religious Ethics,* 1982; **10:** 335–50.

Plato. Euthyphro. In: Hamilton E, Cairns H. eds; Cooper L, translator. *Plato: The Collected Dialogues.* Princeton: Princeton University Press, 1989; pp. 169–185.

Quinn P. *Divine Commands and Moral Requirements.* Oxford: Clarendon Press, 1978.

Ryan M. *The Ethics and Economics of Assisted Reproduction: The Cost of Longing.* Washington: Georgetown University Press, 2001.

Schotsmans PT. Equal care as the best of care: a personalist approach. In: Engelhardt HT Jr, Cherry MJ, eds. *Allocating Scare Medical Resources: Roman Catholic Perspectives.* Washington: Georgetown University Press, 2002; pp. 125–39.

Seifert J. Towards a personalistic ethics of limiting access to medical treatment: philosophical and catholic positions. In: Engelhardt HT Jr, Cherry JM, eds. *Allocating Scare Medical Resources: Roman Catholic Perspectives.* Washington: Georgetown University Press, 2002; pp. 96–124.

Shoenig R. Christians and Abortion. In: Baird RM, Rosenbaum SE, eds. *The Ethics of Abortion.* New York: Prometheus Books 2001; pp. 224–30.

Simmons PD. Personhood, the Bible and abortion. In: Baird RM, Rosenbaum SE, eds. *The Ethics of Abortion.* New York: Prometheus Books, 2001; pp. 207–23.

Taboada P. What is appropriate intensive care? A Roman Catholic perspective. In: Engelhardt HT Jr, Cherry MJ, eds. *Allocating Scare Medical Resources: Roman Catholic Perspectives.* Washington: Georgetown University Press, 2002; pp. 53–76.

Westmoreland R. Two recent metaphysical divine command theories of ethics. *Int J Philos Religion* 1996; **39:** 15–31.

15

Judaism and Medicine: Jewish Medical Ethics

FRED ROSNER

BACKGROUND

In the beginning of Jewish history, religion and healing were inseparable because the priest and the physician were one and the same person, administering healing with divine sanction. The advent of scientific medicine in the middle of the nineteenth century nearly completely separated medicine from religion. Nevertheless, Jewish physicians traditionally consider their vocation to be spiritually endowed and not merely an ordinary profession. Ethical standards for the practice of medicine among Jews have always been high. Jews have always held physicians in great esteem.

Throughout history, Jews have exerted a tremendous influence on the development of medical science. They have and continue to excel in medical practice, teaching, administration and research. Over 20% of all Nobel Prize winners for medicine are Jewish.

The importance of medicine among the Jews is best seen in the long line of rabbi–physicians, which started during the talmudic period (Mar Samuel being the most famous example) and continued through the Middle Ages (Examples include Maimonides, Nachmanides and Judah Halevi). Various factors were responsible for this combination of professions which continues to this day. Medicine was sanctioned by biblical and talmudic law and had an important bearing upon religious matters. Teaching or studying the Torah or word of God for reward was not considered ethical since God taught Torah to Moses and the Israelites for nothing and we should emulate God by not receiving a fee for teaching Torah. Therefore, the practice of medicine was most often chosen as a means of livelihood. This trend was further strengthened by the fact that during the greater part of the Middle Ages, Jews were excluded from almost all other occupations, including public office, and medicine was one of the few dignified occupations by which they could earn their living (Munter, 1971).

INTRODUCTION

The emergence of Jewish medical ethics as a distinct subspecialty within Jewish thought and Jewish law is a relatively recent phenomenon. The late Rabbi Lord Immanuel Jakobovits' doctoral thesis entitled 'Jewish Medical Ethics', submitted to London University in 1955 and published by New York's Philosophical library in 1959, was the first use of that phrase. This landmark monograph was perhaps a revolutionary publication, not merely because the term or concept of Jewish medical ethics was unknown at that time, but the subject itself had been entirely unexplored and left without any literary or scholarly expression in any western language. Physicians, medical students and other interested parties had no writings to consult to familiarize themselves with Jewish views even on such elementary subjects such as abortion, contraception, euthanasia, autopsy and their like. Only a handful of people, mostly rabbis, could consult the original Hebrew and/or Aramaic sources scattered in rabbinic writings, often in highly technical terms, covering many centuries of legal casuistry and creativity.

Yet we are reminded that the study of Jewish medical ethics is not a twentieth century phenomenon. The Jewish people have been studying, writing about and practising Jewish medical ethics for thousands of years. The Jewish tradition, which dates back to Sinai, is perhaps the longest unbroken tradition in bioethics that is still followed by its adherents.

Principles of Health Care Ethics, Second Edition   Edited by R.E. Ashcroft, A. Dawson, H. Draper and J.R. McMillan
© 2007 John Wiley & Sons, Ltd

Throughout the millennia, Judaism and medicine have marched hand-in-hand as allies, not as rivals. The mainstream of Jewish tradition has placed an enormous value on human life and health, has given human beings an obligation to preserve life and health, and has pursued a dual track of encouraging recognized medical therapy together with faith in the Almighty. Judaism has also, for the most part, rejected all varieties of dualism and rivalries between the body and the spirit, maintaining rather that spiritual progress can be enhanced by a healthy body. Our ancients already had insights, as well, into preventive medicine and behavioral medicine (Glick, 1997).

Because Judaism and medicine enjoy historical and intellectual kinships, it is only natural that Jewish law is best qualified to apply its reasoned pragmatic rules of morality to the practice of medicine. In the words of Rabbi Jakobovits, 'for many centuries, rabbis and physicians, often merging their professions into one, were intimate partners in a common effort for the betterment of life. The perplexities of our age challenge them to renew their association in the service of human life, health and dignity. Indeed, they challenge Judaism itself to reassert its place as a potent force in the moral advancement of humanity' (Jakobovits, 1959).

Jews, to whom questions of medical ethics are quests not only for applicable humanitarian principles but also for divine guidance, must, of necessity seek answers in the teachings of the Torah. *The Torah of God is perfect*, (Psalms 19:8) and in its teachings the discerning student can find eternally valid answers to even newly formulated queries. As physicians and patients turn to rabbinic authorities for answers, Jewish scholars seek to elucidate and expound the teaching of the Torah in these areas of profound concern.

Judaism is guided by the concept of the supreme sanctity of human life and the dignity of man created in the image of God. The preservation of human life in Judaism is a divine commandment. Jewish law requires physicians to do everything in their power to prolong life but prohibits the use of measures that prolong the act of dying. The value attached to human life in Judaism is far greater than that in the Christian tradition or in Anglo-Saxon common law. In order save a life, all Jewish religious laws are automatically suspended; the only exceptions are those prohibiting idolatry, murder, and forbidden sexual relations such as incest.

In Judaism, the practice of medicine by a physician does not constitute an interference with the deliberate designs of Divine Providence. A physician does not play God when he practises medicine. In fact, a physician not only has divine licence to heal but he is obligated to heal. A physician in Judaism is prohibited from withholding his healing skills.

Judaism is a 'right-to-life' religion. This obligation to save lives is not only individual but also communal. Certainly a physician, who has knowledge and expertise far greater than that of a layperson, is obligated to use his medical skills to heal the sick and thereby prolong and preserve life. It is erroneous to suppose that having recourse to medicine shows lack of trust and confidence in God, the Healer. The Bible takes for granted the use of medical therapy and actually demands it. Although it is permissible but not mandatory in Jewish law to study medicine, once a person becomes a physician, he is obliged to use his skills and knowledge to heal the sick.

In Judaism, not only is a physician obligated to heal, but a patient is obligated to seek healing from physicians rather than relying on faith healing. The Talmud states that no wise person should reside in a city that does not have a physician. The 12th century Jewish scholar and physician Moses Maimonides rules that a man is obliged to accustom himself to a regimen that will preserve his body's health and heal and fortify it when it is ailing.

The extreme concerns in Judaism about the preservation of health and the prolongation of life require that a woman's pregnancy be terminated if her life is endangered by the pregnancy, that a woman use contraception if her life would be threatened by pregnancy, that an organ transplant be performed if it can save or prolong the life of a patient dying of organ failure and that a postmortem examination be performed if the results of the autopsy may provide immediate information to rescue another dying patient. Judaism prohibits cruelty to animals, but it sanctions experimentation on animals to find cures for human illnesses as long as the animal experiences no pain and suffering.

Judaism also allows patients to accept experimental medical or surgical treatments when no standard therapy is available and the experimental therapy is administered by the most experienced physicians whose intent is to help the patient and not just to satisfy their academic curiosity.

In Judaism, the infinite value of human life prohibits euthanasia or mercy killing in any form. Handicapped newborns, mentally retarded persons, psychotic persons and patients dying of any illness or cause have the same right to life as anyone else, and nothing may be done to hasten their death. On the other hand, there are times when specific medical or surgical therapies are no longer indicated, appropriate or desirable for a patient who is irreversibly, terminally ill. Under no circumstances, however, can general supportive care, including food and water, be withheld or withdrawn to hasten a patient's death.

Thus, in Judaism each human being is considered to be of supreme and infinite value. It is the obligation of individuals and society to preserve, hallow and dignify human life to care for the total needs of all persons so that they can be healthy and productive members of society. This fundamental principle of the sanctity of life and the dignity of man as a creation of God is the underlying axiom upon which all medical ethical decisions are based (Rosner, 1995).

THE PHYSICIAN'S MANDATE TO HEAL

The basic principles in Judaism governing the practice of medicine, whether in the doctor's office or over the telephone or on the Internet are based on the premise that in Jewish tradition a physician is given specific divine license to practice medicine. The biblical verse *and heal he shall heal* (Exodus 21:19) is interpreted by the talmudic sages (Baba Kamma 85a) to teach us that authorization is granted by God to the physician to heal. In Jewish law, a physician is not merely allowed to practise medicine but is in fact commanded to do so if he has chosen to become a physician. This biblical mandate is based upon two scriptural precepts. *And thou shalt restore it to him* (Deuteronomy 22:2) refers to the restoration of lost property. Moses Maimonides, in his Commentary on the Mishnah (Nedarim 4:4), states that 'it is obligatory from the Torah for the physician to heal the sick, and this in included in the explanation of the scriptural phrase *and thou shalt restore it to him,* meaning to heal his body'. Thus, Maimonides as well as the Talmud (Nedarim 38b) state that the law of restoration also includes the restoration of the health of one's fellowman. If a person has 'lost his health' and the physician is able to restore it, he is obligated to do so.

The second scriptural mandate for the physician to heal is based on the phrase *neither shalt thou stand idly by the blood of thy neighbor* (Leviticus 19:16). The passage refers to the duties of human beings to their fellowmen and the moral principles which the Sages expound and apply to every phase of civil and criminal law. If one stands idly by and allows one's fellow man to die without offering help, one is guilty of transgressing this precept. A physician who refuses to heal thereby resulting in suffering and/or death of the patient is also guilty of transgressing this commandment.

If one asks why did God grant physicians' licence and even mandate to heal the sick, one can offer the following explanation. As already mentioned, a cardinal principle of Judaism is that human life is of infinite value. The preservation of human life takes precedence over all commandments in the Bible except three: adultery, murder and forbidden sexual relations. Life's value is nearly absolute and supreme. In order to preserve a human life, the Sabbath and even the Day of Atonement may be desecrated, and all other rules and laws save the aforementioned three are suspended for the overriding consideration of saving a human life. 'He who saves one life is as if he saved a whole world' (Sanhedrin 37a). Even a few moments of life are worthwhile.

Jewish law also requires a physician to be well trained and licensed by the local authorities (Karo, 1984). An unlicensed physician is liable to pay compensation to the patient for unintentional errors or side effects. A negligent physician is obviously culpable even if he is licensed. However, he is not liable for misjudgements or side effects or a bad outcome if he acted responsibly. This topic is discussed extensively elsewhere (Fruchter, 1993). Judaism protects physicians from undeserved liability but stresses that the physician recognize the limits of his abilities and demands that physicians consult with more experienced colleagues in situations of doubt.

A physician is entitled to reasonable fees and compensation for his services (Rosner & Widroff, 1997). In talmudic times when physicians, rabbis, teachers and judges served the community on a part-time basis only and had other occupations and trades, their compensation was limited to lost time and effort. Nowadays, however, when physicians have no other occupation, they can charge for their expert medical knowledge and receive full compensation. Excessive fees are discouraged but are not prohibited if the patient agrees to the fee in advance. Indigent patients should be treated for reduced or no fees at all. These principles are applicable both to a salaried physician as well as a physician in private practice who charges fee-for-service.

These Judaic principles, therefore, require that physicians place the interests of their patients first and advocate for any care they believe will materially benefit their patients. Physicians must practice good medicine, eliminate that which is unnecessary and be conscious of the need to contain costs. Physicians must also practice within the areas that they are credentialed and do so in the best interests of their patients.

THE PATIENT'S RESPONSIBILITY TO STAY HEALTHY

The prevention of illness and the avoidance of dangers to life are mandated in Jewish law. The maintenance of one's health requires Jews to avoid harmful foods and activities and to prevent danger wherever possible. Preventive medicine has been the centrepiece of the Jewish system for more than two thousand years. The Jewish view emphasizes prevention over treatment.

An entire chapter in Moses Maimonides' famous Code of Jewish Law (Maimonides) is devoted to hygienic and medical prescriptions for healthy living and for the prevention of illness. Among the many subjects discussed are normal bodily excretory functions, recommended times for eating, amounts and types of food to be consumed, beverage imbibition, exercise, sleep habits, cathartics, climatic and weather effects on eating habits, detrimental and beneficial foods, fruits, meats, vegetables, bathing, bloodletting, sexual intercourse and domicile.

One must also be concerned about ecological and environmental factors such as clean air and sunshine which may impact upon one's health. One must observe rules of personal hygiene such as hand washing before eating. Diet, exercise, sex and bodily functions must all be tended to as outlined by Maimonides. He concludes his exposition as follows:

> I guarantee anyone who conducts himself according to the directions we have laid down that he will not be afflicted with illness all the days of his life, until he ages greatly and expires. He will not require a physician, and his body will be complete and remain healthy all his life unless his body was defective from the beginning of his creation, or unless he became accustomed to one of the bad habits from the onset of his youth, or unless the plague of pestilence or the plague of drought comes onto the world (Maimonides).

Maimonides cites exceptions to the goal of preventing rather than treating illness. Genetic diseases and certain epidemics of diseases cannot be prevented. For this reason, the final paragraph in Maimonides' chapter on the regimen of health states that a person should not reside in a city that does not have a physician. A similar pronouncement is found in the Talmud (Sanhedrin 17b). Maimonides supports the adage 'An ounce of prevention is more valuable than a pound of cure'. More evidence for this thesis is found in his medical writings (Rosner, 1998).

THE PATIENT'S RESPONSIBILITY TO SEEK HEALING WHEN ILL

The Bible tells us to *take heed to thyself, and take care of thy life* (Deuteronomy 4:9) and *take good care of your lives* (Ibid 4:15). These biblical mandates make it clear that patients are obligated to care for their health and life. Man does not have full title over his body and life. He must eat and drink to sustain himself and must seek healing when sick.

In the Western world, citizens are endowed with a variety of legal rights. People have the right to die, the right to refuse treatment, the right not to be resuscitated, the right to abortion and many others. Rarely does one hear about responsibilities and obligations of citizens. Judaism requires everyone to do what is proper in order to be healthy. It is an obligation in Judaism to be healthy. Hence one should accept appropriate medical advice, whether given in person, over the telephone, by fax, e-mail or over the Internet. One should not smoke, one should eat properly and not excessively, one should exercise regularly, sleep adequately, only engage in proper and legitimate sexual activities and lead an overall healthy life style. These are more obligations and legal imperatives in Judaism.

Thus, while much of the modern secular ethical system is based on rights, Judaism is an ethical system based on duties and responsibilities. The late Rabbi Lord Immanuel Jakobovits eloquently articulates the Jewish view as follows:

Now in Judaism we know of no intrinsic rights. Indeed there is no word for rights in the very language of the Hebrew Bible and of the classic sources of Jewish law. In the moral vocabulary of the Jewish discipline of life we speak of human duties, not of human rights, of obligations, not entitlement. The Decalogue is a list of Ten Commandments, not a Bill of Human Rights (Jakobovits, 1989).

MEDICINE ON THE INTERNET

A new bioethical issue in the field of medicine is the Internet, which is a magnificent scientific tool to provide health education of high quality to masses of people. It is an unparalleled information source whose use Judaism supports because of its potential to inform people about healthy living to prevent or to mitigate illness. Primary prevention activities can deter the occurrence of a disease or adverse event. Smoking cessation reduces the risk of lung cancer. A variety of prevention strategies (e.g. aspirin, exercise, weight, blood pressure and lipid control, etc.) can reduce the risk of a heart attack. Judaism requires communities to not only provide for the medical and social needs of their citizens but also to alert people about drug recalls, epidemics and the dangers of substance abuse. Judaism thus responds to modern technology by harnessing it for the benefit of mankind.

Electronic mail between physicians and patients offers substantial promise as a way to improve access to health care, to let physicians reach out to patients and to increase the involvement of patients in their own care. Elderly patients can consult their physicians by 'electronic house call' to record their vital signs and discuss their condition. Prescription refills, lab results, appointment scheduling and reminders, insurance questions, routine follow up inquiries and reporting of home health measurements such as blood pressure and glucose are well suited to e-mail. Highly confidential information or medically urgent or emergent situations should not be communicated by e-mail.

Jewish concerns about potential dangers of the indiscriminate use of the Internet must be addressed. Pornographic and other prurient and/or defamatory material must be blocked out to avoid violating the biblical and rabbinic laws concerning immorality. The placing of misleading or potentially harmful information, medical or otherwise, violates the prohibitions against deception (Chullin 94a) and against placing a stumbling block before the blind (Leviticus 19:4). 'Cursed is he who leads the blind astray' (Deuteronomy 27:18). The addictive qualities of the Internet result in sleep deprivation for many people who spend more time online than they intended. Such addiction may take its toll on one's health, school grades, employment, marriage, Torah study, and so forth.

The Internet is a wonderful scientific and technological advance with enormous beneficial potential for mankind. Its use must certainly be sanctioned in Jewish law. However, good often is not pure good, but may contain potentially dangerous elements.

CONFIDENTIALITY AND THE INTERNET

Patients have the right and perhaps the obligation to use the Internet to prevent and to treat illnesses. For some patients the Internet may be an absolute necessity. Patients with very rare conditions or diseases can 'talk' to physicians and experts all over the world about their cases. Lay people who need sources of help such as support groups, medical care and specialists can obtain such assistance and information on the Internet. For physicians, the Internet is an indispensable tool for continuing medical education, for patient care and patient education and for information exchange with colleagues. For the general Jewish public, accurate medical information is crucial for healthy living and disease prevention. Confidentiality of medical information is one of the major concerns relating to the Internet. There are no major ethical difficulties if physicians provide generic medical information on the Internet. However, patients' private medical information transmitted by e-mail from patient to physician and vice-versa is accessible to many people with computer expertise, and therefore requires special and careful consideration. Patients must be told that the Internet is not a secure means of communication since Internet messages can potentially be intercepted, viewed and altered by unauthorized individuals. 'Deleted' may still be recoverable. Therefore, sensitive information should not be sent over the Internet. Furthermore, the Internet should not be used for urgent or emergency medical conditions. Direct communication with the physician or ambulance service should then be used.

Other than clerical or administrative communications such as billing, appointments and insurance matters, all e-mail communications related to patient care should be considered sensitive and confidential. Patients must also consider the security of their own home or office computers in regard to the confidentiality of their medical information. The challenge to preserve confidentiality must be pursued and met by the adoption of technologically secure means of data transmission.

The obligation to maintain confidentiality is one of the cornerstones of medical ethical practice and is clearly stated in the Oath of Hippocrates and many subsequent deontological oaths and declarations. This obligation is based on the general ethical principles of doing good for others (beneficence), not to harm others (nonmaleficence), patient autonomy and the right to privacy. This obligation is also based on the trusting relationship between patient and physician and the need to protect and preserve that relationship by not disclosing to others private and personal information about the patient.

Maintaining professional confidentiality is a subject which Jewish thought and literature have dealt with extensively over centuries (Cohen, 1984). In Judaism, the rights of privacy of an individual are balanced against the rights of others and society as a whole (Tendler, 1989). Jewish law regards as inviolate the privacy of personal information that a person does not wish to disclose to others. Jewish law demands that confidences be respected not only by professionals with whom one has entered into a fiduciary relationship but also by friends and acquaintances and even strangers to whom such information has been imparted (Bleich, 2000). The obligation of confidentiality in Judaism is far broader than that of any other legal, religious or moral system (Bleich, 1999).

There is no specific term in Jewish law for professional confidentiality since this topic is subsumed under the general obligation or prohibition against tale bearing and evil gossip (Leviticus 19:16; Proverbs 25:9; Psalms 34:14).

According to these laws, a physician may not share privileged information with his colleagues, his family or anyone else if no benefit to the patient would result therefrom (Steinberg, 1994). However, if the maintenance of confidence might cause harm to another person, the latter may be informed. If the individual's right to privacy conflicts with the need of society to prevent harm to others, the prohibitions against tale bearing and evil gossip are waived and the information must be disclosed to protect other people. The disclosure must be factual, accurate and not exaggerated.

Specific medical situations where disclosure is required include the possible transmission of illness to another person, the presence of a serious medical condition in a potential spouse, and the reporting of certain infectious diseases to public health authorities. The overriding obligation to protect the lives of others requires that confidential information be disclosed if the withholding of that information might lead to serious harm to someone else. Judaism thus balances the obligation and duty to maintain confidentiality with the obligation and duty to protect others.

THE FUTURE OF JEWISH MEDICAL ETHICS

According to Lord Jakobovits, Jewish medical ethics is built on rulings given by leading experts on Jewish law which, when collected and published, are known as 'responsa'. By definition, these rulings are reactive rather than proactive and meet a demand for guidance by patients, physicians, scholars or others who seek to practice Judaism according to traditional teachings. The rulings become normative and assume the force of law by virtue of the universal recognition accorded to their authors. These conditions show every sign of remaining a permanent feature of Jewish medical ethics (Jakobovits, 1997).

A second crucial factor determining the future course of medical ethics will be the development of medicine itself. Most important point from a Jewish point of view will be where to draw the line between the 'blind march to mechanical perfection and the capacity to control the forces science and technology can now generate at our bidding for the exploitation of nature's infinite energies' (Jakobovits, 1997).

In some areas, halachic issues raised by modern medical technology are still unresolved and subject to heated controversy. One such example is the definition of death. Within the next few years, one hopes that this dispute will be resolved – if only by the preponderance of halachic verdicts one way or the other. The decision depends on facts, and facts are bound to emerge convincingly in the end. When heart transplants began, the procedure was condemned by most halachic authorities. The increasing success rate (80% survival for five years) has been accompanied by increasing permissive rulings, which now seem to predominate.

Areas of Jewish medical ethics which require additional study and research are professional ethics such as secrecy, confidentiality, truth telling and the public good; genetics including genetic screening, gene therapy, gene surgery and cloning; mental health issues such as sex therapy, homosexuality, drug addiction, alcoholism, and their like.

A large area that has to date been inadequately discussed and which is bound to engage ever increasing attention is the distribution of scarce resources and the allocation of limited funds. Among the limited resources is the Jewish source material. This need, too, will eventually be met by intensified search for precedents in earlier statements of principles and decisions.

Finally, the significant growth of Jewish medical ethics, both for practical guidance and as an academic discipline of ever-greater sophistication, will call for the more intensive training of experts proficient in Jewish law and medicine alike. Such professional specialists are beginning to emerge, both practising rabbis and practising physicians. Some are both rabbis and doctors in the spirit of famous talmudic and medieval physician–rabbis. All these modern Jewish bioethicists are indebted to and many were stimulated by the pioneering work in this field of the late Rabbi Lord Immanuel Jakobovits. That is why he is more correctly identified today not as the father of Jewish medical ethics but the grandfather of Jewish medical ethics 'through the disciples who now themselves have raised generations of scholars devoted to this field' (Jakobovits, 1999).

SUMMARY AND CONCLUSION

The attitude towards healing in Judaism has always been a positive one. A physician is obligated to heal and is given divine licence to do so. A physician must be well trained and licensed in his discipline. A physician must apply his skills for the benefit of the patient and be careful not to do harm. Thus, the ethical principles of beneficence and nonmaleficence are deeply rooted in Judaism. A patient is also obligated to seek healing since one must be healthy in order to serve the Lord by doing His will in the service of mankind.

A second cardinal principle of Judaism is the infinite value of human life. The preservation of life takes precedence over all biblical and rabbinic commandments except three: murder, idolatry and forbidden sexual relations such as incest or adultery. The Talmud states that all lives are equal since one person's blood is not redder than that of another person (Pesachim 25b).

Preventive medicine is a centrepiece of the Jewish system. The Jewish view towards the practice of medicine emphasizes prevention over treatment. Prevention of danger and thereby the preservation of life and health are biblical mandates. One must observe rules of personal hygiene such as hand washing before eating. Diet, exercise, sex and bodily functions must all be properly tended to. Preventive medical services and patient responsibilities are fully consonant with Judaism. Thus, emphasis on prevention of illness, as well as personal responsibility, are deeply rooted in Judaic teaching and tradition.

With regard to the Internet, Judaism views any new technology or scientific advance with favour if it is used for the betterment of mankind, such as the prevention and treatment of illness. Such harnessing of the natural sciences is not considered an encroachment upon divine prerogatives. On the contrary, God gave us dominion over the world to use nature to subdue the earth (Genesis 1:28) by transforming its secrets into products and technology to benefit mankind. The Internet is a wonderful tool to accomplish this purpose with some caveats as discussed above.

These principles of Judaism guide the Jewish physician in his practice of medicine. As new Jewish bioethical questions arise, rabbinic decisors will provide answers based on the expert medical and technical information provided by physicians and scientists. Such answers must be consonant with the physician's ability to practice medicine, using the most up-to-date advances in medical science and biomedical technology. However, such answers must also remain true to traditional Judaic teachings as transmitted by God to Moses and the children of Israel.

REFERENCES

Bleich JD. Rabbinic confidentiality. *Tradition.* 1999; **33**: 54–87.
Bleich JD. Genetic screening. *Tradition.* 2000; **34**: 63–87.
Cohen AS. On maintaining a professional confidence. *J Halacha Contemp Soc*, 1984; **VII**: 73–87.

Fruchter J. Doctors on trial: a comparison of American and Jewish legal approaches to medical malpractice. *Am J Law Med* 1993; **19**: 453–95.

Glick S. Foreword. In: Rosner F, ed. *Pioneers in Jewish Medical Ethics*, Northvale, NJ: Jason Aronson, 1997; pp. XV–XXI.

Jakobovits I. *Jewish Medical Ethics – A Comparative and Historical Study of the Jewish Religious Attitude to Medicine and its Practice.* New York: Philosophical Library, 1959; p. VIII.

Jakobovits I. *The Timely and the timeless: Jews, Judaism and Society in a Storm-Tossed Decade.* New York: Bloch, 1989; p. 128.

Jakobovits I. Future trends and currents in Jewish medical ethics. In: Rosner F, ed. *Pioneers in Jewish Medical Ethics* Northvale, NJ: Jason Aronson, 1997; pp. 231–4.

Jakobovits I. Personal communication. 1999.

Karo J. *Code of Jewish Law (Shulchan Aruch)*, Section *Yoreh Deah* 1984; 336.

Maimonides M. *Code of Jewish Law (Mishneh Torah)*, Section *Deot*, Chapter 4:1 ff.

Muntner S. Medicine. In: Roth C, ed. *Enclyclopedia Judaica*, Vol. 11. Jerusalem: Keter, 1971; pp. 1178–95.

Rosner F. Jewish medical ethics. *J Clin Ethics* 1995; **6**: pp. 202–17.

Rosner F. Moses Maimonides and preventive medicine. *J Hist Med* 1998, **51**: 313–24.

Rosner F, Widroff J. Physicians' fees in Jewish law. *Jewish Law Annu* 1997; **12**: 115–26.

Steinberg A. *Encyclopedia Talmudit Refuit.* (Encyclopedia of Jewish Medical Ethics), Vol. 4. Jerusalem: Schlesinger Institute of the Shaare Zedek Medical Center, 1994; pp. 613–42.

Tendler MD. Confidentiality: a biblical perspective on rights in conflict. *Natl Jewish Law Rev* 1989; **4**: 1–7.

16

The Search for Islamic Bioethics Principles

ABDULAZIZ SACHEDINA

The earlier edition of *Principles of Health Care Ethics* (1994) included an article providing Islamic equivalents of the Four Principles of Western-American bioethics, namely, autonomy, nonmaleficence, beneficence (including utility) and justice expounded by Tom L. Beauchamp and James F. Childress in *Principles of Biomedical Ethics* (4th edition, 1994). For several reasons the article failed to provide Muslim assessment of the principles and arguments for specifically Islamic principles of bioethics in the Muslim cultural context. First and foremost, it is indispensable to assess the intellectual context of the Four Principles, including the secular and democratic political philosophy that informs much of the principle-based bioethics in the West. No enunciation of the bioethical principles is possible without articulating the presuppositions of the Islamic tradition about human action, its ontology, its ethical evaluation and the roles of moral reasoning and scriptural resources in resolving a practical quandary. There is a critical need to understand moral epistemology in Islam before searching for the equivalents of the secular bioethics in the Islamic legal ethics.

Muslim legal theorists were thoroughly aware of moral underpinnings of the religious duties that all Muslims were required to fulfil as members of the faith community. In fact, the validity of their research in the foundational sources of Islam (the Qur'an and the Tradition) for solutions to practical matters depended upon their substantial consideration of different moral facets of a case that could be discovered by considering conflicting claims, interests and responsibilities in the precedents preserved in these authoritative sources. What ensured the validity of their judicial decision regarding a specific instance was their ability to deduce the universal

moral principles like 'there shall be no harm inflicted or reciprocated' (*lā ḍarar wa lā ḍirār*)[1] that flowed downward from their initial premise to support their particular conclusion without any dependence on the circumstances that would have rendered the conclusion circumstantial at the most. In their appraisal of a network of conflicting moral considerations in the new case that required a legal solution, theoretical arguments embedded in primary sources to derive a resolution functioned more as *ratio legis* ('*illa*) or the attribute common to both the new and the original case. The rule or the principle (*qā'ida* or *aṣl*) was attached to the original case, which due to similarity between the two cases was transferred from that case to the new case. As such, more attention was paid to the original rule and the *ratio legis* that also became the source of much debate among Muslim jurists and formed important part of the procedures used to resolve earlier problems and reapplying them in the new problematic situations (Hallaq, 2001). Practical solutions based on earlier precedents carry the burden of proof on how closely the present case resemble those of the earlier paradigm cases for which this particular type of argument was originally devised. However, the power of these conclusions depended on the ethical considerations deduced from the rules that were operative in the original cases and the agreement of the scholars about analogical deduction that sought to relate the new case to the original rationale as well as rules.

In Islamic jurisprudence ethical values are integral to the prescriptive action guide that the system provides to the community. No legal decisions are made without meticulous analysis of the various factors that determine the rightness or the wrongness of a case under consideration. The universal major premise provided by the scriptural sources – the

---

[1] Literally, the principle translates: There shall be no harming, injuring, or hurting, [of one person by another] in the first instance, nor in return, or requital, in Islam (See: Lane EW. *An Arabic–English Lexicon*. Part V, p. 1775). In this work I will refer to this principle as the principle or the rule of 'No harm, no harassment'.

Principles of Health Care Ethics, Second Edition   Edited by R.E. Ashcroft, A. Dawson, H. Draper and J.R. McMillan
© 2007 John Wiley & Sons, Ltd

Qur'an and the Tradition (*sunna*) – that serves as known is part of the divine commandments regarding the good that must be obeyed and the evil that must be avoided. There is an inherent correlation between God's command in the revelation and the moral reasoning that undergirds the command that is acknowledged by reason as being good. The metaphysical backdrop of the Sharī'a – the religious law of Islam – is the discovery of God's purposes for humanity. Human reason is God's endowment to enable human intellect to fathom the supernatural by exploring the meanings of the revealed message through the Prophet.

Whereas I am a believer in universal moral values that have application across cultures, human conditions in specific social and political culture demand searching for principles and rules that provide cultural-specific guidance in Muslim societies to resolve practical quandaries. My working assumption in this chapter is that praxis precedes search for principles and rules. Customarily, when faced with a moral dilemma deliberations are geared towards a satisfactory resolution in which justifications are based on practical consequences, regardless of applicable principles. For instance, in deciding whether to allow dissection of the cadaver to retrieve a valuable object swallowed by the deceased, Muslim jurists have ruled the permission by simply looking at the consequence of forbidding such a procedure. The major moral consideration that outweighs the respect for the dignity of the dead is the ownership through inheritance of the swallowed object for the surviving orphan. Dissection of the cadaver is forbidden in Islam, and, yet, the case demands immediate solution that is based on consequential ethics. Or, in the case of a female patient who, as prescribed in the Sharī'a must be treated by a female physician, in emergency situation the practical demand is to override the prohibition because the rule of necessity (*ḍarūra*) extracted from the revealed texts outweighs the rule about the sexual segregation extracted from rational consideration. Hence, the rule of necessity determines the teleological solution and provides the incontestable rationale for the permission granted to a Muslim female patient to refer to a male physician not related to her. There are numerous instances that clearly show the cultural preferences in providing solutions to the pressing problems of health care in Muslim societies in which highly rated principle of autonomy in the West takes a back seat, while communitarian ethics considers the consequence of any medical decision on the family and community resources.

Contemporary moral discourse has been aptly described as 'a minefield of incommensurable disagreements'. Such disagreements are believed to be the result of secularization

marked by a retreat of religion from the public arena. Privatization of religion has been regarded as a necessary condition for ethical pluralism. The essentially liberal vision of community founded on radical autonomy of the individual moral agent runs contrary to other-regarding communitarian values of shared ideas of justice and of public good. There is a sense that modern, secular, individualistic society is no longer a community founded on commonly held beliefs of social good and its relation to responsibilities and freedoms in a pluralistic society (Heyd, 1996). To provide the fundamentals of the Islamic ethical discourse which ultimately must guide our search in the complexity of bioethical pluralism in the Muslim world, in this chapter I intend to explore distinctly Islamic, and yet cross-culturally communicable, principle-rule based deontological–teleological ethics[2] that is operative in the Muslim legal–moral culture in assessing moral problems in Islamic biomedical ethics.

ISLAMIC ETHICAL DISCOURSE

When one considers the normative Islamic tradition for standards of conduct and character it becomes obvious that besides the scriptural sources like the Qur'an and the Tradition ascribed to the founder of Islam, which prescribe many rules of law and morality for humans, Muslim scholars recognized the value of decisions derived from specific human conditions as equally valid source for social ethics in Islam. Early on, the theologian-jurists conceded that the scriptural sources could not easily cover every situation that might arise, especially when Muslim political rule extended beyond the Arabian peninsula, and required rules for urban life, commerce and government in advanced countries. But how exactly was human intellectual endeavour to be directed to discover the *ratio legis* ('*illa*), the philosophy and the rationale behind certain original rulings (known as *aṣl*, plural *uṣūl*) provided in God's commandments, in order to utilize these to formulate rational deductive principles for future decisions?

The question had important implications for the administrators of justice who were faced with practical necessity to make justifiable legal rulings, which could be defended against accusations of making arbitrary decisions. There was a fear of reason in deriving the details of law. The fear was based on the presumption that if independent human reason could judge what is right and wrong, it could rule on what God could rightly prescribe for humans. In other words, human reasoning could arrogate the function that was in large measure within the jurisdiction of the revealed

---

[2]Deontological ethical norm determines the rightness (or wrongness) of actions without regard to the consequences produced by performing such actions. By contrast, teleological norm determines the rightness (or wrongness) of actions on the basis of the consequences produced by performing these actions. Deontological norms can further be subdivided into objectivist and subjectivist norms: objectivist because the ethical value is intrinsic to the action independently of anyone's decision or opinion; subjectivist because the action derives value in relation to the view of a judge who decides its rightness (or wrongness). Hourani (1985) introduces the latter distinction in deontological norms.

texts. However, it was admitted that although the details of the revealed law can be known through reason and aid human beings in cultivating the moral life, human intelligence was not capable enough to discover what the rationale for a particular law is, let alone demonstrate the truth of a particular assertion embedded in the divine commandment. In fact, as these theologian–jurists asserted that the divine commandments, to which one must adhere if one is to achieve specific end prescribed in the revealed law, are not objectively accessible to human beings through reason. Moreover, judgements of reason were arbitrary, as demonstrated by the fact of their contradicting each other, and reflected personal desire of the legal expert confronted with conflicting claims and interests.

Besides the problem of resolving substantive role of reason in understanding the implicit rationale of a paradigm case and elaborating the juridical–ethical dimension of revealed text as it relates to the conduct of human affairs in public and private spheres, there was a problem of situating the credible religious authority empowered to provide validation to the ethical–legal reasoning associated with the derived philosophy behind legal rulings. On the one hand, following the lead of the Sunnī jurists like Muḥammad b. Idrīs al-Shāfiʿī and Aḥmad b. Ḥanbal in the tenth and eleventh centuries C.E., Sunnī Islam located that authority in the revealed texts – Qur'an and the Tradition. These scholars represented the predominant schools of Sunnī theology that held that in deciding questions of Islamic law one could work out an entire system based on juridical elaboration of Islamic revelation and the Tradition. On the other hand, following the line of thought maintained by the Shīʿite Imams, Shīʿite Islam located that authority in the rightful successors of the Prophet. The Shīʿite Imams maintained that there was an ongoing revelatory guidance available in the expository ability of human reason in comprehending the divine revelation exemplified by the solutions offered by the Shīʿite leadership.

In general, Muslim theologian-jurists paid more attention to the nature of God's creation and human beings' relation to God as the Creator, Lawgiver and Judge. They were also interested to understand the extent of God's power and human freedom of will as it affected the search for a right prescription for human behaviour. In the final analysis, in view of the absence of the institutionalized religious body (resembling the church in Christianity) that could provide the necessary validation of the legal–moral decisions on all matters pertaining to human existence, the problem of determining the Sacred Lawgiver's intent behind juridical–ethical rulings that had direct relevance to the social life of the community was not an easy task. The entire intellectual activity related to Islamic juridical–ethical tradition can be summed up as a jurist–theologian's attempt to relate specific moral–legal rulings (aḥkām, singular ḥukm) to the divine purposes expressed in the form of norms and rules preserved in the original cases in the Qur'an and the Tradition, not without ambiguities though. In view of incomplete state of their knowledge about present circumstances and future contingencies of human conditions, in most cases of ethical judgement, the jurists proceeded with a cautious attitude on the basis of what seemed most likely (ẓann) to be the case. Such ethical judgements were normally appended with a clear, pious statement that the ruling lacked certainty (ʿilm or qaṭʿ) because it was only God, who being aware about the circumstances and consequences affecting human beings, was the most knowledgeable about the true state of affairs.[3]

In due course, the jurists were able to identify two methods for understanding the justification behind a legal–ethical decision. Sometimes the rationale that discovered the rulings was derived directly from the explicit statements of the Qur'an and the Tradition that set forth the purpose of legislation. At other times, human reason discovered the relationship between the ruling and the effective cause, in order to provide sound theoretical basis for jurisprudence. However, the jurists admitted and determined the substantive role of human reasoning in making valid legal or moral decision. Moreover, it depended upon the jurist's comprehension of the nature of ethical knowledge and the means by which humans can access information about good and evil. In other words, it depended upon the way the human act was defined in terms of human ethical discernment about good and evil and the relation of human act to God's will. In an important way, any advocacy of reason as a substantive rather than formal source for procuring moral–legal verdicts required authorization derived from revealed texts like the Qur'an and the Tradition. In the Qur'an, a teleological view of human beings with the very ability to use reason to discover God's will is possible to maintain, more particularly when the revelation itself endorses reflection on the reasons for revealed laws as well as obeying them. It is important to keep in mind that all the jurist–theologians, belonging to the Sunnī or Shīʿite schools of thought, maintained that without the endorsement of the revelation reason could not become an independent source of moral–legal decisions.

This precautious attitude towards reason has its roots in the belief that God's knowledge of the circumstances and of the consequences in any situation of ethical dilemma confronted by human existence is exhaustive and infallible. In fact, there were a number of the rulings in the Qur'an and the Tradition which were expressed simply as God's

---

[3] The usual practice among Muslim jurists is to end their judicial opinion (fatwā) with a statement allāh ʿālim, that is 'God knows best', indicating that the opinion was given on the basis of what seemed most likely to be the case (ẓann), rather than claiming that this was an absolute and unrebuttable (qaṭʿ) opinion, which could be derived only from the revelatory sources like the Qur'an and the Traditions.

commands which had to be obeyed without knowing the
reasons behind them. The commandments were simply part
of God's prerogative as the Creator to demand unquestioning
obedience to them. To act in a manner contrary to divine
commands is to act both immorally and unlawfully. The
major issue in legal thought, then, was related to the defining
of the admissibility and the parameters of human reasoning
as a substantive source for legal–moral decisions. Can reason
discover the divine will in confronting emerging legal–
ethical issues without succumbing to human self-interest?

THE RATIONALIST AND TRADITIONALIST
ETHICAL REASONING IN THE REVELATION

The use of 'rationalist' and 'traditionalist' in this section
conforms to the general identification of the two major
trends in Islamic theological–ethical discourse above. Based
on their admittance of or cautious attitude towards reason
as a substantive source for ethical–legal judgments, the
Sunnī Mu'tazilites and the Shī'ite fall under the 'rationalist'
group, and the Sunnī Ash'arites fall under the 'traditionalist'
group. The process of formulating the methodology for
deriving sound ethical–legal decision was undertaken with
a clear view of providing principles and rules for deriving
predictable judgements in all matters of interpersonal
relationship. Central to this discussion was the analytical
treatment of the twin concepts of justice ('adāla, usually
defined as 'putting something in its appropriate place') and
obligation (wujūb, sometimes defined as 'promulgation of
divine command and prohibition'). The concept of justice
provided a theoretical stance on the question of human
obedience to divine commands and the extent of human
capacity in carrying out the moral–religious obligations
(takālif shar'iyya). The concept of obligation defined the
nature of divine command and provided deontological
grounds for complying with it. The commandments have
reasons of their own that can be explained in terms of the
function they fulfil for the good of humankind.

Gradually, two responses emerged from the pressing
need of providing consistent and authentic guidance in
the matter of social ethics. Some prominent jurists of the
tenth and 11th centuries C.E. maintained that in deciding
questions on which there was no specific guidance available from the normative sources of Islamic law and ethics,
judges and lawyers had to make their own rational judgements independently of the revealed texts. This was certainly the case when the law, being stated in general terms,
did not provide for the peculiarity of situations. This was
the rationalist group. Other jurists disapproved of this rational method not adequately anchored in the normative
sources, and insisted that no legal or moral judgement
was valid if not based on the authoritative religious texts,
both the Qur'an and the Tradition. There was no way for

humanity to know the meaning of justice outside the revealed texts. In fact, they contended, justice is nothing but
carrying out the requirements of the revealed law. This was
the traditionalist camp. In addition, they argued that it was
the revealed law, the Sharī'a, that provided the scales for
justice in all those actions that were declared as morally and
legally obligatory (wājib, farḍ). At the end of the day, the
latter group's traditionalist thesis became the standard view
held by the majority of the Sunnī Muslims. Some Sunnī
and the majority of the Shī'ite Muslims, on the contrary,
maintained the rationalist thesis with some adjustment in
conformity to their doctrine about supreme religious authority of the Imam.

However, the role of ethical norms in deriving moral
judgements was articulated in greater detail by the theologians who, too, were divided on the same lines as the
jurists: those who supported the substantive role of reason
in knowing what is right and obligatory, and those who
argued in favour of the Tradition as the primary source
of ethical knowledge. In other words, moral reasoning
was placed under the authority of the revealed texts that
provide the justification for doing or avoiding a particular
task. Ethical objectivism or deontological theory, with its
thesis that human beings can know much of what is right
and wrong because of the intrinsic goodness or badness
of actions, is connected with the rationalist theologians,
that is, the Mu'tazilite and the Shī'ite; whereas ethical voluntarism, the traditionalist ethics, which denied anything
objective in human acts themselves that would make them
right or wrong, is connected with Ash'arite theologians
(Hourani, 1971).

The traditionalist reactions to the rationalist ethics corroborated the jurists' apprehension of reason in deriving judicial decisions. The arbitrariness of human reason, as the
traditionalists pointed out, could not guarantee a right solution to the complex moral dilemmas faced by human beings
in everyday situation. Moreover, if reason was capable of
reaching right ethical judgement unaided by the revelation,
then what is the need for God's guidance through the revelation? Hence, according to the upholders of traditionalist ethics, it was more accurate to maintain that God's command
in the form of revelation is not only the primary source of
the moral–religious law; it is also the sole guarantee for
avoiding contradictions that stem from reason's arrogation
of the function of revelation (Madkur, 1960).

This cautious and even negative evaluation of reason
in the traditionalist ethics had a parallel in the systematization of juridical theory among the Muslim jurists. The
ethical–legal problem-resolving device was in search of a
fundamental principle that could function as a template for
the formulation of emerging ethical–legal decisions. The
expansion of Muslim political rule beyond Arabia raised
questions about the application of the rulings provided by
the revealed sources. The jurists were quick to realize that

such absolute application without considering specific social and cultural context of these rulings was not without a problem. After all, the rulings provided by the revelation brought into focus specific human conditions related to custom, everyday human behaviour and ordinary language used to convey moral precepts and attitudes to life in the Arabian society. In other words, even when the moral law is wholly promulgated through divine legislation in the form of the Qur'an and the Tradition, such a law is objective because of the diversity that can be observed among human beings.

Very early on scholars of jurisprudence were led to distinguish between duties to God ('ibādāt ='ritual duties') and duties to fellow human beings (mu'āmalāt = 'social transactions'). 'Ritual duties' were not conditioned by specific human conditions, and hence were absolutely binding. 'Social transactions' were necessarily conditioned by human existence in specific social and political context, and, hence, adjustable to the needs of time. It was in the latter sphere of interpersonal relations that the jurists needed to provide fresh rulings generated by the changing human conditions. The entire area of social ethics in Islam falls under the mu'āmalāt sections of jurisprudence. However, authoritative decisions in matters of social ethics could not be derived without first determining the nature of human acts under obligation (taklīf). The divine command, understood in terms of religious–moral obligation (taklīf), provided the entire ethical code of conduct and a teleological view of humans and the world. More pertinently, violation of divine command, as Muslim jurists taught, is immoral on the grounds that it interferes with the pursuit of human goal of achieving perfection that would guarantee salvation in the Hereafter. Ultimately, human salvation is directly connected with human conduct – the subject matter of legal–theological ethics.

ISLAMIC PRINCIPLES OF BIOETHICS

There was no unanimity among the representatives of four major Sunnī legal thought (Mālikī, Ḥanafī, Shāfi'ī, and Ḥanbalī) regarding the principles nor that these principles were derived from foundational, rationalistically established moral theories from which other principles and legal–moral judgements were deduced. Rather scholars from different legal schools identified several principles extracted from original cases, often but not always the same ones. Since the language of Sharī'a is the language of obligation or duty the primary principles (qawā'id uṣūl) and rules (qawā'id fiqhī) in Islamic ethics are stated as obligations and their derivatives, respectively. Some jurists have identified principles to encompass both principles and rules and have indicated the primary and the subsidiary distinction in their application to particular cases.

Two such intellectual sources in Muslim jurisprudence were istiḥsān (prioritization of two or more equally valid judgements through juristic practice) and istiṣlāḥ (promoting and securing benefits and preventing and removing harms in public sphere). These represented independent juristic judgement of expedience or public utility. However, the legitimacy of employing these reason-based sources depended upon their assimilation into the textual sources.

Thus, for instance, the duty to avoid literal enforcement of the existing law, which may prove detrimental in certain situations, has given rise to the principle of 'juristic preference' (Kamali, 1991). This juridical method of prioritization of legal rulings taking into account the concrete circumstances of a case at hand has played a significant role in providing the necessary adaptability to Islamic law to meet the changing needs of society. However, the methodology is founded upon an important principle derived from the directive of 'circumventing of hardship' stated in the Qur'an in no uncertain terms: 'God intends facility for you, and He does not want to put you in hardship'(2:185). This directive is further reinforced by the tradition that states 'The best of your law (dīn) is that which brings ease to the people'. In other words, the principle of 'juristic preference' allows formulating a decision that side steps an established precedent in order to uphold a higher obligation of implementing the ideals of fairness and justice without causing unnecessary hardship to the people involved. The obvious conclusion to be drawn from God's intention to provide facility and remove hardship is that the essence of these principles is their adaptability to meet the exigencies of every time and place on the basis of public interest. In the absence of any textual injunction in the Qur'an and the Tradition, the principle of 'Necessity (ḍarūra) overrides prohibition' furnishes an authoritative basis for deriving a fresh ruling.

The limited scope of the chapter does not permit us to undertake to identify all the principles that are applied to make juridical decisions in various fields of interpersonal relations in Islamic law. What seems to be most useful and feasible is to identify a number of fundamental Islamic principles that are in some direct and indirect ways discerned through the general principle of maslaha, that is, 'public good'. This principle is evoked in providing solutions to the majority of novel issues in biomedical ethics. The rational obligation to weigh and balance an action's possible benefits against its cost and possible harms is central to social transactions in general and biomedical ethics in particular.

The principles to be elaborated in this chapter are not necessarily the same in priority or significance as recognized, for instance, in the Western bioethics, namely, respect for autonomy, nonmaleficence, beneficence (including utility) and justice. In comparison, Islamic principles overlap in important respects but differ in others. For instance, the two distinct obligations of beneficence and nonmaleficence in some Western systems are viewed as a single principle of nonmaleficence in Islam on the basis of the overlapping between the two obligations in the principle of 'No harm, no harassment'. Moreover, the principle of 'Protection against distress and constriction' ('usr wa al-ḥaraj) applies to social relations and transactions which although, they must be performed in good faith, are independent of religion. There are also a number of rules based on some precedents in the revealed texts, which are important parts of the Islamic system that are usually underemphasized in the Western secular bioethics. Thus the rule of consultation (shūrā) as part of the Islamic ethics functions as a substitute for the dominant principle of autonomy based on the liberal individualism.

Moreover, although this research is based on the bioethical rulings compiled from four major Sunnī and one Shī'ite legal schools, I have attempted to identify only the most commonly referred principles or rules in the biomedical jurisprudence without necessarily attributing them to one or the other school except when there has been fundamental disagreement on their inclusion in one or the other legal theory. These are the principles that have provided resolutions to the moral quandaries in bioethics by seeking to identify and balance risks and benefits to derive probable conclusions in order to protect the society from harms. In the last two decades jurists belonging to all the Muslim legal schools have met regularly under the auspices of the ministry of health of their respective countries to formulate their decisions as a collective body. Some of these new rulings have been published under the auspices of Majmaʿ al-fiqhī al-islāmī (Islamic Juridical Council). A close examination of the juridical decisions made in this council reveal the balancing of likely benefits and harms to society as a whole. In addition, these decisions indicate the search for proportionality (tanāsub) between individual and social interests of the community and the need, in certain cases, to allow collective interests to override individual interests and rights. The inherent tension in such decisions is sometimes resolved by reference to a critical principle regarding the right of an individual to reject harm and harassment ('No harm, no harassment'), which constrains unlimited application of the principle of common good.

THE PRINCIPLE OF PUBLIC INTEREST/ COMMON GOOD (MAṢLAḤA)

Consideration of public interest or common good of the people has been an important principle utilized by Muslim jurist–ethicists for accommodating and incorporating new issues confronting the community. Maṣlaḥa has been admitted as a principle of reasoning to derive new rulings or as a method of suspending earlier rulings out of consideration for the interest and welfare of the community. However, its

admission as an independent source for legislation has been contested by some Sunnī and Shī'ite legal scholars. To be sure, maṣlaḥa is based on the notion that the ultimate goal of the Sharī'a necessitates doing justice and preserving people's best interest in this and the next world. But who defines justice and what is the most salutary for the people? Here theological ethics defines the parameters of maṣlaḥa.

Looking at the majority of the Muslims who belong to the Sunnī-Ashʿarī school of thought in its understanding of God's plan for humanity, one needs to understand the Ashʿarite view of what is the best for people. The Ashʿarites, who maintained the divine command ethics (the theistic subjectivism), confined the derivation of maṣlaḥa strictly from the revealed texts. Abū Ḥāmid al-Ghazzālī (d. 1111), as an Ashʿarī theologian–jurist, elucidates this position in his legal theory:

> Maṣlaḥa is actually an expression for bringing about benefit (manfaʿa) or forestalling harm (maḍarra). We do not consider [maṣlaḥa] in the meaning of bringing about benefit or forestalling harm as part of [God's] purposes for the people or [God's] concern for the people, in order for them to achieve those purposes. Rather, we take maṣlaḥa in the meaning of protecting the ends of the Revelation (al-sharʿ). The ends of the Revelation for the people are five: To protect for them: (1) their religion, (2) their lives (nufūs), (3) their reason ('uqūl), (4) their lineage (nasl) and (5) their property (māl). All that guarantees the protection of these five purposes is maṣlaḥa, and all that undermines these purposes is mafasada (a source of detriment) (Ghazzā).

Hence, justice, according to the Ashʿarites, lies in the commission and application of what God had declared to be good and the avoidance of that which God had forbidden in these sacred sources. Moreover, ruling an action good or evil depends on the consideration of the general principles derived from the original cases in the revealed texts. Consequently, human responsibility is confined to the course ordained by God by seeking to institute what God declares good and shunning what God declares evil. In addition, as far as the solution to the new cases is concerned, the Ashʿarites maintain that the principle of maṣlaḥa is internally operational in the rulings that show with certainty that in legislating them God has the welfare of humankind in mind (Shāṭibī).

In contrast, the estimation of the Muʿtazilite Sunnī thinkers, who maintained objectivist rationalist ethics, was understandably at variance with the Ashʿarites. Their thesis was founded upon human reason as capable of knowing maṣlaḥa – the consideration of public interest that promoted benefit and prevented harm. For them, maṣlaḥa was an inductive principle for the resolution of the new cases in the area where the scriptural sources provided little or no guidance at all, and where judgements had to balance different claims, interests and responsibilities by acknowledging conflicting considerations involving human situations.

In the context of matters connected with social ethics, which deal with everyday contingencies of human life, it is important to keep in mind that regardless whether the principle of common good originates internally in the primary religious sources or externally through intuitive reason, no jurist questions the conclusion that legal–ethical judgements are founded upon concern for human welfare and in order to protect people from corruption and harm. In other words, they maintain that God provides the guidance with a purpose of doing the most salutary for people, even when the exact method of deducing this general principle is in dispute (Subkī).

THE TYPES OF ISSUES COVERED UNDER THE PRINCIPLE OF PUBLIC GOOD

In view of the above explanation about public good the principle comprises each and every benefit that has been made known by the purposes stated in the divine revelation, (Muḥammad Said), and because some jurists have essentially regarded public good as safeguarding the God's purposes for humanity, (Ghaza) the jurists have discussed the principle both in terms of types and the purposes they serve. Some have classified public good in terms of types, while others have resorted to purposes for classification. For instance, among the Sunnī jurists, Shāṭibī has treated the principle and its corollaries in great detail in his legal theory by pointing out that religious duties have been imposed on the people for their own good in view of the fulfillment of God's purposes for them. These purposes are discussed under three headings in that order:

1. *The Essentials or the Primary Needs (al-ḍarūriyāt):* These are things that are promulgated for the good of this and the next world in such a way that without them one cannot acquire the benefits such as providing healthcare to the poor and downtrodden in society (Ibn Amīr).
2. *The General Needs (al-ḥājiyāt):* These are things that enable human beings to improve their life and to remove those conditions which lead to chaos in one's familial and societal life in order to achieve higher standards of living, even though these necessities do not reach the level of essentials (*Al-Muwāfiqāt*).
3. *The Secondary Needs (al-taḥsīnāt):* These are the things that are commonly regarded as praiseworthy in society, which also lead to the avoidance of those things that are regarded as blameworthy. They are also known as 'Noble Virtues' (Shāṭibī).

In terms of the principle's application a number of beneficial or corruptive aspects converge or public good and corruption appear in the same instance. In such cases the balancing of the conflicting considerations becomes indispensable for a just solution about the common good. For example, one of the issues in the Muslim world is relating to prenatal genetic diagnosis (PGD), which inevitably leads to sex selection. Because of cultural or financial reasons, some Muslim parents prefer one sex above the other. Some jurists have argued in favour of sex selection, as long as no one, including the resulting child, is harmed. However, others have disputed the claim that no harm will be done. They point to violations of divine law, natural justice, and the inherent dignity of all human beings. More importantly, permitting sex selection for nonmedical reasons involves or leads to unacceptable discrimination on grounds of sex and disability, potential psychological damage to the resulting children, and an inability to prevent a slide down the slippery slope towards permitting designer babies. In such cases, it becomes critical to assess the important criteria for the public good, or to prioritize criteria that lead to public good or corruption, and provide the requisite ruling.

THE PRINCIPLE OF 'NO HARM, NO HARASSMENT'

'No harm, no harassment'" has a long history in Islamic jurisprudence. The principle is anchored in the primary sources going back to the Prophet himself. 'No harm, no harassment' is regarded as one of the most fundamental principles for deducing rulings dealing with social ethics in Islam. Muslim jurists have discussed and debated on the validity of this principle because it is regarded as one of the critical proofs in support of numerous decisions involving resolution of cases that involve conflict of interests, claims, and responsibilities. However, what renders the principle authoritative in such cases is its ascription to the Prophet himself. Hence, whether from the point of its transmission or from the congruity in the sense conveyed by it, the jurists have endorsed its admission among the principles that are employed in making all decisions that pertain to social and political life of the community. In fact, the Shāfiʿī-Sunnī jurist, Suyūṭī regards the tradition in which the principle of 'No harm, no harassment' is embedded as one of the five major traditions on which depended the derivation of legal–ethical decisions in the Sharīʿa (Suyūṭ). In addition, he affirms that the majority of juridical rubrics were founded on the rule of 'No harm, no harassment', and that closely related to this rule are a number of other rules among which is: 'Necessities make forbidden permissible, as long as it does not lead to any detriment (Suyūṭ)' The rule has played a major role in Islamic jurisprudence when one considers the way jurists have taken up the 'No harm, no harassment' as a general principle that speaks clearly about no harm should be inflicted or reciprocated. Some jurists include it among the five major principles that have extracted from the original cases that can be possibly utilized to deduce the new rulings in the area of interpersonal relations. These five principles are as follows:

1. 'Action depends upon intention'. This rule is deduced from the tradition related by the Prophet: 'Indeed, actions depend upon intentions'.
2. 'Hardship necessitates relief'. This rule is inferred from the tradition that says: 'The best of your law (*dīn*) is that which brings ease to the people'.
3. 'One needs certainty'. To continue an action requires linking the present situation with the past.
4. 'No harm should be inflicted or reciprocated'. This rule is deduced on the basis of the need to promote benefit and institute it in order to remove causes of corruption or reduce their harmful impact upon the possibility of having to choose the lesser of the two evils.
5. 'Custom determines course of action'. The rule acknowledges the need to take local custom into account when making relevant rulings (Shahīd).

'No harm, no harassment' functions both as a principle and a source for the rule that states 'hardship necessitates relief'. As such, it connotes that there can be no legislation, promulgation or execution of any law that leads to harm of anyone in society. For that reason, in derivation of a legal–ethical judgement the rule is given priority over all primary obligations in the Sharī'a. In fact, it functions as a check on all other ordinances to make sure that their fulfilment does not lead to harm. In case of dispute in any situation, the final resolution is derived by applying the rule of 'No harm, no harassment'. For instance, the primary obligation of seeking medical treatment becomes prohibited if it aggravates the affliction suffered under certain medical condition.

In the Sharī'a, definition of harm and harassment in negative sense depends upon custom (*al-'urf*), which determines its parameters. Custom also establishes whether harm to oneself or to another party has been done in a given situation. If custom does not construe a matter to be harmful, then it cannot be admitted as such by applying the principle itself, nor can it be considered as forbidden according to the Sharī'a, even if the matter is lexically designated as 'harmful'. It is important to keep in mind that ultimately it is the Sacred Lawgiver who defines the parameters of harm. However, if custom regards something to be harmful for which there is no specific evidence from the revealed texts, the harm in that situation becomes more broadly defined as conditions that mediate injustice and violation of someone's rights. Moreover, harm differs in accord with causes that include self-harming conditions as well as the actions of another party. Hence, one's social status, culture and time in which one lives play a role in defining harm. Harm is relative to the person who experiences it. Therefore, what appears to be wrong *prima facie* and is regarded by one party as a harmful act may not be considered wrong or unjustified by another. Human experience, although subjective, attains considerable importance in the evaluation of the kind of harm that is to be rejected in the rule of 'No harm, no harassment'. The context in which the Prophet gave the rule clearly leaves the matter of harm to be determined by the situation. In the report that speaks about the harm caused by an inconsiderate neighbour who violated the privacy of his neighbour, it was a case of harmful invasion by one party of another's interest. To be sure, the principle of 'No harm, no harassment' allows for the ruling that one must reject becoming a cause for harm.[4]

The application of the ruling to reject harm has no bearing on the assessment of the actual situation when a person is going through the setbacks to his interests. Nor does the Lawgiver's admission of harm in certain situations as a mediating causation for some rulings that require reparation or compensation render harm as a valid claim. In the final analysis, it is the personal assessment of harm that functions as an important consideration in determining related obligations. Hence, for instance, when a person is sick, she determines whether she can keep the fast of Ramadan as required by the Sharī'a in consideration of the harm that fasting can cause. Regardless of the criteria one applies to determine the level of harm, whether it is less or more, once custom establishes its existence then the Sharī'a endorses it as equally so, even when there might be a difference of opinion whether some forms of harm are more detrimental than other. In any case, when such a difference of opinion occurs, the law requires following the decision that leads to least harm and that causes the least damage to one's total well–being. Hence, in the case of a terminally ill patient, if the decision to prolong life leads to more harm for the patient and his immediate family, then to continue to insist on keeping him on life-saving equipment is regarded as causing further harm to the patient's and his family's well-being and hence, forbidden.

REFERENCES

Al-Muwāfiqāt, Vol. 2, p. 9. Other jurists have mentioned these categories in different order, with different examples in each category. See, for instance: al-Ghazālī, *al-Mustaṣfā*, p. 175.

Hourani (1985) introduces the latter distinction in deontological norms.

[4]There is a sustained discussion among jurists about the nature of harm that this tradition conveys. Undoubtedly, *ḍarar* refers to general forms of harm that include setbacks to reputation, property, privacy, and specific ones that include setbacks to physical and psychological needs. See: 'Alī al-Ḥusaynī al-Sīstānī, *Qā'ida lā ḍarar wa lā ḍirār* (Qumm: Lithographie Ḥamīd, 1414/1993), pp. 134–141.

Ghaza.li., *Mustaṣfa.*, Vol. 1, p. 286–7.

Ghaza.li., *al-Mustaṣfa.*, p. 174.

Hallaq WB. *Authority, Continuity and Change in Islamic Law.* Cambridge: Cambridge University Press, 2001; pp. 131ff. Lists the manner in which preponderance was determined in terms of which rule or rationale had the force of settling the dispute about the probable outcome of the quandary.

Heyd D, ed. *Toleration: An Elusive Virtue.* Princeton: Princeton University Press, 1996.

Hourani GF. *Islamic Rationalism: The Ethics of ʿAbd al-Jabbar.* Oxford: Clarendon Press, 1971. Calls the Muʿtazilite theory of ethics 'rationalist objectivism' because natural human reason is capable of knowing real characteristic of the acts, without the aid of revelation. Fakhry M. *Ethical Theories of Islam.* Leiden: E. J. Brill, 1991; pp. 35–43 regards this as quasi-deontological theory of right and wrong in which the instrinsic goodness or badness of actions can be established on purely rational grounds. Hourani calls the Ashʿarite theory of ethics 'theistic subjectivism' rather than 'ethical voluntarism' because the value of action is defined by God as the judge and observer. However, since it is the divine will that is the determinant of right and wrong it would be more meaningful to retain 'voluntarism' in this particular type of divine command ethical theory. See: Fakhry M. The Muʿtazilite view of man. *Philosophy, Dogma and the Impact of Greek Thought in Islam.* Varior: um, 1994, pp. 107–21, and his *Ethical Theories*; pp. 46–55. Further refinement in specifying the Ashʿarite theory on the basis of Fakhry's discussions is provided by Frank RM. Moral obligation in classical muslim theology. *J Religious Ethics* 1983; **II**: p. 207, where he regards Ashʿarite ethics 'a very pure kind of voluntaristic occasionalism'.

Hourani GF. *Reason and Tradition in Islamic Ethics.* New York: Cambridge University Press, 1985; p. 17.

Ibn Amīr Ḥāj, *al-Taqrīr wa al-taḥbīr*, Vol. 3, p. 213; Shāṭibī, *al-Muwāfiqāt*, Vol. 2, pp. 7-8. Regards performance of all duties under the category of God-human relationship (*ʿibādāt*) as fulfilling the need to protect one's religion; eating and drinking as fulfilling the need to protect one's life; performance of all duties under the category of interhuman relationship (*muʿāmalāt*) as fulfilling the need to protect future generation and wealth; and implementation of penal code and laws of retribution and restitution as fulfilling the need to protect all five essentials.

Kamali MH. *Principles of Islamic Jurisprudence.* Cambridge: Islamic Texts Society, 1991; Chapter 12.

Madkur MS. *Mabahith al-hukm ʿinda al-usuliyyin*, Vol. 1. Cairo: Dar al-Nahda al-ʿArabiyya, 1960; p. 169.

Muḥammad Saʿīd Ramaḍān al-Būṭī, *Ḍawābit al-maṣlaḥa fī al-sharīʿat al-isl āmiyya* (Beirut: Muʾassasa al-Risa.la, 1410/1990), Vol. 3, p. 288

Shāṭibī, *al-Muwāfiqāt.* Vol. 2, pp. 4–5. Believes that essentially legislating laws and promulgating religions have the welfare of humanity as their main purpose. Furthermore, he maintains that even when theologians have disputed this doctrine pointing out, as the Ashʿarite theologian Rāzī has done, that God's actions are not informed by any purpose, the same scholars in their discussions on legal theory have conceded to the notion, however in different terms that divine injunctions are informed by God's purpose for humanity. Shāṭibī clearly indicates that deduction of divine injunctions provides evidence about their being founded upon the doctrine of human welfare, to which Rāzī. and other Ashʿarites are not opposed.

Shāṭibī, *al-Muwāfiqāt*, Vol. 2, p. 9.

Shahi.d Awwal, *al-Qawāʿid*, Vol. 1, pp. 27–28.

Subkī, *al-Ibhāj fī sharḥ al-minhāj.* Beirut: Dār al-kutub al-ʿilmiya. 1404/19, Vol. 3, p. 62.

Suyūṭī, *Tanwīr al-Ḥawālik: isʿāf al-mubattaʾ bi-rijāl al-Muwaṭṭaʾ* (Beirut: al-Maktaba al-Thiqāfi.ya, 1969), Vol. 2, pp. 122, 218.

Suyūṭī, *al-Ashbāh wa al-naẓāʾir fi. qawāʿid wa furuʿ fiqh al-Shāfiʿīya* (Mekkah: Maktabat Niza.r Muṣṭafa. al-Bāz, 1990), p. 92.

17

Buddhist Bioethics

JAMES HUGHES

Describing anything as 'Buddhist', including in this case a distinctively Buddhist bioethics, is fundamentally problematic from both a historic and Buddhist point of view. Historically, the Buddhist tradition has evolved in dozens of countries for 2500 years, with no one tradition having clear doctrinal authority over the others. Internally, even if a common Buddhist ethics was implicit in the practices of the dozens of Buddhist cultures or the exegetics of their traditions, the core philosophical insight of Buddhism is that all things are empty of essential, authentic being, including the Buddhist tradition. So, starting from the understanding that there is no authentic Buddhist bioethics to explicate, and only a constellation of practices and ideas related to medicine and the body among Buddhists throughout history, which may or may not be tied to core ideas of the Buddhist tradition, we can interrogate the tradition for the lessons it may hold for contemporary bioethics.

BUDDHIST ETHICS

There is a vigorous debate among Buddhist scholars about the correspondence of Buddhist ethics to the ethical traditions of the West, and three traditions have the strongest resonances: natural law, virtue ethics and utilitarianism.

The Western natural law tradition holds that morality is discernible in the nature of the world and the constitution of human beings. In the Buddhist cosmogony all sentient beings cycle through multiple rebirths, influenced by their past moral behaviour, *karma*. When the Buddhist properly understands the structure of mind, the effects of immoral behaviour in creating suffering in this life and the next, and the importance of *sila* or moral discipline as the basis for release from suffering, morality is the only rational choice. In this sense, Buddhist ethics are grounded in the natural

law of the universe, and the acts that lead to bad karma, such as killing, stealing, lying, sexual misconduct and intoxication, are clearly spelt out.

The problem with Buddhist ethics as natural law is that the soteriological goal is one of liberating oneself from the constraints of karmic causality to become an enlightened being. The traditional anthropological explanation of this paradox has been to ascribe the natural law ethics of *kammic* reward and punishment to the laity and the *nibbanic* path of escape from natural law to the monastics (King, 1964; Spiro, 1972). More recent scholars (for instance, Keown, 1992; Unno, 1999) have challenged this dichotomy and argued that monastic ethics have always revolved far more around the exchange of accumulated merits for alms than the goal of enlightenment.

Nonetheless, the Buddhist ethical tradition does argue for an escape from all mundane karmic constraints, and the illusions of material existence, to achieve a state of perfect wisdom and compassion. Damien Keown, (1995) the leading Western scholar explicating Buddhist bioethics, calls this a 'teleological virtue ethics'. As in Aristotelian virtue ethics, Buddhists are to strive for the perfection of a set of moral virtues and personality attributes as their principal end, and all moral behaviour flows from the struggle to perfect them. But unlike the Aristotelian tradition, the ethical goal for Buddhists is teleological because they generally believe that a final state of moral perfection can be achieved. As virtue ethics, Buddhist ethics focuses on the intentionality of action, whether actions stem from hatred, greed and ignorance, or insight and empathy.

In the Mahayana tradition the being who embodies these virtues is the *bodhisattva*, who strives to relieve the suffering of all beings by the most skilful means (*upaya*) necessary. As the bodhisattva is supposed to be insightful enough to understand when ordinarily immoral acts are necessary to alleviate suffering, and it is either willing to assume the karmic consequences or is not subject to the karmic consequences of such acts, the consequentialist utilitarian tradition is also especially compatible with Buddhist ethics. The utilitarianism of J.S. Mill is most resonant with this interpretation of Buddhist ethics because Mill emphasized distinctions between coarse and fine states of mind, weighting the contentment of the refined mind more heavily in the utility calculus than base pleasures. From a utilitarian approach, Buddhist moral precepts can be considered 'rule utilitarian' general guides to action, but not deontological absolutes.

Some writers have also explored the compatibility of Buddhism with the 'ethics of care' articulated by Carol Gilligan (1982). Gilligan argues that women are more likely to draw on compassion in their moral reasoning, whereas men are more inclined to employ ethical principles. Gilligan's work is very resonant for those who see Buddhism as a 'situation ethics' relying on direct intuition and empathic sensitivity for appropriate behaviour, as teachers in the Zen tradition often do (Curtin & Curtin, 1994).

BUDDHISM AND MEDICINE

From the outset the Buddhist tradition presents itself as a clinical diagnosis of the cause of human suffering, and a prescription for its alleviation (Duncan et al, 1981; Soni, 1976). The tradition does not set out divine commandments but simple statements about the dis-ease (*dukkha*) afflicting human life, and the way the dis-ease can be treated. Although the emphasis is on a spiritual cure, Buddhism specifically rejects ascetic mortification of the flesh and accepts that medicine is necessary for monks and laity. Although the monastic code forbad monks and nuns from practising medicine, they were instructed to provide medicine to one another and to keep it at hand (Keown, 1995). The use of medicine for a longer, healthier life is in no way seen as incompatible with spiritual practice, but rather is seen as an aid for it.

Buddhism has blended with the medical traditions of each country in which it has taken root. Zysk (1991) and Mitra (1985) discuss links between early Buddhism and the Indian medical tradition of ayurveda, and in China and Tibet Buddhism mixed with traditional medicines and magic to create distinctive psycho-spiritual healing practices and meditations. In the West, Buddhist-influenced clinicians, such as Jon Kabat-Zinn and his Center for Mindfulness in Medicine, Healthcare and Society at the University of Massachusetts, are exploring the health benefits of Buddhist meditation. The Dalai Lama, the exiled monarch of the Tibetan kingdom and head of the Gelugpa sect of Tibetan Buddhism, has been distinctive among religious leaders in embracing the application of the scientific method to the spiritual experience and in

asserting that beliefs and practices that are shown to be unscientific and not empirically supported should be set aside (Gyatso, 2005).

NO-PERSONHOOD ETHICS AND REINCARNATION

A basic, and nearly unique, aspect of Buddhist philosophy is its emphasis on the nonexistence of the self, *anatta*. Consequently, one of the most fundamental Buddhist contributions to be made to contemporary medical ethics will be in the debates over personal identity.

The thrust of the no-self doctrine is complicated within the Buddhist tradition, however, by the doctrine of reincarnation. If there is no self, what reincarnates? The traditional answer has been that the evolving constellation of mental substrates, the *skandhas*, causally encoded with karma, pass from one body to another but lack any anchor to an unchanging soul, just as a causal chain connects a flame passed from one candle to another even though it cannot be said to be the same flame. (The five *skandhas* are the body, feelings, perceptions, will and consciousness.) Buddhist humanists and sceptics, most notably Stephen Batchelor (1997), have argued that the doctrine of reincarnation is not essential to Buddhist spiritual practice and that Buddhists have explicit doctrinal authorization to remain agnostic on reincarnation and on all beliefs without empirical support. Buddhist agnostics note that, in the context of Buddhism's rejection of Hindu beliefs in an eternal soul, the teaching on no-self is actually a *negation* of the importance of reincarnation.

Nonetheless, most Buddhists profess belief in reincarnation, and belief in reincarnation shapes Buddhist practices and beliefs around abortion and dying. Interruption of the instantiation or transmigration of the reincarnating being, through abortion or cadaveric organ transplantation, is therefore potentially as harmful, and has as weighty karmic implications, as murder.

ABORTION

Certainly abortion has been generally disapproved of in Buddhist culture on the grounds that it is a form of murder. Traditional Buddhist beliefs about the exact timing of the instantiation of the reincarnating being in the embryo or foetus are not doctrinal, however, but drawn from latter exegetical texts.

Some contemporary, and especially Western, Buddhist writers on abortion have argued for a more tolerant position, on a number of grounds. First, if the moral status of the embryo and foetus are contingent on the instantiation of a sentient being, then current neurophysiological evidence that suggests that sentience only emerges late in foetal development would validate abortion up to that point (Barnhart, 1998; Hughes, 1999). Keown (1999) argues against this point of view, emphasizing the moral importance of the creation of just the first of the five *skandhas,* the embryonic body. However, as Barnhart (1998). makes clear, the scriptures emphasize that a sentient being is created only when *all five* of the elements, including consciousness, are present.

Moreover, insofar as Buddhism is similar to a utilitarian ethics towards general happiness, or an ethics of care, or an ethics of virtuous intent, then the immorality of the abortive act of violence can be outweighed by the intentions of the mother and the greater suffering that it may prevent to mother, potential child and society. The Dalai Lama has argued, for instance, that although abortion is generally inappropriate, it may be permissible in cases of severely handicapped foetuses that may suffer in life; 'the main factor is motivation' (quoted in Tsomo, 1998). Additional considerations would be the degree to which the mother had become pregnant and aborted carelessly, without sufficient attention to the gravity of the act (Tworkow, 1992). Depending on Buddhists' beliefs about the importance of consciousness to the moral status of the embryo and foetus, the intentionality of the actor and the consequences of the action, some Buddhists will therefore come to different conclusions on derivative issues such as the use of embryos in cloning and stem cell research (Schlieter, 2004).

Much attention has also been paid to the Japanese Buddhist *tatari* rituals for aborted foetuses (*mizuko*) which acknowledge and expiate the mother's karmic debt (Lafleur, 1992). For some Western Buddhists the ritual for aborted foetuses is a way to acknowledge the moral weight of the choice while accepting its occasional appropriateness (Aitken, 1984).

BRAIN DEATH AND ORGAN TRANSPLANTATION

The debate about the importance of consciousness for moral standing also shapes Buddhist approaches to brain death, the permanent vegetative state and organ transplantation. Keown (1995) argues, for instance, that Buddhists should adopt the 'whole brain' theory of brain death, which requires evidence that all brain function, including brain stem activity, has ceased, rather than the 'neocortical' view that only the irreversible cessation of consciousness should be adequate for declaring death and removing life support. Keown cites Buddhist scriptural sources that imply that death only occurs when vitality, heat and consciousness have all left the body. (This would seem to support

the heart-death standard instead, but Keown embraces the whole-brain argument that brain stem death will quickly cause all other bodily functions to cease.) The neocortical view, on the contrary, would apply to people in the 'permanent vegetative state' such as the Florida *cause celebre* Terri Schiavo. In *Buddhism and Death: The Brain-Centered Criteria,* John-Anderson Meyer (2005) argues that the neocortical understanding of death is 'most in conformity with general Buddhist doctrine'.

Some Buddhists reject even the whole brain definition of death, and resist any organ transplantation, on the grounds that tampering with the corpse in the critical days after death may interfere with the transmigration of the *skandhas* to their rebirth. The Japanese only adopted brain death standards after a protracted debate, with resistance partly due to Buddho-Confucian veneration of ancestors (Lock and Honde, 1990; Lock, 2001). Other Buddhists have defended organ transplantation on the grounds that it is the final compassionate act (Lecso, 1991; Tsomo, 1993) and even a means to acquire merit for a better rebirth (Hongladarom, 2006).

SUICIDE, EUTHANASIA AND THE GOOD DEATH

Buddhism has been seen by many Westerners to be indifferent to death, or even to nihilistically valorize suicide. This misconception is perpetuated by images of self-immolating Vietnamese monks and disgraced samurai committing *seppuku* (ritual suicide). Some scriptures even appear to show the Buddha condoning the suicide of enlightened monks (Gethin, 2004; Keown, 1996).

Buddhist meditation does include many contemplations of the inevitability of death and the stages of the decomposition of the corpse. There are also many stories of Buddhist monks, and the Buddha himself, accepting their deaths with equanimity and even humour. But, in fact, Buddhist scripture and tradition, like most religions, holds that suicide and euthanasia are forms of murder. As with abortion, however, consequentialist and compassion-based moral reasoning may legitimate suicide and euthanasia on the grounds that they alleviate suffering and permit a 'good death'.

The 'good death' is especially important for the Buddhist who believes that their state of mind at death will be partly determinative of the quality of rebirth they achieve in the next life. This view is expressed in the Tibetan tradition through the *bardo* meditations which are chanted for the dying and dead to remind them of the 49 days of difficult visions they will traverse as they transition to their next life. Consequently, Buddhists may prefer to be as awake and aware at the moment of death as possible, even if they must endure pain (Levine, 1982). On the contrary, appropriately

PRINCIPLES OF HEALTH CARE ETHICS

calibrated pain medication can allow for greater focus during terminal care, and there is no necessary reason for a Buddhist to embrace pain when it can be medicated (Anderson, 1992). There is a growing literature on Buddhist approaches to end-of-life care and counselling exploring these issues from Tibetan (Rinpoche, 1994; Sachs, 1998), Zen (Kapleau, 1989; Levine, 1982) and Vipassana (Smith, 1998) perspectives.

Beyond death, emerging technologies suggest that memories and consciousness may eventually be transferred to new bodies or to computers. As technological reincarnation becomes a possibility, the Buddhist understanding of the transmigration of our illusory, personal identity will become even more relevant (Hughes, 2004). Indeed the Dalai Lama has opined that human consciousness could be instantiated in a sufficiently advanced computer (quoted in Hayward and Varela, 1992, p. 152).

SPECIESISM AND THE HUMANE TREATMENT OF ANIMALS

Buddhist doctrine holds that animals are part of the reincarnate chain of being, being potentially both former and future human beings, and moral subjects whose behaviour accrues karma. Many of the Jataka tales, about the Buddha's previous lives, concern his lives as a courageous and self-sacrificing animal; for instance as a deer that convinces a king to stop his hunt. The murder of animals is therefore karmically unskilful, and Buddhists have considered vegetarianism praiseworthy, opposed hunting and animal sacrifice, and frowned on butchery and leatherworking as inappropriate occupations. The monastic code allows monks to eat meat that is offered as alms but not to drink water that might contain living creatures. The *Cakkavattisihanada Sutta* says that the righteous ruler will provide for wild beasts and birds. The most famous example of a Buddhist code of humane animal treatment are the edicts of the first Buddhist emperor, Asoka, which include numerous decrees that various species not be hunted and that their habitats should be protected. In India and China, Buddhists released captive animals as a means of acquiring merit.

Although the Buddhist tradition is clearly less anthropocentric than the Abrahamic faiths, in which only human beings are ensouled, Buddhist rulers only rarely advocated an 'animal rights' legal code forbidding the killing of animals, which would be consistent with a belief in the full equality of human and animal life (Waldau, 2002). Vegetarianism was seen as an extreme form of asceticism in the Tibetan tradition, and the Dalai Lama like most Tibetan monks eats meat, although he counsels that those who can should become vegetarian. Nonetheless, some Buddhists are beginning to argue that Buddhism should adopt a more consistent vegan and animal rights position (Phelps, 2004).

CONTRACEPTION, SEXUALITY, GENETIC ENGINEERING AND REPRODUCTIVE TECHNOLOGY

Buddhism is decidedly indifferent to whether people have children or not. Buddhist laity are enjoined to avoid sexual misconduct, but not to be fruitful and multiply. Buddhist monks were forbidden to perform weddings or bless babies, although they eventually developed ceremonies that functionally do both. In the last fifty years Buddhist countries like Sri Lanka, Japan and Thailand have aggressively embraced contraception, and their birth rates are among the lowest in Asia, to the consternation of some Buddhist nationalists.

More fundamentally, Buddhism rejects any notion of a 'natural' and inviolate human body or procreative act which needs protection from 'artificial' contraception, genetic engineering or reproductive technologies (Loy, 2003). The important questions from Buddhist ethics are the intentions of the would-be (non)parents, and the consequences of their actions. Concerns about children not knowing who they 'really are', when they are products of artificial reproduction or cloning, are foreign to Buddhism which does not recognize an 'authentic self' to begin with (Falls et al. 1999).

This tolerance of the 'unnatural' extends to homosexuals and the transgendered. Although homosexuality, as sex outside of marriage, has always been seen as a violation of the precept against sexual misconduct, it is seen as no worse than heterosexual misconduct. Although the monastic code bars the ordination of gay men and eunuchs, the Buddha permitted some transgendered males to ordain and live with nuns and transgendered females to ordain and live with monks (Jackson, 1998). Thailand has an active and tolerated gay and transgender subculture, and it is an international centre for transgender surgery (Jackson, 1998). Gay and transgender people are welcome in the Sri Lankan and Thai armies. Male homosexuality was common among the Buddhist warrior caste samurai and monastic culture of Japan (Jñanavira, 2005), and gay and transgender images are pervasive in contemporary Japanese culture. The largest sect of Japanese Buddhism, the Jodo Shinshu, performs gay wedding ceremonies.

BRAIN SCIENCE, PSYCHOPHARMACOLOGY AND THE MYTH OF THE AUTHENTIC SELF

Brain science and psychology have eroded the idea of an autonomous, continuous and authentic self, in ways quite compatible with Buddhist psychology. Bioethics is just beginning to grapple with the implications. Do anti-depressants, stimulants or pain medications create an inauthentic self, or a more authentic self? How can we respect patient autonomy when preferences change in illness and pain, and from moment to moment? Within Western philosophy Derek Parfit's (1984) *Reasons and Persons* posed the most radical challenge by arguing, parallel to Buddhism, that personal identity is only statistically related over time. After a certain point we share as much with all future people as we do with our future selves. This Parfitian/Buddhist view may, for instance, legitimate the delegation of health care decision-making for the incapacitated to family, friends and society (Kuczewski, 1994), and support a general regard for social welfare over individual self-interest.

Buddhist meditation teachers, and most famously the Dalai Lama, have embraced the emerging field of neurotheology, which explores the neurophysiology of the meditative experience. Some Buddhist neuroscientists, such as James Austin in *Zen and the Brain*, have explored the many neurophysiological bases for meditative experience (Austin, 1999). The collection *Zig, Zag, Zen: Buddhism and Psychedelics* (Badiner, 2002) documents how many Western Buddhists found their way to Buddhism through the use of psychedelic drugs, which many still consider possible adjuncts to spiritual growth.

But anti-depressants in particular pose a challenge for Buddhists (Chambers, 2001), since the beginning of the Buddhist path is embracing the fundamental unhappiness of life (*dukkha*), whereas the idea of 'happy pills' would suggest a short-circuiting of spiritual growth. In other words, is Prozac cheating? Most Western Buddhist psychologists have articulated the view that there should be a distinction between the fundamental dissatisfactoriness of ego-bound life, which is present for the depressed and happy alike, and the immobilizing depression of the chemically unbalanced mind. For people with clinical depression anti-depressant therapy is a necessary adjunct to spiritual growth, returning their capacity for compassion, mindfulness and energy (Hooper, 1999). Just as Buddhists have generally accepted stimulants such as tea as helpful in maintaining mindfulness during meditation, this approach would presumably also apply to other drugs that enhance capacities for empathy or attention, such as stimulant medications for attention-deficit disorder.

Conversely, Buddhists are enjoined to avoid mind-altering substances that interfere with spiritual growth, such as alcohol, narcotics and opiates, and warned that absorption into blissful states is a spiritual dead-end. If and when true 'happy pills' are available, these would be more problematic for Buddhists.

HEALTH CARE ACCESS AND HUMAN RIGHTS

Richard Florida (1994) has explored the compatibility of Buddhist ethics with the four 'Georgetown mantra' principles of medical ethics articulated in the classic work of Beauchamp and Childress (1983) – autonomy, nonmaleficence, beneficence and justice. Florida concludes that Buddhist ethics, being centrally concerned with compassion, is strongly compatible with the nonmaleficence and beneficence principles, but that there is no Buddhist doctrinal basis for an egalitarian social order or the defence of individual liberty. Although Buddhism, like all the world's ancient faiths, developed before the European Enlightenment and has only recently entered into dialogue with democratic and humanist ideas, Florida appears unaware of an extensive literature on the implicit egalitarianism and individualism of the Buddhist tradition.

A classic work that explicates the latent, revolutionary egalitarianism of early Buddhism is the *The Buddha* by Trevor Ling (1973). Ling points to the radical democratic structure of the Buddhist monastic order and ideals of Buddhist governance and to the many dialogues of the Buddha which disparage the Hindu caste system and the emerging monarchism and mercantilism of his time, which together suggest a Buddhist strategy for liberal and egalitarian social reform. The Buddha's story of the origin of governance is of a social contract between citizens and their chosen rulers to protect public order, similar to the Hobbesian view. One of the obligations of the righteous Buddhist king is to ensure that citizens do not fall into poverty, from which all other social ills are said to flow. In *Inner Revolution* Tibetan Buddhist scholar Robert Thurman (1999) argues that the social welfare measures enacted by the Buddhist Asokan monarchy prefigured modern social democracy. In the twentieth century Buddhists have developed these strains into Buddhist-socialist syncretism, most notably the Buddhist socialism of U Nu in Burma (Sarkisyanz, 1965) and Bandaranaike in Sri Lanka, the Dhammic socialism of Bhikkhu Buddhadasa (Buddhadasa, 1986), the Buddhist feminist movement (Gross, 1992), and the myriad ongoing activities of the 'engaged Buddhism' movement (Kotler, 2005; Queen, 1996, 2000). Whether social democracy is validated by doctrinal and historical Buddhism, there is clearly a stronger case for universal health care provision in Buddhism than for a system based on unequal market access.

The case for a Buddhist 'human rights' doctrine is more complicated, however, because Buddhism"s first move is the deconstruction of the autonomous individual on which the Western rights tradition is based. Like contemporary socialist (Sen, 1999), feminist (Binion, 1995; Sherwin, 1998) and communitarian (Glendon, 1993) critics of the Lockean autonomous individual, a Buddhist approach to human rights emphasizes the embeddedness of the elusive individual in a web of interconnectedness, and that human rights are not immutable laws of nature but social norms that encourage respect and compassion. The key Buddhist idea here is 'co-dependent origination' (*paticcasamuppada*); all people and things come into their (temporary, illusory) existence through their relations with other (temporary, illusory) people and things (Traer, 1988). Although monks lived under numerous strict codes of conduct, they were self-chosen to the degree that monks were allowed to form new communities if doctrinal disagreements emerged. The laity was enjoined to acquire merit through fulfilling the reciprocal obligations of parent and child, husband and wife and employer and worker, but there is no model for these moral codes to be enforced by law, as in Islamic Sharia.

Despite this emphasis on social embeddedness over liberal individualism, the soteriological goal, individual enlightenment, is not found through fulfilling social obligations but through letting go of social ties. This rejection of obligations to family and the state brought Buddhism into conflict with more authoritarian cultures, especially the Indian caste system, the Chinese Confucian veneration of family and imperial Shintoism in Japan. Buddhist doctrine, with its pacifism and suggested but not mandated codes of conduct, is more consistent with the respect for individual freedom of choice, thought and action than traditions based on divine, infallible commandments.

REFERENCES

Aitken R. *The Mind of Clover: Essays on Zen Buddhist Ethics*. San Francisco: North Point Press, 1984.

Anderson P. Good death: mercy, deliverance, and the nature of suffering. *Tricycle* 1992; **2**(2): 36–42.

Austin J. *Zen and the Brain: Toward an Understanding of Meditation and Consciousness*. Cambridge MA: MIT Press, 1999.

Badiner, AH, ed. *Zig, Zag, Zen: Buddhism and Psychedelics*. San Francisco: Chronicle Books, 2002.

Barnhart MG. Buddhism and the morality of abortion. *J Buddhist Ethics* 1998; **5**: 276–97.

Batchelor, S. *Buddhism Without Beliefs: A Contemporary Guide to Awakening*. New York: Riverhead, 1997.

Beauchamp TL, Childress JF. *Principles of Biomedical Ethics*, 2nd edition. New York: Oxford University Press, 1983.

Becker CB. Buddhist views of suicide and euthanasia, *Philosophy East and West* 1990;**40**(4): 543–55.

Binion G. Human rights: a feminist perspective. *Human Rights Q* 1995; **17**(3): 509–26.

Buddhadasa B. In: Swearer DK, translator and ed. *Dhammic Socialism*. Bangkok: Thai Inter Religious Commission for Development, 1986.

Chaicharoen P, Ratanakul P. Letting-go or killing: Thai Buddhist perspectives on euthanasia. *Eubios J Asian Int Bioethics* 1998; **8**: 37–40.

Chambers T. Should the Buddha have taken Prozac? Religious implications of SSRIs. *Park Ridge Center Bull* 2001; **19**.

Curtin P, Curtin D. Mothering: moral cultivation in Buddhist and feminist ethics. *Philos East West* 1994; **44**(1): 1–18.

Duncan AS, Dunstan GR, Welbourn RB. Buddhism. *Dictionary of Medical Ethics*. London: Darton, Longman and Todd, 1981.

Falls E, Skeel JD, Edinger W. The Koan of cloning: a Buddhist perspective on the ethics of human cloning technology. *Second Opin* 1999; **1**: 44–56. http://www.parkridgecenter.org/Page169.html

Florida RE. Buddhism and the four principles. In: Gillon R, Lloyd A, eds. *Principles of Health Care Ethics*. Chichester: John Wiley & Sons, 1994; pp. 105–16.

Gethin R. Can killing a living being ever be an act of compassion? The analysis of the act of killing in the Abhidhamma and Pali commentaries. *J Buddhist Ethics* 2004; **11**: 168–202.

Gilligan C. *In a Different Voice: Psychological Theory and Women's Development*. Harvard University Press, 1982.

Glendon MA. *Rights Talk: The Impoverishment of Political Discourse*. New York: Simon and Schuster, 1993.

Gross, R. *Buddhism After Patriarchy: A Feminist History, Analysis, and Reconstruction of Buddhism*. Albany: SUNY Press, 1992

Gyatso HH. Dalai Lama Tenzin. Our Faith in Science. *New York Times*, November 12, 2005. http://www.iht.com/articles/2005/11/13/opinion/edgyatso.php

Hayward JW, Varela F. *Gentle Bridges: Conversations with the Dalai Lama on the Sciences of the Mind*. Boston: Shambhala, 1992.

Hongladarom S. *Organ Transplantation and Death Criteria: Theravada Buddhist Perspective and Thai Cultural Attitude*. 2006. http://homepage.mac.com/soraj/web/Organ%20Transplantation-Buddh.pdf

Hooper J. Prozac and Enlightened Mind. *Tricycle* 1999; **Summer**.

Hughes J. Buddhism and abortion: a western approach. In: Keown D. *Buddhism and Abortion*, Macmillan. http://www.change-surfer.com/Bud/Abortion.html.

Hughes J. The Death of Death. In: Machado C, Shewmon DA, eds. *Brain Death and Disorders of Consciousness*. Kluwer, 2004; pp. 79–88. http://ieet.org/index.php/IEET/articles/hughesdeath/.

Jackson PA. Male homosexuality and transgenderism in the Thai Buddhist tradition. In: Winston L, ed. *Queer Dharma: Voices of Gay Buddhists*. Gay Sunshine Press, 1998.

Jñanavira D. Homosexuality in the Japanese Buddhist tradition. *Western Buddhist Review* 2005; **3**. http://www.westernbuddhistreview.com/vol3/homosexuality.html

Kapleau P. *The Wheel of Life and Death*. New York: Doubleday, 1989.

Keown D. *The Nature of Buddhist Ethics*. New York: St. Martin's Press, 1992.

Keown D. *Buddhism and Bioethics*. London: Macmillan/New York: St. Martins Press, 1995.

Keown D. Buddhism and suicide – the case of Channa. *J Buddhist Ethics* 1996; **3**: 8–31.

Keown D. Buddhism and abortion: is there a middle way? In: Keown D, ed. Buddhism and Abortion. London: Macmillan, 1999.

King W. *In the Hope of Nibbana*. La Salle: Open Court, 1964.

Kotler A, ed. *Engaged Buddhist Reader*. Berkeley: Parallax Press, 2005.

Kuczewski MG. Whose will is it anyway? A discussion of advance directives, personal identity and consensus in medical ethics. *Bioethics* 1994; **8**(1): 27–48.

LaFleur W. *Liquid Life: Abortion and Buddhism in Japan*. New Jersey: Princeton University Press.

Lecso PA. The Bodhisattva ideal and organ transplantation. *J Religion Health* 1991; **30**(1): 35–41.

Levine S. *Who Dies? An Investigation of Conscious Living and Conscious Dying*. New York: Doubelday, 1982.

Ling, Trevor. 1973. *The Buddha: Buddhist Civilization in India & Ceylon*. Gower Publishing.

Lock M, Honde C. Reaching consensus about death: heart transplants and cultural identity in Japan. In: Weisz G, ed. *Social Science Perspectives on Medical Ethics*. New York: Kluwer, 1990; pp. 99–119.

Lock M. *Twice Dead: Organ Transplants and the Reinvention of Death*. Berkeley and Los Angeles: University of California Press, 2001.

Loy DR. Remaking the world, or remaking ourselves? buddhist reflections on technology. In: Hershock P, Stepaniants M, Ames R, eds. *Technology and Cultural Values: On the Edge of the Third Millennium*. Honolulu: University of Hawaii, 2003; pp.176–87. http://ccbs.ntu.edu.tw/FULLTEXT/JR-MISC/101792.htm

Mettanando B. Buddhist ethics in the practice of medicine. In: Fu CW, Wawrytko SA. *Buddhist Ethics and Modern Society: An International Symposium*. New York: Greenwood Press, 1991; pp. 195–213.

Meyer, J-AL. Buddhism and death: the brain-centered criteria. *J Buddhist Ethics* 2005; **12**: 1–24.

Mitra J. *A Critical Appraisal of Ayurvedic Materials in Buddhist Literature (with special reference to Tripitaka)*. Varanasi: The Jyotirlok Prakashan, 1985.

Parfit D. *Reasons and Persons*. Oxford: Oxford University Press, 1984.

Phelps N. *The Great Compassion: Buddhism and Animal Rights*. New York: Lantern Press, 2004.

Pryor FL. A Buddhist economic system–in practice. *Am J Econ Soc* 1991; **50**(1): 17–33.

Queen C, ed. *Engaged Buddhism: Buddhist Liberation Movements in Asia*. Albany: SUNY Press, 1996.

Queen C. *Engaged Buddhism in the West*. Somerville: Wisdom Publications, 2000.

Ratanakul P. *Bioethics: An Introduction to the Ethics of Medicine and Life Sciences*. Bangkok: Mahidol University, 1986.

Rinpoche S. The Tibetan book of living and dying: a spiritual classic from one of the foremost interpreters of Tibetan Buddhism to the West. San Francisco: Harper, 1994.

Sachs R. *Perfect Endings: A Conscious Approach to Dying and Death*. Rochester: Healing Arts Press, 1998.

Sarkisyanz E. *Buddhist Backgrounds of the Burmese Revolution*. The Hague: Maninus Nijhoff, 1965.

Schlieter J. Some observations on Buddhist thoughts on human cloning. In: Roetz H. (Hg.), ed. *Cross-Cultural Issues in Bioethics – The Example of Human Cloning*. Amsterdam: Rodopi, 2004.

Sen A. *Development as Freedom*. Oxford: Oxford University Press, 1999.

Sherwin S. et al., eds. *The Politics of Women's Health: Exploring Agency and Autonomy*. Philadelphia: Temple University Press, 1998.

Smith R. *Lessons from the Dying*. Wisdom Publications, 1998.

Soni RL. Buddhism in relation to the profession of medicine. In: Millard DW, ed. *Religion and Medicine*, Vol. 3. London: SCM Press, 1976; pp. 135–51.

Spiro M. *Buddhism and Society*. New York: Harper Paperbacks, 1972.

Thurman R. *Inner Revolution: Life, Liberty, and the Pursuit of Real Happiness*. New York: Riverhead Books, 1999.

Traer R. Buddhist affirmations of human rights. *Buddhist Christian Stud* 1988; **8**: 13–9.

Tsomo KL. Opportunity or obstacle: Buddhist views of organ donation. *Tricycle* 1993; **Summer**: 30–5.

Tsomo KL. Pro-life, pro-choice: Buddhism and reproductive ethics. *Feminism Nonviolence Stud* 1998; **Fall**: 1998. http://www.fnsa.org/fall98/tsomo1.html

Tworkov H. Anti-abortion/pro-choice: taking both sides. *Tricycle* 1992; **Spring**: 60–9,

Unno MT. Questions in the making – review essay on Zen Buddhist ethics in the context of Buddhist and comparative ethics. *J Religious Ethics* 1999; **27**(3): 509–36.

Waldau P. *The Specter of Speciesism: Buddhist and Christian Views of Animals*. Oxford: Oxford University Press, 2002.

Zysk, KG. *Asceticism and Healing in Ancient India: Medicine in the Buddhist Monastery*. Oxford: Oxford University Press, 1991.

18

South Asian Approaches to Health Care Ethics

HAROLD COWARD

South Asian approaches to health care ethics are rooted in a culture that is common to Hindus, Jains, Buddhists and Sikhs originating in the Indian sub-continent. Common to all these groups is the principle of *ahimsa* or 'do no harm'. Although this ancient moral virtue is not challenged by modern medical ethics, questions do arise when *ahimsa* is applied in clinical situations such as the withdrawal of life-saving therapy, the discontinuance of life support systems or when limited resources are allocated to a person with a better chance of survival (Crawford, 2003, p. 4). These questions are as much at issue for modern medicine in its goal to promote health and life as they are for the ancient South Asian attitudes towards the maintenance of good health, the cure of illnesses and the approach to death with its attendant suffering. Religion and medicine are inevitably brought into dialogue when confronted with beginning of life issues such as procreation, abortion, contraception and birth, or when end of life questions around ageing, suffering, pain and dying are dealt with. For Hindu, Sikh or Jain patients, these questions are often thought of very differently from modern European-based bioethics because of their quite unique South Asian cultural worldview with its own presuppositions.

THE SOUTH ASIAN WORLDVIEW AND HEALTH CARE ETHICS

South Asian Health Care Ethics deals with the ethics inherent in the *religion and culture* of Hindus, Jains and Sikhs. In these traditions, there is no great distinction between religion and culture. In contrast to the contemporary secular approach to bioethics, which is predominantly rights based, South Asian Bioethics is, in the main, a duty-based

approach. Indeed there is no word for 'rights' in traditional Hindu, Jain and Sikh language. Traditional teachings deal with the duties of individuals and families to maintain a healthy physical and mental lifestyle (Coward, 2005). However, after living in Europe and North America for a while, South Asians quickly acculturate to the dominant 'rights-based' approach of modern Western society. This will be the case with most second and third generation individuals and families. But newly arrived immigrants and older first generation people will usually maintain a traditional 'duty-based' approach when considering treatment options. This duty-based approach flows from three basic principles of Indian philosophy and religion: '(1) the transcendent character of human life, expressed through the principles of the sanctity of life and the quality of life; (2) the duty to preserve and guard individual and communal health; (3) the duty to rectify imbalances in the processes of nature and to correct and repair states that threaten life and well-being, both of humans and nonhumans' (Crawford, 2003, p. 6).

Hindu, Jain or Sikh health care ethics take seriously the presuppositions of the South Asian worldview and the implications of that worldview for ethical decision-making duties. What is this South Asian worldview? Although there are strong metaphysical differences between the Hindu, Jain and Sikh religions and considerable diversity within them, these traditions were born on the same South Asia continent and share a common culture and worldview which includes: ideas of *karma* and rebirth; collective (extended family) versus individual identity; a strong culture of purity; a preference for sons (for religious and cultural reasons). We will comment on each briefly.

Ideas of *karma* and rebirth are very important when ethical issues surrounding birth and death are considered.

Principles of Health Care Ethics, Second Edition   Edited by R.E. Ashcroft, A. Dawson, H. Draper and J.R. McMillan

Fundamental to the South Asian worldview is the idea that each person is being continually reborn, in order to purify the soul so that it will ultimately be able to join the divine cosmic consciousness (Radhakrishnan 1968). What a person does in each life conditions the circumstances and predispositions that will be experienced in future lives. This is the notion of *karma*. Briefly put, the concept of *karma* runs as follows. Every time you perform an action or think a thought a memory trace is laid down in the unconscious. A good action or thought leaves behind its trace, as does an evil action or thought. When you find yourself in a similar situation in the future, the memory trace rises up in consciousness as an impulse to perform an action or think a thought similar to the earlier one. Note that this is merely an impulse (a disposition or desire) and in itself does not force us to repeat the good or evil action or thought. We still have free choice. By the exercise of free choice, as each karmic impulse arises into our consciousness, we either nurture or uproot the memory traces in our unconscious. In theory, then, every impulse I experience in this life should be traceable back to actions and thoughts since birth. But *karma* theory does not assume a *tabula rasa* or blank mind at birth. Our unconscious contains memory traces not only of all actions and thoughts since birth but also of those from the life before that, and so on, backward infinitely (as *karma* theory rejects any absolute beginning and assumes life has always been going on). Consequently, each of us is thought to have a huge store of memory traces from previous lives that were transferred to us at birth and, with the additions and deletions we will make by our free choices in this life, will occasion our rebirth in our next life (Woods, 1966). The Hindu, Jain or Sikh view of life is a circular one (birth–life–death, birth–life–death) in contrast to the Jewish–Christian–Muslim linear view of life. All of this has important ethical consequences regarding birth considerations in that from a *karma* perspective what we are dealing with is the rebirth, at the moment of conception, of a fully developed person who has lived many previous lives. Termination by abortion basically sends the soul back into the karmic cycle of rebirth.

Another major difference in the South Asian worldview has to do with the question of identity – who is the ethical agent in decision-making, the individual or the extended family? Here we encounter a collective rather than individualistic conception of personhood. Unlike the modern Western assumption that the person as the ethical agent is the isolated individual, in *Ayurveda* (traditional South Asian medicine) a person is a combination of mind, soul and body in the context of family, culture and geography (Kakar, 1982). Thus the person is not seen as an autonomous individual but rather as one who is intimately integrated with extended family, caste group and geographical locality, necessitating a wholistic approach, for example in

matters of consent. Even the religious or spiritual dimension is included.

Purity practices and considerations are also very important in the South Asian worldview (Madan, 1985). This aspect is more cultural than religious. In the classical Indian tradition there are two terms translated as 'purity'. *Suddha* (or *Shudh* in Punjabi) evokes the image of the human body or elements of nature (e.g. the Ganges River) in its most pure, perfect and desired state of being. *Sauca* (*Sucha* in Punjabi) also means pure, but relates more specifically to one's own personal cleanliness. The most impure (*asauca* or *jutha* in Punjabi) substances are the discharges of one's own body. Women, because they have more discharges (e.g. menstruation) than men, are seen as being necessarily more impure. Only after menopause or before puberty does a female approach the standard of purity of a male. But the matter is even more complex in that the purity–impurity axis in daily life is bisected by the auspicious/inauspicious axis (*subha/asubha*). In daily life, for example, childbirth is auspicious if it occurs under the right circumstances of persons, family and nature. But even if all circumstances relating to auspiciousness are favourable, the act of childbirth itself, involving the discharge of bodily fluids, renders the mother impure (*asauca*). The baby is also impure. But this impurity pales into insignificance in the joy of the auspicious character of childbirth, particularly the birth of a son, which is duly celebrated through ritual performance and social ceremonies during the following eleven days, culminating in the ritual of purification (Coward, 1989).

There is a general bias in favour of males over females in South Asian culture. The roots of this bias are twofold. In some religions (e.g. Hinduism) an eldest son is required to perform yearly rituals for the well being of the father in the afterlife and light the funeral pyre. The eldest son is also the head of the extended family and has the responsibility to protect and provide for his mother and sisters – including a moral obligation to protect the virtue and virginity of daughters and sisters. On a purely monetary level, sons at marriage receive a dowry with their wife and thus add to the family wealth. Daughters in taking a dowry with them do the reverse. Also the male responsibility to provide for and protect the women in an extended family context means that there is often a strong male dominance when matters of consent are considered.

The above aspects of the South Asian worldview and the duties required are representative but not exhaustive. There is great regional diversity among Hindus, especially. But the above approaches do give one an idea of some of the quite different assumptions and duties at play when ethical decisions are to be made.

WHY ARE SOUTH ASIAN HEALTH CARE ETHICS IMPORTANT?

The ethical theories employed in health care today assume, in the main, a modern Western philosophical rights-based framework, which is then applied to issues such as abortion, euthanasia, consent and so on. Yet the diversity of cultural and religious assumptions regarding human nature, health and illness, life and death and the status of the individual demands that doctors be sensitive and respectful of the worldview of their patients in ethical decision-making (Coward & Ratanakul, 1999). South Asian (Hindu/Jain/Sikh) patients are a major minority in the British, Canadian or American ethnic diversity and need to be understood in their own terms which include a strong sense of family, social and religious duty. There are more than one billion South Asians in the world population, with many living in diaspora communities (Coward, 2000). One should keep in mind that in many South Asian patients, there will be an attachment to traditional medicines (e.g., Ayurveda and Siddha) which may be used together with modern biomedicine (Azariah, 1954).[1] Thus cultural beliefs about health, disease and treatment often vary significantly from standard Western medical practice. Diet also differs, from full vegetarian practice (no meat, fish or eggs), if orthodox Hindu, Jain or Sikh, to a rejection of beef but acceptance of chicken or fish. Rather than bringing or sending an ill person flowers, the tradition favours the frequent visits of extended family members and friends so as to offer support – thus, groups of visitors will be more numerous and frequent than the usual pattern.

When dealing with Hindu/Jain/Sikh South Asian patients, the very different worldview and religious/cultural practices must be understood and respected. Otherwise, miscommunication is very likely. Also, there is diversity within the South Asian Hindu/Sikh population. An individual's reaction to a particular clinical situation will depend on whether he/she is first, second or third generation, or a recently landed immigrant. Furthermore, the level of education attained (from illiteracy to postdoctoral), rural versus urban roots, socio-economic status and religious stance (fundamentalist versus moderate) will also influence behaviour and decision-making. Extended families are common and they provide individuals with social support and financial security. Elderly members of the ex-tended family are accorded respect; they help with childcare and provide advice. The family spokesperson (with whom consent issues will have to be negotiated) is usually the most financially established senior person in the family; however, should such a person lack the language skills required, then a younger person may fulfil the communication role for the family. By keeping all of these factors in mind the health care provider can avoid the mistake of *either* treating the South Asian patient the same as an average European or North American *or* a stereotyped South Asian with predictable reactions in biomedical ethical situations.

In situations of ethical decision-making, communication issues are very important. Every effort should be made to find trained and impartial interpreters for South Asian patients not fluent in English. This is particularly important in issues of consent to ensure that information given to or received from the patient is not being censored or altered by the interpreter. South Asian women patients need trained female interpreters who are familiar with the traditions and culture of origin. Women patients will also exhibit a strong preference for a same-sex physician, especially for uro-genital examinations. Due to their deep sense of modesty (along with the sense of purity described above), South Asian women will not feel comfortable with a male physician or interpreter. There is a strong reticence to expose the body, especially to someone of the opposite sex. Although family members such as a teenage daughter may function well as an interpreter for minor day to day problems, an older trained South Asian woman who understands technical medical language, and is not a family member, will make the best interpreter, especially in uro-genital matters. Confidentiality is very important. In a severe bind, a female relative or the husband may serve as an interpreter, but this is not the preferred approach. In addition to interpretation issues, the style of communication to be used with South Asian patients should be different. By planning for a longer interview and adopting an indirect conversational approach, the physician or health care worker will learn more. Also, the physician needs to be alert to nontranslatable Hindu or Punjabi words commonly used to express psychosomatic symptoms – for example *dil* (heart), *kirda* (fragmenting), *dubda* (sinking), which an interpreter or the person may express in English as 'a sinking heart' implies tremendous anxiety which may result from a headache, nausea, stomach pain (especially

---

[1]Ayurveda is the traditional South Asian science of living to a ripe old age. The term is semantically significant: 'Ayur' implies that the ancient Indian doctor was concerned not only with curing disease, but also with promoting health and long life; the second term, 'veda', has religious overtones, being the term used for the most sacred scriptures of Hinduism. It is specifically associated with the Atharva Veda. See Basham AL,. *The Wonder that Was India*. New York: Grove Press, 1954, p. 20. Some basic Ayurveda principles include all living organisms are regulated by pleasure and pain; the yearnings for happiness and freedom from suffering are universal; all living beings have been created for health; disease is an impediment to the fulfilment of all human goals, including the spiritual; the ultimate goal of medicine is the relief of suffering.

epigastric) or generalized malaise. The physician should rule out organic disease, such as a vitamin B12 deficiency (due to genetic causes) common in South Asians, and screen for this before adopting a psychosomatic treatment approach. The physician should also be alert for the term *nazar* (the evil eye) accompanied by a black mark behind the ear or a black thread around the wrist to protect one from the evil eye curse (from someone who, out of envy perhaps, wishes to do them harm).

SOME APPLICATIONS OF THE SOUTH ASIAN APPROACH TO HEALTH CARE ETHICS

CONCEPTS OF HEALTH AND DISEASE

Modern Western medicine sometimes adopts a statistical approach to health and disease, especially in respect to changing figures as to what is 'normal'. New studies often offer new definitions as to what is normal or abnormal. Ayurveda cautions 'all ideas of statistical normalcy to the extent that they fail to give primacy to the particular constitution of the individual'. *In Ayurveda, 'normal' and 'abnormal' are not general but specific measurements* that fully take into account the total makeup of the person (Crawford, 2003, p. 97). This includes the anatomy, biochemistry, age, gender, genetics and environment of the person. Nor is health simply understood as the absence of disease, as is often the approach in the West. Ayurveda rejects this negative approach and instead defines health as a positive, dynamic state that involves the whole person as well as the environment. Indeed, Ayurveda is in many ways closer to what is today referred to as 'environmental medicine'. But Ayurveda goes further still and includes the spirit (*atman*) in any consideration of health. According to Ayurveda it is when one goes beyond psychosomatic states of health and disease and lives in a higher state of spiritual consciousness (*prajna*) that one is ensured health and happiness; in lower states one becomes prey to disorders (Crawford, 2003, p. 100).

THE BEGINNING OF LIFE

When one focuses on the start of life situations, it is crucial that any ethical consideration takes account of the strong pro-natal stance of the South Asian tradition. The South Asian ethics perspective that the foetus is not developing into a person but is a person from the moment of conception needs to be engaged with the cultural demand for a son in counselling the patient. And the 'patient' here might not be just the pregnant mother but the collective extended family. For Hindus, Jains and Sikhs (who all affirm *karma* and rebirth) the single most important ethical consideration surrounding the start of life is their belief that the rebirth of a fully developed person, who has lived many lives, occurs at the moment of conception. Abortion at any stage of foetal development is thus judged to be murder. However, abortion is accepted by Hindus, Jains and Sikhs if it is essential to preserve the life of the mother (Coward, 1993). The distinction between a human being and a human person made in some Western discussions, with its implication of the permissibility of at least early abortion, does not occur in the South Asian religions. Personal moral status is granted to the embryo/foetus from the first moment of conception and throughout pregnancy. In addition to relating to concepts of *karma* and rebirth, this approach to abortion is further grounded in the great respect for the principle of *ahimsa* ('do no harm') that is maintained by these religious and cultural traditions.

If we look to India, a modern secular state in which Hinduism is the majority religion, we find that abortion is permitted by law under certain circumstances, but the topic of the moral status of the unborn and of abortion has been little discussed. In public, the topic is a taboo. Yet it is clear that illegal abortion has a long history and continues today.[2] Although the texts dealing with religious law and ethics are very clear in condemning the wilful killing of a foetus, it is also true that these texts have very limited bearing on daily life. Many people are not even aware of them; others quite easily and happily ignore them. The texts simply do not have the compelling authority that scripture may have in some other religious traditions.

Abortions are done fairly regularly in India for a number of reasons, and in recent years the principal ones seem to be related to sex selection or family planning. As boys are valued more than girls in many communities, sonograms/amniocenteses are performed and female foetuses are aborted. Statistics available from the state of Maharashtra show that in recent years there has been

---

[2]My informant, Dr. Vasudha Narayanan, states that according to both religious texts and popular practice in the Hindu tradition(s), the embryo/foetus has life and, in some rare cases, is even capable of hearing the conversations that take place around it and learning from them. It is clear that the fetus is an entity: people do not bow before pregnant women, because in the Hindu tradition one can only bow down and pay respect to people older than oneself. Since there is a young child, a real entity, within a pregnant woman, bowing before her would mean one is paying respect to the baby also and this should not be done. It would therefore be logical and correct to say that killing the embryo is tantamount to murder. Despite this fundamental belief, abortions have been conducted legally and illegally in many places in India, without much apparent guilt on the women's part about the process. My statement here is only based on impressions and conversations with women doctors from India, but I suspect that a full-fledged study may verify them'.

a dramatic drop in the number of live births of girls (Bumiller, 1990). In the past (about 30 to 40 years ago), students in many medical schools in India had the general impression that abortions could only be done in some 'Christian' clinics (the name given to Western-style clinics) but not in government hospitals or by Indian doctors. Now, many hospitals in India carry out these procedures fairly routinely, and most of the clientele is apparently Hindu.

Infertility (or even the lack of a son) has been considered justification for some form of surrogacy practice. Often this has been accomplished by allowing polygamy. In Hinduism, there has also been the practice in which a man marries the childless widow of his deceased brother. Surrogacy by natural means and under certain circumstances seems to be allowable within the boundaries of the family. The integrity of the extended family is of ultimate importance, since it forms the essential 'self' from which all individual family members receive meaning and identity. The idea of someone from outside the extended family being involved in some kind of surrogacy practice would seem unlikely to receive acceptance by the cultures involved. From this perspective, the very idea of single motherhood (or for that matter fatherhood) by choice is unlikely. In this extended family context, all discussions of new reproductive technologies (NRTs) will be approached with respect to not only the wife involved but also the husband and the family as a whole. The autonomous, individualist approach to moral questions that typifies the modern West is very foreign to members of the Hindu tradition, even after the family has lived in Europe or North American for two or three generations.

Perhaps even more important than notions of *karma*, on the popular level great importance is placed on biological descent; therefore, artificial insemination with sperm other than the husband's would not be tolerated. In higher castes, there is a notion of keeping the purity of one's caste and clan (*gotra*), and artificial insemination from a sperm bank would be intolerable. (For similar reasons, even adoption of an unknown child would be unacceptable for many Hindus.) A Hindu woman in India carrying a child other than her husband's would be likely to incur family and community ostracism or, at the very least, disapproval. However, if a woman could be artificially inseminated with her husband's

sperm and the child carried to term, a childless couple would definitely accept the procedure; there would not be any taboo against unnatural technological intervention. Urban Hindu men and women have generally been accepting of Western medical procedures, and medical help in this regard would be welcomed rather than rejected. Many childless couples from India come to Western countries for advanced tests and help with reproductive technology without prejudice.

The question of IVF is a complicated one when seen from the perspective of Hinduism. Fertility is important, especially the conception and birth of a son. IVF appears attractive to wives and husbands who are having difficulty in conceiving and giving birth to children. Modern India seems to be using IVF enthusiastically. When it is considered by scholars, however, it becomes a very serious issue as the destruction of any embryo would be considered murder. IVF poses a serious dilemma unless all fertilized embryos are implanted. However, in practice, abortions are performed regularly, so for many members of the general population the destroying of embryos may not present a great moral dilemma.[3]

In Hinduism, there are certain religious rituals that must be performed by a son if one's afterlife is to be secured, and the dowry practice makes sons a source of wealth for the family and daughters a drain on family fortunes. Thus, any offering of medical services that allow both sex selection and abortion will introduce severe social and moral pressures into these families. The conflict between the desire for sons (and the possibility for ensuring them through the new technologies) and the proscription against abortion will place severe moral strains on some families, especially upon the mothers involved. In Hindu ritual practice, there are rituals designed to aid in giving birth to a son, but these rituals never involve abortion.

The issue of commercialization is also of concern to the family units of the Hindu religion. Although the religion would not condone the opportunities for commercialization NRTs might spawn, the family and social structure might well encourage such developments. One has only to look at what has happened in the area of organ transplants (with special flights to India where organs of all kinds can be obtained for money by Westerners) to think of possible NRT parallels. It is not simply that the poor are selling their

---

[3]Dr. Narayanan observes, 'Myths in Hindu epics and puranas are filled with supernatural or 'unnatural' means of conception and giving birth. In the *Mahabharata* we encounter the story of a hundred embryos being grown in pots by Gandhari. In other texts, we see an embryo being transplanted from one woman to another (Krishna's brother Balarama was said to have been transplanted into another womb when still in an embryonic stage); divine potions are consumed and children produced fairly regularly; deities are invoked and 'fertilize' the woman if the husband is not capable of procreating, and so on. However, as far as I know, none of these tales have been invoked as authoritative or legitimating instances in connection with NRTs. What we have to recognize is that despite notions of embryonic life, *karma*, *et cetera*, decisions on abortions and NRTs are more likely to be made based on how badly a child, especially a boy, is wanted by the couple or family or, in the case of abortion, how badly a child is *not* wanted by the woman.'

organs, but that at times even a husband volunteers to sell an organ of his wife. The prospect of earning money from paid surrogacy is surely not far removed, given the presence of the requisite technology.

Regarding the Sikh tradition, presuppositions of *karma* and rebirth mean abortion will be seen as the murder of a human person and be unacceptable except for the purpose of preserving the mother's life. Personal moral status is granted to the embryo/foetus from the moment of conception and throughout the pregnancy. In addition to *karma* and rebirth, this approach to abortion is further grounded in great respect for the principle of *ahimsa*, or nonviolence. In Sikh thinking, human life is a gift from God and no individual has the right to alter or destroy this state in any way.

Sikh religious leaders are trying to grapple with the issues raised by the use of NRTs. It is to the *Rehat* that Sikhs often turn when they have to decide on issues of social ethics. There is nothing on NRTs in the Sikh *Rehat*, which is hardly surprising considering that the present authoritative version of the *Rehat* dates back to the 1950s, when there was hardly any discussion on what challenge NRTs pose for the Sikh society. With the increasing availability of NRTs, particularly to the members of the Sikh diaspora, some thought has been given to this issue, and the resolutions that are offered are all drawn from what the Sikh normative tradition has to say.

The actual practice in South Asian cultures, including that of the Sikhs, has been known to depart from the normative. Female infanticide and illegal abortion have been practised. In Sikh cultures, sons have been valued over daughters, and thus, there are temptations to use NRTs for sex selection so as to ensure the reproduction of sons. When the Government of India made abortion legal, there was no sustained opposition to this law on the part of Indian religious communities. Today, abortion clinics are common in Punjab, the original home for most of the Sikh population in Europe and North America.

It is impossible to make any blanket statements on artificial insemination or IVF in Sikhism. Theologically, these practices would be viewed as interfering with the *hukam*, the order of God, a central feature of the Sikh worldview. However, once again these procedures are tolerated in practice. Some Sikh couples have decided to use IVF. Since the norm disallows abortion, it also would not accept aborted foetal tissue for research purposes.

On the commercialization issue, sections of the Sikh population resident in Canada have firmly and very vocally opposed the use of ultrasound scanning techniques for the purpose of identifying the sex of a foetus. They fear that this sex-determination technology will lead to predominantly male selection.

THE END OF LIFE

In South Asian culture and religion, ageing and dying is approached quite differently from modern Western society. Within the extended family, parents and other seniors (aunts and uncles) are venerated and treated with respect. It is expected that they would be cared for within the extended family, likely in the home of the eldest son, and not required to live in a seniors facility or alone in their own home or apartment. Having fulfilled their householder duties of having married, had children and earned money to support the family, the parents, when skin wrinkles, hair turns white and grandchildren appear, are expected to withdraw from worldly life into more spiritual pursuits (Crawford, 2003, pp. 183 ff). It is now up to children to assume responsibility for supporting the young children and the seniors. In the last stages of life, it is expected that seniors may wish to disengage from worldly life and seek to realize ultimate release from rebirth or *moksa*. This is the spiritual goal and may involve leaving the family for periods of intellectual study and yoga in a forest ashram with a teacher or *guru*. This may prove to be especially the case for widows or widowers. Life in such ashrams is simple with vegetarian food, daily exercise and study along with sharing in the chores. It is not required that seniors follow such a path as they age, but many do. If one is content to live the worldly life at home in the comfort of the extended family and wait until the next life to make more spiritual progress towards *moksa*, then that too is quite acceptable.

When it comes to death, South Asians, like most others, hope that death can be held off in favour of a long life. From ancient times, human nature has been understood as composed of three parts: a soul, a subtle body and a physical body (Crawford, 2003, pp. 190 ff). The self, soul or *atman* is the divine portion (usually described as pure being, pure consciousness and pure bliss). The physical body is the locus of all experience arising from the external world and is the seat of consciousness in its wakeful states. It is composed of the five elements (earth, water, fire, wind and space). In death, the body returns to its source, namely, the material elements. '*Death only refers to the dissolution of the physical body* (Crawford, 2003, pp. 191 ff).' The subtle body, however, does not dissolve at death and carries one's *karma* from this life to the next. The subtle body is so-called because it is composed of elements finer than those of the physical body and make up the mind, intellect, five vital breaths (infusing the heart, the anus, the navel, the throat and the whole body), the five organs of action (speech, hands, feet, anus and the sexual organ) and five organs of knowledge (ear, skin, eye, tongue and nose). 'Thus the subtle body is a composite coordination of a person's chief functions – vital, mental and intellectual. The presence of the essential self [or soul] and its direct awareness makes all of this happen. Hence the subtle body is the *linga* or characteristic symbol of the proximity of the self (Crawford, 2003, pp. 191 ff).

In South Asian thought, the subtle body provides a person's continuity from this life to the next and carries the *karma* one has created for oneself (by free choice) from one body to the next. 'It conserves the moral consequences of a person's life, which then impact the direction of the person's rebirth ⋯[and] fix the type of physical body and environment the person will inherit in his or her next birth; and in terms of indirect impact, moral consequences condition the individual's propensities for behaviour (Crawford, 2003, pp. 191 ff). Vedic scripture describes the actual disengagement of the subtle body (resulting in death) as a 'fading out' first of the eye, then of the nose, tongue, voice, ear and mind – all withdraw from the physical body and unite with the subtle body as the dying process continues. Finally, the intellect becomes united with the subtle body and it is said, 'He does not know'. With all of this in mind, it is important that health care workers working with South Asians be able to sense when the dying process has begun and do nothing to block the natural process. The person should be allowed to die in peace surrounded by the extended family and if possible at home. Because the focus is wished to be on providing a good exit for the subtle body from the physical body, the person's physical state should not obscure his or her state of spiritual consciousness. Scripture suggests that whatever state of being one remembers at the moment of death, to that one attains (Gita 9:25). Thus the person should be kept as comfortable as possible so as to have good final moments. As Crawford puts it, 'The quality of one's state of consciousness at the terminus of life sets the stage for the exit of the subtle body from the physical body and also directs its future trajectory' (Crawford, 2003, p. 192). The ultimate goal sought in the afterlife is union with the divine and release from rebirth (*moksa*).

On the basis of the above outline of the South Asian approach to ageing and dying, we can summarize the implications for health care ethics as follows:

- Death is the end of the body. Death occurs with the dissolution of the subtle body from the physical body.
- Death is not the opposite of life; it is the opposite of birth.
- Death and life are not opposites to each other but facets of an ongoing seemingly endless cycle.
- Belief in the eternal *atman* or soul and the ongoing subtle body reduces helplessness in the face of death.
- *Karma* connects a person with past, present and future dimensions of his or her life and gives moral meaning to all events and actions.
- *Karma* and rebirth are answers to questions patients ask, such as 'why me?'
- Death in response to age is considered natural. Only untimely death is profoundly mourned.
- Quality of life is valued more than the length of days.
- A good death is one that happens at home and over which a person has control.
- Death is an important social event when the whole extended family comes together to express love and grief while the patient is alive and through ritual devotion after the person has died.
- The dead are cremated because fire purifies and returns bodies to their original form. Children's bodies are not cremated as they are considered pure as are the bodies of those who live holy lives in the forest (Crawford, 2003, pp. 195–6).

The Ayurveda puts the emphasis on death with dignity. 'Just as it is natural for a ripe fruit to release itself from its bonds, so also the end is inevitable for one whose life is spent' (Crawford, 2003, p. 192). At such a time the role of physician or nurse is to help the person and family live out a good death together.

REFERENCES

Azariah J, ed. *Bioethics in India: Proceedings of the International Bioethics Workshop in Madras*, University of Madras, 1998. Web address: http://www.mit.csu.edu.au/learning/eubios/books.htm.

Bumiller E. *May You Be the Mother of a Hundred Sons: A Journey Among the Women of India* [reports on many clinics specializing in these procedures in Bombay]. New York: Random House, 1990.

Coward H. World religions and reproductive technologies. In: *Social Values and Attitudes surrounding New Reproductive Technologies*, Vol. 2. Ottawa: Royal Commission of New Reproductive Technologies, Research Studies, 1993; pp. 454–63

Coward H, Hinnells JR, Williams RB, eds. *The South Asian Religious Diaspora in Britain, Canada and the United States*. Albany: State University of New York Press, 2000.

Coward H. Are there human rights in hinduism? In: *Human Rights and the World's Major Religions: The Hindu Tradition*. London: Praeger, 2005; pp. 19–30.

Coward H, Ratanakul P, eds. *A Cross-Cultural Dialogue on Health Care Ethics*. Waterloo: Wilfrid Laurier University Press, 1999. (See Chapter 1, Introduction, by Coward H, Ratanakul P, pp. 1–11. I acknowledge the assistance of Dr. Tejinder Sidhu, a practising Sikh physician, in the writing of this section.)

Coward HG, Lipner JJ, Young KK. *Hindu Ethics: Purity, Abortion and Euthanasia*. Albany: State University of New York Press, 1989; pp. 10–11.

Crawford SC. *Hindu Bioethics for the Twenty-First Century*. Albany: State University of New York Press, 2003.

Kakar S. Indian medicine and psychiatry: cultural and theoretical perspectives on ayurveda. *Shamans, Mystics and Scholars*. Boston: Beacon Press, 1982; pp. 219–51.

Madan TN. Concerning the categories of *subha* and *suddha* in Hindu culture. Carman JB, Marglin FA, eds. In: *Purity and Auspiciousness in Indian Society*. Leiden: E.J. Bull, 1985; pp. 11–29

Radhakrishnan S, ed. *The Principal Upanisads*. London: Allen & Unwin, 1968; pp.113–45.

Woods JH, translator. *Yoga Sutras of Patanjali II*: 12–14 & IV: 7–9. Varanasi: Motilal Banarsidass, 1966; Harvard Oriental Series, Vol. 17.

19

The Specious Idea of an Asian Bioethics: Beyond Dichotomizing East and West

JING-BAO NIE

There is already much of the East in the West and vice versa, as the 'twain' of East and West met long ago – including the discipline of health care ethics. Despite its apparent American origin and the continuing US domination of the field, bioethics as a new and expanded form of an age-old medical ethics has been a global phenomenon from the beginning. Unfortunately, the local complexity and richness and the global significance of medical ethics in non-Western societies are far from being well recognized and documented. And the encounter of East and West in the field of bioethics – including the real and potential fusion of horizons and the nature of their real and potential conflicts – are far from being well understood. Even more unfortunately, the old habit of dichotomizing East and West as not only radically different but also in a state of perpetual conflict still haunts the young discipline, cross-cultural bioethics in particular.

Clearly, bioethics exists in Asia as an academic field and especially as a socio-political discourse. Yet, is there an *Asian* bioethics and what, if anything, constitutes the peculiar characteristics of bioethics as practised in Asia? We are hardly in a position to give adequate answers to these questions as our knowledge of bioethics in the various countries and regions of Asia is very limited at present. In fact, few, if any, systematic and in-depth comparative studies have appeared on bioethics across Asian nations, on the different Asian medical ethics traditions, and on any one major Asian medical ethics tradition in different regions. However, a widespread stock answer – a long-rooted stereotype in my view – exists to these complex questions. It characterizes Asian bioethics as communitarian, collectivist or family-centred, in contrast to Western bioethics which is portrayed as individualistic in essence.

As Asia has been playing an increasingly active role in world affairs, bioethics or health care ethics in Asia

is attracting increasing attention from the international community. This essay, nevertheless, is not intended to be a review of recent developments in bioethics in Asia (de Castro et al., 2004). Rather, it focuses on what can be called 'the Asian bioethics debate' and offers a critical examination of the idea of an *Asian* bioethics as opposed to a *Western* bioethics and the underlying dichotomizing of East and West that this distinction presupposes. I argue that, although this concept has grown out of serious and important concerns or issues such as opposition to imperialism and the desire to develop a bioethics based on Asian cultural traditions and sensitive to the Asian context, the notion itself is empirically problematic, conceptually flawed and politically contentious. There are a series of ironies involved in this specious idea which, for convenience of discussion, I will call 'the Asian bioethics approach'. An effective cross-cultural bioethics must first of all challenge this concept and its dichotomizing way of seeing East and West.

THE IDEA: ITS ROOTS, DISSEMINATION AND MODES OF EXPRESSION

In 1958, the distinguished author of *The Logic of Scientific Discovery* and *The Open Society and its Enemies* delivered a public address in Zürich entitled 'What does the West believe in?' For Karl Popper, the West properly believes in its own values: rationalism, progress, democracy as the least evil and thus the best form of government and, most importantly, pluralism of ideas. In his words, 'we can say proudly that we in the West believe in many and different things, in much that is true and in much that is false; in good things and in bad things' (Popper 1994, p. 212). Popper hints that, contrary to the West, where this diversity of ideas is not only a prominent feature

Principles of Health Care Ethics, Second Edition   Edited by R.E. Ashcroft, A. Dawson, H. Draper and J.R. McMillan
© 2007 John Wiley & Sons, Ltd

but also an ideal to be pursued, the East (as represented by Communism) is characterized by a monolithic unity of ideas and thus lacks diversity. Although the 'Cold War' political context of Popper's speech was historically unique and his hostile attitude to the 'East' is no longer widely shared, this way of dichotomizing East and West is still commonplace.

Indeed, the demarcation between the Orient and the Occident is an ancient and a persistent theme in Western civilization and literature. It was manifested in the *Iliad* of Homer, *The Persians* of Aeschylus, *The Bacchae* of Euripides and *The Politics* (1327b18–35) of Aristotle. It has been a cornerstone of modern Western approaches to the Orient. As Edward Said has pointed out,

> Orientalism is a style of thought based on an ontological and epistemological distinction between 'the Orient' and (most of the time) 'the Occident.' Thus a very large mass of writers, among whom are poets, novelists, philosophers, political theorists, economists, and imperial administrators, have accepted the basic distinction between East and West as the starting point for elaborating theories, epics, novels, social descriptions, and political accounts concerning the Orient, its people, customs, 'mind,' destiny, and so on. (Said,1994[1979], pp. 2–3).

Moreover, the discipline of anthropology has for a long time regarded it as its mission to discover the peculiar features and determining patterns of non-Western cultures in terms of their differentiation from Western cultures. From the start, the fundamental difference between the West and the non-West has been assumed. Interestingly, although many anthropologists have evaluated non-Western cultures positively and postmodernist discourse has reversed the negative stance of modern Orientalists towards the East, the belief of these fundamental differences remains.

This is not just a Western sin. The basic distinction between East and West has been an essential part of academic and political discourse in China, Korea, Japan and other Asian countries ever since the twain met. As a dramatically intensified version of the old debate on the differences between Chinese and foreigners and how to deal with them (*huayi zhi bian*), the controversy over Chinese and Western cultures has been a salient theme of the cultural and political life of 20th-century China, especially in the New Culture Movement of the first decades of the century and in the 'cultural browsing' (*wenhua re*) of the post-Mao reform era. China's intellectuals – whether advocates of antitraditionalism and wholesale Westernization such as Hu Shi or cultural conservatives such as Liang Shuming – have too often based their arguments on the assumption of a fundamental difference between China and the West, involving a collectivist or authoritarian China versus the individualistic West. Other popular oppositions include spiritual (China) versus materialist (West), static and ordered versus active and changing, conservative versus progressive, dependent versus independent and controlled by nature versus conquering nature.

Unfortunately, this long-rooted habit of thinking has also come to dominate discussions on bioethics in East and West. It has been too often asserted that there is a distinctive Asian or non-Western bioethics in contrast to the Western discipline, in line with similar simplistic evaluations of non-Western societies and cultures in both academic discourse and popular discussion. Western and Chinese scholars alike have characterized the differences in Chinese and Western or American perspectives on abortion in such a way (see Nie, 2005). As the following citations from prominent advocates of this notion show, the idea of an Eastern versus a Western bioethics consists of a series of shared assumptions and claims.

The first is the *difference* thesis. It asserts that, as a result of the peculiar socio-historical backgrounds of East and West, a series of differences can be detected between Eastern and Western cultures, moral traditions and health care ethics. These differences are often characterized as communitarianism versus individualism, the primacy of the state and the collective versus individual interests, a family-centred emphasis versus individual autonomy, holism versus reductionism, the concept of duty and obligation versus freedom, and so on. Japanese bioethicist Hyakudai Sakamoto, founding president of the East-Asian Association of Bioethics (later the Asian Association of Bioethics), expressed the idea clearly in a keynote speech at the 4th World Congress of Bioethics:

> Generally speaking, Asians hold a holistic way of thinking instead of the European individualistic way. Therefore Asian people put a higher value on the holistic happiness and welfare of the total group or community to which they belong rather than on their individual interest (Sakamoto, 1999, p. 194).

The characteristics of 'the Asian worldviews and general ways of thinking', all defined by contrast with the so-called Western way of thinking, include 'a higher estimation on total and social 'well-orderedness' [rather] than on individual interests and individual rights and dignity'; a fundamental naturalism in which 'there is no antagonism or clear cut dichotomy between nature and human beings'; and a disinclination 'to believe or pursue any 'invariance' or 'eternity' (Sakamoto, 1999, p. 194–6). One political implication of emphasizing these fundamental differences is that such presumed 'Western' norms as human rights, patients' rights and informed consent are not applicable to the Asian context.

Two Filipino bioethicists, Angeles Alora and Josephine Lumitao, have edited a volume entitled *Beyond a Western Bioethics* with the aim of exploring 'the radically different character that bioethics takes in the developing world' (Alora & Lumitao, 2001, p. 3). Their presentation focuses on the dichotomy of a Filipino bioethics and Western bioethics:

The very character of ethics in the West contrasts with ethics in the Philippines not just in terms of the issues and solutions, as well as the context in which each is embedded, but also in the very language and character of moral concern. The focus of Western bioethics is individual; elsewhere it focuses on social units. Western bioethics often is oriented to principles; Filipino bioethics, on the other hand, is not articulated primarily in principles but in lived moral virtues. Whereas Western bioethics is almost always expressed in discursive terms, Filipino bioethics is part of the phenomenological world of living experience. For the West, bioethics is a framework for thought, a conception system. For the Philippines it is a way of life, an embodied activity of virtue (Alora & Lumitao, 2001, p. 4).

Furthermore, because Filipinos treat the family as 'the social unit of greatest value',

> the primary locus of assessment of the good is not the individual but the family . . . Maintenance of harmony within the family and among peers take precedence over other concerns for social justice or honesty, which from this perspective appear to be anonymous formal principles that are disengaged from concrete moral community life (Alora & Lumitao, 2001, p. 7).

Consequently, given a strong family-centred and community-centred ethos, 'Western ideals of individualism and self-reliance have little purchase in the Filipino culture' (Alora & Lumitao, 2001, p. 8). Notably, Alora and Lumitao extend without hesitation these general statements on Filipino ethics to bioethics in the developing world as a whole.

For Chinese bioethicist Ruiping Fan, there exist two bioethical 'principles of autonomy', one Western and the other East Asian:

> Other things being equal, the Western principle of autonomy demands self-determination, assumes a subjective conception of good and promotes the value of individual independence, whilst the East Asian principle of autonomy requires family-determination, presupposes an objective conception of the good and upholds the value of harmonious dependence (Fan, 1997, p. 309).

These two principles 'differ from each other in the most general sense and basic moral requirement[s]'. For Fan, the principle and practice of family sovereignty in East Asian societies was traditionally based on the Confucian understanding of the nature of the family and of individuals. In another article, he shifts the focus from East Asian versus Western principles of medical ethics in general to the West versus China, and Aristotelianism versus Confucianism (Fan, 2002, p. 346). He holds that not only contemporary models of surrogate medical decision-making, but also the entire medical ethics traditions of China and the West are fundamentally different, that is individualistic versus familial. The contemporary patterns of medical decision-making in China and the West are derived from Confucian and Aristotelian perspectives on human life and ideal human

relationships, which are the representatives of the Chinese and Western moral traditions.

This leads us to the second popular thesis regarding Asian bioethics, that of *essence*. The above citations have suggested a belief that, underlying these allegedly opposed cultural characteristics, there are two totally different kinds of ethos, essence, patterns of culture and fundamental ways of thinking or mentality. In the words of Sakamoto, 'a possible Asian Bioethics or bioethical way of thinking . . . is supposed to be essentially different from the European one' (Sakamoto 1999, p. 194). In contrast to the modern European inclination to dualistic individualism, 'a holistic harmony' constitutes 'the essence of the Asian ethos' and of Asian bioethics as well.

The third proposition, the *incommensurability* thesis, goes even further to claim that all the posited differences, especially the fundamental ones, are totally incompatible. They are, as the title of Fan's controversial article (Fan, 1997) puts it, 'incommensurable'.

Asian scholars are not unique in characterizing bioethics in Asia and the West in such a dichotomizing fashion. This habit is widely shared in the West as well. Shortly after China reopened her doors to the outside world, two American sociologists/bioethicists, Renée Fox and Judith Swazey, made a research trip to China. Based on their 6 weeks of fieldwork, primarily in a highly modernized hospital in the city of Tianjian in 1981, they reported their findings on 'medical morality' (a term for medical ethics then current in China) in comparison with bioethics in the United States and concluded as follows: 'it is amply clear that medical morality is not bioethics. It is as Chinese as bioethics is American . . .. In the final analysis, . . . American bioethics and Chinese medical morality are so culturally dissimilar that they are not sufficiently related to form a yin–yang (opposing, but complementary) pair' (Fox & Swazey, 1984, p. 349). According to Fox and Swazey, the Chinese worldview and the 'medical morality' rooted in Chinese culture stress dynamic complementarity, the collective, the larger and vital whole, the relationship of the individual with others, personal virtues, and so on. In stark contrast, 'Individualism is the primary value-complex on which the intellectual and moral edifice of [American] bioethics rests' (Fox & Swazey, 1984, p. 352). Most importantly, rather than making any systematic and careful study of medical ethics in China, Fox and Swazey use the perceived 'Chineseness' of medical morality as a 'beating stick' to criticize the alleged 'Americanness' of bioethics, particularly its individualistic tendencies.

H. Tristram Engelhardt Jr., one of the best-known Western bioethicists in China, apparently subscribes to this popular notion as demonstrated in his articulation of the differences and similarities between Japanese and Western bioethics (Engelhardt, 1997). More significantly, he promotes the idea of Asian or non-Western versus Western bioethics by cultivating his Asian colleagues and students in what has been called the 'Engelhardt circle', which includes Fan, Alora and Lumitao. Besides contributing chapters to collective works, he has had an active involvement in the making of several volumes published in the influential series 'Philosophy and Medicine' (e.g. Hoshino, 1997, Quiz, 2004) and other publications (Alora & Lumitao, 2001) which promote the dichotomizing of bioethics along East–West lines. Such approaches gain attraction because the assumed radical differences between Western and Asian or other non-Western cultures apparently provide strong empirical evidence for a key concept of Engelhardt's bioethical theory that 'moral strangers' can never share what he calls a 'contentful' moral life (Engelhardt, 1996). In fact, his vision of a bioethics for the postmodern world needs and is based on the radical differences in belief systems – whether religious or secular – and cultures.

THE SPECIOUSNESS OF THE IDEA

There are of course critics of the Asian bioethics approach. Aware that the very question might be 'blasphemous' for some, Filipino bioethicist Leonardo de Castro has asked poignantly: 'Is there an Asian bioethics?' (de Castro, 1999). He points out two requirements which must be met for a bioethics to be 'Asian'. 'Firstly, Asian bioethics must be peculiar (or contain feature that are peculiar) to Asia. Secondly, Asian bioethics must be common to Asians' (de Castro, 1999, p. 227). However, both these criteria of peculiarity and commonality can hardly be met, if at all. de Castro has also noted that the real issue seems to be 'that of identity.' He warns that '[i]n the attempt to assert an Asian identity, one must be careful not to commit the mistake of universalizing (among Asians) a single Asian perspective' (de Castro, 1999, p. 227). Moreover, he believes that '[i]n the face of pluralism and multiculturalism, there is some room for a kind of universalist ethic that is founded on a collage of culturally inspired perspectives rather than a single standard of morality' (de Castro, 1999, p. 227).

For Gerhold Becker, founder of the Centre for Applied Ethics at Hong Kong Baptist University, the ethical approach to Asian values has 'the real danger of overlooking some simple facts' (Becker, 1995, p. 31). For instance,

> There is no such thing as 'the' Western values which would neatly define human practice in countries from the Urals to the Rocky Mountains. The 'West' too is not a monolithic entity but embraces a variety of value-laden cultures and traditions (Becker, 1995, p. 31).

Also,

> '[i]n all their differences cultures still share, and always will, the common denominator of being human; true

incommensurability seems only to apply to what separates human kind from the realms of other creatures' (Becker, 1995, p. 32).

Recently, German sinologist and bioethicist Ole Döring (2004), author of *Chinas Bioethik Verstehen*, has offered a thoughtful and critical review essay of several volumes on Asian bioethics published in Engelhardt's book series 'Philosophy and Medicine':

> Altogether, the conceptual frame and cultural outlook in this volume [Qiu 2004] reiterates a tradition of these discussions of pan-Asian cultural essentialism with some chauvinistic overtones. Most of these discussions do not seem to serve well the purpose to develop a culturally sensitive, empirically sound and conceptually satisfying bioethics 'from Asian for Asians.' Their main flaw is that marginalization and distortion of the potential of Asian and other cultural resources for responding to the challenges of biomedical modernisation, which are, indeed, grave (Döring, 2006).

Döring goes on to cite Heiner Roetz, author of the work *Confucian Ethics of the Axial Age*, who argues that 'the logic of the arguments towards the "Third Way" in bioethics (and thereby, in biopolitics) merely transforms the political rhetoric of the Cold War.'

Ruth Macklin, an American bioethicist with enormous international experience, has criticized Ruiping Fan's idea of the two incommensurable principles of cultural autonomy, one East Asian and the other West, as a relativist position. For her, Fan's approach 'merely replaces the puzzling with the obscure'(Macklin, 1999, p. 98). In general, she defines the debate as a part of an old and probably perpetual battle in ethics, that is, relativism versus universalism and absolutism. Other eminent American bioethicists, such as Tom Beauchamp (1997), have also taken a universalist approach to bioethical issues in Japan and the United States, setting it over against relativism. However, Fan (1997) has rejected that he is a relativist. For Sakamoto (1999), what is needed now is 'to unite East and West bioethics in one whole "Global Bioethics"' based on the holistic Asian model rather than the individualistic European model. This is not a relativist position. The exponents of the notion of Asian bioethics, including Fox and Swazey with regard to Chinese medical ethics, do not necessarily argue that one cannot make meaningful moral judgements and ethical criticism of the norms and practices of other societies or cultures.

Macklin has urged that 'philosophy should seek to explain and clarify, not to obfuscate and muddy'(Macklin, 1999, p. 98). In my view, defining the idea of Asian bioethics as relativist (and thus erroneous) from the perspectives of universalism obfuscates and muddies the issues that are really at stake. For framing the debate in this way conceals the serious empirical and conceptual problems of the

Asian bioethics approach, whether presented as relativist or universalist. Logically, the Asian bioethics approach can adopt universalist viewpoints by arguing that, normatively, Asian values are the 'right' moral norms in a universal sense.

Dichotomizing bioethics in terms of communitarian versus individualistic values has oversimplified and distorted the reality of bioethics and culture in both West and East. Elsewhere, I have shown how the widely accepted contrast of American bioethics and Chinese medical ethics as individualistic versus communitarian underestimates the great variations in the discipline within the two societies, especially in China (Nie, 2000). For neither American nor Chinese medical ethics is dominated by a single approach. Rather, bioethics in China, the United States or anywhere else on this planet has always been plural and diverse. My own empirical study of the diverse views and experiences of Chinese regarding abortion and foetal life provides a compelling illustration of this point (Nie, 2005a).

To say that Western, even American, bioethics is dominated by individualism is problematic to say the least. Just as communitarianism has had a place in Western political philosophy since classical times and has come into prominence since the early 1980s, a communitarian or nonindividualistic approach was present at the birth and development of bioethics in the United States (e.g. the works of the co-founder and current president of the Hastings Centre, Daniel Callahan and Thomas Murray; the former and current president of the US President's Council of Bioethics, Leo Kass and Edmond Pellegrino; Ezekiel Emmauel, Carl Elliott, Renée Fox herself, and so on). From the very beginning, the theological approach (e.g. the works of William May and Stanley Hauerwas), a major force within bioethics as a discipline and public discourse, has greatly stressed family values and the importance of a flourishing community. Simplistic generalizations have also ignored the contribution of feminism to bioethics (e.g. by Susan Sherwin and Rosemary Tong), which, if not always opposed to individualism, can hardly be characterized as individualistic. Interestingly, it is the secular bioethics of Engelhardt that is libertarian and highly individualistic.

Especially and most unfortunately, the great internal diversity of health care ethics in Asian societies has been seriously downplayed in the cultural dichotomizing of East and West. For, until a few decades ago, little effort was put into documenting and studying the enormous diversity of non-Western societies in modern Western academic discourse, even in anthropology. The East, and especially China, has been too long treated as a homogenous entity in contrast with the West, the United States in particular. As John Koller noted in the case of India,

In light of this continuous pattern of change and diversity, it would be exceedingly rash and unwise to claim that there is one unchanging way of thinking and acting that is exclusively and uniquely Indian. Such a claim would represent an implicit attempt to reduce the rich and changing diversity that is India to a single simple formula that would reveal next to nothing of the wide range of changing living ideas that constitute the great traditions of Indian thought (Koller 1982, p. 12).

Using Chinese views and experiences of abortion as an illustration, I have argued that China's internal diversity must be taken seriously if the West and China are to open a fruitful cross-cultural dialogue (Nie, 2005a, Chapter 8).

It is ironic that, in their quest for moral and cultural diversity, the supporters of the Asian bioethics approach have often ignored the internal diversity exhibited by every society and culture, especially non-Western examples. However, its exponents occasionally touch on the question of internal diversity as well as cross-cultural similarities. For instance, for Fox and Swazey, while Chinese medical morality and American bioethics have 'very different cosmic outlooks' which are totally alien to each other, the Chinese approach has 'more in common' and is 'compatible with the conceptual and methodological framework' in which they as sociologists 'observe, analyze, interpret and evaluate' (Fox & Swazey, 1984, p. 339). As for bioethics in America, 'the individualism of bioethics constitutes an evolution away from older, less secularized and communal forms of American individualism' (Fox & Swazey, 1984, p. 358). Similarly, Alora and Lumitao have not forgotten the basic fact that 'Filipino culture is a complex blend of Eastern and Western influences' (Alora & Lumitao , 2001, p. 6)because – from the religious standpoint – the Philippines is both a Christian and a Muslim nation and, historically, it has been a colony of both Spain and the United States and has retained its own East Asian traditions. However, for them this internal moral diversity counts for little.

There is a further irony in the Asian bioethics approach. A major concern or drive underlying this approach is opposition to imperialism and Western domination. But it remains under the spell of Orientalism by accepting the stereotypes and the general descriptive claims developed by Orientalism, the intellectual foundation of Western imperialism in the East.

For Asian scholars, the urge to develop an Asian (more specifically, an Indian, Pakistani, Chinese, Japanese, Korean, Vietnamese, Indonesian or Filipino) bioethics is a part of the search for identity. Nevertheless, to allow the politics of identity to dominate academic inquiry has its own traps. For instance, ironically, the Asian bioethics approach continues to define Asians and Asian cultures as the 'radical Other' of the West, rather than in their own terms.

One further irony is concerned with ways of resisting the Western model of bioethics (which exists only as a cultural construct, as hinted above) and developing a bioethics culturally sensitive to the Asian context. From the start, the Asian bioethics approach assumes the existence of a radically differentiated Asian culture and, consequently, the need for a radically different Asian bioethics. But by defining Asia as the 'radical Other' of the West, by paying scant attention to the internal moral diversity of the various Asian societies, by simplifying and ignoring the local richness and complexity of bioethics in Asia, the Asian bioethics approach as currently proposed would be incapable of formulating a genuine Asia-centred bioethics. Elsewhere, in discussing how a Chinese feminist bioethics might be developed, I have proposed three major elements (Nie, 2004, pp. 81–4). Besides learning from the West and exploring indigenous moral and ethical traditions for new insights, I argue that it is crucial for Chinese feminist bioethics in particular, and Chinese bioethics in general, to focus on native problems and concerns by attending to the lived experiences and voices of not only the well-educated, urban and privileged, but also the poor, rural residents, the underprivileged and the oppressed. To treat Asian or Chinese bioethics as the 'radical Other' does not help the task of identifying what really matters morally for people in Asia.

Another serious problem with the Asian bioethics approach is that it shortcuts or even abolishes the moral arguments on the different roles of the individual, the family and the community in health care ethics by the problematic empirical claim on certain cultural practices. Its key moral reasoning goes like this:

(1) the communitarin, collectivist or familistic perspective is the Asian or Chinese way of bioethics;
(2) therefore, the communitarian, collective or familistic perspective is morally justified and should be respected.

Even if the premise is empirically right, the conclusion does not follow. For it assumes that whatever is authentically Asian or Chinese is ethical. Interestingly and ironically, this reasoning is against the most fundamental principle of such Asian moral traditions as Confucianism and Daoism (Taoism) on the primacy of morality; that is, one should follow what is morally right and desirable, rather merely his or her own cultural traditions, whatever it is.

The Asian bioethics approach is an extension of the well-known 'Asian values' approach to human rights and democracy, which defines authoritarianism as the Asian way of life as opposed to the Western emphasis on individual freedom and liberty. Together with the 'Asian values' approach, the Asian bioethics approach is misleading and even politically dangerous. It tends to reject anything Western, even if it is morally sound, and

glorify anything Eastern, even if ethically problematic. The exponents of the specious concept of Asian bioethics almost unanimously reject such notions as human rights and informed consent as not applicable to Asia. Elsewhere I have pointed out the intellectual flaws in this position (Nie, 2001, 2004, 2005b).

Bioethics has to take cultural differences seriously. But, as the Asian bioethics approach shows, some popular misconceptions of culture persist in bioethics. To take culture seriously, it is essential to treat it as being always pluralist, historically complex, full of contradictory elements and open to change. Here I want to use the example of medical truth telling about terminal illness in China to illustrate my point (Nie, in press). In the name of the patient's good, most physicians in contemporary China, along with the patient's family members, do not tell the truth directly to patients suffering from terminal illness. Anticipating the current norm in the West by at least two and half millennia, however, such great medical sages as Yi Huan, Yi he, Bian Que (the 'father of medicine in China' according to some historians) and Hua Tuo (the 'father of surgery in China') always straightforwardly told their patients the whole truth about their condition, even when it was diagnosed as terminal. And physicians were financially rewarded by patients for telling the hurtful truth. According to the biographies of thousands of physicians, as well as pre-19th century fictional works, it was the norm for doctors to tell the truth about terminal illness. The dominant contemporary approach – failing to disclose the facts directly and fully to the patient – is probably a reflection of the old-fashioned Western biomedical model articulated in the influential 1847 Code of Ethics of the American Medical Association – a code which underwent radical change in the West in the 1960s and 1970s. Contrary to the common wisdom in both China and the West, therefore, it is simply wrong or historically groundless to see the contemporary standard practice in China – concealing the truth from patients – as *the* Chinese way, as an intrinsic part or logical development of traditional Chinese culture and medical morality. More and more patients and medical professionals are making efforts to reform the current mainstream practice.

To summarize, the most serious problem of the Asian bioethics approach is that its presuppositions of a communitarian East and a individualistic West make it impossible to properly study and identify the genuine cultural differences manifested by bioethics as practised in Asia. Cultural differences between Asia and the West are far more complicated, subtle, fascinating, difficult to discern and describe than what the over-simplified clear-cut contrasts can indicate. In this sense, more than just its relativist tendency, the current Asian bioethics approach is obfuscatory and muddy. Cross-cultural bioethics will do better without this notion or stereotype.

Together with advocates of the Asian bioethics approach, I too look forward to the development of a genuine Asian bioethics. But my vision is a very different one. For me, an Asian bioethics should be what Zhuang Zi (Chuang Tzu), a founder of Daoism (Taoism), called the music of Heaven (*tianlai*): 'Blowing on the ten thousand things in a different way, so that each can be itself – all take what they want for themselves.' Zhuang Zi, like Karl Popper, believed in pluralism and considered a spurious unity of ideas and the rejection of different ways of living and thinking as contrary to the Dao and the worst nightmare for human beings.

ACKNOWLEDGMENTS

I thank John McMillan for his kind invitation with an enticing suggestion of the topic, the editors for their patience and encouragement, Dr Neil Pickering for his characteristically thoughtful comments, the participants at my presentation on this work at the Student Research Forum of the Bioethics Centre of the University of Otago for their stimulating questions and suggestions, and Dr Paul Sorrell for his professional help with the English language.

REFERENCES

Alora AT, Lumitao JM. An introduction to an authentically non-Western bioethics. In: Alora AT, Lumitao JM, eds. *Beyond a Western Bioethics*. Washington DC: Georgetown University Press, 2001; pp. 3–21.

Beauchamp T. Comparative studies: Japan and America. In: Hoshino K, ed. *Japanese and Western Bioethics: Studies in Moral Diversity*. Kluwer Academic Publisher: Dordrecht, 1997; pp. 25–48.

Becker G. Asian and western ethics: some remarks on a productive tension. *Eubios J Asian Int Bioethics* 1995; **5**: 31–3.

Döring O. *Chinas Bioethik Verstehen*. Germany: Abera Verlag, 2004.

Döring O. Confucinism's Asian Ethos? Essentials of the Culture of East Asian Bioethics. *East Asian Science, Technology and Medicine* 2006; **25**: 125–147.

de Castro L. Is There an Asian Bioethics? *Bioethics* 1999; **13**(3&4): 227–35.

de Castro LD. Sy PA, Alvarez AA, Mendez RV, Rasco JK. Bioethics in the Asia-Pacific region. In: Bergstrom P, ed. *Ethics in Asia-Pacific*. Bangkok: UNESCO Asia and Pacific Regional Bureau for Education, 2004.

Engelhardt HT Jr. *The Foundation of Bioethics*, 2nd edition. New York: Oxford University Press, 1996.

Engelhardt HT Jr. Japanese and western bioethics: studies in moral diversity. In: Hoshino K, ed. *Japanese and Western Bioethics:*

Studies in Moral Diversity. Dordrecht: Kluwer Academic Publisher 1997; pp. 1–10.

Fan RP. Self-determination vs. family-determination: two incommensurable principles of Autonomy. *Bioethics* 1997; **11**(3&4); 309–22.

Fan RP. Reconsidering surrogate decision making: Aristotelianism and Confucianism on ideal human relationships. *Philos East West* 2002; **52**(3): 346–72.

Fox RC, Swazey JP. Medical morality is not bioethics – medical ethics in China and the United States. *Perspect Biol Med* 1984; **27**(3): 337–60.

Hoshino K, ed. *Japanese and Western Bioethics: Studies in Moral Diversity*. Dordrecht: Kluwer Academic Publisher, 1997.

Koller JM. *The Indian Way*. Upper Saddle River, NJ: Prentice Hall, 1982.

Macklin R. *Against Relativism: Cultural Diversity and the Search for Ethical Universals in Medicine*. New York: Oxford University Press, 1999.

Nie JB. The plurality of Chinese and American medical moralities: toward an interpretive cross-cultural bioethics. *Kennedy Inst Ethics J* 2000; **10**(3): 239–60. [A modified Chinese version, Jin W, Rongxia C, translator was published in *Chinese and International Philosophy of Medicine*, Vol. 3, No 4 (Dec 2001): 135–158.]

Nie JB. Is informed consent not applicable to China? intellectual flaws of the cultural difference argument. *Formosa J Med Humanit* 2001; **2**(1&2): 67–74. Also available online: http://www.csmu.edu.tw/genedu/public_html/journal-2.htm. [A modified Chinese version, translated by Zhao Mingjie, was published in *Med Philos* 2002; **23**(6): 18–22.]

Nie JB. Feminist bioethics and its language of human rights in the Chinese context. In: Tong R, Donchin A, Dodds S, eds. *Linking Visions: Feminist Bioethics, Human Rights and the Developing World*. Boulder, CO: Rowman & Littlefield. 2004; pp. 73–88.

Nie JB. *Behind the Silence: Chinese Voices on Abortion*. Boulder, CO: Rowman & Littlefield Publishers, 2005a.

Nie JB. *Medical Ethics in China: Major Traditions and Contemporary Issues*. Washington DC: Georgetown University Press, in press.

Nie JB. Cultural values embodying universal norms: a critique of a popular assumption about cultures and human rights. *Developing World Bioethics* 2005b; **5**(2): 251–7.

Popper K. *In Search of a Better World*. London: Routledge, 1994.

Qiu RZ. *Bioethics: Asian Perspectives: A Quest for Moral Diversity*. Dordrecht: Kluwer Academic Publishers, 2004.

Said EW. *Orientalism*. New York: Vintage Books, 1994 [1979].

Sakamoto H. Toward a new global bioethics. *Bioethics* 1999; **13**(3&4), 191–7. [A somewhat expanded version: (2004) Globalization of Bioethics – from the Asian Perspective. In: Macer DRJ, ed. *Challenges for Bioethics from Asia*. Christchurch: Eubios Ethics Institute. Also available online: http://www2.unescobkk.org/eubio/abac5bk.htm]. [Another slightly different version: Sakamoto H. The foundation of a possible Asian bioethics. In: Qie RZ, ed. *Bioethics: Asian Perspectives: A Quest for Moral Diversity*. Kluwer: Dordrecht, 2004.]

20

Narrative Ethics

HOWARD BRODY

INTRODUCTION

I suggest that anyone who thinks that stories do not matter in medicine try the following experiment:

1. Gather a group of physicians or other health professionals
2. Tell the beginning of a case report
3. Try to escape alive from the room without revealing 'how the story turned out'.

This example may seem too trite to illustrate any important truths. That appearance is deceptive. This example illustrates, even if only in rudimentary form, how we use stories to create order in and to impose meaning on the world (Bruner, 1986). Stories are therefore *ethically* important.

In this chapter I will describe in outline form some aspects of what has come to be called 'narrative bioethics'. I must begin with a qualification. If narrative bioethics is to live up to the claims made for it, we need to proceed by telling and analysing stories in great detail. These stories must be full and rich accounts, what ethnographers call 'thick descriptions' (Davis, 1991). A single such narrative could occupy the entirety of this chapter – leaving no room for any counter-narratives which, as we will see, are part and parcel of the narrative approach to ethics. The very nature of narrative bioethics therefore dictates that 'doing' ethics in this way requires a different format from the usual academic monograph or anthology. In a chapter such as this, therefore, the best one can do is a sort of gesture in the direction of narrative bioethics. I still hope to be able to say enough to show that the subject is worthy of more extensive study, even if our understanding of it today remains preliminary.

A BRIEF HISTORY AND DESCRIPTION

Let us for purposes of argument date the start of modern bioethics in 1945–46 with the trials of the Nazi doctors and with the development of what became the Nuremberg Code, an effort to explain what was wrong with the experiments the Nazis conducted on concentration camp inmates. From that date until the mid-1980s, bioethics in the United States and England was dominated by what came to be called a 'principlist' approach. Principlism is a form of what Thomas Murray has called 'top-down' reasoning, in which one derives judgements about specific cases from the application of general abstract principles. The principles are taken to be the ultimate source of ethical wisdom (Murray, 1987).

Most physicians imagine that medicine is, or ought to be, scientific; and also imagine that in science, one applies general laws to specific cases in order to deduce practical truths. Many physicians were attracted to principlism in bioethics because it appeared to be comfortably analogous to deductive reasoning in the sciences.

Starting in the late 1980s, several authors began to address narrative as a new way of thinking about medicine. Books appeared in which the experiences of patients who were ill were depicted as stories (Brody, 1987; Kleinman, 1988), and in which the diagnostic reasoning processes of physicians were analysed as narratives (Hunter, 1991). Once it was suggested that medical activities might have a narrative structure, others began to argue that moral reasoning in medicine might be directly aided through narrative modes of understanding. Books and journal articles appeared laying the groundwork for the notion of narrative bioethics (Charon, 1994; Frank, 1995; Nelson, 1997; Jones, 1999; Nelson, 2001; Charon and Montello, 2002; Brody, 2003).

Narrative bioethics exemplifies what Murray called a bottom-up approach to ethics. In this approach, wisdom might reside in the careful study of the practical, concrete setting or context in which a moral problem arises. Narrative ethics, I would propose, is neither top-down nor bottom-up exclusively. The arrow is double-headed. We sometimes derive wisdom from very abstract and general concepts – some of which may take a narrative form. We sometimes derive moral wisdom from a thoughtful sifting of particulars, especially when we compare one story to other, similar stories we are already familiar with. We gain wisdom the most when we work both ends against the middle, shifting our perspective as required from the abstract to the particular and back again. In utilizing bottom-up approaches to ethical insights, at least in part, narrative bioethics takes a place alongside other ethical approaches such as casuistry and feminist bioethics.

I submit that narrative bioethics involves one or both of the following claims:

(1) We can gain ethical wisdom and apply ethical knowledge directly through narrative.
(2) Even when we use ethical norms and principles, we rely in some way and at some level on narrative.

By contrast, the following are, I would contend, *not* narrative bioethics:

(a) Using case studies as a way of making an ethics course more palatable to students.
(b) Using narratives as illustrations for the application of moral principles and concepts.

Both of these latter practices are consistent with a totally top-down mode of reasoning and discount narrative as an independent source of ethical insight.

NARRATIVE 1

Melanie Begay is a 5-year-old girl living on the Navajo Indian reservation in the southwestern United States. She is brought to the Indian Health Service hospital with acute abdominal pain. The surgeon, Lori Arviso Alvord, who also belongs to the Navajo tribe, diagnoses appendicitis and recommends immediate surgery. Melanie's legal guardian is her grandmother, Bernice Begay, who refuses consent for the operation. She offers several reasons – uncertainty as to the diagnosis; distrust of a white medical system which has a long history of exploiting the Navajo. Her main reason, however, involves the Navajo cosmology and its ideal of natural harmony. A child's body is sacred, and invasion by a surgical knife would defile what had been an intact and balanced whole, disrupting the natural rhythms that are essential for healing.

Dr Alvord has a certain degree of sympathy with this cosmological view and also wishes to demonstrate respect for Bernice as the decision-maker. Despite the risk of perforation, she agrees to delay the surgery while engaging in further discussions with Bernice. The hospital social workers take a different tack and try to contact the local court to get a judge's order to overrule Bernice and approve the surgery.

The story has a happy ending. Bernice, perhaps won over by Dr. Alvord's willingness to respect her judgement, changes her mind and consents to surgery. The appendix is removed before it perforates and Melanie makes an uneventful recovery (Alvord, 1999 as recounted in Frank, 2004).

Arthur Frank's analysis of this case focuses on the following question:

> What the 'right thing' [to do] is... depends on the prior question of who Melanie is. Is she, as in the Western medical view, an independent physical body that has a right to receive lifesaving treatment? Or is she, as in the Navajo view, a whole that is integral to a larger whole, and that larger whole might be violated if some natural process in her body is disrupted?... Alvord's decision, as I understand it, is that Melanie *is* Navajo. She has a right to be treated within those values, with all the risks and benefits... that involves (Frank, 2004, p. 98).

Frank's analysis suggests in turn a view of levels of narrative as nested within one another, which may be of general value in applying narrative to medical situations and to bioethical issues. Figure 20.1 depicts an inter-nesting of four narrative levels.

The narrative level that is present in virtually every medical encounter, and that is most immediately visible to the practitioner, is the story of the patient's illness. Most patients, if invited and not interrupted, will present a reasonably complete and coherent narrative of how they came to be sick, what symptoms followed in what order and any events to which they attribute causality. If the practitioner inquires further, the patient will also be able to place this narrative about the illness within the context of the next-level narrative, the patient's life story. The patient will be able to explain how this illness episode does or does not disrupt normal life activities, what fears she may have for the future if this illness is not resolved and what past events in her life this illness echoes or reminds her of.

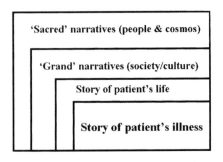

Figure 20.1 Four Levels of Narrative in Medicine.

Less visible to the practitioner, but still accessible to the techniques of the social and behavioral sciences, are the more abstract and general levels of narrative on which the more particular narratives are dependent. Our society and culture teach us a number of model narratives which could be called 'grand' narratives. As a rule we master these as children and reach adulthood knowing implicitly that particular narratives that conform to the general form or genre laid out in the grand narratives will be accepted by our fellows as meaningful, while narratives that fail to conform to the grand patterns will usually be rejected as incoherent and threatening (possibly as a sign of mental illness). For example, one grand narrative influential in American society depicts good people taking personal responsibility for their prior actions and bad people attempting to evade responsibility. A patient who explains a current episode of illness by citing past dietary or lifestyle indiscretions and characterizes the present illness as the inevitable punishment earned as a result of these past actions is therefore working comfortably within this 'grand' narrative framework and can be reasonably confident of a sympathetic hearing (Johnson, 1993; Linde, 1993).

Grand narratives are themselves nested within our culture's (or subculture's) 'sacred' or cosmological narratives. These are the transcendental stories of how human beings relate to the natural world and the cosmos, of where we came from and where we are going as a people, or our relationship to whatever supernatural forces we may believe in. According to a 'grand' narrative, to extend the above example, an illness may be a punishment for past dietary indiscretions; according to a sacred narrative, it may be a punishment for past sins.

Figure 20.2 now applies this schema of the four internested narratives to the case of Melanie Begay. Melanie may be too young to tell much of her own story, so Bernice emerges as the major storyteller. The appendicitis is viewed within the context of the family story of Melanie, her grandmother and other central figures in the family circle; this story in turn is interpreted within the grand narrative of the Navajo experience in the United States and the historical treatment of the Indians by Whites. Finally, arching above, is the Navajo cosmological narrative of the harmonious interconnectedness of the natural world, with humans as part of and not as superior to nature.

Figure 20.2 is actually an overly simplistic depiction of the narrative features of the 'case'. Let us review how Dr Alvord may have gone about making her decisions. Is it merely good luck that Bernice relented before the appendix burst? Or was the outcome of the case at least in part the result of some shrewd clinical decisions? Did Dr Alvord make some guesses, well informed by previous clinical experience, about how sick Melanie was and how far advanced she was in the natural progression of acute appendicitis? Did she make some equally well-informed guesses about what was motivating Bernice in her recalcitrance, how amenable Bernice might be to influence by a physician who was a fellow tribe member, and the relative impact on Bernice of two courses of action (pressing her for an immediate decision versus giving her more time)? How many other stories of sick little girls and of angry and scared family members could Dr Alvord tell, if pressed for the grounds for her decisions?

So Frank may be too hasty in suggesting that this case was 'about' Melanie-as-Navajo. Instead, this case may be 'about' the intersection of three different stories of the ways of trying to be a Navajo in the present world. Figure 20.3 depicts the possibility that Dr Alvord may have approached this case from the standpoint of her own narrative as a Navajo surgeon intersecting with the narratives of Melanie and Bernice Begay.

We can better appraise the notion of the intersection of the three narratives if we ask what would have been meant by failure. Suppose that Melanie's appendix had perforated and that she had either died or had suffered from a serious and prolonged crisis followed by a slow convalescence.

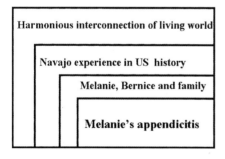

Figure 20.2 Four Levels, Applied to Case of Melanie Begay

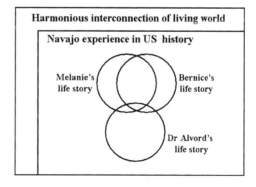

Figure 20.3 Intersection of Life Narratives in the Case of Melanie Begay.

What implications would this outcome have had for the Navajo ideal of harmony? At some point, Bernice would have had to confront the possibility that a septic abdomen in a young child is a *greater* disharmony than a surgical incision would have been. And Dr Alvord would have had to confront the possibility that she was called upon to do surgery and yet allowed her Navajo 'self' to have too much influence over her surgeon 'self'. In short, we find out more about the meaning of the narratives by asking how they might have ended differently than they did – by constructing counter-narratives.

A PRINCIPLIST REJOINDER

Those committed to a principlist approach would argue that the Melanie Begay story really proves their main point – that so-called narrative ethics is either disguised principlism or it is not ethics at all. Ethics, to be worthy of the name, requires judgements according to accepted standards. Such standards must take the form of abstract moral concepts that apply to many different individual cases with relatively equal force. Particular narratives must therefore, according to this rejoinder, be supplemented by moral abstractions, or else can provide no reliable moral guidance.

A principlist retelling of Melanie's narrative might go like this. Melanie, as a 5-year-old, lacks the capacity for autonomous choice. Bernice is obligated to exercise her own autonomy on behalf of Melanie as the latter's proxy. Those who would wish to overturn Bernice's judgement and operate immediately are invoking the principles of beneficence and nonmaleficence as the standards by which to judge Bernice's adequacy as the child's proxy. Bernice should seek to provide maximal benefit for Melanie and to minimize the risk of harm. From the medical viewpoint, only a decision for immediate surgery would conform to that set of standards.

On the contrary, one could infer from Dr Alvord's initial hesitancy to operate a different sort of appeal to principles. Perhaps Dr Alvord is imagining Melanie later as a grown up and as an adult, capable of full autonomy. She may picture that imaginary Melanie looking back on the decision Bernice is now making for her and being asked retroactively to approve or disapprove her grandmother's decision. The statement, 'Melanie *is* Navajo', is a way of claiming that this future imaginary Melanie would retrospectively endorse Bernice's initial refusal of surgery, even knowing what risks that were placed upon Melanie as a child. From the point of view of Melanie-as-Navajo, the surgery would be viewed as a maleficent action, even though it was beneficently intended.

For the principlist, there might be no quick and easy way to choose one of these weightings of principles over the other. That would explain fully, for the principlist, why the case represents a hard case. Hard cases are hard; and it is no reflection on an ethical theory or approach that it cannot change hard cases into easy ones. From all this the principlist concludes that the final outcome in Melanie's case represents an ethical set of actions *because* the eventual decisions made are consistent with the appropriate ethical principles. There is nothing about the narrative of the case that could have allowed us to arrive at this normative conclusion, absent the set of abstract principles to which to appeal.

In response, some advocates for narrative ethics will freely admit that narrative supplements principles without supplanting them (Charon, 1994). In my view, these folks give away the store too readily. Narrative ethics loses whatever 'bite' it might have, and frankly ceases to be of much real interest to bioethics, if it is a *mere* supplement and if principles do all the heavy lifting.

A better response, I argue, is that the principlist and the narrative ethicist are looking at events from different time perspectives. *After the fact*, the principlist can review the case description at leisure, sift through 'the facts of the case', apply various principles and argue that the principles do or do not support certain actions. But we do not, as human beings in the world, have the luxury of living our lives and making our ethical decisions solely through hindsight. *As events are unfolding*, what leading occurrences will later be picked out by the ethicist as 'the facts of the case' might be much harder to discern. Principlism errs seriously by suggesting that one begins to 'do' ethics *only after* 'the facts of the case' have been assembled and selected and thereby ignores the considerable moral work that has already gone into deciding what 'the facts of the case' *are*. In real time, as events are unfolding, we seek indicators of what to do next. We look to narratives to give meaning to, and to assemble and coordinate, both what has already happened and what might happen next. What we choose to do may be heavily influenced by that narrative understanding of what is happening to us, what options we have and what their implications are for us and for those to whom we feel responsible. I might claim (though this chapter will not allow a detailed argument to defend the claim) that the narrative understanding of events is in fact morally primary, and the later, retrospective analysis in terms of principles is a secondary phenomenon.

NARRATIVE 2

Mrs. Shalev is 83 years old. She was born in Poland and escaped to the United States in the early years of the Second World War. She married and raised her family in Brooklyn. Five years ago she moved in with her daughter, Becky Putnam.

Two years ago Mrs. Shalev suffered a severe stroke and since then has been cared for in a hospital and in a nursing home. She is now back in the hospital with a list of medical problems, described by her physician as 'short-term survivable but long-term terminal'. She goes in and out of lucidity.

A dispute has arisen over management of her increasingly severe pressure sores. Treatment of these ulcers is very painful for Mrs. Shalev, and the nursing staff wish to increase her analgesia to provide greater comfort while they do wound care. In general, the nursing staff would rather treat Mrs. Shalev more as a candidate for palliative care and focus on comfort and symptom management rather than on extending her life.

Becky Putnam, who has remained very involved with her mother's care throughout, has a different viewpoint. She opposes any increase in the doses of analgesics because her mother would be less lucid (as she knows from prior experience). She is in full agreement that the long-term outlook is very poor, but nevertheless insists on continuing aggressive life-prolonging therapy. She is resistant to discussing options for limiting care. She views even raising this subject as disrespectful to her mother and says with some asperity, 'In my family these things would never be talked about'. She also tells the staff how many times she remembers hearing her mother say, 'Pain, schmain!' when others would express concern for her or offer pain relief. She is quite sure that her mother would prefer to be lucid enough to recognize family members when they visit, rather than have higher doses of analgesics.

The nursing staff has requested a consultation from the hospital ethics committee. They are concerned about futile and inhumane care and wonder if Ms. Putnam is in fact engaging in elder abuse (adapted from Nelson, 2000).

What should the ethics committee recommend? A more or less standard approach based on widely accepted principles of bioethics would note that Mrs. Shalev has lost the capacity to make autonomous choices and has left no clear advance directive. The question, then, is whether Ms. Putnam is properly engaging in substituted judgement – reflecting for the staff what Mrs. Shalev's own wishes would be, were she able at this time to state them clearly with a full awareness of her present condition, prognosis and therapeutic options.

The nursing staff is arguing that the treatment plan demanded by Ms. Putnam represents an unfavourable benefit-burden ratio for her mother. The continued invasive treatments seem very burdensome to her and the benefits (as measured in the long-term) seem disproportionately meager. By contrast, better pain management would seem to provide a very high benefit for the patient with relatively little burden. Some caregivers might add here that Ms. Putnam's demands interfere with their own conscientiously felt ethical duties as health professionals. They are not supposed to let patients suffer from treatable pain, and they are not supposed to continue interventions that appear futile. Ms. Putnam could perhaps justify her requests by appealing to clear evidence that she was representing Mrs.

Shalev's own previous wishes, but she has not met this burden of proof – she has, to the contrary, avoided even engaging with the staff in any such dialogue.

In sum, the approach based on principles – at least as interpreted by the staff – appears to paint Ms. Putnam as the villain of this melodrama. We might ask whether an approach based more on narrative would arrive at any different conclusions.

A good starting point would be the account of 'moral responsibility' offered by Margaret Urban Walker (Walker, 1998). Walker suggests that ethics, especially as practised among family members and close friends, has more to do with responsibility and less to do with rights and duties. To decide when and whether a person is acting responsibly, we may consult three interconnected narratives, which Walker calls narratives of *relationship, identity* and *value*.

In this case, the narratives of relationship and identity nearly merge. Becky Putnam is Mrs. Shalev's daughter and this relationship defines a great deal of who Becky takes herself to be. She interprets what she is now obligated to do for her mother as the question of what logically follows the narrative of their relationship that has already unfolded over these many years. It deeply offends her that others, who have known her mother only since her recent stroke, somehow feel better suited to make decisions for Mrs. Shalev than Becky with her lifetime of knowledge of her mother and their relationship.

The narrative of value has to do with how Mrs. Shalev lived her life in order to demonstrate for Becky and the rest of her family what truly mattered. It is not enough to invoke virtues such as courage, patience and loyalty as abstractions; rather Becky is concerned to make decisions based on how Mrs. Shalev interpreted these virtues, and the demands they placed on her, within the concrete context of her own life. By recalling comments such as 'pain, schmain!' Becky draws conclusions about how much her mother valued pain relief within her overall set of priorities. Becky also uses past family patterns and practices as indicators of what sorts of discussions are respectful or otherwise. She recalls, for example, that when her mother was getting weaker five years ago, it was simply understood that Becky and her family would take her into their own home. No discussion or negotiation was needed. This intuitive, non-negotiated stance seems to Becky to represent an important value within her family.

We can, at this point, draw two tentative conclusions. First, Becky Putnam believes herself justified in seeking a certain sort of care for her mother *on narrative grounds*. Second, if the hospital staff is to work productively with her and to try to suggest alternatives, they probably need to work with her and to try to engage her *on a narrative level*.

It would make no sense to refer to a practice as narrative *ethics* if one could tell any old story and automatically 'win' any ethical discussion or debate. If narratives are to function in a system of ethics, they must be corrigible. There must be better and worse narratives that one can tell about events, and one must have some means of judging which is which. We do not have space here to discuss those means in great detail, but a few suggestive comments can be made.

Consider first how the staff might go about engaging Ms. Putnam in a useful dialogue. Given the impasse that has arisen thus far, it is very likely that Ms. Putnam has, at one level or another, heard the staff saying to her things such as 'We think you may be guilty of elder abuse', or, 'Let's talk about things that you and your family always thought it improper to talk about'. If those were the messages that she received, it is not too surprising that she and the nurses are at loggerheads. Imagine, instead, how she might now react if asked something like 'Let's talk more about your mother's life story up to this point, and let's try to explore together how your mother would ideally want the next chapter of her life story to unfold' (Yarborough, 2005).

Two common ways to use narrative in making everyday ethical decisions are what we might call 'keeping faith' and 'trying on' (Brody, 2003). Becky Putnam so far has emphasized almost exclusively the task of keeping faith. It is very common for a person using this mode of reasoning, when challenged, to say something like 'My mother would never forgive me if I were to…' Hardly ever does such a statement arise from any explicit promise made to the person in question. Rather, the statement reflects a general sense of the values held as important by the other and the role that those values ought to play in the life of someone who values the relationship with the other and who defines her own identity at least in part according to that relationship. Thus keeping faith points towards an intersection among the narratives of relationship, identity and value.

The staff, by contrast, might wish Becky Putnam to do a bit more trying-on. They would like to work with her to tell alternative stories of Mrs. Shalev's possible futures. They would like her to reflect more on which of these possible stories best coheres with the unfolding (but soon to end) narrative that has been Mrs. Shalev's life. The phrase 'trying on' suggests an analogy of looking into a mirror while trying on clothes. I may admire a suit of clothes hanging on the rack, only to decide, upon trying it on, that it looks all wrong *on me*. Similarly, we may never realize what it would truly be like for us to take an action in the future unless we can construct a narrative of ourselves in the future – to see the action and its likely consequences vividly, in the context of our own lives. Only then might we decide that an action that seems to be required by some rule or principle might actually appear on reflection to be quite wrong *for us*. The action might be out of character, or at odds with some important virtue to which we aspire, or contrary to some deeply held value.

How might the staff go about implementing such an approach? After spending more time listening to what Ms. Putnam had to say about Mrs. Shalev's earlier life, how the relationship between mother and daughter has unfolded so far and how responsible Ms. Putnam feels for her mother's well-being, it might be appropriate to ask questions such as these: 'Could your cherished memories of how strong and courageous your mother was in the past, when she settled in a new land, learned a new language and raised a family with great difficulty, be clouding your vision of what your mother needs right now? How sure can we be that your mother would still say, "pain, schmain!" if the pain was unrelenting and severe, and if the things left for her to do in her life are in fact very limited? Perhaps put more starkly, could it be that you are greatly saddened and distressed to see your mother in her present state, and wish rather if at all possible to remember her as she used to be in the past – and could that be leading you to make decisions which would have been quite appropriate for your mother at those earlier stages, but less appropriate for her now?'

Ms. Putnam might or might not be brought around by such a conversation to rethink her demands for Mrs. Shalev's care. In an extreme case, if she did not alter her views, health professionals might feel bound as a matter of conscience to refuse to provide treatment for Mrs. Shalev under the conditions dictated by Ms. Putnam. As we saw in the case of Dr Alvord, ethical decisions in patient care represent an intersection of our own life narratives with those of the patient and family members, and we have moral responsibility for how our own life narratives unfold, too.

But several points could be made in favour of this more narrative approach. It seems to represent a better job of addressing Ms. Putnam and her key moral concerns at her own level and within the frame of reference from which she is herself operating. As such, it is a more effective way of presenting for her consideration various counter-narratives, which ultimately form the only valid rebuttal to a morally charged narrative. Moreover, the narrative approach seems in this instance to better treat Ms. Putnam with respect and dignity. And treating those whom we encounter in health care with respect and dignity is arguably a minimal ethical duty.

CONCLUSION

Much more needs to be said to show how far ethical reasoning and ethical conclusions can be justified by narrative appeals and to reply to a variety of other objections that principlists and others might raise. More also needs to be said to explore how narrative bioethics relates to other particularist or bottom-up approaches such as casuistry.

Some of what still remains to be said in explication of narrative bioethics have been stated elsewhere, but a good deal remains to be written. Narrative studies in bioethics are in their infancy. I have succeeded in this chapter if I have shown that the approach is promising enough, and captures enough of our common-sense view of how ethical thinking occurs in real life, to make further exploration worthwhile.

REFERENCES

Alvord LA, Van Pelt EC. *The Scalpel and the Silver Bear: The First Navajo Woman Surgeon Combines Western Medicine and Traditional Healing*. New York: Bantam, 1999.

Brody H. *Stories of Sickness*. New Haven, CT: Yale University Press, 1987.

Brody H. *Stories of Sickness*, 2nd edition. New York: Oxford University Press, 2003.

Bruner J. *Actual Minds, Possible Worlds*. Cambridge, MA: Harvard University Press, 1986.

Charon R. Narrative contributions to medical ethics: recognition, formulation, interpretation, and validation in the practice of the ethicist. In: DuBose ER, Hamel RP, O'Connell LJ, eds. *A Matter of Principles? Ferment in U.S. Bioethics*. Valley Forge: Trinity Press International, 1994; pp. 260–83.

Charon R, Montello M, eds. *Stories Matter: The Role of Narrative in Medical Ethics*. New York: Routledge, 2002.

Davis DS. Rich cases: the ethics of thick description. *Hastings Center Report* 1991; **21**(4): 12–17.

Frank A. *The Wounded Storyteller: Body, Illness, and Ethics*. Chicago: University of Chicago Press, 1995.

Frank AW. *The Renewal of Generosity: Illness, Medicine, and How to Live*. Chicago: University of Chicago Press, 2004.

Hunter KM. *Doctor's Stories: The Narrative Structure of Medical Knowledge*. Princeton: Princeton University Press, 1991.

Johnson M. *Moral Imagination: Implications of Cognitive Science for Ethics*. Chicago: University of Chicago Press, 1993.

Jones AH. Narrative based medicine: narrative in medical ethics. *BMJ* 1999; **318**: 253–6.

Kleinman AF. *The Illness Narratives: Suffering, Healing, and the Human Condition*. New York: Basic Books, 1988.

Linde C. *Life Stories: The Creation of Coherence*. New York: Oxford University Press, 1993.

Murray TH. Medical ethics, moral philosophy and moral tradition. *Soc Sci Med* 1987; **25**: 637–44.

Nelson HL, ed. *Stories and Their Limits: Narrative Approaches to Bioethics*. New York: Routledge, 1997.

Nelson HL. Feminist bioethics: where we've been, where we're going. *Metaphilosophy* 2000; **31**: 492–508.

Nelson HL. *Damaged Identities, Narrative Repair*. Ithaca, NY: Cornell University Press, 2001.

Walker MU. *Moral Understandings: A Feminist Study in Ethics*. New York: Routledge, 1998.

Yarborough M. Deciding for others at the end of life: storytelling and moral agency. *J Clin Ethics* 2005; **16**: 127–143.

21

Empirical Approaches to Health Care Ethics

JEREMY SUGARMAN, ROBERT A. PEARLMAN, HOLLY A. TAYLOR

INTRODUCTION

Conducting empirical research in the field of health care ethics can be an important tool for improving scholarship in health care ethics as well as the health care enterprise itself. Nevertheless, it is essential that it be properly conducted. In this chapter, we present a basic introduction to empirical research in health care ethics. First, we define empirical research in health care ethics. Second, we describe how empirical research methods can be valuable to the field of health care ethics. Third, we discuss how to conduct empirical research in health care ethics, beginning with the identification of a suitable research question and method and ending in a formal presentation of findings. This information is critical for those conducting, reviewing, sponsoring or reading empirical research conducted on topics in health care ethics.

DEFINING EMPIRICAL RESEARCH IN HEALTH CARE ETHICS

Empirical research in health care ethics involves the application of research methods to quantitatively measure or qualitatively explore or assess, among many other possibilities, attitudes, behaviours, beliefs, costs, practices, procedures, processes or policies encountered in health care. Data collected during an empirical research project are used to *describe* the phenomenon under study, which may facilitate understanding and interpretation of the phenomenon. As such, empirical research can help illuminate theory and identify other ethical problems worthy of attention as well as assess how particular policies and procedures are working to accomplish their ethical goals (Sugarman and Sulmasy, 2001).

In contrast to empirical research which is a form of descriptive ethics, theoretical (or normative) research in ethics attempts to delineate what *ought to be* the case (see Sugarman and Sulmasy, 2001). For example, a normative research project in health care ethics might seek to provide a conceptual justification for how a particular scarce health care resource (such as organs for transplantation) ought to be allocated, whereas an empirical research project might document how it is currently allocated. By providing reliable and valid data, empirical research can test, modify and support normative conclusions about ethical problems in health care and it can reify philosophical ideas. Thus, there is an iterative relationship between empirical research and normative conclusions, and neither can exist alone (Brody, 1993). Nonetheless, as Hume warned, just because something 'is' does not imply that it 'ought' to be. While normative research is unquestionably an invaluable pursuit in health care ethics, the remainder of this chapter will highlight the value of empirical research and the necessity for such research to be well designed to maximize its contribution to the field of health care ethics.

CURRENT TRENDS IN EMPIRICAL METHODS IN HEALTH CARE ETHICS

In a recent review of reports of empirical research in bioethics published in the academic literature, Sugarman (2004) identified two noteworthy trends. First, the amount of empirical research in bioethics as a subset literature on bioethics generally is on the rise. As compared to a review of bioethics literature published between 1980 and 1989 (Sugarman et al., 2001) that found that 3.4% of bioethics articles represented reports of empirical data collection, using a similar but expanded search, Sugarman (2004) found that 25% of bioethics articles represented empirical research reports. Borry, Schotsmans and Dierickx (2006) conducted a review of empirical research reports published in nine peer-reviewed bioethics journals and found similar results. Specifically, they found that the proportion of empirical research reports has increased steadily over the last decade (a three-fold increase from 1990 to 2003). Second, the review conducted by Sugarman (2004) highlights the fact that topics in 'traditional' health care ethics (e.g. informed consent, end-of-life care) are well represented in the academic literature. Although these trends are positive in our view, 'good empirical research is contingent upon knowing what questions are worth asking and how to investigate and measure them' (Sugarman, 2004, p. 228). In addition, we would encourage those interested in and conducting empirical research in health care ethics to consider expansion beyond the 'traditional' into the ethics of the everyday practice of clinical medicine.

CONDUCTING EMPIRICAL RESEARCH IN HEALTH CARE ETHICS

Determining what constitutes well-conducted empirical research can be challenging given the range of methods that can and should be employed to address particular issues or problems because each method has a set of strengths, limitations, subtleties and metrics of quality. Furthermore, those engaged in conducting empirical research in health care ethics also need to be familiar with the health care enterprise and its ethical underpinnings to be sure that the research is framed appropriately and is sensitive to conceptual models that inform the field. Thus, it is not surprising that good empirical research in health care ethics often requires interdisciplinary collaborations. Nevertheless, regardless of the topic or method that is ultimately selected, research tends to follow a set of steps, beginning with the identification of a suitable research question and method and ending in a formal presentation of findings. Recognizing these steps can facilitate the useful shaping of proposed projects. With this in mind, we describe these steps briefly in the hope of providing a systematic approach to conducting empirical research in health care ethics. In suggesting this approach, we realize that it may be simplistic to the experienced methodologist while challenging to those without extensive research experience who may be quite familiar with the health care enterprise. We hope that experienced methodologists may find value in taking a broad view of the field of empirical research in health care ethics and the many methods that contribute to the field so

they might identify appropriate collaborators and projects to enhance their work.

SPECIFYING THE TOPIC OF INTEREST

The research process starts by choosing a topic, performing a detailed review of the literature, identifying a research question and framing an investigation. Motivations for choice of topic may range from a need to develop a policy, to personal interests, to training requirements. Specification of the topic is crucial to characterize relevant issues for a careful literature review. That is, it is as important for the researcher to map the terrain that ought to be explored (e.g. normative ethics, sociology, health policy, law, etc.) as it is to not miss existing work that will contribute to the identification and refinement of a research question.

REVIEWING THE LITERATURE

Reviewing relevant literature is crucial to establishing what is already known, whether a new study is worthwhile and what methods have been used in past work. A careful literature review involves a thorough retrieval of relevant citations. However, the interdisciplinary nature of health care ethics often makes literature retrieval a difficult task. First, it is important to create a comprehensive list of terms, or keywords, that are related to the topic area. These keywords can then be used in web-based databases or when seeking the assistance of an experienced information retrieval specialist. The process is iterative. As relevant materials are identified, the terms used and the headings by which they are indexed should be used to modify search terms. In addition, the citation index and the reference sections from these materials can be used to identify other publications. This approach has been used to identify empirical research on informed consent (Sugarman, 1999).

Before accepting the conclusions offered in research reports, it is essential to critically appraise each study. Central questions in critical appraisal include: Is this a good study? Were the assumptions valid? Were the methods validated? Were the methods appropriate? Did the researchers use reliable and reproducible measurements? Is the analysis thorough, sound and well grounded? Were proper statistical tests correctly used where applicable? Are the results of the study valid and meaningful, in the real world? Are the findings generalizable or otherwise applicable to the settings of interest?

Critically appraising scholarship requires practice, and slightly different approaches to critical appraisal are needed depending on the empirical research methods used such as surveys, case-control studies, cohort studies and randomized controlled studies (see Sackett et al., 1991); quasi-experimental and experimental designs (see Campbell and Stanley, 1963); qualitative research (see Inui and Frankel, 1991; Cohen and Knafl, 1993; Patton, 1999; Mays and Pope, 2000).

CHOOSING THE APPROPRIATE METHODOLOGICAL APPROACH

Choosing whether to use a qualitative, quantitative or mixed-method approach when designing a study is predicated largely by the research question. Formal research questions are not merely restatements of the content areas of interest, but rather are expressions that capture what the investigator wants to learn specifically by way of the proposed study. A well-formulated research question is essential to any research endeavour. Whether one ought to take a single or mixed method approach when designing a study is largely determined by one's individual skill set or the skill set of the research team.

If little is known about a topic, a qualitative approach using techniques such as focus groups or conducting direct observation is a good way of generating important hypotheses. Then, cross-sectional surveys can be used to delineate knowledge, attitudes and beliefs and to test hypotheses about whether particular subject characteristics or attributes predict knowledge, attitudes and beliefs. Alternatively, data from a cross-sectional survey could be used to identify sub-sets of subjects that share particular knowledge attitudes and beliefs and lead to a purposeful sampling strategy to conduct qualitative, in-depth interviews. In turn cross-sectional data may help generate a prospective study such as a longitudinal cohort study conducted to measure the change in individuals' attitudes or behaviours. Alternatively, an intervention might be examined in a randomized controlled trial to assess whether something, such as patients' ability to provide a meaningful informed consent, can be improved.

A full description of the array of study design and data collection techniques used in qualitative or quantitative research, their strengths and their limitations is obviously beyond the scope of this chapter. Therefore the following section includes simply a description of basic methods and data collection techniques. Thus, those designing a study should seek further guidance from individuals with experience in empirical research and from relevant texts on methodology.

QUALITATIVE RESEARCH

Qualitative research emphasizes the accumulation of data that are derived in large part from participants' personal experiences and ideas. The methods are typically open-ended and inductive, where the researcher attempts to describe what is true about the phenomenon under study rather than manipulate the environment to test a particular hypothesis. Although qualitative data collection techniques are simple in structure, they are difficult and time-consuming to do well. Furthermore, reporting this type of work is challenging, especially in medical journals where quantitative methods have historically been more welcome. Three important qualitative research techniques for health care ethics are focus groups, semi-structured interviews and direct observation. Ethnography is introduced as an approach that incorporates a number of qualitative research techniques.

Focus groups typically involve 6–10 persons. A trained focus group moderator leads the group through a semi-structured conversation about a particular set of issues. Having a *group* discuss such issues is often synergistic where comments from one member of the group may trigger responses in other members of the group (Krueger, 1988). Focus groups are an efficient way to collect multiple perspectives on a limited number of topics. Focus groups are not generally recommended when the topics of interest require disclosure of sensitive personal information. Kalvermark et al., (2004) used focus groups to explore 'moral distress' among health care professionals. The investigators were interested in finding out whether the concept of moral distress in response to ethical tensions in the health care system, originally identified as a phenomenon among nurses, was relevant to other health care professionals. Three focus groups were conducted: two with staff from two different clinical departments and one with staff from the pharmacy. The investigators found that moral distress was expressed by all members of the focus groups and therefore recommended that the phenomenon be revised conceptually to apply to all health care professionals.

Semi-structured interviews can be a means of gathering rich information from respondents who can explain in great detail their experiences about a particular topic; these details would likely be missed if one asked for a closed-ended response in a survey. Carlisle et al. (2004) used semi-structured interviews to find out from adolescents their beliefs and attitudes about the confidentiality of personal health information. Their goal in conducting open-ended, in-person interviews rather than using closed-ended questionnaires was to enable the respondents to express themselves more easily. During the interviews adolescents were asked about their concerns about the privacy of sensitive information (e.g., sexually transmitted infections, illegal drug use) in the third person so that the adolescents would not feel their own lives were under scrutiny. Eighteen adolescents and their parents were interviewed. Parents were interviewed separately and only if the adolescent agreed. The researchers found that the adolescents had given the issues of confidentiality of health information little thought prior to being interviewed. This highlights the utility of taking a qualitative approach to a topic. If given a closed-ended questionnaire, adolescents would have answered from a naïve perspective. Qualitative data collection techniques allow for the introduction of the topic tailored to the respondents' knowledge base. While the adolescents affirmed the principle that the privacy of health records should be maintained, a number of them endorsed the idea that it would be reasonable to disclose information about a serious health condition to their parents. Their preference was to have the physician encourage, and perhaps facilitate, this disclosure by the adolescent rather than the physician making the disclosure in the absence of such encouragement.

Van Kleffens and Van Leeuwen (2005) conducted semi-structured interviews with 30 cancer patients to find out why they refused standard treatment (either before or after treatment recommendations). Interviews were also conducted with their physicians (n = 16) to find out how they felt about their patients' choice. The researchers found that patients' decisions rely on personal values or experiences rather than a measured assessment of the pros and cons from a medical perspective. Patients and their physicians agreed that there are good reasons to refuse treatment but their reasons did not always overlap. The researchers concluded that Weber's concepts and definitions of 'value oriented rationality' and 'goal oriented rationality' apply in this setting. This is an example of qualitative researchers drawing on extant theory to frame their analysis.

Conducting good semi-structured interviews requires skill and training. Interviewers must be able to cover the domains or areas of interest in a conversational manner, offering unbiased probes throughout the interview. Such techniques affect not only the process, but also the outcomes of a semi-structured interview study. Much like focus groups, however, the semi-structured interview is not a good way of generating quantitative information such as how many, or what section of people share the interviewees' experiences.

Observation is a qualitative research technique that involves the observation and recording of naturally occurring events or activities. There are two common forms of observation: *participant* observation and *direct* (or non-participant) observation. As the language implies, participant observation allows the investigator to actively engage with the subjects in the event or activity under study. Participant observation is a mainstay of cultural anthropology where the investigator joins a community to observe its traditional culture and values. An example from the health care setting is that of Byron Good, a medical anthropologist who joined a class of Harvard students during their first year of medical school to provide an insider's perspective on the process of becoming a physician (Good, 1994). In contrast, direct observation is characterized by disengagement from the event or activity under study and mere observation. Given that the presence of the direct observer may influence the event or activity taking place, the direct observer attempts to become as unnoticeable as the circumstances allow. A variation on direct observation has been adopted by a number of researchers who audio or video record physician–patient interactions for future analysis (Beach et al., 2004).

Ethnography, an approach derived largely from cultural anthropology, usually includes at least two qualitative data collection techniques such as direct or participant observation and in-depth interviewing. An ethnographic approach has been used by a number of researchers in the field of health care ethics. Ethnographic work could be done to prospectively examine a particular health care ethics question or the results of ethnographic work could be used to inform such questions. For example, Orfali (2004) compared parental health care decision-making on behalf of their children in neonatal intensive units in the US and France. She employed participant observation, in-depth interviewing with clinicians and parents, and chart reviews. The product is an integrated, comprehensive view of the phenomenon under study. Ethnography takes a lot of time and patience but can provide a wealth of information about how people act in specific situations. Good ethnographic work requires measures to assess validity, sometimes referred to as 'trustworthiness'. These measures include sustained exposure by the investigator, in-depth discussions with key informants and group feedback with local informants.

QUANTITATIVE RESEARCH

Quantitative methods aim to produce numerical answers (e.g., the proportion of persons who hold a particular belief, the number of times information should be repeated to assure that someone understands it, and is X better than Y?), suitable for statistical analyses. Statistical methods include descriptive and inferential techniques. Descriptive techniques help to illustrate the nature of a population or of responses, while inferential techniques are used to determine whether there are significant differences between groups and to estimate how such differences might pertain to a general population and generalize to other sample groups.

Surveys can identify baseline exposure to and/or knowledge, attitudes and beliefs about a particular topic. Although surveys make up a good proportion of published empirical work in health care ethics, good surveys are difficult to design and conduct. DuVal et al. (2004) conducted a national cross-sectional survey of general internists, oncologists and critical care physicians in the US to document their experiences with ethical issues and when and how often they sought ethics consults. They sent their survey to 344 physicians and found that critical care physicians were more likely to report having participated in an ethics consult and that 20% of physicians reported that they did not have access to ethics consults in their primary practice site. In addition, a substantial minority of physicians reported negative attitudes about ethics consultations, noting that they believed the consult would be too time-consuming or make the situation worse. Important aspects of a good survey include the following: the proper phrasing of items (i.e., survey questions) so that each item is directed at only one piece of information; pilot testing to assure that respondents understand the questions and can follow the instructions; assessing reliability of the survey instrument to assure that on re-testing the respondents would give the same sort of response; choosing a sampling frame such that the data obtained will be generalizable to appropriate settings; obtaining a response rate that is high enough to ensure that results are not biased by over-representation of a subgroup with atypical feelings about a topic; using the correct statistical techniques to analyse the survey results; and accurately reporting the data to avoid overstating what has been learned in the study. Useful resources for designing survey research include books by Fowler and Dillman (Fowler, 1993; Dillman, 2000).

Case control studies assess differences between individuals who have had a particular outcome ('cases') and those who have not had that outcome ('controls') to discover what factors might account for the outcome. For each case, a control is sought that matches in other characteristics such as age, gender or disease. Case control studies are particularly useful when the outcome is rare. Alexander et al. adopted a traditional case control methodology in a survey of physicians engaged in 'concierge' or 'retainer' practice (n = 83 cases) and physicians not engaged in 'concierge' practice (n = 231 controls) to document differences in physician, patient and practice characteristics (Alexander et al., 2005). By including a contemporary 'control' population in their survey, they were able to make direct comparisons with their 'case' group and thereby strengthen the power of their results. That is, if they had conducted a survey only of those practising 'concierge' medicine, they would have had to rely on data provided by previous surveys to make their comparisons, diluting the quality of their results. The investigators found that physicians in 'concierge' practice had smaller patient panels and that they cared for fewer minority patients and patients with public insurance coverage. In addition, concierge physicians were more likely to make house calls, accompany patients to visits with specialists and provide 24-hour direct access. Although case control studies are relatively inexpensive to conduct, they have many limitations. For instance, because case control studies are retrospective (after-the-fact) they cannot randomly assign unspecified factors and may misattribute the reasons why the outcomes occurred. A case control study is an appropriate alternative when a randomized controlled trial is impossible or the phenomenon of interest is not one that could have been anticipated well enough in advance to conduct a cohort study.

Cohort studies examine prospectively a group of patients who have a certain condition and/or receive a particular treatment as well as a control group not affected by the condition or treatment. A good cohort study addresses a clearly focused issue (well-defined population, risk factors and/or outcomes). Kapo et al. (2005) used a retrospective cohort design to track outcomes among patients who chose to leave hospice care. Given that hospice care is used less by African-American patients, the investigators were interested in following all patients who chose to leave hospice care to find out if African-American patients were less likely to return to hospice care after their discharge. In a review of the 358 medical charts of patients discharged after their first admission, the researchers found that African-Americans were less likely to return than non-African-Americans (p = .005) as were those with lower socio-economic status (p = .037). While not conducted or reported with an ethics framework, the results of this study clearly contribute to the policy debate regarding ethnic health disparities in access to end-of-life health care options. To provide valid results, the method of case and control selection in cohort studies must avoid bias and represent the target population. Where possible the measurements should be objective and validated. Confounding factors must be carefully considered and countered. The duration and detail of follow-up must be sufficient to accurately identify outcomes.

Experimental studies enable the researcher to prospectively assign individuals or groups to different treatments or interventions. The risk of hidden contributions of confounding factors can be substantially eliminated by randomization: whatever effects are not explicitly managed are distributed in such a way they should have a similar impact in all groups and, thus do not influence outcomes. Moreover, it is often possible to blind, or mask, investigators and participants to whether particular participants are receiving an intervention or not, further lowering the impact of bias. In a typical randomized trial, a hypothesis about whether a particular intervention influences an outcome can be tested directly. A randomized trial was used by Pearson et al. (2006) to assess the effect of a disclosure letter about how group practice physicians are compensated on patients' knowledge, attitudes and beliefs regarding financial conflicts of interest. The researchers found that patients who received the letter were better able to indicate how their physicians were compensated and reported a higher level of confidence in their ability to judge the influence of incentives in the health care system. However, the disclosure had a mixed effect on patients' trust. Although in aggregate almost a quarter of patients indicated that the letter increased the level of trust they had in the physician, 5% of patients reported a reduced level of trust. Though randomized trials have many advantages, they can be expensive to conduct.

Quasi-experimental studies examine events in real life that mimic a prospective cohort study or a randomized trial. For instance, the enactment of a new law that is designed to influence some aspect of health care ethics enables a quasi-experimental study comparing outcomes in the same group before and after, or comparing one group who is affected by the new law to an otherwise similar group that is not affected. Baker et al. (2003) looked at the influence of the Patient Self-Determination Act (PSDA) on the use of Do-Not-Resuscitate (DNR) orders among Medicare beneficiaries diagnosed with serious medical conditions (e.g. stroke) in the state of Ohio. The PSDA was meant to increase the role of patients in decision-making near the end of their lives. The investigators chose the outcome measure of DNR orders filed as a proxy measure that a discussion about end-of-life preferences had taken place between the physician and patient (or family member(s)). Baker et al. (2003) reviewed data from one year before followed by six years after implementation of the PSDA. The researchers found that there was a demonstrable increase in DNR orders written when comparing 1991 and 1992 data. However, on closer inspection they found that the increase in orders indicated a trend in DNR orders being written for patients early during hospitalization ('early' DNR orders) as compared to those written when patients entered a nursing home ('late' DNR orders). That is, the researchers found that the increase in evidence of DNR orders immediately after the passage of PSDA was accounted for by an increase in 'early' DNR orders, whereas the number of 'late' DNR orders remained constant (with the exception in a slight increase among patients with chronic obstructive pulmonary disease). On the basis of these results one might argue that although the overall number of DNR orders has not increased, physicians are not having conversations that lead to the placement of a DNR order in the more acute setting.

Health services research includes an array of quantitative methods largely derived from clinical epidemiology. Health services research often evaluates the characteristics and use of health services, such as outpatient visits or hospitalizations, using medical records and large databases as the substrate for analysis. Health services research is based on the relationship of persons to health services, thereby potentially missing confounding factors, particularly any events that occur outside of the health care environment. Relevant outcomes can be difficult to pick and measure, limiting the range of situations in which health services research is appropriate for ethics research.

PRACTICAL LIMITATIONS

There is no such thing as a 'quick and easy study'. Although some research questions can achieve relatively rapid resolution with a carefully designed study, this is not the norm. It takes a lot of time to review the literature properly, frame research questions, pick appropriate methods, design and conduct a study, analyse the data and interpret and formally report the findings. Practical constraints on time and money available must be considered.

The needed resources (people, time, data access and money) to conduct a well designed study can be relatively modest in some instances (e.g. a survey in one institution of investigator's knowledge of research regulations) or quite elaborate (e.g. incentives to participants in a randomized trial with a long follow-up time). Thus, in designing a study it is critical to estimate all costs accurately.

Local institutional funding might be requested if the research question is part of an established educational programme (such as a research training fellowship) or if the research question itself is of direct importance to an institution. For example, does the hospital have an ethics consultation service? Are the content of those ethics consults tracked? Are the consumers (e.g. physicians, families, etc.) of the ethics consult service satisfied with the outcomes facilitated by the ethics consult service? Could data from the ethics consults be fed back into continuing education efforts?

Other sources of financial support for health care ethics include local and federal governments, corporate funding and private foundations. In each of these cases funding is usually forthcoming only if the research question meshes with the mission of the funding source. Thus, after formulating a research project that requires financial support, an important subsequent step is to identify funding sources that might be interested in the same or similar questions.

CONCLUDING COMMENTS

Empirical research in health care ethics is a challenging and difficult endeavour that requires time, expertise, money and energy. The material presented in this chapter is meant to serve as an introduction to this challenging endeavour. Those interested in pursuing empirical research are encouraged to seek additional information and guidance so that the work they do has an increased likelihood of informing the field and ultimately improving the health care enterprise.

AUTHORS' NOTE

The authors appreciate the important suggestions of Steve Miles, MD, Justin Pearlman, MD, ME, PhD, Joan Sieber, PhD and Joan Teno, MD on earlier drafts of this chapter. Some of the ideas offered appear in Sugarman and Sulmasy (2001) to which Drs Pearlman and Taylor each contributed to a chapter. However, this manuscript has not been published elsewhere.

REFERENCES

Alexander GC, Kurlander J, Wynia MK. Physicians in retainer ('concierge') practice. A national survey of physician, patient and practice characteristics. *J Gen Intern Med* 2005; **20**: 1079–1083.

Baker DW, Enistadter D, Husak S, Cebul RD. Changes in the use of do-not-resuscitate orders after implementation of the Patients Self-Determination Act. *J Gen Intern Med* 2003; **18**: 343–349.

Beach MC, Roter D, Rubin H, Frankel R, Levinson, W, Ford, DE. Is physician self-disclosure related to patient evaluation of office visits? *J Gen Intern Med* 2004; **19**(9): 905–910.

Borry P, Schotsmans P, Dierickx. Empirical research in bioethics journals. A quantitative analysis. *J Med Ethics* 2006; **32**: 240–245.

Brody BA. Assessing empirical research in bioethics. *Theor Med* 1993; 14: 211–229.

Byron GJ. *Medicine, Rationality, and Experience. An Anthropological Perspective*. Cambridge: Cambridge University Press, 1994.

Campbell DT, Stanley JC. *Experimental and Quasi-Experimental Designs for Research*. Chicago: Rand McNally, 1963.

Carlisle J, Shickle D, Cork M, McDonagh A. Concerns over confidentiality may deter adolescents from consulting their doctors. A qualitative study. *J Med Ethics* 2004; **32**: 133–137.

Cohen MZ, Knafl KA. Evaluating qualitative research. *NLN Publ* 1993; **19**(2535): 476–492.

Dillman DA. *Mail and Internet Surveys: The Tailored Design Method,* 2nd edition. New York: John Wiley & Sons, 2000.

DuVal G, Clarridge B, Gensler G, Danis M. A national survey of US internists' experiences with ethical dilemmas and ethics consultation. *J Gen Intern Med* 2004; **19**: 251–258.

Fowler FJ. *Survey Research Methods,* 2nd edition. Newbury Park, CA: Sage Publications, 1993.

Inui TS, Frankel RM. Evaluating the quality of qualitative research. *J Gen Intern Med* 1991; **6**(5): 485–486.

Kalvermark S, Hoglund AT, Hansson MG, Westerholm P, Arnetz B. Living with conflicts - ethical dilemmas and moral distress in the health care system. *Soc Sci Med* 2004; **58**: 1075–1084.

Kapo J, MacMoran H, Casarett D. Lost to follow-up: ethnic disparities in continuity of hospice care at the end of life. *J Pallia Med* 2005; **8**(3): 603–608.

Krueger RA. *Focus Groups: A Practical Guide for Applied Research*. Newbury Park: Sage Publications, 1988.

Mays N, Pope C. Assessing quality in qualitative research. *Br Med J* 2000; **320**: 50–52.

Orfali K. Parental role in decision-making: fact or fiction. A comparative study of ethical dilemmas in French and American neonatal intensive care units. *Soc Sci Med* 2004; **58**: 2009–2022.

Patton MQ. Enhancing the quality and credibility of qualitative analysis. *Health Serv Res* 1999; **34**(5): 1189–1208.

Pearson SD, Kleinman K, Rusinak D, Levinson W. A trial of disclosing physicians' financial incentives to patients. *Arch Intern Med* 2006; **166**: 623–628.

Sackett DL et al. *Clinical Epidemiology: A Basic Science for Clinical Medicine,* 2nd edition. Boston, MA: Little, Brown, 1991.

Sugarman J, McCrory DC, Powell D, Krasny A, Adams B, Ball E, Cassell C. Empirical research on informed consent. An annotated bibliography. Hastings Cent Rep. 1999 Jan-Feb;29(1): S1-S42.

Sugarman J, Sulmasy D, eds. *Methods Med Ethics*. Washington, DC: Georgetown University Press, 2001.

Sugarman J. The Future of Empirical Research in Bioethics. *American J Law, Med & Ethics* 2004; **32**: 226–231.

Sugarman J, Faden R, Weinsten J. A decade of empirical research in medical ethics. In: Sulmasy D, ed. *Methods in Medical Ethics*. Washington, DC: Georgetown University Press, 2001, Chapter 2.

Van Kleffens T, van Leeuween E. Physicians' evaluations of patients' decisions to refuse oncological treatment. *J Med Ethics* 2005; **31**: 131–136.

22

Medical Sociology and the Redundancy of Empirical Ethics

ADAM HEDGECOE

The relationship between medical ethics (at least in its wider conception as bioethics) and social science is not an easy one and, despite numerous attempts to bring these two schools of thought together (usually under the rather leaky umbrella of 'interdisciplinarity'), there is little sign of tension easing. Perhaps best described as 'contentious and adversarial' (Campbell 2003, p. 44, cited in De Vries, 2003), relations could be caricatured with bioethicists long suspecting social scientists of 'Baiting Bioethics', of mounting 'broadside attack[s]' and 'tendentious polemic[s]' (Gorovitz, 1986, p. 364) and accusations of 'ax grinding' (de Wachter, 1998, p. 41). For their part, social scientists claim that bioethics ignores the multicultural nature of modern society, 'solv[ing] practical puzzles for a world that does not exist' (Turner, 2003, p. 113), that it 'generally has a simple, not to say simpleminded, notion of what can be done to bring about social change' (Jennings, 1990, p. 271) and that in important institutional and intellectual ways, modern bioethics is subservient to the biomedical establishment that it set out to challenge (Stevens, 2000; Evans, 2002).

Though such debates are good knockabout fun, they do little to help the aim of this chapter and answer the question: 'In what ways might social scientific research be relevant to health care ethics?' Over the years a number of approaches have been suggested, which vary in the dominance they give to the different sides (social scientific or philosophical) of the equation. The most obvious way to connect empirical social science data and bioethics is in what James Lindemann Nelson has called the 'linear model', whereby social scientists gather data on bioethical topics, for example, 'How many people are willing to make out advance directives? How do chronically ill people experience their illnesses' (Nelson, 2000, p. 13)? These data are then given

to bioethicists as the raw material for their analysis, the 'target' upon which bioethical theory operates.

There is admittedly 'something rather appealing about this linear view. At least in outline, it is simple, straightforward and has the virtue of not raising anxieties about committing naturalistic fallacies: "is" and "ought" remain on their respective sides of the fence' (Nelson, 2000, p. 13). This approach to the relationship between bioethics and the social sciences is appealing enough to attract the support of senior figures such as Tony Hope (1999) and Daniel Callahan (1999). Yet it is badly undermined by the weight of empirical work that questions the reality of the fact/value distinction (e.g. Alderson, 1990; Kaufman, 1997; Lock, 1998). As Nelson points out, the 'notion that salient facts about the natural world, or about pattern of social interaction ... are just there, waiting to be scooped up by neutral forms of inquiry, is hotly contested' (Nelson, 2000, p. 13). In addition to complaints about the unsophisticated naivety of the linear model, on a more prosaic level, given that this approach relegates social scientists to a rather subservient position in relation to bioethicists, there is understandable scepticism about the usefulness of this approach (Zussman, 2000).

In contrast to the linear model there is an approach that we might call the 'social science critique', which comes in a variety of strengths. At one end of the scale is the philosopher Barry Hoffmaster who suggests that ethnography will 'save the life of medical ethics' (Hoffmaster, 1992, 1994) by rooting its reasoning in the actual context of medical decision-making rather than an empirical philosophical theory. At the other end, there are authors like Erica Haimes (2002) or Hedgecoe (2004) who have proposed models for integrating social science data into medical ethics. And in between there are a number of authors, from both the social sciences (DeVries and Conrad, 1998; Kleinman, 1999;

Principles of Health Care Ethics, Second Edition   Edited by R.E. Ashcroft, A. Dawson, H. Draper and J.R. McMillan
© 2007 John Wiley & Sons, Ltd

Zussman, 2000; López, 2004) and more philosophical backgrounds (Häyry and Takala, 2003; Holm and Jonas, 2004), who offer critiques of modern medical ethics and recommend the adoption of at least some elements of social science research. But one obvious problem for medical ethicists faced with this approach is that the polemical, hectoring style which characterizes some of it is rather off-putting and understandably does little to generate the kind of positive attitude towards social science that would be required were medical ethicists to adopt this approach.

But in parallel with this literature is a move from within philosophical bioethics, an 'empirical turn' (Borry et al., 2005) that would seek to combine traditional philosophical medical ethics with empirical research, an approach that 'presents challenges to the very core of bioethics … [that] …shakes the bioethical world and compels bioethics to disentangle the empirical ethical knot' (Borry et al., 2004, p. 3). A range of authors write about such 'evidence based ethics' (Goldenberg, 2005), but perhaps the most fully worked out approach is that of 'integrated empirical ethics'.[1] Such an approach moves beyond simplistic uses of empirical data by ethicists (for example, to test the conclusion of consequentialist reasoning), accepts the implicit normativity of empirical data collection and presumes 'that there is no fixed epistemological gap between "fact" and "value"' (Molewijk et al., 2003, p. 88). This approach trumps the work of most ethicists and social scientists working in this area in terms of the considerable thought that has gone into creating genuine links between empirical and philosophical work (see Molewijk et al., 2004). Yet despite this, it is not clear that 'integrated empirical ethics' constitutes a genuinely novel discipline 'with its own premises, theories, topics and methods' as its supporters propose (van der Scheer and Widdershoven, 2004, p. 72). In fact, as Mairi Levitt has pointed out, it is not clear that 'integrated empirical ethics' does anything that the social sciences do not already do (Levitt, 2004). In response to this claim, Van der Scheer and Widdershoven 'admit that the methodology … is actually derived from the social sciences. Yet the results are clearly normative.' Thus the project in question, presented as an example of 'integrated empirical ethics', 'focuses on the structure of social life as moral practice'. They accept that 'social science does not exclude such explicit references to moral attitudes, but neither is the inclusion of such reference typical of social science' (van der Scheer and Widdershoven, 2004, p. 89).

It depends of course on one's choice of social science, but, as the rest of this chapter shows, in the case of medical sociology this is manifestly not the case. Part of the problem seems to be that, despite proponents' claims to the contrary, integrated empirical ethics maintains social scientists in a subordinate position to philosopher-ethicists. To some

extent it is the terminology. Social scientists are 'descriptive scientists' as opposed to 'prescriptive scientists' (i.e. ethicists). Some authors, although aware of these terminological problems (see Molewijk et al., 2004, endnote 17), are still unable to place social scientists on an equal footing with ethicists when it comes to normative thinking. Others ascribe the role of trying to 'formulate guidelines for further action' arising out of such research to 'ethical researchers' rather than social scientists (van der Scheer and Widdershoven, 2004).

Thus there seems to be a curious blind spot regarding the social sciences on the part of supporters of empirical bioethics. This is most obviously the case in Borry and colleagues' useful quantitative survey of empirical research in bioethics journals. They note that the amount of this research has increased over the past ten years and provide an astute breakdown of publications according to journal and topic. Yet for a social scientist this article ends on a very odd note, since having noted that similar research needs to be carried out on a wider range of bioethics journals (this study looked at just nine), these authors also point out that:

> ethics related empirical research is published in other medical journals, which number over 40,000 worldwide. Further research should address the presence and characteristics of empirical research in bioethics and medical ethics in the context of these publications (Borry et al., 2006, p. 245).

Yet curiously there is no suggestion that social science journals focusing on medical topics, such as *Social Science and Medicine*, might publish any empirical studies which might address topics of bioethical interest. For these authors, empirical work with normative power would only be published in bioethics or medical journals.

The rest of this chapter examines two examples of medical sociology which clearly undermine the idea that social science does not explicitly deal with moral attitudes, and that a new discipline is required to explore this area. Medical sociology provides thoroughly socially, culturally and politically embedded explanations for the values and actions of health care professionals. Thus if medical ethicists are interested in the lived experience of the social world of modern medicine, an obvious solution would be to read some medical sociology, rather than look towards developing a new discipline. This focus on sociology is for reasons of specialization, brevity and because it is, perhaps, the most troublesome social science for ethicists (De Vries, 2003). And rather than provide a review of possible relevant examples (see Zussman, 1997. For similar articles on anthropology, see Marshall, 1992; Muller, 1994), the approach I take in this chapter is to narrow my focus and

---

[1]Although there are disagreements among users of this term over exactly what it entails: Molewijk (2004).

provide an in-depth analysis of two pieces of medical sociology to see how they might contribute to thinking in health care ethics.

Any sociologist can point in the direction of works that one simply *must* read. My grounds for choosing these two examples, Renee Fox and Judith Swazey's *Spare Parts: Organ Replacement in American Society* and Charles Bosk's *All God's Mistakes: Genetic Counseling in a Pediatric Hospital*, are equally partial; I think these are wonderful books telling moving and disturbing stories with style, verve and impressive control of data. To steal from a review on the back of Bosk's book, these works provide 'good example[s] of what a sophisticated, intelligent social scientist can teach us about an ethically difficult medical setting'.

ORGAN REPLACEMENT

Spare Parts is the last in a series of publications from these authors that extend back to Fox's 1959 classic *Experiment Perilous*. Although the focus of that book was a range of clinical trials, one of the topics Fox dealt with was kidney dialysis, and this began an interest in organ replacement technologies that with Judith Swazey led to 1974's *Courage to Fail: A social view of organ transplants and dialysis*. The themes of this book, 'uncertainty, gift-exchange, and the allocation of scare material and nonmaterial resources', are for these authors now even more urgent than in the early 1970s, and thus underpin *Spare Parts*.

In many ways *Spare Parts* is an uneven read. It splits into two clear halves, with the first section serving, in many ways, as a straightforward update of *Courage to Fail*, covering the 'boom' in organ transplants that took place in the wake of the development of Cyclosporine and other immunosupressants, the role of the concept of 'the gift' in organ donation and the impact of market forces on the idea of transplantation as a form of 'medical commons'. What this section serves to do is detail these authors' 'deepening disquietude about the directions of modern medicine', a concern that is 'both sociological and moral' and which 'has been forged, above all, by our views about the nature of the organ replacement endeavour during the past decade' (p. 92).

Methodologically, an ethicist might look at this first section of the book and shrug their shoulders; it draws on the published literature, both newspapers and technical journals. Apart from the occasional use of ethnographic data gathered in previous studies, it is not obvious what is so sociological about this discussion. Why could it not have been written by a medical ethicist? Obvious responses to this question lie in the way in which these authors deal with both the concept of the gift and their treatment of the broader social context of transplantation in American

society. The theme of 'the gift', derived from the work of the French sociologist Mauss, is one that 'remain[s] intrinsic to the dynamics and meaning of transplantation' (p. 31). A gift involves the triple obligations of offer and give, receive and accept, and seek to repay.

In terms of organ transplantation these themes help explain the pressure tissue-matched family members feel in the case of live donation, the reluctance people sometimes feel to accept a donation (because of their inability to repay the debt), surgeons' resistance to the use of non-related live donors and the sometime damage caused to close familial relationships by the 'tyranny of the gift'. Fox and Swazey trace the impact of the transplantation explosion of the early 1980s on the way the concept of the gift was both suppressed (on the grounds that transplantation was a relatively commonplace intervention) and singled out through the increasing need for families of cadaveric donors to meet the recipients. The authors make clear that one of the forces driving these changes was the increasing concern over a shortage of transplantable organs. The same concerns increasingly raised the possibility of commercializing organ transplantation. In turn, 'the persistence of a gift framework for organ transplantation surprised and perplexed some of the market-orientated economists and policy analysts' (p. 31).

The second theme that marks this book out, I think, from a bioethical approach, is the authors' broader societal concerns. At the end of the first half of the book, they review the politically charged debates that took place in the US in the 1980s over the allocation of organs for transplant. They document how transplant surgeons and their teams, the wider medical community and health policymakers have largely ducked a series of vital questions concerning 'how the financial and human resources invested in organ replacement endeavors bear on our society's ability and willingness to meet other need in the medical commons' (pp. 83–4). Thus for Fox and Swazey, one of reasons they have found themselves drawn back to research is that they 'see transplantation as epitomizing many of the issues of what promises to be *the* health policy battle in the United States in the coming years ... the core battle is about rationing' (p. 89). The focus on developing newer and more costly experimental transplantation techniques, at the expense of broader health care provision, leads to the call for 'a penetrating change in our collective, societal perspective about the ends of medicine'. Although they admit to having 'no clear vision of the exact contours of a redefined understanding of the meaning of medical progress and how it would restructure medical care', they are quite clear that the current direction of US medicine is profoundly unethical (p. 92).

In contrast to the broad sweep of the first four chapters, the second half of the book provides a detailed analysis of a series of experiments in the use of an artificial heart, called the Jarvik-7, carried out between 1982 and 1990. Using the traditional ethnographic tools of participant observation and recurring interviews, Fox and Swazey trace the development of the Jarvik-7 at the University of Utah in the late 1970s, its championing by a young, charismatic heart surgeon called William DeVries and the four transplants he undertook with the artificial heart between 1982 and 1985. They detail the personal, institutional and financial issues that led DeVries to move from Utah to Louisville, Kentucky following the first transplant, the transplants and deaths of the next three patients and the critical coverage of these experiments in the medical press. They close their history with the FDA's decision in 1990 to withdraw approval for use of the Jarvik-7 'either as a permanent device or as a temporary bridge in patients awaiting transplant' (p. 148).

Yet this detailed, and sometimes deeply disturbing, history is only the backdrop to an incisive analysis, both of the 'American-ness' of the story of the Jarvik-7 and of the way in which the different levels of the regulatory system failed in allowing these experiments to continue as long as they did. Fox and Swazey place the story of the artificial heart transplants within the context of 'an American morality tale ... in which cardinal aspects of the American dream and of American tragedy were publicly enacted ... on a nationwide scale' (p. 154). They note the classic immigrant story of Willem Kolff who came to the US from Holland after the second world war to found the artificial heart unit at the University of Utah: 'a place where his machines, bold, innovating and indomitable spirit were compatible with the technological evangelism, utopianism and hubris of American social thought' (pp. 155–6). They describe the surgeon William DeVries' 'glamorously folkloric appearance', his habit of speaking in homely American aphorisms ('If you don't make the first step you never get there') and draw comparisons with American literary characters such as Melville's Billy Budd and Miller's Willy Loman (p. 156). Perhaps most intriguingly, they unpack the role of Mormonism in creating the right environment for the Jarvik-7 experiments at the University of Utah, located in Mormonism's 'capital', Salt Lake City. They show how 'Mormonism's historical and spiritual identification with the American West – with the manifest destiny of the pioneers who explored and settled it . . . – influenced these statements about the trail-blazing significance of the artificial heart project' (p. 164).

What Fox and Swazey present is a thoroughly socially, culturally and politically embedded explanations for why these experiments took place and the ethical debates around them. They clearly point out the significant concerns about the Jarvik-7 (particularly in animal tests) felt in the wider (non-Utah) transplant community and they show that the answer to the question 'why was such testing launched?'

lies in factors such as declining NIH funding in this area, the need for personal and international prestige, cultural beliefs about the heart as an organ, medicine's belief that life is always better than death and the Mormon values of Salt Lake City (p. 174). They show how such a combination of factors undermined the normal system of checks and balances that regulate such research. Leaving aside the experimenters' fervent belief in the value of the artificial heart, it is clear that the Institutional Review Board (IRB) at Utah was 'buffeted from within and without by pressures from the heart's proponents, their medical center and university, and the Salt Lake City community to approve and support the experiment' (pp. 179–80). Such pressures were repeated following DeVries' move to Kentucky, where the IRB concerned, far less experienced in reviewing such advanced research, 'were aware of the importance that the hospital's owners ... attached to work on the Jarvik heart going forward under their aegis ... [as well as feeling] .. enormous personal, institutional, and community pride at the presence of the celebrated surgeon and his work in "little old Louisville" (p. 182). The authors suggest that the FDA panel involved in licensing the Jarvik-7 did so despite considerable deficiencies in DeVries' submissions to it following the first transplant and serious concerns among some members of the panel itself. They also note that despite their own second thoughts, administrators in both the hospitals involved and senior NIH officials did not oppose the commencement of these trials.

Although Fox and Swazey accept that some mechanisms of social control did work in this case (they cite experts in health law, ethics and medical specialists outside the transplantation community), overall such mechanisms were:

> weakened and compromised by the zeal with which the quest for a viable mechanical heart was pursued ... To a chastening degree, some of the most valued characteristics of American society and culture contributed to the dangerous excesses and forms of misconduct associated with the Jarvik-7 experiment (p. 193).

Two points could be pulled out of this work and highlighted as being of particular relevance to medical ethics. The first is that cutting through this book is a tension between experimenting with new techniques and technologies and their normal clinical use. The authors emphasize that

> therapeutic innovation, rather than being conceptualized and discussed in dichotomous and static terms as either "experiment" or "therapy", should be viewed as a dynamic process or continuum ... physicians do not have standardized, clear-cut terms to designate the developmental stages of a new therapy and why they often use elaborate, equivocal, emotionally charged language to characterize its clinical status (p. 9).

If this is the case, then how we think about the differing ethical requirements for research and clinical practice needs to come under significant scrutiny. If therapeutic innovations move smoothly between research and clinical settings and if how these technologies are viewed is dependent upon context (for example, the availability of health insurance), then the conventional ethical position that requires significantly higher standards for research in terms of informed consent, say, may make little sense in practice.

The second point of relevance is broader and is more of a warning. What this book rigorously demonstrates is the 'embedded' nature of decisions: how social, cultural and political factors shape decisions that come about. As a result, it is difficult to pick such a 'seamless web' apart to identify the 'ethical' factors. Of course one could use this book, or at least the second half of it, as an extended case study to analyse in classic medical ethics terms (Was DeVries wrong or right? In what terms? Did he infringe patients' autonomy?), but this would be to miss the point of *Spare Parts*. If this book is to be taken seriously by medical ethics, then it requires a broadening of the kinds of issues that are normally taken to 'count' in ethical debate, up to and including the 'meaning' of modern medicine. Fox and Swazey themselves quote Daniel Callahan on a regular basis, particularly in the first half of the book. But Callahan, however iconic his role as a co-founder of the Hastings' Center, is far from being a typical medical ethicist in terms of his broadly social outlook and his concerns. If medical ethics were to take this book seriously, then this would turn back to an older way of thinking about these issues, more in keeping with founders of the discipline like Paul Ramsey.[2] But care would be needed. This book does not provide any answers. As Fox and Swazey note, 'Recognizing and understanding these patterns . . . does little to resolve the disturbing issues of moral agency they raise' (p. 193).

GENETIC COUNSELLING: THE DARK SIDE OF PATIENT AUTONOMY

Compared to the chronological and sociological sweep of *Spare Parts*, the second book I wish to discuss, Charles Bosk's *All God's Mistakes*, seems an intimate, almost introverted work. In 1976, the medical sociologist Charles Bosk was asked to begin observations in the genetic counselling unit of an elite paediatric hospital in the US. The request to start work was made by the counsellors themselves 'because of their sense that as a sociologist trained to observe behavior as it naturally occurs, I would have something useful to

add about how best to manage the myriad of social problems that trailed in the wake of new clinical developments' (Bosk, 1992, p. 3). Between Autumn 1976 and Autumn 1980 Bosk spent around two years in the field, attending the weekly pre- and post-clinic conferences in the unit as well as sitting in on individual meetings between counsellors and the parents they advised. His approach was to adopt the rules of the sociologist of work Everett Hughes, to pay attention to 'the neutralization of dirty work and everyday troubles within the context of routines and emergencies . . . [and] . . . a systematic attention in the analysis of the rough edges of professional practice: those places where professional and lay expectations about service are most problematic' (p. 21).

Many of Bosk's concerns in this book are perhaps of more relevance to other ethnographers than ethicists. He writes of his unease in the field, both because of the topic of the fieldwork and because of the level and extent of access he was granted. He frets about failures to gain formal informed consent from patients undergoing counselling, often at the instruction of counsellors. He baulks at being used by members of the counselling team to 'spy' on their colleagues in cases where there is disagreement over what is to be done. And, in a complementary piece written after this book was published, he outlines the impact publishing a detailed ethnography has on one's relationships with research subjects (Bosk, 2001).

But there is much in this book that will interest the medical ethicist, mainly the way that counsellors, through trying to respect patients' autonomy, through the doctrine of non-directiveness end up failing to provide the sort of moral and emotional support that such patients desperately seek. Bosk presents the problem in stark terms:

> genetic counselors preserved the autonomy of outpatients . . . when they most fervently asserted that parents were autonomous, that they had to make their own decisions, the genetic counselors used such a stance to retreat from engaging the emotional issues with which couples struggled. The dark side of patient autonomy is abandonment (Bosk, 1992, p. 158).

For Bosk, highlighting the way his approach is rooted in the sociology of work, part of the problem is a procedural one, which extends beyond this context to professions as a whole. He notes that:

> The genetic counselors evaluated their performance in terms of the story that they told parents. They judged the stories (Did they reflect the current state of genetic knowledge?), but not the storytelling. Whether the stories they fashioned acted as effective moral parables, as guides to patient action, remained a mystery . . . The emphasis on the telling and not

---

[2]For an explanation of how bioethics got from its original form to its current state, see Evans (2002).

the hearing is itself an example of a more general tendency of professionals to evaluate their work in terms of process not outcomes (p. 123).

And this broadening of focus can be found throughout the book. To some extent this relates to the nature of ethnography itself. In his subsequent discussion of this work, Bosk points out that what ethnographers 'do is take a group's sense of its specialness and inspect it; and while inspecting it, we show how ordinary, commonplace, and self-serving it really is' (Bosk, 2001, p. 213). The way that counsellors' provision of service inevitably trivializes 'the meaning of momentous moments in everyday life' has to be seen in the context of all professionalization, where 'the emergencies of laypersons are transformed in the routines of professionals' (Bosk, 1992, p. 146). Thus Bosk is careful not to suggest that

> counselors alone are guilty of using autonomy as a warrant for abandonment. I am not singling out counselors as the solitary abandoners of patients amongst all the medical profession. Instead I am using counselors to show how rather extensive patient abandonment can occur under the banner of more perfect patient autonomy (p. 11; footnote 6).

In setting autonomy in context, Bosk shows how this most pre-eminent of bioethical values (at least in the US setting) cannot be viewed as an unalloyed good, that we must accept that there are costs to be paid in the exercise of autonomy and that these are most often paid by patients. The book explores the role of autonomy further by comparing the way counsellors treat outpatients, who arrange appointments directly with the unit, to how they treat inpatients, who are asked to give an opinion by other specialisms within the hospital. Following a detailed ethnographic vignette, Bosk notes how one of the counsellors, 'Bill Smith', reacted:

> Evident in the handling of this patient is Bill Smith's distress at the way that Marceau [a neonatologist, seeking advice from Smith] managed the Doughertys. At no time in the conference did he suggest an alternative to Marceau's plan for the treatment of the Doughterys' child...here their [i.e. counsellor's] lack of intervention serves to undermine patient autonomy, the very value that neutrality was adopted to protect (p. 76).

Genetic counsellors' reluctance to intervene on colleagues' 'turf', even though they may have superior technical knowledge, is a recurring theme in *All God's Mistakes*. As Bosk stresses repeatedly, 'Genetic counselors are as nonintrusive with the decision making of their colleagues as they are with their patients...[as a result]...their nonjudgemental stance contributes to procedures and treatments they believe to be unwarranted' (p. 74).

One of the factors underpinning this reluctance is a second lesson that is of value to medical ethics: power. In this hospital, genetic counsellors were a relatively powerless professional group, with low status because of the lack of medical interventions they could offer: 'having nothing special to offer save talk and elective abortion, and having no primary care responsibilities for patients' (p. 58). One consequence of this was the way that counsellors fought to avoid being seen simply as an emotional 'mop-up service' for the parts of the hospital. Other professional groups, such as paediatricians, tended to refer parents to the genetics unit, to get the counsellors to break bad news, 'a referral tactic which allowed these paediatricians freedom to focus on the positive in their dealings with the family' (p. 150). Sometimes the counsellors fought back. Bosk tells the story of when one counsellor, Samuels, deferred telling a couple that their child had only a short time to live by suggesting that they ought to discuss the prognosis with the surgeons treating their child:

> Samuels did not avoid telling the Castleberrys the full story because he was unaware of it, but because of his sense that such momentous bad news should be conveyed by treating physicians...he was at once and the same time reassuring them that it was a legitimate question, while trying to force his colleagues to live up to their role obligations (p. 70).

Although such reversals happened, Bosk makes clear that they are the exception rather than the rule. Thus the book delicately navigates the complex issues that surround the topic of genetic counselling to show how the division of medical labour and the principle of non-directive counselling combine to over-emphasize autonomy for outpatients and under-emphasize it for inpatients to the detriment of both.

Clearly one obvious problem for this book, if it is to be relevant to current medical ethics, is the potentially outdated nature of its data; as Bosk himself points out, 'All ethnography becomes social history'. But at the same time, although:

> Much has changed in applied human genetics...New technologies have made for increasingly refined diagnosis of *in utero* defects...the process of counseling appears static...the way information is transferred, how decision-making responsibility is allocated, and what issues are considered as part of the calculus for exercising responsibility – all of these appear unchanged (p. xx).

Writing in the early 1990s, Bosk looks to the future, suggesting that 'As each part of the human genome is more carefully mapped, as we gain more precise knowledge...we should not expect clinicians/researchers to adopt the nondirective, value-neutral position of genetic counselors' (p. 56).

Although Bosk regards genetic counsellors as imperfect protectors of patients' interests, he also worries that developments in human genetics in the wake of the human genome project may erode what little protection is afforded. Whether these concerns mean that *All God's Mistakes* no longer tells us anything about the ethical dilemmas of modern clinical genetics is hard to say. What is clear is that Bosk raises issues about medical practice and context that move beyond this particular medical speciality and this specific time and place.

Thus this work highlights the importance of power relations in medical organizations and their impact on the ethics of decision-making. If you are at the bottom of the clinical hierarchy, as these counsellors are, your range of action is limited. Although there might be strong ethical arguments in favour of intervening in colleagues' cases, where one has superior knowledge and where unnecessary interventions are proposed, the power differential present in the medical setting may make such a choice, however ethical, unrealistic. Thus power is an important consideration in medical ethics: what might be right in one situation may not be suitable in another, depending on the relationships among individuals.

The second theme of interest is that of autonomy. Bosk's work complements the considerable amount of social science research that has explored the topic of autonomy, highlighting in particular the practical difficulties involved in gaining informed consent. The irony in the case of autonomy as abandonment is that non-directiveness, the feature of the counselling session that is meant to allow patients to do what they want, undermines what these people desire: moral guidance and emotional and spiritual support. The theoretical principle of autonomy is shown to conflict with patients' wants and needs. Of course there is no easy answer to the dilemmas raised by this work: Bosk is not suggesting that counsellors should tell patients what to do. What he does is document the real-world problems caused by the implementation of an ethical concept.

CONCLUSION: AVOIDING THE LINEAR MODEL

To assume that the lessons of these two detailed sociological studies can be directly interpreted and digested by medical ethics is to fall into the trap of the 'linear model'. These authors would oppose such a use of their work, a statement that can be made with some confidence once we realize that Fox and Swazey and Bosk are not bystanders in the debates over the relationship between sociology and medical ethics, but rather have been engaged in a close debate with bioethics and medical ethics for a number years. These authors have challenged the assumptions of modern western medical ethics

(Fox and Swazy, 1984), and have critiqued the tendency of bioethics to underplay sociologists' contribution to debates in this area (Bosk, 2000a). They have used bioethics as a site for sociological research, exploring the role of religious conviction in American bioethics (Messikomer et al., 2001) and questioning the discipline's steady 'professionalisation' (Bosk, 2002). But they have also engaged with bioethics in a less overtly critical way, bringing their expertise to bear on thinking about how to reform PhD training (Fox and Swazey, 2005)and using wider sociological literature to reflect on what might count as success or failure in a clinical ethics consultation (Bosk, 2000b). So these are not innocent authors when it comes to medical ethics, and it would do them, and their work, an injustice to assume that their results can simply be fed into ethical calculation, the handle turned and the right answer produced.

Thus the use of works like *Spare Parts* and *All God's Mistakes* by medical ethicists must necessarily be oblique. But that said, even a cursory glance at current debates in the ethical literature shows how empirically impoverished thinking in these areas is. Taking just the case of organ donation, if one reads medical ethicists' solutions to the problems surrounding a lack of available cadaveric organs, one reads about the need for a regulated market in living donor organs to make up the shortfall (e.g. Erin and Harris, 2003; Hippen, 2005), the need to conscript cadaveric organs (Hippen, 2005), or the potential value of a communitarian approach to this shortfall – 'shaming' people into leaving their organs in the event of their death (Etzioni, 2003). Yet at no point in these discussions is there a mention of why it is that people choose to donate, something that seems fairly relevant to thinking about how to increase donation levels. Nor is there a discussion of the broader cultural impact that the perceived 'need' for organ transplantation has on health care and society as a whole, not even in the contribution of the communitarian Amitai Etzioni. It is not clear how this material would be incorporated by these medical ethicists, although Fox and Swazey do go some way towards explaining how the gift relationship undermines the 'marketisation' of human organ donation. Yet what is clear from reading this work is that medical ethicists are talking about organ donation in the same terms as they discussed it in the 1970s and 1980s. It is not clear how productive this sort of intellectual stagnation is.

That ethical decisions around transplant surgery are shaped by social and political context does not mean that such debates are not real and do not count. That patients can experience genetic counsellors' respect for their autonomy as abandonment does not mean that autonomy as a principle should be struck from the ethical lexicon. What these books, and medical sociology as a whole, should teach as medical ethics is humility. Stories are almost always more complex than they first seem, and telling these stories in detail may take a huge amount of intellectual and emotional effort (the authors of both these books complain of ethnographic 'burnout'). Most importantly, there is rarely a right answer to the question 'what should I do?'.

Thus the empirical information provided by medical sociologists may not prove useful to those ethicists who feel that it is their role to impose their will on social reality, rather than the other way round. Yet for ethicists interested in incorporating empirical research into their work, these two case studies have hopefully shown two things. The first is that we do not need a new discipline, 'empirical ethics', to think empirically about ethical issues. We already have at least one discipline that does that: medical sociology. As Charles Bosk has pointed out: 'the contribution of sociologists to topics bioethical is as remarkable as it is unappreciated...the sociological involvement with these issues predates bioethics as either an organized domain of inquiry or an emergent professional occupation' (Bosk, 2000a, p. 398). It is not that the supporters of empirical ethics are wrong when they speak of the need for ethical debate to pay attention to empirical research, but they are wrong when they suggest that integrated empirical ethics 'is exceptional since it cannot be characterized as either wholly prescriptive or as wholly descriptive' (Molewijk et al., 2004, p. 57). If such a combination makes this form of empirical ethics exceptional, then, as this chapter has shown, medical sociology and, I would argue, the majority of the social sciences are equally 'exceptional'. What is needed from medical ethicists is a willingness to read and engage with medical sociology as it is, rather than develop a discipline to replace social science.

The second, less helpful, concluding point is that it is not at all clear what form this engagement should take. I have suggested elsewhere that ethicists who wish to take social science seriously should approach work in this area with a view to challenging theory, with a reflexive awareness of their own context and with a politely sceptical point of view (Hedgecoe, 2003). Yet this is too vague to provide a programme of work and it remains to be seen whether medical ethics' relationship with empirical social science can successfully sail between the simplicity of the linear model on one side and the redundancy of empirical ethics on the other.

REFERENCES

Alderson P. *Choosing for Children: Parent's Consent to Surgery.* Oxford: Oxford University Press, 1990

Borry P, Schotsman P, Dierickx K. *Empirical Ethics: A Challenge to Bioethics* vol. **7**, 2004; pp. 1–3.

Borry P, Schotsman P, Dierickx K. The birth of the empirical turn in bioethics. *Bioethics* 2005; **19**(10): 49–71.

Borry P, Schotsmans P, Dierickx Empirical research in bioethical journals. A quantitative analysis. *J Med Ethics* 2006; **32**: 240–245.

Bosk CL. *All God's Mistakes: Genetic Counseling in a Pediatric Hospital.* Chicago: University of Chicago Press, 1992.

Bosk CL. The sociological imagination and bioethics In: Bird CC, Conrad P, Fremont AM, eds. *Handbook of Medical Sociology.* 5th edition, New Jersey: Prentice Hall, 2000a.

Bosk CL. Margin of error: the sociology of ethics consultation. In: Rubin SB, Zoloth L, eds. *Margin of Error: The Ethics of Mistakes in the Practice of Medicine.* Hagerstown: University Publishing Group, 2000b.

Bosk CL. Irony, ethnography, and informed consent. In: Hoffmaster B, ed. *Bioethics in Social Context.* Temple University Press: Philadelphia, 2001.

Bosk CL. Now that we have the data, what was the question? *Am J Bioethics* 2002; **2**(4): 21–23.

Callahan D. The social sciences and the task of bioethics. *Daedelus* 1999; **128**: 275–294.

de Vries R. How can we help? From "Sociology in" to "Sociology of" bioethics. *J Law, Medicine Ethics* 2003; **32**(2): 279–292.

DeVries R, Conrad P, 1998. Why Bioethics needs Sociology. In *Bioethics and Society: Constructing the Ethical Enterprise.* R. DeVries & J. Subedi, eds. New Jersey. Prentice Hall: 233–257.

de Wachter MAM. Sociology and bioethics in the USA. *Hastings Center Rep* 1998; **28**(5): 40–42.

Erin CA, Harris J. An ethical market in human organs. *J Med Ethics* 2003; **29**: 137–138.

Etzioni A. Organ donation: a communitarian approach. *Kennedy Inst of Ethics J* 2003; **13**(1): 1–8.

Evans JH. *Playing God? Human Genetic Engineering and the Rationalisation of Public Bioethical Debate.* Chicago: University of Chicago Press, 2002.

Fox RC, Swazey JP. Examining American bioethics: its problems and prospects. *Cambridge Q Healthcare Ethics* 2005; **14**: 361–373.

Fox RC, Swazey JP. Medical morality is not bioethics – medical ethics in China and the United States. *Perspect Biol Med* 1984;**27**: 336–360.

Fox RC, Swazey JP. *Spare Parts: Organ Replacement in American Society.* New York: Oxford University Press, 1992.

Goldenberg MJ. Evidence-based ethics? On evidence-based practice and the "empirical turn" from normative bioethics. *BMC Med Ethics* 2005; **6**: 11. http://www.biomedcentral.com/1472-6939/6/11

Gorovitz S. Baiting bioethics. *Ethics* 1986; **96**: 356–374.

Haimes E. What can the Social Sciences Contribute to the Study of Ethics? Theoretical, Empirical and Substantive Considerations. *Bioethics* 2002; **16**: 89-113.

Häyry M, Tuija T. *Scratching the Surface of Bioethics.* Amsterdam: Rodopi, 2003.

Hedgecoe A. 'Critical Bioethics: beyond the Social science critique of Applied Ethics' *Bioethics* 2004, 18(2): 120–143.

Hippen BE. In defense of a regulated market in kidneys from living vendors. *J Med Philos* 2005; **30**: 593–626.

Hoffmaster B. Can Ethnography Save the Life of Medical Ethics? *Social Science and Medicine* 1992; **35**: 1421–1431.

Hoffmaster B. The Forms and Limits of Medical Ethics. *Social Science and Medicine* 1994;**39**: 1155–1164, p. 1155.

Holm S, Jonas MF. *Engaging the World: The Use of Empirical Research in Bioethics and the Regulation of Biotechnology.* IOS Press: Amsterdam, 2004.

Hope T. empirical medical ethics. *J Med Ethics* 1999; **25**: 219–220.

Jennings B. Ethics and ethnography in neonatal intensive care pp. 261–272 in Weisz G. (ed,) *Social Science Perspectives on Medical Ethics* (Philadelphia: University of Pennsylvania Press).

Kaufman SR. Construction and practice of medical responsibility: dilemmas and narratives from geriatrics. *Culture, Med Psychiatry* 1997; **21**: 1–26.

Kleinman A. Moral Experience and Ethical Reflection: Can Ethnography Reconcile Them? A Quandary for 'The New Bioethics'. *Daedelus* 1999; 128: 69–97,

Levitt M. Complementarity rather than integration *Medicine, Health Care and Philosophy* 2004; **7**: 81–83.

Lock M. Perfecting society: reproductive technologies, genetic testing, and the planned family in Japan. In: Lock M, Kaufert PA, eds. *Pragmatic Women and Body Politics.* Cambridge: Cambridge University Press, 1998; pp. 206–239.

López José. How sociology can save bioethics...maybe. *Sociol Health Illness.* 2004; **26**(7).

Marshall PA. Anthropology and bioethics. *Med Anthropol Q* 1992; **6**(1): 49–73.

Messikomer CM, Fox RC, Swazey JP. The presence and influence of religion in American bioethics. *Perspect Biol Med* 2001; **44**(4): 485–508.

Molewijk AC, Stiggelbout AM, Otten W, Bupuis H. M, Kievit J. Implicit normativity in evidence-based medicine: A plea for integrated empirical ethics research. *Health Care Anal* 2003; **11**(1): 69–92.

Molewijk AC, Stiggelbout AM, Otten W, Bupuis HM, Kievit J. Empirical data and moral theory. A plea for integrated empirical ethics. *Medicine, Health Care and Philos* 2004; **7**: 55–69.

Molewik B. Integrated empirical ethics: in search for clarifying identities. *Med Healthcare Philos* 2004; **7**: 85–87.

Muller, JH. Anthropology, bioethics, and medicine: A provocative trilogy. *Med Anthropol Q.* **8**(4): 448–467.

Nelson JL. Moral teachings from unexpected quarters. *Hastings Center Rep* 2000; **30**(1): 12–17.

Spital A. Conscription of cadaveric organs for transplantation: Neglected again. *Kennedy Inst Ethics J* 2003; **13**(2): 196–274.

Stevens ML. *Bioethics in America: Origins and Cultural Politics.* Baltimore: The Johns Hopkins Press, 2000.

Turner L. Bioethics in a multicultural world: medicine and morality in pluralistic settings. *Health Care Anal* 2003; **11**(2): 99–117.

van der Scheer L, Widdershoven G. Integrated empirical ethics: Loss of normativity? *Med Health Care Philos* 2004; **7**: 71–79.

van der Scheer L, Widdershoven G. A Response to Levitt and Molewijk. *Med Health Care and Philos* 2004; **7**: 89–91.

Zussman R. Sociological perspective on medical decision-making. *Annu Rev Sociol.* 1997; **23**: 171–189.

Zussman R. The contribution of sociology to medical ethics. *Hastings Center Rep* 2000; **30**: 7–11.

23

The Use of Thought Experiments in Health Care Ethics

ADRIAN WALSH

INTRODUCTION

One striking feature of much philosophical debate in health care ethics is the extensive use of thought experiments, many of which are highly fanciful. Think, for instance, of James Rachels' defence of euthanasia which involves a hypothetical story concerning two different men, Smith and Jones, both of whom wish to see a cousin killed. In the first case Smith drowns his cousin. In the second, Jones walks into the bathroom with the intention of drowning his cousin, but at the very moment he intends to do so the cousin bumps his head and drowns without Jones laying a finger on his cousin. Both intend to actively terminate the life of their respective cousins, but only one needs to do so. Or for a more fantastical example, think of Judith Jarvis Thomson's article 'A Defense of Abortion' in which some forms of abortion are justified through a series of thought experiments involving, amongst other things, people-seeds that grow in one's carpet and rapidly expanding infants who crush their mothers to death. The use of these stories is particularly striking when one considers the practical nature of the discipline. Indeed, one might well argue that there is something odd about the extensive reliance upon thought experiments in areas of intellectual inquiry that are so obviously oriented towards practical life.

Somewhat surprisingly, there has been little detailed methodological examination of their use in health care ethics or, for that matter, applied ethics more generally. This is somewhat anomalous, especially if we consider other areas of philosophical inquiry, such as the philosophy of science or discussions of theories of personal identity, where there has been significant exploration of the role of thought experiments.

This is not to suggest that in this area of inquiry thought experiments are without their critics. A number of objections have been raised; thought experiments are variously held to be irrelevant, loaded, frivolous and even morally obnoxious. Do they have a legitimate place, then, in health care ethics? Should we agree with Henry Shue's more general suggestion that artificial cases make bad ethics (Shue, 1978)?

In this chapter I explore a number of questions concerning the legitimacy of their use in health care ethics. I begin by considering what a thought experiment is, the very different ways in which thought experiments are employed in arguments and then suggest a taxonomy based on these different uses. I then consider two blanket objections to thought experiments, neither of which I believe succeeds. My response to these objections is that thought experiments have a number of important clarificatory, analytic and explanatory roles to play in health care ethics. At the same time, this is not to say that their usage is always legitimate. Their legitimate uses are determined not so much by the modal content of any actual thought experiment itself, but by the extent to which the argument in which it is nested follows basic tenets of informal logic and respects the fundamental contingency of problems in health care ethics.

THOUGHT EXPERIMENTS AND ARGUMENTS

What exactly is a thought experiment? They are obviously a species of example, but what distinguishes them from, say, a story of derring-do from long ago or a literary example from one of the great novels? Tamar Gendler, examining thought experiments in the philosophy of science, suggests that '[t]o conduct a thought experiment is to make

Principles of Health Care Ethics, Second Edition   Edited by R.E. Ashcroft, A. Dawson, H. Draper and J.R. McMillan
© 2007 John Wiley & Sons, Ltd

a judgement about what would be the case if the particular state of affairs described in some imaginary scenario were actual' (Gendler, 1998, p. 398). Following Gendler's lead, we might define a thought experiment in ethics as involving making a judgement about what would be the case morally if the particular state of affairs described in the imaginary scenario were actual. We are asked to determine the moral status of that state of affairs. In this way thought experiments are distinct from what we might call 'illustrative examples' which simply illustrate or explain a preceding point. The thought experiment has a bigger role to play for it is intended to be part of our deliberative processes.

A further contentious question concerns the role of thought experiments in arguments. In the philosophy of science there has been considerable debate about whether or not a thought experiment is an argument. On one hand, John Norton argues that thought experiments are really just dressed-up arguments (Norton, 1991). But as Rachel Cooper notes in 'Thought Experiments', there are many thought experiments where this cannot be true (Cooper, 2005). Think of Hume's missing shade of blue. Hume asks us to consider whether someone could imagine what a missing shade of blue would look like without ever having seen it (Hume, 1978).

However, whatever is true in the philosophy of science, in ethics thought experiments are not arguments. Think of James Rachels' example of *Smith and Jones* (Rachels, 1975). As it stands this is nothing more than a story and without the background context of the debate over the moral status of active euthanasia, it might just appear like an ironic tale of two people's different fates. It is certainly not an argument. However, in some cases thought experiments function as premises of an argument or lead one to a premise in an argument. Admittedly, sometimes we might infer some conclusions from a story that is told to us, but that will be because of the surrounding context. In such cases we might think of the thought experiment as being the only explicitly articulated element in an enthematic argument. In other cases, a thought experiment functions as a mechanism for framing an argument.

Given this view that thought experiments function either as elements of an argument or to frame an argument, it follows that thought experiments go wrong in two ways. First, they go wrong when they are employed in arguments where conclusions drawn from them are unwarranted on the basis of the evidence provided by the thought experiment and surrounding premises.

Second, they go wrong when they frame the argument in a misleading way. Thought experiments can have remarkable rhetorical effects and often they lead one to lose sight of what was originally at issue.

In either case we might say that the thought experiment is *illicit*. Here it is important that we distinguish 'being illicit'

from *imaginative failure*. For a thought experiment to fail in this way is for it not to have any imaginative grip. For instance, if I am asked to imagine a square circle, I do not know what I am imagining. Rachel Cooper cites Bernard Williams' thought experiment concerning people that split like amoebas as an example of a thought experiment that fails because 'we are unable to answer the necessary "what if" questions' (Cooper, 2005, p. 342). She notes that we can ask the question 'What if people split like amoebas?', but we are unable to answer it. In the moral realm, equally there will be some scenarios for which we cannot determine what we think morally. Our interest, however, is not in cases of *imaginative failure*, but in cases where the use of thought experiments is illicit or pernicious (Gale, 1991). The use of a thought experiment will be illicit when the conclusions drawn from it are not warranted inferentially or when it frames the question in a misleading manner. It is not that any specific kind of thought experiment will be essentially illicit, but rather it will depend upon the argumentative context.

In considering the issue of the role of thought experiments in arguments, we should note the *rhetorical function* of bizarre thought experiments. Often the very strangeness of these thought experiments obscures the role that they are playing in an argument. One struggles just to get one's head around what to think morally in many of these cases, let alone to work out how exactly it might bear on the topic under discussion. The strangeness then hinders us in exercising the critical faculties we might otherwise employ. Similar points can be made about the over-use of thought experiments in an ethical debate. If an interlocutor presents numerous variants of a case, all involving minor changes, then this can sometimes lead the point of the discussion to be lost. Not only are such discussions tedious, but they can also lead participants to lose any sense of the nature of the topic under examination or of what their intuitions might be. Thought experiments should not be the whole method, but rather should be treated as but one tool at the disposal of the health care ethicist.

FOUR DISTINCT WAYS IN WHICH THOUGHT EXPERIMENTS ARE USED

If I am right that thought experiments are typically employed as elements within arguments or in framing the context of an argument, then we should be able to categorize them in terms of the different roles that they do play. I suggest we can distinguish four main types of role in the taxonomy below. (I make no pretence that the list is exhaustive.)

First, some thought experiments function as *clarificatory* devices. Perhaps the most common of these are what we might call *commitment cleavers* where thought experiments are used to enhance understanding by teasing apart distinct but potentially conflated principles. This, I suggest, is the very point of Plato's *Ring of Gyges* example (Plato, 1974), where he discusses what would motivate one to act justly when in possession of a ring by which one can escape detection and hence disapprobation. The point is that one might agree that it is right to act justly and yet it is not clear whether one endorses this as a rule of prudence or as a fundamental moral obligation. By having Glaucon discuss a ring that makes the bearer invisible, Plato provides a device for determining what principle underpins any claim for the necessity of acting justly. Is it prudence or the intrinsic rightness of acting justly? As C.L. Ten notes, such thought experiments help us to 'decide whether a particular principle is fundamental or subordinate' (Ten, 1987, p. 21). In doing so they increase our ability to deal with complicated normative issues.

Second, there is what I want to call *re-imagining*. This is where we use a thought experiment as a device to reframe or refocus a debate. There are a number of reasons why we might wish to do so. For instance, there will be cases where over-familiarity with an ethical issue might lead us no longer to engage in a genuine dialogue with opponents. Abortion debates might well be a case in point. This a topic about which most people will have an opinion. Often the views on either side are so entrenched that those debating the topic are unable to interact in a meaningful way. In such cases, to avoid intellectual stalemate, thought experiments function to reopen debate. Judith Jarvis Thomson's violinist would be a case in point. Thomson asks the reader to imagine that you awake to discover that you have been kidnapped by a group of music lovers and attached to a famous violinist. If you detach yourself from the violinist then he will surely die. The idea is that the case is analogous to a woman who finds herself pregnant after being raped. The fantastical example is intended to make us reassess our views on abortion.

Such reimaginings can also function as mechanisms for avoiding irrelevancy. Often philosophical discussion of ethical issues can be sidetracked by debates over irrelevant legal, historical or technical detail. Imagine that one is involved in a debate over whether it is ever permissible to use weapons of mass destruction. Here one might be tempted to raise the deployment of the atomic bomb on Hiroshima as an example. However, in some instances, such a discussion can turn into an historical debate over the reasons why the bomb was in fact dropped and questions about the normative legitimacy of this kind of action become obscured. In this case it would have been better to have used an imaginary example – even perhaps a highly improbable science fiction example – in order to maintain focus on the questions of general principle. We might call this the 'Star Wars solution'. Discussing a wrong act that is a long way from us often makes it easier to discuss the general principles. Thought experiments are often used for such purposes.

Third, some thought experiments function as *counter-examples* and *reductios*. For instance, one philosopher might present a theory or a definition which is intended to be either necessarily or universally true. In response, the person's opponent provides a counter-example or shows that the theory has absurd consequences (Gale, 1991). These are what Roy Sorenson calls 'refuters', and it goes without saying that not all refuters involve thought experiments (Sorenson, 1992). In ethics these are very common. One writer claims that it is always wrong to steal and in response an interlocutor tells a story of a starving orphan child whose only way of feeding herself is by thieving bread from the rich. This obviously is an example intended to refute the general moral claim.

Finally, there are what I want to call *intuition pumps*. This term has some currency in the literature, though, with no standardized meaning (Sorenson, 1992). Indeed in ethics it often functions simply as a synonym for 'thought experiment'. Herein I define it stipulatively to refer to a particular class of thought experiments in the moral realm that aim to lead us to some general kind of conclusion from our reactions to a single thought experiment. We might think of it as a form of inductive reasoning. One can read Rachels' *Smith and Jones* example here as an intuition pump that aims to convince us that there is no intrinsic moral difference between active and passive euthanasia.

These then are the four main ways in which thought experiments, as a *matter of descriptive fact*, are used in health care ethics. But is their employment legitimate? Are there grounds for thinking that some thought experiments are always illicit in this context? I want to consider now two objections which make such a case.

THE OBJECTION FROM MODALITY

One obvious objection to the use of thought experiments in health care ethics is that they are illicit when they involve modally bizarre cases. Let us call this the 'Objection from Modality'. This is not an objection to *all* thought experiments, but rather to those that involve fanciful examples. The idea is that there are specific kinds of thought experiments – namely the modally bizarre – that are intrinsically inadmissible.

A prime target for this objection would be Judith Jarvis Thomson's people-seeds thought experiment where, in the context of the debate over the morality of abortion, she asks us to imagine a world in which people-seeds float freely about. If we do not keep our windows closed those people-seeds will settle in our carpets and begin to grow into children. She asks whether we would have any moral obligations to provide for such beings and whether it would be permissible to rip out any growing plants that we find in our carpets.

According to the Objection from Modality, this experiment would count as illicit since it involves counter-factuals that invoke possible worlds very distant from our own. On this line of argument, thought experiments in applied ethics can be legitimate, but only in so far as they do not involve modally remote worlds.

Is proximity to our world a way of differentiating between the licit and the illicit? I believe that we should reject this way of drawing the distinction. First, there will be occasions where bizarre examples provide useful re-imagining devices. If we take the abortion debate it is quite clear that, in many instances, the discussants are no longer engaged in a genuine dialogue, for the positions on each side are so fixed. The advantage of a thought experiment like Thomson's is that it allows for dialogue to begin again.

Second, the objection overlooks the role that general moral principles play in discussions by philosophers of topics such as just war, abortion and euthanasia. In attempting to determine the rightness or wrongness of a case, philosophers often appeal to some kind of ethical universal. These principles are presented as universal truths and, indeed, part of their argumentative force comes from their status as moral universals. For instance, pacifists in discussions of just war might appeal to a principle that says killing is always wrong. In considering the merits of the argument, it is quite legitimate to ask, given its presentation as a universal, whether the premise that 'killing is wrong' is true in all possible worlds. Are there any counter-examples to the case? These are legitimate questions to ask. Thus, although applied ethics deals with real-world cases, if an argument regarding such a case relies on a universal moral principle, then it is quite acceptable to test it against possible scenarios, bizarre or otherwise.

This is not to suggest that bizarre thought experiments cannot be illicit. I suggest that legitimacy or otherwise depends upon what role the thought experiment is playing in an argument. There will be cases where the modally bizarre are inappropriate, but this is not because the story is bizarre. Instead, in these cases the bizarre are illicit because the 'evidence' does not warrant the conclusions drawn provided by the thought experiment. There will also be cases where the bizarre over-stretch our intuitive competence and give rise to 'imaginative failure'. Indeed, one might well feel that it is difficult to determine whether it would be wrong, in one of Thomson's case, to pull people-seeds out of one's carpet.

Conversely, on these grounds there will also be more quotidian cases that fail because of the structure of the argument in which they are embedded. Here I think that on one reading of the argument, James Rachels' *Smith and Jones* experiment would be a case in point (Rachels, 1975). Rachels' story, if we accept that there is only the bare difference between actively bringing about X – as opposed to not intervening to prevent X (and no genuine moral difference) – would demonstrate that there is not always a moral difference to be had between the active and the passive. But much more work would be required to show that the difference between active and passive does not hold in the case of euthanasia or does not hold in a wide range of other cases. All that is refuted here is any argument that says that *there is an intrinsic moral difference between active and passive euthanasia because killing is always morally distinct from letting die*. It does not, however, show that there is no intrinsic difference between active and passive euthanasia, as one reading of Rachels' argument would seem to suggest. But this would simply represent a failure of informal reasoning.

When distinguishing legitimate thought experiments from the illegitimate ones we should examine the role that any thought experiment plays in the argument in which it is embedded. It is the relevance of the example to the argument and not the modal distance that is the key here.

THINGS WE SHOULD NOT THINK?

It might also be argued that there is something *morally objectionable* about the use of thought experiments in the context of issues as important as abortion, euthanasia and cloning. We find this attitude famously expressed by G.E.M. Anscombe when she contemptuously writes of the methods of Oxford philosophers. She claims that the examples they use are either banal or fantastic – and of the fantastic she writes that they ask such things as the ones that follows:

> . . . what you ought to do if you had to move forward, and stepping with your right foot meant killing twenty-five fine young men while stepping with your left foot would kill fifty drooling old ones.

She continues:

> Obviously the right thing to do would be to jump and polish off the lot (Anscombe, 1957, p. 267).

Clearly, the point here is that such thought experiments treat morally serious issues in a frivolous manner.

Anscombe would presumably be equally horrified by a great deal of contemporary health care ethics, for there the literature abounds with examples that might be thought to be morally frivolous. Think, for instance, of Michael Tooley's super-kittens case (Tooley, 1983, p. 191) in which cats are given a drug so that they have the rational capacities of persons. It might well be argued that in these thought experiments the content is such that they encourage us to think about non-trivial issues, such as abortion or euthanasia, in a highly insouciant or casual manner. It might even be argued that the very act of engaging with these kinds of examples is morally corrupting in itself:

it would be a case of having 'one thought too many'. One collaborates with vice simply by contemplating the frivolous scenarios raised by such thought experiments.

One might also think that the content of many thought experiments is morally objectionable because they are so structured as to foreclose on any genuine moral engagement with the issues they are intended to illuminate. We might label this the 'Objection from Moral Creativity', and it involves the idea that the highly artificial construction of many thought experiments leaves little space for genuine choice and accordingly we should not have any truck with them since they do not develop our moral sensitivities. Such an objection would most plausibly be directed at our intuition pumps. In these thought experiments, a single case is constructed with the aim of leading us to some more general conclusion and it does so by asking us to choose between the experimenter's favoured choice and some entirely unpalatable alternative. In offering us only Hobson's Choice, the thought experiment fails to foster genuine moral engagement. This is presumably John Stuart Mill's point when he writes that 'A test of right and wrong must be the means, one would think, of ascertaining what is right and wrong, and not a consequence of having already ascertained it' (Mill, 1972, p. 2).

However, I do not believe that either of these objections provides grounds for the complete repudiation of thought experiments, bizarre or otherwise. Let us begin with the accusation of moral frivolity. This objection accords a great deal of moral significance to what it is we imagine. This strikes me as a mistake for it is our genuine and considered moral attitudes that are of greatest importance, and what we imagine is conceptually distinct from those attitudes. For the objection to bite, we require to have a causal connection between the tone of what it is we imagine and our moral modes of regard. But this overestimates the fragility of many of our genuine moral attitudes – merely talking in a frivolous manner about an issue like abortion is unlikely, by itself, to lead us to treat it with a lack of due seriousness.

Further, there will be cases where obtaining some distance from our ingrained moral views – if need be through a slightly jocular tone – is necessary if we are genuinely to *attend* to the case. When dealing with ethical issues, such as euthanasia and stem-cell research, which most of us take to be of great import, a lack of moral seriousness is rarely the problem. The real problem is our dogged unwillingness to engage in a genuine dialogue with those who hold differing views. If a thought experiment through its jocular tone allows us to stand back from the case and re-examine our views in the light of reason, then this can only assist in a genuine moral engagement.

In response to the Objection from Moral Creativity, I would suggest that this objection only has any grip if one views thought experiments as having apodictic force.

On this strong view it is assumed that by engaging with a thought experiment that is highly loaded, one automatically provides one's interlocutor with a 'knockdown argument'. But this is a mistaken view: engaging with a thought experiment – no matter how loaded – does not mean that one has to accept the conclusions drawn by the thought experimenter. There are a number of ways of responding. If we take Thomson's violinist example, one might agree that in this case it would be justifiable to unhook oneself from the violinist, but then argue that there are a number of important *disanalogies* between this case and that of the woman who falls pregnant through rape. Alternatively, one might offer in response a different but related case where our intuitions seem to run in the other direction. The point is that so long as we do not regard the thought experiment as the final word, but rather as an opportunity for continual dialogue, then imagining what it is the thought experimenter wants us to imagine need not stifle our moral creativity.

I would conclude then that these objections do not give grounds for abandoning the use of thought experiments. To be sure, there are other objections one might raise to the use of thought experiments; and space does not permit that we cover even all of the extant ones let alone the possible ones. However, the preceding discussions should provide some indication of possible ways of responding to abolitionist critiques that would eliminate their use altogether. I would suggest that they provide us with extremely valuable intellectual resources and any plausible criticism would need to demonstrate that its concerns outweigh the intellectual benefits that thought experiments bring. Further, given the highly divergent variety of uses to which they are put, it is hard to imagine a criticism that could successfully demonstrate all the different varieties as illicit. I suggest that any genuine criticisms would be of particular uses not their use in general.

THE CONTINGENT CONTEXT OF HEALTH CARE ETHICS

So far in defence of the continued use of thought experiments in health care ethics, I have focused on their usefulness, suggesting that there is nothing intrinsically wrong with their employment. At the same time, I have also stressed that on some occasions their use is illicit. The primary way in which such use is illicit is when they fail to provide the inferential basis for the conclusions which philosophers intend them to support. But notice this: such a constraint could apply to the use of thought experiments in any area of philosophy. I want to add a further constraint that is specific to applied ethics, for there is something special about our deliberative processes in health care ethics that arises out of the very *contingency* of the problems with which such ethicists deal. Although bizarre thought experiments are not illegitimate when they tell us something about the principles we employ, the arguments in which they are 'nested' need to respect the contingency of the context of health care ethics. In this area of inquiry we aim to determine the rightness and wrongness in very particular sets of circumstances. Given that context, our ethical claims do not need to be true in all possible worlds in order to be legitimate. This is not to rule out the possibility that some ethical claims will be true in all possible worlds, but simply that they need not be.

Here we need to exercise some caution, for this might sound rather like a repudiation of the defence of the bizarre in the previous section. The difference here is between the *content* of a thought experiment and the *argumentative context*. It is not that the modal content of the thought experiment fails to respect the contingency of applied ethics, but that the argument in which it is nested does so.

Perhaps an illustration would be helpful at this point. Imagine a debate between a vegetarian and a carnivore on the morality of eating meat. Suppose that the vegetarian says that eating meat is wrong because it involves killing. To this the carnivore responds that he can imagine a scenario in which various cuts of meat are grown in chemical solutions and that no live being is killed in the production of this meat. Is this a legitimate counter-example? It depends upon what our vegetarian is arguing. If the claim is that meat-eating is intrinsically wrong because it always involves killing then this strikes me as a legitimate counter-example. However, if the claim is more muted and the vegetarian simply defends the view that, as it stands, meat-eating involves killing and killing animals is wrong, then I do think the thought experiment is illegitimate. The vegetarian need not be opposed to meat-eating in the hypothetical scenario. Here we also see the rhetorical powers of thought experiments, for the counter-example distracts us from the fundamental question which concerns whether or not killing animals for food is morally justifiable.

Equally, in health care ethics we are dealing with very particular contexts. We are typically asking whether an action in *this particular context* is right or wrong. To answer that question by showing other contexts in which it is permissible will often involve *changing the subject*. For instance, if the topic under discussion was the question of whether it is morally permissible to incarcerate human beings without trial, it would be changing the subject to point to creatures that did not mind being incarcerated. Here we are assuming that the prisoners in question do not differ substantively in terms of their philosophical anthropology from us and do not wish to be in jail.

The wider point is that in health care ethics the *contingent details* of the decision-making context are vitally important,

and thought experiments which overlook these are pernicious. In such cases we stop talking about the rightness or wrongness of a decision in one particular circumstance and end up talking about the moral status of a far broader class of circumstances. To do so is to change the subject. Note that this line of criticism certainly does not rule out bizarre thought experiments, but simply advises us to be cautious of those which lead us to change the topic under discussion. What it involves is simply a repudiation of the philosophical nostrum that any genuine ethical claim, in order to be genuine, must hold true in all logically possible worlds (Jacquette, 1997).

CONCLUDING REMARKS

One common – and entirely understandable – response to the thought experiments employed by many health care ethicists is to refuse absolutely to engage with any of them. This response is most marked when readers are confronted by bizarre imaginary cases such as Thomson's. However, any such response which would have us rule out all thought experiments – or even all bizarre ones – is ultimately mistaken, for it would deny us a very important intellectual resource. Thought experiments have a legitimate role to play in discussions of health care ethics, in focusing our attention on the morally salient features of a moral problem, providing counter-examples to general moral claims and allowing us to re-imagine moral problems that for various reasons have become stale.

This is not to suggest that our use of thought experiments in health care ethics cannot go wrong. First, they are illicit when they are elements of invalid arguments. In addition, there is a second way of going wrong that is specific to both health care ethics and applied ethics. When thought experiments fail to respect the *contingent context* of problems in health care ethics, then here too their use is illicit. On this line of reasoning, legitimacy or illegitimacy is not a property of any thought experiments in itself, but depends upon the argumentative context in which it is embedded.

The upshot of this approach is that if one finds a particular thought experiment wrong-headed, the proper response is not to reject it entirely or to refuse to engage with it. Instead the proper course of action is to seek to discover exactly where the argument goes wrong or why the framing of the argument might be misleading. It would be a genuine mistake for us to stop imagining.

REFERENCES

Anscombe GEM. Does Oxford moral philosophy corrupt youth? *The Listener.* 14 February, 1957; pp. 266–271.
Cooper R. Thought experiments. *Metaphilosophy* 2005; **36**: 328–347.

Gale RM. On some pernicious thought-experiments. In: Horowitz T, Massey G, eds. *Thought Experiments in Science and Philosophy*. Lanham, MD: Rowman & Littlefield, 1991.

Gendler T. Galileo and the indispensability of scientific thought experiment. *Br J Philos Sci* 1998; **49**: 397–424.

Hume D. *A Treatise of Human Nature*. Oxford: Clarendon Press, 1978, first published in 1739.

Jacquette D. Wittgenstein on the transcendence of ethics. *Aust J Philos* 1997; **75**(3): 304–324.

Mill JS. In: Acton HB, ed. *Utilitarianism*, London: JM Dent and Sons, 1972.

Norton J. Thought experiments in Einstein's work. In: Horowitz T, Massey G, eds. *Thought Experiments in Science and Philosophy*. Lanham, MD: Rowman & Littlefield, 1991; 129–148.

Plato. *The Republic* (Translated by Lee D). Harmondsworth: Penguin, 1974.

Rachels J. Active and passive euthanasia. *N Engl J Med* 1975; **292**(2): 78–80.

Shue H. Torture. *Philos Public Aff* 1978; 7(2): 124–143.

Sorenson R. *Thought Experiments*, New York: Oxford University Press, 1992.

Ten CL. *Crime, Guilt and Punishment*. Clarendon Press: Oxford, 1987.

Tooley M. *Abortion and Infanticide*. Clarendon Press: Oxford, 1983.

24

Deliberative Bioethics

MICHAEL PARKER

Our public men have, besides politics, their private affairs to attend to, and our ordinary citizens, though occupied with the pursuits of industry, are still fair judges of public matters; for unlike any other nation, we regard the citizen who takes no part in these duties not as unambitious but as useless, ... instead of looking on discussion as a stumbling-block in the way of action, we think it an indispensable preliminary to any wise action at all (Thucydides II.40).

INTRODUCTION

Bioethics is, in all its manifestations, political. It is most clearly and explicitly so in the deliberations of international bodies such as CIOMS or the World Medical Association, national bioethics commissions such as the President's Council on Bioethics, governmental advisory groups such as the UK's Human Genetics Commission and national organizations of other, related kinds such as the Nuffield Council on Bioethics. Bioethics is also political when it concerns the regulation of medical research through the deliberations of IRBs and the regulation of medical practice, whether through formal bodies such as the Human Fertilization and Embryology Authority and the General Medical Council, professional associations such as the American Medical Association, and less formal mechanisms such as clinical ethics committees and clinical ethicists or through the education of medical students and practising health professionals. Bioethics is also political when it manifests itself in the development of policy by health care organizations (for example, in their criteria for eligibility for treatment, referral criteria for intensive care and so on) and in the making of clinical decisions in day-to-day health care practice.

Bioethics is in all its manifestations political, above all, because it concerns the normative analysis of social institutions and practices and the negotiation of normative relationships between the private and the public and between the social and the biological and by virtue of the fact that these relationships, structures and practices concern key moments and features of human (and animal) life: such as the relationships between the public and the private, sexuality, death and birth. Bioethics is political because in all its manifestations it is constituted by clusters of normative, value-driven activities with implications for people's lives and their environment.

This chapter discusses approaches to bioethics in which the political is foregrounded, in which it is argued that public discussion should be central to the identification and analysis of bioethical issues, and which call for the development of approaches based on the concept of an inclusive deliberative democracy, contrasting these to approaches addressing ethical issues through other democratic methods, or applying deontological analysis or consequentialist calculation by experts *ex situ*.

WHAT IS DELIBERATIVE DEMOCRACY?

Deliberative approaches to bioethics draw upon concepts with their origins in theories of deliberative democracy in political philosophy. These two concepts, 'democracy' and 'deliberation', are, as shall be seen below, contested. However, the deliberative and democratic approaches also have much in common. The concept of 'democracy' in both political philosophy and bioethics arises out of the belief that decisions affecting people's lives should be made by those people themselves or their representatives rather than by, for example, bioethicists. The 'deliberative' part of

Principles of Health Care Ethics, Second Edition   Edited by R.E. Ashcroft, A. Dawson, H. Draper and J.R. McMillan
© 2007 John Wiley & Sons, Ltd

deliberative democracy relates to the ways in such decisions are to be reached. There are two main democratic methods by which the preferences of people might be reflected in decision-making. The first of these is through the aggregation of preferences, that is, by means of voting, bargaining or some combination of the two. Deliberative approaches to democracy are by contrast based on the belief that democratic decision-making should be pursued not through the aggregation of preferences but through their transformation in deliberation. Advocates of deliberative democracy hold that democratic decision-making is legitimate only to the extent that it is the result of argument and the use of public reason by free and equal citizens (Bohman, 1996).

Bringing these two ideas together, John Elster defines deliberative democracy as follows:

> . . . collective decision-making with the participation of all who will be affected by the decision or their representatives: this is the democratic part. Also, all [proponents of deliberative democracy] agree that it includes decision making by means of arguments offered by and to participants who are committed to the values of rationality and impartiality: this is the deliberative part (Elster, 1998, p. 8).

In addition to requiring that deliberation be free and equal, advocates of deliberative democracy place a number of further constraints on what is to count as legitimate decision-making. The first of these constraints is, as the quotation above suggests, that deliberation should involve the transformation of preferences through the use of persuasion or reason by participants who are committed to impartiality and rationality, and not by methods involving coercion or deception.

> Deliberation as a social process is distinguished from other kinds of communication in that deliberators are amenable to changing their judgements, preferences, and views during the course of their interactions, which involve persuasion rather than coercion, manipulation, or deception (Dryzek, 2000, p. 1).

Additional constraints typically include the requirement that deliberation be transparent, accessible to all and ideally take place in public; the requirement that deliberation be based in appeal to principles that people who are committed to finding fair terms of co-operation would accept; the requirement that when consensus is not possible deliberation should aim to find solutions that minimize conflict; and the requirement that the decisions should be for a limited time period only and should be open to revision.

Those who advocate deliberative democracy claim that it has a number of advantages over aggregative approaches such as voting. First, the use of deliberation and of public reason involving those who will be affected, especially where this results in consensus, lends decisions greater legitimacy than other methods, for example, voting or bargaining. Second, the fact that deliberation takes place in public among all who will be affected encourages the use of particular modes of justifying and expressing demands. Third, public deliberation leads to the generation of new ideas, arguments and options that would not be possible in private deliberation (Fearon, 1998). Fourth, the use of public reason can draw people out of narrow, personal or parochial interests and encourage them to see the merits of broader public and community concerns. Relatedly, and fifth, public deliberation reveals private information and the views of marginal groups that would otherwise not be taken account of in decision-making. Sixth, some deliberative democrats argue that deliberation makes it more likely that a broad consensus will be achieved. Seventh, deliberative democrats argue that decisions made as a result of the use of deliberation will in most cases be better in many respects including, for example, in relation to distributive justice. Eighth, it is argued that deliberation leads to the correction of false beliefs and invalid arguments. Finally, and importantly, it is argued that deliberative approaches promote respectful decision-making (Elster, 1998).

TYPES OF DELIBERATIVE DEMOCRACY

I have suggested that the key concepts in deliberative democracy are contested, and I shall return to some of the detail of these contestations in a moment. But first, following Gutmann and Thompson, I set out some of the key broad areas of methodological difference within deliberative approaches (Gutmann and Thompson, 2004).

INSTRUMENTAL OR EXPRESSIVE?

Some of the advantages claimed for deliberative approaches set out above are instrumental in nature, for example, decisions will be less subject to error because they will have been tested publicly. Many advocates of deliberative democracy argue that its value lies not in substantive reasons but solely or primarily in the fact that deliberation leads to better and more justified decisions of these kinds. These are *instrumentalist* approaches. Other advocates argue that whilst it may well be true that deliberative democracy leads to better and more justified decisions, the key reason why deliberative approaches are of value is because they embody a recognition of respect for persons, that is, people should be treated not simply as the objects of legislation but as autonomous, if socially embedded, agents capable of taking part in the governance of the societies within which they live their lives. The deliberative approach is valuable on this account because it is a manifestation of the value of mutual respect. These are *expressive* approaches.

These two approaches can on occasion overlap; for example, it may be argued by some that it is the fact that such processes express mutual respect that enables them to lead to better decisions.

PROCEDURAL OR SUBSTANTIVE?

Some approaches to deliberation are *procedural*. That is, although they specify the procedures by which decisions should be made, for example, that such decisions should be made in public, they do not attempt to prescribe or limit the outcomes of such deliberation. One of the criticisms sometimes made against procedural approaches is that they can offer no guarantee that procedures will not lead to unjust or unethical decisions. Those who adopt *substantive* approaches to deliberation (often also those who adopt expressive positions) argue that unjust and unethical decisions should not be possible on any adequate account of democracy, and for this reason substantive approaches to deliberation will place constraints on the legitimate outcomes of deliberation, often justifying these constraints in terms of consistency with the underlying expressive approach.

CONSENSUAL OR PLURALIST?

Many approaches to deliberation are based on the idea that deliberation offers the possibility of achieving some level of *consensus* in an increasingly pluralist and complex world. This consensus may take the form of agreement about the substance of the decisions made, or about the mode of decision-making. The claim here is that consensus should be sought wherever possible, and where it is not possible decisions should be made in ways that are both open to revision and also accepted as made fairly, by those who would have chosen otherwise. *Pluralist* approaches resist the push to consensus and argue that the aim of deliberation should be to find fair and inclusive ways of living with diversity. The pursuit of consensus is on the pluralist account both tyrannical and futile in contemporary societies. Consensualists criticize pluralist approaches on the grounds that if deliberation is to be justified at all it must, at least in part, be by appeal to some core even if minimal set of universal values, for example, respect for persons.

CRITIQUES OF DELIBERATIVE DEMOCRACY

Deliberative approaches to democracy and bioethics of these various types have been subject to a number of more specific critiques. Many of these have been the result of internal debate between advocates of deliberation who adopt different positions in relation to the above broad distinctions. Some have been external. In what follows, the key critical themes are identified and related to the broad areas of contestation described above.

DELIBERATIVE DEMOCRACY SACRIFICES MORAL PRINCIPLES SUCH AS JUSTICE TO DEMOCRACY

An important criticism of approaches to moral decision-making based on democracy, and in particular, of those based on procedural variants of deliberative democracy, is that they sacrifice important moral principles to democracy or to agreement. The fact that a decision has been made by those who will be affected does not, it is argued, make it right, nor does the rightness of a decision increase with increasing proximity to unanimity or to consensus (Nino, 1996). Substantive and expressive approaches are less susceptible to such criticism than procedural accounts because they are based on moral claims which constrain the outcomes of deliberation, but such approaches are vulnerable to another critique which is that if substantive principles can be established prior to deliberation and as a condition for its possibility, is not deliberation redundant? (Raz, 1998).

THE DELIBERATIVE APPROACH IS 'CIRCULAR'

The critique from redundancy relates to another, that of *circularity*. Deliberation requires, for deliberative democrats, the involvement of free and equal citizens. We do not live in just societies where people are free and equal and this suggests that deliberative approaches will not be possible until such societies have been established. A just society can, from a deliberative perspective, only be established through the deliberations of free and equal citizens and this is, to complete the circle, impossible because we live in societies which are neither just nor free. One response to this criticism would be to adopt a developmental approach wherein the creation of societies in which deliberation is possible is achieved by the progressive inclusion of people in decision-making in ways which approximate as closely as possible to situations of free and equal deliberation.

IT IS NOT POSSIBLE TO EXCLUDE POWER FROM DELIBERATION

Notwithstanding the difficult question of how in practice it might be achieved, the deliberative approach to democracy does depend, ultimately, upon the possibility of the free and equal involvement of citizens. Some critics of deliberative approaches argue that free and equal deliberation is an incoherent and unrealistic fantasy. Such critics argue that it is not possible to exclude bias and power from deliberative forums not only because of existing structural social inequalities but also because deliberative discourse is itself the very expression and embodiment of the power it purports to neu-tralize (Shapiro, 1999). In addition to this broad sociologi-cal critique, of which more later, three related practical cri-tiques are often made of deliberative approaches: that some people are less able to participate, that some people will be excluded from deliberation, and that some modes of expres-sion will be excluded.

SOME PEOPLE ARE LESS ABLE TO PARTICIPATE

Many who would agree with the democratic imperative that decisions should be made by those who are to be affected, nevertheless draw attention to the fact that even if it were in fact possible to ensure that everyone who was subject to a decision was able to participate in the deliberative process, it would inevitably be the case that some would find this easier than others. Deliberation and the use of argument in a de-liberative setting are, it is argued, elitist and more suited to seminars than to the kinds of settings and discussions with which most people are familiar and comfortable. This means that even if everyone were in a position to participate, the arguments of the more educated and articulate would still be likely to carry the day. Some citizens are simply better than others at articulating their views and concerns, and this means that the proposed benefits of deliberation, for ex-ample, that a diversity of voices would be heard and taken seriously and that all perspectives would be included, is highly unlikely to manifest itself in practice. Whilst every-one might be present, the usual groups, that is, those from ethnic minorities, women, the poor and the children, would be likely to be overlooked. Furthermore, there is very good empirical evidence that, quite apart from their abilities at de-liberation, the perspectives of some citizens are systemati-cally privileged in public discourse and the perspectives of others systematically suppressed (Sanders, 1997). The fact is that some people will be ignored no matter how good their reasons are. Furthermore, there is danger too for the delibera-tive approach in the persuasive power of rhetoric and of the charismatic speaker (Plato, 1971). To what extent in practice will the exercise of free and equal reason rather than rhetoric, deception or manipulation carry the day?

SOME MODES OF EXPRESSION ARE EXCLUDED

To what extent *should* reason carry the day? Just why is it that arguing is thought to be a better way of making deci-sions than other ways? Many critiques of deliberative ap-proaches, both internal and external, criticize deliberation on the grounds that it excludes modes of expression of other kinds that might also be capable of inducing reflection, of expressing otherwise un-witnessed perspectives and of capturing important and potentially neglected testimony

(Bohman, 1996). Deliberative approaches to democracy, it is argued, exclude, by definition, modes of expression that are passionate, extreme, fragmentary, non verbal, 'unrea-sonable' or the product of particular narrow interests. Is it always and necessarily the case that such modes of expres-sion are undermining rather than enriching of public reason and decision-making?

> Nor should deliberative theories be considered one-sidedly rationalistic. Many different 'self-governing capacities are necessary if citizens are to participate effectively in public deliberation and dialogue, including understanding, imagining, valuing, desiring, storytelling, and the use of rhetoric and argumentation (Bohman, 1996, p. 7).

The emphasis, indeed the insistence, on reason and argu-ment, it is argued by critics, is not only a failure of democ-racy but also potentially an epistemological/ontological failure of the deliberative approach because the exclusion of certain modes of expression and voices of certain kinds leads inevitably to the exclusion of certain views, beliefs, opinions, concerns and values, which may be of profound ontological and epistemological significance (Nino, 1996).

EXCLUDES SOME PEOPLE

The previous sections have highlighted critiques of delib-erative approaches which suggest that explicit power struc-tures and implicit or informal norms lead to the exclusion of the voices of some and privileges of others. It is also likely, however, that deliberative processes will exclude some citi-zens from deliberation altogether. This might occur as bias in representation and participation as a result of working arrangements, childcare availability, the times and location of meetings, poverty and so on. This suggests that there may be structural inequalities in societies which lead to greater participation among some groups than others.

DELIBERATION IS NOT PRACTICAL

In addition to criticisms based on concerns about justice, some proponents of alternative approaches to democracy criticize deliberative approaches for being unrealistic and impractical and for failing to take account of the actual practice of real democracy (Bohman, 1996). This criticism is often particularly aimed at highly idealized procedural approaches to deliberation. Many advocates of procedural approaches to deliberation do so, at least in part, on the grounds of the failure of other models to deal with the complexity of modern life.

> Under modern conditions of life none of the various rival traditions can claim prima facie general validity any longer. Even in answering questions of direct practical relevance, convincing reasons can no longer appeal to the authority of unquestioned traditions (Habermas, 1993, p. 151).

Whilst advocates such as Habermas argue that deliberation is needed just because such diversity exists, the fact that societies are pluralistic can also present a significant obstacle to processes of public reason however and critics question the practical feasibility of deliberative approaches in modern pluralistic and complex societies. The critique here is that even if deliberation might work in some cases, this is likely to be in relatively homogeneous groups and societies.

Another practical reason why deliberative approaches might fail, even if the above problems were to be addressed, is because of public disaffection with democracy and politics, reluctance to get involved or lack of interest in participation (deliberation fatigue) (Dolan, 1999; Litva et al., 2002).

What these 'practical' critiques suggest is that a workable and coherent approach to deliberation is only going to be possible where it is grounded in a good understanding of key empirical facts concerning the nature of pluralism and social complexity, public attitudes to and experiences of deliberation, mechanisms of social exclusion, structures and mechanisms of inequality and the most effective and inclusive models of deliberation (Abelson et al., 2003).

WHAT IS THE SCOPE OF DELIBERATIVE DEMOCRACY?

If decisions affecting people's lives are legitimate to the extent to which they have been subjected to public deliberation by all of those who will be affected, this raises the question of what ought to be the scope of deliberation? Many decisions affecting people's lives are currently considered 'private' or 'familial'. To what extent can, and ought, this distinction be maintained within the context of a deliberative theory? The boundaries between the public and the private are in practice socially constructed, neither fixed for all time nor clearly demarcated. Some aspects of what was formally thought of as private, for example, aspects of human reproduction, have increasingly become subject to the public gaze and public policy in recent years. To what extent should deliberation be a feature of all decision-making permeating all aspects of social life? To what extent should it be solely a feature of governments and other public institutions? (Gutmann and Thompson, 2004, p. 46). Such questions are of particular importance to bioethics which often deals with highly 'personal' or 'familial' decisions and the boundaries between the public and the private.

DEEP SCEPTICISM: DELIBERATIVE DEMOCRACY AS A MECHANISM FOR DOMINATION AND CONTROL

The prospect of the increasing intrusion of deliberation into the nooks and crannies of all aspects of human life,

particularly when combined with concerns about the exclusion of certain voices and modes of expression discussed above, raises another, Foucauldian, concern about deliberative approaches which is that the call for deliberation is nothing more than the disguised exercise of power, the broadening imposition of liberal egalitarian preferences and values on increasingly pluralistic, complex societies, and the production of relationships and self-identities of particular, problematic kinds (Fish, 1999). Stokes, for example, refers to a number of *pathologies of deliberation* (Stokes, 1998). These include the possibility that deliberative approaches can promote the inculcation of beliefs promoting vested interests and undermining the well-being of those who are involved and the possibility that once participants buy into the rules of the game of deliberation they may already have taken on ideas that will make them worse off both politically and materially (Przeworski, 1998). Stokes also argues that the exclusion of modes of expression other than reason has the potential to undermine the sense of identity and self-worth of people, leading to changes in their identities which may in some cases, most likely in those who are already at the margins of societies, reduce their sense of capability and increase their vulnerability further still. Furthermore, when considered against a background of gross inequality in wealth, capabilities and representation, it is sometimes argued that the pursuit of the common good and of compromise around liberal ideals must be seen as a form of domination. Indeed, as Sanders argues, in situations of gross inequalities to power and status, calling for compromise comes close to requiring the suppression of the perspectives of minority groups (Sanders, 1997). Relatedly, it is argued that the deliberative approaches to decision-making which focus on the achievement of consensus or agreement on the terms of co-operation based upon the creation of methods of communication across difference have the potential to lead to the erasure of difference or to give the impression that difference about fundamental values is essentially provisional or unimportant.

AN AGENDA FOR A DELIBERATIVE BIOETHICS

I have described the main principles underpinning deliberative democracy and its incorporation into bioethics and some of the main criticisms of such approaches. In what follows I consider how an advocate of a deliberative approach to decision-making in bioethics might respond to these critiques of deliberative democracy. In doing so, I describe five techniques for the development of a substantive and pluralist model of deliberative bioethics, grounded in, and constrained by: respect for persons; reflexivity; focusing on listening to and capturing marginalized voices, modes of expression and overlooked narratives; resisting the erasure of difference; the importance of 'thick description'; and adopting a critical perspective.

REFLEXIVITY

Recognition of the political dimensions of bioethics and of the potential dangers of deliberation demands, of those who practise it, reflexivity about the political and social roles of bioethics itself. The bioethical is political because it 'shares in the power of the professional complex of medicine', and reflexivity requires of bioethicists that they be aware of and explicitly question the political and social role of bioethics and their own practice (Dzur, 2002).

FOCUS ON LISTENING TO AND CAPTURING MARGINALIZED VOICES, MODES OF EXPRESSION AND OVERLOOKED NARRATIVES

The criticisms mentioned above highlight a possible tension between the democratic and deliberative impulses informing deliberative democratic approaches to bioethics. Although the deliberative imperative calls for the impartial use of reason and justification, the democratic imperative demands the inclusion of diverse voices and marginal modes of expression. This suggests that any coherent account of deliberative democracy in bioethics is going to require a trade-off between these two concerns. The need for reflexivity suggests that the nature of any trade-off and the grounds for it should be made explicit. The limits of this trade-off will be determined on one hand by the need to rule out domination/coercion and on the other by the need to include as diverse a constituency as possible.

> A more tolerant position, which I favour, would allow argument, rhetoric, humour, emotion, testimony or storytelling, and gossip. The only key condition for authentic deliberation is then the requirement that communication induces reflection upon preferences in non-coercive fashion. This requirement in turn rules out domination via the exercise of power, manipulation, indoctrination, propaganda, deception, expressions of mere self-interest, threats (of the sort that characterize bargaining), and attempts to impose ideological conformity (Dryzek, 2000, p. 1).

RESISTING THE ERASURE OF DIFFERENCE

The criticism mentioned above also suggests that in addition to its overemphasis on reasoning and rationality, deliberation is also in danger where it focuses too much on the achievement of consensus and agreement at the expense of inclusivity. Some space needs to be preserved for disagreement,

conflict and difference if the benefits, both democratic and epistemological, of deliberation are to be gained (Bohman, 1996). This suggests the need for an explicitly and self-consciously pluralistic approach.

> ...deliberative democracy should be pluralistic in embracing the necessity to communicate across difference without erasing difference, reflexive in its questioning orientation to established traditions (including the tradition of deliberative democracy itself), transnational in its capacity to extend across state boundaries into settings where there is no constitutional framework, ecological in terms of openness to communication with non-human nature, and dynamic in its openness to ever-changing constraints upon and opportunities for democratisation (Dryzek, 2000, p. 3).

THE IMPORTANCE OF 'THICK DESCRIPTIONS'

The previous two sections, on the need for awareness of difference and the requirement to listen to marginalized voices, have each suggested the need for a rich empirical dimension to bioethics (Bohman, 1996). Furthermore, criticisms of deliberative approaches highlighting the requirement for bioethics to capture marginalized voices, respect difference and encourage diversity of modes of expression suggest that this empirical dimension ought to be concerned, in major part, with what Clifford Geertz calls 'thick description' and will perhaps best be achieved through the incorporation of ethnographic methods into bioethics (Geertz, 1973).

Supporting this view, Dzur also argues that bioethics should draw upon ethnographic research in order to locate persons more fully and richly and to make sense of their moral reasoning and their modes of expression in relation to their context.

> Methods of ethnography like participant observation, close reading and interpretation of informants' narratives can provide a 'thick description' of ethical contexts (Dzur, 2002, p. 198)

> Ethnography means two things here: an inquiry into the life, relationships, and beliefs of patients needing consultation and an inquiry into the very construction of ethical choices in the medical domain. Together, these focus bioethnography on the normative expectations of pluralistic sensitivity and micro- and macro-level attentiveness (Dzur, 2002, p. 196).

In relation to the possible dangers arising out of the exclusion of marginal groups, one of the key values for deliberative bioethics of ethnographic approaches is that they also offer the possibility of describing,

> ... as thickly as possible how ethical problems are ignored, unattended, recognized, managed, and resolved in medical settings (Bosk, 1999, p. 64).

Arthur Kleinmann offers a four-stage model for ethnographic approaches to ethics along something like these lines. He argues that an ethnographic bioethics will involve self-reflexivity, thick description, deliberation and debate (Kleinmann, 1999). Kleinmann's 'stages' provide a reminder that description alone, no matter how thick, cannot lead to the deliberative resolution of normative questions in bioethics and suggest that an ethnographic bioethics requires in addition the creation of ethnographically oriented deliberative forums.

ADOPTING A CRITICAL ORIENTATION

In addition to the incorporation of emphases on reflexive practice and on the use of high quality ethnographic research methodologies, a bioethics that is concerned to resist the marginalization of different voices, perspective and modes of expression will, if it is to induce reflection and generate deliberation, need to adopt a constructive but self consciously critical approach to established, agreed and uncontested practices, attitudes and beliefs.

> ... a defensible theory of deliberative democracy must be critical in its orientation to established power structures, including those that operate under the constitutional surface of the liberal state, and so insurgent in relation to established institutions (Dryzek, 2000, p. 2).

> I have argued that the promise of democratic authenticity held by the deliberative turn can only be redeemed to the extent of a critical orientation to established power structures. Recall that the authenticity of deliberation requires that communication must induce reflection upon preferences in non-coercive fashion. This means, to begin, an emphasis on the contestation of discourses in the public sphere, rather than exclusive reliance on the deliberative institutions of the liberal state (Dryzek, 2000, p. 162).

CONCLUSION

In this chapter I have described some of the key features of theoretical and practical considerations informing deliberative approaches to bioethics. I have also discussed some of the most important criticisms of such approaches and have, in the light of these critiques, proposed five techniques which offer the possibility of the development of a bioethic which is empirically rich, deliberative, democratic and radical.

REFERENCES

Abelson J, Forest PG, Eyles J, Smith P, Martin E, Gauvin FP. Deliberations about deliberative methods: issues in the design and evaluation of public participation processes. *Social Sci Med* 2003; **57**(2): 239–251.

Bohman J. *Public Deliberation – Pluralism, Complexity and Democracy*. Cambridge, MA: The MIT Press, 1996.

Bosk C. *Professional Ethicist Available: Logical, Secular, Friendly*, vol. 128. Daedalus, 1999; pp. 47–68.

Dolan P, Cookson R, Ferguson B. Effect of discussion and deliberation on the public's views of priority setting in health care: focus group study. *Br Med J* 1999; **318**: 916–919.

Dryzek J. *Deliberative Democracy and Beyond: Liberals, Critics, Contestations*. Oxford: Oxford University Press, 2000.

Dzur A. Democractizing the hospital: deliberative-democratic bioethics. *J Health Polit Policy Law* 2002; **27**(2): 177–211.

Elster J, ed. *Deliberative Democracy*. Cambridge: Cambridge University Press, 1998.

Fearon JD. In: Elster J, ed. *Deliberation as Discussion*, 1998; pp. 44–68.

Fish S. Mutual respect as a device of exclusion. In: Stephen M, ed. *Deliberative Politics*. Oxford University Press, 1999.

Geertz C. *The Interpretation of Cultures*. New York: Basic Books, 1973.

Gutmann A, Thomson D. *Why Deliberative Democracy?* Princeton, NJ: Princeton University Press, 2004.

Habermas J. *Justification and Application: Remarks on Discourse Ethics*. Oxford: Polity, 1993.

Kleinmann A. *Moral Experience and Ethical Reflection: Can Ethnography Reconcile Them?* vol. 128. Daedalus, 1999; pp. 69–98.

Litva A, Coast J, Donovan J, Eyles J, Shepherd M, Tacchi J, Abelson J, Morgan K. The public is too subjective: public involvement at different levels of health-care decision making. *Soc Sci Med* 2002; **54**: 1825–1837.

Nino CS. *The Constitution of Deliberative Democracy*. New Haven, CT: Yale University Press, 1996.

Plato. *Gorgias*. London: Penguin Books, 1971.

Przeworski A. In: Elster J, ed. *Deliberation and Ideological Domination*, 1998; pp. 140–160.

Raz, J. Disagreement in politics. *Am J Jurispr* 1998; **43**: 25–52.

Sanders LM. Against deliberation. *Political Theory* 1997; **25**(3): 347–376.

Shapiro I. Enough of deliberation. In: Stephen M, ed. *Deliberative Politics*. London: Oxford University Press, 1999.

Stokes S. In: Elster J, ed. *Pathologies of Deliberation*. 1998; pp. 123–139.

Thucydides. Peleponnesian War, vol. II (Translated by Lattimore S). Indianapolis: Hackett, 1998; p. 40.

25

Law, Ethics and Health Care

SHEILA A.M. McLEAN

INTRODUCTION

The growth of 'ethics talk' in health care is a relatively recent phenomenon. It has now been widely recognized that ethics means considerably more than 'professional ethics' or 'etiquette'. At the same time, there has been a significant growth in an extent to which the law regulates practices which would in the past have been left broadly within the remit of health care professionals. Legislation such as the Human Fertilisation and Embryology Act 1990, the creation of regulatory bodies such as NICE and, of course, the Human Rights Act 1998 have circumscribed the capacity of individual health care practitioners to deliver services in certain areas based purely on their professional judgement. Oddly, however, beyond recognition of the so-called litigation explosion, it is common to elide law and ethics, with ethics often seemingly given centre stage.

THE RELATIONSHIP BETWEEN LAW AND ETHICS

The leading UK textbook on medical law and ethics (Mason and McCall Smith's Law and Medical Ethics) has over the years used a quotation from an elderly legal case as a form of introduction to the relationship between law and ethics or morals. Quoting Lord Wilberforce in the case of *R v Instan*, the authors (Mason and Laurie, 2006) – presumably with approval – use his description of this relationship:

> It would not be correct to say that every moral obligation involves a legal duty; but every legal duty is founded on a moral obligation.

With respect, this characterization may have been appropriate in the nineteenth century, but it is arguably of little purchase in the twenty-first century. It is all too easy to think of legal duties which are only tangentially (if at all) linked to a moral obligation. For example, the law requiring the licensing of motor vehicles would not seriously be argued as being based on a moral obligation. To be sure, it may serve a pragmatic social function, but the obligation to register as a vehicle owner, or to pay road tax, is an artefact rather than a truly moral obligation. We must, therefore, look beyond Lord Wilberforce's definition.

It is also important to note that law is not one homogeneous monolith; it comes in a variety of shapes and sizes and the extent to which it informs or is informed by ethical evaluation may well differ (Montgomery, 2003; McLean, and Mason, 2003). For example, it is possible to create legislatively a structure or system which has purely pragmatic – even self-serving – aims. One example might be the council tax. We pay this as an obligation to the state, but arguably there is no over-arching, underlying moral principle associated with it; rather, it is a device to ensure that services can be paid for irrespective of whether or not we believe these services are to be based on morality and irrespective of whether or not we approve of them. Of course, some legislation does seem to have a clear ethical basis – the Human Fertilisation and Embryology Act, for example, was based on a report which took clear views on the ethics of assisted reproduction and embryo research. Equally, the recent report from the House of Commons Select Committee on Science and Technology, Reproductive Technologies and the Law (2005) takes a clear ethical stance in its recommendations on the future legal regulation of assisted reproduction services.

Perhaps the link between ethics and the law is most evident, however, in the common law. Common, or judge-made, law – unlike legislation – depends on an iterative process; that is, when faced with novel situations, judges will seek historical support for a particular position, but must

Principles of Health Care Ethics, Second Edition   Edited by R.E. Ashcroft, A. Dawson, H. Draper and J.R. McMillan
© 2007 John Wiley & Sons, Ltd

also on occasion work from basic principles which – in the area of medical law at least – will often be clearly ethical in nature. In the case of *Airedale NHS Trust v Bland* ((1993) 12 BMLR 64), for example, Lord Browne-Wilkinson said, 'behind the questions of law lie moral, ethical, medical and practical issues of fundamental importance to society' (1993, p. 124).

Indeed, such is the growth of new and complex decisions confronting the courts that some judges have expressed their concern that they are increasingly being invited to make decisions which contain significant ethical questions; matters which, for at least some of the judiciary, should be decided by Parliament rather than by courts.

For example, in the case of *R (on the application of Pretty) v DPP* ((2001) 63 BMLR 1), Lord Bingham in the House of Lords said:

> In discharging the judicial functions of the House, the appellate committee has the duty of resolving issues of law properly brought before it, as the issues in this case have been. The committee is not a legislative body. Nor is it entitled or fitted to act as a moral or ethical arbiter.

One of the most important debates on the relationship between the state (as personified by the law) and the ethical dimensions of individual behaviour was that between Hart (1963) and Lord Devlin (1965), which focused on the report of the Committee on Homosexual Offences and Prostitution (the Wolfenden Committee) (Cmd 247/1957). Although it is not intended to provide an in-depth analysis of this debate here, a couple of comments from it serve to highlight the important issues raised in this context. The question related to the extent to which the law – in this case the criminal law – should be used to constrain practices felt to be immoral. Lord Devlin, for example, said 'the question is not how a person is to ascertain the morality which he adopts and follows, but how the law is to ascertain the morality which it enforces (1965, p. x).' This is an extremely important assertion as it leaves open the possibility that even behaviour of which we morally disapprove may not be an appropriate subject for law or criminalization. Equally, the mere fact that there is an identifiable, common moral position may not be sufficient to render its translation into law appropriate, even in societies which pride themselves on democracy or majority rule. As Hart said:

> It seems fatally easy to believe that loyalty to democratic principles entails acceptance of what may be termed moral populism: the view that the majority have a moral right to dictate how all should live...The central mistake is a failure to distinguish the acceptable principle that political power is best entrusted to the majority from the unacceptable claim that what the majority do with that power is beyond criticism and

must never be resisted. No one can be a democrat who does not accept the first of these, but no democrat need accept the second (Hart, 1963, p. 79).

Thus, although disagreeing on some matters, both Hart and Devlin agree that law need not always be involved in matters which are based on morality; that some aspects of life, even if disapproved of by the majority, should be left outside of legal regulation or scrutiny. This was echoed in the US case of *McFall v Shimp* ((1978) 127 Pitts Leg J 14), in which a man refused to agree to make a potentially life-saving donation to a relative. As the court said:

> Morally, this decision rests with the defendant, and in the view of the court, the refusal of the defendant is morally indefensible. For our law to *compel* the defendant to submit to an intrusion of his body would change every concept and principle upon which our society is founded. To do so would defeat the sanctity of the individual...

The ultimate conclusion that the state should not seek to constrain private (im)morality reflects the views of thinkers such as J.S. Mill (and is interestingly highly influential in the House of Commons Report mentioned above). It is, however, not universally followed, as we shall see. For example, in the case of *R v Brown*, a group of homosexual men engaged, in private, in sado-masochistic sexual practices. They were charged and convicted under the terms of the Offences Against the Person Act 1861. Mason and Laurie note that the decision was hotly debated in the academic literature (for discussion see Mason and Laurie 2006, para 2.16). For present purposes, what is important is that this conviction, which was upheld in the European Court of Human Rights (*Laskey, Jaggard and Brown v United Kingdom* ((1997) 24 EHRR 39), seems to suggest that the criminal law is *in fact* closely intermeshed with morality; that our disapproval of behaviour which harmed only the participants was sufficient to render consensual, private – albeit injurious – behaviour reached the standard required for being a criminal offence, although this was subsequently rejected in a later, similar case (*ADT v United Kingdom* (2001) EHRR 33). As Mason and Laurie say, this is a question that tests the role of the criminal justice system, which they describe as 'society's most overt commitment to the protection of its citizens..' at para 2.14 Although jurisprudence in this area has at times been unsatisfactory, recent cases involving the knowing transmission of sexually transmitted diseases seem to have clarified the extent to which society will take action against someone whose behaviour is essentially immoral by bringing the forces of the criminal law to bear on it (*R v Dica* [2004] 3 All ER 593).

MORALS OR LAW IN ACTION?

From what has gone before, we can see that the relationship between ethics and law is complex. Manifestly, they do not need to equate to or inform each other, but in some cases the impact of moral values on the law is clear. Although it might be anticipated that this would be for the good, in fact when morality intrudes into the law's development, the result can sometimes be perverse. The area of 'maternal/ foetal conflict' is one such example.

As was true in the case of *McFall v Shimp* referred to above, we might morally disapprove of certain behaviour, but the question remains as to whether or not we should impose that moral intuition by law; in other words, should we, in Lord Wilberforce's words, equate a moral obligation to a legal duty? This question became very real when the law began to intervene in the management of pregnancy and labour.

In the United States, for example, some women were compulsorily detained because of their 'inappropriate' behaviour during pregnancy and because of the perceived risk to the foetuses they were carrying (Kolder et al., 1987). Moreover, at the moment of birth, non-consensual caesarean sections were carried out in some cases, perhaps most significantly in the case of a young woman called Angela Carder. Ms Carder had suffered from leukaemia which had gone into remission. She married and became pregnant, but sadly in the course of the pregnancy her leukaemia returned and she became terminally ill. At first, she rejected certain treatment for herself in order – hopefully – to bring the pregnancy nearer to term, thereby increasing the chances of the foetus surviving *ex vivo*. However, at about 26 weeks into the pregnancy she became very ill and her doctors decided that she should undergo a caesarean section to deliver the foetus. This she refused.

The hospital summoned a judge, who heard the arguments (albeit without Ms Carder being represented) and concluded that the interests of the foetus in possible survival were greater than the interests of Ms Carder. The caesarean section was carried out against Ms Carder's wishes (and incidentally against the wishes of her husband and family) and the baby survived for a matter of hours and Ms Carder for about two days. This tragic story highlights very clearly the possibility of perverse outcomes deriving from the moral view that women should do everything in their power to benefit their foetus, despite the fact that the foetus has no legal standing until it is born. Annas claims that the court in this case:

> treated a live woman as though she were already dead, forced her to undergo an abortion, and then justified their brutal and unprincipled opinion on the basis that she was almost dead and her fetus's interests in life outweighed any interest she might have in her own life and health (Annas, 1988, p. 25).

The judgement was reversed on appeal, but this was obviously too late for Ms Carder.

Such interventions are not, however, confined to the United States. The general rule about the provision of treatment is, of course, that it depends (save in exceptional and clearly defined circumstances) on the provision of a voluntary 'informed' consent: theoretically, this derives from both ethical and legal considerations. For example, in the case of *Re T (adult: refusal of medical treatment)* ((1992) 9 BMLR 46) Lord Donaldson stated the law's position in this way:

> An adult patient who . . . suffers from no mental incapacity has an absolute right to choose whether to consent to medical treatment, to refuse it or to choose one rather than another of the treatments being offered (p. 50).

However, at the end of this statement he proposed a qualification which has arguably been the source of a series of highly contentious decisions which have had the result of constraining women's reproductive liberty. He suggested that '[t]he only possible qualification is a case in which the choice may lead to the death of a viable foetus'. This exception was used in a number of cases to enforce major surgery on unwilling women. For example, in the case of *Re S (adult: refusal of medical treatment)* ((1992) 9 BMLR 69) an English judge authorized a forced caesarean section on a woman who had refused it on religious grounds. The judge, influenced by the Angela Carder judgement, but apparently without knowing that that judgement had been overturned, took account not only of the risk to the woman's life if the caesarean was not performed but also of the welfare of the foetus. It was, in his very brief judgement, clear that the foetal interests were of considerable importance, even though – as has been said – the foetus, even at term, has no legal rights. In other words, the moral status accorded to the viable foetus was sufficient to override the actual rights of the existing woman.

As Lew says:

> Conflicts between a woman's needs and those of her fetus are vexing because they pit powerful cultural norms against one another; the ideal of autonomy and the ideal of maternal self-sacrifice. Parents who make sacrifices for their children should be encouraged, even lauded, but the law should not require such sacrifices. Self-sacrifice is a gift. Forcing a pregnant woman to sacrifice her health for her fetus is simply slavery (Lew , 1990, pp. 621–622).

Equally, as Draper says, 'it is one thing to show what a woman ought to do in relation to her unborn child and quite another thing to say that this obligation ought to be enforced (Draper, 1992, p. 13).

Interestingly, this case and those that followed it flew directly in the face of the words of one judge in the earlier case of *Re F (in utero)* [1988] 2 All ER 193:

> If the law is to be extended in this manner, so as to impose control over the mother of an unborn child, where such control may be necessary for the benefit of that child, then under our system of parliamentary democracy it is for Parliament to decide whether such controls can be imposed and, if so, subject to what limitations or conditions (p. 200).

Finally, in this context, the judgement of Butler-Sloss LJ in the case of *Re MB* (38 BMLR 175 (1997)) is worth noting as it seems to signal a shift in emphasis, taking the moral questions out of the equation and basing the outcome firmly in the legal arena. As she said:

> The foetus up to the moment of birth does not have any separate interests capable of being taken into account when a court has to consider an application for a declaration in respect of a caesarean section operation. The law does not have the jurisdiction to declare that such medical intervention is lawful to protect the interests of the unborn child even at the point of birth (1997, p. 186).

It is now arguable (McLean, 2002) that pregnant women will be treated in the same way as other non-pregnant people, whose rights were described by Lord Mustill in the case of *Airedale NHS Trust* v *Bland* (12 BMLR 64 (1993) as follows:

> If the patient is capable of making a decision on whether to permit treatment and decides not to permit it his choice must be obeyed, even if on any objective view it is contrary to his best interests. A doctor has no right to proceed in the face of objection, even if it is plain to all, including the patient, that adverse consequences and even death will or may ensue (1993, p. 136).

Indeed, in the subsequent case of *Re F (in utero)*, ([1998] 2 All ER 193), the court was prepared to declare that '[i]n such a sensitive field, affecting as it does the liberty of the individual, it is not for the judiciary to extend the law' (1998, p. 201).

ETHICS OR LAW?

Ultimately, therefore, irrespective of the 'ethical' views of decision-makers – legal or medical – there are rules under which they must operate, like it or not. Whether or not they are based on 'moral obligations' as Lord Wilberforce would have it, they nonetheless are superior (in practical terms) to the outcome predicted by adherence to one ethical school of thought or another. Of course, the law may also take different approaches. On the one hand, it may (as it has traditionally done) defer not to the ethical but to the professional. That is, the behaviour of health care professionals may be adjudicated upon based on its conformity with accepted medical practice. This approach was traditionally utilized most often in respect to matters of operational negligence, but it has also been extended into other, more contentious areas.

One example of this can be found in cases involving the treatment of babies and young children born with impairments or disabilities. As long ago as 1981, two cases brought this firmly into the public domain; one heard in a criminal court and one in a civil court. In the case of *R v Arthur* (1981) 12 BMLR1), the parents of a child born with apparently uncomplicated Down Syndrome indicated that they did not wish it to survive. The consultant, Dr Leonard Arthur, accepted their wishes and prescribed 'nursing care only'. The child died some hours later and Dr Arthur was charged with murder. This charge was subsequently reduced to attempted murder following the findings of the paediatric pathologist that the infant in fact suffered from a range of other conditions which could in the event have caused his death. Dr Arthur was acquitted of this charge, following direction from the judge that, amongst other things, the jury should be reluctant to conclude that Dr Arthur, and his colleagues who testified that they would have done the same thing, had developed a professional practice which was criminal. In other words, the fact that other doctors agreed with Dr Arthur's practice was sufficient to acquit him of a crime.

The second case, which was heard in a civil court before Dr Arthur's trial, is the case of *Re B (a minor)* ((1981) reported in [1990] 3 All ER 927). In a similar way, the child was born suffering from Down Syndrome and required relatively minor but life-saving surgery. The parents refused to permit the operation to go ahead, and the case reached the English courts. In this case, however, the judge was disinclined to respect the parents' views, arguing that unless the child's life could be shown to be 'demonstrably awful' she should not be condemned to die. Here, the morality utilized was not derivative from what doctors might do (assuming that this is a moral position *in se*), but rather from the infant's inherent right to life, even with disabilities.

THE HUMAN RIGHTS ACT 1998

Superimposed on the modern relationship between law, ethics and health care is the Human Rights Act 1998. Although its provisions translate into law a series of commitments which are broadly ethical and its jurisprudence is complex, yet, as with our last example, it is the terms of this legislation that must be adhered to irrespective of the ethical or moral view of the individual decision-maker. Moreover, those interpreting the provisions of the legislation will do so within the bounds, not of ethics but of law, including the legal devices used to reach a decision. Many people undoubtedly anticipated that when the European Convention on Human Rights was incorporated into UK law by the Human Rights Act there would be a significant impact on individual freedom. The terms of the Convention seem to offer (or perhaps more accurately reinforce) individual rights. However, it is arguable that it has been the process-based requirements (for example, the right to a fair trial/hearing) rather than the choice-based rights of the Convention which have had the biggest impact. That the 1998 Act was not to be a route to permit people to have their individual morality (or ethics) guaranteed by law became very clear in the case of Diane Pretty. It will be remembered that Mrs Pretty was in the late stages of motor neurone disease and wished the Director of Public Prosecutions to declare in advance that her husband would not be prosecuted if he assisted her to die at a time of her choosing. The DPP refused to issue any such statement, and Mrs Pretty took her case through the courts of the United Kingdom and ultimately to the European Court of Human Rights (*Pretty v United Kingdom* (2002) 66 BMLR 147).

The concept of human rights has played an extremely important role in social and political discourse, particularly since the end of the second world war when the appalling abuse of individuals and communities became clear. The European Convention on Human Rights was one of a number of international human rights treaties promulgated in the years after the war had ended and incorporates basic ethical principles which can loosely be equated with concepts such as respect for persons and autonomy or self-determination in thought and deed, and privacy.

Mrs Pretty's case is noteworthy for present purposes because of the range of human rights she claimed applied to her case and the manner in which her arguments were dealt with by the Court of Human Rights. She first argued that the terms of the Convention guaranteed her a 'right to die', deriving this claim from article 2 of the Convention which guarantees the right to life. She argued that 'The right to die is not the antithesis of the right to life but the corollary of it, and the state has a positive obligation to protect both' (2002, p. 155). This she based on the fact that some Convention rights imply their opposite – for example, the right to join a trade association also includes the right not to do so. However, the court was unconvinced by this argument, basing its decision in large part on the ethical principle of the sanctity of life, saying:

The article protects the right to life and prevents the deliberate taking of life save in very narrowly defined circumstances. An article with that effect cannot be interpreted as conferring a right to die or to enlist the aid of another in bringing about one's own death (2002, p. 196).

The second strand to her argument involved article 3 of the Convention, which prohibits inhuman and degrading treatment. Mrs Pretty argued that

(1) Member states have an absolute and unqualified obligation not to inflict the proscribed treatment and also to take positive action to prevent the subjection of individuals to such treatment . . . . (2) Suffering attributable to the progression of a disease may amount to such treatment if the state can prevent or ameliorate such suffering and does not do so . . . . (3) In denying Mrs Pretty the opportunity to bring her suffering to an end the United Kingdom . . . . will subject her to the proscribed treatment . . . . (4) Since . . . . it is open to the United Kingdom under the Convention to refrain from prohibiting suicide, The . . . [DPP] . . . can give the undertaking without breaking the United Kingdom's obligations under the Convention (2002, pp. 159–160).

For the court, however, it was legal, rather than ethical, issues which were determinative of this argument. That is, the question was focused on whether or not the United Kingdom had a procedural rather than an ethical obligation to respect Mrs Pretty's wishes. As was said:

it could not in my view be said that the United Kingdom is under a positive obligation to ensure that a competent, terminally ill person who wishes but is unable to take his or her own life should be entitled to seek the assistance of another without that other being exposed to the risk of prosecution (2002, p. 162).

One of the central commitments of the Convention is what has been called the right to self-determination which is derived from article 8 – the right to private and family life. Unlike article 3, this article is subject to acceptable derogations based, for example, on the need to protect public morals. Mrs Pretty argued that this article should be interpreted as including 'a right to choose when and how to die so that suffering and indignity can be avoided', concluding that it was therefore 'for the United Kingdom to show that the interference meets the Convention tests of legality, necessity, responsiveness to pressing social need and proportionality' (2002. p. 162).

The Court, however, although accepting that the burden of proving that limitations on behaviour required to be justified by the state, was satisfied that this burden had been met.

Mrs Pretty also sought to make a case under article 9 of the Convention, which guarantees freedom of thought and expression. The court, however, said:

One may accept that Mrs Pretty has a sincere belief in the virtue of assisted suicide. She is free to hold and express that belief. But her belief cannot found a requirement that her husband should be absolved from the consequences of conduct which, although it would be consistent with her belief, is proscribed by the criminal law (2002. p. 169).

Finally, Mrs Pretty referred to the non-discrimination provisions in article 14 of the Convention. Basically, she argued that as she was physically unable to commit suicide (which would not be a crime), she was being discriminated against because of her disability if she were not permitted to gain assistance in committing suicide. However, as none of her Convention rights had otherwise been breached, this article could not be used.

CONCLUSION

It can be seen that the rather simplistic description of the relationship between morals (ethics) and the law provided by Lord Wilberforce has a limited relevance in the modern delivery of health care. Perhaps the issues have changed; perhaps society has. What is clear, however, is that it is necessary to adopt a more sophisticated and nuanced analysis when considering modern health care. Commitment to a particular ethical position may not be sufficient to guide practice, particularly when there are legal rules which differ from it or which require that other values are more important. Ethics and law are ultimately both interlinked and separate. Those entering the health care professions increasingly need an awareness of both the limitations of ethical argument and its strengths. In the modern world, however, they also require an understanding of the legal issues which underpin or prescribe their freedom to practice, particularly since we have seen that ethics and law are not always obviously the same.

REFERENCES

Annas G., 'She's going to die: the case of Angela C', *Hastings Center Report*, Vol. 18, No. 1, 1988, 23, at p. 25.

Devlin P. *The Enforcement of Morals*. London: Oxford University Press, 1965.

Draper H. *Women, Forced Caesareans and Antenatal Responsibilities*, vol. 1 (Working Paper no. 1). University of Liverpool: Feminist Legal Research Unit, 1992.

Hart HLA. *Law Liberty and Morality*. London: Oxford University Press, 1963.

Kolder VE, Gallagher J, Parsons MT. Court-ordered obstetrical interventions. *N Engl J Med* 1987; **316**: 1192–6.

Lew JB. Terminally Ill and pregnant: state denial of a woman's right to refuse a caesarean section. *Buffalo Law Rev* 1990; **38**: 619.

Mason JK, Laurie GT. *Mason and McCall Smith's Law and Medical Ethics*, 7th edition. Oxford University Press, 2006.

McLean SAM, Mason JK. *Legal & Ethical Aspects of Healthcare*. London: GMM, 2003 (particularly chapter 1).

McLean SAM, Ramsey J. Human rights, reproductive freedom, medicine and the law. *Med Law Int* 2002; **5**(4): 239–58.

Montgomery J. *Health Care Law*, 2nd edition. Oxford: Oxford University Press, 2003 (particularly chapter 1).

26

Medical Humanities: An Overview

MARTYN EVANS

Rarely are the humanities in medicine assessed for what they are – neither educational flourishes nor panaceas but indispensable studies whose everyday use is as important for the quality of clinical decisions as the basic sciences are now presumed to be (Pellegrino, 1974, p. 4).

Although 'medical humanities' has, in 2007, a still-fashionable ring to it, the concerns it denotes are not new; the lament above was penned in 1974 by physician-philosopher Edmund Pellegrino, responding to what he took to be a re-grettable but well-established neglect of the humanities in medicine. Exploring the nature, scope and situation of med-ical humanities is our concern in this chapter, in the course of which we shall need to note its relation to medical ethics. But where to start? If patriotism is the last refuge of the scoundrel, then armchair etymology might be thought the first resort of the too-timid philosopher. Certainly, some-where in what follows I am going to have to say what I think medical humanities actually *is*, where it is found, what goes on when it happens, why anyone might bother and so forth – and I promise that I will do so. But when exploring an idea that, like medical humanities, is still somewhat unfa-miliar (and still rather lacking in gravitas or 'street-cred') it is difficult to start without a little reconnaissance. The field of medical humanities is still young enough, at least in the UK, for there to be different viewpoints concerning the field's nature, scope and research agenda. (The expres-sion 'medical humanities' derives from the United States where it largely refers to the incorporation of material from selected humanities disciplines within the teaching of medicine (Sirridge and Welch, 2002)).

Furthermore, even at this early scene-setting stage, the beliefs and attitudes of the observer colour his report, again along lines reflecting his academic discipline and back-ground. That ought not to be a problem, for faced with a variety of conflicting reports about what geology is, we can ask which of them are supplied by geologists, and prefer those. But to ask whether any accounts of medical humani-ties have been supplied by medical humanists is already to plunge into contested territory and, on at least one view of medical humanities, to make an elementary mistake. So I have to ask the reader both to indulge a review of terms, and to suppress the urge to ask for my professional credentials: I may not have any, because – depending on the view one takes – there may be none to be had.

So, to proceed: the phrase 'medical humanities' is an awkward one; it invites various interpretations, not all of them helpful. This is particularly apparent in the context of the ambiguity of the similar phrase 'medical ethics'. 'Medical ethics' has come to denote both a set of questions or enquiries (which quite quickly accreted to produce an academic specialism) and a broad set of practical and pro-fessional obligations (whose precise content and realization are of course just as contested as are obligations anywhere else in moral life). This same ambiguity beckons in the phrase 'medical humanities', but the corresponding denota-tions are less easy to establish to general satisfaction.

On one hand the phrase seems to suggest a branch of that area of thought collectively dubbed 'the humanities' that specially belongs to or is concerned with medicine and things that are medical. Although this is partly right, it is not the whole story, and in any event it requires that we say clearly what we take the humanities to be. On the other hand the phrase may suggest a set of practical and profes-sional attitudes, a *modus operandi* for doing clinical medi-cine, that is practising humanely and with due concern for the humanity of the patient (Pellegrino, 1974). Of course one could hardly complain at someone's working like this, but it might be thought to be so intrinsic to the practice of

Principles of Health Care Ethics, Second Edition   Edited by R.E. Ashcroft, A. Dawson, H. Draper and J.R. McMillan

medicine as to make such an interpretation of 'medical humanities' a platitudinous truism.

Whether humane practice is indeed internal to the idea of medicine is an interesting question – paralleled, of course, by the question of whether *ethical* practice is internal to the idea of medicine. If it is, then the practical or professional sense of 'medical ethics' is similarly vulnerable to collapsing into truism. Those who, like Cassell (1991), regard essentially humane concerns such as the relief of suffering as being *internal* goals of medicine seem committed to the idea that, properly conceived, medicine in practice must be both ethical and humane by definition; departures from this mode of medicine are thus departures from the idea of medicine as such.

There are other similarly named activities whose scope is constrained by the term 'medical': for instance, medical physics, medical anthropology medical statistics. Modern medical technology (and perhaps modern physiology) relies on the knowledge and techniques of physics, but in 'doing medicine' one is not 'doing physics' except in a very contrived sense. On the other hand, medical anthropology artfully captures much that is interesting and important about the dynamics of health and medicine, but it is more plausibly the name of a study *of* medicine than of a way of *doing* medicine. Perhaps medical statistics represents an intermediate case: many doctors will have to integrate statistical knowledge into their treatment decisions (and statistical method into their research). But we need not resolve these questions here. Both medical ethics and medical humanities have at least one denotation – intellectual and practical enquiry – that would remain unaffected by the collapse of either ethical or humane practice into contingent *modes* of medicine that were logically external to it.

Other senses of the phrase 'medical humanities' can be considered. Some retain an affiliation to medical ethics. The field's early exponents in the United States flourished within medical curricula, where their presence was most readily justified in terms of teaching literary immersion and analysis to hone the sensitivities of would-be doctors to the fine grain of interpersonal understanding and communication with patients (Montgomery, 1991; McLellan and Hudson Jones, 1997). This approach is maintained in much contemporary teaching of literature in British medical schools and elsewhere, (Calman et al., 1988; Glasser, 1999) and to this may be added the widespread encouragement of literary habits in both reading and writing as resources for the hard-pressed clinician beset by the demands of professional life (Graham-Pole, 1996). The cathartic benefits of producing reflective, expressive writing, autobiographical narratives and even formal poetry are claimed to benefit not only clinicians but patients as well, particularly when facing life-threatening or life-changing illnesses or disabilities (Bolton, 1999).

The medico-ethical objective of such endeavours is obvious and admirable. Indeed one could generalize, from the rather obvious thought that 'humane' is itself a term of ethical applause, to the only slightly less obvious thought that to explore the human concerns of medicine is in effect to explore the ethical concerns of medicine, albeit on a broader and less closely specified canvas (Evans, 2001).

Less overtly tied to ethics are the views, reported in Greaves (2001), that medical humanities concerns all the non-scientific (though not unscientific) aspects of medicine, or even simply all that concerns 'the human' within medicine.

In sum, then, there are several different viewpoints upon medical humanities, not all of them consistent with each other. This chapter is written from one such viewpoint: it arises from a considered commitment to a particular, and largely philosophical, perspective reflecting my own background as a philosopher. To set out this conception of the medical humanities, I will briefly put forward a number of questions that a puzzled onlooker might reasonably ask, and I will suggest responses to each of them in turn. These questions concern the nature and identity of medical humanities as a field of enquiry and, following this, how one might do research in medical humanities and what research questions one might pursue.

A FEW QUESTIONS FROM THE PUZZLED ONLOOKER

THE PHRASE 'MEDICAL HUMANITIES' MEANS WHAT?

Many humanities subjects or disciplines could be said to have in common that (i) they are concerned with recording, understanding and interpreting human experience at the individual level, and (ii) (in contrast perhaps to scientific and many social-scientific disciplines) they take individual subjectivity seriously – allowing as valid, and sustaining an interest in, the detail of what differentiates particular people and particular experiences from another. Literature, history and philosophy all seem to me clear examples that do this with regard to experience(s) generally.

If we grant this, then 'medical humanities' could be simply a particular application of humanities: familiar disciplines, doing what they are typically good at, but with particular regard to experiences and subjectivities within a particular context of medicine (taking 'medicine' to include many forms of clinical care) and of the conditions to which medicine pays special attention: health, illness, disease, disability and suffering. This also suggests that the identity and nature of any contributory humanities discipline within 'medical humanities' is pretty much what it is in any other context or application. (We may here recall that medical ethics is, among other things, the special application of ideas that are more widely familiar than within medicine alone; medical ethics is part of ordinary reasoning thinking about ordinary moral life, but carried out in the particular context of medicine.)

We might therefore at this point suggest that a piece of work – thinking, writing, reflecting – would constitute work in the medical humanities if

> (i) it illuminates the practice of medicine using distinctive insights normally associated with thinking in the humanities or social sciences; or it illuminates the human, experiential, side of medicine in a way that is not usually accessible through scientific descriptions and explanations.

There is more to be said than this, of course. How do these familiar disciplines combine within medical humanities? Are there any more of them than the three I have suggested as examples? Let us attend to this now.

WHICH DISCIPLINES CONTRIBUTE TO MEDICAL HUMANITIES?

I have suggested some central candidates above, and they all have 'allied trades' that could contribute to medical humanities, such as historiography, literary criticism and critical theory, comparative religious study and so on. There seems also a clear role – alongside the study of literature, for instance – for the study of fine art and music. This is still a modest list, and to it we might add some slightly less central humanities subjects such as journalism, drama, media studies and perhaps linguistics, even law. Beyond these, it brings us to the least generalizing of the social sciences (for instance, anthropology and ethnography) and to some forms of the study of psychology, but at this point it is clear that we can encounter controversy in the form of 'boundary disputes' concerning the scope and nature of individual subject disciplines. (Some psychology departments' evolution has reflected sharp differences between social and biological psychologists, the latter at times asserting their subject as a form of natural science).

Let us here add another provisional component to the specification for work falling within medical humanities, namely that

> (ii) it is a self-conscious engagement of one (or more) *disciplines*, from a list of characteristic humanities or social sciences disciplines, with medicine. (Let us also allow that 'medicine' refers equally to concerns with health care, health, illness, disability, etc.)

Any particular list of contributory disciplines is bound to be to some extent stipulative. Moreover any given list will also tend to reflect its author's view on another contested question, namely, 'Which, if any, discipline is central to medical humanities?' If asked this question, my own answer (unsurprisingly) would be that it is philosophy. (I confess that I tend to think that philosophy is also central to biomedical ethics.) Medicine is an enquiry into our bodily selves; the humanities together form an enquiry into our rational and experiential selves; and philosophy offers ways of describing, analysing and connecting both enterprises. In other words, philosophy of medicine is a natural, necessary and in some ways inevitable conversation between the two disciplines, as co-enquirers into human nature. Philosophy of medicine is the most apparent form of medical humanities, as by much the same token biomedical ethics is the best known form of philosophy of medicine (and the first to reach a popular audience). So when I write within medical humanities, I believe that I am writing philosophy of medicine, but with the broader agenda and perhaps the greater informality of method that are made possible on a larger canvas. This does not mean that all forms of enquiry in medical humanities – or, for that matter, in medical ethics – need constitute philosophical enquiry but, on the view that I propose, philosophical enquiry is never far away.

HOW IS 'MEDICAL HUMANITIES' CONSTITUTED?

How do these various disciplines (literature studies, history, theology, philosophy, law, psychology, anthropology, music, fine art studies, drama and so on) actually *constitute* medical humanities as a field of enquiry? Are they no more than a list or collection? Are they a procession of staged contributions, each with its allotted role, its job to perform? Or do they somehow provide a *fusion* of their respective insights (or methods, or enquiries, or characteristics)?

This is a difficult question because it presupposes a view on whether such cross-disciplinary fusion is possible – that is, on whether genuine *interdisciplinarity*, as distinct from the less ambitious *multi*-disciplinarity, is actually attainable in this context (or, indeed, ever!). So as well as being difficult, it is also very important for our view of how ambitious and novel it is possible for medical humanities enquiries to be. As this is a question about the forms of, and limits to, knowledge in the various contributing disciplines, then it is also an irreducibly philosophical one. The distinction between multi-disciplinarity and interdisciplinarity hinges on what we think is required to understand the world from a disciplinary viewpoint other than our own – how other disciplines *see and name* the objects in their world and to what extent we can view that world with them. This shows how ambitious claims of interdisciplinarity really are.

There seems no doubt that interdisciplinarity is sometimes achieved, but so far the more convincing examples to my mind come from outside medical humanities. A good example is arguably constituted by chemical process technology (Evans and Macnaughton, 2004).

I would suggest that interdisciplinarity ought to be possible – and it ought to be our goal – in medical humanities. As such, I will suggest that work in medical humanities can be characterized insofar as

(iii) it illuminates the human side of medicine in a way that is not usually accessible through enquiry in an *isolated* humanities or social sciences discipline.

When Stephen Toulmin described medical knowledge of individuals in terms of 'the intersection of nature and history' he was appealing precisely to the fusion of different forms of knowledge and different epistemologies (Toulmin, 1993). This strikes me as a good litmus test for interdisciplinarity. I would also suggest two further characteristics or signs (perhaps even criteria) of interdisciplinarity: (i) the presence of *emergent* questions that could not be asked, let alone answered, by single contributory disciplines in isolation (as is serially apparent in the case of chemical process technology); and (ii) the availability of shared metaphors across disciplinary boundaries (something that is important to the engagement of, for instance, historians or philosophers with the discourses of particle physics, where terms such as 'colour' seem to the outsider to have their roots in metaphor).

WHERE DOES MEDICAL HUMANITIES SIT IN RELATION TO MEDICAL PRACTICE AND MEDICAL KNOWLEDGE?

This is rather like the question of whether ethical practice or 'humane' or 'humanistic' practice is somehow internally bound up with what it is to practise medicine at all. In particular, do insights, knowledge or understanding that might arise from medical humanities enquiries belong *within* the body of knowledge and understanding that is called medicine? Is medical humanities an integral part of medical practice, or is it an added (perhaps optional) part? Do humanities, methods and enquiries supplement the conduct of medicine in practice, or alternatively, do they have an *intrinsic intellectual place* within medical practice (or even medical theory)? Typically, views divide (Macnaughton, 2000).

The question is distinctly a philosophical one because at stake are rival conceptions of the nature of medicine as a body of theory and knowledge, most especially concerning our organic embodied nature, the nature of health, illness and disease, and what we think causation is in medicine. Furthermore, different scales of ambition for the humanities are at stake in this question – therefore it is institutionally and functionally important, as well as intellectually so.

Not surprisingly I favour the view that as patients are 'experiencing subjects' as well as dynamic physio-anatomical objects, clinical medicine is as concerned with understanding and working with patients' subjectivities as it is with their biological generalities. As I have put the point elsewhere,

patients are 'meat with a point of view' and medicine is as inherently concerned with the 'point of view' as with the 'meat' (Evans, 2002). This suggests that medical humanities could indeed contribute to medical knowledge and understanding and belong within medicine's practice and theory, broadly conceived.

Let us formalize the attention to subjectivity in medical humanities, by declaring that work within medical humanities

(iv) helps us to understand one or more 'subjectivities' within the experience of medicine, or of health, illness, suffering or disability.

IS MEDICAL HUMANITIES ANY DIFFERENT FROM 'ARTS-IN-HEALTH'?

Probably the influences of arts and humanities upon organized health care are most publicly apparent when fine art and music are incorporated into the ways that hospitals are experienced by patients, visitors and health professionals (Loppert, 2006). The therapeutic and even diagnostic uses of art and music in the health care arena are also fashionably reported (Anon, 2005; Ghosh, 2006). It seems but a simple extension of this to include the therapeutic uses of creative writing and expressive self-reflection.

Even so, I strongly believe that arts-in-health and medical humanities are indeed different and that they are related to one another as the observed is to the observer. Arts-in-health is best thought of as a valuable extension of clinical medicine's therapeutic (and perhaps public health's preventative) repertoire of *resources*, something that can be offered and undertaken clinically (be it as art therapy, cathartic creative writing or self-expression) or in the community (health education through drama presentation and so on) (White, 2006). Some will contest this account as too narrow, but I think it can be enlarged without negating the essential contrast with medical humanities.

By contrast, medical humanities is a repertoire of *enquiry* (usually in an academic context) into the whole range of medical knowledge, acts, contexts and therapeutic resources. These include arts-in-health. Medical humanities can draw attention to why arts-in-health is important and attempt an understanding of how, when and why it can be effective – through attempting a richer account of health and illness and of medicine's claim to be a 'science of the human'.

The possible extent of medical humanities' 'repertoire of enquiry' will concern us shortly.

DO THE MEDICAL HUMANITIES BELONG WITHIN MEDICINE OR WITHIN THE HUMANITIES?

The answer I will suggest is 'neither' – but, first, why ask the question? It might look arcane or 'theological', but it is important for two reasons: it could influence whether particular researchers will think it worth their while to undertake medical humanities enquiries, and – closely connected to this – it could influence which funders of research will think that medical humanities falls within their remit. This is, I freely admit, a question of most concern to university academics, but in the long run it bears directly upon the capacity of medical humanities enquiries to make any worthwhile difference to clinical practice.

We can make a distinction between two views on the question, namely between (A) medical humanities as placing humanities at the service of medicine; and (B) medical humanities as naming an intellectual co-engagement between medicine and the humanities. The first of these views seems to offer a sense of security to academic researchers within humanities departments, but it makes it less apparent why humanities should 'bother' with medical humanities; it also leaves open the possibility of a certain smugness on the part of humanities and resentment on the part of medicine. If, alternatively, we prefer the second view, then researchers within the humanities can feel not only comfortable in but also excited by the prospects for research in medical humanities; and (to allow a prudential consideration to intrude momentarily) both the humanities funding bodies and medical funding bodies can take a legitimate interest in medical humanities research.

But simply preferring a view is not enough. To decide whether (A) or (B) is the more plausible view, we need to consider the goals of medical humanities enquiry. A number of these are apparent – though my suggestions here are far from exhaustive. Some point towards view (A), the humanities in the service of medicine, and are relatively conventional, much in the spirit of the General Medical Council's publication *Tomorrow's Doctors* (General Medical Council Education Committee, 1993). But others point towards (B), an intellectual co-engagement between medicine and the humanities and are more radical. We can set them out like this:

(A) Conventional goals:
1. taking values seriously including ethical values;
2. helping clinicians (and students) to develop their own personal values;
3. providing personal resources for the demands of clinical life;
4. developing interpretative sensitivity and skills of listening and communication.

These certainly seem worthwhile goals, and I think that they would readily be recognized within the study of biomedical ethics. Any and all of these should also pay off in terms of effective health care. As such, these goals ought to be recognized in acknowledging, within the larger compass of medical humanities endeavour, work that

(v) makes a specific educational contribution, characteristic of a humanities discipline and not normally expected from a scientific education, to preparing doctors for the human side of clinical medicine.

Even so, such essential educational goals are important because their underlying ideas are important, and these are better captured in other ways, ways that are necessarily more abstract, general and – like it or not – sounding rather high-flown, viz.:

(B) More radical goals:
1. taking subjectivity seriously both in practice and in theory;
2. stimulating and encouraging a sense of wonder at embodied human nature;
3. asking how technological medicine's picture of human nature/the human condition contributes to our self-understanding, and whether other pictures are available (for instance, from the humanities);
4. from this, asking whether technological medicine spurs humanities disciplines to extend (or revisit) their own research agendas;
5. exploring disciplinarity, interdisciplinarity and the varying nature of knowledge and evidence in medicine, sciences and humanities.

These goals too should pay off in terms of individual clinical practice, but they also invite – and support – sustained reflection on the nature and goals of medicine, reflection that should impact upon the agendas for medical education, practice and research.

It seems clear that both sets of goals are worthwhile. Those listed under (B) are more radical, more ambitious, more philosophical and – I suspect – more likely to attract the attentions of adventurous and original researchers in medicine and the humanities alike than are the more education-oriented goals listed under (A). It will be apparent nonetheless that I would choose where possible to promote the more radical goals, so I will include them in the accumulating (though provisional) specification of medical humanities work, which

(vi) specifically uses some aspects of medicine (health care, etc.) to achieve some gain in our understanding of the human condition, or of embodied human nature.

WHAT MIGHT COUNT AS RESEARCH IN THE MEDICAL HUMANITIES?

A relatively simple way of approaching this question is to look at what has in fact been regarded as recent research in the medical humanities. The principal non-US journal in the field is *Medical Humanities*, a twice-yearly special edition of the *Journal of Medical Ethics*, now in its sixth year. As one of the journal's co-editors throughout that time, I must again submit a disclaimer: the journal's conception of the field obviously to some extent reflects my own conception. As against that, any influence on my part is tempered by the varying views of my co-editors, associate editors, editorial board and our substantial panel of independent reviewers of submitted manuscripts. In that context, and given that there are relatively few other prominent places in which medical humanities research can be published *under that name*, then a review of the contents of the journal's first 11 issues (and some 92 selected research papers, not counting editorials or special sections) may be taken to be a reasonable representative of a field that is, after all, still in its infancy.

A very small proportion of these papers are concerned to explore arts-in-health or the benefits of creative writing. *Pace* our observations above on the distinction between arts-in-health and medical humanities, these papers count as medical humanities research in proportion as they are also reflective and analytic regarding why and how arts-in-health has a therapeutic role, or why and how creative writing properly belongs in the arena of health care, as this in turn requires reflection on the kind of medicine that is appropriate to our conjoint biological/existential nature. (From a philosophical perspective, work that simply reported on what was done and whom it helped would seem less interesting.)

These are a minority of papers in the journal to date. The substantial remainder offer a range that bridges two poles – the concrete particular and the abstract general. To take the concrete particular first, accounting as it does for the majority of the journal papers in question, we find here work pursuing the more conventional goals listed above, including such enquiries as the human cost to doctors of first-hand experience of anatomical dissection (Francis and Lewis, 2001), the role of (quasi-biblical) lament in patients' communications and expressions (Bub, 2004), the relation between evidence-based medicine and clinical freedom (Parker, 2005), the relation between literature and the body in the work of physician-poet Thomas Beddoes (Bamforth, 2004) or whether literature can be taken seriously as literature yet remain of instrumental value in medical education (Pickering, 2000).

The more abstract and general category of work is only incompletely addressed by the remaining research papers of those reviewed. This category for me includes work that promotes the 'conversational' engagement between medicine and the humanities, including: work that promotes their co-enquiry into our understanding of our embodied human nature; work exploring the nature of interdisciplinarity; and work that looks at what medicine might contribute to the humanities' own research agendas and – for that matter – to our larger cultural and intellectual resources. This is a substantial

agenda, and the smaller number of relevant papers (whose enquiries include the relationships among surgery, aesthetics and intention (Holm, 2000), the relations between narrative and ethics (McCarthy, 2003), the fundamental positioning of science and art in medicine (Saunders, 2000) and the intertwining of physical and cultural notions of lightness in a radical understanding of anorexia (Giordano, 2002)) address it only partially. This may be because many would-be medical humanities researchers are nervous of such questions, or because research funders are, or because the questions simply do not yet have much currency. (It is worth observing, in a context somewhat related to that of the public understanding of science, that the 'meta-questions' of the relations of medicine to the humanities generally are themselves representatives of a still larger – and for a long time neglected – set of questions about the re-engagement between sciences and humanities.)

There is one more thing, perhaps, to be said about research in medical humanities: its fruits should *cohere* – we should aim at an accumulated understanding of what we as embodied, experiencing patients have in common as well as of what makes us irreducible individuals. A collection of essentially unconnected insights will be valuable for the individuals concerned, but from the viewpoint of understanding ourselves and the medical practice that we as patients need, we shall require more than a heap: we shall require a structure. I suggest then that we formalize this by noting that the most valuable medical humanities work:

> (vii) is *transferable* to our understanding of other subjectivities: we gain something which we can meaningfully relate to other insights gained on other occasions of comparable enquiry, allowing us to be systematic, albeit in a rudimentary way.

ARE THERE ANY METHODS OR PRINCIPLES SPECIFIC TO MEDICAL HUMANITIES?

Generally speaking, I shall presume that the answer to the question of whether there are distinctive *methods* is 'no'. In terms of their detail, such methods as might be appropriate to work conducted in medical humanities are likely to derive from what is acknowledged as proper and scholarly within their respective contributing disciplines: to judge the success of bringing methods of literary criticism to bear upon our understanding of embodied illness, it seems we should look at how those methods are used well (or badly) in their more familiar contexts, such as (for example) the understanding of the development of individual personalities more generally. Philosophical reflection upon medicine and upon the experiences of ill-health and medical intervention ought, one senses, to be judged by the same lights as those by which one might judge philosophical reflection upon the more general features of experience, knowledge and perception. I see no reason to expect anything fundamentally different in other disciplines, but authority here belongs to scholars of those disciplines.

Having said this, there might nonetheless be other features of medical humanities research that, whilst not exactly constituting *methods*, do mark out medical humanities research independently of its particular subject matter. It would be difficult to do medical humanities research well, I am suggesting, if one were uninterested in the contributions likely to be available from disciplines other than one's own and particularly difficult if one were devoted to reductionist approaches yielding results of maximum generality with regard to patients in general, but minimum penetration into the subjective consciousness of individual patients. One must not of course make a fetish out of subjectivity, still less descend into subjectiv*ism*, but still it would be odd to maintain a credible interest in the medical humanities as an exploration of human experience, whilst paying sustained attention only to the generalities of human physical constitution – to attend to the meat rather than to the point of view; to the clay rather than that by which it is 'impassion'd'.

Are there, then, any usable guiding 'principles' of medical humanities enquiry? In a gentle homage to the four 'principles' of biomedical ethics with which this volume is substantially concerned, I am tempted to suggest at this point four (rough) principles of conduct and approach in medical humanities enquiry. These would, I think, be good ways by which to proceed, at the same time illuminating something of the content of the field's most important areas, yet without constraint as regards one's central or 'home' discipline. (If they are plausible, then they may be plausible also in the context of thinking about interdisciplinary work *per se*, but a verdict on this must remain beyond the scope of this chapter.) Here they are:

Principle of disciplinary openness – 'always remain open to (and where coherently possible, incorporate) insights, ways of seeing and metaphors proper to disciplines other than one's own'.
Principle of humility – 'always be ready to recognize the value of aspects of enquiry (and specific questions) that are simply not amenable to one's own discipline, and be ready to stop and ask, rather than proceed recklessly'.
Principle of subjectivity – 'always think, judge and analyse with a respect for individual subjectivity – that is, so as to take the subjectivity of experience seriously'.
Principle of wonder – 'always remain open to, and be reverent towards, that which is or contains something of wonder'.

These are, of course, sketches and nothing more; I have space neither to explore nor to illustrate them. They might usefully guide enquiries within medical humanities as I have described the field here, but an adequate demonstration (or even a test) of this would require a separate discussion.

Meanwhile, and because the nature, scope and research aims of medical humanities as a field of enquiry are still very much open to discussion, let me summarize the position of this chapter by collecting together the connected but distinguishable features that, I suggested above, individually and together mark out work that falls clearly within the field. I offer the claim that a serious enquiry genuinely works within medical humanities as described here if:

(i) it illuminates the practice of medicine using distinctive insights normally associated with thinking in the humanities or social sciences; or it illuminates the human, experiential side of medicine in a way that is not usually accessible through scientific descriptions and explanations;

or if

(ii) it is a self-conscious engagement of one (or more) *disciplines* from a list of characteristic humanities or social sciences disciplines, with medicine. (Let us also allow that 'medicine' refers equally to concerns with health care, health, illness, disability, etc.);

or if

(iii) it illuminates the human side of medicine in a way that is not usually accessible through enquiry in an *isolated* humanities or social sciences discipline;

or if

(iv) it helps us understand one or more 'subjectivities' within the experience of medicine, or of health, illness, suffering or disability;

or if

(v) it makes a specific educational contribution, characteristic of a humanities discipline and not normally expected from a scientific education, to preparing doctors for the human side of clinical medicine;

or if

(vi) it specifically uses some aspects of medicine (health care, etc.) to achieve some gain in our understanding of the human condition, or of embodied human nature;

or if

(vii) it is *transferable* to our understanding of other subjectivities: we gain something which we can meaningfully relate to other insights gained on other occasions of comparable enquiry, allowing us to be systematic, albeit in a rudimentary way.

This is an eclectic but still, I hope, a coherent list of candidates. An emerging field of enquiry – or, better as well as more truthfully, of many enquiries – can afford much eclecticism; it can afford only a very little incoherence. This is a significant responsibility for those who engage in the field's early development.

REFERENCES

Anon. 'Music therapy on hospital wards', BBC Radio 4 News, 26th January 2005.

Bamforth I. Pickled essence of Englishman: Thomas Lovell Beddoes – time to unearth a neglected poet. *J Med Ethics: Med Human* 2004; **30**(1): 36–40.

Bolton G. *The Therapeutic Potential of Creative Writing*, London: Jessica Kingsley, 1999.

Bub B. The patient's lament: hidden key to effective communication; how to recognise and transform. *J Med Ethics: Med Human* 2004; **30**(2): 63–69.

Calman KC, Downie RS, Duthie M, et al. Literature and medicine: a short course for medical students. *Med Educ* 1988, **22**: 265–269.

Cassell E. *The Nature of Suffering and the Goals of Medicine*. Oxford: Oxford University Press, 1991.

Evans HM, Macnaughton RJ. Should medical humanities be a multidisciplinary or an interdisciplinary study? *J Med Ethics: Medical Humanities* 2004; **30**(1): 1–4.

Evans M. Philosophy and the medical humanities. In: Evans M, Finlay IG, eds. *Medical Humanities*. London: BMJ Books, 2001; pp. 250–263.

Evans, M. Reflections on the humanities in medical education. *Medical Education* 2002; **36**: 506–507.

Francis NR, Lewis W. What price dissection? Dissection literally dissected. *J Med Ethics: Med Human* 2001; **27**(1): 2–9.

General Medical Council Education Committee. *Tomorrow's Doctors*. London: General Medical Council, 1993.

Ghosh P. 'Music "aids the healing process"', BBC Radio 4 News, 19th July 2006.

Giordano S. *Qu'un souffle de vent*: an exploration of anorexia nervosa. *J Med Ethics: Med Human* 2002; **28**(1): 3–8

Glasser B. *Indian-Camp*—a story by Ernest Hemingway. *Educ General Pract* 1999; **10**: 209–214.

Graham-Pole J. Children, death and poetry. *J Poetry Ther* 1996; **9**: 129–141.

Greaves D. The nature and role of the medical humanities. In: Evans M, Finlay IG, eds. *Medical Humanities*. London: BMJ Books, 2001; pp. 13–22.

Holm S. Changes to bodily appearance: the aesthetics of deliberate intervention. *J Med Ethics: Med Human* 2000; **26**(1): 43–48.

Loppert S. 'Don't mock: art really does help the sick', *The Guardian*, 17th November 2006.

Macnaughton J. The humanities in medical education: context, outcomes and structures. *J Med Ethics: Med Human* 2000; **26**(1): 23–30.

McCarthy J. Principlism and narrative ethics: must we choose between them? *J Med Ethics: Med Human* 2003; **29**(2), 65–71.

McLellan F, Hudson Jones A. Why literature and medicine? *Lancet* 1997; 348: 109–111.

Montgomery Hunter K. *The Narrative Structure of Medical Knowledge*. Princeton, NJ: Princeton University Press, 1991.

Parker M. False dichotomies: EBM, clinical freedom and the art of medicine. *J Med Ethics: Med Human* 2005; **31**(1): 23–30.

Pellegrino ED. *Humanism and the Physician*. Knoxville: University Tennessee Press, 1974; p. 4.

Pickering N. The uses of poetry in health care ethics education. *J Med Ethics: Med Human* 2000; **26**(1): 31–36.

Saunders J. The practice of clinical medicine as an art and as a science. *J Med Ethics: Med Human* 2000; **26**(1): 18–22.

Sirridge M., Welch K., Body image and the innocent eye. *J Med Ethics: Med Human* 2002; **28**(1): 35–40.

Toulmin S. 'Knowledge and art in the practice of medicine: clinical judgement and historical reconstruction' in C. Delkeskamp-Hayes & M.A. Gardell Cutter (eds), *Science, Technology and the Art of Medicine*, Dordrecht: Kluwer Academic Publishers 1993; 231–249.

White M. *What Might the Health Trainer Role Look Like in Practice?* Durham: CAHHM., Durham University, 2006.

27

Reflective Equilibrium as a Method in Health Care Ethics

THEO VAN WILLIGENBURG

INTRODUCTION

Reflective equilibrium is a philosophical method that was introduced by John Rawls in his *A Theory of Justice* (Rawls, 1971). Rawls elaborated the method as an argumentative device for developing and justifying theories and principles of justice. Subsequent work has shown that the reflective equilibrium approach may be successfully used for other purposes too, for instance as a method of reflection about practical moral problems. Reflective equilibrium has become popular, especially in bioethics, health care ethics and clinical ethics.

The basic idea behind the reflective equilibrium method is that, in developing and justifying moral theories and in seeking answers to practical moral problems, we bring to bear – in some ordered way – all kinds of moral and non-moral beliefs and theories. A reflective equilibrium process pays attention to our moral and non-moral beliefs at various levels of reflection and abstraction, like particular intuitions, moral rules or principles and abstract theories. For instance, in their textbook *Principles of Biomedical Ethics* (1983/1994), Beauchamp and Childress describe their method as an interplay – a 'dialectical reasoning' – between theories, moral principles and judgements about cases. In a process of mutual confrontation and adjustment of our beliefs and theories (which on all levels of abstraction may need to be refined and revised), one seeks coherence among the widest possible set of beliefs that are arguably relevant in establishing a moral theory, in formulating moral principles or in deciding on a specific moral problem.

This basic idea has been developed in various ways, in answer to the epistemological criticisms about the model of justification used. In this chapter, I will analyse reflective equilibrium as a coherentist and at the same time weakly foundationalist method of ethical reflection and justification.

My analyses will lead to an example of the way in which the method may be deployed in health care ethics. This example will reveal four characteristics of the process of reasoning according to the reflective equilibrium method.

COHERENTISM

The reflective equilibrium approach is usually presented as a coherentist, clearly non-foundationalist method of ethical reflection and justification. Coherentism holds that a belief p is justified insofar as it coheres with a coherent set of beliefs. It is important to note that coherence is more than *logical consistency*. Coherence is also a positive function of (1) the *probabilistic relation* and (2) the number and strength of *inferential connections* between beliefs. If p1, p2 and p3 make p6 more probable than p7, and if p6 follows from p4 and p5, whereas p7 only follows from p4, then p6 better coheres to p1, p2, p3 than p7. Moreover, coherence is a negative function of (3) the extent to which parts of one's belief system are *unconnected* (e.g. what you morally believe has no connection to your religious worldview) and (4) the presence of unexplained *anomalies* in your beliefs (e.g. strong convictions that are unsupported by the rest of what you believe).

The reflective equilibrium method of ethical survey deploys a coherentist, non-foundationalist epistemology, because it does not start from unquestionable axiomatic beliefs upon which one's moral beliefs may be based. According to the reflective equilibrium approach, a warranted solution to a practical moral problem is reached by questioning the tenability and relevance of all sorts of beliefs, none of which is immune to revision. If a person's well-considered judgement regarding what is to be done in a particular case

Principles of Health Care Ethics, Second Edition   Edited by R.E. Ashcroft, A. Dawson, H. Draper and J.R. McMillan
© 2007 John Wiley & Sons, Ltd

is in conflict with the deliverances of applying some general moral principle, then, according to the method of reflective equilibrium, it is an open question whether the judgement or the principle should be retained. Coherentism holds that, in the end, neither the generality nor the abstractness of a belief nor the intuitive appeal of a well-considered judgement gives it special credibility. The justification of one's conclusion rests upon 'the mutual support of many considerations, of everything fitting together into one coherent view' (Rawls, 1971, pp. 21, 579).

THE CIRCULARITY REPROACH

Coherentist as this approach claims to be, however, reflective equilibrium cannot dispense with some weak form of foundationalism. The reflective equilibrium method must deploy a coherentist epistemology, while at the same time allowing for certain beliefs to have a non-inferential initial credibility. Such initial beliefs can function as provisional foundations of the reflective equilibrium process of deliberation and justification. The reason that we need to incorporate a weak form of foundationalism is that this is the only way to counter a powerful epistemological criticism on coherentism as a method of justification. The critique is that coherentism suffers from a serious circularity in justification. The circularity reproach says that the fact that many considerations support each other does not add to their justification. A coherent set of mutually supporting prejudices still is a set of prejudices. Some have suggested that reflective equilibrium brings us nothing more than a neat systematization of our biases (Brandt, 1979; Gibbard, 1995).

A possible strategy to counter this criticism is to enlarge the circle of considerations that play a role in the reflection process. If the circle is large enough, the circularity will be less disturbing or even cause no problem at all. If everything we believe hangs together in a justificatory way, then there will be a circularity in our belief system, but there is no reason to be bothered about that. We must only be concerned with the degree of coherence of our belief set because the degree of justification of any belief in that set is a function of the degree of coherence of the set. A belief system S^1 that is closer to the most perfectly coherent system of beliefs provides for a better 'circle of justification' than a system S^2 that is less close to the most perfect one. This means that one is only justified in accepting a new belief p, if inclusion of p results in a system that is closer to the most perfectly coherent belief system.

However, the problem with widening the 'circle of justification' in this way is that it would be very odd if every time you were asked, 'Why do you accept p?', you replied, 'Because it fits into everything else I believe.' Not only is this hardly an illuminating answer, but it is also difficult to

believe that this really is the reason for you to accept p. That p coherently fits into your entire belief system cannot be the reason for which you believe p. Actual justification involves challenging and supporting specific beliefs by providing specific reasons for doubt or support. This means that the coherence we are looking for must be local, not global.

But, if relevant coherence is always local, it seems that the justification for our beliefs is always only partial justification. A believe p may cohere with the relevant part of one's belief system, but that does not mean that it may not be in tension with other beliefs one has or would have, if one were to think further. It is always possible to challenge the believer to show that local coherence really provides for the kind of justification that entitles one to hold a particular belief. Partial justification is always provisional: the partial set of beliefs is always open to revision. What makes us think, then, that such a partial justification has brought us any closer to knowing what is morally right and true?

The answer of the reflective equilibrium theorist might be that the method invites us to throw in any consideration that makes one think that the local coherence which provides for partial justification does not bring us closer to moral truth, and to use this consideration to test the provisional equilibrium reached. Any reason for being suspicious about the local coherence set and any reason for thinking that the coherence set is just an amalgam of cooked-up prejudices may be used to scrutinize one's consideration. If one's beliefs survive such a test they will have gained credibility. If certain beliefs do not stand up to the test, one will abandon those beliefs, which will lead to an improved equilibrium set of beliefs (Nielsen, 1988). This is a default-and-challenge strategy. We may trust what we think, until we are challenged to think further and possibly improve our belief set. Our provisional moral convictions are justified until proven guilty. When proven guilty, we may alter them or even abandon them and so move closer to what is right and true.

COHERENTISM NEEDS WEAK FOUNDATIONALISM

However, the success of such a default-and-challenge approach rests upon the soundness of an important presupposition, that is, the presupposition that we are justified to take our present system of beliefs (the present provisional equilibrium) as a reliable point of departure of reflection and justification. For the default-and-challenge approach takes it that reasonably rejecting or incorporating a critical consideration will lead to an improvement of the provisional equilibrium: we move gradually in the direction of a correct or true moral view. But this presupposes that we can trust our starting point. It presupposes that we are warranted in taking our present system of beliefs as the point of departure for all justification, if it has a sufficient degree of coherence. The relevant system must, therefore, possess an *initial credibility*. For if one were to begin with a system of beliefs without any initial credibility, making it all fit together and increasing the level of coherence could not introduce credibility. Coherence is not the philosopher's stone which turns lead into gold. We have to assume that the members of the current coherent system of beliefs have some initial credibility, if they are to function as starting point of successful further reflection.

The question is what grounds one has for thinking that the beliefs we start with have initial credibility, especially because many of those beliefs arise spontaneously, without a sound backing. We know from experience that people can spontaneously come to believe odd things. It seems wrong to say that a person is justified in believing something just because it strikes her as plausible. Even so, there may be some reason to put initial trust in our current beliefs, even in our spontaneous beliefs. We are warranted in taking our current beliefs as the start of our quest for justification, if our current beliefs encompass also a number of epistemic norms about evidence gathering, about a minimal measure of mutual support of beliefs and about the conditions in which one has formed a belief.

One may compare spontaneous moral beliefs to perceptual beliefs, which we trust, if the circumstances in which they were formed are not abnormal and if they fit into the rest of what we believe. If these conditions are fulfilled, we are justified in holding our spontaneous beliefs until they are proven guilty. This comparison is inspired by the way Rawls originally modelled reflective equilibrium on scientific method, which sees theory construction as proceeding from observation reports (Gutting, 1982). According to this approach, moral principles and theories have to be tested against spontaneous moral beliefs, just as in science theoretical conjectures are tested against the facts as they appear in observation reports. Rawls does not speak about spontaneous beliefs, however, but about 'considered moral judgements': '[T]here is a definite if limited class of facts against which conjectured principles can be checked, namely our considered judgements in reflective equilibrium' (Rawls, 1971, p. 51). Considered moral judgements are 'considered' because of the circumstances under which they were formed. They are given 'under conditions favourable for deliberation and judgement in general' (Rawls, 1971, p. 48).

The analogy with scientific method goes back to Rawls' early article 'Outline of a decision procedure in ethics' (Rawls, 1951). In this article, he articulated a method for validating and invalidating proposed moral principles. The main part of that article consisted of an elaboration of criteria on the basis of which a judgement may be called 'considered', and, thereby, function as one of the moral 'data'

against which principles are tested. Rawls formulated various conditions on the nature and emergence of considered judgements, but also defined a limited set of 'competent' judges (characterized by a certain requisite degree of intelligence, knowledge, sympathy and 'moral insight'). Only the considered judgements of such competent judges may count as reliable data for decision-making and theory construction. In *A Theory of Justice*, this idea of a limited set of competent judges is abandoned. An appeal can be made to the considered judgements of 'bienpensants' generally. The criteria for calling a judgement considered are now predominantly circumstantial: 'Considered judgements are simply those rendered under conditions favourable to the exercise of the sense of justice, and therefore in circumstances where the common excuses and explanations for making a mistake do not obtain' (Rawls, 1971, p. 50).

The other difference from his 1951 article is that in *A Theory of Justice*, Rawls more clearly embraces a coherentist epistemology. It may be that considered judgements are the moral 'data' against which principles and theories are tested, but these data may be distorted, even when they are collected in 'optimal' circumstances. For, even in such circumstances, prejudices may arise. The 'data' for which the moral theory has to account may themselves need to be adjusted, rectified or even rejected as prejudiced, in the light of some convincing principles, theoretical framework or background idea. Therefore, there is no one-way accommodation but 'mutual adjustment', a concept which Rawls adapted from Goodman's inductive account of inference (Goodman, 1955; Rawls, 1971, p. 20, note 7).

Spontaneous moral beliefs, even if they are well considered given the circumstances in which they arise, can only be assigned a modest foundational role. Spontaneous beliefs are where our quest for further support and justification begins. This is different from the traditional intuitionist conception of spontaneous beliefs. For the traditional intuitionist, moral intuitions had a kind of self-evidence, which gave them certainty, or at least a degree of justification sufficient to give them axiomatic status. According to *weak foundationalism*, spontaneous moral beliefs possess an initial credibility, which warrants counting them as epistemic assets. But such spontaneous beliefs can always be rejected if they fail to achieve further justification through their inferential links.

Even so, our spontaneous beliefs have special importance because they determine in a sense the direction in which we reflectively proceed. They are the provisional foundations on which the edifice of further deliberation and argument rests. This is why the reflective equilibrium method cannot only be concerned with the epistemic quality of belief systems, but also with the circumstances in which the spontaneous judgements are made and with the quality of the inquirer's abilities and faculties for making moral judgements, constructing arguments and developing a well-founded moral outlook. Typically, a person can acquire the ability to make relevant discriminations in spontaneous judging and further arguing only after considerable experience. Deliberation along the lines of the reflective equilibrium method should not only be thought of as affecting our beliefs and arguments, but should also be expected to cause 'changes in a person's judgemental faculties, so that these faculties no longer function in the same way, yielding the same beliefs as they previously did' (DePaul, 1986). This means that reflective equilibrium thinking may demand the expansion of one's range of experiences – be they 'real life' or vicarious experiences, for example through case-stories and literature – in order to refine and possibly revise one's judgemental faculties and 'gut feelings'.

REFLECTIVE EQUILIBRIUM AND THE DEVELOPMENT OF SPONTANEOUS MORAL BELIEFS

The picture of the reflective equilibrium method of moral survey that results from the above analysis is this: reflective equilibrium is a specific method of systematizing one's moral beliefs and judgements in a connected and well-ordered structure. Spontaneous moral beliefs may determine in what direction the process of reflection proceeds, as long as such spontaneous beliefs arise in conditions favourable for deliberation and judgement in general, and as long as these spontaneous beliefs are available for scrutiny by principles and theories bearing on the moral issue to be decided. The actual decision reached is developed and supported by going back and forward between beliefs and impressions on different levels of abstraction – correcting, adjusting, pruning and perhaps rejecting some of these beliefs and impressions until a reflective equilibrium is reached.

The reflective equilibrium method combines coherentism with weak foundationalism. According to the method, a belief is justified as long as it coheres with a coherent reflective equilibrium set of beliefs (coherentisn). But the method also allows for spontaneous moral beliefs, like moral intuitions, to function as a temporary foundation and starting point of the process of reflection (weak foundationalism). The model *can* allow for this because the equilibrium it is looking for is always temporary and local. The equilibrium reached is never definite; it is always open for further correction, refinement and *enlargement*. Enlargement means that we move from more particular and immediate insights (intuitions) to more general and mediated stances (in terms of principles and general convictions). Practical reflection aims at structuring and enlightening our beliefs, which requires the formulation of general views that provide for insight into the purport of a complex

manifold of judgements and the diverse relations between these judgements. We have to try to understand the purport of our spontaneous beliefs in more general terms. Part of the reflective equilibrium method, therefore, consists in the rational development of our moral intuitions.

EXAMPLE: REFLECTION ABOUT GROUNDBREAKING BIOMEDICAL TECHNOLOGIES

Think, by way of example, about the spontaneous beliefs people have in view of groundbreaking developments and possibilities in health care. Biotechnological breakthroughs have opened the way to genetic therapy and genetic enhancement. Take one of the most challenging and frightening fantasies of the future: the possibility of cloning people. Such possibilities evoke not only horror (*The Boys from Brazil*) but also ideas about possibly salutary applications. Think of the parents who have just lost a young child, and who are offered the possibility to have a clone of their beloved child created out of cell material that has been stored. In this way they could have a replacement baby. Is this something we should immediately repudiate and reject as morally horrible, or is there also something to be said in favour of such a possibility? Most people feel strong revulsion and even fear in view of the possibility that these technologies might become reality. One way to understand this fright is to rationalize the intuitive images and ideas upon which it rests. Intuitions and worries about biotechnological reproduction of human life can be systematized and rationalized by connecting them to more general ideas and beliefs. An implicit, but very powerful idea in the background is that these technologies give humans too much power. If biotechnology gives us the possibility to create human life according to our own image and liking, then we will be taking responsibilities that humans cannot bear. If man starts to act as if he were omnipotent (playing God), then this 'hubris' will soon be destructive and result in gruesome possibilities. Procreation will be 'instrumentalized' and further denaturalized. We will finally create monsters that might destroy us. The intuition that certain new technologies in biomedicine are morally dangerous can be rationalized by connecting it to the idea that there are borders one should not transgress, because transgressing these borders opens possibilities that go beyond the range that humans can grasp and control.

The challenge of ethical reflection is to clarify and develop this idea and to see whether one can derive from it some critical and applicable criteria for assessing new medical technologies. The 'hubris' objection is connected to our self-image as actors. To understand ourselves and others as actors we need to ascribe to ourselves and others responsibility for certain 'happenings' that are the product of our activity. This ascription of responsibility takes place, even if we are aware that we are susceptible to 'moral luck'. For instance, our *character*, source of many of our choices and actions, has been formed by factors most of which are not under our control. And we know that very often the *circumstances* determine the outcome of our choices and actions (think of Oedipus and his tragic fate). In spite of these factors which we cannot control, we take and assume responsibility. We need to presuppose a realm in which we are in charge. And just as we need to presuppose such a realm where we are in control and responsible for our actions, we need a realm of happening, of things given – the 'givenness' of which functions in the background of what we do. This is not just a psychological need. It is not that we would not be able to live with the idea that everything is the result of our choices and actions. It is a metaphysical need: we cannot understand action and control, but against a background of happenings beyond control. On the one hand, we cannot understand ourselves and what we do as completely determined by the circumstances (we are agents, not patients). On the other hand, we cannot understand ourselves as the cause of everything, as if everything that happens is related to human choice. Just as determinism threatens agency, so complete voluntarism threatens to undermine our self-understanding as actors.

Such a metaphysical need is the reason for speaking about the 'natural' and the 'unnatural'. *Nature* is understood as that which is not touched by human hands. One may understand this in a normative way as 'that which is unspoiled by human hands'. Or one may understand it in a metaphysical way as 'that which is not our creation'. We need such a metaphysical understanding of the natural versus the artificial more than we need the normative understanding.

The above rationalization of the intuition that biotechnological reproduction of human life gives us responsibilities we cannot bear does not preclude the intervention in things that were up to now beyond human control. It means that we always need time and effort to reconstruct our self-understanding in terms of what we are responsible for and what not, given developing technological possibilities. Again and again, we need to reconstruct the border between actions and happenings. We need to delineate the domain of 'givenness' in contrast with the domain in which we are in charge. We need to sort out what we can take responsibility for and what not. The idea that we need to do so, in order to have a workable self-understanding as actors, may help to put our 'gut feelings' in view of groundbreaking biomedical technologies in a context where we can understand their import *and* their limitations. This may provide a basis for developing moral principles and rules that may have a say in regulating groundbreaking developments in medicine and health care. Such principles may prescribe, for instance, a certain level of caution, while at the same time encouraging

particular ways of enlarging the span of human control over life, death and procreation.

FOUR CHARACTERISTICS OF THE REFLECTIVE EQUILIBRIUM METHOD

The above example reveals four important characteristics of reflective equilibrium as a method of ethical deliberation and justification in health care ethics.

First, the example makes clear that the method takes the spontaneous moral beliefs and judgements of people seriously. In the context of health care ethics, this means that the reflective equilibrium method takes seriously the intuitions and moral judgements of doctors, nurses and patients. Reflective equilibrium not only aims at the rationalization of the moral intuitions of the public in general, but also specifically aims at a critical reconstruction of the views of those who are most directly concerned with the issue at stake. Such views are not taken for what they are. They are critically scrutinized and developed. Still, the answers arrived at via the reflective equilibrium process will be recognized as originating from the views and experiences of those most directly involved in the moral issues that require a decision and response.

Second, the above example shows that in our attempts to rationalize initial moral beliefs and 'gut feelings' we need to appeal not only to well-considered judgements and moral principles, but also to background considerations such as theories of action and theories of the person. Though the reflective equilibrium we are striving for is a local, not a global equilibrium, this equilibrium needs to expand the set of considerations that are relevant for the issue reflected upon, including non-moral ideas and non-moral theories. This is in line with the distinction Norman Daniels has made between narrow and wide reflective equilibrium. Narrow reflective equilibrium is a coherence of considered moral judgements and moral principles fitting together and mutually supporting each other. Wide reflective equilibrium introduces background theories and strives for coherence and mutual support between judgements, principles and a set of relevant moral and non-moral theories in the background. This means, as Daniels has phrased it, that wide reflective equilibrium allows for 'far more drastic *theory-based* revisions of moral judgements' (Daniels, 1979). In order to rationalize our spontaneous moral beliefs and intuitions we need to appeal to complex background theories relevant to the issue. Such background theories may clarify and systematize our initial beliefs, but they may also radically revise and modify them.

The third characteristic of wide reflective equilibrium thinking is the way it tries to rationalize and justify our spontaneous moral beliefs, by explaining and clarifying those spontaneous beliefs, putting them in a broader context. We may call this *justification by explanation*. This connects to Rawls' idea of his theory of justice as a systematization and elucidation of our 'sense of justice'. Wide reflective equilibrium seeks to provide a characterization and conceptualization of our moral sensibility with regard to questions of justice, a sensibility which is part of what Rawls called our 'moral capacity'. An important way to increase the number and strength of inferential links within a body of belief is to formulate principles and background ideas that provide for an explanation of the normative gist and power of the beliefs held. This is what we do if we try to elucidate our 'gut feelings' by invoking philosophical ideas about how we must understand ourselves in the world in which we live. Explanation which enlarges our understanding always involves generalization. We cannot elucidate the complex and opaque by referring to something that is even more complex and opaque. We explain our spontaneous beliefs and intuitions by putting them in a broader context where they make sense.

The fourth characteristic of the wide reflective equilibrium method has to do with the type of coherency justification that it provides. After accepting my analysis of the importance of rationalizing one's spontaneous moral beliefs and 'gut feelings' by invoking principles and background theories, one may still think that the circularity objection is undefeated. It seems that, even if spontaneous moral beliefs are rationalized by putting them in a broader context, prejudices cannot fully be excluded. A coherent set of prejudices still remains a set of prejudices. The objection ignores, however, that justification can grow by having beliefs participate in networks of other beliefs that may support or undermine those initial beliefs, as the coherentist recommends. The richer the inferential connection in a set, the stronger the credibility of the beliefs in that set. The idea is that if belief p1 and p2 are both to some degree justified, their joint justification is greater if p1 supports p2 and vice versa. It is like having two independent pieces of evidence for, say, the fact that Peter has committed a crime, and then finding out that these pieces of evidence also provide evidence for each other. One may think of two witnesses who not only have seen the crime committed but also have seen each other witnessing the crime. The confidence in their testimony about the crime increases because they have witnessed each other. Similarly, justification is amplified if more inferential connections are established in one's network of beliefs. If an intuition can be rationalized and modified by putting it in the broader context of a background theory, and if this rationalization implies particular moral principles which connect well to other principles we already hold, or which clarify some of our well-considered judgements in concrete cases, we will have increased the overall level of credibility of our beliefs.

CONCLUSION

In this chapter, I have presented reflective equilibrium as a coherentist and, at the same time, weakly foundationalist argumentative method for developing moral theories, formulating moral principles and reaching decisions on specific problems. Reflective equilibrium is a method of adjusting, clarifying and systematizing one's moral beliefs by connecting moral intuitions to theoretical insights, confronting principles with well-considered moral judgements and bringing, in this way, all sorts of belief to bear on each other, until a maximal coherence between one's relevant convictions is reached. The justification of one's conclusions rests, as Rawls famously phrased it, on 'the mutual support of many considerations, of everything fitting together into one coherent view' (Rawls, 1971, pp. 21; 579). It is like a tree that is held up, not by one deeply reaching tap root, but by a myriad of bigger and smaller roots, a complex root system.

Reflective equilibrium combines such a coherentist epistemology with a weak form of foundationalism, according to which our spontaneous moral beliefs, our intuitions or 'gut feelings' may function as provisional foundations that give direction to further reflection, deliberation and argument. Reflective equilibrium takes seriously the spontaneous moral views of patients, nurses, doctors and the public in general, by critically developing such views. This is done by using background theories and ideas that put those spontaneous views in a broader context, where we come to understand their import and their limitations. We, therefore, always seek a wide reflective equilibrium that allows for theory-based revisions of our moral judgements.

The reflective equilibrium method sees justification of beliefs as an incremental process. By increasing the number and strength of the connections between one's convictions on various levels of reflection (from intuitions to theoretical complexes), the overall credibility of one's beliefs is amplified. Such a growth of credibility is usually reached by seeking reflective connections that help us to understand why certain beliefs have moral import and how our moral views are connected to our self-understanding as actors and as social creatures. Reflective equilibrium aims at illuminating the opaque, and, in this way, increasing our understanding of the morally right and the morally good.

REFERENCES

Beauchamp TL, Childress JF. *Principles of Biomedical Ethics*. Oxford: Oxford University Press, 1983/1994.

Brandt RB. *A Theory of the Good and the Right*. Oxford: Clarendon Press, 1979; p. 93.

Daniels N. Wide reflective equilibrium and theory acceptance in ethics. *J Philos* 1979; **76**: 256–282; 266.

DePaul MR. *Balance and Refinement: Beyond Coherence Methods of Moral Inquiry.* London: Routledge, 1986; p. 211.

Gibbard A. Why theorize how to live with each other. *Philos Phenomenol Res* 1995; **55**: 2; 323–343; 331.

Goodman N. *Fact, Fiction, and Forecast.* Cambridge, MA: Harvard University Press, 1955; pp. 65–68.

Gutting G. Can philosophical beliefs be rationally justified? *Am Philos Q* 1982; **4**: 315–330.

Nielsen K. In defence of wide reflective equilibrium. In: Odegard D, ed. *Ethics and Justification.* Edmonton, AL: Academic Printing and Publishing, 1988; pp. 19–37.

Rawls J. *A Theory of Justice.* London: Oxford University Press, 1971.

Rawls J. Outline of a decision procedure in ethics. *Philos Rev* 1951; **60**: 177–197.

28

Hermeneutic Ethics between Practice and Theory

GUY A.M. WIDDERSHOVEN, TINEKE A. ABMA

INTRODUCTION

The Greek verb *hermeneuein* means interpreting. According to hermeneutic philosophy, human life is essentially interpreting the world and giving meaning to it. In ordinary life, people know what to do because they know how to interpret the situation. They know what to do at home, at work or with friends, because these situations are meaningful. This knowledge is embodied in stories people tell about their life. It is refined through communication and deliberation about proper ways of behaving towards the world and towards each other. Processes of interpretation in stories, communication and deliberation are related to moral issues and moral responsibilities. Should parents be lenient towards their children or strict towards them? Should colleagues at work take over from one another and be supportive or put their own work and career first? Should a friend be warned against making unwise decisions or should she be free to make them and learn from them?

Hermeneutic ethics is a theoretical enterprise, aiming to elucidate the role of interpretation in human life. It is also a practical endeavour, trying to foster processes of interpretation in concrete social settings. In hermeneutic ethics, theory and practice are interwoven. Theoretical notions of interpretation are developed through experience with practical interpretation processes. Practical interventions are elaborated on the basis of theoretical conceptions of interpretation and meaning-making.

In this chapter we will present hermeneutic ethics as an intertwinement between practice and theory. We will start from practice, focusing on an example of a story of a psychiatric patient. The story was told in a patient group, which was part of a project on coercion in psychiatry. We will show that the patient's story gives insight into several central concepts of hermeneutic philosophy. Finally, we will return to the practical impact of the story in the project and discuss some consequences of our theoretical analysis for the practice of hermeneutic ethics.

STARTING FROM PRACTICE

Between 1998 and 2004, a national project on coercion in psychiatry was set up in The Netherlands. The project was started by a group of psychiatrists and ethicists, who were worried about the high number of coercive interventions in Dutch psychiatric hospitals, in comparison to other countries in Europe. The national organization of Dutch psychiatric hospitals supported the project. The project was grounded in a responsive approach to evaluation. In this approach as many stakeholders as possible were engaged in a dialogue about issues that mattered to them in order to enhance their mutual understanding (Guba and Lincoln, 1989; Abma and Widdershoven, 2005).

The project consisted of two phases. The first phase (1998–2000) aimed at developing a framework for dealing with coercion in a responsible way. In six hospitals, groups of patients, psychiatrists, nurses and family members were formed. Participants were invited to tell stories about their experiences with coercion. Patients told about their feelings of anxiety and loneliness in the isolation cell. Staff told about their ambivalences. Should they intervene early, in order to prevent future problems, or give the patient a chance to calm down by himself? On the basis of these discussions, a document was drafted, containing guidelines for dealing

Principles of Health Care Ethics, Second Edition   Edited by R.E. Ashcroft, A. Dawson, H. Draper and J.R. McMillan
© 2007 John Wiley & Sons, Ltd

with coercion. The guidelines were drafted by researchers with a background in ethics, making use of quotations from the stories in the discussion groups. The draft recommendations were discussed in a national group, consisting of representatives of the six local groups. Participants in this group were very concerned about the proper way of describing the recommendations and making them concrete. After a process of adjusting the draft, the recommendations were accepted by the national organization of Dutch psychiatric hospitals in 2000.

In the second phase of the project (2001–2004), the focus was on implementation of the guidelines in twelve psychiatric hospitals (five out of the first six and seven new ones). In each hospital, a local group was formed in order to make an implementation plan. In this group, various staff members, patients and family members participated. The group was supervised by a local coordinator, in co-operation with an ethicist. The local coordinators met in a national group to exchange experiences. A national group of patients was formed to talk about experiences and develop methods for including patients in the implementation process. The aim was to share experiences and to learn from one another. At the end of this phase, a book was edited with examples from practice in each of the participating psychiatric hospitals.

One of the participants in the national patient group told how she regained control over her life. The story has been included in the book about the project. In the story, Jenny, a person suffering from manic depression, describes how she is put in isolation during the early phase of her disease. She tells about her feeling of not being treated as a human being. Later on, she is helped by an effective treatment with medication. She describes how she finally gets out of the hospital again. The story of Jenny had a powerful effect on the patient group. Other patients recognized her experiences, and hence, Jenny's 'I' story turned into a 'we' story. The listeners commented upon the story and helped it to unfold. They learnt that it is good to tell others about difficult phases in one's life. They felt that Jenny's story would help them to cope with future problems. We think the story had this powerful effect because it expressed crucial aspects of hermeneutic experience. In the following section we will make explicit these aspects.

MEANING-MAKING AND MOODS

From a hermeneutic perspective, meaning is related to lived experience. The meaning of a situation is felt, rather than consciously constructed. According to Heidegger (1927) human existence is characterized by moods. Human existence is being related to the world and finding oneself

being moved by the world. The fundamental role of moods in life shows that meaning is bestowed upon us. Events are experienced as thrilling or dull, before we even think about what is going on. Every interpretation is based upon primary feelings and emotions. Yet, our reactions are not merely caused by the feelings we have. They are oriented towards the future. In our response to the situation, we understand what to do and how to handle it. In the process of interpretation, we actively shape the world. This does not mean that we consciously plan what to do. Interpreting is not primarily knowing what to do, but knowing how to do.

Jenny describes the importance of moods in her life. In the beginning of the disease, she was taken into care in a psychiatric hospital. She felt ill at ease and was hot-tempered. She says:

> I could be very angry, because I felt powerless. I would be warned, and this would make me feel rebellious. If a nurse said: 'Do not put your cigarette out in that plant', I would not see this as reasonable, and I would become more and more rebellious.

As a result, Jenny was often put in an isolation cell. The cell makes her feel uncomfortable.

> It is not humane to be in a cell without a toilet. These cardboard chamber pots are very awkward.

After a while the medication starts to work. Yet, she is anxious about the risk of becoming numbed by it. Luckily, this does not occur.

> I was really worried that I would not have any feelings any more. Well, it did not turn out that way.

She is hesitant about leaving the hospital and returning home. In the end, she is forced to go. At home she often feels down and lonely.

> I stayed in the hospital for three years, and then I had to go home. I went home one day and never returned to the hospital. I experienced a lot of anxiety and loneliness. I felt abandoned by the hospital. I often called the emergency line.

The process depicted by Jenny is charged with emotions. They are in part the result of her illness, which makes her feel excited and rebellious at some times and anxious and lonely at other times. Yet, her moods are also crucial for the process of learning how to live with the disease. Jenny's story shows that emotions are important, in that they make clear what matters and what really needs attention. Emotions are not unreliable compared to conscious calculations; they are often more reliable (Nussbaum, 1990). Jenny found ways of dealing with her problems by taking her emotions seriously. The story shows that Jenny is a person who is able to endure her fate and to find ways of coping with it, not by discarding her emotions, but by acting upon them.

PERSPECTIVE AND DIALOGUE

From a hermeneutic perspective, understanding is always partial. One can never fully grasp the meaning of a situation, just as one cannot see an object totally (Merleau-Ponty, 1945). The possibility of various perspectives is not primarily something we consciously conclude. It is forced upon us, when we realize that the object is different from what we presupposed, for instance when a seemingly placid dog turns on us and tries to bite. Because understanding always takes place within a specific perspective, it can be enlarged by a change of perspective. This change again is not something we primarily decide; it is something we go through when our expectations are not being met. By being confronted with an aggressive dog, we come to understand that we have to be more careful. According to Gadamer (1960) hermeneutic understanding means extending one's perspective, or broadening one's horizon. In a conversation, we can be confronted with unexpected statements or utterances. Gadamer distinguishes hermeneutic understanding from two other kinds of knowledge of the other, namely, law-like explanation and understanding the other as a unique person (Gadamer, 1960). If one understands the expression of the other by categorizing it under some general law, one is not really open to what the other has to say. If one understands the other as unique, one empathically tries to enter into the perspective of the other, by leaving behind one's own horizon. Even if this were possible, it would not result in really understanding the other because one would not relate the other's perspective to that of oneself. In contrast to these two modes of knowledge of the other, hermeneutic understanding means being open to what the other has to say, which means being prepared to accept it as relevant and valid for oneself.

In Jenny's story, limitations of perspective are clearly visible, for instance, when she talks about medication. She is convinced that she will lose her feelings when she takes drugs. After a discussion with her physician, she changed her perspective.

> First I had a drug that did not work well. I thought I might need another one. I discussed this with my psychiatrist. He said: 'we can add another drug, because you might need support from both'. I was really frightened, thinking I would lose all my feelings. Well, it turned out not to be the case. I can still feel everything.

Jenny describes a similar experience when she talks about the phase of leaving the hospital and going home. Her initial perspective is that the hospital is safe. She wants to stay there and remain secure. In line with the policy of de-institutionalization, she is forced to leave. She does not like it at all.

> I had to go home because of a change in the law. I had been in the institution for three years, nicely hospitalized. From one day to the next, I was home, and I never returned.

In the end, she agrees that she is better off at home. Yet, she still remains angry about the way in which she was discharged from the hospital. She describes how she expressed her indignation to a staff member from the emergency service.

> On one occasion, I was very aggressive towards the lady on the emergency telephone. She said: 'You are really angry, but I know a lot of people who have gone home, and for whom it has turned out well'. But I felt left abandoned by the hospital. My anger was not taken enough into account.

This passage in Jenny's story touches upon a crucial point in dialogical ethics; namely, the reciprocity between all parties involved in a dialogue. Although Jenny is open to the views of the caregivers, it appears that they are not that open to hers. The reaction of the professional at the emergency phone shows that she does not take Jenny's anger seriously. She is told to consider that many other patients have done well after being discharged. This is an example of classification, not of hermeneutic understanding. Evidently, it is not easy for caregivers to be really open to the patient and change their own point of view. Dialogic hermeneutics requires that all parties are open to one another and prepared to listen and change (Widdershoven, 1999).

The crucial element of reciprocity is taken up by another patient in the group. After hearing Jenny's story about the discharge procedure, she comments that the hospital has not treated Jenny well. Jenny suspects that the attitude of the hospital has to do with giving up on people.

> Maybe patients are regarded as even more hopeless nowadays. They have a disease, and nothing can be done about it, apart from trying some medicines. There is no attention paid to the person or her history. A person's anger can be understandable from her life history.

We may conclude that hermeneutic understanding requires a change of perspective, not only on the side of the patient but also on the side of the staff. This is in line with Gadamer's conception of hermeneutics: 'To reach an understanding in a dialogue is not merely a matter of putting oneself forward and successfully asserting one's own point of view, but being transformed into a communion in which one does not remain what one was' (Gadamer, 1960, p. 360).

DELIBERATION AND NEGOTIATION

In medical ethics and medical law, the interaction between physician and patient is ideally conceived in terms of informed consent. The role of the physician is to provide information and present treatment options. The physician should not bring any values to the discussion with the patient. From a hermeneutic perspective, this view is one-sided. Health care implies helping people to protect their vulnerability. This requires not only assistance in knowing technical options but also support in dealing with questions concerning the good life. In this process, values are not given, but are in need of investigation and exploration. A hermeneutic perspective on values is in line with the deliberative model of the physician–patient relationship (Emanuel, 1992; Widdershoven, 1999). According to this model, the physician's role is to help the patient to clarify and elaborate her values. Autonomy is not regarded as the right to choose without interference, but as a process of moral development.

Moody proposes to replace the notion of informed consent by that of negotiated consent (Moody, 1992). Moody follows Habermas (1980) in conceptualizing communicative action as negotiation about the definition of the situation. According to Moody, a physician confronted with a patient's refusal should not simply accept it, but should start a process of negotiation. The aim of this process is to investigate why the patient refuses and to see what options might be acceptable to the patient. The physician should not give up his perspective, but try to find an opening in the perspective of the patient. From a hermeneutic point of view, negotiation will only work if the physician is prepared to open his own perspective. The physician should not only try to persuade the patient but also be prepared to be persuaded.

In Jenny's story, deliberation and negotiation play a role around her discharge from the hospital. Although Jenny herself prefers to remain in the secure environment of the psychiatric hospital, she is not allowed to stay. The policy of deinstitutionalization is based upon the perspective that living in society is more valuable than feeling safe in an institution. This clearly entails a view of the good life: living in the community is crucial to human life. Jenny not only has to accept this as a fact but she is also expected to share this view. Jenny should learn to see that living at home is good for her. Although she experiences a lot of problems after discharge, Jenny actually becomes convinced that living at home is better than staying in the

hospital. In this respect, her values change. In the end, she concludes that endorsing this view has enabled her to keep going.

> Two things really helped me. One is my medicine, and the other is my desire to live on my own. The latter made it worthwhile to try and learn to live with my disease.

The history of Jenny's discharge shows that it was necessary for her to change her view of the good life. In the end, patient and staff agree that living at home is a crucial aspect of the good life; yet they still disagree about how to deal with emotions in the process of leaving the institution. Jenny seems not to be allowed to have any positive feelings about the institution. The view that she is losing something valuable (her security) is not accepted. A truly hermeneutic process of moral development would have included awareness on the side of the care providers that institutions have some value too. Deinstitutionalization is not the only good in the world, and awareness of its relative value might make the policy of deinstitutionalization both more acceptable and more humane.

MORAL EXPERIENCE AND PHRONÈSIS

Hermeneutic ethics is based on the assumption that interpretation is not a matter of theoretical insight, but of practical moral experience. In line with Aristotle, hermeneutic ethics claims that one can only come to know what is right by dealing with moral problems in practice. Moral insight requires experience with moral issues in real life. That is why, according to Aristotle, moral insight, or phronèsis, cannot be found among young people (Aristotle, *EN* 1142a). The notion of phronèsis in Aristotle combines knowledge and practice. A person with phronèsis knows what is good because she has learnt through experience and exercise. The knowledge in this case is essentially practical itself. It says what should be done in a concrete circumstance. In Aristotle's ethics, medicine is often mentioned as an example of phronèsis (see Widdershoven, 2002; Svenaeus, 2003). A good doctor needs to have moral insight. According to Aristotle, a competent physician is able to see what is the right treatment for the individual patient in the concrete situation (Widdershoven, 1987; Benaroyo, 2000; Svenaeus, 2003). He is a *phronimos*, a person who knows in a specific situation what is the right thing to do at the right time.

The physician advising Jenny to add another drug to her regime had the right insight into her needs. The staff setting in motion the process of dehospitalization considered themselves wise. Yet, Jenny's reaction shows that their insights were limited. It may be good in general for psychiatric patients to leave hospital once they are more stable, but this general rule did not simply apply to Jenny at that specific time, as her anger shows. Jenny should have been supported in overcoming her anxiety and doubts, as she was in the case of the medication. She needed help to develop the skills and habits necessary in her new situation. Because the staff overlooked this, their intervention missed adequate insight. Jenny's history shows that phronèsis is not a visionary power on the side of the physician. It is actually the ability to be open to the reaction of the patient. A morally competent care-giver shows responsiveness in case the care is not well received (Tronto, 1993).

In the philosophy of medicine, the Aristotelian notion of phronèsis is normally reserved for the physician. It is, however, relevant for the patient too (Benaroyo and Widdershoven, 2004). Just as a moral teacher has the aim to develop moral skills in the pupil, so a responsible physician will try to teach the patient how to live well. He succeeds in this, if the patient acquires insight into what is the right thing for her to do at the right time in a specific situation. Patients always have some knowledge about their situation. They know from experience about risks and opportunities. Their knowledge is, however, not always correct. As the story of Jenny shows, her insights into the risks of medication were wrong. Medication may make people numb in general, but this appeared not to be so in her case. The physician taught Jenny to see this. After being discharged, Jenny lacked the skills to know how to behave towards others. Jenny explains how she was helped by behaviour therapy.

> When I phoned the emergency team, I got very angry. The lady on the telephone said to me: 'You should try behaviour therapy'. My general practitioner did not know much about it. Therefore I went to see my psychiatrist. He said: 'You can join a group'. In the group, I felt safe. The therapist was very good. He told me things I was already waiting for for a long time. For instance, that I should tell people what I needed. I always tended to think that other people were mean to me, and so remained silent and turned inwardly, instead of telling them what I needed. Therapy was not easy. You notice at first that you are very afraid of other people. You think they will see that you are a patient. But you have to learn to behave differently. Talking to one another in a group is really helpful in this respect.

Jenny's experience shows that behaviour therapy provided her with phronèsis. Most behaviour therapists will not interpret their own activity as raising the patient's moral awareness and skills. They will define the effects of therapy in terms of mental health, not in terms of living a good life. Jenny's story makes clear that the value of behaviour therapy for her was that it helped her to acquire hermeneutic skills, enabling her to understand her own situation, engage with other people and live her life in a meaningful way. She expresses this thus:

> Now I can live and be at home in a normal way. I think: you have gone through a lot, you should take it in. That is what I do, and I get a lot of support from others in doing so.

FROM THEORY BACK TO PRACTICE

Jenny's story has enabled us to present some important elements of hermeneutic ethics. The story shows the importance of emotion in life in a concrete way. Jenny is moved by fears and hopes, which motivate her to try to find a way to live with her disease. It is often a painful process and it has a rather erratic (versus linear) character (Abma, 1998; Deegan, 1988). During this process, she broadens her perspective on the use of medicine and on the value of living at home. This change of perspective is the outcome of a dialogue with her care-givers. Through deliberation and negotiation, a process of moral development takes place in which Jenny comes to regard her life differently. Her life does not become easy. She is often lonely, but at crucial moments she calls for help and is open to advice. Behaviour therapy specifically provides her with the moral skills necessary to live in the community. Her story can be regarded as a successful history of recovery, not because she has finally overcome all problems, but because she has enough motivation, openness and skills to deal with them in a more or less satisfactory way.

Jenny's story draws an ambivalent picture of the health care system. On one hand, the caregivers help her to find new ways of dealing with her problems. On the other hand, they often impose their views upon her and neglect her worries. The reaction of other patients in the group shows that they recognize these ambivalences in the current health care system. They all experience that health care providers can help to change the moral views of patients, but are not open to moral issues themselves. Jenny's story and the group's reaction to it show that moral learning by health care professionals is not easily achieved. Although they use words like patient-oriented care and demand-driven care, health care providers are not very open to patient views. In spite of the dominant informed consent model, health care providers still feel the need to educate patients and to stimulate them to change their view of the good life. From a hermeneutic perspective, this is good. It shows that care-givers have a moral commitment and consequently try to convince their patients of the importance of fundamental human values. Their approach is, however, one-sided. They are willing to challenge patients to change their view, but they are much less willing to broaden their own perspective.

How can we make the theoretical insights of hermeneutic ethics useful in practice? What can we do to change health care into a process of shared moral learning? One way is to write down the conclusions from our theoretical analysis and make (future) health care professionals study them. The relevance of written documents should not be underestimated. From a hermeneutic perspective, texts are powerful media. Yet, if it comes to finding concrete new ways to further moral learning in health care practice, we should also look for other methods. One such method is clinical case deliberation (Steinkamp, 2003). In this approach, concrete moral problems are discussed with practitioners in the institution. It is based on real cases, inviting participants to share concrete experiences. A problem in clinical case deliberation is how to give a voice to the patient (Reiter-Theil, 2003). Therefore, we started to use patient' stories as input for moral deliberation within groups of professionals (Abma and Widdershoven, 2006). In the implementation project, patient stories, like the story of Jenny, were presented to professionals. Quotations from the stories were used to elicit comments and to develop new ideas about practice improvement. We did not want to answer such questions as moral experts, but give new input to and function as mediators in the conversation in practice (Walker, 1993). When confronted with patient' stories expressing concrete experiences, professionals were able to be more aware of the nature and impact of their actions. They learned to see patients' perspectives. Finally, they reached better self-understanding and were more motivated to improve practice.

Hermeneutic ethics aims to develop theoretical notions from practical experience and to translate these theoretical insights into practical learning processes. The basic idea behind this is the hermeneutic circle (Gadamer, 1960). In order to understand the meaning of notions such as dialogue, deliberation and negotiation, one has to start from actual experiences in health care practice. A theoretical analysis of stories from participants may make visible both the strong and the weak sides of the way in which the notion of dialogue is realized in current practice. Such an analysis requires method and rigor (Koch, 1996; Abma and Widdershoven, 2005). In our case, the analysis showed that in psychiatric practice, the fundamental notion of reciprocity is underdeveloped. By elaborating the notion of reciprocity, we came to understand better what is really necessary for a hermeneutic dialogue. We used this as input for the group discussion with practitioners. By listening to the patient's story and discussing it with each other, practitioners became motivated to change practice, in order to realize the notion of dialogue more fully. They developed concrete views on the way in which this could be done; for instance, by changing the equipment of the isolation room and paying attention to resistance to and providing more support during the processes of deinstitutionalization. The hermeneutic circle proved to be a practical movement, starting from stories of participants in practice, subsequently making experiential knowledge explicit through theoretical analysis and finally using resulting theoretical notions to further practical learning processes and changes.

REFERENCES

Abma TA. Storytelling as inquiry in a mental hospital. *Qual Health Res* 1998; **8**(6): 821–838.

Abma TA, Widdershoven GAM. Sharing stories. Narrative and dialogue in responsive nursing evaluation. *Eval Health Prof* 2005; **28**(1): 90–109.

Abma TA, Widdershoven GAM. Moral deliberation in psychiatric nursing practive, *Nursing Ethics* 2006; **13**(5): 546–547.

Aristotle, *Nicomachean Ethics* (*EN*).

Benaroyo L. The contribution of philosophical hermeneutics to clinical ethics. In: Thomasma DC, Kissel JL, eds. *The Health Care Professional as Friend and Healer. Building on the Work of Edmund D. Pellegrino*. Washington, DC: Georgetown University Press, 2000.

Benaroyo L, Widdershoven G. Competence in mental health care: a hermeneutic perspective. *Health Care Anal* 2004; **12**, 295–306.

Deegan P. Recovery: the lived experience of rehabilitation. *Psychosoc Rehab J* 1988; **11**(4): 11–19.

Emanuel EJ, Emanuel LL. Four models of the physician–patient relationship. *JAMA* 1992; **267**: 2221–2226.

Gadamer H-G. *Wahrheit und Methode*. Tübingen: J.C.B. Mohr, 1960.

Guba EG, Lincoln YS. *Fourth Generation Evaluition*. Beverly Hills: Sage, 1989.

Habermas J. *Theorie des kommunikativen Handelns*. Frankfurt am Main: Suhrkamp, 1980.

Heidegger M. *Sein und Zeit*. Tübingen: Max Niemeyer Verlag, 1927.

Koch T. Implementation of a hermeneutic inquiry in nursing: philosophy, rigour and representation. *J Adv Nursing* 1996; **24**: 174–184.

Merleau-Ponty M. *Phénoménologie de la perception*. Paris: Gallimard, 1945.

Moody HR. *Ethics in an Aging Society*. Baltimore, Ms: Johns Hopkins University Press, 1992.

Nussbaum MC. *Love's Knowledge. Essays on Philosophy and Literature*. Oxford: Oxford University Press, 1990.

Reiter-Theil S. Balancing the perspectives. The patient's role in clinical ethics consultation. *Med Health Care Philos* 2003; **6**: 247–254.

Steinkamp NL, Gordijn B. Ethical case deliberation on the ward. A comparison of four methods. *Med Health Care Philos* 2003; **6**: 235–246.

Svenaeus F. Hermeneutics of medicine in the wake of Gadamer. The issue of *phronesis*. *Theor Med* 2003; **24**: 407–431.

Tronto JC. *Moral Boundaries. A Political Argument for an Ethic of Care*. New York/London: Routledge, 1993.

Walker MU. Keeping moral space open. New images of ethics consulting. *Hastings Center Rep* 1993; **23**: 33–40.

Widdershoven GAM. Care, cure and interpersonal understanding. *J Adv Nursing* 1999; **29**: 1163–1169.

Widdershoven GAM. Technology and care from opposition to integration. In: Gastmans C, ed. *Between Technology and Humanity. The Impact of Technology on Health Care Ethics*. Leuven: Leuven University Press, 2002.

Widdershoven-Heerding I. Medicine as a form of practical understanding. *Theor Med* 1987; **8**: 179–186.

29

Paternalism in Health Care and Health Policy

JAMES F. CHILDRESS

When, if ever, may or should a health care professional withhold a diagnosis of a serious disease from a patient? Or downplay the seriousness of that disease? Or refrain from mentioning the likelihood of imminent death? Is it justifiable for a health care team to continue treating a severely burned young man against his wishes in order to prevent his death, in the belief that he will later be glad to be alive? Under what conditions may and should a clinician seek to have a patient involuntarily hospitalized because of risks of self-harm or suicide? When, may or should policy-makers seek to develop laws to control the risks people take when there are no risks, costs or burdens to other people or to the society? In short, and more abstractly, when, if ever, are paternalistic actions and policies ethically justified?

Controversies surround the meaning and justification of paternalistic actions in health care and paternalistic public policies related to health. Despite extensive and intensive critiques of paternalism, particularly from the standpoint of respect for personal autonomy, it persists and remains common and important in both contexts. Indeed, it has even gained new appreciation and new momentum in recent years. For instance, in health-related policy, neopaternalists have offered arguments for government policies that, at a minimum, seek to protect or benefit individuals through shaping or steering their choices without, in fact, limiting or coercing those choices (Sunstein, 2004). Similarly, in health care, arguments have emerged that the physician should take a leading role in helping patients select the goals of care, instead of merely presenting in a neutral way 'a laundry list of means and insist[ing] that patients choose for themselves' (Loewy, 2005).

This chapter will examine the nature of paternalism, particularly by discussing its moral foundations and limits and drawing several distinctions that bear on its interpretation and justification, consider circumstances in which it may be justified and finally, explore the new paternalism, based on recent studies in behavioural economics and psychology, that plays a role in proposals for health-related public policies.

WHAT IS PATERNALISM?

Paternalistic actions display at least two features: they aim at protecting or promoting the welfare of individuals themselves and they do so by not acquiescing in the preferences, choices or actions of those individuals. Paternalism invokes a metaphor of the relationship between father and child as depicted in the late nineteenth century when the term emerged. Even before the term itself, the metaphor functioned in the language, for instance, of 'paternal government' that Mill (1976) and others used to criticize governmental policies. The metaphor is problematic because it expresses gender roles. However, there are reasons, some feminists argue, for retaining the gendered language of paternalism because it highlights the link between a father's privileges in a patriarchal family and a physician's privileges in a hierarchical medical system (Sherwin, 1976). Nevertheless, both 'parentalism' (Kultgen, 1995) and 'maternalism' – as well as the 'nanny state' and various other terms – have been used to cover beneficence-based actions that do not acquiesce in the preferences, choices and actions of individuals for their own benefit. Each of these terms also has social and cultural baggage. In the final analysis, the term paternalism still remains the most appropriate because of common usage, tradition and philosophical debates.

Both medical paternalism and governmental paternalism have a moral foundation in the principle of beneficence and/or the virtue of benevolence (Childress, 1982; Beauchamp and Childress, 2001). In pure paternalistic actions, the intended beneficiary must be an individual whose own

Principles of Health Care Ethics, Second Edition Edited by R.E. Ashcroft, A. Dawson, H. Draper and J.R. McMillan
© 2007 John Wiley & Sons, Ltd

good is sought (or for health-related policies, classes of individuals whose own good is sought). Philosopher Gerald Dworkin (2006) has defined paternalism as 'the interference of a state or an individual with another person, against their will, and justified by a claim that the person interfered with will be better off or protected from harm'. (The agent need not be limited to the 'state' or an 'individual' but can include an institution or a group of individuals in specific roles.)

Dworkin's definition captures the beneficence/benevolence foundation of paternalism, but there is more debate about how to understand the means employed by paternalists. Specifically, how should we understand 'interference' and is it the best term? A broad interpretation of interference is non-acquiescence in the preferences, choices and actions of others (Childress 1982; Beauchamp, 2001). More limited interpretations focus on interference with liberty. Still others focus on infringement of certain moral rules and so forth. What is involved in 'interference' is important for determining whether and why paternalism is ethically problematic and when, if ever, it can be ethically justified. For instance, efforts to persuade an individual to act in certain ways for his or her own welfare are rarely problematic from an ethical standpoint, whereas coercion always stands in need of ethical justification. Interferences are most problematic and even *prima facie* wrong when they infringe the principle of respect for autonomy and/or specific rules such as liberty or freedom, privacy and confidentiality.

Still another distinction may illuminate paternalistic acts in health care. Dworkin's term 'interference' captures much *active* paternalism, which occurs, for example, when clinician intervenes, perhaps by providing information or treatment against a patient's request. But 'interference' may be too interventionist and too strong to encompass *passive* paternalism. Consider a health care professional's refusal to perform an action requested by a patient on the grounds that it would not benefit and would even be harmful to that patient. For example, a physician refuses to perform a request for permanent sterilization because of his or her judgement that it would not be in the sexually active, 20-year-old requester's best interests in the long run. Or a physician declines to participate in assisted suicide in a jurisdiction where it is legal because he or she does not believe it would be in that patient's best interest. Or a physician elects not to provide a futile treatment requested by the patient. In passive paternalism, then, a person refuses to be an agent for the requester, while leaving open the possibility that the requester could find someone else to carry out the request. Other things being equal, it is easier to justify passive paternalism than active paternalism, and the remainder of this chapter will focus largely on active paternalism.

WEAK AND STRONG PATERNALISM

In the moral analysis and assessment of paternalistic actions or policies, one of the most prevalent and important

distinctions is between *weak* and *strong* paternalism, first formulated by Joel Feinberg (1971) and subsequently elaborated by many others. In strong paternalism, the intended beneficiary is deemed to be an autonomous or substantially autonomous person whose preferences, choices and actions appear to damage or threaten to damage his or her best interests. A strong paternalistic action will, at a minimum, infringe the intended beneficiary's autonomy, an infringement of an important moral principle of respect for autonomy. It may also infringe other moral principles and rules. The burden of justification for strong paternalism is heavy, though not impossible to meet.

By contrast, in weak paternalism, the intended beneficiary is deemed to be non-autonomous or substantially non-autonomous. As a result, his or her preferences, choices and actions do not carry the same weight as those of an autonomous person. Indeed, in the absence of patient autonomy, the principle of beneficence encounters no tension with and no resistance from the principle of respect for autonomy. For instance, an incompetent patient – that is, one who lacks the mental capacity to provide informed consent or refusal – may nonetheless oppose a particular treatment the clinician believes is necessary. In such a case, the principle of beneficence towards the patient does not conflict with the principle of respect for autonomy because the patient lacks substantial autonomy. Hence, there would be a clear and easy justification for overriding the patient's opposition to the treatment in question, especially if it is necessary to produce a major health benefit. Various means that would otherwise be morally problematic could also be justifiable, such as non-disclosure of information. An example might be non-disclosure of diagnosis of Alzheimer's disease to a patient who already has advanced symptoms.

Is weak paternalism even a form of paternalism? One important conceptual question is just this: is weak paternalism even paternalism at all, at least in any morally interesting and significant sense, if the intended beneficiary of a beneficent/benevolent deed lacks substantial autonomy? (Beauchamp 2001, 1984). Answers to this question clearly affect the pattern of justification for non-acquiescence or interference in a patient's preferences, choices and actions. However, it is helpful to use the term 'paternalism' for beneficence-based actions targeting the patient's own best interests when they are in apparent conflict with the patient's preferences, choices and actions, even if the patient is substantially non-autonomous.

There is a presumption that adults can form their own preferences and choose to act with substantial autonomy. In health care that presumption provides a starting point from which clinicians address any conflict that emerges. In doing so they may determine that it is justifiable to disqualify the patient as a decision-maker, for example, because of his or her incompetence and hence lack of autonomy. Caution is needed because judgements of incompetence – and other failures of autonomy – are not merely scientific and technical; they sometimes mask value conflicts. Hence, it is more illuminating and useful to screen actions, including possibly paternalistic actions, in the light of the relevant moral principles and the available evidence about the relevant benefits and harms to the patient and about his or her autonomy. Nevertheless, if the patient is not substantially autonomous, beneficence triumphs easily because the principle of respect for autonomy offers no resistance in those circumstances. Weak paternalistic actions are thus easily justified, but are not uncontested instances of paternalism.

By contrast, strong paternalistic actions are clearly instances of paternalism, but are not so easily justified, if, indeed, justifiable at all, in part because, as Dworkin (1977) notes, they are disrespectful, demeaning and insulting to the autonomous beneficiary. The most plausible approach, in my judgement, is not only to keep the door slightly ajar to the justification of some strong paternalistic acts but also to recognize that we should rarely open that door all the way. Beyond the principle of respect for autonomy and related conceptions, John Stuart Mill and others have provided utilitarian reasons for deep suspicion of paternalistic interventions, stressing the odds that the paternalist will be mistaken. According to Mill, (1976), '[t]he strongest of all the arguments against the interference of the public with purely personal conduct, is that when it does interfere, the odds are that it interferes wrongly, and in the wrong place.' Here Mill (1976) offers a more specific utilitarian argument than his broadly utilitarian argument that rules of liberty, where the agent's action do not put others at risk without their consent, contribute to human fulfilment.

Nevertheless, strong paternalistic actions may sometimes be ethically justifiable. By and large, such actions have a significant moral presumption against them, particularly in a liberal society that emphasizes the principle of respect for autonomy and related principles and rules. Nevertheless, theoretically, both beneficence and respect for autonomy are *prima facie* binding and their respective weights can only be determined in specific situations. What conditions need to be met in justifying strong paternalistic actions that infringe the principle of respect for autonomy because the intended beneficiary is substantially autonomous? Following are several important conditions for justifying strong paternalistic acts in health care; these conditions both modify and expand the conditions presented by Beauchamp and Childress (2001):

1. A patient is at risk of a significant, preventable harm.
2. The paternalistic action will probably prevent the harm.
3. The paternalistic action is necessary to prevent the harm.

4. The anticipated benefits of the harm prevention to the beneficiary outweigh the risks of the intervention to the beneficiary.
5. The anticipated benefits of the harm prevention to the beneficiary outweigh the principle of respect for autonomy in this case.
6. The paternalistic action involves the alternative that least restricts the beneficiary's autonomy while still securing the benefits for him or her.

These conditions specify for strong paternalistic actions the broader, more general conditions for overriding any *prima facie* principle in order to maintain another one (see Beauchamp and Childress, 2001).

Earlier I noted that physicians might decline, on grounds of weak paternalism, to disclose a diagnosis of Alzheimer's disease to a patient with *advanced* symptoms. A more difficult ethical question is whether physicians should tell patients in the *early* stages of Alzheimer's disease their diagnosis. In one case, a man in his sixties was brought to the physician by his son who suspected that his father had Alzheimer's disease because of his apparent problems in interpreting and handling what used to be normal day-to-day activities (see Drickamer and Lachs 1992; Beauchamp and Childress 2001). But the son also asked the physician not to tell the father if she confirms a diagnosis of Alzheimer's. After the appropriate tests, the physician believes that she has a firm diagnosis of Alzheimer's disease and discusses with a nurse and a social worker the son's 'impassioned plea' not to tell his father the diagnosis.

The nurse notes that there is now a settled and fairly strong consensus that patients who have cancer should be told their diagnosis – truthful disclosure is required because beneficence usually does not outweigh the respecting of the patient's autonomy in these cases. (Of course, beneficence should structure how the information is disclosed – a point that is often overlooked.) Nevertheless, the physician wonders just whether and how the principles and precedents regarding the disclosure of cancer illuminate the case of the patient diagnosed with early Alzheimer's disease. After all, there are some important differences between patients diagnosed with cancer and those diagnosed with Alzheimer's disease. First, in contrast to most cancers, the diagnosis of Alzheimer's disease lacks certainty (though over 90% of these diagnoses are confirmed by autopsy). Second, in contrast to many cancers, the course of Alzheimer's disease is uncertain for patients. Third, while therapeutic options have greatly increased for patients with many kinds of cancer, the therapeutic options for patients with Alzheimer's disease are still quite limited even though they are improving. Fourth, patients with Alzheimer's disease face an inevitable erosion of their decision-making capacity, which may not occur for most patients with cancer.

The physician in this case also has a specifically paternalistic concern. She worries that telling the patient would harm him because patients with Alzheimer's disease tend to have limited coping mechanisms, perhaps because of the neurobiological effects of the disease and disclosure could lead to functional decline, depression, agitation or paranoia – perhaps even suicide. Recently, however, investigators have begun to stress the potential positive benefits of disclosure to patients with early Alzheimer's disease because, for example, they can usually still participate in important decisions about their present care and in advance for their future care. Although the available evidence indicates that most patients with cancer want to know their diagnosis, the data are less clear for patients with Alzheimer's disease even though they suggest that more patients now want to know their diagnosis, particularly in the early stages.

In view of this range of arguments, clinicians (and family members) of goodwill may be quite unsure about the right course of action in these circumstances – as they affirm beneficence and non-maleficence, as well as respect for autonomy. There is no reason to believe that this patient diagnosed with early Alzheimer's disease is substantially non-autonomous. Hence, if the physician determines that disclosure would not be in the patient's best interest, the rationale would be strong paternalism. In view of the range of arguments just summarized about the disclosure of a diagnosis of early Alzheimer's disease and the facts of this case, it would be difficult, in my judgement, to justify non-disclosure as an act of strong paternalism.

PURE AND IMPURE PATERNALISM

Suppose the professional's or policymaker's motives are mixed – suppose he or she seeks to benefit particular individuals, to protect the public health, to avoid burdens to third parties and so forth. How should we characterize actions that express such a variety of motives? Debates about pure and impure or mixed paternalism surface in deliberations about both clinical actions and health-related policies. Consider a clinical case in which a mentally retarded teenager's parents and health care professionals are trying to determine whether it would be appropriate to have her sterilized because she has become sexually active. They concentrate on the young woman's best interests, but also consider the impact a pregnancy might have on several other parties, including potential offspring, the family and the society. If they elect for sterilization, their primary rationale might be paternalistic (the young woman's best interests), but the other concerns also may have been significant in

their decision. Hence, the decision might be characterized as impure or mixed rather than pure paternalism.

Rarely are governmental interventions in a liberal society, which professes the value of personal liberty, defended as purely paternalistic. Most often their supporters appeal to the protection of other individuals or of the society, sometimes because of threats to public resources. In contrast to the mid-nineteenth century when Mill was penning *On Liberty*, a justification based on public resources is much more plausible. In the context of public expenditures on health care and other goods and services, claims arise about the societal impact of individuals' actions that appear to harm only themselves. Hence, relevant third-party effects that justify non-paternalistic or mixed paternalistic actions include not only the traditional public health threats to others through infectious diseases, violence and so on, but also excessive burden on public resources.

A pure paternalistic justification would focus solely on the harms prevented or reduced or on the benefits provided to the affected individuals. For instance, a paternalistic campaign targeting obesity would feature the welfare of potentially or currently obese individuals. However, most campaigns, whether against obesity, cigarette smoking and so on explicitly invoke both paternalistic and non-paternalistic justifications, often with an emphasis on the latter because they are more palatable to the public in a society committed to individualism. It is appropriate to describe such campaigns as impure paternalism or mixed paternalism because the warrant is directed at both the individuals affected and at the impact their actions have on other individuals or on the society.

In debates about legislation to require motorcycle helmets, some arguments in support of mandatory helmet laws are clearly paternalistic – the legislation is intended, at least in part, to protect the motorcyclists themselves. Other arguments strain to show that unhelmeted motorcyclists increase the risks of harm to others, for instance, in creating hazards to passing vehicles and in imposing unfair burdens on ambulance drivers, emergency teams, nurses and neurosurgeons, as well as on the public, who, in an interdependent society, may pick up part or all of the costs of the motorcyclist's care. Exempting motorcyclists who internalize the financial costs, perhaps through mandatory health insurance, could reduce some of the externalities. But even so here, as in debates about governmental policies to reduce obesity, a contemporary source of major health problems for so many people, the line between what Mill (1976) called self-regarding and other-regarding acts and effects may be unclear.

Paternalistic actions often masquerade, at least in part, as protection of others or of the society, rather than the individual himself or herself, again because these justifications can be more easily accommodated within a liberal framework. Hence, it is important to consider, in the light of the best available evidence, the respective roles and merits of different arguments focused on protecting individuals' best interests, the public health and the public treasury. For example, as public health returned to centre stage in recent years because of newly emergent infections, the possibility of pandemic influenza and the threat of bioterrorist attacks, the temptation has been to hijack the language and norms of public health to cover private harms and thus to invoke public health rather than paternalism to justify proposed interventions.

SOFT AND HARD PATERNALISM

A similar issue arises with respect to soft and hard paternalistic interventions by the government, what Mill (1976) called a 'paternal government' or what in Britain has been called 'the nanny state, a protective but intrusive matriarch, coddling citizens for their own good' (Economist, 2006). In debates about paternalism, the terms hard and soft have been used in different but overlapping ways. On one interpretation, soft paternalism appeals to values that the beneficiary actually holds, but cannot realize because of problems of limited rationality or limited self-control (Childress, 1982). The individual's preferences, choices and actions are unwise even by his or her own standards. By contrast, in hard paternalism, the intended beneficiary does not accept the values that the paternalist uses to define his or her own best interests. Although soft paternalism reflects the intended beneficiary's conception of his or her best interests, hard paternalism reflects the benefactor's conception of the beneficiary's unrecognized best interests. According to Glen Whitman (2006) hard paternalists, as representatives of the old paternalism, say: 'We know what's best for you, and we'll make you do it', while soft paternalists, as representatives of the new paternalism, say: 'You know what is best for you, and we'll make you do it'.

The relations between the two sets of distinctions are complex – hard and soft paternalism on the one hand, and strong and weak paternalism on the other hand. The soft paternalist usually claims that limited rationality and/or limited self-control compromise the intended beneficiary's autonomy and thus prevent them from realizing their own recognized best interests. By contrast, the hard paternalist may hold either a weak or a strong conception of paternalism: the intended beneficiary may be viewed as a substantially autonomous agent who has selected and acts on the wrong values or as a substantially non-autonomous person who suffers from encumbrances in reasoning, willing or acting.

A related but distinguishable conception of hard and soft paternalism focuses instead on the *means* used to achieve the paternalistic goal. These distinctions are connected because the kinds of means used in soft paternalism generally presuppose greater compatibility with the beneficiary's

own beliefs and values, not yet realized or implemented because of inadequate rationality or inadequate self-control. Hard paternalistic interventions generally ban or prescribe or regulate conduct in ways that coerce individuals' actions to secure the desired result. These often involve clear trade-offs, as in 'sin taxes' directed at harmful conduct such as smoking cigarettes. By contrast, soft paternalistic means tend to influence, shape or steer individuals' choices without undermining their freedom to choose – for instance, they often frame information in certain ways while still being truthful and honest. Soft paternalists characterize their means as relatively weak and non-intrusive (Sunstein and Thaler, 2003).

In the light of this second version of the distinction between hard and soft paternalism, we can now qualify Whitman's earlier striking characterization of soft paternalism. Rather than saying, 'You know what is best for you, and we'll make you do it,' the new soft paternalist says, 'You know what best for you, and we'll *enable* you to do it without curtailing your liberty.' Along these lines, some proponents of soft paternalism even label their position 'libertarian paternalism' in order to underline the compatibility between liberty and this kind of paternalism (Sunstein and Thaler, 2003). Drawing on recent literature in psychology and behavioural economics, Sunstein and Thaler (2003) write: 'The idea of libertarian paternalism might seems to be an oxymoron, but it is both possible and desirable for private and public institutions to influence behaviour while also respecting freedom of choice.' As soft or as minimal – another term is 'minimal paternalism' – as it is, what they propose is still paternalistic because of the 'claim that it is legitimate for private and public institutions to attempt to influence people's behaviour even when third-party effects are absent' (Sunstein and Thaler, 2003).

The new soft paternalists focus on two major limitations on the intended beneficiary's preferences, choices and actions that may justify interventions to benefit him or her. These two limitations also show the convergence between versions of soft paternalism (in both senses) and of weak paternalism. The limitations are what Sunstein and Thaler (2003) call 'bounded rationality' and 'bounded self-control'. The conception of bounded rationality focuses on the bounds of rational decision-making that lead to departures from the 'economic assumption of unbounded rationality' (Jolls and Sunstein 2006). For instance, different default rules on the same action will lead many people to make different choices, or techniques of debiasing may correct biases such as the optimism bias that leads many people to underestimate the risks of some actions for themselves, even if they accurately estimate the risks to the population in general. In the presence of bounded rationality, the state may intervene, softly, in several ways, on paternalistic grounds, that is, enable individuals to choose and act in accordance with their overall best interests over time. As Jolls and Sunstein (2006) note, if the available evidence were to establish that smokers discounted the risks of smoking because of an 'optimism bias', among other factors, 'it is hardly obvious that government would violate their autonomy by giving a more accurate sense of those risks, even if the best way of giving that accurate sense were through concrete accounts of suffering'.

If private individuals are limited in their decision-making by bounded rationality, is there any reason to believe that governmental officials are exempt from this limitation? And if they are not exempt, then their policies may be unwise, ineffective or counterproductive. As Glaeser (2006) contends, 'flaws in human cognition should make us more, not less, wary about trusting government decision-making', which may be more flawed than private decision-making.

Some proponents of soft paternalism argue that, in any event, the government cannot avoid using soft paternalism, for instance, in framing the information it presents. After all, any presentation of information involves some standpoint or perspective and hence some framing because pure neutrality is impossible. However, in my judgement, neutrality should remain an important critical idea even if ultimately unrealizable for many, though not all situations in which the government discloses information about health-related risks. Others contend that soft paternalism is not only unavoidable but it is also justifiable, at least in some circumstances. Even though it can sometimes be justified, there are good reasons for sounding a cautionary note or warning about the recent wave of support for soft paternalistic policies.

Several arguments undergird this suspicion (see Glaeser 2006), but I will focus here only on a few important points. One apparent advantage of soft paternalism may turn out to be a serious ethical disadvantage from the perspective of social and political philosophy. Recall that this paternalism is soft – that is, it reflects many values that individuals would realize or implement themselves if they did not encounter internal limits of rationality and of control, and the means employed shape and steer without thwarting free choice. As a result, specific paternalistic policies may face little opposition and resistance and evoke few calls for or efforts at monitoring their implementation and effects. Indeed, these policies may even generate their own social and political support. All of this may happen without the transparency and publicity needed for public assessment, in part because some forms of soft paternalistic actions may be incompatible with transparency and publicity – once they are disclosed, explained and justified, they may be rendered ineffective.

At least, hard paternalistic interventions that involve coercion or serious and explicit trade-offs will be transparent and public, and opponents can mount counter arguments and resistance. Hence, it is plausible to suspect that soft paternalistic governmental policies may also be susceptible to abuse in part because of their lack of transparency. Furthermore, government decision-makers may single out some conduct for correction not only or primarily because it involves self-harm over time but also because it displays some moral flaws (e.g. lack of self-control). Not only may such moralistic judgements lead to the selection of some conduct for correction, among the wide range of acts that involve self-harm, but they may also intensify efforts to censure the conduct and ensure the correction.

Other related ethical concerns also arise. One focuses on stigmatization of conduct that breaches the social norms invoked in soft paternalistic policies. There is evidence that stigmatization can change behaviour, but there are also concerns about its psychosocial costs. Proponents of stigmatizing health-related policies usually insist that they target acts, not persons. However, in practice, it is easy to slide from stigmatizing certain conduct to stigmatizing people who engage in that conduct. For example, this has happened in the United States where, over time, stigmatization has played an increasingly explicit and important role in private and public efforts to curtail smoking: 'the antitobacco movement has fostered a social transformation that involves the stigmatization of smokers' (Bayer and Stuber, 2006). The slide from stigmatization of acts to stigmatization of people who engage in those acts can lead, as Glaeser (2006) reminds us, to hostility and even hatred for population subgroups. Again, cigarette smoking may be an example especially as smoking is now more common among lower socio-economic groups in the United States. As Bayer and Stuber (2006) stress, the ethical concerns become 'all the more pressing as stigmatization falls on the most socially vulnerable – the poor who continue to smoke'.

Another possible or even probable slippage provides yet another reason for suspicion of soft paternalism. The acceptance of soft paternalistic interventions, as Glaeser (2006) suggests, can prepare the way for and even lead to hard paternalistic interventions. One reason is that soft paternalistic interventions succeed in part by increasing support for the social values and norms that undergird the use of those interventions. The campaign against cigarette smoking again provides an instructive example – the movement from disclosure of information to sharper warnings and to hard paternalistic measures such as ever-increasing taxation of cigarettes (Viscusi, 2002–2003).

CONCLUSIONS

Paternalism is here to stay, in both health care and health-related public policies. Yet, that statement is uninformative without a more nuanced analysis of the many different kinds of paternalism this chapter has attempted to identify. Not all paternalistic acts are the same, and they need and receive different justifications and face different limits and constraints. Not all of them, for instance, infringe the principle of respect for personal autonomy. Hence, weak paternalistic acts are more readily justified than strong paternalistic acts. Other distinctions are also important: active and passive paternalism; pure and impure or mixed paternalism; and hard and soft paternalism. Although each type of paternalistic act or policy can be justified under some circumstances, the burden of proof is the heaviest for pure, strong, active and hard paternalism, but other forms, such as soft paternalism, also need close ethical scrutiny for reasons this chapter has identified.

REFERENCES

Bayer R, Stuber J. Tobacco control, stigma, and public health: rethinking the relations. *Am J Public Health* 2006; **96**(1): 47–50.

Beauchamp TL, Childress JF. *Principles of Biomedical Ethics*, 5th edition. New York: Oxford University Press, 2001.

Beauchamp TL, McCullough LB. *Medical Ethics: The Moral Responsibilities of Physicians*. Englewood Cliffs, NJ: Prenctice-Hall, 1984.

Childress JF. *Who Should Decide? Paternalism in Health Care*. New York: Oxford University Press, 1982.

Drickamer MA, Lachs MS. Should patients with Alzheimer's disease be told their diagnosis? *N Engl J Med* 1992; **326**: 947–951.

Dworkin G. Paternalism. In: Zalta EN, ed. *The Stanford Encyclopedia of Philosophy*, 2006; online http://plato.stanford.edu/entries/paternalism/ (last accessed 24 June, 2006).

Dworkin R. *Taking Rights Seriously*. Cambridge, MA: Harvard University Press, 1977.

Economist, The state is looking after you. *The Economist*. April 6, 2006; http://www.economist.com/opinion/displaystory.cfm?story_id56772346 (Accessed 23 June, 2006).

Feinberg J. Legal paternalism. *Can J Philos* 1971; **1**: 105–124.

Glaeser EL. Symposium: homo economicus, homo myopicus, and the law and economics of consumer choice: paternalism and psychology. *Univ Chicago Law Rev* 2006; **73**: 133–157.

Jolls C, Sunstein CR. Debiasing through law. *J Legal Stud* 2006; **33**: 199–237.

Kultgen J. *Autonomy & Intervention: Parentalism in the Caring Life*. New York: Oxford University Press, 1995.

Loewy EH. In defense of paternalism. *Theor Med Bioethics* 2005; **26**: 445–468.

Mill JS. In: Himmelfarb G, ed. *On Liberty*. Harmondsworth: Penguin Books, 1976.

Sherwin S. *No Longer Patient: Feminist Ethics and Health Care*. Philadelphia: Temple University Press, 1992.

Sunstein CR, Thaler RH. Libertarian paternalism is not an oxymoron. *Univ Chicago Law Rev* 2003; **70**: 1159–1202.

Viscusi WK. The new cigarette paternalism. *Regulation* 2002–2003; 58–64.

Whitman G. Against the new paternalism: internalities and the economic of self-control. *Policy Anal* 2006 (No. 563).

30

Need: An Instrumental View

ANTHONY J. CULYER

Health care is a commonly cited example of a service that ought to be distributed according to need. In this chapter I shall briefly review some of the approaches that have been taken by people who have thought about what this might mean and develop an approach that seems to be appropriate for the analysis of social policy (especially health policy). The general context is, I shall assume, one of fairly high-level resource allocation decisions – that is, levels like those of governments, professional organizations, managed care organizations and third party payers, above one-to-one decision-making in the professional–patient relationship. I shall use the words 'allocation' and 'distribution' as synonyms for 'rationing', which brings baggage in the form of associations with arbitrariness, ration coupons and the paraphernalia of wartime civilian privation. My conclusion will be that there are helpful and not so helpful concepts of 'need' but that none is particularly helpful in making resource allocation decisions.

Talk of 'need' is important for a number of reasons (I shall use scare quotes for 'need' only when I am referring to the word itself). One is simply that one ought to be as clear as possible about what one means, especially when using nouns that resonate strongly. Another is that 'need' has been and is used both in the slogans used by politicians, patient interest groups and ideologues and in more careful academic discourse, but it seems unlikely that the same meaning and significance attach to the word in each of these contexts. Yet another is that the word is commonly used by those actually involved in the process of managing and delivering health care but, again, one doubts that each profession attaches quite the same meaning and significance to it. Finally, need is often advocated and, indeed, accepted as an appropriate moral basis for prioritizing choices about resource allocations within health care systems, so one talks of meeting needs efficiently and meeting them equitably or fairly. The last of these uses requires precision and even

quantification to be practically useful, and it is that usage with which this chapter is primarily concerned: what is a need and how ought need be interpreted and used (if at all) in matters of health care resource allocation?

The existence of a need seems always to imply an absence of something, together with an implication that the something that is lacking is not trivial either on account of the severity of the deprivation, which is exemplified in the frequent coupling of 'poor' with 'needy', or, possibly, of the extreme attractiveness of the state achieved if the need is met. However, mere absence is plainly not enough, for there is a wide gap between what we generally imply when using the word 'need' compared to our use of 'demand', yet 'demand' is no less a response to the absence of something. This chapter therefore concentrates on what seems to be special about 'need'.

The distinction between satisfactory (according to canons of fairness and efficiency) allocations of *health care* to people (not just patients but also whole populations, especially in programmes of primary prevention) and satisfactory distributions of *health* is fundamental. It is a common carelessness to assume that there is a one-to-one correspondence between health care (or, more narrowly, medical care) and health. It takes little thought, however, to realize that the one is the hoped-for product of the other and that there is no automaticity about the relationship (for example, Rachlis and Kushner, 1989). Health care can be harmful to health; it can be irrelevant; it can be effective but only at prohibitive cost (when it is more satisfactory to devote resources to other forms of health care – or, indeed, to something altogether different, like programmes to develop regional sports facilities). There are large variations in the rates of medical intervention, not only between different health care systems but also within them (for example, McPherson et al., 1982; Wennberg and Gittesohn, 1982; McPherson, 1988; Sanders et al., 1989). These variations often reflect

Principles of Health Care Ethics, Second Edition   Edited by R.E. Ashcroft, A. Dawson, H. Draper and J.R. McMillan
© 2007 John Wiley & Sons, Ltd

what has become known as a 'surgical signature' in which the uncertainties, subjective judgements and preferences of particular physicians vary. They are sometimes indicators of wasteful use of resources and at best suggest that in practice there may be considerable empirical uncertainty as to what really is needed.

The concept of 'need' has commanded the attention of philosophers, most significantly Barry (1965), Braybrooke (1987), Daniels (1985), Flew (1977), Gillon (1986), Liss (1993), Miller (1976), Thomson (1987), Weale (1978) and Wiggins (1987). Some have taken an extremely simple idea of need as 'absence'. For example, both Williams (1962) and Gillon (1986) suggest that people who are more ill than others have greater need. While it is obvious that they have a relative absence of health, it is not altogether clear *what* it is that they need other than 'something that will fix their health for the better'. What if that 'something' does not exist, or if 'it' (whatever it may be) would make only a tiny improvement to their condition? Even if there is a 'something', there may be considerable argument about its efficacy (that is, the way it works under ideal, usually experimental, conditions) and even more argument about its effectiveness (that is, the way it can be expected to work in practice), for which indications it ought to be used (even those for which, if it is a drug, it has been licensed) and for which patients.

The identification of need at the aggregate level of whole communities with either morbidity or mortality (absolute or relative) has been common amongst economists (for example, Le Grand, 1978; O'Donnell and Propper, 1991; Wagstaff et al., 1991) and raises similar issues to those just mentioned.

'NEED' VERSUS 'DEMAND'

An early attempt to distinguish 'need' and 'demand' was made by Matthew (1971). He argued thus:

> The 'need' for medical care must be distinguished from the 'demand' for care and from the use of services or 'utilization'. A need for medical care exists when an individual has an illness or disability for which there is an effective and acceptable treatment or cure. It can be defined either in terms of the type of illness or disability causing the need or of the treatment or facilities for treatment required to meet it. A demand for care exists when an individual considers that he has a need and wishes to receive care. Utilization occurs when an individual actually receives care. Need is not necessarily expressed as demand, and demand is not necessarily followed by utilization while, on the other hand, there can be demand and utilization without real underlying need for the particular service used (p. 27).

This approach has been characterized by Williams (1978) as a 'supply' concept. As Williams puts it: 'a "need" exists

so long as the marginal productivity of some treatment input is positive' (p. 33). It is plain that the marginal product in question is not to be equated with the usual underlying maximand of demand theory (that is, 'utility') but something else – not quite defined by Matthew (1971) but apparently health or at least some outcome which someone (again not identified precisely) considers 'effective and acceptable'.

Bradshaw (1977) adopted a more synthetic approach. He developed a four-fold classification of need:

Normative need – that which the expert or professional, administrator or social scientist defines as need in any given situation. A standard is laid down and is compared with the standard that actually exists, the difference being what is needed.

Felt need – people who do not have something are asked whether they feel they need it. It is an expression of hypothetical demand.

Expressed need – felt need expressed by behaviour, as when a consultation is sought or when one is placed on a waiting list; need turned into action.

Comparative need – the difference between two individuals or groups who are otherwise the same, but one of which is receiving a service and the other not, the latter being 'in need'.

Each of these definitions is descriptive and empirical, and each clearly captures something of the 'absence' element of 'need', essentially based on a 'with and without' comparison, but, in 'comparative need', having the additional twist of comparing people with and people without. The definitions are not philosophically normative. Their 'truth' is tested by asking for the opinions of either professional groups or patients, or by looking at their behaviour. Having these characteristics, need is devoid of persuasive power – there is no particular ground offered, for example, for distinguishing it from 'demand' and, indeed, Bradshaw's concept of 'felt need' is similar to the idea of demand used in studies of contingent valuation and willingness to pay (for example, Bateman et al., 2002). So the question arises: why ought we to feel impelled to meet any of the needs thus described?

This question takes us beyond the descriptive, technical relationship between health care (input) and health (outcome) (or changes in the one and consequential changes in the other) into the matter of the valuation of the outcomes. It also raises the question of who ought to be deciding such matters. Plainly, it does not follow, just because doctors, nurses and other clinically qualified professionals like physiotherapists may be relatively expert at predicting the consequences for health of various inputs into the process of health care, that they are also expert at assessing the worth of the outcome and of outcomes forgone. If the 'productivity' approach addresses need essentially from the supply side, the valuation of outcomes is plainly a demand-side matter. It is a characteristic of the concept of 'need' suggested here that a useful concept will entail both a supply-side and a demand-side element: supply-side because what is needed must be productive in terms of promoting health, and demand-side because productive effects have value and we must address the question, 'how much value?' Of course, not all care is equally productive nor is all equally productive care equally valued. One must tread carefully here for the standard economic theory of value is built on the idea of 'preference'. Whether the analysis is positive (explanatory) or normative (prescriptive), 'preferences' are the fundamental sources from which value is derived (see, for example, Boadway and Bruce, 1984). In the case of need, the source of value is far more ambiguous, though it is plainly not mere 'preferences', and it will need careful examination, particularly in a context that often asserts that needs trump demands. The idea that some considerations 'trump' others is frequently found in non-utilitarian philosophical literature. It goes against the grain of economic thinking on the grounds that it denies the possibility of trade-off. For example, it entails the view that the meeting of the least of needs ought invariably to dominate the meeting of the greatest of demands and, should there be a hierarchy of needs, that the least of a high order need ought to be met before the greatest of a lower order need. This form of lexical prioritization is well suited to the organization of telephone directories but unattractive and unhelpful in practical policy discussions of 'what shall we do?'

'NEED', ABSOLUTE AND RELATIVE

Some usage of 'need' is not only categorical, like Bradshaw's typology or the identification of need with morbidity or mortality, but also absolute, with the implication that the need described ought therefore to be met absolutely and regardless of any other claims there might be on resources. One difficulty with absolutism over need is that health is not itself absolute. It is a variable, for example, in functioning, activities of daily living, experience of pain, mobility and longevity, mental state and it is also largely culturally determined – both with regard to the pathologies regarded as detrimental to living in a particular community at a particular time and with regard to the social construction of 'living'. An extreme example of this is pinta, a bacterial skin disease so prevalent among some South American tribes that it was not regarded as a disease at all: the few single men *not* afflicted were regarded as pathological to the point of being excluded from marriage. So in such tribes' culture there can be no *need* for a treatment for pinta; that would not be the case, however, in Scotland (if pinta were ever to arise there).

Another sort of extremism to which an absolute approach is prone is illustrated by Harris (1987): 'life saving has pri-

ority over life-enhancement and . . . we should first allocate resources to those areas where they are immediately needed to save life and only when this is done should the remainder be allocated to alleviating nonfatal conditions' (p. 120). Thus the smallest possibility of the shortest extension to the most miserable of lives is to receive priority over the most sure and massive improvement in the quality of a life already expected to be long.

'NEED' INTERPRETED INSTRUMENTALLY

The peculiar power of 'need' resides in the combination of two elements, one empirical and the other ethical. The empirical element is the idea of 'necessity'. If something is to be said to be needed, then it must be necessary for some purpose. This is an empirical matter because it is a matter of fact whether the thing in question really is necessary. In medical research, the generally accepted gold standard for knowing whether something is necessary (though it is not a standard that can always be achieved) is the randomized controlled trial, a scientifically designed method for testing the link between an intervention and its alleged effects and for minimizing the intrusion of confounding variables which might bias the attribution of cause and consequence both as to its sign (positive or negative) and to its effect size (large or small). In popular parlance, the question is 'does it work?' A positive answer to that question does not, however, imply that the intervention in question is *necessary*. After all, there may be other interventions that also 'work', or that work even better than the one on which we are currently focusing, or that work much the same but at a much lower cost. In such cases we plainly cannot describe the one in question as 'necessary' because there are substitutes for it which may actually be the intervention of choice. 'Necessity' is nonetheless about the productivity of health care in terms of health outcomes. It is a supply-side concept.

The ethical element concerns values (as does 'demand') and derives from the association of need with the moral idea that needs *ought* to be met, at least in part. Now the 'oughtness' of need might be fixed in a number of ways. One view might be to locate it in the ethical character of the end served by meeting it. Thus I, the author, may cheekily assert that I have a need for an SL-Class Mercedes Roadster in order to promote a dashing image (and impress my students) but this object carries little moral weight, even if it is true that my image would become more dashing and that my students would be suitably impressed. But if, instead, the end served is better health, and I would escape from a bed-bound and pain-racked life, and there is indeed a procedure that will deliver me in the way described, then the ethics of the claim about need changes in a way that depends not only on the empirical truth of the link between the thing needed and the outcome of the need being met but also, and critically, on the value of the outcome, so it is the significance of the end that distinguishes need from preference. This is a demand-side concept, though there is no particular reason to suppose that the value appropriately to be attached to an outcome is based (or solely based) on a person's preferences. The coupling of something being necessary for something else to happen with the ethical desirability of that consequence is what I mean by the instrumental idea of need.

The view that need is an instrumental concept has been strongly argued by Barry (1965) and Flew (1977). It has been opposed by others (for example, Miller, 1976; Thomson, 1987) on the grounds that some statements using the word 'need' are intrinsic and elliptical, or imply an objective which would be trivial to make explicit. For example, the statement: 'surgeons need manual dexterity' is hardly elucidated by asking 'why', for the answer might well be that 'surgeons need manual dexterity in order to be surgeons'. Similarly the statement: 'Anthony needs open heart surgery' is hardly elucidated by adding: 'if he is to live'. But this is to use trivial examples to cast doubt on the usefulness of the concept. It is easy to think of nontrivial examples that are still service- and person-specific and these usually require that one adds prepositions: something (like a specific medical act) has to be needed (is necessary) *for* something else to be accomplished. We must ask also *for what* it is needed (necessary). And we must also ask *for whom* it is needed (necessary). The first requirement is crucial in health care, for it directs attention towards the crucial question of whether *in fact* (or whether it *is probable that*) the act in question will have the effects (for the better) expected. As so much in medical (and health) care is of unknown effectiveness (or is even of known ineffectiveness), directing attention in this way alerts one to the possibility that someone may even be seriously ill without there being any reasonable prospect of medical care effectively changing their characteristics for the better. In such cases, whatever else they need, they do not need the sort of health or medical services that might be available. Too many unsubstantiated assertions of need *assume*, rather than *enquire* whether, the acts in question really are necessary. The 'reasonable prospect' I have in mind is one judged by people, including scientific experts, who have examined the matter via, say, randomized controlled trials, overviews or meta-analyses.

One should ask *for what* it is needed because there ought to be some more ultimate good from which the need in question derives its moral force. It should be person-specific or, at the planning and management level, group-specific as one must be able to identify who it is that needs whatever is asserted to be needed. One can trivialize these requirements

as in the cases of Anthony and the surgeon, but the more precise statement 'I need prophylactic lignocaine following my heart attack' may be false if I fear the risk of early mortality more than I value the prevention of arrhythmias (Yadav and Zipes, 2004). And the statement 'I need intragastric hypothermia for my gastric ulcer' is plainly false; for gastric freezing will do me no good at all and may do me harm (Edmonson, 1989).

A major objection to unsubstantiated assertions of need is therefore that they assume that, rather than inquire whether, the thing needed really is necessary. Modern technology may indeed make surgery less dependent on manual dexterity. Therefore, if we are to stipulate the skills surgeons ought to have, it becomes important to be explicit in determining how surgeons should be trained – and re-trained. Or, if we are deciding on Anthony's treatment, we really do need to know whether open heart surgery is appropriate for him, what the risks are, what the probability of success is, and what alternative actions might be taken. Moreover, these assertions assume that the objective really is the one sought. If the operation is likely to extend Anthony's life, will it do so only at the cost of a much lower quality of life? Or, how small must the probability of perioperative death be before Anthony judges the risk worth taking? The assertion that this or that is needed, even though its effectiveness may be disputed or unknown and even though the end sought may rank low in the priorities of those allocating resources or receiving services, is a commonplace of medical politics.

EFFECTIVENESS OR COST-EFFECTIVENESS?

It is rare to have a fixed and unique technology of treatment. It seems absurd to suppose that, of two procedures, each with the same expected resource implications but one with a much better expected outcome available, the one with the poorer outcome is as equally needed as the other. Conversely, of two procedures having the same expected outcomes but differing in the amount of resources used, it seems no less absurd to consider the costlier one as equally needed as the other. It makes more sense to say in the former case that the less productive procedure is no longer necessary (needed) because another, more effective and no more costly one is available and, with regard to the latter, that the more resource-intensive procedure can hardly be said to be necessary (needed) when there is an alternative that will achieve the same outcome but with fewer resources.

It is not absurd to talk of a need for an effective procedure that does not exist – people may have a disease for which there is no treatment of any kind, or they may have acquired a chronic resistance to the only effective treatment there is. Such people have needs and we know the character of the things that are needed but they do not have needs that can be met (yet) and they do not pose an issue in resource allocation (apart, possibly, from resource allocation to research).

I conclude from this that the only procedures that can be truly judged to be needed are those judged to be cost-effective.

NEED AND THE FLOURISHING LIFE

Even if health care is indeed effective, it hardly follows that the need ought to be met, let alone provided for, at public expense. Whatever is morally compelling about a need comes from the end served. A need for health services exists only if there are grounds for believing that these services will promote health, restore it, prevent ill-health or postpone death. These are the principal benefits sought from health care (less critical benefits include reassurance, legitimization of status for purposes of receipt of benefit and hotel services), and it follows that a need for health care can exist only when there is a capacity to benefit in one or more of these ways. More specifically, the need is for the service that might generate the benefit and the nature of the benefit must be sufficiently weighty, ethically speaking, to justify the use of so persuasive a term as 'need' rather than, say, 'preference' or 'demand'.

One can conceive of a hierarchy of goals, especially in the context of health care. One may, for example, speak of *health* as being needed. The weighty end served by this means might be a 'flourishing life' (Wiggins, 1984), or a 'vital purpose' (Nordenfeldt, 1984) or realizing one's 'life's projects' (Williams, 1973), or being able to operate within the 'normal opportunity range' (Daniels, 1985). But if one speaks, as we do in this chapter, of *health care* being needed, the principal goal in question then becomes the improvement of health. What then gives health the special ethical character to warrant the use of 'need' rather than 'demand' for health care?

Le Grand's (1991) answer to this is that people demand health care because they fall ill and that, since whether or not they fall ill is not within their control, the demand for health care is qualitatively different from the demand for other commodities where ethical considerations do not feature prominently if at all. It is for this reason, contends Le Grand, that the term 'need' is applied to health care but not to, say, televisions. But this does not seem to get to the heart of the distinction sought. There is, to be sure, a large stochastic component to the demand for health care. But individuals' health – and hence their demand for health care – is also affected by their behaviour. Once this is accepted, it becomes hard to use this line of argument to draw a meaningful distinction between health care and other commodities whose demand is also subject to uncertainty.

An individual's demand for automobile spares, for example, is also highly stochastic, but it is also influenced by the way the individual drives and how carefully they look after the vehicle.

Tobin (1970) thought that services like health care seem to be different in that they are more fundamental to the good life than others, which begins to make the beginnings of an ethical grounding for 'need'. Insofar as health is necessary for (or at the least conducive to) the more ultimate human good of 'flourishing', and insofar as health care is necessary for health, then the ethicality of the ultimate objective becomes transferred to the activity that can contribute to producing the ultimate good. It is that which differentiates the ethical status of health care from that of televisions.

We have now arrived at a point at which it may be seen that there are two necessary conditions that should be met when we speak of a need for a service. One is that the service in question should be cost-effective; the other is that it should be necessary for achieving a high ethical aim. Health care fits both. But not all health care fits. Ineffective care is not needed. Cost-ineffective care is not needed. Cost-effective care that meets mere demands without serving the higher ethical end is not needed. The definition has an ethical element (it must contribute to an ethical end) and a technical element (cost-effectiveness – which also involves ethical judgements, for example ones to do with appropriate measures of outcome that stand in operational terms for 'health' or 'change in health').

NEED AND ALLOCATION PRINCIPLES

If we consider resource allocation in the context of a publicly funded or a managed care system, almost any definition of 'need' carries the implication that a service that is not needed probably ought not to be provided. Beyond that, however, need turns out *not* to be an especially useful way of developing allocation criteria.

The claim that health care ought to be distributed according to need comes in two versions due essentially to Aristotle: a horizontal version (persons in equal need should be treated the same) and a vertical version (persons in unequal need should be treated in proportion to the inequality in need). These principles do not imply that all needs ought to be met but, rather, stipulate the manner in which resources and needs ought to stand in relation to one another. I shall assume that resource constraints prohibit the meeting of all needs and also the meeting of any single need completely. I shall also assume that we have a well-calibrated and uncontroversial measure of 'health' in order that we may focus on the implications of the principles without becoming entangled in the complexities (and controversies) about the validity of the construct 'health' and its measurement.

NEED AS ILL-HEALTH

Horizontal equity requires persons having like ill-health to be treated in a similar fashion. It would plainly be silly to interpret this as requiring each to have the same resource, partly because having the same degree of ill-health does not mean each has the same disease or, even if they did, that the appropriate treatment for each would be the same.

As far as vertical equity is concerned, similar considerations apply. Unless there were a coincidental correlation between ill-health and the cost of the procedures for addressing those needs, and a further correlation between ill-health and individuals' capacity to benefit from medical care (which is by no means the case, especially *in extremis*), the application of a formula using the principle would again cause any actual health gain to the population to be less than the potential health gain (assuming equal weights to be attached to the gains accruing to different people). The full potential is realized if provision differentially favours those needing low-cost procedures and those with high capacity to benefit from the procedures most appropriate for their condition.

The difficulty with both the horizontal and vertical equity implications of considering need as ill-health arises because it is hard to see why a group that is sick can sensibly be said to need health care irrespective of its ability to improve their health. They may need medical research, they may need comfort, and they may, most fundamentally of all, need health, and they *may* (or *may not*) need health care.

A related idea is Daniels' (1985) definition of health in terms of an individual's impairment within what he calls the 'normal opportunity range' for a person's life plans. In his view, need depends not only on the ability of health care to restore the range or compensate for its curtailment but also on the magnitude of the existing curtailment. By this definition, someone can need health care even though health care can make no contribution to the restoration or expansion of the range. According to the definition advanced here, a need exists over the whole range of cost-effective health, wherever the marginal product of care is positive in terms of health. Imagine that the capacity of a population to benefit from health care is ordered so that the person with the highest capacity to benefit is placed first in a parade, the person with the next highest capacity is placed second and so on until individuals with zero capacity are reached. Only the individuals ahead of those with zero capacity are in need. Or, considering a single individual, imagine that by the application of one 'unit' of health care, a given 'pile' of health can be obtained and that we order incremental units

in such a fashion that the biggest pile per unit is placed on the left, the next biggest immediately to its right, and so on until the piles have become tiny. Need exists only in the range where the piles are visible.

NEED AS CAPACITY TO BENEFIT

Capacity to benefit is the difference between what a person's health is predicted to be over a period of time with and without care. It is not a before and after but a with and without comparison. On the face of it, capacity to benefit is a more attractive allocation principle than the mere fact of ill-health. It is not subject to the objection that it could entail allocating health care resources to people who cannot benefit from them (at least in terms of their health). It also implies that care is needed only if it is a necessary condition for the more ultimate goal to be attained. Capacity to benefit is therefore a condition for a need for health care to exist. It does not itself amount, however, to need.

Despite this, capacity to benefit could plainly – at least in principle – be used as a principle for allocating health care. But it is not immediately apparent that this is an attractive criterion. It will favour those with relatively high capacities to benefit, even if they are already relatively healthy. Conversely, in a situation where people start off with equal health, it will generate health inequality. These considerations cause one to dig deeper into the real distributional concern that may underlie talk about need. If, for example, that concern actually relates to the distribution of health, or ill-health, in the community, then the appropriate allocation rule would be to allocate resources neither in proportion to the prevailing distribution of ill-health nor in proportion to capacity to benefit, but in relation to the contribution made to redressing health inequalities. That contribution will depend in part on the initial distribution of ill-health and in part on capacities to benefit, but neither alone suffices. The need is for disproportionately more health for those with low health and the 'derived need' for health care will flow from the effectiveness of the technologies that are available.

NEED AS HEALTH CARE EXPENDITURE

A technological breakthrough which makes it possible to treat a particular condition at a fraction of the previous cost clearly leaves a person's capacity to benefit the same (in the sense that the improvement in health achieved by treatment is the same) whereas the amount of resources the individual needs is much reduced. This suggests that the definition of need for health care for which we seek is best conceived as *the resources (or the expenditure on them) required to effect the maximum possible health improvement*. In more general terms, the amount of any service that is needed is that which is sufficient to exhaust capacity to benefit. Equivalently, the expenditure required to reduce the individual's capacity to benefit to zero is what is needed. If marginal capacity to benefit is zero, need is, accordingly, also zero. Where marginal capacity to benefit is positive, assessment of need requires an assessment of the amount of resource required to reduce capacity to benefit to zero.

This definition captures the instrumental nature of need by defining it in terms of what is needed – resources. It also relates the need for resources to the ethical objective sought – health to enable 'flourishing' – which is what gives need its special ethical status. It also defines a finite quantum of need (namely, that which exhausts capacity to benefit) without building in distributional values about *how much need ought to be met*, a question still to be resolved. This definition is also not subject to the objection that it could entail allocating health care resources to people who cannot benefit from them. Like the capacity to benefit concept of need, it implies that care is needed only if it is a necessary condition for the more ultimate goal to be attained. Unlike capacity to benefit, it specifies that it is health care resources that are needed. But again it is not immediately apparent that this is an attractive criterion. It will favour those whose marginal capacity to benefit falls to zero only after very large expenditures have been incurred. The application of such a distributional rule could, as in the previous cases, increase the inequality of the distribution of (ill-) health and, again, does not address what may be the real underlying concern of distributive fairness in health care – that is, promoting a fairer distribution of health.

None of the three allocation principles discussed here is in conflict with the principle of efficiency, in the sense of using resources to maximize the impact of health care on the health of those receiving it (see Culyer and Wagstaff, 1993; Culyer, 2006). The conflict in question arises in health care policy chiefly if one (a) seeks to apply the efficiency criterion across individuals in the manner of classical utilitarians and (b) makes the value-laden assumption that increments of health, however measured, count for the same whoever gets them. Assuming this is to make a very strong distributional value judgement. It is this judgement that creates the conflict with other distributional criteria.

FIVE IMPORTANT IMPLICATIONS OF 'NEED'

The instrumental approach to 'need' has several important and potentially radical implications, not only for the way we speak about need but also for the ways in which we use it in resource allocation decisions.

First, 'need' and 'ill-health' are not synonyms and therefore one should not imagine that in measuring the latter, one is also measuring the former. The only kind of health care that can be held to be needed is that which promotes health, reduces or postpones deteriorations in health, or extends life.

Second, capacity to benefit is not identical to need. On the one hand, capacity to benefit is defined in terms of outputs (improved health compared to what would have happened without the health care intervention). On the other hand, need is defined as the resources required to exhaust capacity to benefit. It is possible, in a comparison of two individuals, that their capacities to benefit will differ but be exhausted by the same resource expenditure on each. Hence the need for resources is the same, even though capacity to benefit is not.

Third, need is forward-looking rather than backward-looking. It is prospective rather than retrospective. It emphasizes what can be done for people rather than what has previously happened to them or what their current situation is. Past and present are important only in so far as they may affect what can be done. The inadequacy of a definition of need based only on past or current sickness, impairment or disability is thrown into sharp relief (although a long history of suffering might be held to be a ground for weighting one person's need more highly than another's); so too is the need for evidence about effectiveness.

Fourth, it will usually be both efficient and equitable for some needs to go unmet. This implication arises out of resource constraints. If resources are insufficient to exhaust all capacities to benefit and if it is deemed efficient, equitable and otherwise desirable not to divert resources from other (non-health) uses, then the question arises as to what is the most equitable way of distributing existing resources across the range of needs. Some individuals may receive none and those who receive some may not receive all they need. Either can be compatible with equitable resource allocation, whether directed at achieving an allocation proportionate to need or one that will be conducive to a more equal distribution of health.

Fifth, need, even when it relates directly to a need for health care derived from the technological possibilities and an acceptable set of social value judgements, is probably at root not an appropriate criterion for resource allocation. In any version of it that can be linked to resources, it bears no systematic relationship to distributions of health that are likely to be considered to be equitable. It has no bearing on desert and it has no systematic bearing on health equality; indeed, its application might both reward the undeserving (if desert matters at all) and enhance social inequalities.

CONCLUSION

I conclude that 'need' is most usefully construed in an explicit way as being a need for resources when individuals have a capacity to benefit, the resources are used in a cost-effective way and the benefit is a part of a socially determined ethical objective. It is sharply to be differentiated from 'demand' by virtue of the source of its value content, 'demand' being a function, *inter alia*, of preferences rather than moral values that are independent of individuals' preferences. This does not necessarily place any specific need higher in an ethical hierarchy than any specific demand. If the objectives of health services include having maximum impact on the community's health and doing so in an equitable fashion, then need is not a helpful guide and can, indeed, be a mischievous one. Focus in that context is more appropriately directed to establishing the cost-effectiveness of services with resource allocation designed to increase equality in the distribution of health.

REFERENCES

Barry B. *Political Argument*. London: Routledge & Kegan Paul, 1965.

Bateman IJ, Carson RT, Day B, Hanemann WM, Hanley N, Hett T *et al. Economic Valuation with Stated Preference Techniques*. Cheltenham Edward Elgar, 2002.

Boadway R, Bruce N. *Welfare Economics*. Oxford: Basil Blackwell, 1984.

Bradshaw J. The concept of social need. In: Gilbert N, Specht H, eds. *Planning for Social Welfare*. Prentrice-Hall: New Jersey, 1977; 290–296.

Braybrooke D. *Meeting Needs*. Princeton, NJ: Princeton University Press, 1987.

Culyer AJ, Wagstaff A. Equity and equality in health and health care. *J Health Econ* 1993; **12**: 431–457.

Culyer AJ. The bogus conflict between efficiency and equity. *Health Econ* 2006; **15**: 1155–1158.

Daniels N. *Just Health Care*. Cambridge: Cambridge University Press, 1985.

Edmonson JM. Gastric freezing: The view a quarter century later. *J Lab Clin Med* 1989; **114**: 613–614.

Flew A. Wants or needs, choices or commands? In: Fitzgerald R, ed. *Human Needs and Politics*, Pergamon Press: London, 1977; 213–228.

Gillon R. *Philosophical Medical Ethics*. New York: Wiley, 1986.

Harris J. QALYfying the value of life. *J Med Ethics* 1987; **13**: 117–123.

Le Grand J. The distribution of public expenditures: the case of health care. *Economica* 1978; **45**: 125–145.

Le Grand J. *Equity and Choice*. Harper Collins: London, 1991.

Liss P-E. *Health Care Need*. Aldershot: Avebury, 1993.

Mathew GK. Measuring need and evaluating services. In: McLachlan G, ed. *Problems and Progress in Medical Care*, 7th Series, Oxford University Press: London, 1972; 27–46.

McPherson K, Wennberg J, Hovind O, Clifford P. Small area variation in the use of common surgical procedures: and international comparison of New England, England and Norway. *N Engl J Med* 1982; **307**: 1310–1314.

McPherson K. *Variations in Hospitalization Rates: Why and How to Study Them*, London: King's Fund Institute, 1988.

Miller D. *Social Justice*. Oxford: Clarendon Press, 1976.

Nordenfeldt L. On the circle of health. In: Nordenfeldt L, Lindahl BIB, eds. *Health, Disease and Causal Explanations in Medicine*. Dordrecht: Reidel, 1984.

O'Donnell O, Propper C. Equity and the distribution of UK National Health Service resources. *J Health Econ* 1991; **10**: 1–20.

Rachlis M, Kushner C. *Second Opinion: What's Wrong with Canada's Health Care System and How to Fix It*. Toronto: Harper and Collins, 1989.

Sanders D, Coulter A, McPherson K. *Variations in Hospital Admission Rates: a Review of the Literature*. London: King's Fund Institute, 1989.

Thomson G. *Needs*. London: Routledge & Kegan Paul, 1987.

Tobin J. On limiting the domain of inequality. *J Law Econ* 1970; **13**: 263–278.

Wagstaff A, van Doorslaer E, Paci P. On the measurement of horizontal equity in the delivery of health care. *J Health Econ* 1991; **10**: 169–205.

Weale A. *Equality and Social Policy*. London: Routledge & Kegan Paul, 1978.

Wennberg J, Gittlesohn A. Variations in medical care among small areas. *Sci Am* 1982; 246: 100–111.

Wiggins D. *Need, Values, Truth*. Oxford: Basil Blackwell, 1987.

Wiggins D. Claims of need. In: Honerich T, ed. *Morality and Objectivity*. London: Routledge & Kegan Paul, 1984.

Williams A. 'Need' – an economic exegesis. In: Culyer AJ, Wright KG, eds. *Economic Aspects of Health Services*. London: Martin Robertson, 1978; pp. 9–31.

Williams B. *Utilitarianism: For and Against*, Cambridge: Cambridge University Press, 1973.

Williams B. The idea of equality. In: Laslett P, Runciman WG, eds. *Philosophy, Politics and Society*. Oxford: Basil Blackwell, 1962.

Yadav AV, Zipes DP. Prophylactic lidocaine in acute myocardial infarction: resurface or reburial? *Am J Cardiol* 2004; **94**: 606–608.

31

Rights

JAMES G. S. WILSON

We are all familiar with assertions of rights: we talk of the right to confidentiality, the right to health care and, more controversially, the right to die. But beneath this surface familiarity lies a heap of difficulties about what it is to have a right, how we should go about determining which assertions of rights are genuine and what role (if any) rights should play in our broader moral thinking. This chapter aims to offer a guide through these perplexities.

THE CONCEPT OF A MORAL RIGHT

The most basic distinction we must make is between *legal* and *moral* rights. Legal rights are those rights that exist under a given legal system, whereas moral rights are those rights that morality requires us to recognize. Moral rights are more fundamental than legal rights, for we turn to an account of moral rights to determine the acceptability of a given set of legal rights, rather than vice versa. When a given legal system does not protect all the moral rights we think persons are entitled to, then we say that the legal system is *unjust* (Steiner, 2005).

HOHFELD'S TAXONOMY OF RIGHTS

In thinking through the concept of a moral right, it is helpful to start with Hohfeld. Hohfeld (1919) argued that there were four separate conceptions of rights used in the legal discourse of his time and that failure to disentangle these frequently led to fallacious reasoning: what was a right on one conception would be asserted, and a conclusion would be drawn based on a *different* conception. Although Hohfeld's work focused on legal rights, thinking through the distinctions he makes is a vital first step in sharpening up our understanding of moral rights.

Hohfeld's four conceptions of rights are claim rights, liberty rights (Hohfeld referred to these as 'privilege rights', but his terminology is misleading), power rights and immunity rights. A claim right entitles its holder to the fulfilment of a duty by a third party. This could be either a special duty – created by the voluntary actions of individuals, as in the case of contracts – or a general duty – which holds independently of any voluntary actions by persons, as in the case of the duty not to assault persons on the street. But whether special or general, all claim rights presuppose correlative duties: there cannot be claim rights without duties.

A liberty right gives the holder permission to *do* something. But the sense in which it gives the rightholder permission to do something is quite minimal: a person has a liberty right to do something if and only if that person has no duty *not* to do that thing. Having a liberty right does not put anyone else under a duty: so it follows from the bare existence of a liberty right neither that anyone else must help you to do the thing you have a liberty to do, nor that it is wrong for others to attempt to interfere with your doing what you have a liberty to do.

Power rights and immunity rights are *second-order* rights: they are rights which relate not to actions (as claims and liberties do) but to claims and liberties themselves. A power right authorizes the power right holder to alter the legal situation either of themselves or of others. For example, a person's legal right to consent to participate in a clinical trial contains a Hohfeldian power: by exercising this power the person authorizes the researcher (that is, grants the researcher the liberty) to behave in certain ways, such as administering an untried drug to the participant, which the researcher would otherwise have had a duty not to.

Principles of Health Care Ethics, Second Edition   Edited by R.E. Ashcroft, A. Dawson, H. Draper and J.R. McMillan
© 2007 John Wiley & Sons, Ltd

Immunity rights afford the immunity holder protection against having their legal situation changed in certain ways. The World Medical Association's *Declaration of Helsinki* asserts an immunity when it says: 'The subject should be informed of the right to abstain from participation in the study or to withdraw consent to participate at any time without reprisal' (World Medical Association, 2000, paragraph 22). The immunity asserted is that the subject's claim right to withdraw without reprisal cannot be changed by anything the subject or the researcher is able to do, and so cannot, for example, be signed away by the subject. (For a more detailed exposition of Hohfeld's scheme, see Wellman, 1985, Chs 1 and 2; Sumner, 1987, Ch. 2; Kramer, 1998; Wenar, 2005a, 2005b).

Once we have drawn these distinctions between claims, liberties, powers and immunities, it is clear that many of the assertions of rights we customarily make do not assert a single Hohfeldian right, but rather amount to the assertion of a complex bundle of Hohfeldian rights. For example the legal right of a competent adult to refuse treatment, as it exists under most jurisdictions, seems to be composed of the following Hohfeldian rights:

- The liberty to refuse any particular treatment offered.
- The claim right not to be treated against the rightholder's will.
- The power to consent to treatment, which when exercised *authorizes* the relevant health care professional to proceed (that is, it accords the health care professional a *liberty* that they did not previously have).

It should now be clear why it is that there is ample scope for confusion in talk about legal rights. Claims, liberties, powers and privileges each have different implications, and until we start thinking in Hohfeldian terms, we can easily fall prey to simple errors such as assuming that the fact that we have a liberty right to do something implies that someone else owes us a duty in respect of this right (Wenar, 2005b). In response to these potential confusions Hohfeld argues that we should reserve the term 'rights' for claim rights and refer to the others as privileges, powers and immunities. Any such move is prone to charges of arbitrariness, but one reason to think that we should adopt Hohfeld's approach is that claim rights are fundamental to our conception of why rights are important and valuable in a way that liberties, powers and immunities are not. For the value of having a liberty, power or immunity seems to depend in very large measure on its being accompanied by a claim right not to be interfered with in the exercise of it (for example, a liberty to walk in the street is not worth much, unless it is accompanied by a claim right preventing others from interfering with my attempts to do so) (Hart, 1982). However, claim rights (say, for example, the right not to be enslaved) do not

seem to depend for their value on having a relevant liberty, power or immunity.

I shall suggest that we should also take claim rights to be the core of the concept of moral rights. Working out how best to cash out the idea of moral rights will occupy the next subsection.

FROM HOHFELDIAN RIGHTS TO MORAL RIGHTS

We can transfer Hohfeld's framework to the moral realm and make distinctions between *moral claim rights, moral liberties, moral powers* and *moral immunities*. So, a moral claim right would be something that entitled the claim right holder to the fulfilment of a moral duty by a third party. A moral liberty would be something that entitled its holder to a moral permission to do something. A moral power would be something that entitled the power right holder to alter the moral situation of themselves or someone else, whereas a moral immunity would be something that entitled the immunity holder *not* to have her moral situation altered by another.

I shall assume that, following what we said about legal claim rights, we should take moral claim rights to be the core of our concept of moral rights. In other words, no combination of Hohfeldian moral rights that does not contain a moral claim should count as a moral right. I shall now argue that moral claims are the *only* essential element of moral rights: in particular, it is possible to have a moral right to do something without having a liberty to do that same thing; and it is conceptually possible to have a moral right without having a moral power to waive or annul that right.

RIGHTS TO DO WRONG: WHY MORAL RIGHTS DO NOT ENTAIL MORAL LIBERTIES

Does having a moral right to do X imply that one has a moral liberty to do that same thing? It is important to see what is at stake here: if every moral right to do Y contains within it a moral liberty to do Y, then it follows that if X has a moral right to do Y, then X's doing Y must be morally permissible. On the contrary, if moral rights and moral liberties are separable, then it will at least sometimes be the case that moral rights protect people in the pursuit of morally wrong choices.

There is reason to think that we should prefer a conception of moral right in which moral rights do not imply moral liberties. This is because there do seem to be clear cases where we would want to be able to say *both* that X had a right to do Y *and* that it was wrong for X to do Y. If the concept of a moral right prevented us from saying this, then we would have to deal with such cases either by denying that the person had the moral right in question, or by denying that what they did was wrong. (Two cases where we might want to say someone acts wrongly despite having a moral right to do what they do are (a) where 'a voter casts a ballot for a racist candidate'; or (b) 'where an athlete ridicules an obese person struggling to board a bus' (Edmundson, 2004, p. 135; see also Waldron, 1981).

MORAL RIGHTS DO NOT CONCEPTUALLY ENTAIL MORAL POWERS

Clearly, many moral rights entail moral powers: we take it to be part of the practice of promising that the promisee has the moral power to release the promisor from their duty. But should we take such powers over the duties that others owe to be an *essential* component of having a right? *Will* (or *choice*) theorists of rights argue that we should. According to will theorists, the purpose of rights is to grant the right holder the freedom (within a particular domain) to *control the duties that others owe to him*. In H. L. A. Hart's words, it views the right holder as 'a small-scale sovereign' in the area in which the duty is owed, 'able to waive or extinguish the duty or leave it in existence' (Hart, 1982, pp. 183–4). (Prominent expressions of the Will Theory include Austin 1832; Hart, 1982; Steiner, 1994, 1998; Simmonds, 1998; Wellman, 1995) *Interest* or *benefit* theorists deny this and argue that the purpose of rights is to *protect or promote interests*, and so argue that there is nothing incoherent about the idea of rights which the right holder does not have the moral power to waive or annul. (Prominent expressions of the Interest Theory include Bentham, 1970; MacCormick, 1977; Raz, 1986; Kramer, 1998). I shall suggest that the conceptual claims about rights that will theorists are committed to are highly dubious, and that whether or not we should accept the Interest Theory as an account of moral rights, we should certainly reject the Will Theory.

The Will Theory as a conceptual analysis of moral rights claims suffers from two serious problems. First, the theory claims that rights by definition must be under the control of the right holder, and hence that a necessary condition of having a right is having sufficient competence to be able to waive or annul that right. But this rules out large swathes of human beings whom we standardly attribute moral rights to (or at least think it reasonable to attribute rights to) from having any rights at all. For example, 'foetuses, minors, the comatose, the mentally disabled, the dead and members of future generations – to say nothing of the members of virtually all known species – must lack all Will Theory rights' (Steiner, 1998, p. 259). This is, to say the least, rather difficult to square with ordinary conceptions of rights: what are we to make of a conception of rights under which a child does not have a right to be free from sexual abuse? (Kramer, 1998, p. 69).

Second, according to the Will Theory, if you have a claim right to X, then by definition you also have the power right to waive or annul your claim right to X. But it seems to be a mistake to adopt a conceptual analysis of rights which

by definition rules out inalienable rights, given that many people do in fact think that there are at least some such rights (for example, the right not to be enslaved, or the right not to be tortured): if we are to show that there are no inalienable rights, surely this will require substantive moral arguments, rather than mere stipulation (Wenar, 2005b).

The Interest Theory fits better into our ordinary understanding of rights. First, it seems to provide a good explanation for a wide variety of cases in which we want to attribute rights: many of the central rights we wish to attribute, such as the right to life, the right to liberty or the right to refuse treatment can very plausibly be thought to further the interests of their right holders. Second, it does not prejudge too much about what rights there are and what kinds of entities can be right holders: it requires of potential right holders only that they should have interests that are worthy of protection. And so according to the Interest Theory there is nothing in the very nature of what it is to have a right that would prevent for example, foetuses, chickens, future generations or ethnic groups from having rights. Whether or not such entities have rights will depend on the results of a substantive argument about whether each of the different types of entities have interests in the relevant way, and if so, whether the interests are sufficiently important to be worthy of protection by rights.

But on closer inspection the thesis that all rights protect or further the interests of right holder also looks too narrow. For there seem to be clear cases where we usually say that there is a right, but where either (a) it seems wrong to say that the right exists to benefit the right holder (the power right that a judge has to pass a sentence, does not seem to have the function of protecting the judge's interests) or (b) the interest that the right holder has does not seem to be sufficiently strong to explain a right of the stringency we in fact think holds. (The interest that the journalist has in keeping her sources secret does not seem sufficiently strong to justify her stringent claim right not to divulge them.) Interest theorists have a number of ingenious solutions to these types of problems (see, for example, Raz, 1986, Ch. 7; Kramer, 1998; Kramer and Steiner, forthcoming); but it remains unclear whether such solutions can ultimately be successful, and so recently there have been a number of attempts to go beyond the apparent stand-off between the Will and Interest Theories (Wenar, 2005b, Sreenivasan, 2005). Whatever the results of this new debate, I suggest we do best to at least allow for the possibility of inalienable rights.

THE ROLE OF RIGHTS IN MORAL THINKING

I have suggested that we should think of moral rights as moral claim rights, which need not be accompanied by either moral liberties or moral powers. It is now time to consider what the role of moral rights thus conceived should play in broader moral thinking.

HOW DO WE DECIDE WHAT RIGHTS THERE ARE?

What justifies us in saying that an alleged moral right is genuine? There are two basic approaches to the justification of rights claims: intrinsic and instrumentalist. Intrinsic conceptions of rights hold that there are rights because of the moral status that human beings already have prior to anything we do: as Warren Quinn puts it, 'It is not that we think it fitting to ascribe rights because we think it is a good thing that rights be respected. Rather we think respect for rights a good thing precisely because we think people actually have them–and . . . that they have them because it is fitting that they should' (Quinn, 1993, p. 173). On the intrinsic conception of rights, we justify the claim that a particular moral right exists, and that this right should have one content rather than another by doing first-order moral thinking about what is permissible and what impermissible to do to human beings. (See, for example, Thomson, 1990; Kamm, 1993, 1996).

For the rights instrumentalist, rights are tools whose purpose is to promote morally valuable goals. Rights instrumentalists argue that, given various plausible assumptions, we will tend to bring about a morally better world if we recognize the existence of at least some moral rights. There are two types of rights instrumentalists: some see recognizing rights as a *means* to a further goal of bringing about the most good (Sumner, 1987, 2000; Mill, 1998 on some interpretations) and those who think that rights being respected *just is* a morally good consequence that we should be trying to bring about (Scanlon, 1977; Sen, 1982; Dworkin, 1977, 1984; Mill, 1998 on other interpretations.)

The intrinsic and instrumental approaches presuppose radically different conceptions of the terrain of morality: intrinsic approaches to rights require us to take rights as the basis of morality, whereas instrumental approaches to rights seek the basis of morality elsewhere. Serious thinking about moral rights will require us to take some sort of stance on this question. I shall not attempt to do so here because doing so would require the defence of a full moral theory. I shall instead attempt to elucidate the issue at stake by examining two sorts of problems that will arise whether or not we take rights to be the basis of morality: first, rights will need to be specified, and second, rights will conflict with the pursuit of other morally valuable goods, including potentially respecting other rights.

SPECIFYING RIGHTS CLAIMS

A moral right consists of a relationship between first, the *holder* of the right, second, the *content* of the right (what the right the right is a right *to do,* or a right to *have done*) and third, those *against whom* the right is held. Each of these will need to be specified, and each way we specify the right will require further moral argument. (On the idea of specifying principles, see Richardson, 1990)

Suppose we agree that there is a moral right to refuse treatment. To be able to know what follows from the existence of this right, we would need first to specify *who* counts as the holder of this right: should the right be restricted to competent adults? And if so, why?

Next we would have to specify the content of the right – that is, what the right allows the right holder to do, and what it requires those against whom the right is held to do or refrain from doing. What counts as treatment? What, if anything, does the right to refuse treatment imply about the amount of information that health care professionals must give to patients? How fine-grained a control should the right give the right holder? (Does it give the right holder the right to refuse each and every sub-step in a treatment plan, however minute, or does it extend only to the treatment plan as a whole?)

Finally, we would need to specify which person(s) or institution(s) has the duties correlative to the claim right. In the case of the right to refuse treatment it seems clear that the duty not to impose treatment must fall on everyone, not just on health care professionals. (It would be equally as much a violation of the right for a private citizen to force treatment on someone as it would be for a health care professional to do so.) But in other cases (such as a moral right to health care) it can be markedly less clear against whom a moral right is held, and establishing this can take substantive moral argument.

Specifying rights is morally problematic for two reasons. First, moral rights by their nature conflict with the pursuit of broader moral goods such as increasing welfare or avoiding suffering. For all moral rights either contain *constraints* on maximizing the good or *options* for agents not to maximize the good (Summer, 2000). Hence, all rights have moral costs: in positing a moral right we are *ipso facto* limiting our ability to pursue the good. Second, depending on how we specify a given moral right, we may find that it conflicts with other moral rights. I shall briefly address each worry.

CONFLICTS BETWEEN RIGHTS AND GOODS

There are two options we could adopt in our approach to conflicts between a given moral right and broader moral goods: either we claim that the moral right always trumps considerations of broader moral good (that is, there is no amount of broader moral good that would justify us in infringing the right) or we claim that the right at least sometimes does not. If we say that the right does not always trump considerations of broader moral good, then we are committed to the claim that there is *some* threshold (the threshold may be very high) at which the claims of broader moral good are able to override that claim of moral right. It is plausible to think that whether there is such a threshold, and if so where we should draw it, will depend in large part on how fundamental we think the moral right in question is, and how important the goods in question are. Thinking schematically, we can imagine four types of cases. (I assume without argument that there is not a *moral right* to be happy.)

1. Where the moral right to be infringed is a fundamental right, such as the right not to be tortured, and the good to be obtained is trivial, though very widely spread. (Torturing one person to death allows 10 minutes of mild pleasure for 1,000,000 people.)
2. Where the moral right to be infringed is a fundamental right and the good to be obtained is valuable, though not something they have a right to. (Torturing one person to death allows 100 to find true happiness.)
3. Where the moral right to be infringed is less weighty (such as a right that someone keep their promise) and the good to be obtained is trivial, though very widely spread. (Breaking one promise allows 10 minutes of mild pleasure for 1,000,000 people.)
4. Where the moral right to be infringed is less weighty and the good to be obtained is valuable, though not something they have a right to. (Breaking one promise allows 100 to find true happiness.)

We can stipulate for the purposes of the argument that in each case more good will be done overall if we infringe the right than if we do not. Many will wish to claim that in cases such as (1) *no* amount of mild pleasure could possibly justify someone being tortured to death. On the contrary, many will claim that in cases such as (4) we clearly ought to infringe the moral right for broader moral goals. Cases (2) and (3) are more controversial: is there an amount of true happiness that could outweigh the wrong of torturing someone to death? Is there a degree of mild pleasure that could outweigh the obligation to respect a promise? Reflecting on our answers to these questions will, I think, send us back to the more fundamental question of whether the correct account of rights is an instrumental or an intrinsic one.

CONFLICTS BETWEEN RIGHTS

Just as we can envisage conflicts between rights and other goods, so we can envisage conflicts between any single right and other rights. It seems that there can be circumstances where, unless we infringe one person's right, another person's right will be infringed. So, for example, if someone has a deadly infectious disease, but refuses to isolate himself voluntarily, we might be faced with a choice between in-fringing his right to liberty and allowing the general population's right to life and right to security to be infringed.

Theorists reply in two ways to such situations. Specificationists deny that rights can conflict. For the specificationist, apparent conflicts of moral rights are in fact failures of specification (Steiner, 1994). On this view, the process of specification will ensure that all rights are 'compossible': 'rights fit together like pieces in a jigsaw puzzle, so that in every circumstance there is only one right which determines what is permitted, forbidden or required. Each right is absolute within its own area, but the area in which each right prevails is elaborately gerrymandered' (Wenar, 2005a).

However, such a view cannot make room for an important feature of our usual understanding of rights: the permissible infringement of rights in the service of other rights. For example, suppose I have promised to take Johnny to the zoo, but stop to help at an emergency on my way home and end up breaking my promise. Let us assume that stopping at the emergency is the right thing to do. What, then, becomes of Johnny's moral claim right to be taken to the zoo? Steiner's specificationist model seems to be committed to the claim that a right that is defeated in this way was never really a right after all. But as Thomson (1990) points out, this sits badly with our usual understanding of these sorts of cases: we usually assume that there is a 'moral residue' when a moral right is defeated in this way. (I should take myself to be under a subsidiary duty to make amends to Johnny in some way.) Hence our intuitions about rights conflict with this form of specificationism, and rather imply that there can be conflicts of rights.

Given these problems, it seems sensible to admit the possibility of conflicts of rights. How, then, should we handle them? Rights instrumentalists will tend to be drawn to the idea that we should adopt what Nozick (1974) refers to as a 'utilitarianism of rights', namely, that we should *minimize* the number and extent of rights violations.

Intrinsic rights theorists argue that things are a lot more complex than this. They argue that it may often not be permissible to perform the action that would end up with fewer people having their rights infringed. For the intrinsic rights theorist, rights are a response to our intrinsic moral status, and they entail duties *to each person* not to treat that person in certain ways. By treating one person's rights as easier to infringe in order to prevent others' from being violated, we imply that the first person (and by extension everyone) is less inviolable than they would have been had it been impermissible to do so. But it is not clear that it is morally permissible for us to make such choices: as Kamm puts it, 'what it is impermissible to do and the associated degree of inviolability is not legislated by our choosing any given morality: we do not make people violable. They either do or do not deserve to be inviolable. If they do, we should act in accord with this' (Kamm, 2002, p. 507). Just how intrinsic rights theorists *should* think about the permissible infringement of rights is an open question. Thomson (1990) and Kamm (1993, 1996) have championed an approach that places a great deal of emphasis on testing intuitions through subtly differentiated thought experiments: but an increasing body of work suggests that this methodology is far less reliable as a way of doing moral thinking than Thomson and Kamm think it is (See, for example, Unger, 1996; Sunstein, 2005.)

THE FUTURE OF RIGHTS

We have clarified the conceptual nature of moral rights and the role of rights in moral thinking. It remains to reflect briefly on the role that rights should play in our broader political discourse. The years since the Universal Declaration of Human Rights in 1948 have seen a massive expansion in the role of rights claims in political thinking. To the extent that these claims embody genuine moral rights, clearly, we should welcome them as signs of moral progress. But it is hard to believe that all the claims made which purport to assert moral rights are genuine.

One reason that we should be suspicious is that the special status we accord to moral rights brings with it a strong temptation to continually expand their scope:

> To claim a right to something is not just to say that it would be nice to have it or generous of others to provide it: rather, one is entitled to expect or demand it, others are obliged to provide it, it would be unjust of them to deny or withhold it. Once a right has been invoked on one side of an issue it must therefore be countered by a weapon of similar potency on the other. But then if one interest group has built its case on an appeal to rights none of its competitors can afford not to respond in kind. Like any other weapons, once they have appeared in the public arena rights claims will tend to proliferate and to escalate (Sumner, 2000, p. 298).

There are three main reasons why we should be worried by this proliferation of rights claims. First, in the long run it will tend to devalue and undermine rights discourse as a whole: for if *everything* is an issue of moral rights, nothing will have the special protection that we think genuine moral rights deserve.

Second, overreaching in our claims of rights will be morally counterproductive. As we have seen, all moral rights have moral costs: every moral right provides either constraints on maximizing the good or options not to do so. So the more moral rights we recognize and the more stringent we allow these moral rights to be, the more we hamstring our attempts to pursue other socially valuable moral goals.

Third, our current over-extension of rights claims may lead to a general crisis of confidence in rights discourse as a whole, as happened after rights' first high-water mark at the end of the eighteenth century (Waldron, 1987, and Edmundson, 2004 provide good overviews of this period).

In the face of these problems with rights discourse, O'Neill (2000, 2002) argues we should abandon our current rights-based rhetoric for a duty-based one. Her argument is three-fold: first, claim rights and duties are correlative – so by definition if we work out what our duties are, we will also have worked out which rights are implied by these duties. Second, talk about duties is more concrete and thus more likely to actually lead to necessary actions than assertions of rights. Third, talk of duties is inherently more sober and less inflammatory than talk of rights: hence duty talk does not leave itself wide open to abuse.

It is worth reflecting in conclusion about what if anything would be lost if we were to follow O'Neill's advice and replace rights with duties at the centre of our political thinking. It seems to me to bring us back to the fundamental question of whether an intrinsic or an instrumentalist view of rights is correct. For if the best account of rights makes rights mere tools, then it seems O'Neill is correct that nothing would be lost and much gained by placing duty-based thinking at the heart of things. But if (as I suspect, but have not argued here) an intrinsic account of rights is correct, then we would miss something of moral significance by replacing rights with duties. For, on the intrinsic view, rights are a fitting response to the moral status human beings in fact have, and human beings have the duties corresponding to these rights *because of* this moral status; starting from duties would be akin to looking at the shadow rather than the person who casts it.

REFERENCES

Austin J. *The Province of Jurisprudence Determined*. Cambridge: Cambridge University Press, 1995 [1832].

Bentham J. In: Hart HLA, ed. *Of Laws in General*. London: Athlone Press, 1970.

Dworkin R. *Taking Rights Seriously*. Cambridge, MA: Harvard University Press, 1977.

Dworkin R. Rights as trumps. In: Waldron J, ed. *Theories of Rights*. Oxford: Oxford University Press, 1984; pp. 153–167.

Edmundson W. *An Introduction to Rights*. Cambridge: Cambridge University Press, 2004.

Hart H. *Essays on Bentham: Studies in Jurisprudence and Political Theory*. Oxford: Clarendon Press, 1982.

Hohfeld W. In: Cook W, ed. *Fundamental Legal Conceptions*. New Haven, CT: Yale University Press, 1919.

Kamm F. Rights. In: Coleman J, Shapiro S, eds. *The Oxford Handbook of Jurisprudence and Philosophy of Law*. Oxford: Oxford University Press, 2002; pp. 476–513.

Kamm F. *Morality, Mortality, Volume 1: Death and Whom to Save From It*. Oxford: Oxford University Press, 1993.

Kamm F. *Morality, Mortality, Volume 2: Rights, Duties and Status*, Oxford: Oxford University Press, 1996.

Kramer M, Steiner H. Theories of rights: is there a third way? *Oxford J Legal Stud*, in press (doi:10.1093/ojls/gqi039).

Kramer M. Rights without trimmings. In: Kramer M, ed. *A Debate over Rights*. Oxford: Oxford University Press, 1998; pp. 7–112.

MacCormick N. Rights in legislation. In: Hacker P, Raz J, eds. *Law, Morality and Society: Essays in Honour of H.L.A. Hart*. Oxford: Oxford University Press, 1977; pp. 189–209.

Mill J. In: Crisp R, ed. *Utilitarianism*. Oxford: Oxford University Press, 1998 [1871].

Nozick R. *Anarchy State and Utopia*. New York: Basic Books, 1974.

O'Neill O. *Bounds of Justice*. Cambridge: Cambridge University Press, 2000.

O'Neill O. *Autonomy and Trust in Bioethics*. Cambridge: Cambridge University Press, 2002.

Quinn W. *Morality and Action*. Cambridge: Cambridge University Press, 1993.

Raz J. *The Morality of Freedom*. Oxford: Oxford University Press, 1986.

Richardson H. Specifying norms as a way to solve concrete ethical problems. *Philos Public Affairs* 1990; **19**: 279–310.

Scanlon T. Rights, goals and fairness. *Erkenntnis* 1977; **II:1**; 81–94 (reprinted in Waldron, 1984).

Sen A. Rights and agency. *Philos Public Affairs* 1982; **11**: 3–39.

Simmonds N. Rights at the cutting edge. In: Kramer M, ed. *A Debate over Rights*. Oxford: Oxford University Press, 1998; pp. 113–232.

Sreenivasan G. A hybrid theory of claim-rights. *Oxford J Legal Stud* 2005; **25**: 257–274.

Steiner H. Moral rights. In: Copp D, ed. *The Oxford Handbook of Ethical Theory*, Oxford: Oxford University Press, 2005.

Steiner H. *An Essay on Rights*. Oxford: Basil Blackwell, 1994.

Steiner H. Working rights. In: Kramer M, ed. *A Debate over Rights*. Oxford: Oxford University Press, 1998; pp. 233–302.

Sumner L. *The Moral Foundations of Rights*. Oxford: Oxford University Press, 1987.

Sumner L. Rights. In: LaFollette, ed. *The Blackwell Guide to Ethical Theory*. Oxford: Basil Blackwell, 2000.

Sunstein C. Moral heuristics. *Behav Brain Sci* 2005; **28**(4): 531–573.

Thomson J. *The Realm of Rights*. Cambridge, MA: Harvard University Press, 1990.

Unger P. *Living High and Letting Die: Our Illusion of Innocence*. Oxford: Oxford University Press, 1996.

Waldron J. A right to do wrong. *Ethics* 1981; **92**: 21–39.

Waldron J, ed. *Theories of Rights*. Oxford: Oxford University Press, 1984.

Waldron J, ed. *Nonsense upon Stilts: Bentham, Burke, and Marx on the Rights of Man*. London: Methuen, 1987.

Wellman C. *A Theory of Rights*. Totowa, NJ: Rowman and Allanheld, 1985.

Wellman C. *Real Rights*. Oxford: Oxford University Press, 1995.

Wenar L. Rights. In: *The Stanford Encyclopedia of Philosophy*, Winter 2005 edition, 2005a; http://plato.stanford.edu/archives/win2005/entries/rights/.

Wenar L. The nature of rights. *Philos Public Affairs* 2005b; **33**: 223–253.

World Medical Association (WMA). *Ethical Principles for Medical Research Involving Human Subjects*, 2000; http://www.wma.net/.

32

Exploitation in Health Care

ALAN WERTHEIMER

The avoidance of exploitation is not one of the four canonical principles of health care ethics (which need not be restated here), although many violations of those principles also involve exploitation. Indeed, there is only one index citation to exploitation in the first edition of *The Principles of Health Care Ethics*. At the same time, discussions and critiques of health care practices frequently do or could invoke the concept of exploitation. Consider the following examples, where it *is* or *could* be said that a practice is exploitative. (I am decidedly *not* suggesting that all of these claims are true.)

Surrogacy. Commercial surrogacy involves the exploitation of the surrogate mothers.

Psychotherapy. Psychotherapists who have sexual relations with their patients are engaged in exploitation.

Kidneys. The sale of bodily organs, such as kidneys, involves the exploitation of impoverished persons.

Elderly. Health care providers sometimes exploit the elderly, particularly those who suffer from dementia.

Unnecessary procedures. Physicians exploit their patients when they propose unnecessary procedures.

Interns. Hospitals exploit interns by requiring them to work long hours for relatively low pay.

Brain drain. Affluent nations are engaged in exploitation when they recruit physicians and nurses from underdeveloped societies to the latter's detriment.

Animals. Medical research involves the exploitation of animals.

Tissue. Parents who conceive children so that their tissue or organs can be used for the benefit of a sibling are exploiting them.

Inducements. Medical researchers exploit subjects when they offer (undue) inducements to participate in research.

Vaccine. A doctor would be exploiting his patients if he were to inject a potential vaccine into patients (without their knowledge) in order to test its efficacy or side effects.

AZT. The Burroughs-Welcome Company, which produced AZT, was exploiting people with AIDS by charging high prices for a life-saving drug.

Prisoners. The use of prisoners in medical research involves exploitation because the environment of prisoners is inherently coercive or because the offer of perquisites or a reduction in sentence is 'too good to refuse'.

Risk-pooling. Medical insurance, which involves risk-pooling, involves the exploitation of those at low risk by those at higher risk.

Cost-shifting. When people consume more medical care than is necessary because they are insured, they exploit other insured persons by shifting the cost of their medical care to others.

Trust. Doctors exploit their patients' trust or position of dominance when they get their patients to agree to procedures without much questioning, even when the procedures are medically indicated.

Stem cells. Stem cell research treats 'nascent human life as raw material to be exploited as a mere natural resource' (Kass, 2002, p. 2).

HMOs. HMOs exploit patients when they fail to provide indicated medical care in order to increase their profits.

Manipulation. Children exploit their parents' love when they convince them to forgo medical treatment by appealing to their desire not to use up resources that would otherwise be inherited.

Clinical research. Clinical research in underdeveloped societies exploits the subjects who agree to participate because it is their only chance to receive therapeutic care.

Principles of Health Care Ethics, Second Edition   Edited by R.E. Ashcroft, A. Dawson, H. Draper and J.R. McMillan
© 2007 John Wiley & Sons, Ltd

Let us refer to the statement that a practice is (or is not) exploitative as an *exploitation claim*. Although we frequently claim that some act, practice or transaction is exploitative, the concept of exploitation is typically invoked without much analysis or argument, as if its meaning and moral significance were self-evident. They are not. Thus, the first task of a theory of exploitation is to provide the truth conditions for an exploitation claim. The second task is to consider the *moral force* of exploitation. In particular, we need to ask whether we should interfere with transactions just because they are exploitative. Many people implicitly or explicitly endorse what I shall call the *exploitation argument*, to wit

(1) if a practice is exploitative, it should not be permitted;
(2) some practice, X, is exploitative;
(3) therefore, X should not be permitted.

The exploitation argument moves too quickly, for even if (2) is true, it does not automatically follow that X should be prohibited.

In what follows, I do the following. First, I provide an analysis of the concept of exploitation. Second, I distinguish between harmful non-consensual exploitation and mutually advantageous consensual exploitation. Third, I will discuss the arguments for prohibiting or interfering with exploitative transactions. Fourth, I apply this analysis to the now prominent argument exemplified by Clinical Research.

THE CONCEPT OF EXPLOITATION

We sometimes use the verb 'to exploit' in a morally neutral sense, in which we simply mean 'to make use of'; for example, 'the surgeon exploits his natural manual dexterity'. We are interested in the morally charged sense of exploitation, in which to say that A exploits B is to imply that A acts wrongly. There are two ways in which this can occur. First, A can wrongfully exploit B because A makes use of B when A simply should not make use of or interact with B at all, as (perhaps) in *Animals* and *Stem cells*. Second, and more importantly, A can wrongfully exploit B when A takes 'unfair advantage' of B, as in many of the examples above. One problem with such a broad account is that there will 'be as many competing conceptions of exploitation as theories of what persons owe to each other by way of fair treatment' (Arneson, 1992, p. 350). We can gain a somewhat sharper view of the issues that we must confront if we consider a sampling of the accounts that appear in the literature.

1. '[T]o exploit a person involves the *harmful, merely instrumental utilization* of him or his capacities, for one's own advantage or for the sake of one's own ends' (Buchanan, 1985, p. 87).

2. 'Exploitation [in exchange] demands . . . that there is no reasonably eligible alternative [for the exploitee] and that the consideration or advantage received is incommensurate with the price paid. One is not exploited if one is offered what one desperately needs at a fair and reasonable price' (Benn, 1988, p. 138).

3. 'Exploitation of persons consists in . . . wrongful behavior [that violates] the moral norm of *protecting the vulnerable*' (Goodin, 1988, p. 147).

4. 'Common to all exploitation of one person (B) by another (A) . . . is that A makes a profit or gain by turning some characteristic of B to his own advantage . . . exploitation . . . can occur in morally unsavory forms without harming the exploitee's interests and . . . despite the exploitee's fully voluntary consent to the exploitative behavior . . . ' (Feinberg, 1988, pp. 176–179).

5. 'Persons are exploited if (1) others secure a benefit by (2) using them as a tool or resource so as (3) to cause them serious harm' (Munzer, 1990, p. 171).

6. 'An exploitative exchange is . . . an exchange in which the exploited party gets less than the exploiting party, who does better at the exploited party's expense . . . [T]he exchange must result from social relations of unequal power . . . exploitation can be entered into voluntarily; and can even, in some sense, be advantageous to the exploited party' (Levine, 1988, pp. 66–67).

7. '[E]xploitation forms part of an exchange of goods and services when (1) the goods and services exchanged are quite obviously not of equivalent value, and (2) one party to the exchange uses a substantial degree of coercion' (Moore, 1973, p. 53).

8. '[E]xploitation is a psychological, rather than a social or an economic, concept. For an offer to be exploitative, it must serve to create or to take advantage of some recognized psychological vulnerability which, in turn, disturbs the offeree's ability to reason effectively' (Hill, 1994, p. 637).

There are some important differences between these accounts. Only some accounts explicitly or implicitly suggest that exploitation requires that the exploiter gains (1, 2, 4, 5, 6). Whereas some accounts state that the exploited party must be harmed (1, 5), others explicitly or implicitly allow that the exploited party may gain from the transaction or relationship (2, 4, 6, 7). With respect to consent, one account says that the exploited party must be coerced (7), whereas another says that exploitation involves a defect in the quality of the exploitee's decision-making capacity (8), and yet other accounts maintain that the exploitee can give voluntary consent (4, 6).

We should not put rigid constraints on what counts as exploitation. Although some exploitative transactions are harmful to the exploitee, we often call exploitative cases in which the exploitee seems to gain from the transaction, as in this garden-variety example of exploitation.

> *Rescue.* B's car has broken down on a rural road late at night. A stops and ascertains that it will take him 5 minutes to fix the car. A offers to fix B's car for $100.

In my view, the concept of exploitation would be of little theoretical interest if only harmful transactions counted as exploitative. It is trivially true that it is wrong for A to gain from an action that unjustifiably harms or coerces B. By contrast, it is more difficult to explain when and why it might be wrong for A to gain from an action that benefits B and to which B voluntarily consents. And it is certainly more difficult to explain why society might be justified in interfering with such transactions or refusing to enforce some such agreements.

For these reasons, it will be useful to make two sets of distinctions. First, we can distinguish between *harmful exploitation*, where A gains by harming B, and *mutually advantageous exploitation*, where the exploitee gains from the transaction as well as the exploiter as in *Rescue* or the following case.

> *Unfair surgery.* B needs life-saving surgery. A is the only surgeon available. A proposes to perform the surgery for $20,000 when the normal fee is $5000. B agrees.

We can similarly distinguish between *non-consensual exploitation* and consensual exploitation. In cases of non-consensual exploitation, the exploitee does not token consent at all (as in *Cost-shifting*) or fails to give appropriately valid or voluntary consent, as when the consent is compromised by coercion, deception or incompetence (as in *Psychotherapy*). By contrast, in cases of *consensual exploitation*, the exploitee makes a voluntary, informed, competent and rational decision to agree to the transaction.

Although the two sets of distinctions are not equivalent, most cases of harmful exploitation are non-consensual and most cases of consensual exploitation are mutually advantageous. So, for present purposes, let us distinguish between harmful non-consensual exploitation and mutually advantageous consensual exploitation.

THE ELEMENTS OF EXPLOITATION

In this section, I shall identify three dimensions of exploitative transactions.

BENEFIT TO A

A cannot take *unfair* advantage of B unless A gets some *advantage* from B. We can see the relevance of this element

of exploitation by contrasting exploitation with other forms of wrong-doing, such as discrimination, neglect and paternalism. Let us say that A discriminates against B when A wrongly deprives B of some opportunity or benefit because of some characteristic of B that is not relevant to A's action. Although A acts wrongly if A refuses to provide medical care to B solely because of B's race, it would be odd to say that A exploits B for A does not gain from the wrong to B. Consider neglect. Let us say that A neglects B when A has an obligation to provide for B and fails to do so. Although neglect is a serious problem, it would be odd to characterize it as exploitative unless (as in *HMOs*) someone gains by not providing that which they ought to provide. Let us say that A is wrongfully paternalistic to B (a competent adult) if A acts so as to promote B's interests without B's informed consent. Although paternalism may be wrong, it does not typically involve exploitation because A does not necessarily gain from his paternalism.

Now the benefit to A from an exploitative transaction can take several forms. For example, A may gain financially as in *Unnecessary procedure* or may gain sexual pleasure as in *Psychotherapy*. More interestingly, A's gain may be somewhat altruistic or benign, as when A seeks to further scientific research by exploiting potential subjects (as in *Prisoners* or *Animals*). As the latter case illustrates, the ultimate beneficiaries of exploitation may not be parties to the transaction. Even if the citizens of affluent nations benefit from clinical research in underdeveloped societies, they do not participate in and have not authorized the research.

THE EFFECT ON B

A engages in harmful exploitation of B when A gains by harming B; A engages in mutually advantageous exploitation when A gains wrongly or unfairly from a transaction with B that also benefits B. The distinction between harm and benefit is not always transparent. First, we must adopt an *all things considered* point of view. There are, after all, negative *elements* in virtually all beneficial transactions. Paying money for a good that is clearly worth the price is still a negative element in the transaction. It would be better to get it for free. So in deciding whether a case of alleged exploitation should be classified as harmful exploitation or mutually advantageous exploitation, we must look at its *net* effect on B. From that perspective, the sale of a kidney may or may not be harmful to B.

Second, in assessing the effects of a transaction on B, we should generally adopt an *ex ante* rather than an *ex post* point of view. Suppose that A enters into a type of business transaction with B, where B expects (*ex ante*) to gain 80 per cent of the time and lose 20 per cent of the time, as when A sells B land on which B hopes to find oil. We would not regard a transaction in which A does not find oil as harmful in any morally significant way because B's *ex ante* utility is clearly positive. So if a woman can expect, *ex ante*, to benefit from being a surrogate mother and then even if B is harmed in a particular case, all things considered, I would regard it as a mutually advantageous transaction.

Third, in determining whether B benefits from or is harmed, we need a baseline against which to evaluate the transaction. Consider this case.

> *National Health Service.* A works for the National Health Service and is obliged to provide care for B at no cost. Seeing that B needs medical care and that there are no other providers available, A tells B that he will provide the care if, but only if, B pays £500.

As contrasted with the *status quo baseline* in which B receives no medical care, the transaction is beneficial to B. As contrasted with a *moral baseline* defined by what A has an obligation to do for B, we can say that the transaction is harmful to B. For present purposes, I believe that we should evaluate a transaction against the *moral baseline*, in which case this would be harmful exploitation.

Finally, just as A may not be the ultimate beneficiary of an exploitative transaction, the ultimate exploitee may not be a party to the transaction. The physician may not be exploiting her patient in *Unnecessary procedures* so much as she is exploiting the third party payer, be it the government (or B's fellow citizens) or the insurance company (or its premium payers).

Let us assume that a transaction or interaction between A and B is mutually advantageous. A transaction is (wrongly) exploitative only if the outcome is (in some way) unfair to B, or A wrongfully uses B. This is not merely definitional. It may be thought that a transaction is exploitative whenever it takes advantage of B's vulnerabilities or desperate situation to strike a deal. That is false. For if A makes a *reasonable* proposal that B has no alternative but to accept given the desperate situation of B, it would be silly to say that A exploits B.

But what makes a transaction unfair? It is frequently suggested that a transaction is exploitative when A gains much more than B from the transaction. This cannot be right. If we measure the parties' gains by reference to the utility they receive as compared with the baseline in which there is no transaction, the exploitee typically gains *more* than the exploiter. If A charges four times her standard fee for a procedure, as in *Unfair surgery*, B has still gained much more than A. Indeed, on closer inspection, the exploiter's power over the exploitee stems precisely from the fact that the exploiter does *not* stand to gain too much. The exploiter can easily walk away from the transaction, whereas the exploitee cannot.

This suggests that we cannot evaluate the fairness of a transaction by comparing utility gains. Rather, we must measure the fairness of their gains against a *normative standard* as to how much the parties *ought* to gain, and that baseline is not easy to specify. A promising but not unproblematic candidate is to measure the parties' gains against what they would have gained in a 'hypothetical competitive market' where there was relatively complete information (Wertheimer, 1996). Although I cannot produce a non-problematic theory of fair transactions, I will simply assume that some mutually advantageous transactions are unfair by reference to an appropriate normative standard and that A exploits B when A gains more than A should (or B gains less than B should) from the transaction.

I say 'from the transaction'. In my view, exploitation is transaction-specific. Suppose that B agrees to serve as a surrogate mother because society does not provide an adequate 'safety net' for her family. Although A's proposal has traction only because B's background conditions are unjust, it does not automatically follow that A's proposal is unfair to B given that A bears no responsibility for B's unjust background condition nor does A have an obligation to repair those conditions. To put the point slightly differently, just because A takes advantage of unfairness to B, it does not follow that A takes unfair advantage of B.

CONSENT

Let us assume that a transaction is mutually advantageous, although unfair, and hence exploitative. It is still important to distinguish between consensual and non-consensual exploitation because there may be reason to prohibit non-consensual exploitation but *permit* consensual exploitation. So when is a transaction consensual? There are some instances of alleged exploitation in which the issue of consent does not seem to arise, as in *Tissues*, *Stem cells* or *Cost-shifting*. By contrast, B tokens consent in one way or another in most of the examples. The question there is whether B's consent is 'valid'. B's consent is valid only if it is sufficiently voluntary, informed and competent. Each of those criteria is the subject of a long and complicated story that we cannot adequately tell here. A few words will have to suffice.

We generally say that consent is voluntary when it is not coerced. In my preferred view, A coerces B to do X only if A proposes (threatens) to violate B's rights if B chooses not do X (Wertheimer, 1987). At the same time, A does not coerce B into consenting if A makes an offer to B, that is, if A does not propose to violate B's rights if B should reject A's proposal. If A gets B to pay A $100 per week by threatening to bomb B's store if he does not pay up, then A coerces B into paying $100 a week. By contrast, if A gets B to pay A $100 per week by proposing to clean B's store each night, then A has made a non-coercive offer to B. If this is right, A does not coerce B *Kidneys* or *Surrogacy* because A does not propose to worsen B's situation if B rejects A's proposal.

Some say that B's consent is coerced when B has no reasonable alternative but to consent. I disagree. Consider this case.

> *Amputation.* B has gangrene and will die unless she agrees to have a leg amputated. A proposes to amputate B's leg and B consents.

We are inclined to treat B's consent as valid, even though B has no reasonable alternative but to agree. We would certainly not say that A had performed surgery without B's consent.

Voluntariness is not enough. B's consent may not be valid if B does not have the requisite information or if B lacks the competence to give valid consent. Because these are standard issues in health care ethics, I shall not say much more about them here. Suffice it to say that many cases of exploitation in health care involve defects in information or competence. For example, we may regard sexual exploitation in psychotherapy as non-consensual even if the patient tokens consent and is not coerced because we think that the process of psychotherapy itself distorts the patient's decision-making capacities. There are other ways in which B's decision-making capacities can be compromised, as in *Trust* or *Manipulation*.

What I call *seductive offers* can also compromise B's competence to consent. A makes a seductive offer when A's proposal contains such great short-term benefits that it causes B to excessively discount the long-term costs and to make a decision that does not serve her long-term interests. B's consent in *Kidneys* may not be valid if B is unable to make a reasonable judgement, and there is some evidence that kidney donors systematically overestimate the economic benefits of donation and underestimate the long-term costs.

All that said, there are numerous cases of alleged exploitation where B would not have agreed to the transaction with A under better or perhaps more just background conditions, but where B is making a voluntary, competent and informed choice under the circumstances in which she finds herself. This might be true in *Surrogacy, Kidneys, Prisoners* or *Clinical research*. There may be something terribly wrong with the background conditions that make it rational for B to consent to certain proposals and those transactions may well be exploitative, but we should not presume that B's consent is invalid on grounds of coercion, information, competence or rationality, just because we think the transaction is morally objectionable.

JUSTIFYING INTERFERENCE

Let us assume that a transaction is properly described as a case of mutually advantageous consensual exploitation. Could we be justified in interfering with such transactions? Reconsider *Rescue*. Suppose that the following represents the parties' utility gains from various options.

	A's pay-off	B's pay-off
No transaction	0	0
Unfair transaction ($100)	5	5
Fair transaction ($20)	2	8

Note that a fair transaction does not yield equal utility gains. Because being rescued is important to B, she gets as much utility in the unfair transaction from being rescued as does A from $100. And if she were rescued for only $20, she would get much more overall utility than A. Two points are to be considered. First, even if A is under absolutely no obligation to transact with B, we might still think A has moral reason to be fair to B given that A benefits from the interaction with B. Second, even if A's behaviour is wrong in such transactions, it might still be argued that it would be wrong to interfere with or prohibit transactions which are beneficial to both parties and to which both parties consent. Suppose A proposes (2), and B counters that they should agree on (3), that A rejects (3) and tells B that it is either (1) or (2). If B is willing to accept (2), its unfairness notwithstanding, what, if anything, would justify not allowing B to do so?

A paternalistic argument for interference simply does not apply in the present context because we cannot justify intervention on paternalistic grounds if B fully understands her interests, if the exploitative transaction is advantageous to the exploitee and if interference is not likely to result in a transaction that is more beneficial to B.

We might interfere with mutually advantageous and consensual transactions because they cause harm to others. For example, even if commercial surrogacy were beneficial to the participants directly involved, such activities might diffuse negative effects on the way in which we think about mothers and children. There are three points about this line of argument. First, if intervention prevents harm to others, the case for intervention is relatively easy to make. Second, it is an empirical question as to whether interfering with a practice would actually avert harm to others. Third, this line of argument for intervention actually has *nothing* to do with the exploitation of surrogate mothers *per se*.

In my view, what I call the *strategic* argument for intervention is the strongest argument for interfering with or prohibiting mutually beneficial and consensual exploitative transactions. That argument maintains that if we disallow an unfair transaction, we render it more likely that a fairer transaction will occur. In *Rescue*, A can make a credible threat to opt for (1) (no transaction) rather than (3) (fair transaction) and so get B to agree to (2) (unfair transaction). Yet if we *prohibit* A from entering into an unfair transaction (2) with B, it is likely that A will propose a fair transaction (3) rather than refusing to transact with B (1). After all, A benefits from a fair transaction with B (3), and so has no reason to refuse to transact with B if the unfair transaction (2) is taken off the table.

Suppose, however, that the strategic argument does not apply. What I shall call the *Permissible Exploitation Principle* (PEP) maintains that it is wrong to interfere with an exploitative transaction: (1) if A is under no obligation to transact with B on any terms; (2) A proposes terms that are unfair to B; (3) if we prevent A from transacting with B on unfair terms, then A would choose not to transact with B at all; (4) B consents to the transaction; (5) the transaction is worse for no one else. In my view, there is a very strong presumption in favour of accepting this principle. Although I do not think it *incoherent* to claim that there might be deontological reasons to reject PEP, it is not equivalent to the utilitarian principle that we should allow any action that has better aggregate consequences, where the advantages to some outweigh the losses to others. Rather, PEP says that we should allow a transaction whenever it would be better for all parties to the transaction and worse for no one else. Moreover, because PEP precludes intervention only when the parties consent to the transaction, one cannot easily reject PEP on the Kantian grounds that it allows A to use B as a mere means to his own ends. For it is at least plausible to maintain that A does not treat B as a *mere* means if B's valid consent is a necessary condition of any transaction between A and B.

EXPLOITATION IN CLINICAL RESEARCH

Let us now apply this analysis to a case of alleged exploitation. Consider this case.

> *The Pharma Trial.* An American drug company, Pharma, wants to test a new drug Q for disease X. There is a standard treatment, T, for X, but Q is cheaper to produce and Pharma wishes to discover whether it is equally effective. Pharma could try to run an active controlled trial (ACT) in the United States, where it tests Q against T, but it prefers to run a placebo controlled trial (PCT) in, say, Ecuador, because a PCT requires a smaller sample and produces cleaner statistical results. Because virtually no one in Ecuador can afford T, people are willing to enrol in a trial for which they have at least a 50% chance of receiving treatment.

Many bioethicists have claimed that this sort of clinical research in underdeveloped societies is vulnerable to the charge of exploitation. Here are some typical statements.

1. 'Unless the interventions being tested will actually be made available to the impoverished populations that are being used as research subjects, developed countries are simply exploiting them in order to quickly use the knowledge gained from the clinical trials for the developed countries' own benefit' (Annas and Grodin, 1998, p. 561).
2. 'If the knowledge gained from the research in such a country is used primarily for the benefit of populations that can afford the tested product, the research may rightly be characterized as exploitative and, therefore, unethical' (CIOMS, 2002).
3. 'Residents of impoverished, postcolonial countries, the majority of whom are people of colour, must be protected from potential exploitation in research. Otherwise, the abominable state of health care in these countries can be used to justify studies that could never pass ethical muster in the sponsoring country' (Lurie and Wolfe, 1997, p. 855).

Should we seek to prohibit Pharma from conducting its trial? The Declaration of Helsinki states that 'in any medical study, every patient – including those of a control group, if any – should be assured of the best proven diagnostic and therapeutic method'. *The Pharma Trial* seems to be incompatible with this principle, unless one fudges with the notion of the 'best proven . . . method' by arguing that we should adopt a 'local' standard, under which the best proven method is no treatment at all. But the real question is not whether *The Pharma Trial* is compatible with the principles of the Declaration of Helsinki or other similar documents, but whether we should accept those principles in the first place. If Pharma proposed to run an ACT in the United States or Great Britain, thereby providing no care to anyone in Ecuador, the principles of the Declaration of Helsinki would not be violated. So if Pharma is not required to provide *any* care at all to Ecuadorians, why should we insist that it provide at best a proven method of care to all participants in the study?

We can consider the best proven care principle in terms of the *strategic argument* for intervention. If we insist that ACTs be used in the developed world whenever a standard therapy exists, there is little risk that the research will simply go away. Although the drug companies might prefer PCTs, the potential subjects in the developed world may be collectively helped by rules that force researchers to treat them better than they otherwise might. By contrast, the strategic argument may or may not work in the developing world. On one hand, it is possible that such constraints will prevent a 'race to the bottom' among developing nations that are competing for the benefits of being used for such research. On the other hand, it is also possible that – given such constraints – the researchers will decide that they might as well use ACTs in their own nations. There is little reason for Pharma to run an ACT in Ecuador when it could run such a trial in the United States. If that is right, interference cannot be justified as the best strategy for improving the lot of potential research subjects in developing nations. In any case, it is an *empirical* question as to whether disallowing PCTs such as *The Pharma Trial* works to the advantage of potential subjects in Ecuador. This will not be solved by philosophical discussion.

Nonetheless, it may be thought that there is something particularly morally obnoxious about a practice in which the affluent entice the poor to provide a service which will primarily benefit the rich. Perhaps, but it is arguable that there is no reason to regard medical research as particularly different from a wide variety of practices in which the affluent directly or indirectly hire the less affluent to provide manufactured goods at low prices or to do dirty or dangerous things for them, such as hiring nannies, gardeners and domestics. And we cannot say, 'But those are not life-threatening situations,' because the affluent also effectively hire others to engage in dangerous occupations such as coal miners, construction workers or volunteer (professional) soldiers.

I have, of course, been assuming that the participants in studies such as *The Pharma Trial* actually give valid informed consent. And that may be false. For example, many subjects may not understand that they are consenting to participate in a PCT as opposed to consenting to medical treatment. It may or may not be feasible to resolve these sorts of cognitive deficiencies, but, if not, it is also possible that a proxy or surrogate, such as the government or its representatives, can supplement the subjects' consent by insisting that participation in the study actually serves their interests just as parents serve as surrogates for their children who are not capable of giving informed consent.

Assuming that consent is adequately informed, would it be voluntary? It may be said that impoverished persons who would ordinarily have no medical care available to treat X may have no choice but to participate in a study in which they have a chance of obtaining medical care for them and that their consent is consequently involuntary. I argued in an earlier section that we should resist this line of argument. The central fact is that Pharma did not propose to violate a potential subject's rights should a potential subject decide not to participate.

Still, it might be argued that *The Pharma Trial* represents a 'seductive offer'. Just as The Council for the International Organization of Medical Sciences worries that the offer of monetary payments may 'induce prospective subjects to consent to participate in the research against their better judgment', a similar worry may arise with respect to the offer of a chance at life-saving therapy. We must, however, be careful to properly interpret the phrase 'against their better judgment'. It is important to distinguish between two claims:

(1) The inducements constitute a seductive offer that motivates subjects to consent to participate and when doing so does not advance their interests.
(2) Given the subject's objective circumstances, the inducements make it rational for the subjects to participate.

Note that in (2), the inducements are large enough to render participation compatible with the participants' better judgement given the objective conditions in which they find themselves. In my view, the real tragedy of poverty is not that poverty renders (1) true, but that it renders (2) true. David Rothman writes that 'abject poverty is harsh enough without people having to bear the additional burdens of serving as research subjects' (Rothman, 2000). But the point could easily go the other way. We might say, after all, that abject poverty is harsh enough without denying people the opportunity to make their lives somewhat less miserable by receiving benefits that they would not otherwise receive.

Interestingly, as the quotations noted above suggest, worries about exploitation in clinical research often focus not on the treatment of the experimental subjects but on the lack of benefits to the community when the study is over. Although the commentators have not been precise, they may be arguing (1) that the research would not be exploitative at all if the products that result from such studies were to be made available to present or future citizens of the host country, or (2) the research would exploit the research subjects, but such exploitation would be counterbalanced and justified if the benefits of the research were made available to the host country. Both arguments are problematic. If, as in (1), the research does not exploit the research subjects, I do not see why it should be necessary that B's fellow citizens will benefit. If, as in (2), it is wrong to ask B to participate in research from which B will not benefit, then it is not clear to me why it becomes permissible just because B's fellow citizens may benefit.

Many commentators have argued, in effect, that to allow a PCT in an underdeveloped society that would not be permitted in a developed society is to countenance moral relativism or a double ethical standard, which would allow 'studies that could never pass ethical muster in the sponsoring country' (Lurie and Wolfe, 1997). If *The Pharma Trial* would not be permitted in the United States, then it should not be permitted in Ecuador. As Marcia Angell puts it, 'Acceptance of this ethical relativism could result in widespread exploitation of vulnerable Third World populations for research programs that could not be carried out in the sponsoring countries' (Angell, 1997). Now a justification for a PCT in an impoverished society need not appeal to ethical relativism or double standards. Rather, it may be argued that one principle – that we should allow clinical trials to which the parties give rational consent – should be universally applied, but that this principle will have different implications in different contexts. If, for example, it would be irrational for Americans to consent to participate in a PCT but it would not be irrational for Ecuadorians to do so, then insisting that only 'rational' consent can be taken as valid will have different implications in the two societies, but there is no relativism or double standard here.

I have just scratched the surface of this debate. The most important point is this. We will not resolve questions as to the justifiability of studies such as *The Pharma Trial* by appealing to the derisive language of exploitation. We will resolve them by the rigorous examination of ethical arguments and by the painstaking study of the relevant data as to the effects of various policies on people's lives.

REFERENCES

Angell M. The ethics of clinical research in the third world. *N Engl J Med* 1997; 847–849.

Annas G, Grodin M. Human rights and maternal–fetal HIV transmission prevention trials in Africa. *Am J Pub Health* 1998; **88**: 560.

Arneson R. Exploitation. In: Becker LC, ed. *Encyclopedia of Ethics*. New York: Garland, 1992.

Benn S. *A Theory of Freedom*. Cambridge: Cambridge University Press, 1988.

Buchanan A. *Ethics, Efficiency, and the Market*. Totowa, NJ: Rowman and Allanheld, 1985.

Council for International Organizations of Medical Sciences. *International Ethical Guidelines for Biomedical Research Involving Human Subjects*. Revised draft, January 2002.

Feinberg J. *Harmless Wrongdoing*. Oxford: Oxford University Press, 1988.

Goodin R. *Reasons for Welfare*. Princeton, NJ: Princeton University Press, 1988.

Hill JL. Exploitation. *Cornell Law Rev* 1994; **79**: 631–699.

Kass L. *Life, Liberty and the Defense of Dignity*. San Francisco: Encounter Books, 2002.

Levine A. *Arguing for Socialism*. London: Verso, 1988.

Lurie P, Wolfe S. Unethical trials of interventions to reduce perinatal transmission of the human immunodeficiency virus in developing countries. *N Engl J Med* 1997; **33**: 855.

Moore B. *Reflections on the Causes of Human Misery*. Boston, MA: Beacon Press, 1973.

Munzer S. *A Theory of Property*. Cambridge: Cambridge University Press, 1990.

Rothman D. The shame of medical research. *The New York Review of Books*, 30 November 2000.

Wertheimer A. *Coercion*. Princeton, NJ: Princeton University Press, 1987.

Wertheimer A. *Exploitation*. Princeton, NJ: Princeton University Press, 1996).

33

Competence to Consent

MONIQUE F. JONAS

INTRODUCTION

A valid consent is generally taken to consist of four key elements: information provision, voluntariness, the opportunity to deliberate and competence (Gillon, 1986; Beauchamp and Childress, 2001). Competence is, in one way, the odd one out amongst this group. The first three components of a valid consent relate to properties of the consent process that are essentially external to the consenting party; namely, the environment in which the consent is sought and the way in which it is sought. The requirement for competence, on the contrary, relates to the properties of the party from whom consent is sought: the consenting party must possess certain capacities for their consent or refusal to be valid.

It is clear that competence serves an essential purpose in legitimating a consent. A consent for a complex surgical procedure gained from an 18-month-old under conditions of perfect voluntariness, information provision and with plenty of opportunity to deliberate would nevertheless fail to serve the purpose that consent is intended to serve. There are two principal reasons to seek consent to a medical intervention: to protect and promote a patient's autonomy and to increase the likelihood that the patient's welfare will be served (on the grounds that individuals tend to be better judges of their own welfare than others, and perhaps because the consent process itself contributes positively to welfare). When consent is sought from an incompetent individual, it is likely that neither of these purposes will be met. Determining that a person is incompetent implies that they are incapable of making an autonomous choice about that decision. An incompetent individual is typically not a good judge of his own welfare either, and although welfare might be advanced by involving incompetent patients in the consent process, these welfare gains must be balanced

against, and will frequently be outweighed by, the welfare considerations associated with the decision itself. Thus, welfare considerations generally also tell in favour of the competence condition.

This is all very uncontroversial, but the requirement for competence is not without its controversies. Problems occur at the levels of both theory and practice. There are difficulties in determining what competence actually entails and difficulties in formulating a reliable method for detecting competence in practice, once this has been established.

There are interesting discussions about whether emotions should be incorporated into accounts of competence (Chadwick, 1998; Charland, 1998) and on the effect addiction might have on competence (see Charland, 2002). The role that values ought to play in assessments of competence is another subject open to debate (Buchanan and Brock, 1990; Applebaum and Grisso, 1995; Draper, 2000).

There are also questions about what should follow from a finding of incompetence: should the wishes of an incompetent patient be factored into decisions in some fashion? Recent moves to encourage or require an incompetent child's assent before involving her in medical research are based upon the view that the preferences of an incompetent individual should not be disregarded and may even be decision-determining. Several regulations and guidelines for research emphasize the importance of obtaining the assent of incompetent children, although the nature of the emphasis varies. Where it is possible to obtain one, The Helsinki Declaration (World Medical Association, 2000) makes the assent of a legally incompetent minor a requirement, in addition to the consent of a 'legally authorised representative' (World Medical Association, 2000, paragraph 25). The Medicines for Human Use (Clinical Trials) Regulations 2004 (the English incarnation of the European Clinical Trials

Principles of Health Care Ethics, Second Edition   Edited by R.E. Ashcroft, A. Dawson, H. Draper and J.R. McMillan
© 2007 John Wiley & Sons, Ltd

Directive (Directive 2001/20/EC) takes a somewhat different approach (The Medicines for Human Use, 2004). It specifies that 'The explicit wish of a minor who is capable of forming an opinion and assessing the information... to refuse to participate in, or to be withdrawn from, the clinical trial at any time is considered by the investigator'. (Schedule 1, Part 4, paragraph 7). This allows that the views of incompetent children may be taken into consideration without being decisive in all cases. The same principle is applied to clinical trials involving 'incapacitated' adults (Schedule 1, Part 5, paragraph 7). Despite their differences, these documents suggest that competence is not the only relevant consideration when assessing how involved a patient should be in decisions concerning them.

This chapter focuses on two of the main debates that occur at the level of the theory of competence. The first relates to whether competence assessments should be decision-relative or global. The second addresses the claim that competence is a risk-relative concept. Before these debates are introduced, however, the prevailing accounts of competence are described.

SEVERAL INFLUENTIAL ACCOUNTS OF COMPETENCE

Competence, or capacity, basically means 'the ability to perform a task' (Beauchamp and Childress, 2001; Culver and Gert, 1990) and in this context, the task at hand is that of making a medical decision, or a series of medical decisions. Some claim that there is a distinction between these terms, and they do have different provenances, competence being a legal term and capacity a medical one. However, they are widely used as synonyms and essentially relate to the same thing (Grisso and Applebaum, 1998).

Although there are a number of competing accounts of what competence to make medical decisions entails, there is substantial agreement amongst theorists, practitioners and the courts about the constituent elements or abilities that characterize competence to make medical decisions. Several influential accounts capture these basic features.

Grisso and Applebaum's account, which draws upon the standards of competence that have been adopted by common law courts, lists the following as the attributes relevant to competence consent to treatment:

(1) The ability to communicate a choice;
(2) The ability to understand relevant information;
(3) The ability to appreciate the nature of the situation and its likely consequences
(4) The ability to manipulate information ration ally (Applebaum and Grisso, 1995, pp. 109–110).

Buchanan and Brock's account is similar. They pick out the following central requirements:

> ...the capacity for understanding and communication, and the capacity for reasoning and deliberation...A third important element of competence is that the individual must have a set of values or conception of the good (Buchanan, Brock, 1990, p. 23).

Beauchamp and Childress offer this account:

> Patients or subjects are competent to make a decision if they have the capacity to understand the material information, to make a judgement about the information in light of their values, to intend a certain outcome, and to communicate freely their wishes (Beauchamp and Childress, 2001, p. 71).

In the United Kingdom, The British Medical Association (BMA) and the Law Society's joint account of competence to consent, which was intended to function as a guide for health care practitioners and lawyers, are widely referred to:

> To demonstrate capacity individuals should be able to:
> –understand in simple language what the medical treatment is; its purpose and nature and why it is being proposed;
> –understand its principal benefits, risks and alternatives;
> –understand in broad terms what will be the consequences of not receiving the proposed treatment;
> –retain the information for long enough to make an effective decision. (BMA and the Law Society, 1995, ch. 10; see also Tan and McMillan, 2004)

Several court cases provide tests of competence that draw upon similar accounts. See, for instance, the test outlined by J. Thorpe in *Re C* (refusal of medical treatment) [1994] 1 All ER 819 (FD) at p. 36: 6 [competence requires] first comprehending and retaining treatment information, secondly believing it and thirdly, weighing it in a balance to arrive at a choice'. (See also *Gillick v. W. Norfolk AHA* [1985] 3 All ER.)

Although these accounts of competence do contain important and interesting differences, they also share a lot of common ground. The components of competence tend to be cognitive, for instance, with understanding and the ability to appreciate and apply information assuming key roles. This section has presented several of the most influential accounts of the *elements* of competence: of those capacities needed to qualify as competent. But there are also questions about the nature of the *concept* of competence itself. The answers that these questions meet with reflect views about what the point of assessing competence is, and different approaches will support different ways of assessing competence.

There is widespread agreement that competence is a threshold concept. It is worth considering why this is so before looking at two features of the concept about which views differ.

COMPETENCE AS A THRESHOLD CONCEPT

Competence can be regarded in one of two ways: it can be seen as all-or-nothing, or as a matter of degree. It is clear that, if accounts of the sort that currently prevail are correct, competence is, in an important sense, a matter of degree. Key elements of competence, such as understanding, appreciation and the ability to manipulate information rationally, are not all-or-nothing matters: it is possible to understand a piece of information to a greater or a lesser degree and to appreciate its application to oneself more or less profoundly. Some people will qualify as highly competent decision-makers, as judged by the accounts referred to above, others will be competent, but to a lesser degree, and still others will fall short of attaining any level of competence at all. But despite the fact that several of the abilities that competence entails are matters of degree, there is a strong preference amongst theorists and practitioners for viewing competence as a threshold concept, which establishes two categories of individuals: those who are competent and those who are not. This preference reflects the very purpose of competence assessments (Buchanan and Brock, 1990).

Competence assessments are undertaken in order to establish whether a given patient has the ability to give or refuse consent at a given time. A valid consent or refusal is, of course, one that is made voluntarily, on the basis of sufficient understanding and appreciation of all the relevant information. Although each of the elements of a valid consent is a matter of degree, the decision about whether or not a treatment should proceed on the basis of the patient's consent is not: either patients should determine their course of treatment or they should not. The all-or-nothing nature of the decision about whether to respect a patient's decision dictates that the test for competence is one that operates a threshold, and thus yields a determinate yes-or-no conclusion about that patient's competence.

For these reasons, competence is held to be a threshold concept, and tools of assessment must establish cut-off points, below which patients do not count as competent. This does not mean that no account can be taken of variations in levels of competence in medical decision-making. The preferences of a person who narrowly fails a competence test may be taken into account by decision-makers to a greater extent than those of someone whose decision-making capacities fall wildly short of the threshold, for instance.

CONTROVERSIES IN THE THEORY OF COMPETENCE: DECISION-RELATIVE OR GLOBAL?

Although there is substantial agreement about various aspects of competence, there are areas of dispute, one of which relates to the breadth of competence assessments. There are two relevant accounts here. First, competence can be seen as 'global', so that competence assessments embrace and apply to every aspect of one's life. One is either competent, and thus entitled to make decisions regarding all aspects of one's life, or incompetent, so that all decisions must be made on one's behalf.

This model of competence has been rejected by the majority of theorists in favour of a task-relative approach. This approach has also been upheld by the courts.

Buchanan and Brock express the thought behind the task-relative approach:

> The statement that a particular individual is (or is not) competent is incomplete. Competence is always competence for some task — competence to do something. The concern here is with competence to perform the task of making a decision. Hence competence is to be understood as decision-making capacity. But the notion of decision-making capacity is itself incomplete until the nature of the choice as well as the conditions under which it is to be made are specified. Thus competence is decision-relative, not global (Buchanan, Brock, 1990, p. 18).

According to the decision-relative approach to competence, competence is contingent upon the particular cognitive skill-set required by a given decision. A person may qualify as competent to make one sort of decision but not another if it calls for a skill, or level of skill, that the patient does not possess. In the case of competence to make medical decisions, the capacities at issue will generally be understanding and appreciation of information (although the same claims apply to the other elements of competence, such as the ability to communicate, to retain information and so forth). The cognitive skills required to make a given decision are dictated by the nature of the information that must be understood and appreciated in order to make it. Due to the kinds of information that they involve, and perhaps to the circumstances in which they must be taken, certain decisions call for a highly advanced level of understanding, a developed ability to reason probabilistically, and so forth, whilst others are much less demanding in these respects. Thus, when adequately informed, an eight-year-old may qualify as competent to decide whether or not to take paracetamol for the pain of a broken arm, whilst being incompetent with respect to a decision about whether or not to participate in a research trial involving a greater level of risk than that associated with standard treatment, but which also boasts the possibility of a greater benefit than standard treatment in terms of certain aspects of the child's condition.

The decision-relative account of competence can operate (albeit uncomfortably) alongside the general presumption that all adults are competent. What it means is that, when reasons to question the competence of a patient to make a decision emerge, the assessment process should focus upon the specific demands of the decision at issue, rather than attempt to establish whether the patient is competent in some more general sense. It also means that conditions that might generally be associated with incompetence, such as mental illness that has led to compulsory treatment under mental health legislation, cannot be taken as an indication of incompetence to make all medical decisions. Although a sectioned patient may be incompetent to make decisions relating to the treatment of the condition for which they have been sectioned, they may fulfil the criteria for competence to make medical decisions unrelated to that condition.

Although the decision-relative approach to competence has achieved wide subscription, it is not without its critics. I will focus on the criticisms presented by Tom Buller, who identifies two competing theories that support the decision-relative account. (See also Abernathy, 1984.) The first is 'internalism', or the idea that decisions vary in the level of cognitive skills that they require of a decision-maker. The second theory is 'externalism', which states that decisions vary in the risks that attach to them and that riskier decisions require a greater level of competence (Buller, 2001). Buller finds both accounts wanting, but this section will focus upon the objections he presents to internalism. Problems associated with risk-relative accounts are addressed below.

Buller outlines the task-relative account of competence in general and claims that competence relates to *types* of actions, rather than to *tokens*:

> When we say that a person is competent to do X but not Y, we mean more than that she is competent to do X at this time under these particular conditions; instead we mean more vaguely that, in the absence of adverse environmental factors, the person is competent to do actions like X under most conditions (Buller, 2001, p. 95).

According to Buller, one need not be utterly infallible at a given task in order to qualify as competent at it, but one does need to be able to succeed at it as a general rule. Buller then turns to the specific activity of making decisions and asks what it would mean for competence to be decision-relative. He concludes that it would suggest that the capacities required to make decisions are largely dependent upon the characteristics of particular decisions: one decision might differ from another in terms of the demands it makes upon the decider in the same way that football differs from figure-skating. The fact that one has mastered the skills required by football does not mean that one is also a competent figure-skater. If competence to decide is decision-relative, it must be because decisions are susceptible to significant variation in the skills that they call for. But Buller questions whether decisions do vary in terms of the capacities they require in the same way that activities differ from each other:

> Whereas it is clear that cooking a meal requires at least some different skills than composing an opera, one can make the argument that exactly the same skills are needed to make financial decisions as educational ones, namely attention to detail, appropriate weighing of options, understanding of implications etc. (Buller, 2001, p. 96).

One response to this is to point to the difference in subject matter that different sorts of decisions concern: people differ in their familiarity with and ability to negotiate different forms of information. But Buller doubts whether such a distinction can support a decision-relative approach to competence, on the grounds that focusing on an individual's existing familiarity with the information relevant to a given decision can lead us down a path of objectionable elitism, too easily dismissing people as incompetent because they require more assistance than others do to understand and appreciate the facts of the matter (Buller, 2001).

This move is unconvincing. It is not clear from Buller's account why decision-relative accounts of competence lead to objectionable elitism or paternalism, and in fact one of the attractions of the decision-relative approach is that it allows individuals who would fail most global assessments of competence to retain some control over aspects of their life. By suggesting that a decision-relative approach would focus on pre-existing knowledge and thereby discriminate against those who enter the decision-making process with limited understanding, Buller attacks a straw-man: what matters is not what the patient understands at the outset, but what she is *capable* of understanding, with guidance.

Although Buller is right to point out that all decisions involve broadly the same sorts of cognitive skills, decisions may call for very different levels of development in those skills, because the information involved in decisions can differ in its complexity. Some decisions relate to matters that do not involve high levels of abstraction, or very complex concepts, for instance, whereas others do. A five-year-old, for example, may be able to understand the information relevant to deciding whether to have a bandage applied to a wound, but lack the requisite cognitive skills to make decisions involving much more abstract information, such as those relating to the programme of treatment that she should receive for acute lymphoblastic leukaemia.

One of the charges that Buller makes against 'internalist' theory is that it must give an account of why life-and-death treatment decisions involve information that requires a higher level of cognitive skills than mundane treatment decisions do (Buller, 2001). This charge misses the mark: nothing commits the 'internalist' to the claim that complexity of information is a function of a decision's effect upon an individual's expected life-span. Decisions about some non-life-and-death matters may require more in terms of capacity to understand and appreciate than some life-and-death decisions do. Buller gives no reason to think that the claim that some decisions require more in terms of cognitive capacity than others do fails. In the absence of arguments that do threaten the 'internalist' theory supporting it, the claim that competence is decision-relative remains a plausible one, and the fact that it allows individuals who might otherwise be considered globally incompetent to make certain decisions for themselves could render it positively attractive.

CONTROVERSIES IN THE THEORY OF COMPETENCE: IS COMPETENCE RISK-RELATIVE?

In recent years the question of whether competence should be thought of as risk-relative has excited more controversy than the question of whether it is global or decision-relative. This debate relates to the issues of where the threshold that demarcates competence should be set and what factors should determine this.

As has been observed above, understanding and appreciation can differ in degree, but to facilitate rulings about whether a patient's decision should be respected, a threshold must be set that specifies the level of understanding that is sufficient for him to qualify as competent to make a given decision. Some theorists claim that the risks that are associated with a given decision should influence threshold-setting. Their claim is that the level of understanding that must be attained in order to qualify as competent to make a risky decision (in that it exposes the patient to more than minimal possibility of harm) should be higher than that required to make a less risky decision.

The risk-relative approach suggests that a person might be competent to consent to a given treatment without being competent to refuse it, if the risks attached to refusing are higher than those attached to consenting. It does not merely claim that risky decisions call for more careful scrutiny of competence, but that the actual level of understanding, appreciation and so forth, must be higher to qualify as competent for riskier decisions.

Against this is the view that risk should not be a factor in determining the level at which competence is set because risks do not necessarily make a decision *harder* in the relevant sense. The claim here is that what matters for competence is whether the decision-maker has adequately understood the information at hand, appreciated it, incorporated it into a decision-making process along with his values and so forth. The level of understanding at which one qualifies as competent should be the same across all decisions, but because some decisions involve more complex information than others, one can qualify as competent to make one decision but not another. The determining factor should not be how risky the decision is, but how complex the information that one must understand to make the decision in a sufficiently informed and autonomous manner is.

Because complexity of information does not always track risk, introducing risk into the process of setting thresholds infects competence assessments with irrelevant considerations and 'fails to strike an acceptable balance between benevolent intervention and personal autonomy' (Cale, 1999, p. 135). This position has been called the 'fixed threshold conception' (Buchanan and Brock, 1990, p. 59).

This section reviews some of the arguments advanced by Buchanan and Brock, and Wilks, in favour of a risk-related threshold. (See the following for critical discussion of the risk-relative approach, and in particular of Wilks' article: Cale, 1999; Wicclair, 1999; Checkland, 2001; DeMarco, 2002).

Buchanan and Brock point out that the account of competence one adopts must avoid two errors that can be made when the values of welfare and autonomy conflict:

> The first error is that of failing adequately to protect a person from the harmful consequences of his or her decisions when the decision is the result of serious defects in the capacity to decide. The second error is failing to permit someone to make a decision...when the patient is sufficiently able to make the decision him-or herself (Buchanan and Brock, 1990, pp. 40–41)

They claim that a risk-related conception of competence (or what they call a 'sliding scale' of competence) is most capable of avoiding these errors. They produce several arguments to support this conception, several of which are worth examining here.

The first is that a risk-related standard is in keeping with the way in which people make competence judgements in everyday life:

> For instance, you may decide that your five-year-old child is competent to choose between a hamburger and a hotdog for lunch, but you would not think the child competent to make a decision about how to invest a large sum of money (Buchanan and Brock, 1990, p. 60).

Buchanan and Brock attribute parental reluctance to accord their young children decision-making authority over matters such as investment to a combination of the complexity of information and the risk involved in such decisions. A proponent of the fixed threshold conception of competence could agree with Buchanan and Brock's ascription of variable competence to five-year-olds with respect to these decisions, but disagree that risk plays the part they attribute to it. The complexity of the information involved in these choices differs enormously: this alone might explain judgements about the child's competence to make each decision. Risk could be factored in on a fixed threshold view insofar as understanding and appreciating risk requires greater cognitive skills, without it assuming independent force. It is likely, however, that risk *does* retain independent force in our considerations about everyday situations such as this. This need not suggest, however, that our tendency to consider risk when authorizing others to make decisions is right: some deeper normative support of the risk-relative standard is required.

Buchanan and Brock also cite the fallibility of competence assessments in support of a risk-related standard. Competence assessments can fail, and they attract deep disagreement. They can fail by imperfectly testing for the standards of competence that are adopted. It is impossible to devise an assessment tool that will track competence perfectly in every case: there will always be false positives and negatives. And they attract disagreement because people differ in the relative emphasis that they place upon the values of welfare and respect for autonomy, and as the implemented standard will balance these values in a particular way, there will always be people who consider that balance to be wrong (Buchanan and Brock, 1990).

Buchanan and Brock claim that, given the fallibility of competence assessments, risk-related standards of competence are preferable to fixed standards. In cases in which a decision carries minimal risk (compared to the alternatives), the level at which competence is set can be fairly low, as this allows autonomy to be served, and little will be lost in terms of welfare if the competence assessment is incorrect. But in cases where risks are high, the level at which a patient qualifies as competent should be higher because welfare interests are more profoundly involved (Buchanan and Brock, 1990).

There are a number of potential problems with Buchanan and Brock's solution to the problem of fallibility (DeMarco, 2002). If one accords autonomy priority over welfare interests, for instance, the loss of autonomy sustained at the risky end of the scale will appear unjustified by possible welfare gains. There are also questions about how risk is assessed: if risk is a function of one's aims and values, perhaps health care professionals and others are ill-placed to identify decisions as highly risky for a given patient. It may be possible to strike a balance between respecting autonomy and protecting welfare *without* imposing higher standards of competence for risky decisions by requiring more *evidence* of competence where risks are greater, whilst retaining a fixed threshold. DeMarco advocates this approach (DeMarco, 2002).

Wilks takes another tack in his defence of a risk-related threshold (Wilks, 1997). He responds to the observation made by Culver and Gert, and Wicclair, that risk-related standards create situations in which one individual qualifies as competent to (for instance) consent to a treatment, but not to refuse that same treatment, when the level of risk attached to consenting and refusing differs (Culver and Gert, 1990; Wicclair, 1991). This seems strange for a number of reasons. First, it makes sense to hold that one must understand and appreciate the relevant information

in equal measure to consent to or refuse a single treatment. If one understands enough to consent, does not that imply that one also understands enough to refuse? Second, there are questions about whether an asymmetry produces real choice: how can one be free to agree to a proposition if one is not free to refuse it? The requirement for a higher standard of understanding for a refusal than a consent (or vice versa, depending on which way the risk falls) to a proposition is taken by Culver and Gert, and Wicclair, to degrade the value of that consent. These theorists advocate what Wilks calls 'the principle of symmetrical competence' (Wilks, 1997, p. 419) described by Culver and Gert in the following way:

> when we are discussing a person's competence to make a decision about his medical treatment…if we regard him as competent to consent to a given medical treatment, then we must regard him as competent to refuse that very same treatment (Culver and Gert, 1990, p. 620).

Wilks uses a number of examples to make sense of the notion that one might be competent to consent to but not to reject a single proposition. The first involves a high-wire act performed with and without a safety net. Wilks imagines a high-wire walker of middling ability, who is able to traverse the wire but not infallibly. Wilks claims that such a person would be competent to cross the wire with the net *in situ*, but would not be considered competent without it (even if the negative influence of anxiety would be avoided by removing the net unbeknownst to the walker). For Wilks, this example illustrates the point that

> Our competence to perform [a] task is easily seen to depend upon how probable it is that we will undertake it in the wrong way…But our competence to perform a task is also dependent upon how negative the consequences of undertaking it in the wrong way are…One is more hesitant to regard a fallible tightrope walker as competent to walk the rope without a net, even though quite competent to walk with one, because of the fact that ill-performance at walking without the net is negatively so much more consequential than walking with it (Wilks, 1997, p. 420).

In this example, Wilks regards the walker as competent to walk the rope with the net *in situ* but not without. This understanding of the situation is contestable, however. As Wilks notes, the walker is just as likely to fall when the net is in place as he is when it is removed; what differs in each situation is how much he is likely to suffer through his failures. But whether this difference supports a finding a differential competence depends on how one describes the task at hand.

If the task is described as traversing the rope without falling, then it is wrong to consider the walker any more competent when the net is *in situ*. If the task is described, however, as crossing the rope without incurring substantial personal injury then, because the risks associated with falling differ in each case, the walker is more competent when the net is in place than when it is absent. But it seems strange to adopt the second description of the task: tight-rope walking is fundamentally about crossing a rope without falling from it; injuries are secondary considerations. Wilks fails to separate the question of how one defines and assesses competence from two further questions: will the person incur harm if she/he performs an act (Cale, 1999) and should a person be allowed to perform (or attempt) that act? If risks are low, there may be reasons to allow an individual to perform a task (or fewer reasons to prevent them) at which he is not competent. Parents, for instance, often allow their children to 'practise' activities that they have not mastered in controlled environments. This does not mean that parents regard their children to be competent in these situations.

The question of whether competence should be risk-related is far from settled in theory. In practice, it is likely that risky decisions will attract competence assessments more readily than decisions involving minimal risk, but the standards that those assessments should apply do not generally take a risk-related form.

CONCLUSION

Competence plays an integral part in valid consents in the health care arena, but precisely what it involves and how it ought to be detected are matters that continue to cause considerable debate. Whether competence is decision-relative or global and whether standards of competence should be risk-related are just two of the questions that exercise theorists and practitioners alike, and the debate that surrounds them is likely to rumble along for as long as informed consent takes a central place in medical ethics.

REFERENCES

Abernathy V. Comparison, control and decisions about competency. *Am J Psychiatry*. 1984; **141**: 53–60.

Applebaum PS, Grisso T. The MacArthur treatment competence study. I: Mental illness and competence to consent to treatment. *Law Human Behav* 1995; **19**(2): 105–125.

Beauchamp T, Childress J. *Principles of Biomedical Ethics*, 5th edition. Oxford: Oxford University Press, 2001.

BMA, the Law Society. *Assessment of Mental Capacity: Guidance for Doctors and Lawyers*. London: BMA, 1995.

Buchanan A, Brock D. *Deciding for Others: The Ethics of Surrogate Decision-Making*. Cambridge: Cambridge University Press, 1990.

Buller T. Competence and risk-relativity. *Bioethics* 2001; **15**(2): 93–109.

Cale G. Risk-related standards of competence: continuing the debate over risk-related standards of competence. *Bioethics* 1999; **13**(2): 131–148.

Chadwick R. Commentary on is Mr Spock mentally competent? *Philos Psychiatry Psychol* 1998; **5**(1): 83–86.

Charland L. Is Mr Spock mentally competent? Competence to consent and emotion. *Philos Psychiatry Psychol* 1998; **5**(1): 67–81.

Charland L. Cynthia's dilemma: consenting to heroin prescription. *Am J Bioethics* 2002; **2**(2): 37–47.

Checkland D. On risk and decisional capacity. *J Med Philos* 2001; **26**(1): 35–59.

Culver CM, Gert B. The inadequacy of incompetence. *Milbank Q* 1990; **68**: 619–643.

DeMarco J. Competence and paternalism. *Bioethics* 2002; **16**(3): 232–245.

Department of Health. *Reference Guide to Consent for Examination and Treatment*. London: Department of Health, 2002.

Drane J. The many faces of competency. *Hastings Center Rep* 1985; **15**.

Draper H. Consent and midwifery. In: Frith L, ed. *Ethics and Midwifery*. Oxford: Butterworth Heinemann, 1994; pp. 17–33.

Draper H. Anorexia nervosa and respecting a refusal of life-prolonging therapy: a limited justification. *Bioethics* 2000; **14**(2): 120–133.

Elster J. *Solomonic Judgements: Studies in the Limits of Rationality*. Cambridge: Cambridge University Press.

Gillick v. W. Norfolk AHA 1985; 3 All ER.

Gillon R. *Philosophical Medical Ethics*. London: Wiley, 1986.

Grisso T, Applebaum PS. *Assessing Competence to Consent to Treatment: A Guide for Physicians and Other Healthcare Professionals*. New York: Oxford University Press, 1998.

Grisso T, Applebaum PS, Mulvey E, Fletcher K. The MacArthur treatment competence study. II: Measures and abilities related to competence to consent to treatment. *Law Human Behav* 1995; **19**(2): 127–148.

Nozick R. *The Nature of Rationality*. Princeton, NJ: Princeton University Press, 1993.

Re C (Refusal of Medical Treatment) 1994; All ER 819 (FD) 36: 6.

Tan J, McMillan J. The discrepancy between the legal definition of capacity and The British Medical Association's guidelines. *J Med Ethics* 2004; **30**: 427–429.

The Medicines for Human Use (Clinical Trials) Regulations. London: HMSO, 2004; Also available at http://www.opsi.gov.uk/si/si2004/20041031.htm

Wicclair M. Patient decision-making capacity and risk. *Bioethics* 1991; **5**(22): 91–104.

Wicclair M. The continuing debate over risk-related standards of competence. *Bioethics* 1999; **13**(2).

Wilks I. The debate over risk-related standards of competence. *Bioethics* 1997; **11**(5): 413–426.

World Medical Association. *Declaration of Helsinki: Ethical Principles for Medical Research Involving Human Subjects*, 2000; http://www.wma.net/e/policy/17-c_e.html 2000.

34

The Doctrine of Double Effect

SUZANNE UNIACKE

INTRODUCTION

The Doctrine or Principle of Double Effect arises from the application of moral theory to some difficult moral problems. The Doctrine is applied across a range of issues in practical ethics, where it is held to be relevant to the morality of particular types of actions and practices that have both good and bad effects. The term 'double effect' refers to the two effects that can follow from one and the same action: a good or desirable effect which the agent intends, and a bad or undesirable effect which the agent foresees but does not intend. The Doctrine is relevant where the foreseen bad effect of such an action is morally serious in nature; it is thought especially significant when the bad effect amounts to causing or allowing a person's death. The Doctrine draws a moral distinction between cases in which a person's death is a foreseen, incidental effect, as opposed to cases in which a person's death is intended. The Doctrine is often referred to in contemporary health care ethics. It is frequently invoked, for example, in distinguishing the permissible use of opioids in palliative care of the terminally ill for the purpose of pain relief, where this also has the effect of hastening a patient's death, as opposed to active euthanasia for which the patient's death would be the intended outcome. The distinction drawn by the Doctrine of Double Effect between an intended as opposed to a (merely) foreseen effect of an action is sometimes a fine one. (Many people regard it so, for instance, in the example just mentioned.) Nonetheless, advocates of the Doctrine maintain that this distinction is important to the morality of various actions and practices.

The Doctrine applies a strict notion of what it is for an agent to *intend* an effect: a person is said to intend an effect of his action only if he aims to bring it about either as an end or instrumentally as a means of achieving his end in the circumstances. The Doctrine contrasts an effect that is intended in this sense with an effect which, although it might be a certain or highly probable outcome of a particular action, is incidental to what a person aims to achieve in acting as he does. The Doctrine invokes the moral significance of this particular distinction between an intended effect of an action, as opposed to an effect that is (merely) foreseen, in certain practical contexts and under a set of conditions.

ORIGINS AND MORAL CONTEXT

The Doctrine of Double Effect originates in St Thomas Aquinas's account of permissible homicide in self-defence. Aquinas held the view that it is morally impermissible for a private individual (i.e. someone not acting with political authority or under its command) to kill any person intentionally. Does this imply that as a private person I cannot legitimately use lethal force in self-defence against an unjust attack, even when this is necessary to save my own life? Aquinas thought not. He maintained that homicide in self-defence need not violate a prohibition against intentional killing. This is because, he argued, the use of necessary force in warding off an attack can have the 'double effect' of both self-protection (a good effect that I intend in acting in self-defence) and also killing the attacker (a bad effect which I foresee but do not intend). Aquinas maintained that as the attacker's death is unintended, the use of lethal force in self-defence can be permissible because self-preservation is a legitimate aim and a person who is unjustly attacked has a greater duty to preserve his own life than he has to preserve the life of the attacker (Aquinas, 1966, IIa, IIae. 64, 7).

Aquinas's notion of an act of double or two-fold effect, where a good effect is intended and a concomitant bad effect is (merely) foreseen, is central to what became the Doctrine of Double Effect (DDE). The DDE was subsequently developed in Catholic moral theology as a guide to

Principles of Health Care Ethics, Second Edition   Edited by R.E. Ashcroft, A. Dawson, H. Draper and J.R. McMillan
© 2007 John Wiley & Sons, Ltd

morally permissible action in a range of contexts (Mangan, 1949). For any moral theory that holds that certain types of intentional actions are always impermissible difficult practical decisions will arise where in acting for a legitimate end (a good effect) in very pressing circumstances a person foresees that she cannot avoid also bringing about a bad effect of a type that it is impermissible to intend. Faced with this problem in relation to homicide in self-defence, Aquinas characterized it as permissible, unintended killing. Many people who accept that intentional killing is always impermissible believe, *contra* Aquinas, that this prohibition applies not to all persons but only to the intentional killing of *innocent* persons. Those who accept this latter, more qualified absolute prohibition might, then, regard an unjust attacker as outside its impervious protection and justify homicide in self-defence as an instance of permissible intentional killing. (Those who accept that the intentional killing of innocent *persons* is always impermissible can also disagree about whether it applies, for example, to foetuses (abortion) or to those in a persistent vegetative state.) But other questions for the application of an absolute prohibition against the intentional killing of innocent persons will arise. For instance, a long-standing question of political ethics is whether it is ever permissible to kill innocent civilians in fighting a war. Just War Theory, which also has its origins in the ethics of Augustine and Aquinas, prohibits the intentional killing of noncombatants. The traditional Just War conditions of *jus in bello*, which govern legitimate action within war, include the principle of noncombatant immunity, which says that hostile action must not be *directed* against innocent people. Given this principle, could strategic bombing of a genuinely military target be permissible where this would also involve, as a foreseen, incidental effect, the killing of civilians who are in the vicinity of the target? The DDE has been invoked as relevant to moral decision-making in relation to this question. Long-standing applications of the DDE in medical contexts include the withdrawal of treatment where a patient's death is a foreseen outcome, and cases of abortion which arise from the removal of a pregnant woman's cancerous womb. In another context, at the level of personal action, we might ask whether, for example, it would be morally permissible for a motorist to swerve his car in order to avoid hitting some children who have run out on the road (good effect), when he foresees that if he swerves he will knock down a pedestrian who has stepped out from the curb (bad effect). A similar type of example and numerous variations of it are discussed in great detail in the philosophical literature on the DDE as 'the Trolley Problem' (Foot, 1978; Thomson, 1986; Kamm, 2000).

In many cases of actions of double effect, both the intended good effect and the (merely) foreseen bad effect can occur. This is true of all of the examples mentioned above.

However, the DDE is arguably also applicable to actions in which the intended good effect would be incompatible with the occurrence of the unintended bad effect (Duff, 1990). For instance, a surgeon might engage in highly risky organ transplantation surgery in a desperate attempt to save a patient's life. In this case, the surgeon acts with the intention of saving the patient; in so acting, the surgeon might also foresee that the patient will probably die from the surgery or its effects. For those who believe that intentional killing is always impermissible, it is insufficient simply to characterize actions of this type as instances of justified risk-taking (if and when indeed they are) without reference to the fact that, while foreseen as highly probable and perhaps by far the more likely outcome, the bad effect (the patient's death) is unintended.

According to the DDE, an act of double effect can be morally permissible provided certain conditions are met (these conditions are outlined below). The DDE arises from a position of moral absolutism – the view that some types of intentional actions are always morally impermissible. Such acts, it is said, cannot be justified instrumentally, even as necessary means of achieving a good or legitimate aim. For example, if a person acts with the intention of killing another, innocent person as a means of saving a number of other people's lives, this intention is sufficient to make that particular action morally impermissible, irrespective of the agent's motive and irrespective of what good the action might also achieve. (Here we might think, for example, of the infamous legal case of *Dudley and Stephens* in which after 20 days adrift in an open boat, two sailors killed and ate the (by then unconscious) cabin boy so that they and a third man might survive to be picked up and rescued. The jury in the case accepted that if Dudley and Stephens had not acted as they did, the cabin boy would not have survived long enough to be rescued, and all four in the boat would have died.) Given the emphasis on absolute moral prohibitions in many expositions of the DDE, it is important to remember that as traditionally conceived the DDE is embedded in a complex morality which also condemns acts of malicious and gratuitous harm, and which includes a positive obligation of charity, for instance. Moral absolutism does not hold that it is always impermissible to intend harm. (Punishment of the guilty is justified, for instance.) Nor does moral absolutism maintain that it is permissible for a person to cause a foreseen bad effect provided that particular effect is unintended. (Killing as a result of negligence, or from indifference to another person's life, or from morally indefensible priorities, is wrong.) Application of the DDE assumes that acts of double effect are morally well motivated (McIntyre, 2001). It assumes that the agent is not indifferent to causing the foreseen bad effect and that he does not desire or welcome it, opportunistically, from malice or from an improper, ulterior motive.

THE DOCTRINE'S CONDITIONS

Contemporary accounts of the DDE usually encompass four conditions under which an act of double effect can be permissible. The *New Catholic Encyclopedia* (Connell, 1967) states these conditions as follows:

> (1) The act itself must be morally good or at least indifferent. (2) The agent may not positively will the bad effect but may permit it. If he could attain the good effect without the bad effect he should do so. (3) The good effect must flow from the action at least as immediately (in the order of causality, though not necessarily in the order of time) as the bad effect. In other words, the good effect must be produced directly by the action, not by the bad effect. Otherwise the agent would be using a bad means to a good end, which is never allowed. (4) The good effect must be sufficiently desirable to compensate for the bad effect. In forming this decision many factors must be weighed and compared, with care and prudence proportionate to the importance of the case. Thus, an effect that benefits or harms society generally has more weight than one that affects only the individual, and an effect sure to occur deserves greater consideration than one that is only probable; an effect of a moral nature has greater importance than one that deals only with material things …

As traditionally explained, this set of conditions is strict. This means that fulfilment of each of the four conditions is necessary for the permissibility of an act of double effect. The strictness of the conditions does not mean, however, that taken together they are intended to work like a formula that always produces a definitive answer. Although the DDE is sometimes said to give a 'ruling' in morally difficult cases, it was explicitly developed as a *guide* to the moral permissibility of acts of double effect. Interpreted as a guide to moral decision, fulfilment of conditions 1–3 would establish that a particular act of double effect could be morally permissible; it would establish that such an act is not morally out of question.

Contemporary philosophical discussions of the DDE often expect great precision and certainty from its set of conditions; they assume that the plausibility and moral significance of the DDE depends on its ability to yield a definitive answer for all problem cases of double effect (including highly fanciful ones). Arguably this is a reasonable assumption in relation to conditions 2 and 3, in particular, because the DDE's insistence that an agent may foresee but must not intend the bad effect is held to be crucial to the permissibility of acts of double effect. (I shall discuss more about this requirement in the following section.) Condition 4, however, invokes a requirement of proportionality, and it is clearly meant to outline the sort of considerations that are relevant to making a sound judgement about whether the intended good effect is sufficiently morally important to permit causing the foreseen bad effect. This condition is highly significant because a well-intentioned action can

be wrong if it causes disproportionate harm. (It would be wrong, for example, to intervene to prevent the loss of someone's umbrella, if in so doing one would risk causing a traffic collision.) Condition 4 will clearly be met in some cases, and in other cases it will clearly not be met. Nonetheless, in some factual circumstances this condition can also admit a degree of uncertainty about whether a particular act of double effect is morally permissible. (In the above example, would swerving the car to avoid hitting the children be sufficiently desirable to permit knocking down and killing the pedestrian?) Some acts of double effect might be a 'close call' in terms of condition 4.

A further important clarification of the DDE's requirement of proportionality is that, contrary to what some philosophers claim, this condition is not 'consequentialist' in nature. Consequentialist moral theories, such as utilitarianism, maintain that the rightness or wrongness of an action depends entirely on its overall outcome. Moreover, according to consequentialism, an action that, from amongst the alternative actions available to the agent, will be optimal in terms of its overall balance of good consequences is positively the right action to perform in the circumstances, such that not to perform this particular action would be wrong. (There might be rare cases in which alternative actions would have equally optimal outcomes.) To the extent that the DDE takes comparative outcomes and requirements of proportionality into account in judging the moral permissibility of an action of double effect, it is not thereby appealing to consequentialist considerations. Nor is condition 4 meant to establish that an act of double effect would be morally right, such that refraining from that particular action would be wrong. An action that clearly meets the DDE's four conditions is said to be morally permissible. It does not follow from this alone that there is an obligation to perform that action.

It is appropriate at this point also to clarify three other aspects of the DDE that are often misunderstood. First, the DDE does not maintain that under its set of conditions the agent is not morally responsible for the foreseen bad effect, for example, the death of an innocent person. The agent is morally responsible for a foreseen effect that he voluntarily brings about, in the sense that he must justify having caused or allowed the effect. Second, the DDE's distinction between an intended effect as opposed to a foreseen one does not coincide with a distinction between positive and negative action. The DDE does not itself draw a conceptual or a moral distinction between what a person does, as opposed to what he allows to happen. (Some statements of the DDE, such as the one from the *New Catholic Encyclopedia* quoted above, might lead to confusion in this regard by characterizing the foreseen bad effect as something the agent 'permits'. But here the contrast with an effect that an agent 'permits' is an effect that he 'positively wills' (intends), not with an effect that he brings about.) The DDE can sometimes be applicable to foreseen bad effects that a person allows to occur. For example, in setting priorities for the treatment of a large number of severely injured people in a major emergency, medical personnel working with limited resources can foresee, but they do not intend, the deaths of some critically injured people who are allowed to die because they do not receive treatment immediately. In this case, priorities are set that allow particular people to die, and these deaths are foreseen. It is important also to note that according to the DDE there are circumstances in which an *intended* effect can arise from negative action, from what a person deliberately does not prevent. For example, a person could intend the death of someone whom he fails to rescue, where he lets someone die whose life he could easily save because he stands to benefit personally from that person's death. Moreover, as far as the DDE is concerned, an effect that is (merely) foreseen, as opposed to intended, can result from positive action. In the example above, knocking down the pedestrian would be a foreseen, unintended effect of the motorist's positive act of swerving the car to avoid hitting the children.

INTENTION AND ITS MORAL RELEVANCE

The most important issue for a critical appraisal of the DDE is undoubtedly that of intention. There are two distinguishable questions to be addressed in this regard. The first is whether the DDE invokes, or can be made to invoke, a defensible distinction between the intended (good) effect of an action, as opposed to a (bad) effect of that action that is (merely) foreseen. The second question is whether if a defensible distinction of this nature can be maintained, it has the moral significance that the DDE takes it to have.

According to the traditional DDE, we intend an effect of our action, *x*, if we aim to achieve *x* either as an end or as a means of achieving an end in the circumstances. In many contexts we distinguish between those effects of actions and practices that are intended in the sense that they are (part of) what we aim to achieve, either as an end or instrumentally, in acting as we do, as opposed to effects that we (merely) foresee. For example, nausea and hair loss are foreseen effects of chemotherapy, but they are not intended effects of this type of cancer treatment. Chemotherapy is not administered for the purpose of causing nausea or hair loss. Nor are nausea and hair loss means of achieving the intended effect of killing cancer cells. This is why, although foreseen, nausea and hair loss are commonly referred to as side-effects of chemotherapy. It would not, of course, be morally impermissible to intend to cause nausea or hair loss if, contrary to fact, these effects of chemotherapy were actually instrumental in bringing about the other, desirable

effects of chemotherapy. The point here is simply that the distinction between effects that are intended, as opposed to effects that are (merely) foreseen as certain or highly probable, is one that we commonly acknowledge.

On what basis do we draw this particular distinction? To what do we intuitively appeal in judging that a particular foreseen effect is intended as opposed to incidental? Here a so-called 'test of failure' has been invoked in the context of applying conditions 2 and 3 of the DDE. According to this 'test', a person does not intend a foreseen bad effect of his action if he can sincerely answer 'yes' to the question: 'Would my intention in acting as I do be achieved if, contrary to expectation, this bad effect does not occur?' In many contexts, this 'test' can be a good guide to what an agent intends. In the above examples, for instance, the motorist can sincerely say that his intention to avoid hitting the children by swerving the car would be achieved if the pedestrian somehow manages to get out of the way; the surgeon who engages in highly risky surgery can honestly say that his intention would be achieved if the patient does not die (especially so in this case because achieving the intended outcome is incompatible with causing the foreseen bad effect). Application of this 'test of failure' can also distinguish between administering morphine for pain relief where this will also hasten a terminally ill patient's death, as opposed to the administration of a lethal dose of morphine as an act of euthanasia. In the latter case (euthanasia) the agent intends to the cause the patient's death as a means of relieving suffering, and this particular intention will be achieved only if the patient dies.

The claim that these two cases of morphine use are distinguishable in terms of their respective intentions can serve to highlight two important considerations. The first is that the question posed by the 'test of failure' must be answered in the light of the agent's beliefs at the time of action (Duff, 1990). If, for instance, I administer what I believe to be a lethal dose of morphine, believing that an act of 'mercy killing' is necessary to relieve the subject's suffering, and, contrary to all expectation, the subject survives and is cured, I cannot then claim in the light of this actual outcome that in acting as I did, I did not intend to kill. (Even with this proviso about the agent's beliefs at the time of action, some commentators maintain that the 'test of failure' can be an inadequate means in distinguishing between intended and incidental effects (Kamm, 2000; McIntyre 2001).) The second consideration is that the 'test' must assume what the DDE's condition 2 explicitly states, namely that if the agent can bring about the good effect without the bad he should do so. Fulfilment of this can be an important indication that the foreseen bad effect is incidental, as opposed to intended. McIntyre (2001) points out, for example, that adequate pain relief can now be administered for many terminal patients by methods that do not slow respiration or hasten death. If a morphine drip which includes a lethal dose is chosen when other methods adequate for pain relief are available, it is disingenuous to claim that hastening the patient's death is not part of the intention.

The DDE's condition 3 requires that the good effect must flow from the action at least as immediately (in the order of causality, though not necessarily in the order of time) as the bad effect. This means that the foreseen bad effect must be incidental both to the aim of action and to the way in which the good effect is achieved. Traditional accounts of the DDE hold that the bad effect is intended if it is a means to achieving the good effect in the actual circumstances. One way of elaborating condition 3 is to say that in any case of double effect, it must be possible to describe the agent as having performed two distinct acts based on the one more basic act, with one of the two acts having been intended and the other not. The intended act will have been the agent's reason for doing the unintended act; the unintended act must not explain why or how the intended act was done (Uniacke, 1994). (For example, the motorist swerves his car (more basic act), and thereby both avoids the children (act) and also knocks down a pedestrian (act). The motorist does not swerve the car in order to knock down the pedestrian; nor is knocking down the pedestrian a means of avoiding the children. Similarly, by administering morphine (more basic act), a doctor both relieves a patient's pain (act) and also slows respiration (act). The pain is relieved directly by the morphine, not by means of the slowing of respiration.) This interpretation of condition 3 is what the traditional DDE implies. However, Kamm's intricate analysis of variations of the Trolley Problem and her appeal to a distinction between doing something *in order* (or intending) *to* bring about something else, as opposed to doing something *because* something else will be brought about, would allow instances of double effect that fail to meet condition 3 (Kamm, 2000). Undoubtedly, there are cases in which a foreseen bad effect is arguably, although not incontrovertibly, (merely) foreseen as opposed to intended, and vice versa. Some such cases, especially those discussed as variations of the Trolley Problem, can seem very remote from what can reasonably be regarded as an intended effect in actual empirical circumstances.

A defensible account of the difference between an intended effect as opposed to one that is (merely) foreseen must in some cases invoke a criterion that *disallows* a sophistical distinction between, for example, intending to kill someone as opposed to intending (merely) to blow him to pieces (Foot, 1978; Quinn, 1989; McMahan, 1994). Several traditional applications of the DDE can seem dubious in this regard. These include some instances of homicide in self-defence where it is very difficult to maintain that there was no intention to kill (Uniacke, 1994). In cases of ectopic

pregnancy, abortion also seems implausibly characterized as an incidental effect of removal of the fallopian tube, before it ruptures. In such cases the pathological condition of the fallopian tube is due to the presence of the embryo.

On the question of whether the distinction between a bad effect that is intended as opposed to one that is merely foreseen has the moral significance that the DDE takes it to have, it is well to remember that the DDE cannot be called upon to justify the particular moral constraints or prohibitions on which it is based and which give rise to appeal to the DDE in morally difficult circumstances. The rationale of the DDE assumes that some intentional actions are intrinsically morally wrong and impermissible, not the other way around.

Adoption and appeal to the DDE is in fact much more widespread than its origins in Catholic moral theology might suggest. Secularized versions of the DDE (and also of Just War Theory) now have general currency in practical ethics. The DDE is a significant feature of much contemporary ethics that is non-consequentialist in nature. Prominent advocates of the DDE, or of a particular version of it, include Catholic philosophers who can be regarded as institutionally committed to the DDE (e.g. Anscombe, 1981; Finnis, 1991) and also philosophers who are not (e.g. Duff, 1982). The DDE's advocates include those who can be regarded as moral absolutists (e.g. Anscombe, 1981) and also critical exponents of the DDE who are not moral absolutists (e.g. Quinn, 1989; Kamm, 2000). The attraction of the DDE across a range of non-consequentialist positions in contemporary ethics lies in the fact that it is widely taken to represent an important moral insight, namely that there can be a morally significant difference between intending, say, the death of an innocent person as a means to an end, as opposed to causing a person's death as an incidental effect of an act that aims to achieve a sufficiently significant good effect. (Moral absolutists claim that certain types of intentional actions are morally impermissible. Other advocates of the DDE hold that, *ceteris paribus*, it is morally worse to intend an intrinsically bad effect such as the death of an innocent person instrumentally, as a means to an end, than to bring it about as a foreseen, incidental effect of an act of double effect.)

Moral theories that maintain that the *intention* with which a person acts can have an important, sometimes a decisive, bearing in its own right on the morality of what he does are usually referred to as deontological. Such theories contrast with purely consequentialist approaches to the morality of actions, including acts that have both good and bad outcomes. A consequentialist theory such as utilitarianism may take an agent's intention into account in forming a view about his moral character: A person's moral character is relevant in that it can greatly influence his tendency to act in certain ways; an agent's intention can also be relevant to whether he is morally to blame on account of some bad effect that he causes or does not prevent. Nonetheless, for consequentialism, an agent's intention is significant to the morality of his action (what he does) only indirectly, only in as much as it has some bearing on that action's overall outcome. Consequentialist critics will, then, mostly dismiss the DDE as morally irrelevant. Other philosophical critics of the DDE may think that the important insight that the DDE is widely taken to represent, between an intended outcome as opposed to one that is (merely) foreseen, is in fact represented by other morally relevant distinctions and considerations (e.g. McIntyre 2001). Some philosophers who are broadly sympathetic to the DDE are nevertheless critical of some of its interpretations and supposed applications (e.g. Kamm, 2000).

LEGAL APPLICATION

The Doctrine of Double Effect is a moral, not a legal principle. Nonetheless, the notion of an act of 'double effect' would also seem to play a role in distinguishing legally permissible use of lethal doses of opioids in palliative care as opposed to legally impermissible acts of euthanasia (Tur, 2002). The notion of intention that is central to the DDE has also featured in legal decision-making about, for example, the separation of conjoined twins where the death of one twin is a certain outcome of the surgery (*Re A Children* (Conjoined twins), 2001). (Whether a distinction between intention and foresight (of death) is applicable to the particular facts of this case is debatable.) Appeal to a distinction between intention and foresight in these particular contexts might seem unsurprising because intention is a necessary element of some crimes and of murder in particular. (In a case of homicide, what a person intends in acting as he does can determine whether his conduct is murder, as opposed, say, to manslaughter.) However, in *other* legal contexts, what the law regards as an intended effect of a person's action can extend beyond what the agent strictly aims to achieve either as an end or instrumentally as a means and include what he foresees as a certain or highly probable outcome of what he does. English law adopts this more inclusive notion of intention in holding that, for example, a person who sets a bomb in a railway carriage in order to kill only one passenger in particular intends the deaths of (and is guilty of murdering)

those other people in the carriage whose deaths he most certainly foresees. This action is not an instance of double effect, of course, because what the agent aims to achieve (the murder of a particular person) is something morally impermissible. Nevertheless, the deaths of the *other* passengers who happen to be in the carriage are incidental to what the bomber aims to achieve, and hence, according to the DDE, these particular bad effects are unintended.

REFERENCES

Anscombe GEM. Modern moral philosophy. In: Anscombe GEM, ed. *Collected Papers*, vol. III. Oxford: Blackwell, 1981.

Aquinas T St. *Summa Theologiae*, vol. 38. Blackfriars edition, London: Eyre and Spottiswood, 1966.

Connell FJ. Double effect, principle of. *New Catholic Encyclopedia*, vol. 4. New York: McGraw-Hill, 1967; pp. 1020–1022.

Duff RA. Intention, responsibility and double effect. *Philos Q* 1982; **32**(126): 1–16.

Duff RA. *Intention, Agency and Criminal Liability.* Oxford: Blackwell, 1990.

Finnis J. Intention and side-effects. In: Frey RG, Morris CW, eds. *Liability and Responsibility.* Cambridge: Cambridge University Press, 1991.

Foot P. The problem of abortion and the doctrine of double effect. In: Foot P, ed. *Virtues and Vices.* Oxford: Blackwell, 1978.

Kamm FM. The doctrine of triple effect and why a rational agent need not intend the means to his end. In: *Proceedings of the Aristotelian Society*, Supplementary volume, vol. 74, 2000; pp. 21–39.

Mangan J. An historical analysis of the principle of double effect. *Theol Stud* 1949; **X**(1): 41–61.

McIntyre A. Doing away with double effect. *Ethics* 2001; **III**(2): 219–255.

McMahan J. Revising the doctrine of double effect. *J Appl Philos* 1994; **11**(2): 201–212.

Quinn W. Actions, Intentions and consequences: the doctrine of double effect. *Philos Public Affairs* 1989; **18**(4): 334–351.

R v Dudley and Stephens. 14 QBD 273, 1884.

Re A Children (Conjoined twins). 4 All ER 961, 2001.

Thomson JJ. The trolley problem. In: Thomson JJ, ed. *Rights Restitution and Risk.* Cambridge, MA: Harvard University Press, 1986.

Tur RHS. The doctor's defense. *Mountsinai J Med* 2002; **60**(5): 317–328.

Uniacke S. *Permissible Killing: The Self-defence Justification of Homicide.* Cambridge: Cambridge University Press, 1994; chapter 4.

35

Ordinary and Extraordinary Means

STEPHEN D. JOHN

In debates over end-of-life decision-making, appeal is often made to the distinction between ordinary and extraordinary means: a physician is obliged to use ordinary means to prolong a patient's life, but she is permitted to forgo the use of extraordinary means (O'Rourke, 2005). There is evidence that physicians often find this distinction helpful (Dickenson, 2000). However, bioethicists have been sceptical of both the cogency of the distinction and its alleged moral significance (Brock, 1993). In this chapter, I shall first set out an account of the distinction between ordinary and extraordinary means, focusing on its use in Roman Catholic moral theology and bioethics. In the second section, I shall outline a dilemma for those who would use the ordinary/extraordinary distinction in secular bioethics. In the third section, I shall investigate some ways in which the ordinary/extraordinary distinction might be rehabilitated within secular contexts.

END OF LIFE DECISION-MAKING: ORDINARY AND EXTRAORDINARY MEANS

Some of the most difficult problems in medical ethics occur in end-of-life cases. Often we must decide whether we ought to attempt to extend a patient's life or whether we ought to let her die. Very few people hold the extreme position that we must always do *everything* we can to keep a patient alive. Rather, it is common to allow that, in some cases, it is permissible to withdraw or to forgo provision of some kinds of medical care. Of course, given the extremely strong moral injunction against killing in general, and the way in which duties of beneficence and non-maleficence are normally understood to structure the doctor–patient relationship, deciding just when it is permissible to let a patient die is no easy task (Beauchamp and Childress, 2001). Appeal to the distinction between ordinary and extraordinary means is sometimes invoked in response to such problems. It is claimed that a physician always has a duty to use all ordinary means to prolong a patient's life, but that it may be permissible to forgo extraordinary means.

To understand the distinction between ordinary and extraordinary means, three points need to be stressed. First, the distinction is not intended to be read in a 'naturalistic' sense. Brock provides a useful list of ways in which we might think to differentiate the 'ordinary' from the 'extraordinary' in medical contexts: in terms of what is (statistically) 'usual' and 'unusual'; in terms of 'low' versus 'high' technology; in terms of 'natural' versus 'artificial'; in terms of invasiveness; in terms of cost; and in terms of the 'normal' versus the 'heroic' (Brock, 1993). He rightly points out that none of these (quasi-) naturalistic distinctions can support a normative distinction between the permissible and the impermissible. Rather than define ordinary versus extraordinary means in terms such as statistical frequency, Catholic bioethicists, according to Brock, define extraordinary treatment as one that is 'excessively burdensome for the patient'. Brock's summary of this claim is slightly over-simplified: Catholic theologians standardly claim that a treatment is extraordinary if the burdens of that treatment for a patient, her family and her community outweigh the benefits associated with that treatment for the patient in question (O'Rourke, 2005). However, he is right that the ordinary/extraordinary distinction does not map neatly onto naturalistic categories.

The second point to emphasize is that the doctrine of ordinary and extraordinary means captures a distinctively religious claim that although human life as a 'divine gift' is of great value, human life is not itself an 'ultimate good', but only important relative to 'spiritual goods' (O'Donnell, 1996). As such, in some circumstances striving to continue life may reflect a confused attitude towards the nature and value of human life. Treatments may legitimately be forgone

Principles of Health Care Ethics, Second Edition   Edited by R.E. Ashcroft, A. Dawson, H. Draper and J.R. McMillan
© 2007 John Wiley & Sons, Ltd

if they offer little hope of enabling enjoyment of spiritual goods. There is, unfortunately, not enough space in this chapter to discuss these topics fully, but it is important to remember that the doctrine of ordinary and extraordinary means, although expressed in terms of a metaphor of balancing benefits and burdens, should not be read in simple, 'consequentialist' terms but against a backdrop of a strong default injunction, based on an understanding of man's relationship to God, against allowing others to die.

I have emphasized two features of the ordinary/extraordinary distinction: it is evaluative, rather than naturalistic, and it should be read against the backdrop of a particular religious viewpoint. A third important point concerns the question of who is to decide whether or not some means counts as 'ordinary' or as 'extraordinary'. Traditionally, defenders of the distinction claim that the decision of whether or not treatment should be forgone is to rest with the patient (or her proxies) rather than with medical or other officials (O'Rourke, 2005). Ultimately, it is a patient, rather than a physician, who is to make a sincere decision about whether burdens outweigh benefits or vice versa.

THE DILEMMA

The distinction between ordinary and extraordinary means was developed within the context of Roman Catholic moral theology and, as such, rests on a particular view of the value of life and of the structure of our moral obligations. However, if bioethicists want to make claims relevant to public policy, then their arguments should be couched in 'public' terms; that is, the claims of bioethicists ought to be claims that can be agreed to by all reasonable citizens of societies characterized by deep religious and moral disagreement (Rawls, 1993). Therefore, we must ask whether a distinction between ordinary and extraordinary means, for example, as the basis of legislation, can make sense in secular contexts. Many philosophers – for example, Dan Brock and Jonathon Glover – have argued against the usefulness of appealing to the ordinary/extraordinary distinction in secular debate (Brock, 1993; Glover, 1997). The problem with appealing to the ordinary/extraordinary distinction in secular debate can be summarized in the form of a simple dilemma: either we adopt a weak reading of the distinction, in which case it introduces an unnecessary terminology into a simple debate, or we adopt a strong reading of the principle, in which case it is ethically partial, and thus unsuitable as the basis for a secular, liberal bioethic.

Liberal-secular bioethicists are standardly committed to the view that if a patient makes an autonomous choice to forgo some life-prolonging treatment, then we ought to respect her wishes. This resembles one way of phrasing the ordinary/extraordinary distinction: if a patient feels the burdens of some treatment outweigh the benefits of that treatment, then it is permissible for a physician to forgo provision of that treatment. However, if all that the ordinary/extraordinary distinction tells us is that if a patient *feels* that the burdens of a treatment outweigh the benefits of that treatment, then we ought to forgo the use of that treatment, it seems simply to add a layer of unnecessary vocabulary, couched in pseudo-scientific terms, to an ethical principle that is at the core of contemporary liberal bioethics.

Of course, defenders of the ordinary/extraordinary distinction might object to the claim that their theory is a restatement of familiar liberal themes. Rather, they might point out that their account of what legitimates the withdrawal of treatment – that to continue such treatment would be to misunderstand the nature of God's gift of life – differs in important respects from the liberal justification framed in terms of patient autonomy for permitting physicians to forgo treatment. However, if the defender of the doctrine of ordinary and extraordinary emphasizes this point, then she may be accused of arguing from a particular religious view of 'the good life' to normative conclusions. This kind of argument would violate the demand that arguments put forward in bioethical debate ought not to rest on contested views of the good for man, such as those of religious doctrine. Of course, no liberal would want to deny that, within some legal framework where patients have the right to forgo life-prolonging treatments, some Roman Catholics might want to reason in terms of the doctrine of ordinary and extraordinary means. However, such tolerance is, obviously, different from the claim that the justification for granting patients a right to forgo treatment in the first place ought to be framed in terms that underpin the ordinary/extraordinary distinction.

Therefore, we seem to be trapped between a 'thin' account of the doctrine of ordinary and extraordinary means, where the doctrine seems, for all intents and purposes, identical to traditional liberal thought, and a 'thick' account of the doctrine which, although tolerable, cannot serve as the basis for policy in a multicultural society. Gillon seems to have welcomed the first result (Gillon, 1986). However, both Brock and Glover suggest that, even if co-extensive with liberal thought, we would do well to lose the confusing terminology of ordinary and extraordinary means in bioethical debate. It is no wonder, then, that the doctrine of ordinary and extraordinary means is rarely appealed to in more recent debates over end-of-life decision-making.

A RESPONSE TO THE DILEMMA

At a procedural level, both the doctrine of 'ordinary/extraordinary' means and liberalism suggest that patients ought to be allowed to forgo treatments if they so choose. However, 'liberalism' – understood in this context as a theory that emphasizes a choice-based account of 'autonomy' as the ultimate moral value in bioethics – is better suited than Roman Catholic theology as a justification for allowing patients the right to choose whether or not to forgo treatment. Therefore, the doctrine of ordinary/extraordinary means is either empty or overly partial. In this section, I shall suggest that this conclusion, close to orthodoxy in bioethics, may be too hasty.

When we ask whether it is permissible to forgo certain sorts of treatments, we can distinguish two ways in which a (potential) patient's wishes are relevant to such a question. We might think that there is no question of right and wrong separate from what a patient chooses: what makes it permissible to forgo some treatment (thus allowing a patient to die) is that this is what the patient wished for. This position, where a patient's judgement is constitutive of what makes a physician's actions acceptable or unacceptable, is central to 'autonomy-based' approaches to end-of-life decision-making. However, this is not the only way in which we might think about these issues. Rather, we might think that there is a fact of the matter, independent of a patient's wishes, whether or not it is permissible to forgo treatment. This is, for example, the position advocated by crude classical utilitarianism: there is a fact of the matter as to whether or not extending a patient's life would maximize happiness, and it is this fact – rather than a patient's autonomous wishes – which justifies continuing or forgoing treatment. One way of understanding the traditional doctrine of ordinary and extraordinary means is as making a similarly 'objectivist' claim: there is a fact of the matter as to whether some treatment's expected benefits outweigh the burdens (for the patient, her family and her community) associated with that treatment, and this fact is what makes forgoing some treatment permissible or impermissible.

Before turning to ask how a patient's wishes relate to this 'fact', it is worth asking whether there could be any 'secular' account of when some individual's life is (or is not) objectively worth living. If not, the difference between the metaethics of liberalism and that of the ordinary/extraordinary distinction may seem empty as the latter cannot be the basis of a public bioethics. One way in which to ground a secular version of the claim that certain sorts of lives are worse than no life at all, without directly appealing to patients' autonomous choices, would be on 'dignitarian' grounds. 'Dignitarians' typically hold that individuals should not be able to exercise certain sorts of rights as exercise of those rights would violate their dignity (see Brownsword and Beyleveld, 2001 for one version of such a theory, and Kass, 2002 for a rather stronger statement of such an approach). There may be an argument that keeping alive human beings who have no chance of recovery via expensive and artificial means is a violation of human dignity. Is 'dignitarianism' a reasonable moral view for a secular bioethics? This difficult

question cannot be answered here (see Ashcroft, 2005 for a useful discussion). However, we can at least make the conditional claim: if we think that certain practices ought not to be allowed even in secular societies, on the grounds that they demean human dignity, then artificially prolonging a painful life may be an example of such a practice.

We can, then, outline secular grounds on which we might distinguish the question of what a patient wants from the question of whether the benefits of treatment would outweigh the burdens associated with such treatment, without collapsing into crude utilitarianism. However, proponents of the doctrine of ordinary and extraordinary means *do* claim that the question of whether or not means are 'ordinary' or 'extraordinary' must, ultimately, be made by the patient. How, then, does this relate to the distinction between a liberal view where choice is constitutive of the rightness of forgoing treatment and an approach where 'facts' other than choices make forgoing treatment (im)permissible? There are two options here. The first would be to stress the 'epistemic primacy' of the patient's perspective in deciding whether or not some treatment counts as 'ordinary' or 'extraordinary'. We could say that the most reliable indicator of whether or not the benefits of treatment outweigh its burdens is the judgement of the patient in question. To say that a patient's wishes are, in this context, a reliable indicator is *not* to say that a patient is more likely than a doctor to be 'right'. Remember that in such a morally charged context, we will be concerned with avoiding a particular kind of error, judging some means to be 'extraordinary', when it is, in fact, 'ordinary'. Given any patient's usual wish to live, we may think that she is particularly unlikely to judge erroneously that the burdens of some treatment outweigh its benefits. Given the epistemic complexities of assessing whether some means is ordinary or extraordinary we ought to err on the side of caution and treat the patient's (partial) judgement as the yardstick of certainty.

This 'epistemic' reading of the importance of patients' judgements to the legitimacy of forgoing treatment may seem too weak. A second approach would be to return to the 'dignitarian' view which, I argue, might provide the bases for an account of 'facts' about ordinary and extraordinary means. The dignitarian might claim that, if we are to respect human life, then we ought to respect the fact that human beings are reasoning creatures, who respond to 'moral concerns'. There is a 'right' and a 'wrong' answer over whether or not care counts as 'ordinary' or as 'extraordinary'. However, even if we could ascertain this fact independently of patients' wishes, such certainty would not suffice to justify forgoing treatment regardless of the expressed wishes of a patient (or her proxy). To ignore these wishes would be to undermine human dignity in a second way, by failing to allow patients (or their proxies) to engage in the activity of reasoning about the ultimate questions of life and death. Therefore, even if there is a 'correct' answer, independently of what we choose, we cannot impose certain options on patients, but rather the very same reason which justifies sometimes withholding treatment – a concern for human dignity – also demands that we are responsive to patients' own understanding of the reasons they have. This line of argument might be developed from the position advocated by Brownsword and Beyleveld (2001), or it might follow from the views expressed by John Harris in his debate with John Finnis over the permissibility of euthanasia (Keown, 1997).

CONCLUSIONS

The suggested secular reinterpretation of the distinction between 'ordinary' and 'extraordinary' means might seem to have little impact on policy. Furthermore, it may seem to rest on the acceptability of a 'dignitarian' bioethic in a secular community. Therefore, it would be overly optimistic to say that appeal to dignitarianism helps proponents of the ordinary/extraordinary distinction to avoid the dilemma as mentioned above. However, it may be that reflection on the distinction does help us to understand better the range of different ways in which we can think of end-of-life decisions, and, as such, reflection on the distinction will remain a feature of bioethical debate.

REFERENCES

Ashcroft R. Making sense of dignity. *J Med Ethics* 2005; **31**: 679–682.

Beauchamp T, Childress J. *Principles of Biomedical Ethics*, 5th edition. Oxford: Oxford University Press, 2001.

Brock D. *Life and Death*. Cambridge: Cambridge University Press, 1993.

Brownsword R, Beyleveld D. *Human Dignity in Bioethics and Biolaw*. Oxford: Oxford University Press, 2001.

Dickenson D. Are medical ethicists out of touch? Practitioner attitudes in the US and UK towards decisions at the end of life. *J Med Ethics* 2000; **26**: 254–260.

Gillon R. *Philosophical Medical Ethics*. Chichester: John Wiley & Sons, Ltd, 1986.

Glover J. *Causing Death and Saving Lives*. London: Penguin Books, 1997.

Kass LR. *Life, Liberty and the Defense of Dignity*. San Francisco, CA: Encounter Books, 2002.

Keown J. *Euthanasia Examined*. Cambridge: Cambridge University Press, 1997.

O'Donnell TJ. *Medicine and Christian Morality*. New York: Alba House, 1996.

O'Rourke K. The Catholic tradition on forgoing life support. *Natl Catholic Bioethics Q* 2005; **5**(3): 537–553.

Rawls J. *Political Liberalism*. New York: Columbia University Press, 1993.

36

Acts and Omissions

TUIJA TAKALA

Traditionally, the doctrine of acts and omissions refers to the idea that (sometimes) actions that result in bad consequences are morally worse than omissions that bring about similar states of affairs (Glover, 1977; Gillon, 1985). For instance, killing a person is thought to be worse than letting the person die. In bioethics the doctrine is most often invoked in discussions concerning euthanasia and being a Bad Samaritan, that is, failing to help others in need.

Although, arguably, it is in accordance with our ordinary moral intuitions to think that we are more responsible for the consequences that our actions bring about (say, bruising on a person we have hit) than of things that could have been different had we not omitted to act (say, failing to help someone who has had an accident) (Gibson, 1998), numerous fictional and factual examples can be presented to challenge the intuition (Glover, 1977). And this is indeed one of the problems in discussing the doctrine of acts and omissions; the whole issue seems to rely on our intuitions. A different kind of problem is whether it is possible to differentiate between acts and omissions in any morally meaningful sense. First of all, most omissions can, with creative use of language, be described as acts, and similarly, most acts can be made omissions. It is also quite possible to say that 'all that X had to do was to do nothing' (Hall, 1989). Another profound problem is that the doctrine of acts and omissions is usually challenged by people subscribing to various forms of consequentialism, whereas its supporters tend to lean towards deontological or Aristotelian theories. Given that the presuppositions of these theories are different, it is unclear whether the criticism ever meets its target.

RECOGNISING ACTS AND OMISSIONS

CAUSALITY

It is sometimes suggested that causal connection could be used to tell acts and omission apart. For instance,

by pulling the trigger of the gun I am holding against someone's head I cause that person's death. This seems straightforward enough. What if I am driving along a straight highway with the cruise control on, when I see someone standing in the middle of the road? If I do absolutely nothing, I will hit the person, and given that I am doing 80 miles an hour, the person will consequently die. I have seen the person well in advance, perhaps even recognized her as my neighbour from hell. All I needed to do was to turn the steering wheel ever so slightly to avoid the collision, but I did not. I seem to be causally responsible for that person's death, yet it seems to be caused by an omission. In medical ethics the most often used example is that of disconnecting life support. To disconnect a machine involves an act, but still, withdrawing life support is often described as causing death by omission. The argument here is that it was not the disconnecting that caused the patient's death, but the underlying condition that made her unable to breathe in the first place. What the doctor did was merely to omit continuation of the artificial breathing. However, it could also be argued that given that the patient was connected to the ventilator, and was alive because of that, it was the action of disconnecting that caused her death.

It would seem that causal connections can be established for both acts and omissions. With the examples above, we are inclined to think that some sort of moral responsibility comes with the causal connection. It is, however, easy to come up with examples where that is not the case. Say that it is a dark night, and the person walking in the middle of the highway is actually there with the intention of killing herself. I do not see her in time because she is deliberately wearing clothes of such colours that it is impossible to see her before it is too late. I had a causal role in her death, but whether I should be morally blamed for it is another matter.

Principles of Health Care Ethics, Second Edition   Edited by R.E. Ashcroft, A. Dawson, H. Draper and J.R. McMillan
© 2007 John Wiley & Sons, Ltd

MORAL BLAME AND INTENTIONS

Those wishing to question the moral distinction between acts and omissions often say that it does not matter whether something followed from our action or from our failure to act, but rather that the morally decisive criteria is what our intention was. James Rachels coined the oft-quoted example of Smith and Jones who both stand to inherit a fortune if their young cousin dies. Smith sneaks into the bathroom of his cousin with the intention of killing him. He drowns the cousin. Similarly, Jones sneaks into his cousin's bathroom with the intention of killing the cousin, but just as he is about to push the cousin's head under water, the cousin slips, hits his head and drowns. Jones could have easily saved his cousin, but instead he just stands by (Rachels, 1975). Even some defenders of the acts and omissions doctrine have claimed that if the reasons for omitting to act are wrong, then the person can be as liable as she would have been had she acted (Stauch, 2000).

When there is an intention to harm someone, it could be argued that whether the desired outcome was brought about by an act or an omission does not alter the blameworthiness considerably. And arguably the same would be true if the intention were to do good. The person could be said to be praiseworthy in these cases – provided that she has chosen the best means to bring about the desired effect, be it an act or an omission. When it comes to euthanasia, it is not obvious what our goals are and what they should be.

ACTS, OMISSIONS AND EUTHANASIA

Thou shalt not kill but needst not strive officiously to keep alive
(Arthur Clough, *The Latest Decalogue*)

Modern medicine makes it possible to keep human beings biologically alive for a very long time. This is not, however, always desirable. The practice of passive euthanasia, letting the patient, who is suffering intolerably or who has no chance of recovery, die has, in certain circumstances, become an acceptable part of end-of-life care. Decisions to withhold or withdraw life-supporting treatments are taken daily in hospitals everywhere. One of the justifications given is the distinction between acts and omissions. Although killing is seen as absolutely forbidden, it is thought that allowing someone to die can sometimes be acceptable. Those wishing to extend the right to die also to active (voluntary) euthanasia often try to make their case by showing that there is no moral difference between acts and omissions.

There is, however, one major problem with this tactic. Although the critics of the acts and omissions distinction usually are, very roughly, consequentialists, and as such hold that the consequences of our actions are of utmost

importance when it comes to moral evaluations, those whom they criticize tend to think that there is more to morality than mere consequences — absolute moral rules, such as 'thou shalt not kill' for instance. Let me illustrate the difficulty with the following dialogue between C (consequentialist) and D (deontologist).

C: Surely you must admit that it is inconsistent to allow passive euthanasia but disallow active euthanasia. Can you not see that there is no clear moral distinction between acts and omission?

D: Well, yes, I suppose, but there is no absolute rule against letting someone die, but there is against killing a person.

C: But if the consequences are the same, and the intention and the circumstances?

D: It is not only about the consequences. There are simply some things you should not do! Also, by allowing someone to die, I am not primarily intending her to die.

C: Surely you would allow a person who is suffering intolerably, has no chance of recovery and who wishes to die to be disconnected from the ventilator that is keeping her alive.

D: In certain circumstances, yes. But that would not be killing. It would be letting the patient die.

C: The act of disconnecting kills the patient!

D: No, it is the underlying illness!

C: Wait a minute here. But if you didn't disconnect the ventilator, the patient would remain alive. Let me try this with an analogy: think of a man who is found in a small floorless cage in the middle of a much larger cage that is occupied by hungry lions. (It does not matter how the man in the cage got there – it could have been a maleficent act by some people or it could have resulted from a freak accident or a small tornado – the point is that he is there.) If someone were to lift the small cage that protects the man, would you not say that they killed that man by lifting the cage and not that they merely let him die?

D: Hmm . . . I suppose that you are right . . . Perhaps we should not allow passive euthanasia either.

This is not where the consequentialist wanted to take the argument, but given the opponent's premises, it is a logical conclusion. It is also compatible with the oft-quoted definitions of acts and omissions doctrine, which all talk about acts and omissions in relation to bad consequences (Glover, 1977; Gillon, 1985). Even if the consequentialist succeeds in convincing her opponent that in certain situations the distinction between active and passive euthanasia is artificial, it does not mean that others will necessarily accept death as a good consequence. If there is no difference between acts and omissions, and euthanasia by omission is accepted, a possible conclusion is that then also euthanasia by act should be accepted. But there is also the other option, namely, that if there is no difference between acts and omissions in certain cases of euthanasia and the act of killing is absolutely forbidden, so should euthanasia by omission be.

ACTS, OMISSIONS AND BAD SAMARITANS

Those who wish to maintain the distinction between acts and omissions sometimes use examples like omitting to give money to charity versus sending poisonous food to those in need. I would assume that everyone would think the latter to be morally worse. Obviously, the consequences of these two actions are not the same because in the latter case more people would suffer; no one would benefit through charity and additional people would die because of the venomous food. Consider a refined example: here the options are not giving money to charity, or giving money to charity and sending poisonous food (Gillon, 1985). Provided that the calculations are done correctly, arguably, equal amounts of suffering would follow. In the first case, some people who would not have died had I sent the money to charity, will die. In the latter case some people will not die because of the money given to charity whereas others will after eating the poisonous food. The aspect that these examples miss is the intention behind the acts and omissions. I find it difficult to imagine how someone with a maleficent intention to have people die would pick 'not sending money to charity' as the method of choice.

Similar problems arise when the concept of a Bad Samaritan is brought to bear on acts and omissions. A Bad Samaritan can be defined as a person who stands in no special relationship to the endangered party, who omits to do something (warn, rescue, help, aid), which she could have done without unreasonable cost or risk to herself and others, and as a result of which the endangered party suffers harm (Feinberg, 1992).

For example, imagine yourself sitting in a lounge chair next to a swimming pool. Suddenly you see a child (not your own) drowning just a few inches away from where you are sitting. You realize that to save her you would only need to put down your drink, reach down and grab her by her swimming suit. She is so light that you would not even have to get up from the chair (Feinberg, 1992). People are likely to hold you morally blameworthy if you do not save the child, but it is unlikely that if you omit to act, you are as responsible for the child's death as you would have been had you drowned the child yourself. But, then again, if you, like Smith and Jones in Rachels' example, attended the poolside with the intention of killing the child, the situation might be different. But most Bad Samaritan examples are not like that. They talk about failing to call for help when you see that your neighbour's house is on fire, failing to stop at an accident site in a middle of nowhere to see if there is something you can do, and also, up to a point, about not

giving money to charity. The difference between acts and omissions and the Bad Samaritan case is that in the latter there is very seldom a comparable act that would lead to similar consequences and involve the same intentions.

MORAL BLAME, KNOWLEDGE AND SKILLS

There is, however, a problem in making intentions part of the ethical evaluation. How do we know what the intention in any given situation is? Many consequentialists are quick to point out the hypocrisy of the principle of double effect, which is sometimes brought to play in end-of-life situations. According to this principle, if there is a neutral act with two consequences, one of which is good and the other bad, and where the good consequence precedes the bad one, we are allowed to do the act provided that our intention was the good consequence and the bad one was merely a foreseen, but unintended side effect (Callahan, 1970). This principle is used, for instance, to justify giving a patient a large dose of painkillers with the intention of relieving her suffering, but with the foreseen side effect that the dose given will shorten her life and, in effect, kill her. The question that is asked here is that if it is known that such an amount of pain-killer will kill the patient, how credible is the claim that this is not the intention?

Similarly, it could be argued that if we know that as a result of our omitting to give money to charity, a number of people who could have been saved will die, we are, in some sense, intending them to die. We may not have maleficent motives, but if we know that these follow from our omission, should we be held as responsible as if it were our uncaring acts that caused the deaths? Somewhat counterintuitively it seems that the more we know, the more moral responsibility we have.

And it is not only knowledge, but also special skills that seem to increase our blameworthiness in terms of things we omit to do. Medical doctors have special responsibilities both on and off duty. If a doctor fails to diagnose a clear case of pneumonia and sends the patient home, she can be blamed for the omission, whereas a layperson could not be blamed for failing to make the diagnosis. If there is a doctor present when someone goes to a cardiac arrest in a public place, the doctor has a duty to provide the necessary emergency treatment. If there are no health care professionals around, anyone with some knowledge of first aid could be said to have a moral duty to help. They could be morally blamed for their omission, whereas people with no relevant knowledge could not be held responsible.

Apart from the criticism from the theoretical frameworks that believe there is more to morality than consequences, the main problem in thinking that acts and omissions often are morally equal is that this would require us to constantly perform supererogatory acts. Or, alternatively, we could try to avoid these by evading knowledge about the pain of others that we could alleviate and by not acquiring skills with which we could do this. It could be the old 'ought implies can' that ultimately makes wide applications of the equal moral importance of acts and omissions impossible. This is not, however, to say that there could be instances where upholding the doctrine of acts and omissions would not be justifiable.

DECISION TIME – THE LIMITED EQUALITY OF ACTS AND OMISSIONS

In this chapter I have described the various uses and difficulties in adhering to the principle of acts and omissions. I have also shown some of the problems that there are in the attempts to challenge the principle. It seems that this discussion can only take place with examples, which will be interpreted differently by different people. Without claiming to know which intuitions are right, some conclusions can still be drawn.

The distinction between acts and omissions is blurred and not helped by the flexibility of the English language. To claim that we are always less responsible for our omissions seems to be wrong and not only because it is not always clear what is an act and what is an omission. Intentions should be taken into account when the morality of our acts and omissions is evaluated, but the way this should be done is unclear. To show that, for instance, in the case of euthanasia acts and omissions are morally equal (if the intention is the same and the circumstances roughly similar) does not necessarily lead to the conclusion that both forms of euthanasia should be accepted.

In the end there are only a handful of cases where the principle of acts and omissions completely falls apart. This is not necessarily so because the principle is particularly strong. I would rather say that it is because it is quite a reliable rule of thumb. It is more often with acts than omissions that we have strong intentions. In cases of omissions, it is also more often unclear who the responsible party is. To say that we are more responsible for our acts than our omissions makes sense in most cases, but not in all.

The 'killing/letting one's elderly relative die because of expected inheritance' cases are the most straightforward examples of situations where we can be equally blamed for our acts and omissions. This is because in these cases the intention and the desired consequences are clear: I want my

relative dead, and it is only about selecting the means to bring about the death. I might decide that withholding medication is the best option or, alternatively, that giving them 100 times their daily dose would 'do the job' better. It is difficult to see how my moral blame would depend on the means I choose.

Euthanasia is an interesting example in that those who are arguing that there is no difference between acts and omissions think that in certain situations death would be a good thing. Although the traditional formulations of the acts and omissions doctrine do not talk about good consequences, it could be argued that the case of euthanasia could be used against the doctrine. If death is the desired end result (because there are no other ways of alleviating the patient's pain), then it would seem that it does not make any difference whether the chosen means include acts or omissions (all other things being equal). Obviously, if death is not the desired end result, different conclusions would follow.

The reason why the principle of acts and omissions is difficult to challenge is that there are very few cases where we could intentionally bring about similar consequences by acts and omissions, and where both would be real options. There is asymmetry even in the example of Smith and Jones, because the opportunity of death by omission is not open to Smith.

REFERENCES

Callahan D. *Abortion: Law, Choice and Morality.* London: Macmillan, 1970.

Feinberg J. The moral and legal responsibility of the bad Samaritan. In: Feinberg J, ed. *Freedom and Fulfillment: Philosophical Essays.* Princeton, NJ: Princeton University Press, 1992; pp. 175–196.

Gibson S. Acts and omissions. In: Chadwick R, ed. *Encyclopedia of Applied Ethics,* vol. 1. San Diego: Academic Press, 1998; pp. 23–28.

Gillon R. *Philosophical Medical Ethics.* Chichester: John Wiley & Sons, Ltd, 1985.

Glover J. *Causing Death and Saving Lives.* Harmondsworth: Penguin Books, 1977.

Hall JC. Acts and omissions. *Philos Q* 1989; **39**: 399–408.

Rachels A. Active and passive euthanasia. *N Engl J Med* 1975; **292**: 78–80.

Stauch M. Causal authorship and the equality principle: a defence of the acts/omissions distinction in euthanasia. *J Med Ethics* 2000; **26**: 237–241.

37

Personhood and Moral Status

AINSLEY J. NEWSON

INTRODUCTION: PERSONS AND HUMANS

Imagine you are on a train. With you are other adult humans, a young infant and a suitcase. If you were feeling mischievous, you might take the suitcase and leave it on the platform at the next station, separating it from its owner. In doing this you have acted inconsiderately, but you have not *wronged the suitcase* by leaving it on the platform. However, if you were to forcibly eject another adult human from the train you will wrong them in some way, as the interests of an adult human are distinct from those of a mere thing. Wronging a young infant may be more problematic, as he or she may not have the same kind of interests as an adult human. The properties, rights and interests of entities like adult humans, infants and suitcases are often tackled using theories of personhood.

Throughout the history of health care ethics, concepts of personhood have shaped debates at the start and end of life and many places in between. It influences the rights we bestow on different beings, the duties they owe us and the obligations we have towards them. To count as a moral agent, with moral status, one has to prove one is a person. Yet this seemingly straightforward and ubiquitous concept is surprising in its lack of theoretical consensus.

What is apparent, however, is that being a *person* is different from being *human*. Although these terms are functionally equivalent in popular use, philosophers have drawn a sharp distinction between them (Tooley, 1972, 1983). A human being is a member of the *homo sapiens* species; distinguished by its genetic and biological characteristics. A person, on the contrary, has a set of metaphysical and psychological properties which go beyond mere 'humanness' and confer moral status. Not all humans will be persons, and not all persons will be human (Singer, 1993). As Dennett states:

> I am a person, and so are you ... I am a human being, and *probably* you are too (Dennett, 1988, p. 145).

Those who establish criteria for personhood have tended to do this by defining cognitive properties which can be ascribed to all and only persons. Such characteristics are those we typically associate with a normal adult human being, although as Harris (1999) has pointed out, there is no reason why aliens, or computers, or even non-living creatures like Mickey Mouse cannot be persons too. Cognitive features make beings persons, not which species they belong to.

The application of personhood within health care ethics is readily apparent. Answers to the question: 'what makes a person?' have been applied to a variety of dilemmas in health care, including abortion, infanticide (and the status of anencephalic infants), reproductive technology, stem cell research, organ donation, dementia, defining death, the use of advance directives, care of those in comas, euthanasia and animal experimentation (Tooley, 1983; Harris, 1985; Steinbock, 1992; Singer, 1993; Warren, 1997; Kuhse, 1999; Lizza, 1999; Borlotti and Harris, 2005). For example, does an anencephalic infant have a right to life? Should we respect the desires of a patient with dementia? Is it ever acceptable to undertake experiments on apes or chimpanzees? A significant problem in health care ethics is whether a being who has never had, or who no longer retains, personhood is deserving of the same respect as persons.

WHY A THEORY OF PERSONHOOD?

Before describing some theories of personhood, we need to ask why we are raising this question in the first place. According to Becker:

Principles of Health Care Ethics, Second Edition Edited by R.E. Ashcroft, A. Dawson, H. Draper and J.R. McMillan
© 2007 John Wiley & Sons, Ltd

The importance of these definitional questions for moral philosophy is obvious. Human beings protect themselves with a thicket of rights they do not grant to other beings . . . (Becker, 1975, p. 334).

The importance of personhood also emerges when we examine its relationship with moral status, which confers a right to life. Warren has defined moral status:

> To have moral status is to be morally considerable, or to have moral standing. It is to be an entity towards which moral agents have, or can have, moral obligations. If an entity has moral status, then we may not treat it in just any way we please; we are morally obliged to give weight in our deliberations to its needs, interests, or well-being (Warren, 1997, p. 3).

Personhood is one aspect of moral status; a necessary but not sufficient criterion (Walters, 2004). Therefore, many who have written on personhood have situated their analysis as one means to understand the value of life and the morality of killing humans and other beings (Tooley, 1972, 1983). Harris, for example, has stated:

> When we ask what makes human life valuable we are trying to identify those features, whatever they are, which both incline us and entitle us to value ourselves and one another, and which license our belief that we are more valuable . . .than animals, fish or plants. We are looking for the basis of the belief that it is morally right to choose to save the life of a person rather than that of a dog where both cannot be saved, and our belief that this is not merely a form of prejudice in favour of our own species but is capable of justification (Harris, 1985, p. 9).

The concept of the person is therefore intimately connected with the value of life. When we denote a being as a 'person', we are claiming that being has a special value or moral importance – it has a 'serious right to life' (Tooley, 1973) and is deserving of respect. Personhood is the link between a full right to life or no rights at all.

To summarize, a theory of personhood is useful as part of our suite of problem-solving tools in health care ethics, as it can help us distinguish morally between persons and other beings, determine when and why certain lives become valuable and ascertain when some human lives may cease to be valuable (Harris, 1985). We can use it to find out whether anencephalic infants, demented patients or chimpanzees have moral status and a right to life. Do we value the lives concerned, and why? It also has relevance for determinations of equality and priority in distributing health care resources and public health priorities (Harris, 1999).

Not all agree on the utility of personhood, however (Beauchamp, 1999; Gordijn, 1999). As will be discussed further below, consensus on the concept of a person might be removed from the practicalities of debates in health care ethics. In response, Harris argues that the concept is still helpful, however uncomfortable it may make us feel (Harris, 1999).

THEORIES OF PERSONHOOD

Most philosophers agree that clusters of properties will contribute to a creature being a person. Agreeing on the nature, scope and application of those properties has, however, proved difficult.

EARLY THEORIES OF PERSONHOOD

Personhood has been discussed throughout the history of philosophy. Aristotle believed that persons are rational animals, capable of socialization and guided by reason. A being with these kinds of qualities should not be used to serve the ends of another.

Unsurprisingly, Kant also discussed what might be required to be a person (Kant, 1785). As one of the first to distinguish persons from mere things, he claimed that any beings who were persons should be treated as ends in themselves, and they had absolute as opposed to instrumental value. Consistent with his deontological stance, Kant identified *rationality* as the basic defining feature of persons; the basis for their unique and privileged moral status. Any rational agent would be self-determining and could command respect as a moral agent; the only kind of agent who could have moral status.

John Locke's works have influenced several modern theorists writing on personhood and the value of life. He offered a species-neutral description of personhood, contending that a person is a rational and self-conscious agent aware of her or his past and future:

> We must consider what person stands for; which I think is a thinking intelligent being, that has reason and reflection, and can consider itself the same thinking thing, in different times and places; which it does only by that consciousness which is inseparable from thinking . . . (Locke, 1690, Book II, Ch 27, p. 333).

RELIGIOUS PERSPECTIVES

Religious perspectives have also had a significant influence on theories of personhood. A common position has been to adopt a vitalist view of moral status and personhood, which emphasizes the wrongness of intentionally taking human life. This position incorporates all humans, regardless of their age or development, and the criteria for personhood are satisfied simply by virtue of being human. Moral status is present from fertilization, and all beings (from an early embryo to a comatose adult) who presently have *or will have* the conditions satisfying personhood are moral persons, deserving of respect.

Joyce is one who adopts this position (Joyce, 1978). A person is a being with the natural capability (whether developed or not) for reasoning, willing, desiring and so on. In arguing for full personhood in the zygote, he claims that the potential to engage in an action in the future (such as demonstrating self-consciousness) must be recognized as an *actual* potential and should be treated now as if it were a functional capability.

Debates over this position critique the validity of *potentiality* – the capability to satisfy conditions for personhood in future. Many theorists such as Becker (1975), Harris (1985) and Tooley (1983) have rejected this concept. Becker, for example, highlights the being/becoming boundary: a caterpillar is clearly not a butterfly, and a foetus is not a human *being*, only a human *becoming* (Becker, 1975).

Harris argues that the claim to actual potential is unfounded as not every fertilized egg will give rise to a new individual; many pregnancies are spontaneously lost (Harris, 1999). There is also a logical difficulty, as a *reductio* will result if potentiality is broadly applied: zygotes have the potential to become embryos, and sperm and ova have the potential to become a zygote – must these entities also command respect as potential persons?

APPROACHES TO PERSONHOOD IN MODERN ETHICS

The majority of approaches to personhood theory have attempted to define an attribute or set of attributes which are collectively constitutive of personhood. Any being who displays or is capable of displaying these attributes can be deemed a person. However, these criteria remain contested and are also dogged by further issues, such as whether these attributes are necessary or sufficient, how to handle 'uncomfortable' consequences, such as sanctioning infanticide, and whether personhood is a matter of threshold or degree. A potentially more serious problem, faced with this longstanding impasse, is whether answering definitions of personhood is required at all. This will be discussed further below. First, however, several theorists' views of personhood will be presented.

Theologian and bioethicist Joseph Fletcher proposed one of the first modern lists for what would now be termed personhood, but which was then termed 'humanhood'. Drawing on the fact that human beings characteristically possess specific capacities, he suggested that self-awareness, self-control, a sense of the future, a sense of the past, the capability to relate to others, concern for others, communication and curiosity were required for a person to show 'real human qualities' and be morally significant (Fletcher, 1972).

Daniel Dennett proposes a list of interdependent conditions for personhood, all of which are necessary: rationality, consciousness, the capability to take and reciprocate a personhood stance towards the being in question, self-consciousness and the ability to engage in verbal communication. His requirements for adopting and reciprocating attitudes towards others and verbal communication are unique in personhood theory. He recognizes the inherent interdependency of these conditions and, given their normative nature, queries whether they can be sufficient as well as necessary for personhood (Dennett, 1988). Although the capability for verbal communication can be demanding, losing this attribute does not mean one will lose a right to life, so long as one can still act as a moral agent.

Michael Tooley's approach to questions of personhood is to ask what properties a thing must have in order to have a right to life (Tooley, 1972, 1983, 1988). In order to be a person with a right to life, an organism must meet the *self-consciousness requirement* and be capable of having an interest in its own existence:

> An organism possesses a serious right to life only if it possesses the concept of a self as a continuing subject of experiences and other mental states, and believes that it is itself a continuing entity (Tooley, 1972, p. 44).

Consistent with other theorists, Tooley also stipulates a broad set of cognitive capacities which can constitute personhood. He states:

> [A]nything that has, and has exercised, all of the following capacities is a person, and . . . anything that has never had any of them is not a person: the capability for self-consciousness; the capability to think; the capability for rational thought; the capability to arrive at decisions by deliberation; the capability to envisage a future for oneself; the capability to remember a past including oneself; the capability for being a subject of nonmonetary interests; the capability to use language (Tooley, 1983, p. 349).

These requirements do not affect sleeping or unconscious people because desires do not always have to be present in our conscious mind. People who are asleep or unconscious have already experienced a sense of self existing over time. If a person becomes permanently unconscious, however, then they will cease to be a person, a contention also advanced by Singer (1993).

Tooley is frank in admitting that his theory is not satisfied by the concept of human zygotes, foetuses and infants, as the potential future holding of the above properties does not preclude destroying an entity (Tooley, 1988).

These beings therefore lack a right to life – they cannot possess actual desires, nor do they have the capability for them.

Like Tooley, John Harris situates the question of personhood within the debate over what makes life valuable (Harris, 1985). All lives are valuable unless a creature loses some feature which entitles it to such valuing. He adopts an impartial and relatively straightforward approach to personhood, contending that any being with 'what it takes' to be valuable has a right to life, whether they are a human being, an alien or a sophisticated computer.

In developing his theory, Harris reflects on Locke's criteria for personhood. However, he observes that such properties all admit of degrees, which could lead to a hierarchy of persons. Although some theorists do believe such a hierarchy is feasible, Harris advances a simpler criterion for determining which lives are valuable. He contends a being's life will have value so long as it is *capable of valuing its own existence*: 'Persons are beings capable of valuing their own lives' (Harris, 1985, p. 16). The reasons why a being values its own life are irrelevant; all that matters is the capability for valuing. Personhood is therefore a threshold concept and cannot admit of degrees.

Locke's characteristics are not irrelevant though, as in order to value one's own life a being will require certain characteristics. A list similar to Locke's might be used, with self-consciousness perhaps being the most important trait:

> To value its own life [and be a person], a being would have to be aware of itself as an independent creature of consciousness, existing over time with a future that it was capable of envisaging and wishing to experience (Harris, 1985, p. 18).

Contrary to some other theorists, however, Harris suggests this capability would have a low threshold, not requiring any sophisticated form of rationality. Any non-persons or potential persons cannot be wronged by death as death will not rob them of anything they can value. But if a being does value its own life, killing it will be wrong (Harris, 1985).

One difficulty with this approach is determining which beings are or are not persons. Harris suggests the most straightforward way of determining this is to ask someone. However, this necessitates some ability to use language or communicate, which some humans and most animals will have difficulty with. Therefore, we must err on the side of caution (Harris, 1985). This may lead to an all-encompassing approach, in which beings that are not actually persons are treated as if they are.

Peter Singer also adopts a non-species-specific view of personhood (Singer, 1993). Although he argues that non-persons who cannot use tools or language do not deserve to suffer, he admits there does seem to be a difference between adult human beings and many animals. Most animals cannot think or reason, nor do they have a conception of themselves as a distinct entity with a past and a future. He proposes to use the term 'person' to denote a rational and self-conscious being, capturing those elements of a human being that go beyond mere membership of the species *homo sapiens* (Singer, 1993).

Many non-human animals can, according to Singer, be persons. He presents evidence to suggest that some animals exhibit elements of self-consciousness and an understanding of past and future events. For example, a chimpanzee named Washoe was taught sign language, and Singer argues that animals like her are entitled to the same valuing and protection as human persons. Further, he argues that killing a chimpanzee is often worse than killing a human being who is not and can never be a person (Singer, 1993; Beauchamp, 1999).

Singer also argues that only persons can have a right to life (Singer, 1993). Compared to a merely sentient creature, a self-conscious and rational being has self-awareness over time, so will have desires about its future. Taking the life of this kind of being will frustrate its future desires. This is different from killing an infant or a snail, as they will not have similar desires (Singer, 1993).

Harry Frankfurt proposed another unique condition for personhood: the ability to generate *second-order volitions* (Frankfurt, 1971). If a first-order desire is something like 'I desire to do X'. a volition of the second order becomes 'I desire to desire X'. To Frankfurt, true freedom of the will (and personhood) exists only when second-order volitions can be effected by moving an agent to action. If this does not take place, then personhood has not been attained.

The ability to hold and act on second-order volitions is, however, not a species-specific criterion. In effect it is limited to more complex creatures. And, as Beauchamp observes, it would also create a greater class of human non-persons (Beauchamp, 1999). Additionally, as most of us do not use second-order volitions all the time, Frankfurt's approach may render many of our actions undeserving of respect.

DOES PERSONHOOD THEORY UNAVOIDABLY LEAD TO 'UNCOMFORTABLE' CONCLUSIONS?

Most theories of personhood have in common a requirement for some form of self-consciousness, whether as a primary threshold (as with Singer) or an underlying requirement (as with Harris). Yet such approaches seem to prove too much. If applied to their logical conclusion, practices many are uncomfortable with may be sanctioned, for example late-term abortion, infanticide and non-voluntary euthanasia.

To circumvent this problem, other theorists have supplemented personhood theory. Engelhardt, for example, accepts the importance of capacities such as self-consciousness and agrees infants have no *fundamental* basic right to life. However, recognizing their social and cultural role, he imputes these beings with a right to life via constructing the utilitarian concept of imputed or *social personhood* (Engelhardt, 1986, 1988).

Engelhardt proposes two alternative but overlapping conceptions of personhood. First, there is *strict personhood*, which is bestowed on those entities who are self-conscious and rational. This incorporates moral agents who bear rights and duties and who make claims deserving of respect. Second, there is *social personhood*, which involves treating beings as if they were persons, even when they do not meet the strict criteria. To satisfy social personhood, a being must have the ability to engage in a minimum of social interaction (thus excluding anencephalic infants and brain-dead adults).

The rationale for social personhood is that some beings, although not persons, have a significant role in family structures and in society more generally. A mother responding to her infant's cries is acting as if her infant held conscious desires for care and nurturing – as if it were a strict person. It allows us to treat these beings with care and respect, imputing a right to life. Embryo research is, however, permissible as embryos represent a form of human biological life, not personal life. Likewise, abortion would be acceptable (as this can have significant utility for women), but infanticide would not be sanctioned.

Another alternative, pluralistic approach to personhood and moral status has been offered by Warren (1997), who describes a multi-criterial theory of moral status. Drawing on common-sense morality, she incorporates intrinsic properties such as life, sentience and personhood, and combines these with social, emotional and biosystemic relationships. Moral status cannot be based on one property, although key cognitive faculties are still necessary, with the capability to have conscious experiences among the most fundamental. She suggests seven common-sense principles of moral status, including respect for life, equality of rights and respecting attributions of moral status. Like Engelhardt, she argues it is acceptable to accord full moral rights to sentient human beings, even when they lack the capability to be full moral agents. Additionally, more than one type of moral status is possible, applying to different kinds of entity, with varying strengths. Moral agents, sentient beings, nonsentient living things and ecosystems all demand some kind of moral consideration, albeit of differing strengths. Only full moral agents will have a full complement of rights, yet moral status is not merely a matter of inherent capabilities. Social standing and relationships are also important.

A concern with incorporating social and relational values to complement personhood is the potential relegation of theoretical personhood into irrelevance. Will we circumvent the rigour of personhood using social criteria way every time a difficult issue arises?

IS PERSONHOOD A MATTER OF THRESHOLD OR DEGREE?

Perhaps some of the uncertainty over theories of personhood and their application to problems like the moral status of infants and embryos arises because the major theorists have tended to see personhood as an 'all-or-nothing' concept, with personhood being a threshold to overcome to obtain moral status. However, not all see personhood in this way – some view it instead as a matter of degree and argue that it can serve as a useful tool in the difficult sphere of health care decision-making (Perring, 1997).

Applying personhood as a matter of degree has a similar effect to Engelhardt's social personhood, but the approach is incorporated into the analytical framework of personhood *per se*. If personhood develops as a matter of degree, it may be possible to accord moral status to some beings that are not yet persons, but who are already showing some signs of personhood. The moral status of such beings will then steadily increase the closer they approach full personhood. Although an embryo is not a person in the same way an acorn is not an oak tree (Thomson, 1971), some acorns must be protected, otherwise no oak trees will grow in future.

Carter is one who has argued for degrees of personhood (Carter, 1980). Although he supports the 'cognitive capability' approach to personhood, he recognizes such capacities as unlikely to develop at once. This gradient of time and attainment makes it difficult to draw a line between persons and non-persons and suggests there can also be *marginal persons*. Every theory of personhood will give rise to tough borderline cases, where a being exists in a 'penumbra region' in which an objective determination is difficult. He states, disapprovingly:

> If the best that can be done in such cases is to draw an arbitrary line between what is, and is not, a person, the lines may be drawn differently in say, New York and Moscow . . . [it] will turn out that whether certain entities have a right to life is something that depends on whether they happen to be located in New York or Moscow.(Carter, 1980, p. 65).

If he is right, it would be possible to say a creature is 'to some extent' a person; a being who may have a right to life but whose rights will not be as strong as those of full persons.

A similar approach is offered by Walters (1997), who advocates a pragmatic and non-principled definition of personhood termed *proximate personhood*. Under this theory, the closer a human or other being is to attaining self-consciousness, the greater that being's claim to moral status will be. To satisfy proximate personhood, a being will need to possess: (1) the potential to develop personal capacities such as self-awareness and an anticipation of the kind of life they will want to lead; (2) some physical development towards becoming a person; and (3) evidence of social bonding with significant others and society (Walters, 1997).

On these views, the logical steps towards infanticide or non-valuing of some human lives are again avoided, although vulnerable beings will not always be designated with moral status. The weakness of some of these theories, however, is a reliance on social consensus and sentiment: some may question whether this less principled approach is a legitimate way to shape argument in health care ethics. However, there does seem to be some degree of room for concepts like social, proximate or degrees of personhood, particularly when health care professionals face difficult decisions in clinical practice.

In summary, no consensus on the properties required for personhood has emerged. However, several authors have drawn conclusions about where consensus may lie. Beauchamp, for example, suggests that the properties may be:

1. Self-consciousness;
2. The capability to act on reasons;
3. The capability to communicate with others by command of a language;
4. The capability to act freely; and
5. Rationality (Beauchamp, 1999, p. 311).

CRITIQUES OF PERSONHOOD

Personhood theory is not without its critics, with several detractors arguing that the concept lacks the requisite rigour for application in health care. Two such critics are Tom Beauchamp (1999) and Bert Gordijn (1999).

Beauchamp's central criticism is that a significant distinction has been ignored: that between metaphysical and moral personhood (Beauchamp, 1999; Dennett, 1988). The term m*etaphysical personhood* can be used to describe the person-defining cognitive properties discussed above. Yet this concept is insufficient for addressing *moral personhood*, which applies to individuals who possess properties like moral agency and moral motivation.

The tendency to draw moral conclusions (such as a right to life) from metaphysical accounts of personhood is thus also unfounded, as cognitive properties do not confer moral

standing. He argues that the current lists of cognitive properties fail to 'capture the depth of commitments embedded in using the language of 'person'' (Beauchamp, 1999, p. 312). Conclusions about moral standing therefore cannot depend on just one concept of personhood.

To solve this problem, we need to explicitly adopt the concept of moral personhood. A creature will be a moral person if: (1) it can make moral judgements about the rightness or wrongness of actions; and (2) it has motives that can be judged morally. Some features of metaphysical personhood will be required to satisfy these criteria, although moral personhood and not metaphysical personhood is sufficient for moral standing. Any being who can meet these two criteria will be a moral agent deserving of respect. On this view, psychopaths may be excluded as moral persons, whereas dolphins or apes may be included. Selected nonmoral attributes can also confer moral standing, such as the ability to experience pain and suffering and the potential for emotional deprivation. Beings can possess these rights even when they cannot be exercised, as representative can exercise them on a being's behalf.

Gordijn shares Beachamp's concern that current theories of personhood are used as an oblique detour for solving substantive moral issues in health care ethics (Gordijn, 1999). Conceptions of personhood are superfluous to our needs for deciding what we should do for newborns, the comatose and animals. The concept has taken on a purely pragmatic role and is used tactically in making arguments rather than addressing substantive normative issues. The result is widespread and shows artificial dichotomies between persons and non-persons and moral status and non-moral status, which fails to reflect the reality of clinical decision-making. As a consensus on criteria for personhood is unlikely to arise soon, Gordijn argues that we can set the concept aside. This will improve the clarity and quality of analysis in health care ethics and will ensure, we think, systematically those properties and capabilities necessary for particular kinds of moral status.

CONCLUSION

Theories of personhood and moral status have influenced a variety of debates in health care ethics, including abortion and euthanasia – two illustrations of the boundaries of these concepts. Yet despite some degree of consensus, theories of personhood are subject to significant variation and contention, with some arguing they should not be used at all.

Faced with these problems, it is reasonable to ask whether it is even worth considering what makes a person. In answering, it is interesting to return to the thought experiment at the start of this chapter. It does seem that being a person has special value and moral importance; an importance which justifies our valuing an adult human's interests over those of a suitcase, or (potentially) an infant. If this is a valid assertion, then concepts of personhood are perhaps the best tools for arguing around the issues arising.

It is, however, necessary to ensure that theories of personhood and moral status are compatible with the realities of decision-making in both applied ethics and health care practice. It may, therefore, be necessary to incorporate some elements of social and moral personhood into existing theoretical frameworks, subject to reasonable limitations. It will also be interesting to undertake further empirical research into cultural differences in perception of personhood (Morgan, 2006). Although this may reduce some of the vigour of personhood theory and may subject it to social fluctuations, its utility and applicability to difficult decisions in health care will be increased. For those wishing to delve into this debate, there is rich thinking to be done.

REFERENCES

Beauchamp TL. The failure of theories of personhood. *Kennedy Inst Ethics J* 1999; **9**: 309–324.

Becker LC. Human being: the boundaries of the concept. *Philos Public Affairs* 1975; **4**: 334–359.

Borlotti L, Harris J. Stem cell research, personhood and sentience. *Reprod Biomed Online* 2005; **10**(Suppl. 1): 68–75.

Carter WR. Once and future persons. *Am Philos Q* 1980; **17**: 61–66.

Dennett D. Conditions of personhood. In: Goodman MF, ed. *What Is A Person?* Clifton, NJ: Humana Press, 1988; pp. 145–67.

Engelhardt HT Jr. Medicine and the concept of person. In: Goodman MF, ed. *What Is A Person?* Clifton, NJ: Humana Press, 1988; pp. 169–184.

Engelhardt HT Jr. *The Foundations of Bioethics*. New York: Oxford University Press, 1986; pp. 115–119.

Fletcher J. Indicators of humanhood: a tentative profile of man. *Hastings Center Rep* 1972; **2**(5): 1–4.

Frankfurt HG. Freedom of the will and the concept of a person. *J Philos* 1971; **68**: 5–20.

Gordijn B. The troublesome concept of the person. *Theor Med Bioethics* 1999; **20**: 347–359.

Harris J. The concept of the person and the value of life. *Kennedy Inst Ethics J* 1999; **9**: 293–308.

Harris J. *The Value of Life*. London: Routledge, 1985.

Joyce RE. Personhood and the conception event. *New Scholast* 1978; **52**: 97–109.

Kant I. *Groundwork of the Metaphysics of Morals*. Cambridge: Cambridge University Press, 1785 (1997).

Kuhse H. Some reflections on the problem of advance directives, personhood and personal identity. *Kennedy Inst Ethics J* 1999; **9**: 347–364.

Lizza JP. Defining death for persons and human organisms. *Theor Med Bioethics* 1999; **20**: 439–453.

Locke J. *An Essay Concerning Human Understanding*. London: T Longman, 1690 (Book II, Chapter 27. Also available on the World Wide Web: http://books.google.com).

Morgan LM. Life begins when they steal your bicycle: cross-cultural practices of personhood at the beginnings and ends of life. *J Law Med Ethics* 2006; **34**: 8–15.

Perring C. Degrees of personhood. *J Med Philos* 1997; **22**: 173–197.

Singer P. *Practical Ethics*, 2nd edition. Cambridge: Cambridge University Press, 1993.

Steinbock B *Life Before Birth: The Moral Status of Embryos and Fetuses*, New York: Oxford University Press, 1992.

Thomson JJ. A defense of abortion. *Philos Public Affairs* 1971; **1**: 47–56.

Tooley M. *Abortion and Infanticide*. Oxford: Clarendon Press, 1983.

Tooley M. Abortion and infanticide. *Philos Public Affairs* 1972; **2**: 37–56.

Tooley M. In defense of abortion and infanticide. In: Goodman MF, ed. *What Is a Person?* Clifton, NJ: Humana Press, 1988; pp. 83–114.

Walters JW. *What is a Person? An Ethical Exploration*. Urbana, IL: University of Illinois Press, 1997.

Walters JW (2004). Moral Status. In Post SG, ed. *Encyclopedia of Bioethics, Third Edition* New York: Macmillan Reference, 2004; pp. 1855–1864.

Warren MA. *Moral Status: Obligations to Persons and Other Living Things*. Oxford: Oxford University Press, 1997.

38

Commodification

STEPHEN WILKINSON

The idea of commodification plays a prominent role in several areas of bioethics. The most obvious is the debate about trading in human bodily parts and products such as kidneys and blood (Erin and Harris, 2003; Wilkinson, 2003; Taylor 2004). The other is reproductive ethics. A recent report by the Human Genetics Commission, for example, notes that some people:

> '... are worried that the introduction of techniques enabling deliberate selection between embryos may lead to children being treated as commodities' (HGC, 2006, para. 4.5).

This chapter is divided into four main sections. The first introduces the concept of commodification. The second and third look at instrumentalization and fungibility (respectively) because these are, I argue, the main constituents of the moral concept of commodification. Finally, I look at the claim that monetary incentives, in some contexts, cause instrumentalization and commodification and hence should be avoided or prohibited. Throughout, my focus will be on the concept's role within bioethics. The term 'commodification' plays other roles in other contexts, notably within the Marxist tradition, and I shall not say anything about these.

INTRODUCING COMMODIFICATION

Our starting point is the idea of *commodity*. Kaveny, while introducing a special issue of the *Journal of Medicine and Philosophy* on commodification, identifies three essential characteristics:

> 'First, every commodity has its price, which a seller will receive for surrendering it and a buyer will part with in order to acquire it . . .'.

> '. . . commodities are typically fungible, which means they are interchangeable with other goods of like type and quality. To use the language of contract law, one 'widget' is as good as any other'.

> 'A third basic feature of commodities is that their value is instrumental, not intrinsic' (Kaveny, 1999, p. 209).

So to treat a thing as a commodity is to treat it as if: (1) it has a price; *and* (2) it is fungible; *and* (3) it has only instrumental value.

The next step is to distinguish descriptive from normative senses of 'commodification'. In the first of these, 'commodification' refers to a social practice and/or legal system under which rights over the thing in question are bought and sold (Alexandra and Walsh, 1997; Resnik, 1998; Wilkinson, 2000). To talk of commodification in this sense is not to make a moral judgement, but merely to point out that, as a matter of fact, certain things are being treated as commodities (Hanson, 1999). In the second (normative) sense to call something 'commodification' is to express moral disapproval and to refer to a distinctive kind of wrong: the wrong of commodification. Consider, as an illustration, the following criticism of organ sale from Brecher:

> 'the possibility of people's buying a kidney represents the further commoditisation [commodification] of human beings, [and] to that extent the practice resembles prostitution, certain forms of surrogacy, and . . . page three of *The Sun* in symbolising, partly constituting, and encouraging a moral climate within which the commoditisation [commodification] of human beings proceeds apace' (Brecher, 1990, p. 122).

Brecher's point here is not merely that permitting organ sale would constitute an extension of *the social practice of* commodification. That claim taken alone would be too obvious

Principles of Health Care Ethics, Second Edition   Edited by R.E. Ashcroft, A. Dawson, H. Draper and J.R. McMillan

to be worth a mention and certainly would not constitute an argument for prohibition, but would be more like a description of what should be prohibited. Instead, his point seems to be that we ought not to permit these practices because doing so would be or cause a specific wrong: the commodification of human beings (Wilkinson, 2000).

It is this normative sense of 'commodification' which is most relevant to bioethics and which is the exclusive concern of the rest of this chapter. The key to understanding it is a distinction between proper and wrongful commodities. Proper commodities are those things that *really are* fungible and only instrumentally valuable; thus there is nothing wrong with treating them as fungible or as merely instrumental, because that is what they are. Wrongful commodities, on the other hand, are things that are treated as if they are commodities despite their not being (really) fungible or merely instrumentally valuable. Thus, the distinctive wrong of commodification is treating something non-fungible and intrinsically valuable as if it were fungible and merely instrumentally valuable.

The idea of commodification is applicable not just to persons but to anything which is (purportedly) non-fungible and intrinsically valuable. Thus, commodification concerns may (for example) be raised about (non-human) animals, artworks, or the natural environment. For reasons of space and focus, however, my exclusive concern here is the commodification of people and people's bodies.

INSTRUMENTALIZATION

The commodification of persons involves two putative wrongs: treating people as merely instrumental and treating them as fungible. In this section, I shall explore the first of these. The classic anti-instrumentalization statement is Kant's:

'Act so that you treat humanity, whether in your own person or in that of another, always as an end and never as a means only' (Kant, 1959, p. 47).

A feature of Kant's principle that is sometimes overlooked is that it does not prohibit, or even claim that there is anything wrong with, treating people as means *per se*. Rather, it asserts that we have a positive obligation always to regard and treat them as ends. So treating people as means is permissible as long as we also treat them as ends. That this is the meaning of the Kantian principle should be unsurprising, because if it ruled out treating people as means altogether, it would have absurdly restrictive implications. For, as Harris notes, in 'medical contexts, anyone who receives a blood transfusion has used the blood donor as a means to their own ends' (Harris, 1985, p. 143).

So which ways of using people are compatible with respecting them 'as ends' and which are not? Some people would want to say, for example, that there is a moral difference between the ways in which doctors, nurses and teachers are used as means by their clients, patients and pupils and the ways in which children working in 'sweatshop' factories, people who sell their kidneys, and sex workers are used. But what is this difference? Why are some uses (apparently) worse than others?

One difference, in these examples, is that the latter three are more likely to be harmful. However, for our present purposes, we need to set aside thoughts about harm. There are two reasons for this. First, these examples are not *necessarily* harmful, even if in the real world they usually are; thus, it is not difficult to construct hypothetical cases in which sex workers or kidney sellers are not harmed, at least once financial benefit is taken into account. Crucially, many would want to claim that wrongful commodification can persist even in the absence of harm: that even if kidney sellers and sex workers do well out the transaction in practical terms, there is a residual moral concern about commodification. Second, even if there is a strong link between wrongful commodification and harm, they are nonetheless distinct moral objections and, because the concern of this chapter is commodification, it is best (for reasons of analytical precision) to sideline questions of harm.

One reason for not using people in certain ways is its effects on our attitudes, either to that person, or more generally. In particular, it may be that certain kinds of using make us inclined wrongfully to disregard other people's status as ends. Consider, for example, Anderson's remark:

'The commodification of sexual 'services' destroys the kind of reciprocity required to realise human sexuality as a shared good. Each party values the other only instrumentally, not intrinsically' (Anderson, 1993, p. 154).

The idea is that, during a commercialized sexual encounter, each party neglects the other's personhood and intrinsic value. For the first party, this is because she/he is interested primarily in using the other as a means of gaining sexual pleasure. For the second, it is because she/he is interested primarily in using the other as a means of obtaining money. Both parties, though, are subject to broadly the same psychological phenomenon: the 'personhood perspective' on the other is *displaced* by a 'use perspective'. This is what I have elsewhere termed *the displacement thesis*, which says that some kinds of use generally displace our intrinsic valuing of persons and our seeing persons as ends (Wilkinson, 2003).

The displacement thesis is empirical and psychological and it is not (or at least it ought not to be) claimed that there is a logical or necessary relationship between particular use-types and failing to regard the persons as ends in". themselves. Thus, we can (for example) imagine possible cases of commercialized sex in which both parties are fully regarded and respected as ends throughout; although conversely we can imagine examples in which someone's utility as a lecturer causes students to treat her as a mere means. So I doubt that there is a list of activity-types which *always* cause instrumentalization (sex work, organ selling, etc.) and another of those that *never* do (accountancy, lecturing, etc.). For much will depend, in each case, on the context within which the use takes place.

One intriguing and difficult question is: why are some use-types generally better than others at coexisting with respect for personhood? I would speculate (and this is only speculation) that those use-types that demand active engagement with the used person *as-a-person* (through communication and interaction with her mental characteristics and personality) are generally less dangerous in terms of instrumentalization. While, at the other end of the scale, use-types which do not involve personal contact and/or which are mainly kinds of using of the other's body are the ones where the risk of instrumentalization is highest. This is one reason why the selling of body parts and commercialized sex are potentially morally problematic (Garrard and Wilkinson, 1996).

An illuminating and well-known example is the case of Manuel Wackenheim. Wackenheim is a (so-called) 'dwarf' who (until a ban was imposed by the local mayor) made a living from being tossed by customers in bars and nightclubs. This tossing formed part of a dwarf-throwing competition – a sport 'in which the aim of the competitors is to fling a dwarf over the furthest distance possible' (Millns, 1996, p. 375; Beyleveld & Brownsword, 2001). Wackenheim appeared keen to pursue his chosen career and did not welcome the ban on dwarf-throwing, saying: 'this spectacle is my life; I want to be allowed to do what I want'.

Wackenheim can be regarded both as intrinsically valuable (as-a-person) and as instrumentally valuable (as-a-projectile). There is no reason in principle why a friend of his could not both respect him as an 'end' and recognize the fact that his body is formed in a way which makes it instrumentally valuable to throwers. But could Wackenheim's friend *actually use him* as a projectile, at the same time respecting his personhood?

As I and others have argued elsewhere (Nussbaum, 1995; Wilkinson, 2003) the key to answering this is the overall context of the relationship, along with other structural features of the situation. It would be extraordinarily hard to argue plausibly that it is *impossible*, in *all* contexts, to use Wackenheim as a projectile at the same time respecting his personhood. For what if he enjoys being thrown, gets paid for it and freely and knowingly consents to it? If for these reasons – if because I want him to get pleasure and money and am certain that it is what he really

wants – I throw him, then there seems no basis for saying that I am failing to respect his personhood. For in such a case, I am deliberately giving him what he wants (and, we can stipulate, wants in a free, informed and otherwise autonomous way) and deliberately benefiting him. How can this be a failure to recognize his status as an end?

It is not, although I should straight away add two qualifications. First, this does not rule out the existence of other separate moral objections to dwarf-throwing. Second, there certainly are contexts in which the practice would constitute wrongful instrumentalization. These include cases in which the people thrown are substantially harmed and cases in which they do not consent or in which their consent is invalid. Indeed, this is the crucial point. What does all the ethical work here is context: in particular issues relating to the existence and quality of the person's consent, and perhaps also those relating to harm and welfare.

Lying behind this way of thinking is one of the following principles (which differ just in that the second, more cautious, principle includes a 'substantial harm' constraint) (Wilkinson, 2003).

> 'If A seeks and obtains valid consent from B to do x to B, then that is sufficient to guarantee that B's status as an end-in-themselves is respected by A.
>
> If A seeks and obtains valid consent from B to do x to B and x is not substantially harmful to B, then that is sufficient to guarantee that B's status as an end-in-themselves is respected by A'.

These principles are driven by the view: (a) that respect for autonomy is either identical with or is the most important part of Kant's anti-instrumentalization doctrine; and (b) that the relationship between autonomy and consent is of the first importance. On this view, A, by seeking and obtaining valid consent, has respected B's autonomy and status as an 'end' – though it must also be the case that *A would not have gone ahead and done x to B if B had not consented*. In other words, what matters is not so much the *existence* of consent than the fact that A *requires* it. It is by *requiring* valid consent that A respects B's autonomy (Wilkinson, 2003).

The word 'valid' is doing a lot of work here. Consent *per se* is relatively insignificant, because an invalid consent, in ethical terms, is often no better than no consent. It is *valid* consent that matters morally. Indeed, what 'valid' *means* here is that the consent in question is morally significant, that it goes at least some way. Towards justifying A's actions. Also, the view that A treats B as an 'end' so long as A requires B's consent does not entail the view that there is nothing to which B could not validly consent: that is, it is entirely compatible with the view that in practice there are certain kinds of use to which no one could validly consent. One may think (for example) that selling parts of one's body or being used as a projectile cannot be validly consented to because only someone whose consent was invalidated by coercion, manipulation, insanity, desperation or whatever would agree to be used in such awful ways.

FUNGIBILITY

The moral wrong of fungibilization is structurally like commodification and instrumentalization in that it comprises treating something that is not (properly or really) fungible as if it were fungible. So, as our main concern is with persons, this raises the question of in what senses (if any) people are non-fungible (non-interchangeable)?

Marshall reminds us that, in many contexts, regarding people as fungible is morally unproblematic.

> 'it is not difficult to see how fungibility can be an aspect of a market relation. One well-trained waiter is just as good as another, one paying customer is just as good as another. There may be nothing wrong with this: to treat people as interchangeable within the market activity need not be in any way damaging. Indeed, it is perfectly possible to imagine that with developments in robotics we could do without waiters altogether without loss' (Marshall, 1999, p. 145).

It seems, then, that I am not obliged to care *which particular* hairdresser or taxi driver or solicitor or ethics tutor provides me with services; although personal engagement with people in these roles may well be desirable, it is not morally required, or at least not beyond a very basic level. So there seems to be a fundamental problem with the moral concept of fungibilization and with the principle that we ought to treat persons as unique, rather than as interchangeable, because (in many respects) people are not unique. At least as role occupants, one customer or hairdresser or waiter is much like another. For these kinds of reasons (and for some more complex theoretical ones for which there is no space to explore here) I have argued elsewhere that the claims about persons being unique, on which the moral concept of fungibilization depends, are deeply problematic. They are either irredeemably vague or trivially true or simply unjustified (Wilkinson, 2003). Thus, when commercial practices are objected to on the grounds that persons are treated as fungible, such claims should be approached with a high degree of scepticism.

I would grant, however, that there are special contexts in which the claim that we ought to treat people as non-fungible makes more sense and should be accorded more weight. In particular, not-treating-as-fungible seems to be an important part of personal friendship. Part of B's

being A's friend is that A cares that the particular person with whom she/he is talking, or going out to dinner, or going on holiday is B, and not merely *someone like* B. In other words, viewing B as replaceable or substitutable is incompatible with true friendship. Perhaps this is because, in the case of friendship, something approaching a meaningful uniqueness claim is plausible, for instance due to friends' shared histories. Or, perhaps the demand for non-fungibility can be explained in terms of other things such as the idea of loyalty, or the fact that (given certain expectations) to treat a friend as fungible (for example, to 'swap' her for another on trivial grounds) would be immensely harmful. Whatever the explanation, it does seem that the idea of treating persons as non-fungible has more applicability in personal relationships than in other contexts. If this is right (and I have only suggested rather than argued for it here), then perhaps the idea of fungibilization will have more relevance to some areas of bioethics than to others. Thus, in the sale of body parts debate, where close personal relationships between vendors and recipients are unlikely, perhaps it has little relevance; whereas, in reproductive ethics, when considering the relationships between parents and children, concerns about fungibility may have more force.

INDUCEMENTS AND CONSENT

In this section, I explore the relationship between monetary incentives, consent, and instrumentalization, using as an illustrative example the Inducement Argument against paying people who supply tissue for research. More detailed discussions of this issue can be found in Wilkinson (2003, 2005).

For commodification to occur, there must be instrumentalization; someone must be used as a mere means. And, for instrumentalization to take place, there must be an absence of valid consent. Monetary incentives, it is sometimes argued, make valid consent difficult or impossible, whilst at the same time encouraging commercial activity. Thus, money plays a dual role in commodification, both making people do (or part with) the thing in question and invalidating their consent. For a consent to be valid, three elements must be present in sufficient quantities: information, competence and voluntariness (Faden and Beauchamp, 1994; Gillon, 1986; Wilkinson, 2003). The Inducement Argument focuses mainly on the last of these: voluntariness. As the Nuffield Council on Bioethics puts it:

> '[a] factor which may affect the voluntary nature of consent to research is any inducements accompanying invitations to participate in research' (Nuffield Council, 2002, p. 76).

Although this is a widely held view, saying why we should believe it is not easy. Here are some of the main possible reasons.[1]

(a) Financial incentives encourage people to do things that they would not otherwise do.
(b) Financial incentives encourage people to do things that are likely to be harmful to them and which go against their 'better judgement'.
(c) Financial incentives can make people's actions and decisions less autonomous, or nonautonomous. (Wilkinson, 2005, p. 28).

(a) and (b) seem to be what the General Medical Council has in mind when it tells doctors:

> 'not [to] offer payments at a level which could induce research participants to take risks that they would otherwise not take, or to volunteer more frequently than is advisable or against their better interests or judgement' (GMC, 2002, s. 14).

(a), however, seems problematic. For the fact that payments encourage people to do things that they otherwise would not do does not, in and of itself, invalidate consent. For, if it did, consent problems would be endemic and would occur every time someone was encouraged by payment to go to work for wages or to surrender property for a price. So although some subjects do only provide tissue because of the money (indeed, if this were not the case then payment would be unnecessary) this fact alone does not invalidate their consent.[2]

(b) is in some ways more plausible. Or at least it is plausible to suppose that we ought not to expose research subjects to more than a certain level of danger and ought not to encourage them, as the GMC puts it, to 'volunteer more frequently than is advisable'. Admittedly, allowing payment (especially generous payment) does make it possible for there to be a class of 'professional' research subjects who take excessive risks (Boyd, 1998; Helms 2005). But the fundamental problem with this is not payment, rather the fact that they are exposed to too much danger. So, provided that we have an adequate way of controlling and regulating risk to research subjects (as we should), this particular worry about payment ought not to arise.

This is backed up by two additional considerations. First, the amount of danger remains the same regardless of whether or not payment takes place. So if people object to paying subjects on the grounds that payment will encourage excessive risk-taking, they ought to object to the research project itself, not just the payment. Imagine people objecting to paying astronauts on the grounds that it encourages them to do something excessively dangerous. Surely we should say to them that, if the objection is danger, they should object to space travel *in general*, not (just) to *paid* space travel. Much of the same goes for paying tissue donors. If the worry is danger, we should object to dangerous research of all kinds, not just the paid variety.

Second, it is by no means obvious that monetary incentives make people act, as the GMC suggests, 'against their better interests or judgement'. Indeed, this is a rather surprising view to take because people trade off monetary gains and losses against other factors on a daily basis; commerce and work require us to do this all the time. So if an adequately informed and autonomous person decides, after deliberation, that it is worth subjecting herself to a given risk in return for £5000, then we should not just assume that she is acting against her better judgement because, for all we know, the £5000 is more valuable to her than avoiding an x% risk of physical harm.

When people debate this issue there is sometimes a tendency to discount or ignore the prospective research subject's (often sensible) desire for money, along with the fact that money is frequently beneficial. This in turn leads to the (mistaken) view that taking part in research is only in accordance with a person's 'better interests or judgement' if she or he would have been willing to participate for free, or if doing so for free would be in the subject's best interests. But this is a curiously demanding criterion to use, not least because it is not one that we apply in other contexts. After all, most people would not go to work if it were not for the pay, but we do not generally say that, for this reason, wages make people act against their 'better interests or judgement' (although obviously *sometimes* they do). Rather, we recognize that monetary gain must be counted as an important benefit to be weighed against the disbenefits of going to work. It seems sensible, then, to take a similar approach to paying people for bodily parts and products.

Finally, we need to look at the idea that financial incentives make people's decisions less autonomous. The main idea is that certain sorts of payment, or payment in certain circumstances, exert 'undue influence on a participant's decision' (Nuffield Council, 2002, p. 14). Accusations of undue inducement almost always occur in one of two different contexts. The first is where the 'victim' of the inducement

---

[1]Another related reason, not discussed here due to lack of space, is that some offers of monetary reward can be coercive. For a discussion of this argument see Wilkinson (2003, pp. 82–98, 116–129).

[2]Following Wilkinson and Moore, (1997), I prefer the term 'subjects' to 'participants'. The latter term is ambiguous among researchers and research subjects. Furthermore, only some kinds of research require the subjects' participation.

is in desperate need of money; the second is where the 'victim' is not desperate, but is offered such a huge amount of money to do X that doing X becomes almost irresistible. We can call these 'desperate offeree' cases and 'enormous offer' cases. One notable thing that these have in common is that there is a huge difference between how well-off the 'offerees' would be if they accepted the offer and the (much lower) welfare-levels that they would endure if they chose to reject it. In desperate offeree cases, this is because the offerees need what is offered and will be substantially harmed if they do not get it, whereas in enormous offer cases, it is because of the offer's sheer size (Wilkinson, 2003).

For our purposes, the important question is: is valid consent possible in these cases? In both scenarios it is terrifically hard for offerees to decline. However, as the following example shows, this does not mean that autonomous and valid consent is impossible:

> 'If the sole alternative to death is some lifesaving treatment . . . this does not rule out autonomous choice of the treatment. All the features of autonomous choice might be present: careful deliberation, correct understanding of the options, no manipulation, and so on. If informed consent is possible, despite the dire choice one faces, it cannot be because one is free to refuse the treatment. It must be because one can nonetheless act autonomously' (Wilkinson and Moore, 1997, p. 377).

So, as Wilkinson and Moore point out, even if we grant that there is a sense in which the recipients of enormous offers and desperate offerees are not free to decline, this does not mean that they cannot autonomously and validly consent. This must be so. Otherwise, it would be impossible for anyone ever to consent validly to lifesaving operations, not to mention lottery 'jackpot' wins or large wage rises; the mere fact that a proposal is tremendously attractive does not mean that it cannot be validly and voluntarily accepted by the offeree.

Given this, the position as regards tissue is as follows. In many cases, the monetary rewards offered to tissue donors are relatively modest and the donors are not in any way desperate. These cases are pretty unproblematic (at least as far as consent is concerned) provided that the other key elements of valid consent (in particular, adequate information and competence) are in place. There may, however, be a few cases which fall into the desperate offeree and/or enormous offer categories outlined above: cases in which the prospective tissue providers are significantly economically disadvantaged and/or where the rewards are unusually large. In these cases, it is certainly advisable to *consider very carefully* whether consent is truly voluntary but, as the lifesaving treatment example suggests, it is possible for the person to consent autonomously and voluntarily to selling her tissue (Wilkinson, 2003) Hence, what was earlier labelled as argument (c) also appears quite weak.

Although this section has discussed specifically people who sell their tissue for research purposes, the same general considerations apply across the board: to all areas of medical practice and research in which the body and its products are contested commodities.

SUMMARY AND CONCLUSIONS

To commodify (in the moral sense) is to treat as commodities things that are not (proper) commodities. This seems to mean treating as fungible and as merely instrumentally valuable things that are non-fungible and non-instrumentally valuable. Thus, commodification arguments in bioethics typically incorporate two distinct claims: one about fungibility and the other about instrumentalization. I have argued briefly here (and in more detail elsewhere) that the supposed obligation to treat people as non-fungible is problematic except perhaps in special contexts such as close personal relationships (Wilkinson, 2003). Thus, the best way of understanding, in a sympathetic way, claims about commodification is to view them essentially as about instrumentalization, about people being treated as mere means. Instrumentalization does seem to me to be a genuine moral wrong (although there has not been space to *argue* for that here). However, deciding which actions constitute treating people as mere means is tricky. I have suggested that one of the main ways in which we fail to treat (autonomous, competent) people as ends is by doing things to them (or that involve them) without requiring their valid consent; conversely, I have suggested that provided that we do require their valid consent (and perhaps also provided that we do not substantially harm them) then instrumentalization will not occur.

Then there is the question of how exactly paying people for (or to do) things is meant to cause commodification and instrumentalization. It is sometimes argued that monetary incentives cause commodification and instrumentalization by encouraging people to sell, while at the same time making valid consent to sell difficult or impossible. One of the main reasons for this (people argue) is that many sellers would be economically disadvantaged and hence their choices may not be autonomous or voluntary owing to their desperate need for money. I have argued here (and elsewhere) that although concerns about valid consent and voluntariness should be taken very seriously indeed, there is no reason *in principle* to believe that valid consent is impossible, even in fairly desperate circumstances (the example of consent to life-saving surgery being decisive here). Thus, we should not be too quick to assume that instrumentalization must be occurring in these situations, although it should, of course, be condemned when it does occur, as indeed should the desperate circumstances (such as extreme poverty) that allow some people to commodify, exploit and harm others.

REFERENCES

Alexandra A, Walsh A. Exclusion, commodification, and plant variety rights legislation. *Agric Human Values* 1997; **14**: 313–323.

Anderson E. *Value in Ethics and Economics.* Cambridge, MA: Harvard University Press, 1993.

Beyleveld D, Brownsword R. *Human Dignity in Bioethics and Biolaw.* Oxford: Oxford University Press, 2001.

Boyd R. A view from the man in the seat opposite. *Br Med J* 1998; **19**: 410.

Brecher R. The kidney trade: or, the customer is always wrong. *J Med Ethics* 1990; **16**: 120–123.

Erin C, Harris J. An ethical market in human organs. *J Med Ethics* 2003; **29**: 137–138.

Faden R, Beauchamp T. The concept of informed consent. In: Beauchamp T, Walters L, eds. *Contemporary Issues in Bioethics*, 4th edition. Belmont, CA: Wadsworth, 1994.

Garrard E, Wilkinson S. Bodily integrity and the sale of human organs. *J Med Ethics* 1996; **22**: 334–339.

Gillon R. *Philosophical Medical Ethics.* Chichester: John Wiley & Sons, Ltd, 1986.

GMC. *Research: The Role and Responsibilities of Doctors.* London: General Medical Council, 2002.

Hanson M. Biotechnology and commodification within health care. *J Med Philos* 1999; **24**: 267–287.

Harris J. *The Value of Life.* London: Routledge, 1985.

Helms R, ed. *Guinea Pig Zero: An Anthology of the Journal for Human Research Subjects.* Philadelphia: Garrett County Press, 2005.

HGC. *Making Babies: Reproductive Decisions and Genetic Technologies.* London: Human Genetics Commission, 2006.

Kant I. *Foundations of the Metaphysics of Morals* (Beck Translation). Indianapolis: Bobbs-Merrill, 1959.

Kaveny M. Commodifying the polyvalent good of healthcare. *J Med Philos* 1999; **24**: 207–223.

Marshall S. Bodyshopping: the case of prostitution. *J Appl Philos* 1999; **16**: 139–150.

Millns S. 'Dwarf'-throwing and human dignity: a French perspective. *J Soc Welfare Family Law* 1996; **18**: 375–376.

Nuffield Council. *The Ethics of Research Related to Healthcare in Developing Countries.* London: Nuffield Council on Bioethics, 2002.

Nussbaum M. Objectification. *Philos Public Affairs* 1995; **24**: 249–291.

Resnik D. The commodification of human reproductive materials. *J Med Ethics* 1998; **24**: 388–393.

Taylor J. *Stakes and Kidneys: Why Markets in Human Body Parts are Morally Imperative.* Aldershot: Ashgate, 2004.

Wilkinson M, Moore A. Inducement in research. *Bioethics* 1997; **11**: 373–389.

Wilkinson S. Commodification arguments for the legal prohibition of organ sale. *Health Care Anal* 2000; **8**: 189–201.

Wilkinson S. *Bodies for Sale: Ethics and Exploitation in the Human Body Trade.* London: Routledge, 2003.

Wilkinson S. biomedical research and the commercial exploitation of human tissue. *Genom Soc Policy* 2005; **1**: 27–40.

PART II

ISSUES IN HEALTH CARE PRACTICE

The aim of Part Two is to provide the reader with a fairly comprehensive overview of the core issues in health care ethics. Sometimes authors refer to legal decisions or procedures, but the reader must bear in mind that authors are generally dealing with the laws of their own country and the main emphasis for the collection as a whole is ethics rather than law.

The first four chapters deal with consent. Manson lays out the reasons why consent is considered to be a vital prerequisite but also argues that whilst standardized and formalized consent procedures are important for patient protection and reassurance, justifications for gaining consent do not entail 'any specific way of achieving consensual action' (p.301). Dresser explores the three ways of dealing with adult patients once it has been determined that they lack decisional capacity: advance treatment directives, substitutive judgement and the best interests standard. She reminds us that as the population in western and developed countries ages, incapacity is an increasing problem with work still to be done on how best to determine the appropriate treatment when people are unable to decide for themselves. Archard looks at how to apply the principle of consent to children with sections devoted to research, saviour siblings and genetic testing. He concludes that 'We can better safeguard the interests of children if they are participants, and they will become better participants if we give their views weight' (p. 315). Finally, Oakley argues that patients are entitled to be informed about an individual surgeon's success rates when deciding whether or not to consent to a surgical procedure. He points out that 'Patients usually consider information about risks to them

in a given procedures ... as more important than information about the risks of this procedure ... for patients generally' (p. 319), and these risks depend not just upon their individual circumstances but also in large measure upon the skills of their surgeon.

The next two chapters deal with confidentiality and truth-telling. Bennett provides a review of the importance of medical confidentiality, but looks specifically at whether the norms for confidentiality cope well with genetic information which is both intensively personal and shared amongst the wider family. She concludes that the solution lies in maintaining the same standard of confidentiality in the case of genetic information but against a background of promoting wider access to genetic testing to lessen the harms that are supposed to be prevented by disclosure. Higgs revisits truth-telling focussing firmly on practice, noting that there is more to truth-telling then telling the truth; it is a skill that takes practice to develop and maintain and also requires time, over time, with the patient.

Jackson and Benn look at the related issues of personal belief and personal conscience. In her chapter, Jackson tries to pin down precisely what the GMC mean when they say that doctors have a duty to ensure that their personal beliefs do not prejudice patient care. Using abortion as an example, she argues that the guidance most likely refers to 'unreasonable beliefs, which we (the GMC) just about put up with' but that in this case the guidance is rather empty unless 'accompanied by some indication as to which beliefs are unreasonable' (p. 342). Benn outlines the problems with, and the desirability of, conscience clauses and demonstrates that conscientious objection in medical practice is most acceptable where the values asserted 'are not too out of kilter with the accepted core values of medicine (p. 350).

It may be wrong to think of a 'standard' health care ethics, not just because it would be hard to be precisely certain what this standard is but also because care-giving happens in such diverse circumstances, and not all of it is given by professional carers. Lindemann demonstrates, for instance, the ways in which orthodoxies in health care ethics are at variance with orthodoxies of family ethics. Because families are ends in themselves, the division of labour is gendered, the relationships are frequently non-consensual, family members are not fungible, families are sites of love, and families help us to maintain our sense of ourselves, especially when we are ill, a different ethic has to apply to health care given in and by families. Braunack-Mayer explores the relationship between primary care and public health and particular ethical issues they raise. Of course, those working in primary care and public health are not the only workers who might have divided loyalties or dual responsibilities. Sommerville and English point out that many health care workers do, but some to a greater degree than others. They argue that being open about the dual nature of these responsibilities is imperative, though they also concede that on occasion the obligation to adhere to professional ethics might be prior to other duties, for example, that of obeying a direct command. Edwards is concerned about how different models of nursing are related to the four principles approach to health care ethics, and ultimately argues that a principles-based approach is surprisingly compatible with the care model. Finally, Behr and Ruddock address the question of how we should respond to violent and abusive patients. They argue that leaning towards uncritical tolerance does not respect their autonomy. They define what it takes for a patient to be considered morally responsible for her behaviour and show that it is not always in the patient's, nor indeed other patients', interests for morally bad behaviour to go unchecked.

There is enormous public and academic interest in the ethical issues that surround human reproduction. This includes not only the perennial problem of abortion but also questions such as 'What children we ought to create?' or 'What is owed to the human foetus?' or 'Can we use pre-implantation genetic diagnosis or abortion to ensure that we have the kinds of children we want?' Large as this collection is, there simply was no space to represent the myriad of questions in reproductive ethics in different chapters. Rather, we chose to commission chapters that could be generalised to address them. Ford, exploring the moral status of the foetus, proposes that the human foetus should be considered a legal person because '...it suffices to be a subject of a rational nature to be a person and that a spiritual soul is required to render human nature rational' (p. 389). Given that the soul is created along with the embryo at conception,

the foetus must be morally significant from the moment of conception. Asch provides a rather unusual look at abortion, asking whether it would be permissible in a world where women's position in society was much more equal. Part of this utopia would be a loosening of the genetic bonds that appear to bind biological parents of both sexes to parental responsibilities. She argues that whilst such a utopia would undoubtedly create a range of choices for both men and women, people should still be left to make their own evaluations about whether their bodies could be used to sustain life. Continuing the theme of what can be expected on the basis of biological relationships, Scott explores what is owed by pregnant women to the foetus they carry or the child it will become, in particular whether there is an obligation to agree to medical treatment for his/her benefit. Murray gives an account of reproductive liberty that argues that it cannot fail to take into account the interests of the child-to-be. Then, there is a pair of papers by Sorell and Shakespeare that present different views about the value of mental or physical impairment. Louhiala's chapter looking specifically at intellectual impairment compliments this pair. Finally, Clarke describes and discusses the range of issues that face genetic counsellors, including – but not limited to – those that arise in prenatal testing and screening. Because of the general nature of these chapters, some overlap is inevitable. Scott, for instance, also looks at the status of the foetus, whilst Sorell, Shakespeare and Clarke, all talk about abortion. Clarke's views on genetic testing in children can be read alongside those of Archard, and his views on the disclosure of genetic information within families alongside those of Bennett.

The next group of chapters discuss ethical issues that arise in mental health care. Bond gives an analysis of trust in the therapist-client relationship. Both McMillan and Matravers discuss compulsory treatment and detention. McMillan argues that antipsychiatry does not really help in determining whether or not compulsory treatment can be justified. Rather, given the imposition of any compulsory treatment, it can only be justified when the risks are high and the degree of involuntariness is severe. Matravers is concerned with the compulsory detention of those with personality disorders, for the protection of others. Giordano gives a distinctive account of anorexia, arguing that the desire to be thin could actually be related to the moral value of thinness rather than to media pressure or mental illness.

From mental health we move in the next chapters towards the end of life. Hughes' chapter introduces the ethical issues that surround the care of older people, and usefully can be read in conjunction with that of Dresser and Lindemann (regarding lack of capacity and care in and by families), and it also explores who the elderly actually are, ageism and risk-taking by and with older people. Next, Price looks at (primarily cadaveric) organ and tissue transplantation issues post Alder Hey and Bristol, whether there can be property in tissue and whether the dead can be harmed. He is followed by Wilkinson who explores the issues facing those engaged in transplanting tissue from live donors, particularly risks, harms and autonomy, incompetent donors and whether conditional allocation of organs in the case of the living justifies conditional allocation by the relatives of the dead. Huxtable provides a beautifully systematic and concise analysis of euthanasia and argues for greater consideration of what he calls the middle ground. Lamb provides a fascinating historical overview of death ending with an argument for a universal and holistic definition.

The final three chapters cover areas that have gained greater prominence since the first edition was produced. Pennings looks at the benefits and problems that arise when individuals seek cross-border medical help and health care workers migrate to wealthier areas in pursuit of more favourable working conditions. Foddy and Savulescu discuss the use of drugs and gene therapies to enhance sporting performance, concluding that it might be better to target resources on evaluating the fitness of athletes to compete rather than detecting enhancement. And in the final chapter of this section, Athanassoulis, using her own experience of developing a medical undergraduate curriculum for ethics, outlines how she thinks ethics should be introduced to, and incorporated within, medical education.

Heather Draper

39

Consent and Informed Consent[1]

NEIL C. MANSON

Informed consent is widely assumed to be a fundamental part of medical ethics. A great deal has been written about informed consent and various problems and dilemmas to do with informed consent (Sugarman et al., 1999). We cannot engage with this large – and ever-growing – body of literature here. The aim here is to clarify what *consent* is, what *informed* consent is, how they differ and why they are ethically important. The stress here will be on the fact that there are a number of different reasons why consent and informed consent are of importance in medical ethics and that any debate about the limits, nature and scope of consent and informed consent should take this fact into account.

CONSENT

Informed consent is a species of consent. But what is consent? We can begin with three very simple examples.

1a. Tom takes some apples from Sue's garden. Sue did not want Tom to take these apples. But Tom did not ask whether he could take the apples; he simply took them.
2a. Sue jumps out at Tom and cuts his thumb with a knife. Tom did not want Sue to do this. But Sue did not ask whether she could cut Tom's thumb; she simply cut him.
3a. Bill forces Tom, at gunpoint, to take part in a medical experiment where he is kept in a room and denied food for 24 hours.

We do not need to avail ourselves of any substantive moral theory to recognize that in each of these simple examples someone does something that is (in the absence of further qualifying details) morally impermissible. Tom *steals* Sue's apples. Sue *assaults* Tom and is guilty of *battery*. Bill *coerces* Tom and *falsely imprisons* him.

All the actions in our examples impinge upon, or otherwise affect, a particular individual. The wrongdoing is done to an individual, and we can readily view these wrongs as, broadly, breaching certain rights of the individual; certain 'negative' rights that the individual has *against* theft, assault, battery, false imprisonment and so on.

Let us now consider a second set of examples.

1b. Tom asks Sue whether he may take some apples from her garden. She says that he may. He takes the apples.
2b. Tom asks Sue whether she would cut his thumb to remove a splinter. She agrees. She cuts his thumb.
3b. Bill tells Tom about a medical experiment where he will be kept in a room and not eat for 24 hours. Tom tells Bill that he would very much like to participate.

Where the first examples involve theft, battery, coercion and so on, the second examples do not. The key difference between the first and second set of examples is that in the second set the affected party – the one whose rights would be breached – does something that effects a *waiver* of those rights. By saying that Tom may take the apples Sue waives her right against theft (by Tom, of the apples). By asking Sue to remove the splinter Tom indicates that he waives his right against battery (at least with respect to the specific action of cutting the thumb). Consent is akin to related

[1]Many of the ideas discussed in this chapter draw upon the ideas of Onora O'Neill, and some are discussed further in a more detailed way in our joint work. (Manson and O'Neill, 2007) I am indebted to Onora for her insights and for many discussions about the nature of consent and informed consent. Any errors or weakness in the arguments expounded here are my responsibility alone.

notions like *agreement, permission, authorization*. We will not be concerned with the many and varied differences between these. What matters for our purposes is that our examples show what consent does. In many contexts, an agent can, if she wishes, *waive* certain rights that she has against others acting in particular ways. This can be achieved in a very wide variety of ways: by nodding the head, by asking for help, by saying 'OK' and so on.

There is, then, a broad class of actions – call them *consent-dependent actions* – that have a distinctive feature; they impinge upon, or affect, an individual in such a way as to constitute a breach of an individual's rights *unless* they are performed with that individual's consent. When a consent-dependent action is performed with consent, it is a *consensual* action. Not all actions are 'consent-dependent'. There are many actions that are impermissible whether or not the agent consents: for example, murder or being sold into slavery. Consent is not sufficient to legitimate certain actions against an individual. For many other actions individual consent is not required and has no role to play (O'Neill, 2003). I do not need your consent to squash an ant or to stand within 10 metres of you in a public space (even if you would prefer not to have me in your view). Consent, then, has a limited application to those contexts where consent is both required and sufficient to waive certain rights that an individual has against others acting in certain ways. Viewed thus, it would seem that consent cannot be a fundamental right because consent plays a 'procedural' role in waiving *other* more basic rights (Brownsword, 2004).

By getting clear about the role that consent plays we can clarify what it is for an act to be consensual. The first point to note is that consent-dependent actions involve, in effect, two 'tiers' of rights. Take the example of theft. Theft involves a breach of a *first-order* right: a negative claim right against others (i.e. that others refrain from certain actions) (Hohfeld, 1919). The person who holds this first-order right also has a second-order right – what legal theorists call a *privilege*, or, less frequently, a *liberty* – to waive her first-order right against others. If the waiver is to be valid, this privilege (or liberty) is one which must be freely exercised. If Tom forces Sue at gunpoint to 'consent' to his taking the apples she does not really consent at all, no matter what she says, and Tom may be guilty of both theft and coercion.

It is essential to consensual action that the various parties involved in a consent transaction know certain things. For example, the person who proposes or intends to perform a consent-dependent action without breaching moral (and perhaps legal) norms needs to know that the agent has exercised her privilege and waived the right in question. But consent – waiving of the right – can be achieved in countless ways. For example, Sue may put up a sign that says 'Apples: help yourself'. Although Sue may not know Tom personally, and Tom may not know Sue, the sign indicates to all parties that the taking of (these) apples is permissible. There are other ways that Tom could come to know of Sue's consent. He might remember a previous occasion when a general consent was given ('Come and pick apples any time you like, Tom'). He might rely on the word of a third party ('Sue says you can have some of her apples'). He might infer that Sue does not mind, given other things that she has said ('Property is theft, Tom, property is theft!'). Suppose, however, that Sue is forced at gunpoint to put up the sign. Here she does not waive her right. Consent must be freely given.

Our simple examples show that consent is not always something that is given reactively (e.g. by way of response to a specific proposal for action). When Sue puts up her sign she consents to actions of a certain kind but not by way of response to someone else's proposal or intention. It should also be clear that consensual action can be achieved in a very wide variety of ways and that some of these ways are more likely to secure legitimate consent than others. For example, Tom may infer that Sue's remark about property being theft implies that Sue does not view her apples as her own property. But Sue might be making a general remark, or a remark about certain kinds of property (owning land or houses), whilst being vehemently opposed to having her apples taken by anyone. Simply inferring (or worse, assuming) that other parties consent is extremely problematic unless the inference is based upon a good deal of reliable evidence.

In most contexts, consent requires certain kinds of *communicative* action (Manson and O'Neill, 2007). This is because consent requires the various parties to know various things, and communication is a way of bringing it about so that the other party comes to know the relevant facts. Those who perform consent-dependent actions need to find out whether consent has been given; those who give consent may need to learn more about what is proposed, or about *who* is to act, and in what context. There are many different kinds of communicative action that can be used to secure, or give, consent. Different kinds of consent-dependent action done by different people to different people, in different contexts, may require more or less consent by way of communication amongst the various parties. For example, actions that breach norms of etiquette may demand nothing more than a modest attempt to secure consent ('Is this seat taken?') especially where the costs and consequences of a failure to obtain consent are unlikely to be great. Actions that breach, say, rights against invasive bodily contact or against theft are likely to be much more significant in terms of their costs and consequences (for all parties) and, as such, it becomes all the more important that the various parties *know* about the proposed course of action in some detail, and that all participants know whether consent has been given. Many – but not all – actions performed in the course of medical research, or medical treatment or diagnosis, are of this latter type, and we shall say more about medical actions in the following section.

INFORMED CONSENT

We have discussed what we might call 'simple' consent in certain everyday contexts. Consent is a way of waiving certain rights, and thus it allows actions to be performed that would otherwise be impermissible. Consent requires the various involved parties to know certain things and, typically, to communicate with one another, but, as we have seen, just what is communicated and how it is known will vary from case to case and from context to context. So much for 'simple' consent. But what about *informed* consent?

Now, in a broad sense, all consent must be 'informed' consent. You simply cannot consent to something without knowing something about it. When Sue puts up a sign saying 'Apples: help yourself', she knows something about the kind of action that she is consenting to, even if she does not know *who* it is that might take the apples, or *when*, or in *what manner*. If we take 'informed consent' in this broad way, then informed consent has long been an essential part of ethically sound medical practice. The reason why it is so is that medical practice involves many actions that *if they were performed without consent* would be impermissible: acts of cutting; invading the body; causing pain; administering material into the body; restricting movement; removing limbs and organs, and so on. Many medical actions breach first-order rights. But these first-order rights can be waived if the patient or research subject knows something about them, and consents to their being done. If a doctor is to gain her patient's consent for, say, a surgical intervention, she has to tell him something, perhaps in loose, vague terms, about what she proposes to do ('I'm going to have to cut out the growth, I'm afraid').

Although all consent is informed consent, the phrase 'informed consent' has come to have a distinctive, specific meaning that goes beyond 'consent' (and from now on, when we refer to informed consent, we'll use it in this restricted sense). Informed consent is consent that is voluntarily given (or refused) in response to a prior, explicit disclosure, detailing the nature, risks, costs, benefits and side-effects of a proposed course of action (perhaps with a specification of the risks, costs, benefits and side effects of alternative courses of action, or of taking no action at all).

But why should ethically sound medical practice require *informed* consent rather than just consent? (which, as we have seen, is always informed to some extent or other). We

have seen that without consent many medical interventions and treatments would constitute morally impermissible actions: assault; battery; false imprisonment. But consent does not require any particular form of communication, nor does consent always require prior, explicit 'disclosure' about a proposed course of action. There are two broad questions that emerge here: first, why should medical practitioners (in a clinical or research context) be obliged to engage in such a specific form of communication when consensual action does not, by itself, require it? Second, why is there an obligation to communicate in just *this* way? (i.e. prior, specific, explicit consent disclosures). In the remainder of this brief overview we will see that, in fact, there are a number of different reasons why the specific kind of communicative action central to informed consent is taken to be of importance for medical ethics.

THE HISTORY OF INFORMED CONSENT

In the large literature on informed consent there is a general consensus about the history of how informed consent came to be a central part of medical ethics (Beauchamp and Faden, 1986). This history cites (i) the medical experiments performed in Nazi Germany upon unwilling prisoners in labour camps and concentration camps; (ii) various 'research abuses' or 'research atrocities' where subjects were harmed, or subjected to risk of harm, and whose participation in such research was obtained via *deception*; (iii) a number of *legal* cases where plaintiffs claim that they were not properly or sufficiently informed about the nature or consequences of a medical intervention, and *had they been* sufficiently informed they would not have consented to the intervention in question; (iv) a history of *paternalism* in medicine, especially paternalistic deception and withholding of information; (v) a more abstract *ethical* argument which seeks to justify contemporary informed consent procedures by making appeal to the centrality of *respect for autonomy* in medical ethics (this is closely related to (iv)).

There is not space here to explore this historical background in any detail. What we can draw attention to, however, is the way that these historical, legal and ethical considerations support, and justify, current informed consent procedures. For example, Nazi medical research atrocities were (and are) ethically wrong not only because they were brutally and obscenely harmful but also *coercive*. The prosecutors of the Nazi doctors at the Nuremberg trials faced the problem of clearly specifying what constitutes ethically permissible medical research. Their findings were presented in 1947 as The 'Nuremberg Code' (Nuremberg Code, 1949). The Code, in its first section, lays a great deal of stress on *consent* and in spelling out what consent involves;

the Code then expands on the idea that the research subject needs 'sufficient knowledge and comprehension of the elements of the subject matter involved as to enable him to make an understanding and enlightened decision' and goes on to offer the kind of description of informed consent that is familiar today: the research subject should know something about 'the nature, duration, and purpose of the experiment; the method and means by which it is to be conducted; all inconveniences and hazards reasonably to be expected; and the effects upon his health or person which may possibly come from his participation in the experiment'.

Histories of informed consent cite other research atrocities and abuses: for example, the infamous 'Tuskegee Study of Untreated Syphilis in the Negro Male' in Alabama, which ran for over 40 years (Jones, 1981). Participants were told, misleadingly, that they were being studied for 'bad blood' and were denied any treatment for their condition. It may seem obvious that, as with the Nazi medical experiments on camp prisoners, the underlying problem here is a failure of informed consent. But note that the Tuskegee participants were *volunteers* (enticed, perhaps, by the offer of free meals, insurance and, without a hint of irony, free medical examinations and burial). The victims of the Nazi doctors were prisoners and not volunteers at all. The ethical deficit in the Tuskegee case is primarily one of *deception*, whilst the failing in the Nazi experiments derives from the brutally *coercive* nature of the experiments (indeed, in such a context there is no need to deceive the victim as her consent or voluntary participation is not being sought).

Nowadays, and this is partly by way of response to the research abuses noted above, informed consent is a central part of medical research ethics and of medical ethics more generally. Informed consent procedures provide a protection for patients and research subjects against coercion, deception, battery, false imprisonment and the like. Although informed consent procedures do not rule out the possibility of morally impermissible actions in the medical sphere, they do, arguably, make such actions less likely. Informed consent is now explicitly specified in most codes of good practice for medical professionals, and this indicates that certain kinds of communicative action are to be expected as a precondition of many medical actions. Such explicit statements of good practice shut down certain avenues of exculpation, where a clinician or researcher might seek to excuse or justify her deceptive or coercive actions by, for example, pointing out that such actions are not expressly forbidden. Such codes rule out a clinician claiming that it is *her* responsibility to exercise professional judgement as to how much her patients or research subjects 'need to know'. Similarly, it becomes harder – but not impossible – to routinely deceive when research subjects *expect* such communication, and might be suspicious if such communication were not forthcoming. Explicit informed consent disclosure documents can provide a reference point should there be a dispute about the outcome or effects of a medical intervention (and we will say more about this in a moment). Such documents are also available to parties *other* than those who are immediately involved in seeking or giving consent: ethics committees, auditors, professional bodies and others who might play a role in monitoring the behaviour of medical practitioners. The adoption of such procedures provides an assurance to patients and research subjects that medical practitioners and medical institutions are committed not just to refraining from coercion and deception but also to monitoring medical actions and sanctioning those who breach codes of good practice. Explicit informed consent procedures may also secure *trust* in the medical profession with the line of reasoning: 'They are not trying to hide anything, so they can be trusted'.

We saw earlier that simple consent, in everyday contexts, is extremely 'open' as to the kinds of communicative transaction that can and do secure consent. The history of research abuses gives us one reason why medical research involves something more specific than this and gives us a sense of why informed consent disclosures take the form that they take. Such disclosures are meant to provide an explicit form of protection for research subjects and to provide evidence that medical research has proceeded in an ethically proper, consensual way. Note that this line of argument is not that medical research constitutively requires this kind of informed consent disclosure. The argument is that in the kinds of institutional and social context in which medical research occurs, it is important that certain kinds of procedure are put in place for the purposes of protecting patients. A research pharmacist might ask a colleague to self-administer a new drug, and the colleague, knowing about the drug and its likely effects, might well agree and participate *without* any explicit informed consent transaction or signed documentation. There is nothing ethically improper about this. But most medical research involves the recruitment of those without medical knowledge or expertise. Researchers and research subjects are likely to be strangers to one another, and thus unable to base decisions on whether to participate on standard everyday criteria such as those derived from shared goals and a long history of mutual interaction which gives a sense of trustworthiness, and so on.

It is also important to note that the medical profession has been radically transformed by developments in information and communication technology, and by changes in how large organizations are managed and structured. There is a tendency (certainly in a vast institution like the UK National Health Service) towards *formalization* and *standardization*. The obtaining of consent has been transformed by these changes in medical bureaucracy. Where consent in an everyday context is obtained in a vast variety of ways without documentation or explicit records being kept, large institutions can use new technologies to produce lengthy standardized informed consent disclosures, which can then be archived and stored. Such changes partly explain the *form* of informed consent interactions.

INFORMED CONSENT AS PROTECTION FROM LITIGATION

Informed consent procedures protect patients and research subjects. But they also serve to protect the interests of medical practitioners, in both research and clinical medicine. Many medical actions would breach core rights if performed without consent. It is thus important for medical practitioners both to *obtain* consent and to be able to *show* that consent has been obtained. Although (in the UK at least) there is no 'law' of informed consent, there is a definite and widespread *fear* of litigation that has gripped the medical profession (Jones, 1999). In the United States, where litigation seems to be a commonplace part of everyday life, matters are even more problematic for the medical profession. Medical interventions typically involve a degree of risk of harm to the patient, and, given that the interventions are upon extremely complex systems (human beings) with largely unknown histories (other than what might appear in a medical record), there is no guarantee that any particular intervention (prostate surgery, say) will always have the same effects and consequences each time it is performed. Explicit informed consent disclosures serve as an invaluable form of legal documentation for the medical profession by showing that the patient (or research subject) was told about the nature of, and risks involved in, a certain course of action and, importantly, that the patient has acknowledged understanding and accepted whatever risks were explicitly mentioned.

To sum up: on the account we have given so far, patients and research subjects have a range of first-order rights against – and medical practitioners have correlative first-order obligations to refrain from – assault, battery, false imprisonment and so on. Consent allows much needed medical actions to be performed without a breach of these first-order rights and obligations. But *informed* consent is something much more specific than 'simple' consent in that it involves specific obligations to inform patients and research subjects about the nature, risks and side effects of proposed courses of action. As we have viewed things so far, this obligation to inform is *derived* from, and has it roots in, the first-order obligations to refrain from battery, false imprisonment and so on. But this derivative obligation is then subject to further constraint and direction, given

that (a) there is reason to provide *explicit* evidence of non-deceptive, non-coercive medical practice; (b) there are reasons to provide assurance that the first-order obligations are being met; (c) there is a perceived need to provide explicit evidence that might be used in the case of medical litigation; and (d) medical practice has become standardized and formalized in such a way as to favour the routine production and storage of standardized documentation.

PATERNALISM AND MEDICAL DECISION-MAKING

So, we have an account of how informed consent emerges out of a recognition and protection of *first-order* rights. There is, however, another line of argument in favour of explicit informed consent procedures which has a very different emphasis. Consent, as we have seen, involves two tiers of rights: various first-order claim rights against battery, false imprisonment, coercion and so on; and a general second-order right – a privilege or liberty – to waive the first-order right. There is a very widely accepted – or, at least, very widely duplicated and cited – line of argument which, in effect, focuses primarily on this second-order right: the right to *decide* whether to consent to, or refuse, a proposed course of action. There are reasons for this selective focus, but it also has far-reaching consequences for how debates about informed consent tend to be framed.

In the past it was widely assumed that the responsibility for medical decision-making (in a clinical context) lay with medical practitioners. Sometimes there may be a clear-cut, obvious course of medical action where great pain or ill-health is avoided without much cost or risk. But in many cases just *which* action to pursue, or *whether* to pursue a proposed course of action or another, will be a difficult decision to make, involving an assessment of probabilities together with a reasoned, subjective weighting of the various outcomes (relative to their likelihood). Medical professionals assumed that they, and they alone, had the experience and expertise necessary to make such decisions.

Such assumptions about who has responsibility for decision-making underpinned a widespread practice of *withholding* information from patients. But the ubiquitous withholding of information in clinical practice – unlike the deception in, say, the Tuskegee Study – was paternalistic. It was assumed that the beneficent withholding of information – about risks, about pain or about diagnoses in cases where no cure or proper treatment is available – was justified by the doctor's duty to act in the patient's interests. For example, withholding information, or other forms of deception, might be necessary to convince a patient to agree to the only course of action that will benefit her.

Are paternalistic actions of this kind *consensual*? We have seen that consent is extremely 'open' as to what is required by way of knowledge and communication. Given that patients typically *trust* their doctors to decide in their best interests, there is no reason to suppose that the actions by paternalistic doctors *need* be non-consensual just because certain information was deliberately withheld. All decisions are – for finite beings such as ourselves – based upon *partial* information. Consent transactions take place within a social context where the various parties have deep-rooted commitments, knowledge and expectations not just about the various courses of action for which consent might be sought, but also about the distribution of rights, privileges and obligations of the various parties. We need not suppose that paternalistic medicine is, necessarily, something that has to be *imposed* upon unwilling participants, as many people – including many sane, 'autonomous' adults in this day – are willing to defer medical decision-making to 'experts' (Schneider, 1996).

Contemporary discussions of medical ethics typically start with the assumption that paternalism is impermissible in – or at least something to be excised from – medical practice. Now, as we have seen, this cannot be because paternalistic actions are non-consensual, for they *can* be consensual. Paternalistic medicine may not breach any first-order rights, but it does seem to put constraints on the exercise of the *second-order* right – the privilege or liberty to waive one's first-order rights. There is a tight connection between deciding whether to waive one's rights and other deliberative activities such as deciding *what should be done*; or deciding *whether* some proposed course of action should be pursued. Those who object to paternalism in medicine argue that decisions about what should be done, or whether some proposed course of action should be pursued, *should be*, properly speaking, the ultimate responsibility of patients and research subjects. The main *complaint* against paternalism – in any walk of life, not just medicine – is that it denies adults the right *to make their own decisions* about how to lead their lives, and about what is to be done for them or to them. By withholding information, so the argument goes, sane, independent adults are treated by doctors as if they were children or as if they were somehow less than the capable adults that they are. Such treatment (and the attitudes that lie behind it) is, ultimately, disrespectful and demeaning. Paternalism interferes with people's freedom to decide how and whether to act (Buchanan, 1978). Non-paternalism is typically framed and justified in terms of notions of respect: for example, respect for 'autonomy' or 'decision-making' or 'freedom' or 'liberty' or 'choice', sometimes in terms of respect for 'persons' or, less commonly, in terms of respect for 'dignity'.

How does the rejection of paternalism support informed consent? In loose form, the argument is that in paternalistic medicine information was routinely *withheld* from patients, whilst in non-paternalistic medicine information ought to be routinely *made available* to patients (and, relatedly, to research subjects in medical research). From this, it seems to follow that medical practitioners are under an obligation to provide patients with the material that is *necessary* for them to make their decisions.

We saw earlier that *all* consent is informed to a greater or lesser degree. But the argument from the rejection of paternalism supports (or at least seems to support) a very specific set of informational obligations: the obligation to proactively provide explicit and specific information about proposed courses of action, their risks, side effects and so on. Correlative to this positive obligation to provide information, then, is a patient's *right* to receive information of certain kinds – that is, about risks, side effects and so on – *from* medical practitioners or researchers.

The rejection of paternalism thus lays particular stress on one specific element of consent: the second-order right (the *privilege* or *liberty* to waive rights by giving consent) in the guise of the *decision-making* of the patient or research subject. Now, insofar as good medical practice has always sought to be consensual, there has always been a limited respect for this second-order right. But from the analysis and account given here, it should be clear that the rejection of paternalism, when coupled with the ethical requirement that medical actions be *consensual*, does not entail a proactive obligation to give a specific 'disclosure' of risks, side effects and so on.

Why not? Consider the fact that autonomous agents vary widely with regard to their informational interests and with regard to the kinds of strategies which they choose to use to reach decisions in complex social contexts. Some people prefer to base their decisions on large volumes of information that they have scrupulously checked themselves, others are happy to *trust others* or to *devolve responsibility* to others. People differ, then, with regard to their informational interests and their decisions about how and whether they want to be informed. Given this variation in informational interests the following question arises: should informational interests, and autonomous decisions about whether to be informed, be respected? Respect for autonomy seems to be distorted, or only partial, if patients and research subjects are denied the option of relying on trust or devolving decision-making. Indeed, it is a common *complaint* of patients that they are 'forced' to read large volumes of information when what they most want is someone expert in deciding what is best (Schneider, 1996). They are, in effect, being coerced into reading information that they have no wish to read, or, perhaps, into (dishonestly) claiming that they have done so.

With regard to those cases where proactive informing is viewed by patients as counter to their informational interests and decisions, there seem to be two options. The first option is that informed consent disclosures are offered, not in response to subjects' *avowed* interests but in response to the interests that they *ought* to have, or in response to what medical institutions conceive of as these subjects' best interests. But this is, obviously, paternalism all over again: informational paternalism. The other option is that, in these cases, such disclosures serve and protect the interests of other parties (e.g. they protect doctors from litigation). Whilst this may be justifiable and proper, it is very far indeed from the standard idea that, somehow, proactive informed consent procedures are automatically in *patients'* interests.

There are various responses to such complaints (e.g. we might argue that a certain kind of information-heavy participation in medical decision-making is not a right, but an *obligation*). Or, we may argue that the proper solution is to tailor informed consent disclosures to an individual patient's standards. Or, more pragmatically, we might argue that mildly paternalistic informed consent disclosures *de facto* are the best way of securing an acceptable level of protection against more problematic forms of paternalism. The account offered here suggests that a simple, widely accepted solution to this problem is likely to be hard to obtain and that any practical solution to this kind of problem will have, at the very least, to negotiate competing sets of interests and a wide variety of arguments that engage with different rights, at different 'levels'. This is because – as we have seen – the obligation to inform is supported and held in place by a wide variety of considerations that come into play in different ways with regard to the complex, structured, normative phenomenon that is consent. On one hand, communication is important as a way of securing consent precisely because many medical actions breach first-order rights against battery, false imprisonment and so on. By itself this does not entail any *specific* way of achieving consensual action. But specific informed consent procedures – perhaps standardized and formalized as part of the administrative structure of modern medical institutions – provide a form of *protection* and *assurance* for patients and research subjects and may provide legal protection for both patients and medical practitioners. On the other hand, the orthodox view in contemporary medical ethics is that there is a right to information; information is the stuff upon which decisions are made and autonomous decisions are the object of *respectful* medical practice. This view rests upon assumptions about how medical decisions *ought* to be made, and reflects a

major shift in thinking (from the early twentieth century, say) about the rights and responsibilities of patients and research subjects with regard to their participation in medical decision-making.

Given that informed consent procedures protect and assure patients, provide legal protection for medical practitioners and have been widely adopted by relatively rigid institutional bureaucracies, it may be that such informational practices are indeed in conflict with individual autonomy, at least with regard to people's *informational* interests. There is nothing odd about this kind of conflict provided that we do not assume that informed consent is solely, or primarily, justified by respect for individual autonomous decision-making. From our brief sketch it should be clear that there is much more to consent and informed consent than this, and any adequate approach to medical ethics needs to be properly attuned to the subtleties and complex structures that constitute the landscape of consent.

REFERENCES

Beauchamp T, Childress J. *Principles of Biomedical Ethics*, 5th edition. Oxford: Oxford University Press, 2001.

Beauchamp T, Faden R. *A History and Theory of Informed Consent*. New York: Oxford University Press, 1986.

Brownsword R. The cult of consent: fixation and fallacy. *King's, College Law J* 2004; **15**: 2.

Buchanan AE. Medical paternalism. *Philos Public Affairs* 1978; **7**(4): 371–90.

Hohfeld WN. *Fundamental Legal Conceptions as Applied in Judicial Reasoning*. New Haven, CT: Yale University Press, 1919.

Jones JH. *Bad Blood: The Tuskegee Syphilis Experiment*. London: Collier Macmillan, 1981.

Jones MA. Informed consent and other fairy stories. *Med Law Rev* 1999; **7**: 103–134.

Manson N, O'Neill O. *Rethinking Informed Consent*. Cambridge: Cambridge University Press, 2007.

Nuremberg Code. *Trials of War Criminals before the Nuremberg Military Tribunals under Control Council Law,* vol. 2, no. 10, 1949; pp. 181–182 (U.S. Government Printing Office: Washington, DC, Web: http://www.hhs.gov/ohrp/references/nurcode.htm).

O'Neill O. Some limits of informed consent. *J Med Ethics* 2003; **29**: 4–7.

Schneider CE. *The Practice of Autonomy*. New York: Oxford University Press, 1996.

Sugarman J et al. Empirical research on informed consent: an annotated bibliography. *Hastings Centre Rep* 1999 (Special Supplement, January–February): 1–42.

40

Treatment Decisions for Incapacitated Patients

REBECCA S. DRESSER

Decisions about treatment, particularly about life-sustaining treatment, often involve patients whose reasoning capacities are impaired. Illness, injury and medication can have effects that compromise patients' abilities to participate in medical decision-making. The proportion of cognitively impaired patients is increasing, too. Advances in medicine make it possible for people in developed countries to live longer lives, often into the eighth and ninth decades. With increasing age comes a greater possibility of dementia and other conditions that reduce or remove the individual's ability to decide whether to accept or reject medical interventions. As a result, clinicians, families and others must cope with making treatment choices at the bedside.

This chapter describes four concepts that become relevant when treatment questions arise for adults with suspected or known cognitive impairments. The first is decisional capacity. Sometimes patients are so obviously impaired that no capacity evaluation is needed. At other times, however, clinicians must evaluate a patient's cognitive abilities to determine whether that person should be regarded as an independent decision-maker or as someone whose choices must be made by another. The remaining three concepts apply when clinicians, relatives, friends and appointed guardians make decisions on behalf of patients who cannot choose for themselves. Health professionals, scholars and policymakers have developed three standards to govern treatment decisions for incapacitated patients. Advance treatment directives, the substituted judgement standard and the best interests standard are the major approaches guiding such medical choices.

DECISIONAL CAPACITY

Two moral principles make capacity determinations central to good medical care. First, people capable of exercising autonomy should be permitted to make their own choices about whether or not to accept medical interventions. Treatments carry with them burdens as well as potential benefits. Except in unusual cases, such as the threat of contagious disease, individuals should be free to decide for themselves whether the gains that treatment makes available justify the physical and psychological costs it could impose. In diverse societies, people have different ideas about how to balance matters such as survival and quality of life. Because the individual patient will be most affected by the decision, that patient ought to be free to choose the treatment approach that best accommodates the individual's personal values and life situation.

Not all patients are capable of exercising autonomy, however. When individuals lack the ability to select the approach that would be most consistent with their values and preferences, it is inappropriate to give them control over their medical care. In these cases, the second principle comes into play. This principle holds that vulnerable persons need the protection of a trustworthy individual to make decisions on their behalf. The capacity evaluation is essential to determine whether autonomy or protection is the appropriate governing principle in particular cases.

Because capacity determinations have significant moral implications, evaluators must strive to avoid mistaken classifications. Treating a decisionally *capable* person as *incapable* leads to a demeaning and unjustified deprivation of that person's right to decide whether treatment would be

Principles of Health Care Ethics, Second Edition   Edited by R.E. Ashcroft, A. Dawson, H. Draper and J.R. McMillan
© 2007 John Wiley & Sons, Ltd

acceptable in the light of her individual beliefs and preferences. Treating a decisionally *incapable* person as *capable* exposes that person to harm from choices that fail to rest on an adequate understanding and appreciation of the treatment situation.

To make autonomous choices, people must have certain abilities. Although no single definition is enshrined in ethics and policy, agreement exists on the basic features of decisional capacity. According to Appelbaum and Grisso (1988), four abilities are central: (1) the ability to communicate a choice; (2) the ability to understand relevant information; (3) the ability to appreciate how this information applies to one's current and future situation; and (4) the ability to give comprehensible reasons for a decision.

Although simple mental status assessments may furnish preliminary guidance, they are insufficient to determine whether someone is able to make autonomous treatment decisions. Instead, clinicians should evaluate decisional capacity in the context of the specific treatment situation at hand. Decision-making capacity should be assessed through a discussion of the facts relevant to the particular choice facing a patient. At minimum, patients should demonstrate the ability to understand the goals, potential benefits and risks of a proposed treatment and of any reasonable alternatives to that treatment (including the alternative of no treatment). The patient should be able to express a reasonably stable choice as well.

Some scholars and health professionals support a sliding-scale approach to evaluate a person's capacity to decide about treatment. According to this approach, capacity standards may be lower when patients are in low-risk situations, where any choice offers reasonable benefit and minimal risk. Conversely, a higher level of decisional ability should be required for decisions with more serious consequences, such as decisions about life-sustaining treatment (Lo, 2000). Others oppose the sliding-scale approach, however, contending that genuine respect for autonomy requires adopting the same capacity standards for all medical decisions, no matter how significant the consequences are (President's Commission for the Study of Ethical Problems in Medicine, 1983).

Assessing a person's decision-making *capacity* goes hand-in-hand with assessing that person's *understanding* of the important treatment information. To make an informed choice, a patient must be cognitively capable of understanding the basic facts about the relevant medical decision. To determine whether a patient has the requisite cognitive capacities, the clinician must disclose these facts and then evaluate the patient's level of comprehension.

The assessment process itself can be conducted using a variety of methods. The simplest method is to ask patients to describe briefly and in their own words the basic information relevant to the treatment choices they are facing.

In questionable cases, a psychiatrist may be asked to examine the patient's cognitive abilities. Some patients are hostile and refuse to talk with a health professional about their treatment situations. In these cases, it may be useful to enlist family members, social workers or religious advisers to encourage the communication necessary to assess the patient's decision-making abilities.

From the legal perspective, persons are presumed competent to make their own medical decisions. Strictly speaking, a judge must determine that a patient is incompetent before others may make decisions on the patient's behalf. In reality, however, few cases are taken to court. Most cases can be adequately addressed in the medical setting. Requiring a legal proceeding in every case would be burdensome, expensive and impractical. To distinguish clinical judgements about decision-making capacity from formal legal determinations, however, contemporary medical ethics discussions usually refer to incapable or incapacitated patients, rather than to incompetent patients.

When the capacity assessment reveals that a patient lacks the ability to choose, someone else must assume responsibility for medical decision-making. In such cases, advance treatment directives, the substituted judgement standard, and the best interests standard move to the forefront.

ADVANCE TREATMENT DIRECTIVES

Most scholars and policymakers regard the advance treatment directive as the preferred approach to treatment decisions on behalf of incapacitated patients. Two types of directives exist. One is the instruction directive, often called the living will. This is a written or oral account by a decisionally capable individual addressing future treatment during a period of incapacity. Instruction directives usually describe the types of treatment that would be acceptable or unacceptable in various illness situations. Sometimes they contain more general statements about the activities or functional abilities that are essential for continued life to have value to the individual. The other type of directive is the proxy directive, also called the health care power of attorney. This is a written or oral statement designating a particular family member or other trusted person to act as a future decision-maker if the individual making the designation becomes incapacitated.

Advance treatment directives were first proposed in the 1960s and 1970s, as modern medicine was developing ventilators and other intensive care procedures that could sustain patients who previously would have died from their conditions. Some people thought that doctors were using the new technology inappropriately and that they lacked good judgement about how to use their expanded power to sustain life. People were afraid that doctors would keep them on life support, rather than allow them to 'die with dignity'.

In response to this situation, professional groups and legal authorities developed two general rules. First, in contemporaneous treatment situations, patients should be empowered to decide, based on their individual values, whether treatment would be worth it. Second, if illness or injury leaves patients unable to choose for themselves, decisions should reflect what they said when they could still think about their choices. Living wills and other advance treatment directives were created so that people could register their preferences about future care.

Support for advance directives rests on the desire to respect individual autonomy. The advance directive is also attractive because it seems to avoid putting treatment decisions in the hands of others. But empirical research on advance directives suggests that there are serious obstacles to putting advance directives into practice.

One problem is that most people fail to issue advance directives, despite public campaigns encouraging them to do so. And many of the people who do issue directives make very general requests such as a wish to forgo 'heroic' or 'extraordinary' measures in the event of terminal illness (Teno et al., 1997). Statements like this offer little guidance to the clinicians and families, who must later settle an actual treatment question. Proxy directives are more common and can be helpful in the clinical setting. Yet proxy decision-makers do not necessarily know how patients would decide and as a result, proxies may face the same uncertainties faced by others attempting to decide on an incapacitated patient's care (Emanuel and Emanuel, 1992).

Some instruction directives set forth an individual's precise treatment preferences, thus providing more information to those at the bedside. These directives raise a different set of concerns, however. Precise directives may not accurately communicate a patient's wishes. For example, a study of dialysis patients with advance directives found that two-thirds of them wanted their families and physicians to have at least some freedom to override the directives (Sehgal et al., 1992).

Some instruction directives may be ineffective in transmitting information, too. In another study, older people were asked to identify the relative they would prefer as their surrogate medical decision-maker if they lost capacity. Investigators then asked the older people whether they would want four different life-sustaining interventions in nine different illness situations. After that, the investigators asked the chosen surrogates how *they* thought the older person would answer the treatment questions. Some surrogates were permitted to review the older person's instruction directive before responding, whereas others simply relied on their existing knowledge about the older person. Surrogates who consulted the older relative's instruction directive were no more accurate than were other surrogates in estimating what the older persons' answers would be. (Both groups were accurate about 70% of the time.) Thus, written evidence of a patient's choices may not supplement the general knowledge that the family members have about each other's medical care preferences (Ditto et al., 2001).

Another problem is that people completing instruction directives may lack adequate information about the choices they are making. Unless they are already ill and face a limited array of likely treatment questions, it is difficult to predict future medical situations. A currently healthy person faces an astronomical number of possible treatment questions. And these questions will arise when dementia or another incapacitating condition significantly alters their experiential lives. An important issue is whether people completing advance directives sufficiently understand what they would want in a future state of dementia or other impairment.

A related problem is that a person's treatment preferences may be different at different times. Research on competent individuals demonstrates both that treatment preferences change and that people overestimate the stability of their preferences (Gready et al., 2000). This research calls into question the idea that a person has certain 'authentic' preferences that should prevail in later treatment situations. It also suggests that individuals whose preferences change may fail to alter their directives because they are unaware of the changes.

Other studies point to additional implementation problems, including difficulties in ensuring that advance directives are delivered to clinicians at the appropriate times (Morrison et al., 1995). Indeed, there is evidence suggesting that the treatment of patients with directives is similar to the treatment of other patients with the same medical problems (Schneiderman et al., 1992; Tulsky, 2005).

The problems with implementing advance directives suggest that future-oriented individual autonomy offers limited guidance for decisions on behalf of incapacitated patients. Two authors reviewing the empirical data concluded that even if one assumes that instruction directives are a desirable method of respecting patient autonomy, they 'do not and cannot achieve [that] goal' (Schneider and Fagerlin, 2004).

Besides the practical problems, certain advance directives present serious ethical conflicts. Sometimes honouring a patient's advance directive would harm the patient as she is now. The conflict situations fall into two categories. In one, the directive refuses an intervention that would make a patient more comfortable or would extend what appears to be a worthwhile life for the patient. In the other, the directive requests an invasive or otherwise burdensome treatment that observers believe offers the patient no material benefit.

Which should take priority, the advance directive or the incapacitated patient's welfare? Writers are divided on this question. Some contend that the advance directive should prevail, based on the judgement that respect for future-oriented autonomy has a higher value than protection of incapacitated patients for this welfare (Dworkin, 1993). Yet the empirical data on instruction directives indicate that advance choices may not be the informed, considered choices that should qualify as autonomous decisions. The real dilemma is how to balance the patient's previous less than ideal decision against the patient's current welfare. Because few individuals complete precise instruction directives and because few of those directives present a clear conflict with the patient's present well-being, legal authorities have not yet taken a stand on this difficult question.

THE SUBSTITUTED JUDGEMENT STANDARD

When advance directives fail to resolve treatment questions, two standards guide patient care. One of them is the substituted judgement standard. According to this standard, the goal is to make the treatment decision that the patient would make if 'miraculously lucid for an interval (not altering the existing prognosis of the condition to which she would soon return) and perceptive of her irreversible condition' (Quinlan, 1976). When patients have not registered their preferences in an advance directive, however, decision-makers must look to matters such as the individual's previous general remarks, religious beliefs and attitudes towards medical care as indicators of what the patient would choose.

Respect for the patient's previous autonomous values and preferences underlies support for the substituted judgment standard. Because very few people complete specific instruction directives that apply precisely to a later treatment situation, substituted judgement is commonly invoked to produce the choice that the patient would make, if able. Yet the evidence underlying a substituted judgement choice is sometimes questionable. For example, a person's comments in response to a relative's illness or a patient in a television show are not necessarily based on serious reflection about the matter. Furthermore, the speaker may not intend for these comments to be taken as explicit instructions for future care. Similarly, a young or middle-aged person's failure to attend to health needs does not necessarily indicate how that person would regard medical care at a later point in time.

These weaknesses in the evidence about patients' personal views generate worries about the quality of the decisions substituted judgement can produce. The standard is flexible enough that proxy and surrogate decision-makers may incorporate their own values and concerns as the basis for decisions purporting to be what the patient would want. Some writers argue that to protect the patient, the range of decisions based on the substituted judgement standard should be restricted: 'the inherently speculative nature of substituted judgment, along with the vulnerable position of the incompetent, require that substituted judgment may not be used to justify a course of action that serves the interests of others at the expense of the ward's basic interests' (Buchanan and Brock, 1989, pp. 117–118).

According to this view, incapacitated patients retain a set of fundamental interests that may not be ignored. To ensure that these interests are recognized, clinicians must examine the patient's current situation and the benefits and burdens that would accompany various treatment decisions (Lowy, 1988). This assessment requires decision-makers to turn to the best interests standard.

THE BEST INTEREST STANDARD

The best interests standard is sometimes called the objective standard or the 'reasonable person' standard. When clear evidence of a patient's past values and preferences is absent, decision-makers turn to this standard. Although advance directives and the substituted judgement standard seek to duplicate the choice an individual patient would make, the best interests standard turns to normative judgements about what is good and bad for human beings. It rests on a societal consensus, or the perspective of "a reasonable person", choosing as most people would choose for themselves' (New York State Task Force, 1992, p. 33).

To apply the best interests standard, decision-makers must evaluate the benefits and burdens that an incompetent patient could experience from different treatment approaches. Examples of benefits and burdens are pleasure, enjoyment, pain and distress. According to the best interests standard, treatment interventions are justified if they are expected to produce a substantial benefit enough to outweigh their risks and burdens.

The best interests standard requires healthy individuals to evaluate incapacitated patients' quality of life. History shows that this sort of evaluation is easily influenced by social worth and economic considerations. Concern about potential discrimination and abuse leads many scholars and legal authorities to prefer advance directives and the substituted judgement standard over the best interests standard. Because advance directives and substituted judgement aim at the choice the patient herself would make, they seem to pose less risk of inappropriate quality-of-life evaluations. But the limitations of advance treatment directives and the substituted judgement standard make it necessary in many cases to turn to the best interests standard. Due to the emphasis on advance directives and the substituted judgement standard, however, the proper content and application of the best interests standard remains unclear.

Several dimensions of the best interests standard present issues. First, to apply the standard, there must be agreement about what should count as benefits and burdens to patients and what combination of benefits and burdens permits a specific treatment choice. But people have different views on the appropriate content of the best interests standard. Although everyone agrees that burdensome treatment may be withheld when it fails to offer a reasonable possibility of extending life, other potential applications of the standard remain controversial.

One contested matter involves applying the best interests standard to patients whose awareness is permanently absent. Concepts such as interests, benefits and burdens are closely tied to a patient's consciousness. Some people think that because unconscious patients are unaware of pain and other negative experiences, it is difficult to argue that treatment could be burdensome to them. Others contend that withholding or withdrawing treatment from permanently unconscious patients is permissible under the best interests standard. The rationale for this position is as follows:

> Patients who are permanently unconscious are unaware of benefits and burdens. The only possible benefit to them of life-sustaining treatment is the possibility that the diagnosis of irreversible unconsciousness is wrong and they will regain consciousness.

> Accordingly, the major considerations are whether a reasonable person in the patient's circumstance would find that this benefit, as well as the benefits to the patient's family and concerned friends (such as satisfaction in caring for the patient and the meaningfulness of the patient's continued survival) are outweighed by the burdens on those loved ones (such as financial cost or emotional suffering) (Hastings Center, 1987, p. 29).

Another conflict concerns what may count as burdens to the patient. Some writers defend what is referred to as the 'sanctity of life' position, which holds that 'burdensomeness should be assessed by focusing on the pain or invasiveness caused by the treatment itself, not by evaluating the quality of life that such medical intervention may sustain' (New York State Task Force, 1992, p. 57). On the other side are those who contend that burdens and benefits may include the kind of life the patient will gain with treatment. According to these writers, 'discontinuing treatment, even if it leads to the patient's death, is consistent with his or her best interests when the treatment is hopeless and serves only to sustain biological existence that is painful or of no benefit to the patient' (New York State Task Force, 1992, p. 58). People holding this position say that the lives of vulnerable persons will be adequately protected as long as

the examination remains focused on the value life holds for the individual patient, as opposed to the value the patient's life holds for others:

> The question is not whether the patient's quality of life is below average, or worse than it used to be, or anything of the sort. Instead, the proper quality of life judgment is only whether the quality of the patient's life with the life-sustaining treatment will be so poor as to be not worth living or worse than no further life at all (Buchanan and Brock, 1989, p. 124).

Yet another hotly debated question is whether the best interest standard should ever consider burdens the patient's care imposes on family members. According to the US President's Commission for the Study of Ethical Problems in Medicine, '[t]he impact of a decision on an incapacitated patient's loved ones may be taken into account in determining someone's best interests, for most people do have an important interest in the well-being of their families or close associates' (President's Commission for the Study of Ethical Problems in Medicine and Biomedical and Behavioral Research, 1983). Another policy group criticized this position, however, questioning whether such 'imputed altruism' should be part of the best interests standard. According to this group, the interests of others should influence treatment decisions only if there is strong evidence that the average person would take such interests into account in making medical choices (New York State Task Force, 1992).

A related issue is whether the best interests standard permits decision-makers to consider the quality of services and facilities available for an incapacitated patient's care. As philosophers Buchanan and Brock observe, 'some would justify withholding life-sustaining treatment from a severely demented elderly individual . . . on the grounds that it would not be in that individual's best interests to live in an inadequately funded state institution...' (Buchanan and Brock, 1989, p. 134). Buchanan and Brock reject this view, arguing instead that the best interests standard calls for remedying deficiencies in the care available to such patients. Yet they also concede that 'neither the interests of others nor the defects of existing institutions can be ignored in determining what is in the incompetent's best interest' (Buchanan and Brock, 1989, p. 134).

Factors such as family burdens and available care options are likely to influence decisions at the bedside. The moral challenge is to keep patient welfare at the forefront. Although most scholars and officials agree that families and other surrogates should ordinarily be empowered to make treatment decisions for their incompetent relatives, they also support some limits on surrogate decision-making. Commentators speak in terms of permitting decisions 'within the range of medically sound alternatives, as determined by appropriate medical standards' (Buchanan and Brock, 1989,

p. 143) or 'a range of plans of care [recognized] as generally acceptable by community and professional standards' (Lynn, 1992, p. 2084).

CONCLUSION

All three approaches to decision-making for incompetent patients raise moral questions and present practical difficulties. It would be foolish to think that a simple formula could supply easy answers to decisions about how vigorously to treat patients who cannot make their own medical decisions. At the same time, there is much room for improvement in the existing ethical and policy framework. In many cases, a patient's previous values and preferences fail to point to a clear treatment approach. More work is needed to develop the best interests analysis that determines appropriate treatment for patients in this situation.

Developing a more rigorous and thoughtful best interests standard will require public and professional debate. It will also require a better understanding of how different treatment interventions can affect incapacitated patients (Dresser and Whitehouse, 1994). The challenges will be especially severe in cases involving patients with Alzheimer's disease and other forms of dementia. For these patients, many years can elapse between the onset of decisional incapacity and the point at which death is inevitable. During much of this time, patients are aware and able to interact with the world. They can be harmed or helped by the medical decisions others make for them. This group is likely to be the focus of ethical analysis addressing incapacitated patients in the years to come.

ACKNOWLEDGEMENT

Portions of this chapter draw on my earlier analyses in Dresser R. Precommitment: a misguided strategy for securing death with dignity. *Texas Law Re* 2003; **81**: 1823–1847; Shapiro M, Spece R, Dresser R, Clayton E. *Bioethics and Law: Cases, Materials and Problems*. St. Paul, MN: Thompson West, 2003.

REFERENCES

Appelbaum P, Grisso T. Assessing patients' capacity to consent to treatment. *N Engl J Med* 1988; **319**: 1635–1638.

Buchanan A, Brock B. *Deciding for Others: The Ethics of Surrogate Decision Making*. Cambridge: Cambridge University Press, 1989.

Ditto P, et al. Advance directives as acts of communication. *Archives Intern Med* 2001; **161**: 421–430.

Dresser R, Whitehouse P. The incompetent patient on the slippery slope. *Hastings Center Rep* 1994; **24**(4): 6–12.

Dworkin R. *Life's Dominion: An Argument about Abortion, Euthanasia, and Individual Freedom*. New York: Knopf, 1993.

Emanuel E, Emanuel L. Proxy decision making for incompetent patients. *J Am Med Assoc* 1992; **267**, 2067–2071.

Gready R, et al. Actual and perceived stability of preferences for life-sustaining treatment. *J Clin Ethics* 2000; **11**: 334–346.

Hastings Center. *Guidelines on the Termination of Life-Sustaining Treatment and the Care of the Dying*. Bloomington, IN: Indiana University Press, 1987.

Lo B. *Resolving Ethical Dilemmas: A Guide for Clinicians*, 2nd edition. Philadelphia: Lippincott Williams & Wilkins, 2000.

Lowy C. The doctrine of substituted judgment in medical decision making. *Bioethics* 1988; **2**: 15–21.

Lynn J. Procedures for making medical decisions for incompetent adults. *J Am Med Assoc* 1992; **267**: 2082–2084.

Morrison S, Olsen E, Mertz K, Meier D. The inaccessibility of advance directives on transfer from ambulatory to acute care settings. *J Am Med Assoc* 1995; **274**: 478–482.

New York State Task Force on Life and the Law. *When Others Must Choose: Deciding for Patients Without Capacity*. Albany, NY: Health Research, Inc., 1992.

President's Commission for the Study of Ethical Problems in Medicine and Biomedical and Behavioral Research. *Deciding to Forego Life-Sustaining Treatment*. Washington, DC: Government Printing Office, 1983.

In re Quinlan. 355 A.2d 647. NJ, 1976.

Schneider C, Fagerlin A. Enough: the failure of the living will. *Hastings Center Rep* 2004; **34**(2): 30–42.

Schneiderman L, et al. Effects of offering advance directives on medical treatment and costs. *Annals Inter Med* 1992; **117**: 599–606.

Sehgal A, et al. How strictly do dialysis patients want their advance directives followed? *J Am Med Assoc* 1992; **267**: 59–63.

Teno J, et al. Do advance directives provide instructions that direct care? *J Am Geriat Soc* 1997; **4**: 508–12.

Tulsky J. Beyond advance directives. *J Am Med Assoc* 2005; **294**: 359–365.

41

Children's Consent to Medical Treatment

DAVID W. ARCHARD

INFORMED CONSENT

In very general terms, the principle of informed consent requires that a patient must give her consent to any course of treatment and a subject must give her consent to participation in any programme of medical research. In the absence of such consent, the actions of the doctor or researcher are considered morally impermissible. The consent in question must be freely given, informed by knowledge of the salient relevant facts, and given by someone competent to consent (Young, 1998).

This principle of informed consent is central to medical practice and is to be found expressed in various key statements of medical ethics. The Nuremberg Code offers a particularly robust and stringent version of the principle:

> The voluntary consent of the human subject is absolutely essential. This means that the person involved should have legal capacity to give consent; should be so situated as to be able to exercise free power of choice, without the intervention of any element of force, fraud, deceit, duress, over-reaching, or other ulterior form of constraint or coercion; and should have sufficient knowledge and comprehension of the elements of the subject matter involved as to enable him to make an understanding and enlightened decision (Nuremburg Code, 1949).

The principle has had two different kinds of warrant (Beauchamp and Childress, 2001). The first is prophylactic: the obtaining of consent serves to protect the individual from harm, exploitation and injustice, or the risks thereof. This source for the principle is easily understood as a reaction to the horrors of enforced experimentation upon prisoners by the Nazis. The second warrant views the principle of informed consent as a positive expression of respect for individual autonomy. Securing consent recognizes the entitlement of each person to determine for herself what shall and shall not be done to her.

In respect of children, the application of the principle of informed consent is obviously problematic. Most children are properly viewed as not competent to give or to withhold their consent. They are, in this respect, like some other groups of humans: the seriously mentally ill and the comatose, for instance (Buchanan and Brock, 1989). But they also differ. Unlike those who are seriously mentally ill or brain-damaged, the incapacity of children is not permanent. Children will normally mature and as adults acquire the ability to consent. Unlike those who are comatose or unconscious, it is not possible to rely on any prior indications of consent. Children are throughout their minority deemed unable to consent.

In the cases of some adults who cannot consent, we may rely on the idea of substituted choice – essentially a hypothetical characterization of what, in the absence of any explicit statement, they would consent to if now competent. This possibility is not open to us in the case of children. For to think of an incompetent child choosing, in the person of a competent adult, what she would wish for is simply to think of somebody far removed – in fact, totally different – from the child in question. Young children in particular do not have settled dispositions, beliefs and values from which we might construct a view as to their life plans.

CHILDREN, PARENTS AND THE STATE

Children usually have parents or guardians, adults entrusted with their daily care and custody. We are disposed to think that these adults can give their proxy consent to medical treatment of their child. Some (Ross, 1998) have offered a good extended defence of according a substantial role for parents in the making of health care decisions about children. Others have written about making such decisions within a family context (Nelson and Nelson, 1995).

Principles of Health Care Ethics, Second Edition   Edited by R.E. Ashcroft, A. Dawson, H. Draper and J.R. McMillan
© 2007 John Wiley & Sons, Ltd

However, clearly there are limits to these powers of consent. Parents could not, we think, consent to their child suffering an unnecessary or superfluous serious harm or the risk of harm; nor could they refuse necessary and risk-free therapeutic treatment of a painful or life-threatening condition. It is also important to acknowledge that the powers of proxy consent do not derive from a more general right of parents to dispose, as they see fit, of their children. Parents do not, as was once thought, own their children. However, it is reasonable to judge that parents are excellent judges of what is in the best interests of their child – both because they know them better than anyone else and because they are normally disposed to do what is best for their own.

There is thus a fundamental distinction between the ways in which parental rights might be justified: from the side of children, it can be argued that it is in their interests or for their good that parents make choices on their behalf; or, from the side of parents, it can be argued that the fact of parenthood grounds entitlements to choose for offspring.

For its part the state has a fundamental duty – that of *parens patriae* – to protect the vulnerable within its jurisdiction, of whom children are the most obvious members. Thus when a parent's choices for her child are seriously inimical to that child's best interests it is entirely appropriate for the state, or its agencies, to intervene to protect the child. The most obvious kind of case within the medical domain will be one – such as it would be with Jehovah's Witnesses objecting to an essential blood transfusion – in which parents refuse life-saving treatment for their child.

Note that if the state does intervene in such circumstances, it does not deny that the parents are disposed to do what they think is in the child best's interests – in the case of the Jehovah's Witnesses, the parents act to safeguard the child's eternal soul. Note further that the state's denial of the parents' view of what is best for the child would not be sufficient reason for the state to act paternalistically in respect of an *adult* Jehovah's Witness who refused blood.

CHILDREN AND COMPETENCE

Children have been characterized as not competent to give and to withhold consent. This assumption needs qualification. In the first place it is proper to distinguish within the broad category of children – whom the law will characterize as anyone below a specified age – between the different age groups. Although it is undoubtedly true that infants cannot give consent, let alone make an explicit statement of their preferences those who are better described as young persons – teenagers – will most definitely have views on what may be done to them and are at least putatively capable of consent.

UK law operates with the very useful idea – formally known as Gillick competence – of a mature minor (Gillick, 1985). Below the age of 16, children are deemed to be minors, and as such incapable of giving consent. However, this presumption is defeasible: a minor may be able to demonstrate sufficient understanding and knowledge of her situation and a proposed course of action to be regarded as mature enough to make her own decisions. It is noteworthy, then, that age as such is not the marker of ability. Rather it is maturity that serves as the legal guide, and it is seen as normally but not invariably associated with attainment of a certain age.

The second qualification concerns the characterization of competence. There are a number of ways in which the putative ability or inability of a child to consent could be appraised. The first would be by means of an index of global competence or general ability to understand matters. A threshold could be specified, and those above it deemed competent to consent. The problem with this manner of assessing capacity is its failure to acknowledge that more complex or more significant matters may require a higher degree of competence.

A second way to appraise ability would be by means of an evaluation of the content of any choice or decision. An unwise choice of action betokens an inability to choose. The problem with this manner of assessing capacity is that imprudence should be evidence for but not constitutive of a lack of ability. After all we do not think the undoubted folly of many adult decisions sufficient warrant for a general paternalistic usurpation of their choices.

The most plausible way to appraise ability, then, is a functional one that measures competence against that in respect of which a choice is being made: the more complex or significant the matter the greater the required degree of ability. It should be noted that complex matters need not be significant, and significant matters need not be complex. The choice of whether or not to have a life-saving operation is in one sense of the term a simple one, as there are only the two possibilities. On the contrary, medical treatment of a minor ailment may be very complicated and multifaceted. More mundanely, consider how complicated, yet relatively insignificant, is the choice of a five-course meal from a large menu.

This leads neatly to a further feature of competence. The Gillick judgement required of a mature minor not only that she retains and have command of the relevant facts, but that she appreciates their significance. Lord Scarman, in particular, argued that in respect of advice about contraception, a mature minor should both understand the nature of that advice and also have 'a sufficient maturity to understand what is involved'. This, he said, broached 'moral and family questions' (Gillick, 1985, p. 424). Thus a 13-year-old may know that unprotected sex risks pregnancy or a sexually transmitted disease, but she may simply fail to recognize or grasp what these would actually mean for her – what having a child or suffering an STD would entail. Similarly, a 14-year-old may know full well that failure to undergo a medical procedure will almost certainly result in her death. But she may be judged insufficiently mature to grasp what death means – its utter finality, for instance.

The test of Gillick competence is consequently a stringent one, and its operation raises a simple issue of equity. It would be unfair if mature minors were required to satisfy a test of competence that adults – or a significant number of them – would fail but are nevertheless not required to satisfy. There is no good reason why children must be more able than their adult counterparts if their consent is to count. This point generalizes to cover all those – including, centrally, the mentally disabled – whose capacity to consent is in doubt.

Any actual evaluation of competence will probably involve a psychological test of some kind or the testimony in court of an expert. But it should be recognized that different tests will yield different results and that no single test can claim authoritative status. Similarly, expert witnesses can and do disagree in their assessments of competence. The contentious nature of evaluations of competence needs to be acknowledged, especially when so much rides on any particular assessment.

A number of further comments about children's consent are appropriate. First, the talk has been of competence to consent. But consent must also be informed and voluntary. Children may be thought of as especially vulnerable to the influences of those closest to them, most obviously parents. If the parents strongly desire a course of treatment and make their wishes known to the child, can the child make a truly free and independent decision? All of us are to a degree subject to the influences of others and inclined in our decision-making to seek the approval of those we are closest to. But children are arguably especially dependent on their parents and guardians, and thus particularly prone to their influence.

Again, a child may not be in a position to give informed consent because she is not informed. Further, she may not be informed because the medical personnel judge that full disclosure of the relevant information would not be in her best interests. Disclosure, for instance, might be thought of as extremely distressing to the child. Care here is needed. There may well be good reasons to withhold information from a patient. But doing so effectively forecloses the possibility of informed consent being given and thus amounts to prejudging of competence. It would certainly be wrong to judge a young person able to make a choice about her treatment but not sufficiently able to receive information on the basis of which such a choice could be made.

In general terms it is important to emphasize that even when a child is not Gillick competent, it remains good medical practice to keep her informed about her situation and any proposed actions. The evidence suggests that children kept in the know about their condition, the treatment and its outcomes are better patients. They cooperate more fully with and are more responsive to the treatment (Alderson, 1993; Mahall, 1995). Moreover, there is a moral obligation on doctors to inform their patients about what they propose to do. This is as true of children as it is of adults. Hence, a paediatrician's actions conform to good practice if she explains to a 7-year-old child what, for instance, a lumbar puncture is and what it involves. This remains the case whether or not she needs that child's consent to the procedure (Mahowald, 1996).

It helps here to note that consent is normally distinguished from assent, just as the withholding of consent is seen as distinct from dissent. The giving of consent is an agreement *to* a proposal, state of affairs or whatever, whereas assent is agreement *with* a proposal and so on. The former is a basic, normatively transformative act, whereas the latter is a state of mind or attitude. Giving consent is something I do, whereas assent is what I feel or think about something. A parallel distinction holds between withholding consent and dissent. An individual can thus give her consent to that with which she disagrees, just as she can withhold consent from that with which she does agree (Archard, 1998).

The relevance to children is as follows. A child may not be competent to consent but, nevertheless, be fully able (and more than prepared) to express agreement or disagreement with a medical proposal. Let us say that a doctor prefers treatment A to treatment B, although both secure the desired state of affairs. This is because both A and B carry slight risks, but A is less risky than B, for instance, or because B involves marginally more discomfort than A, or because B takes a little more time to work than A. The child is not Gillick competent but expresses a strong preference for the second course of treatment, B, over the first, A. Indeed, she loudly and explicitly dissents from A. The doctor has good reason to choose treatment B. The good reason is not that the child withholds consent from A but gives it to B. This is not a good reason because, *ex hypothesi*, the child's 'consent' counts for naught. The good reason is that the child will cooperate with treatment B but not A because it is the former that she agrees with. Such cooperation may help to ensure that the treatment works, that it will involve less distress to the patient and so on.

A final remark about consent is in order. This is that the giving and withholding of consent within the medical context is not likely to be a single, isolated event but rather a process extended over time and subject to negotiation, changing circumstances and new information. This feature of consent is especially important in the case of children. One central reason often given for thinking that children are not able to make their own choices is that they are inconstant, fickle and affectively unstable – expressing a preference one day for that which is rejected the next day, and vice versa. Assessments of a child's competence to consent must thus be made over time and not amount to a single 'snapshot' judgement. It is entirely possible that a child should come to understand her illness and the treatment options open to her and should come to have a clear and settled view about how she would like matters to proceed. She could, in this sense, mature into a state of Gillick competence.

CONSENT TO AND REFUSING TREATMENT

In respect of treatment, some have discerned a fundamental asymmetry between consent to and refusal of treatment. In the case of adults, an ability to give consent is also sufficient to ground any refusal of treatment. An adult can choose to have an operation or choose not to, and no distinction is made in respect of her competence to choose between the two kinds of choice. However, this is not thought so – at least not by the English courts in a series of judgements after Gillick – in the case of children (*Re E,* 1993; *Re L,* 1998; *Re M,* 1999).

Thus, imagine a 15-year-old wants a particular operation but her parents do not. The courts might be satisfied that she is Gillick competent and thus that her parents' right to choose for her cedes to her own right to choose for herself. On the other hand a 15-year-old might refuse a life-saving operation against the wishes of her parents and contrary to the best judgement of the medical personnel. Here the courts might rule that the operation should, nevertheless, proceed.

Now of course it could be that the court determines her not to be Gillick competent. Employing a functional understanding of competence it could judge that her decision to refuse life-saving treatment is much more portentous than a decision to have treatment and, hence, requires a higher degree of ability than she actually displays. Moreover, she is making a choice at variance with that of medical experts who may be assumed to be better placed to know what should be done. Thus, she is making a very unwise decision and that could be taken as presumptive evidence of her incapacity.

However, care is needed. Doctors may indeed have expertise in respect of diagnosis, prognosis and the terms of treatment. But they cannot and should not be assumed to be authoritative in respect of judgements about whether a life is worth living under certain terms, or whether a treatment can be endured. A 15-year-old deemed Gillick competent to choose life-saving treatment is also Gillick competent to refuse such treatment. Either she chooses a difficult life over death, or she chooses death over a life she considers intolerable.

On the other hand the court could deem the 15-year-old who refuses life-saving treatment to be Gillick competent but judge that it has an obligation to act in her best interests which is more pressing than that of respecting her choices. Yet again, however, caution is needed. If it is under such an obligation, it is so also in cases where a mature minor chooses to have treatment, which it considers not to be in her best interests. There is no justification for a simple asymmetry between choosing and refusing treatment, with Gillick competence being determinative of the outcome in the former but not in the latter. Rather a principled distinction must be made between competent choices which do and those which do not significantly harm the interests of the child. However if this is the proper distinction, it is not a justifiable one. If a child is Gillick competent then she is, in all significant respects, the equal of an adult; she should be able to choose *and* to refuse treatment just as an adult can.

The following is an important consideration in cases where a court determines that it is in the best interests of a child that she should have an operation or course of treatment that she, for her part, refuses. This is that the court's judgement may only be enforceable by measures of compulsion such as detention or the use of force. In some cases – for instance, psychiatric treatment – the use of such measures might simply be counterproductive or in conflict with the treatment itself. Again consider cases where a treatment is refused on strongly held religious grounds. Compelling a child to undergo treatment in these circumstances might be thought wrong if the outcome is a child deeply and permanently unhappy with and unable to accept her situation. Thus, although an operation might initially be thought in the child's best interests, enforcing it might not be on balance and, considered in the whole, be in her best interests.

'SAVIOUR SIBLINGS'

Medical interventions intended to benefit not the child but another party need to be considered. This is the case – normally referred to as that of 'saviour siblings' – with tissue donation to a sister or brother. The decision to conceive a child, or to select, pre-implantation, an embryo with a view to the child serving as a tissue donor once born is properly subject to ethical review. But the issues raised by these kinds of case are distinct from those under consideration here. What is relevant in the present context is the putative consent of an existing child to tissue donation. It is appropriate in the first instance to distinguish between the donation of renewable tissue or blood, and the donation of a non-renewable but superfluous organ such as a kidney. Clearly, the latter is a far more serious matter than the former, and any judgement of the donor child's competence to consent must fully be sensitive to these differences. Indeed legal regulations might well be informed by the judgement that donation of non-renewable tissue should never be open to the consent of even a mature minor.

Again although we could judge that a child is generally competent to give or to withhold consent to medical treatment, we might fail properly to acknowledge the extraordinary pressures to which a family member can be subject in these circumstances. Can we really appreciate what it must be like for a child who is asked by her parents to make a tissue donation that represents the only way in which her beloved sibling's life could be saved? When the child agrees to the donation does she really do so willingly? This is the stuff of not just intriguing philosophy but also engaging fiction (Picoult, 2004).

But what should we say when the potential donor child is not competent to consent? Should the operation, nevertheless, proceed? After all it may be the only way in which the life of the sibling can be saved. Even though incapable of consent, the child may express a clear wish to help. In the sense indicated above, she assents to the prospective treatment. Talk of the benefits to the donor child – the psychological and emotional rewards of having saved a family member's life – may well be justified. Or such talk might only amount to a specious rationalization of a procedure whose real justification is a straightforwardly consequentialist one. A life is saved at the expense only of minimal discomfort or pain to the child operated on.

Once again it is not appropriate in this context to appeal to the hypothetical consent a child would, if competent, give to such an operation. A substituted judgement justification is plausible when we can construct one from the settled dispositions and beliefs of a person over time. This is not going to be possible in the case of a child. If the child objects to the operation, then that objection should be a weighty reason against proceeding. This is so even if the child is not competent to withhold consent. Overriding her dissent, and simply factoring it into an estimation of overall costs which also include those of the operation itself, means treating her only as a means to the desired end of the sibling's saved life. It fails to acknowledge the child as the source of wishes and fears; it violates an entirely defensible obligation to protect the vulnerable from exploitation and harm.

CHILDREN'S CONSENT TO RESEARCH

What then of a child's consent to research? The relevant considerations and arguments are many (Montgomery, 2001). Some would make a distinction between therapeutic and non-therapeutic research, the former alone being of potential direct benefit to the subject. Arguments about the permissibility of research on children then turn on this distinction. However, others do not find the distinction entirely helpful. This is in part because it may not always be easy to draw, but principally it is because its use can be thought to distract attention from the nature of the research itself to its aim or purpose. What is actually being done to a child and how she is involved in the research perhaps matter most. Nevertheless, we should always give consideration to the benefits and harms for the subject of any proposed research.

At one extreme is the view that no research whatsoever should involve children. The Nuremberg Code holds that research is only ever permissible if informed consent is obtained, and consent can only ever be obtained from those legally competent to give it. This amounts to an absolute prohibition on research on minors. This position is not credible. It would rule out therapeutic research that might, for instance, be life-saving. It would also rule out any research that held no or negligible risks for the child but carried enormous potential benefits for humanity as a whole.

Consider also the following: if it is not possible to test drugs and procedures on children, then the actual ongoing medical treatment of children will have to be done without the benefit of knowledge gained from any controlled tests. It is not just that children in the future cannot benefit from trials done now; it is also that what is and must currently be medically done for children on a daily basis can have, strictly speaking, no warrant from past trials. Rather, such treatment will simply be a matter of custom and established practice.

A more plausible view then is that there should not be an absolute prohibition on but only a presumption against using children for research. The presumption, in turn, may be thought to derive from the obligation upon us all to protect the most vulnerable members of our society from harm and exploitation. This view does not say that research on children is never justified, but it does demand that good reasons always be provided for proceeding with any such research. Two conditions in particular are frequently, and rightly, insisted upon. The first is that the use of children is essential because it is not possible to obtain the information from adults or by any other means. The second is that any risks to the children meet a threshold requirement of acceptability. If these conditions are satisfied, then research on children may be justified.

Note, first, that no appeal can or should be made to consent. The justification of the use of children who are not Gillick competent in research that does not benefit them directly is not that they would consent under certain hypothetical circumstances. To repeat a point made several times already, there is no space for the idea of the competent adult in whose person the child might choose. Thinking in this way takes us too far from anything that could reason-ably be represented as a choice by this child.

Furthermore, to secure the desired conclusion the adult who would consent to undergo distress and pain in order to benefit others has to be represented in ideal terms. So it is not just a child choosing as a competent adult who would consent to the operation, it is a child choosing as a competent adult who is motivated by an appropriate moral concern for the welfare of others (MacCormick, 1974). The justificatory work in such a form of reasoning is not done by consent. Rather it is done by the good reasons someone would have to make a sacrifice for the welfare of others. Note then that the reason-ing would extend to adults: an adult would, if motivated by a suitable concern for others, agree to take part in research that benefited others. Would the hypothetical consent of his better self constitute any kind of binding agreement on a person to participate in research he actually refuses?

The second comment to make in this context concerns the role of parents. Most agree that non-competent children could not be made to participate in research if their parents objected – even if the research satisfied the two conditions above, and presaged enormous benefits for humanity. How-ever, what role does the proxy consent of a parent play? A parent cannot donate his child to research as a mere exten-sion of his own self. If a parent's proxy consent to the child's participation in the research has force, it can only be inas-much as the parent is considered a good – perhaps the best placed – judge of what is in the child's interests. A parent's consent serves as a guarantee, albeit not an infallible one, that the child's best interests are safeguarded. Once again we see the force of the distinction between a justification that proceeds from a claim about what is good for children and one that is claimed to follow from the mere fact of be-ing a parent.

GENETIC TESTING OF CHILDREN

Finally, there is a form of medical intervention involving children which does not fit into either category of research or treatment, but which does broach issues of consent. This is the predictive genetic testing of children for diseases that will only develop in adulthood and which are resistant to any form of treatment. Such testing may be said to deny to the future competent adult the freedom to take the decision not to undergo the test and thus not to know whether she suffers from the disease. Securing the informed consent of individuals is a way, indeed the principal way within the medical context, in which the autonomy of individuals is respected. Thus, testing children who are not competent to consent removes from the future adults they will become the power of consenting to or withholding consent from the test (Malpas, 2005).

How might the defender of such testing in children respond? He might first point to the many possible interven-tions in children's lives, which remove from the subsequent adults powers of choice over some significant matter. Consider merely baptism, circumcision, vaccination and intelligence tests. In what respects are these significantly different from genetic testing? Indeed, why not think that any form of education shapes an adult's life in such a manner that subsequently some choices are open to her but some others are closed. One might convincingly argue that what really matters is the range and quality of choices an adult is bequeathed by her childhood.

Moreover, autonomous choices are never made in a vacuum. They are made by somebody possessed of a cer-tain character and identity, and within a context of relevant information. Does not the acquiring of genetic information in childhood help to form the nature of the adult? Is not the possession of a disposition to suffer a non-treatable disease an essential part of a person's identity? This would suggest that an adult cannot make genuinely autonomous life choices if she does not know who she is, and awareness of her medi-cal condition, secured through testing in childhood, is an important and ineliminable part of her self-knowledge.

In sum, it is hard to see how the genetic testing of children poses a distinct, particular or significant threat to the autonomy of the future adult. Moreover, the adult herself cannot make autonomous decisions unless she has acquired essential information about herself and is also possessed of a well-formed identity. Crucial to both of these is early genetic testing in relevant cases.

CHILDREN'S RIGHTS

Article 12 of the United Nations Convention on the Rights of the Child accords to 'the child who is capable of form-ing his or her own views the right to express those views freely in all matters affecting the child, the views of the child being given due weight in accordance with the age and maturity of the child' (UNCRC, 1989). Clearly, medi-cal and health matters affect the child, and thus the Article ensures that children should be participants in the processes of decision-taking about these matters. At one extreme the child's consent is required to any intervention inasmuch as the child is already sufficiently mature to be treated as if she was an adult. But when the child is not deemed competent enough to give or to withhold consent, she ought still to be consulted and her views given some weight.

Doing so acknowledges that the child is both a prospec-tive and a partial agent. The child is on the road to be-coming an adult decision-taker. Accordingly, children are given a voice and making them participants in decision-making helps the process of maturation and education whose goal is self-sufficient adulthood. But children are not as yet full agents. Hence, we give their views *some* weight, even when these are not, as they are with adults, entirely determinative of the matter. We can better safeguard the interests of children if they are participants, and they will become better participants if we give their views weight. The world as a whole is better managed, and the overall outcomes are better ones, if we allow children to have some say in what happens to them. This is as true in the medical domain as it is in any other area of children's lives.

REFERENCES

Alderson P. *Children's Consent to Surgery*. Buckingham: Open University Press, 1993.

Archard D. *Sexual Consent*. Oxford: Westview Press, 1998.

Beauchamp TL, Childress JF. *Principles of Biomedical Ethics*, 5th edition. Oxford: Oxford University Press, 2001.

Buchanan AE, Brock DW. *Deciding for Others, The Ethics of Surrogate Decision Making*. Cambridge: Cambridge University Press, 1989.

Gillick v West Norfolk and Wisbech Area Health Authority 1985; 3 All ER (HL) 402.

MacCormick RA. Proxy consent in experimentation situations. *Perspect Biol* 1974; **18**: 2–20.

Mahall B. The changing context of childhood: children's perspectives on health care resources including services. In: Botting B, ed. *The Health of our Children*, decennial supplement. London: Office of Population, Censuses and Surveys, HMSO, 1995; pp. 21–27.

Mahowald MB. On caring for children. In: Thomasman DC, Kushner T, eds. *Birth to Death: Science and Bioethics*. Cambridge: Cambridge University Press, 1996; pp. 85–98.

Malpas P. Predictive genetic testing in children and respect for autonomy. *Int J Children's Rights* 2005; **13**: 251–263.

Montgomery J. Informed consent and clinical research with children. In: Doyal L, Tobias JS, eds. *Informed Consent in Medical Research*. London: BMJ Books, 2001; pp. 173–181.

Nelson HL, Nelson JL. *The Patient in the Family: An Ethics of Medicine and Families*. London: Routledge, 1995.

Nuremburg Code, 1949; Web: http://www.hhs.gov/ohrp/references/nurcode.htm.

Picoult P. *My Sister's Keeper*. London: Hodder and Stoughton, 2004.

Re E (A Minor). Wardship: Medical Treatment 1993; 1: FLR 386.

Re L. Medical Treatment 1998; 2: FLR 810.

Re M. Child: Refusal of Medical Treatment 1999; FLR 753.

Ross LF. *Children, Families, and Health Care Decision-Making*. Oxford: Clarendon Press, 1998.

UNCRC. The United Nations Convention on the Rights of the Child, 1989; Web: http://www.unicef.org/crc/crc.htm.

Young R. Informed consent and patient autonomy. In: Kuhse H, Singer P, eds. *A Companion to Bioethics*. Oxford: Basil Blackwell, 1998; pp. 441–451.

42

Patients and Disclosure of Surgical Risk

JUSTIN OAKLEY

During the recent scandal involving surgeon Dr Jayant Patel at Queensland's Bundaberg Base Hospital, intensive care nurse Toni Hoffman vividly described what happened with one of the patients at the hospital:

> We had a patient who had a caravan roll on his chest. He was one of the other surgeons' patients so he needed to be transferred out. And then Dr Patel came in and just said, 'Oh, this patient doesn't need to go to Brisbane,' very loudly, and put a stop to the transfer. I had actually begged the other surgeon, 'Please transfer this patient out because I'm really afraid he's going to die.' There was the CT scan of the man's chest. They found that he had three litres of blood in his lung. And they decided they would send him to Brisbane . . . I came back in the morning and I met the Director of Anaesthesia outside the lift, and I just said, 'Oh, did Mr Bramich get off all right?' He said, 'No, he died.' I just said to him 'We have to do something about this man. We cannot let this go on any longer' . . . Dr Patel had decided to drain off what he thought was fluid around the man's heart. There was no fluid around the man's heart. He decided that he was still going to do this. And the nurse who was looking after [Mr Bramich] describes a stabbing motion with a very thick needle, around 50 times. And he told Mrs Bramich that she wasn't to cry when her husband died. The image that I have, they had a little girl, and she was standing at the end of the bed, and she was watching And we couldn't do anything. And I think that after that . . . we all . . . thought 'Well, we have to do something' (Australian Story, 2005).

In his account of the widely publicized tragedies in paediatric cardiac surgery at Bristol Royal Infirmary during the 1990s, anaesthetist Stephen Bolsin spoke of his attempts to prevent one of the cardiac surgeons from performing an operation for which the surgeon had a particularly high mortality rate:

> During this time [1990–1992], Mr Dhasmana began performing arterial switch procedures on neonates, with disastrous consequences . . . In late December 1994 . . . I discovered, from the routinely circulated operating list, that Mr Dhasmana intended to undertake one more [arterial] switch operation, in January 1995. The child was 18 months old and had previously undergone palliative surgery. We immediately notified all the clinical and nonclinical managers within the hospital who we thought would be able to influence Mr Dhasmana to cancel the operation, but no one was prepared to help. . . The next day the operation went ahead and the child died on the table (Bolsin, 1998: pp. 370–372).

These two cases highlight the appalling effects that surgical incompetence can have on patients and their families, when rogue surgeons continue to practise without adequate scrutiny. The cases also provide extreme illustrations of a general point which has received little discussion in health care ethics – that the risks of a surgical procedure depend in part on the ability of the surgeon who performs it.

There are risks inherent in any surgical procedure. Coronary artery bypass graft patients, for instance, may risk various post-operative effects and complications, such as wound infection, cognitive impairment, stroke and depression, among other things. These sorts of risks are typically spelled out in general terms by patient information leaflets. Another risk factor in surgery, though not usually mentioned in patient information leaflets, is the level of skill of the particular surgeon who performs the operation. Apart from the outright surgical incompetence seen at Bundaberg and Bristol, there is obviously a range of ability amongst surgeons deemed competent by the standards appropriate to each surgical speciality. Surgical outcomes are, of course, determined by many factors, including the initial condition of the patient, the quality of pre- and post-operative care and the abilities of the surgical team overall, but the skill of the surgeon themselves is clearly a vital factor in producing a successful outcome for the patient. This is a key reason why different surgeons have different success and failure

Principles of Health Care Ethics, Second Edition   Edited by R.E. Ashcroft, A. Dawson, H. Draper and J.R. McMillan

rates for a given procedure. So, a surgeon's track record for a particular procedure can be regarded as simply another type of risk information, just like the risk information gathered from clinical studies of that procedure. Because these various sorts of risks can be matters of interest and concern to patients, the disclosure of surgeon performance data to patients is a good case study of respecting patient autonomy in health care, and of informed consent and its limits.

INFORMED CONSENT AND SURGEON RISKS

Given that one's risks in surgery vary in part according to which surgeon performs the operation, the standard doctrine of informed consent can be applied here straightforwardly. That is, informed consent to a medical procedure is widely thought to require the disclosure and understanding of those aspects which the patient regards as material, or relevant, to their decision about that procedure. Patients typically regard various risks of a procedure as relevant to their decision about whether to consent to the procedure, and some patients view a surgeon's track record as a risk factor worth considering. Not providing this track record to a patient who regards this as relevant information can therefore be seen as a failure to obtain the patient's informed consent, just as not informing a patient about the risks of various side effects and complications is a failure to gain informed consent, where the patient views these factors as relevant (as most patients clearly do) (see Clarke and Oakley, 2004). Clearly, neither the patients who died due to Dr Patel's incompetence at Bundaberg nor the parents of the children who died due to the incompetence of Dr Dhasmana (and another cardiac surgeon) at Bristol gave their informed consent to the procedures undertaken. There was a failure of informed consent in those cases, not because the procedures turned out badly, but because it is obviously relevant to patients and parents to know about the manifest inadequacies of those surgeons. In placing themselves or their loved ones in the hands of these surgeons, they were unwittingly making themselves or their loved ones vulnerable to the lethal consequences of surgical incompetence.

However, some who agree that informed consent requires giving patients the opportunity to know about and avoid rogue surgeons argue that it does not follow that health authorities are therefore obliged to develop and make available to patients a 'league table' on all surgeons' performance. For example, representatives of surgeons' professional organizations sometimes say that an absence of such publicly accessible league tables or other surgeon report cards could not pose a problem for informed consent. Ethical objections to surgeon report cards come from a number of sources (see Clarke and Oakley, 2007). But it is difficult to see how a lack of patient access to surgeon-specific performance information could be thought of as never to pose a problem for giving informed consent to various surgical procedures. For if one accepts that patients are morally entitled to know about the performance of surgeons such as Dr Patel and Dr Dhasmana, why would not patients also be morally entitled to know about the performance and outcomes of surgeons whose mortality rates are lower than those of Dr Patel and Dr Dhasmana?

Looking at this issue only in terms of a scale of mortality rates can skew the debate, by leading health professionals to ask the following question. At what point does a risk become low enough that a patient is not entitled to be provided with information about it? But this question is altogether misguided. Patients' moral entitlement to risk information about a particular medical procedure does not depend upon how high the inherent risks of that procedure are. What creates an ethical obligation to disclose a risk is not the magnitude or probability of the risk itself, but whether that particular risk is material to the patient and whether the doctor could reasonably be aware that this risk was material to this patient. The reason there is usually an ethical obligation to inform patients about risks with high magnitudes and/or probabilities is not because these risks are high, but because patients generally regard high risks as material to their decision (and it is reasonable to expect a doctor to realise this).

AUTONOMY AS CHOICE VERSUS AUTONOMY AS AUTHORIZATION

Enabling patients to give informed consent to a procedure is a way of showing respect for their autonomy. The notion of autonomous decision-making is thus more fundamental than the concept of informed consent. We sometimes decide, perfectly autonomously, that we wish to proceed with certain ventures without having very much information about them, so long as we have the information that we regard as relevant to our decision. Indeed, delegating our decision-making authority to someone else whose judgement we trust can itself be an autonomous decision (where we have good reasons for trusting their advice). So, a decision made without a great deal of information about treatment risks and alternatives could still count as autonomous – it depends how much we really value knowing, in these circumstances.

Those in favour of exposing rogue surgeons but against surgeon league tables sometimes argue that autonomy is all about choice and that although patients should be able to avoid rogue surgeons, the failure to make a surgeon's track record available to patients is no failure to respect patient autonomy because many patients (in countries with national health schemes, such as the United Kingdom and Australia) do not have a choice of surgeon and so would not be able to act on such information. But being in a position where one is unable to act on risk information does not remove one's moral entitlement to it, if one still regards this information as relevant to one's decision. A commitment to respecting patient autonomy is not only about helping patients make informed *choices* between different interventions and therapies, and respecting those choices when made but it is also about helping patients *understand* what it is they are consenting to, even when there is only one option available to them. (As Faden and Beauchamp [1986] put it, informed consent is best understood as a patient's 'autonomous authorization' of the procedure that a health professional proposes to perform on them.) Thus suppose, for instance, that there was only one effective medication available to treat a condition of yours. It would be clearly absurd for a health professional to argue that you are therefore not morally entitled to information about the side effects of this medication. If you consider the side effects of the medication worth knowing about, then being told about those side effects is part of what is involved in your *authorizing* this medication being administered to you. Similarly, the fact that the design of a particular health system precludes patients having the option of choosing a different surgeon from the one allocated to them for the procedure does not entail that patients in that system lack a moral entitlement to information about the risks of this operation when performed by this particular surgeon (and this applies whether the surgery is elective or non-elective). Providing surgeon-specific performance information to a patient who wishes to have this information is helping this patient autonomously authorize the operation upon them in the first place, and so is a key way of respecting this patient's autonomy.

Of course, those emphasizing autonomy as choice could argue that patients still have the choice of refusing the operation, and so any obligation to provide patients with relevant surgeon performance information would still derive from an understanding of autonomy as choice. However, basing the obligation to inform patients on the value of helping them choose between options is misleading because this can lead us to overlook the importance of informing patients to help them understand and assess the various aspects of their decision that matter to them, even if this information would not lead them to choose differently. The idea that information *material* to a patient ought to be made available to them means that they ought to be provided with information that they consider *relevant* to their decision (whether information about possible side effects or about surgeon-specific risks), even if the information is not such as to make them change their mind about having the procedure. For instance, if a patient considers information about the likely size of the scar after their incision has healed as relevant to their decision about having the surgery, then

they ought to be given this information, even if it is unlikely to change their mind about having the surgery (see Faden and Beauchamp, 1986).

What risk information will be material to patients deciding about a particular procedure is difficult to fully specify in advance, as some patients want a great deal of risk information whereas other patients want very little. Just as there are patients who want to know about many of the possible side effects and complications of a procedure (even when these are very remote), there are also patients who want to know how their chances of a successful outcome might be influenced by the surgeon's own characteristics such as the surgeon's track record with the procedure in question (see Robinson and Brodie, 1997; Schneider and Epstein, 1998; Marshall et al., 2000; Kaiser Family Foundation, 2004). For example, a study of patients' consent to various emergency department procedures (like suturing or inserting an intravenous line) carried out by inexperienced medical students found that most patients wanted to know if it was the student's first time at performing the procedure, but the study also found that most patients gave their consent to the student carrying out the procedure, in any case (Santen et al., 2005, cited in Spriggs, 2007).

Also, risk information can be about the average probability of some outcome eventuating from a given procedure, or it could be about the probability of this outcome eventuating for a certain patient, given their specific characteristics. Patients usually consider information about the risks to them in a given procedure or health care decision as more important than information about the risks of this procedure or decision for patients generally – we often especially value attempts to establish where we ourselves might fall on a distribution curve representing the probabilities of a particular outcome occurring across a group of patients. For example, the average probability across a population of having a child with a particular genetic disease may be of some interest to prospective parents, but many of those who have reason for concern about this also want to know the risk that they (together with their partner) will pass on that genetic disease to their offspring. This is the sort of thing some prospective parents discuss with a genetic counsellor. When patients value knowing about their own risks in some procedure more highly than they value knowing the average risks for that procedure, informing them about patient-specific risks is more important for respecting their autonomy than is informing them about the average risks of that procedure.

A similar point can be made about surgeon performance information. Public reporting of hospital outcomes for a given procedure (as seen, for instance, in the UK 'Dr Foster' league tables) is sometimes advocated as a more ethically acceptable alternative by those opposed to surgeon league tables. But, although hospital outcomes data may be of some interest to patients considering a certain procedure, patients will often attach more value to information about surgeon-specific outcomes for that procedure. In such cases then, making surgeon-specific outcome information available to patients best respects their autonomy. Where a patient values having surgeon-specific outcome information for a given procedure, providing them with this information is part of helping them autonomously authorize the procedure being performed on them.

Focusing on hospital data and system-level failures rather than individuals is sometimes advocated as a way of improving safety by encouraging a culture of openness about mistakes. For example, the influential US Institute of Medicine report *To Err is Human* argues that 'The problem is not bad people; the problem is that the system needs to be made safer' (see Kohn et al., 2000, p. 49; see also Leape and Berwick, 2005). But whether or not such a strategy effectively improves patient safety generally, looking *solely* at system errors and hospital-level data hinders the appropriate identification and redress of problems with individual clinicians, as happened in the initial investigations into adverse patient outcomes at Bundaberg (see Davies, 2005, p. 165). For, among other things, one or two surgeons' poor results can be masked in the unit-level data by the excellent results of their colleagues (as was the case at Bristol).

None of this is to underestimate the size of the task involved in developing meaningful comparative performance information, which can be used to help patients understand the significance of their surgeon's mortality rate or other outcomes. Many surgeons have long kept records of their patient outcomes, but meaningful comparisons with other surgeons' outcomes requires establishing a common dataset so that the same types of information are collected, adjusting raw outcomes (e.g. raw mortality rates) to take into account the particular mix of patients a given surgeon operates on (such as whether or not the surgeon has a disproportionate number of high-risk patients), and benchmarking to determine significance levels beyond which results are to be regarded as genuine outliers. Carrying out these tasks properly can take several years, as the recent UK experience in the wake of the Bristol Royal Infirmary inquiry attests. But once adequate comparative surgeon-specific performance information exists, then, as with other forms of risk information, doctors should not wait until a patient asks for this information. Rather, doctors should be proactive by making patients aware that such performance information exists, without patients having to specifically ask for it. Proper respect for patient autonomy requires surgeons to volunteer their track records to patients, in case a patient wishes to see the record. Of course, league tables of surgeon-specific performance data may not be readily comprehensible to patients at first glance. For example, New York State's presentation of each cardiac surgeon's risk-adjusted mortality rate for coronary

artery bypass grafts usually requires some explanation to patients. But health professionals have an ethical obligation to assist patients to understand surgeon performance data, whether for the sake of helping patients make more informed choices between surgeons, or at least (where this choice is not available), in order to help with patients autonomously authorizing the surgery to be performed. Health professionals tend to be rather practically minded individuals and so may see facilitating patient understanding of risk information as important only when patients can *act* upon this understanding. But a conception of autonomy-as-authorization also requires helping patients comprehend the data, for the purposes of properly authorizing the procedure to be performed.

DEFENSIVE SURGERY AND THE VALUE OF PATIENT AUTONOMY

The publication of surgeon report cards raises many other ethical issues, apart from the questions about autonomy, informed consent and risk that I have considered here. The most common objection to publishing individual surgeon performance information is that this makes surgeons unwilling to operate on 'high-risk patients'. As I mentioned earlier, the risks of surgery (and a surgeon's outcomes) depend not only on the surgeon's skills but also on the condition of the patient when they present for surgery: some patients are at greater risk of poor outcomes than others. For example, in cardiac surgery, patients over 65 needing emergency coronary bypass surgery are often classified as high-risk, as such patients tend to have higher mortality rates for this procedure than do other patients. If report cards on cardiac surgeons lead them to avoid high-risk patients, this would be a significant moral objection to report cards, as high-risk patients would then be disadvantaged by an environment where report cards exist. Evaluating this objection involves weighing the autonomy-based interests of individual patients obtaining the risk information they seek against the interests of high-risk patients in finding a surgeon to operate upon them. In closing then, I will briefly consider this 'defensive surgery' objection, since doing so will help clarify what moral weight individual patients' autonomy-based interests should have when compared with other moral considerations.

There is some evidence from New York State and Pennsylvania that lends support to the claim that cardiac surgeon report cards have made some cardiac surgeons more reluctant to operate on high-risk patients. However, this evidence also indicates that there are a significant number of cardiac surgeons who have not become more reluctant to take on high-risk patients due to the introduction of report cards (see Oakley, 2007). So, although this evidence is of some concern, the available empirical studies do not establish a general claim that high-risk cardiac patients cannot find a surgeon willing to take them on. But suppose further studies provided stronger evidence to support such a claim, would this show that publishing surgeon performance data is ethically unjustified, all things considered?

If a widespread defensive surgery reaction to surgeon report cards was more conclusively established, I do not believe the correct response would be to abandon the publication of surgeon performance data. Supporting high-risk patients' access to coronary artery bypass surgery is clearly an important social goal (up to the point where likely outcomes for such patients indicate that subsidizing their access to this costly procedure is still a just allocation of health care resources), but it seems to me implausible to argue that this socially important goal is best achieved by abandoning or preventing the publication of surgeon performance information. We have seen that surgeon performance data can be regarded simply as further information about one's risks in undergoing a particular surgical procedure, and that there is a strong autonomy-based argument for making these data available to patients who see this information as relevant to their decision about surgery. Patients' autonomy-based interests in being informed about medical procedures are not thought justifiably sacrificed in order to promote broader social goals in the case of *other* sorts of currently available risk information (such as information about side effects and complications of surgery), so why should it be any different when the risk information is about individual surgeons' mortality rates? And, if there is no plausible ethical requirement to *abandon* an existing surgeon data publication scheme in order to preserve (or restore) a certain level of access by high-risk patients to a particular surgical procedure, then it seems to me that preserving that level of access by such patients does not constitute sufficient reason to avoid *establishing* such a publication scheme, where one does not already exist. For why should the fact that a public reporting scheme is already in existence itself be a decisive factor here?

Indeed, there is something of a false dichotomy underlying this defensive surgery objection. For the objection seems to assume that any surgeon report card scheme will create a defensive surgery reaction whereby high-risk patients are disadvantaged, and so we must choose between one of these two scenarios. However, it is not clear that any surgeon data publication scheme will inevitably disadvantage high-risk patients. Surgeon performance data need to be properly risk-adjusted to enable fair comparisons to be made in the light of surgeons' varying patient profiles, and this process needs to be carried out in ways that surgeons themselves and their professional organizations have confidence in. Also, assistance needs to be made available to patients to help them interpret and contextualize surgeon data, where necessary, so that they do not jump to the wrong conclusions

if they notice (for instance) that a particular surgeon has a high raw mortality rate for a certain procedure. If steps like these are taken, then it may be possible to publish surgeon-specific performance data without disadvantaging high-risk patients through any defensive reactions by surgeons. So, the ethical significance of concerns about defensive surgery do not overturn the case for informing patients about the performance of individual surgeons (see Oakley, 2007).

CONCLUSION

It is clear that patients' risks in surgery depend not only on their own condition but also on which surgeon operates upon them. I have argued that surgeon data can be viewed as just another sort of risk information, and so the standard ethical doctrine of informed consent can also be applied here. That is, patients who regard surgeon performance information as relevant to their decision about surgery should be provided with this information, so that they can give their adequately informed consent to undergoing the procedure. We have also seen that the role such information can play in patients' decisions highlights an important general point about respecting autonomy in health care. That is, respecting patient autonomy is still meaningful and important when patients have only one option available to them (such as one effective medication, or one surgeon), for in doing so health professionals help patients to autonomously authorize the course of action to be taken, or the procedure to be performed on them. Many patients value having patient-specific and surgeon-specific risk information, and so adequately respecting patient autonomy requires making such information available to them. I also argued that, although the available evidence of a general defensive surgery reaction to report cards is inconclusive, better evidence for such a reaction would still not defeat the case for report cards. Nevertheless, measures can and should be taken to help safeguard high-risk patients' access to surgeons, under an ethically justifiable surgeon data publication scheme.

REFERENCES

Australian Story. ABC television documentary, 26 June 2005; http://www.abc.net.au/austory/content/2005/s1402495.htm
Bolsin SN. Professional misconduct: the Bristol case. *Med J Aust* 1998; **169**: 369–372.
Clarke S, Oakley J, eds. *Informed Consent and Clinician Accountability: The Ethics of Report Cards on Surgeon Performance.* Cambridge: Cambridge University Press, 2007.
Clarke S, Oakley J. Informed consent and surgeons' performance. *J Med Philos* 2004; **29**: 11–35.
Davies G. *Queensland Public Hospitals Commission of Inquiry – Report.* Brisbane: Queensland State Government, 2005; also at: www.phci.qld.gov.au

Faden RR, Beauchamp TL. *A History and Theory of Informed Consent*. New York: Oxford University Press, 1986.

Kaiser Family Foundation and Agency for Health Care Research and Quality. *National Survey on Consumers' Experiences with Patient Safety and Quality Information*. Washington, DC: Kaiser Family Foundation, 2004.

Kohn LT, Corrigan JM, Donaldson MS. *To Err is Human: Building a Safer Health System*. Washington, DC: Institute of Medicine, National Academy Press, 2000.

Leape LL, Berwick DM. Five years after. *To Err is Human*: What have we learned? *J Am Med Assoc* 2005; **293**: 2384–2390.

Marshall MN, Shekelle P, Leatherman S, Brook R, Owen JW. *Dying to Know: Public Release of Information about Quality of Health Care*. Los Angeles: RAND Corporation/Nuffield Trust, 2000.

Oakley J. An ethical analysis of the defensive surgery objection to individual surgeon report cards. In: Clarke S, Oakley, eds. *Informed Consent and Clinician Accountability: The Ethics of Report Cards on Surgeon Performance*. Cambridge: Cambridge University Press, 2007.

Robinson S, Brodie M. Understanding the quality challenge for health consumers: the Kaiser/AHCPR survey. *J Qual Improv* 1997; **23**: 239–244.

Santen S, Hemphill R, Spanier C, Fletcher N. 'Sorry, it's my first time!' Will patients consent to medical students learning procedures? *Med Educ* 2005; **39**: 365–369.

Schneider EC, Epstein AM. Use of public performance reports: A survey of patients undergoing cardiac surgery. *J Am Med Assoc* 1998; **279**: 1638–1642.

Spriggs M. The practical limits and value of informed consent. In: Clarke S, Oakley J, eds. *Informed Consent and Clinician Accountability: The Ethics of Report Cards on Surgeon Performance*. Cambridge: Cambridge University Press, 2007.

43

Confidentiality

REBECCA BENNETT

Medical confidentiality has long been regarded as a fundamental characteristic of the relationship between health care worker and patient. This notion of confidentiality of information passed from patient to health care professional is enshrined in virtually every code of practice relating to health care from the Hippocratic Oath onwards.

THE IMPORTANCE OF MEDICAL CONFIDENTIALITY

It is not contentious to say that medical confidentiality is deemed as important by patients and is generally assumed within the relationship between patient and health care worker. People expect information imparted to the doctors to be safe from disclosure and believe this to be an important characteristic of a medical consultation (Jones, 2003). But why is medical confidentiality important? There are two main reasons for the central role of medical confidentiality.

PRAGMATIC/CONSEQUENTIALIST

Perhaps the most fundamental reason why medical confidentiality is deemed central to the relationship between health care professional and patient is a pragmatic reason that focuses on optimizing this therapeutic relationship. As Margot Brazier explains:

> Doctors, like priests and lawyers, must be able to keep secrets. For medical care to be effective, for patients to be able to trust their doctor, they must be confident that they can talk frankly to him (Brazier, 2003, pp. 56–57).

There is evidence that breaches in confidentiality will affect the level of information imparted by patients (Jones,

2003). Thus, the consequences of breaching confidentiality are likely to result in patients being less candid about the information they divulge to health care professionals, which is likely to have a further consequence of impeding the level of treatment, support or counselling they will receive. The archetypal example of this is found in the treatment and prevention of HIV. Policy and practice relating to HIV and AIDS has emphasized patient autonomy and medical confidentiality. Without this emphasis on confidentiality it is thought that patients would not be frank about their risk behaviour and thus be unable to receive accurate advice and effective counselling, which may not only impact on their own health status but also may not facilitate the behavioural change that is the main focus on public health policy in this area. This reasoning is clear in the influential English case of *X v Y* (1988). This case focused on the issue of whether the names of two HIV-positive general practitioners could be made public. The judge in this case argued that if such exposure were sanctioned, health care professionals might be deterred from coming forward for testing and as a result pose a greater risk to patients. Rose J reviewed the evidence and concluded the following:

> [P]reservation of confidentiality is the only way of securing public health; otherwise doctors will be discredited as a source of education, for future individual patients will not come forward if doctors are going to squeal on them. (*X v Y*, 1988)

Confidentiality is fundamental for pragmatic, therapeutic reasons. The consequences of undermining this duty of confidence would not only be damaging to the individual patient's treatment and health to patients but would be damaging in terms of public health goals.

Principles of Health Care Ethics, Second Edition   Edited by R.E. Ashcroft, A. Dawson, H. Draper and J.R. McMillan
© 2007 John Wiley & Sons, Ltd

RESPECT FOR AUTONOMY

Although the importance of medical confidentiality can be defended adequately on the basis of pragmatic, consequentialist grounds alone, a high regard for medical confidentiality also fits well with modern medicine's focus on respect for individual autonomy.

It is generally accepted that respecting individual autonomy is a fundamental moral principle, enabling individuals to have control over their own lives. This is reflected in legal and social policy as well as ethical doctrine. It is this principle of respect for individual autonomy that justifies the move away from medical paternalism to a setting where the choices of patients are paramount. If one holds that respect for individual autonomy is important, one does so because this freedom to orchestrate one's own life is an important factor in making a life valuable. Thus, respect for individual autonomy dictates that patients should be in control of their medical treatment, emphasizing the importance of informed consent and confidentiality. Medical Research Council expresses this link with the notion of respect for autonomy well saying:

> Keeping control over facts about one's self can have an important role in a person's sense of security, freedom of action, and self-respect (Medical Research Council, 2000, p. 5).

Just as an insistence on informed consent to medical treatment allows patients to make authentic choices about their lives, so medical confidentiality allows patients to remain in control of information about their lives, the disclosure of which may be detrimental.

IMPORTANT BUT NOT ABSOLUTE

While confidentiality is held to be central to the relationship between health care professional and patient there would be very few who would argue that this duty to maintain patient confidentiality should be considered absolute. The reasons for this are clear. The very principles that explain the importance of confidentiality also undermine it. Thus, while consequential reasoning and respect for autonomy generally require that we maintain medical confidences, in some cases the same consequential reasoning and respect for autonomy seem to require that we breach confidentiality. Consider the famous Tarasoff case (1976). In this case, a disturbed man revealed to his psychiatrists that he had homicidal thoughts towards his girlfriend. His confidentiality regarding this information was maintained, and the woman was not warned. The patient murdered her. On both consequentialist grounds and based on a general respect for autonomy, there are good reasons to argue that the confidentiality of a patient with such murderous intentions should be breached in order to warn a third party at risk. While breaching confidentiality in this instance may result in an erosion of trust between patient and psychiatrist, perhaps even result in harm to others as a result, the alternative consequences of failing to prevent murder are severe. Similarly, although a breach of confidentiality undermines the patient's autonomy, removing his control over this information, if respect for autonomy is important in order to allow individuals control over their lives, then not attempting to prevent murder seems inconsistent with this respect for individual lives. Thus, we are left with a scenario where it is typically held that 'confidentiality should be maintained without exception' but also agreed that 'confidentiality should be broken when people were placed at risk' (Jones, 2003, p. 350). This ethical dichotomy is enshrined in law and reflected in professional guidelines. So that while medical confidentiality is regarded as fundamental both ethically and legally, there are clear instances where law and morality either permit or require disclosure of 'confidential' information.

The ethical question of whether confidentiality should be breached is raised in many contexts. For instance, there are questions as to whether confidentially should be breached in order to protect the patient himself from harm (for example, in cases of potential suicide) or whether parents should be informed of their adolescent child's contraceptive prescription, abortion or eating disorder. The answers to these questions, at least in theory, are ethically relatively straightforward. If a patient can be shown to be competent and making what could be considered an autonomous choice, then, if the importance of respecting autonomy is accepted, breaching confidentiality will be ethically unjustifiable. The problematic issue here is not the ethics but the practicality of determining competency to make this decision. Similarly, it is ethically uncontroversial to stress that every attempt should be made to minimize the risk of accidental or careless breaches of confidentiality. This again is a practical problem.

However, an area of confidentiality that is hugely ethically complex and problematic is the issue of when breaching confidentiality is ethically acceptable in order to protect the interests or welfare of third parties. This chapter will attempt to analyse current approaches to this issue and the ethical foundations they are based on, in order to produce some recommendations for policy in this area.

PROTECTION OF THIRD PARTY INTERESTS/WELFARE

As we have already discussed, it is clear that in some instances it is morally acceptable (perhaps even morally required) that we breach confidentiality in order to protect others. The Tarasoff case outlined in the above section is a good example of this type of case. It is this moral requirement to breach confidentiality in order to protect others that provides foundations for the majority of legal duties that require or permit disclosure of patient information. In most jurisdictions, the law allows for breaches of confidentiality only where there are serious and identifiable risks to third parties whether that be as a result of physical attack, impaired driving, communicable diseases or failure to prevent a further outbreak of food poisoning. In this way, the law attempts to deal with the difficult ethical dichotomy that confidentiality embodies, allowing for breaches where serious harm to others is likely to be prevented by this disclosure, but maintaining a requirement for confidentiality in other cases.

This leaves health care workers in a very powerful and ethically complex position. While health care professionals have a general obligation to respect personal autonomy and consequently to maintain medical confidentiality, they also have an obligation to protect the welfare and autonomy of others. An obvious and well-used example here involves disclosure of HIV status, for example:

A man visits his general practitioner (GP) asking for an HIV test. He is worried that he may have become infected as a result of sex with prostitutes on a recent business trip. The HIV test proves to be positive. The GP attempts to persuade the man to disclose his HIV status to his wife (who is also a patient of the GP's). While the man confirms that he does have a sexual relationship with his wife, he refuses to disclose his HIV status to her.

Similar issues are raised in cases where a health care professional is led to believe, from information provided by a patient, that a third party is in danger as a result of sexual, mental or physical abuse or as a result of the consequences of other medical conditions – for example, an epileptic patient who insists on continuing to drive.

In such cases moral and legal duties are not easily distinguished as there are, and can be, no clear legal guidelines laid down in this area. Although it can be stressed that the risk to third parties must be 'serious' (General Medical Council, 2004, para 24), that is, 'risk of death or serious harm' (General Medical Council, 1997, para 19), that attempts should be made to persuade the patient to consent to disclosure (General Medical Council, 2004, para 24), and that ultimately 'the benefits to an individual or to society of the disclosure outweigh the public and the patient's interest in keeping the information confidential' (General Medical Council, 2004, para 22), such guidance leaves a great deal to the discretion of the health care professional. Although the legal/policy guidance that is provided stresses the need for such decisions to be well considered and restricted to cases where the third party is at risk of serious harm, these decisions, for the most part, are left to the *moral* judgements of individual health care professionals.

It is left to the particular health care professional to weigh up the consequences of the two possible courses of action: maintain confidentiality and risk harm to a third party or warn the third party and risk an erosion of trust in the relationship between health care professional and patient. This is not an easy calculation at the best of times. But there are further issues that complicate this calculation. We need to consider how serious the risk needs to be before it warrants this breach, we must also consider how likely the risk of harm is and whether breaching confidentiality is likely to prevent the harm. Although guidance based on past cases can be provided, this guidance will still leave the bulk of the decision-making to the individual health care worker.

The conclusions that are made in these instances, as well as depending on the detail available and the interpretation of this detail in order to calculate as clearly as possible the consequences of each possible course of action, will depend upon the weighting that the individual gives to respect for personal autonomy, and this will vary from person to person. It has been claimed that this weighting is even influenced by areas of practice; for instance, O'Brien and Chantler maintain the following:

For some doctors, particularly GPs and other clinicians, a rights based approach is paramount, perhaps because of their daily contact with, and responsibility for, the care of individual patients. Many other doctors, particularly those who work principally in public health, epidemiology and other research, have a broadly utilitarian approach to confidentiality (O'Brien and Chantler, 2003 pp. 36–37).

The decision made by health professionals in such cases will be shaped largely by their views regarding the relative importance of respect for autonomy versus a notion of the duty to protect others from harm. However, like any other complex ethical decision, there is a danger that this decision will also be influenced by personal beliefs and even prejudices. As Mason and Laurie concur:

In so far as it rests on subjective definitions, the doctor's overriding duty to society represents what is arguably the most controversial permissible exception to the rule of confidentiality. Society is not homogeneous, but consists of groups amenable to almost infinite classification – regional, political, economic, by age and so on. It follows that what one person regards as a duty to society may be anathema to another. Individual doctors are bound to weigh the scales differently in any particular instance . . . (Mason and Laurie, 2005, p. 260).

From this it is clear why such decisions are often controversial. The decisions taken will depend not only on the detail of the situation but also on the personal attitudes of the individual health care worker making this decision. This issue has become a particularly poignant one in the area of genetic testing. It is within this context that we will explore this subject further.

GENETIC TESTING

In recent years, the study of human genetics has enabled testing for a number of familial disease, including breast, ovarian and various kinds of colon cancer (Harris et al., 2005), as well as other disorders including Huntington's disease and Alzheimer's dementia. As genetic testing may provide information not only about the individual tested but also about his genetic relatives, it often raises particularly difficult issues of confidentiality. The issues are clear when we consider a case study, for instance:

> Steve knows that his uncle Geoff died at 42 from familial adenomatous polyposis, a type of colon cancer. This genetic disorder is characterized by the formation of polyps in the colon and without intervention virtually all of those with the disorder will have developed the cancer by the time they are 50-year-old. However, effective treatments are available if the condition is identified early (Giardiello et al. 1993). Steve knows that there is a chance that he is also affected by the disorder and wishes to undergo a genetic test to identify whether this is the case in order to allow early treatment if necessary. A genetic counsellor explains that if the test reveals that Steve is affected then this implies that his father (Geoff's brother) is also affected by the genetic disorder. He is advised to discuss this matter with his father. However, Steve's relationship with his father has broken down and he is adamant that he does not want to tell his father he has been tested or the result of any such test.

Although this case may seem to be very similar to those we have considered that deal with HIV infection, or the risk of harm caused by physical or sexual abuse, there have been calls to treat cases relating to genetic testing differently. These calls exemplify the problems generally associated with disclosure to protect third parties by reflecting the biases of those who propose policy revision. Those for whom respect for autonomy is fundamental to the morality of modern health care argue that confidentiality should never be breached in order to give others unsolicited genetic information, whereas those who believe that the possession of genetic information is a general good argue that policy on confidentiality should be relaxed in the area of genetic information in order to maximize this good. I will consider each side of the argument in turn.

RESPECT FOR AUTONOMY AND GENETIC 'EXCEPTIONALISM'

The term 'exceptionalism' was first used in the health care setting as a description of the novel policy approach to HIV/AIDS (Bayer, 1991). As we have seen, instead of the traditional approach to communicable disease control which may permit coercive testing, treatment and even quarantine, policy relating to HIV and AIDS tends to emphasize medical confidentiality, individual autonomy and informed consent. In recent years, there have been calls for what has been termed 'genetic exceptionalism'; the argument being that, as was the case with HIV/AIDS, 'genetic information is sufficiently different from other health care information that it deserves exceptional treatment' (Ross, 2001, p. 141).

One characteristic of this call for exceptional treatment of genetic information is a call for stricter protection of genetic privacy (Roche and Annas, 2001). The argument here is that genetic information is particularly sensitive information. As a result the damage done by breaching confidentiality relating to genetic information is, it is argued, potentially more damaging than disclosure of other types of medical information. Genetic information can reveal not only a great deal of information about the individual tested but also about their family members, perhaps revealing serious genetic disorders or even false paternity. This information may result in distress, discrimination, stigmatization and even penalties in terms of insurance and employment. Thus, the claim is that as disclosure of genetic information has these potentially widespread and damaging consequences, confidentiality should be protected even more strictly than other kinds of medical information. Roche and Annas express this view, explaining that;

> Some individuals want to know as much of this information about themselves as possible, and might be willing to share this information with their families and others. Others would rather remain ignorant about their own genetic make-up, and thus their risks for future illness, or at least keep others ignorant of such information. We believe that individual choices are best served by policies that place primary control over an individual's DNA and genetic information in the hands of individuals (Roche and Annas, 2001, p. 396).

Thus, here the primary focus of these arguments is the importance of respect for individual autonomy, that is, the importance of allowing individuals to decide for themselves if they wish to receive or disseminate this information about their genetic make up.

THE GOOD OF GENETIC INFORMATION AND 'SHARED OWNERSHIP'

At the other end of this debate are arguments aiming to enable broader disclosure of familial genetic information. Here, it is proposed that instead of considering the information as the individual patient's information, it is considered as belonging to all his genetic relations, thus allowing disclosure of this information to any individuals that may be affected (Wertz and Fletcher, 1991; Loewy, 1991; Sommerville and English, 1999; Weijer, 2000; Doukas, 2001; Parker and Lucassen, 2004).

Taking this type of position Parker and Lucassen argue that we should view the information produced from a genetic test not as personal information but as familial information where 'genetic information is shared by more than one person, much like information about a joint bank account' (Parker and Lucassen, 2004, p. 166). On this 'joint account model' the dilemma regarding whether to warn others of a possible genetic abnormality is

> not about the appropriate limits to confidentiality but is analogous to me asking my bank manager not to reveal information about a joint account to my fellow account holders. The problem the clinician faces is not when to respect confidentiality but what, if anything, would justify excluding others from the joint account. Whereas on the personal account model the default position is an assumption of confidentiality, on the joint account model it is assumed that information should be available to all account holders unless there are good reasons to do otherwise (Parker and Lucassen, 2004, p. 166).

Parker and Lucassen conclude that:

> The joint account model takes seriously the familial nature of genetic information and clinical genetics and offers the possibility of broad access to the benefits of testing, where this does not cause serious harm to the index patient (Parker and Lucassen, 2004, p. 166).

Thus, instead of maintaining confidentiality unless there is risk of serious harm to a third party, the claim here is that this information should routinely be disclosed unless it is thought that this disclosure will cause serious harm to the patient who generated this information.

GENETIC INFORMATION: A GENERAL GOOD?

In order to determine which of these approaches is the most morally appropriate, we need to determine whether the possession of genetic information is such a general good that it justifies the overturning of our usual respect for patient autonomy.

It is clear that for some people knowledge of their genetic make-up and any disorders or potential disorders this might reveal is helpful information that they wish to have to help them make more informed choices about their lives. However, it is clear from the low uptake of these tests that not everyone shares this view (Codori et al., 1999; Meiser and Dunn, 2000). Although allowing broader disclosure of genetic information assumes that this information is a good thing, it seems that at least in terms of public opinion this is not necessarily the case.

But perhaps public opinion about genetic information is not the deciding factor regarding whether this information is a good thing. Many have argued that in order to respect

individual autonomy we need to strive to ensure that people have all the available relevant information when making choices about their lives (Harris and Keywood, 2001). The claim is that without this information their choices cannot be informed and thus be deemed autonomous. In the context of genetic information, according to this argument, this means that not disclosing relevant genetic information to other family members, even where this information was not sought by this individual, would be to undermine an individual's autonomy. As Sommerville and English put it:

> the luxury of informed consent should not be exclusive to the individual in the family who, by luck or judgment, is the best informed about factors affecting all (Sommerville and English, 1999).

This argument is based on a particular formulation of respect for autonomy, a formulation usually attributed as originating with Immanuel Kant. Harris and Keywood explain this, arguing that:

> where the individual is ignorant of information that bears upon rational life choices she is not in a position to be self-governing. If I lack information, for example about how long my life is likely to continue, I cannot make rational plans for the rest of my life . . . Of course it is not necessarily irrational not to want to know one's probable life expectancy and many would be prepared to forgo autonomy rather than face the knowledge of a looming premature death. However, they cannot defend the wish to remain ignorant of a fact like that in the name of autonomy (Harris and Keywood, 2001, p. 421).

Thus, this formulation of respect for autonomy involves much more than enabling individuals' freedom to make choices about their own lives; it focuses on a *duty* to make informed decisions. So, as Häyry and Takala clarify, '[t]he idea seems to be that by concealing any facts from their patients, physicians commit the ultimate offence of forcing other to act immorally' (Häyry and Takala, 2001, p. 411).

It is clear that those who hold this particular formulation of autonomy would support a broader disclosure of the results of genetic tests. So that, in cases like that of Steve (above), the clinician would feel it her duty to disclose this information to relatives who are at risk from this disorder. If people have a moral duty to make informed decisions, then health care workers have a moral duty to enable this by imparting the information they have in their possession.

What also seems clear is that this conception of respect for autonomy would require disclosure in a majority of cases. Thus, although it has traditionally been assumed that confidentially should only be breached where there is a serious risk of harm that could be avoided by disclosure, under this conception of autonomy disclosure is required even where risks are less serious and treatments not available.

Thus, this conception of autonomy provides ethical foundations for proposals such as that put forward by Parker and Lucassen (2004) where the assumption will be that information relevant to others is disclosed apart from those in exceptional circumstances.

RESPECTING AUTONOMY OR UNACCEPTABLE PATERNALISM?

However, it could be argued that basing policy on the assumption that giving unsolicited information to individuals about their health state is a good thing undermines rather than enhances autonomy. If we move away from the Kantian conception of respect for autonomy and towards a conception that is perhaps more in line with our common understanding of this principle, the reasons for this will be clear.

It is normally assumed that respect for autonomy is important to allow individuals control over how they live their lives. Individuals are left to make their own decisions as to what they see as important or beneficial to them. It is usually accepted, ethically and legally, that the only exception is where an individual's actions risk serious harm to third parties. As we have seen, it is not clear that individuals do wish to have this information about their genetic make-up (Codori et al., 1999; Meiser and Dunn, 2000). This attitude to genetic information is particularly understandable in the majority of circumstances where genetic testing will reveal information about a disorder that may not have an effective 'cure' or may never develop. To assume that the reasonable and moral course of action is to disclose this information wherever the health care professional thinks this information is helpful to the individual arguably takes control away from the individual who is informed. This individual has not sought this information and may have good reasons not to do so. The enactment of a policy which includes the assumption of disclosing genetic information where it has not been sought is done on the basis of the 'doctor/health care worker knows best'.

It is difficult to see how taking control of our medical information away from patients and allowing disclosure, not only in extreme circumstances but routinely, is not medical paternalism. Paternalism is something that, in general, we no longer see as acceptable in modern medicine for the good reason that it removes the patient's control about their treatment and their lives. Paternalism is not only rejected as a infringement of individual autonomy but also because it assumes that health care professionals are somehow in a better position to decide what is the best course of action, even though these decisions do not focus on *clinical* decisions but *moral* ones. Thus, as Powers explains, there are

> significant worries about the wisdom of putting the healthcare professional in the role of enforcer of otherwise commendable social goals and of presuming that a decision about what is in the best interests of the family unit is within the scope of their moral authority or in principle a matter about which medical professionals are competent to judge. If one is in the grip of a largely paternalist view of healthcare professionals, one may be easily tempted to see this task as part of one's legitimate professional brief. . . . While medical professionals may have superior insight into the strictly medical aspects of the dilemma, even there we do not ordinarily presume that superior medical insight entitles them to override the purely medical aspects of their patients' decisions. Medical paternalism of this sort has been roundly rejected. That we should presume that healthcare professionals have superior moral insight into whether the expected medical benefits to the recipient of the information outweigh all of the other potential harms that might ensue grants to the medical profession a degree of moral authority that exceeds even that of the widely discredited versions of medical paternalism (Powers, 2002 pp. 374–375).

Although calls to allow wider disclosure of genetic information are undoubtedly well meaning, if accepted there is a danger that they will open the door to a culture of medical paternalism where individual health care professionals' views of their patients' best interests overrule their patients'.

IS GENETIC INFORMATION SO SIGNIFICANTLY DIFFERENT AS TO WARRANT DIFFERENT TREATMENT?

As we have seen, there has been a general trend to attempt to change policy in terms of confidentiality as it relates to genetic information on the assumption that genetic information is so significantly different from other medical information that this exceptional treatment is warranted. The 'special' nature of genetic information is used both as a reason to strengthen the requirement for confidentiality in this area and to relax it. However, unless this uniqueness of genetic information can be established convincingly, any change in policy regarding confidentiality in this area will inevitably bleed into all other aspects of medical care. So before going any further, we need to determine whether genetic information is sufficiently different to warrant this special treatment.

There is a great deal of scepticism as to whether genetic information does constitute a 'special' case (Ross, 2001; Powers, 2002). Whereas those who argue that confidentiality should be strengthened with regard to genetic testing emphasize that genetic tests reveal information that may cause distress, stigmatization and discrimination; this is also true of other diagnostic tests such as HIV or mental illness. Claims are made that there is not the same urgency relating to the 'harm' that is caused by an undiagnosed genetic disorder as there is with a potentially lethal, infectious or psychotic person; a person will be a carrier of a genetic disease whatever action is taken to warn him or her, and it may be many years before any preventative measures are appropriate. But clearly there are cases in which the speed of diagnosis will give patients with genetic disorders a greater chance of effective treatment, and it is difficult to see how information regarding possible genetic disorders relevant to reproductive decision-making does not suffer from delayed disclosure. Further, it is argued that in the cases like that of possible HIV transmission and physical assault the fact that it is these particular individuals that are the agents of the potential harm that distinguishes these cases from those of genetic disorders. The claim here is that, as the agents of harm, these individuals have somehow forfeited their rights to confidentiality. However, making this the basis of a clear distinction between these cases is dubious. First, the supposed aim of breaching confidentiality has nothing to do with punishment of 'wrong doers'; the aim is to prevent avoidable harm. To use forewarning as a sanction for unsavoury behaviour and to give individual health care professionals the role of judge and jury in such matters is to open a whole new layer of ethical problems. Second, if 'blameworthness' is seen as an important factor in breaching confidentiality, then it will be extremely difficult to determine with any accuracy the level of blame involved in this kind of cases. Is a psychotic fully responsible for his psychotic tendencies? Is an HIV-infected individual who takes reasonable precautions to prevent transmission of the virus to 'blame' when his partner becomes infected? On the other side of the argument, while genetic tests reveal information that is relevant to other members of the family, similarly relevant information may be revealed by a psychological assessment that reveals homicidal tendencies or a diagnostic test for a communicable disease.

Although space does not allow a detailed evaluation of these issues, what is clear is that the case for establishing genetic information as a 'special case' is far from proven. If genetic information is not a special case, then it should be treated in line with other medical information. As Ross explains:

> That genetics is non-exceptional also raises major implications for health policy. Genetic information raises important questions about privacy, confidentiality, the legitimate interests of individuals in the medical information of others, and whether health care providers have a duty to warn others who may not know they are 'at risk'.

The policy issues, however, cannot be treated as unique to genetics. Health policies need to be designed to protect all of our health care information and promote all of our health care interests; a patchwork system that gives additional protections only to genetic concerns is not a morally desirable solution (Ross, 2001).

The increase in the availability of genetic testing has stimulated the debate surrounding the issue of medical confidentiality. Although this new context arguably does not raise any novel issues it should be used as an opportunity to re-evaluate our general approach to confidentiality.

A desire to give others information that we feel is important to have is a very understandable and, in some cases, laudable aim. However, we need to be careful at what cost this disclosure comes. Before going down the road of allowing breaches of confidentiality in broader circumstances, the health care worker must consider the reasoning this is based on and the wider consequences of this action. If the result is an erosion of respect for autonomy, a return to paternalism and a decline of the trust between doctor/health care professional and patient, then, however well meaning this aim, it must be avoided. Even if we do not hold respect for autonomy as the most central issue ethical issue in this context, there are good pragmatic reasons for maintaining confidentiality in all but the most extreme cases.

Decisions as to whether confidentiality should be breached are already left, to a great degree, to the discretion of the individual health care professional. Even within a context where the assumption that confidentiality must be maintained except in exceptional circumstances, the nature of these decisions is such that the prejudices, biases and outlooks of the health care professional will greatly influence in which cases he discloses information and in which cases he does not. To widen the remit of these choices and to allow forewarning in other less serious circumstances would not only damage the clinical relationship but also allow much greater scope for the flourishing of prejudices and biases.

While the aim of those who wish to broaden the ability to disclose genetic information is to allow greater access to information about one's genetic make-up, this could arguably be achieved by promoting the availability of genetic counselling and testing and emphasizing the confidential nature of this service. This approach would not only increase the numbers of individuals who were aware of their genetic make-up but it would do so without undermining respect for autonomy by respecting confidentiality and ensuring that those who, perhaps for good reason, do not wish to know about their genetic make-up are not forced to do so simply because others believe this would be in their best interests. Guidance for both health professionals and patients in this complex and difficult area need to be clear, to reduce the scope of paternalism and to reassure patients.

REFERENCES

Bayer R. Public health policy and the AIDS epidemic. An end to AIDS exceptionalism? *N Engl J Med* 1991; **324**: 1500–1504.

Brazier B. *Medicine, Patients and the Law*, 3rd edition. London: Penguin Books, 2003.

Codori A, Petersen GM, Miglioretti DL, Larkin EK, Bushey MT, Young C, Brensinger JD, Johnson K, Bacon JA, Booker SV. Attitudes toward colon cancer gene testing: factors predicting test uptake. *Cancer Epidemiol Biomark Preven* 1999; **8**: 345–351.

Doukas DJ. The family covenant and genetic testing. *Am J Bioethics* 2001; **1**(3): 2–10.

General Medical Council. *Confidentiality: Protecting and Providing Information*. London: General Medical Council, 2004; also available on the World Wide Web: http://www.gmc-uk.org/guidance/library/confidentiality.asp#The%20public%20interest

General Medical Council. *Serious Communicable Diseases*. London: General Medical Council, 1997; also available on the World Wide Web: http://www.gmc-uk.org/guidance/library/serious_communicable_diseases.asp

Giardiello FM, Hamilton SR, Krush AJ, Piantadosi S, Hylind LM, Celano P, Booker SV, Robinson CR, Offerhaus GJA. Treatment of colonic and rectal adenomas with sulindac in familial adenomatous polyposis. *N Engl J Med* 1993; **328**: 1313–1316.

Harris J, Keywood K. Ignorance, information and autonomy. *Theor Med* 2001; **22**: 415–436.

Harris M, Winship I, Spriggs M. Controversies and ethical issues in cancer-genetics clinics. *Lancet Oncol* 2005; **6**: 301–310.

Häyry M, Takala T. Genetic information, rights, and autonomy. *Theor Med* 2001; **22**: 403–414.

Jones C. The utilitarian argument for medical confidentiality: a pilot study of patients' views. *J Med Ethics* 2003; **29**: 348–352.

Loewy E. Families, communities, and making medical decisions. *J Clin Ethics* 1991; **2**(3) 150–153.

Mason JK, Laurie GT. *Mason and McCall Smith's Law and Medical Ethics*. Oxford: Oxford University Press, 2005.

Medical Research Council. *Personal Information in Medical Research*. London: Medical Research Council, 2000; also available on the World Wide Web: http://www.mrc.ac.uk/pdf-pimr.pdf

Meiser B, Dunn S. Psychological impact of genetic testing for Huntington's disease: an update of the literature. *J Neurol, Neurosurg Psychiatry* 2000; **69**: 574–578.

O'Brien J, Chantler C. Confidentiality and the duties of care'. *J Med Ethics* 2003; **29**: 36–40.

Parker M, Lucassen A. Genetic information: a joint account? *Br Med J* 2004; **329**: 165–167.

Powers M. Privacy and genetics. In: Harris J, Burley J, eds. *A Companion to Genetics*. Oxford: Blackwell, 2002; pp. 364–378.

Roche PA, Annas GJ. Protecting genetic privacy. *Nat Rev Genet* 2001; **2**: 392–396.

Ross LF. Genetic exceptionalism vs. paradigm shift: Lessons from HIV. *J Law, Med Ethics* 2001; **29**: 141 [accessed via World Wide Web – no page numbers available].

Sommerville A, English V. Genetic privacy: orthodoxy or oxymoron? *J Med Ethics* 1999; **25**: 144–150.

Tarasoff v Regents of the University of California. 551 P2d. 334, CA 1976.

Weijer C. Family duty is more important than rights. *Br Med J* 2000; **321**: 1466.

Wertz D, Fletcher J. Privacy and disclosure in medical genetics examined in a ethics of care. *Bioethics* 1991; **5**: 212–232.

X v Y. 2 All ER 648 at 653, 1988.

44

Truth Telling, Lying and the Doctor–Patient Relationship

ROGER HIGGS

Tom Cruise (as rookie military lawyer):
  "I demand the truth."

Jack Nicholson (hard-bitten commander from the front line):
  "You can't handle the truth!"

A Few Good Men

Perhaps nobody yet has been truthful enough about what 'truthfulness' is.

Nietzsche, *Beyond Good and Evil*

Physicians should tell their patients the truth about their conditions. Thus runs the thinking and teaching at the present time in western medicine. It is confirmed by official pronouncements and policies and backed up by writers in the area: and it really happens. In the last decade, whenever my family have had to face a serious diagnosis, in conclusion we were given it straight, clearly and usually kindly. This is what was found. This is what needs to be done. The treatment is not nice, but the alternatives are worse. If you agree, please sign here.

Given the justice and security of this position, for all parties, we might now be heading for the shortest chapter in this series, were it not for a few disquieting thoughts. Tinkering with the truth is a regular concern in other walks of life, like advertising or politics, so it is likely to be a problem in health care too. Individuals are often tempted to tell lies and sometimes present apparently good excuses for doing so. Unlike many other issues in medical ethics, where the problems are created by 'frontier' science or extraordinary circumstances, the challenge of whether to be completely truthful is an *everyday* one for clinicians. In addition, the default position here for doctors over thousands of years

seems to have been the opposite of what it has been now in the past few decades. Experience of abrupt changes in human behaviour elsewhere suggests that current best practice might still contain unanswered or even unrecognized questions. The cynic or extreme traditionalist might even dismiss our opening sentence as merely modern fashion, with just as many moral side effects as the old days, only just causing problems for different people or affecting them in different ways. Telling the truth sounds a simple and important idea, but there are clearly many ways of trying to do so, and there are other types of deception, other than straight lying, that may be better options or just as bad.

THE TIPPING POINT

It might be as well to revisit what has happened in scarcely more than a generation. Before this, veracity in health care seemed to be running very much on its own rules. Some of the earliest evidence from classical ancient Greek philosophy offers a picture of doctors using truth 'like a medicine', to be dispensed whenever and in whatever doses the treating physician saw fit. Medical practice was used as the paradigm case of honesty not always being the best policy. Evasion or concealment, non-disclosure as we might say today, was so obviously right on occasions for patients that it was not in question.

The silence about veracity in ancient oaths and more modern codes until near the end of the twentieth century confirms that it was not a troublingly important issue for most doctors at least in what they saw as appropriate circumstances. In 1975 one of my elderly patients, born into working-class London as the nineteenth century closed, told

Principles of Health Care Ethics, Second Edition   Edited by R.E. Ashcroft, A. Dawson, H. Draper and J.R. McMillan

me that she would never expect to get the truth about herself from her doctors. In her view, the oath that new entrants to the profession swore was to keep all these things secret from her. My own medical training in the 1960s would have done little to dispel her anxieties. I only received instruction about veracity once I had qualified. One of my hospital firm chiefs (who later climbed to the highest echelons in medical education) made it clear that as a matter of policy he did not tell patients what was the matter with them and that I as his registrar should do likewise. He obviously had found it troubling and had thought a lot about it, but had made his mind up: it was not a subject open for discussion. With hair longer than the Beatles I clearly symbolized a subversive minority: and patients and students recounting their experiences today indicate that they still meet a subversive and convinced minority who thinks my former boss was right. To this minority, the unspoken statement from doctor to patient mirrors the clip at the chapter head. The voice, at the back of the doctor's mind declares, 'You can't *handle* the truth'.

Studies in anglophone countries, of both physicians' behaviour or intention and of patients' experiences or needs, underline the extraordinary change (Oken, 1961; Radovsky, 1985). They also usually confirm the persistence of minority views on both sides. Some of this change may indeed have been caused by the law, or by physicians' fears about falling foul of the law. Even natural justice can hardly fail to underpin honest communication when a new procedure or treatment is required. Consent is impossible without information as to what one is consenting to and why. Any patient who was not informed or was deliberately misinformed might thus have a case in law. But the reversal in practice must have been built on a broader base. Some of this relates to factual outcomes and changes: treatments even of conditions like cancer have become more effective, and people can see that the treatments work. Non-disclosure is more difficult to control when diagnosis and treatment are delivered by a team rather than just by an individual doctor. But much of the change also relates to a genuine shift in moral thinking and attitudes in society, something that caused the emergence of medical ethics as subject for instruction in medical schools and validated discussion in the wider community. Medical paternalism is no longer acceptable because it is unjust and unfair to infantilize adult patients, and their autonomy should be respected. Historically, in the last half of the twentieth century as the command and control structures of a global war receded, it became increasingly unacceptable in the west for any adult, as a *person*, to be treated as anything less than a *full* person. It was in part the flowering of Enlightenment thinking, both about the importance of individual freedom and about the need for rules to be universal. Thinking based on duties, on rights or on consequences all seemed to combine forces here. Even utilitarians, who might have wished to challenge Kantian

absolutism in the field of veracity, would have to concede that here was an area where one counted for one and no more nor less than one. The post-war western world saw a democratization of all parts of life that medicine could not ignore. Empowerment of those remaining vulnerable and weak in any society, however, is encouraged but not necessarily achieved by the passing of laws, helpful as those may be. Patients, as members of one such vulnerable group, in spite of all the rhetoric, find themselves in the turmoil of the daily struggle to maintain self-determination.

THE REALITY OF BEING A PATIENT

To become ill is to encounter, often without warning, some unpleasant facts beyond the unpleasant facts of the illness itself: that you are not able to function (because you are ill), but also often in addition that you are simply not able to think about or decide what should be done to restore normal function. Tales of mountaineers sawing off trapped limbs, or individuals facing up alone and unaided to the terrors of madness, are stories of heroism and are just that: the exception that can but outline the usual realities. It is like an IT failure: it is not just that the computer crashes and the user does not know what to do, but that the machine is switched off at the wall. Such an analogy is important because health care is often described as if it is a commodity that one chooses, like buying a washing machine, and individuals are urged to 'get over things' as if they had just had a burglary. The potential powerlessness and fear are in reality *sui generis*: even apparently trivial changes or symptoms, a little bleeding, a slight pain, a tiny lump, might herald the beginning of the end and generate a disabling panic. An injury or illness might take away the very skill that is needed to initiate recovery. It is in the face of such onslaughts against practical autonomy, of thought, will or action, that the *respect* of autonomy by professionals becomes such a key concept. Even if function returns, recovery cannot be complete until former autonomy is restored.

To be denied information, to be kept out of the loop of discussion, for a patient is not only insulting and paternalistic but actually like a further wound. It is a double jeopardy; fear made more frightening by the surrounding darkness. The risk now is not just of loss of the power supply at the wall, but of total power failure. As recovery ultimately comes from within the patient, by definition, whatever skills and restoratives medical teams bring to bear, it remains bizarre that so many of these teams (to keep to our metaphor) seem not simply to be failing to restore the power supply of open communication but actively digging up the road and removing the cable. However good an overall outcome may be, for a patient even nowadays to be considered part of a treating 'team' and to be kept regularly within the information loop is not yet, it seems, a common experience.

THE REALITY OF BEING A DOCTOR

Good reasons for this lack of involvement are not hard to find. Diagnosis is seldom a certainty, more an issue of sorting probabilities. Even apparently objective investigations on their own cannot be relied on: each has its interpretation and possible false positive or negative trails. Clinical reasoning is needed to make sense of all this, and this requires time and thought. Keeping a patient fully informed is a gargantuan task in itself. It may not be what the patient really wants. It may massively increase his anxiety and thus cloud the clinical picture even further. The point to declare on a diagnosis may not be obvious. Treatment itself in the individual case will always be its own little experiment, whereas prognosis is even less of a science and will probably always remain so. In the short term deception can be very effective: the placebo effect that has to be accounted for in clinical trials remains witness to this. Clinical practice remains a series of minute and interlocking contextual decisions, however much backed by the scientific evidence base. Does veracity clarify or further confuse?

THE DOCTOR–PATIENT RELATIONSHIP

The complexity of clinical work cannot excuse lack of disclosure, however, if there is no other justification for it. Modern life is full of immensely complex ideas and tasks and most of these have to be explained by professionals to others before decisions are made. Communicating the essentials is a job professionals just have to learn to do properly. A therapeutic relationship has to be based on a degree of trust: unless agreed on at the outset, it would be a very unusual patient who would continue to consult or be effectively treated by a physician whom she knew to be persistently deceiving her. In the long term, deception is almost bound to be destructive. Information is a power that is not simply rhetorical: it is certainly clear that in areas such as pain management, preparative information can be very effective. The power struggles that may occur within the doctor–patient relationship may be intense, but in such situations they are often indications of sickness in themselves (on either side) and require to be addressed. Unlike such battles elsewhere, however, it is not a question of one side gaining by the other's loss: for effective recovery, ideally both doctor and patient need the other to be as powerful as possible in their pursuit of this goal. Whether health care has matured enough to put partnerships here into real practice, however, from available evidence still seems unclear.

What is sometimes seen, in contrast, is a confusion of *role* powerful enough to become a destructive deception. If the physician is, for instance, more interested in advancing her career, in performing poorly explained research or trying to reduce costs as a priority rather than caring for the patient, such mixed motives become perversions in their own right which need to be overtly challenged before it all ends in tears. The doctor may understandably be unaware of what she is up to, or be working in a management structure that hides these conflicts, but self-deception is unlikely to be a helpful trait in strengthening the relationship or moving to a good outcome for the patient. The issue, once the problem is identified, is how to conduct the internal or external dialogue.

CONTRIBUTIONS FROM THEORY IN ETHICS

Although most people would find the Kantian inviolable rule of truthfulness hard to live with, equally most of us, from childhood on, long for people around us to be honest with us, and it no longer seems satisfactory for medicine to sit outside that world. However, the problems arise precisely when honesty conflicts with other similarly important concepts or binding duties. Although it would be possible for Kantians to define more closely the rules in context, veracity feels much more satisfactorily posed as what has been called a *prima facie* duty. There are many other important duties laid on workers in health care. Where confidentiality is vital, enquiries obviously have to be seen off with a suitable form of words. When a patient is confused or dying, clear possibilities exist for doing more harm than good unless the situation is thought through very carefully. Where the person is not afforded full autonomy by society elsewhere, rightly or wrongly, careful judgements will have to be made that pay attention to all the circumstances.

At the other end of the spectrum, it will be important to avoid the obfuscations of some postmodernist thought which might suggest to the unwary that because objective truth really cannot exist, we are all wasting our time worrying. This is at least in part a confusion of truth as an abstract concept with the different and very concrete conception of *truthfulness*. In his last big work addressing both, Bernard Williams looked within truthfulness at the twin questions of *accuracy* and *sincerity* (Williams, 2002). The first is seldom justifiably a problem in medicine. Scientific research provides the gold standard here, and we have already seen that struggling to translate, as it were, such ideas for lay people in terms that suit each person's level and style of understanding is a vital professional skill. It is unlikely ever to feel perfect, but as a human practice it will always need attention and if necessary, iteration. Sincerity is much more likely to be the key issue. In this, it is hard to improve on the question posed by Sissela Bok: do you *intend* your statement to mislead? (Bok, 1980). If you have no such intention, but do mislead, the problem reverts to one of communication; but if you really want to deceive someone by a form of words, for instance in a way that falls short of an outright lie, honesty as a duty suggests that such intentions require justification. What might these be?

PRIVACY

Our general desire for more honesty would seem to be answered by everyone being open about everything. Why do we need so much secrecy and concealment? It is fascinating to see how often open government has been the selling point of a political party in opposition, only to be hastily forgotten once it is in power. Children who hated adult evasiveness suddenly grow into adolescents whose taciturnity becomes impenetrable. It seems that *homo sapiens* must have private space. For patients, the state of sitting in near nakedness in a public ward, with intimate words and normally private functions generally broadcast, is probably more powerful a motivator towards discharge than actual physical recovery. Being asked to spill every bean about one's private life becomes an unjustifiable invasion. With confidentiality a 'decrepit principle' on the ward, most long-term patients get used to thinking twice before owning up. Patients who conceal vital information are the staple of medical soap operas, but more empirical and philosophical work needs to be done on patient veracity as the mirror of what is expected of professionals. The practice of psychotherapy could not exist without what Jung called the *vas bene claustrum*. Likewise a professional would seem to have a good claim to a personal life hidden from patients and from management unless or until there is an issue of harm. This extends to personal attitudes. Professionals have to be able to deal with situations or people that would evoke strong negative feelings in other people. Being a professional cannot help being in a small measure or on some occasions an act.

VIRTUE

The discussion here as elsewhere is helped by a consideration of virtue theory. Not only is there an Aristotelian mean to be found, but also *honesty as integrity*, something that goes 'all the way down' in a person, is more what seems to be the professional virtue sought by patients than *honesty as openness*. Watching a professional at work, we are more likely to be impressed by someone who struggles with truthfulness in context and decides with great reluctance and some shame to conceal or even lie for an apparently good motive than we are by someone who as a reflex reveals all, or, as in some postgraduate clinical teaching that I have come across, advocates dumping complex information on the patient's side of the table and leaving them 'to clear up because it's their business'. Not only does this feel like a betrayal of partnership, it can also look like a perversion of autonomy, deprived as it is of decent respect.

This remains an important issue for educators. The people most deceived in the majority of societies are children, for different reasons, and families vary in their ability to help them mature through this. It is not surprising therefore to find some health care students still struggling with their values and boundaries. Without supervised practice and guidance, neophytes sometimes reduce uncertainty by adopting a rigid extreme: in such cases unwavering honesty can seem as pathological as paternalistic concealment and just as much in need of mentoring help.

HARM

Maturity in clinical practice as elsewhere comes with the somewhat depressing realization that there is usually more than one sort of harm to be taken into account. In most cases the principle can cut both ways. There is no doubt how much harm deception or non-disclosure can bring. In general, it may be a 'poisoning of the wells'. In some individual situations, the manifested harm can be extreme. Some years ago, we described a terminal cancer case where a spouse insisted on non-disclosure and the patient was kept for months in a sort of suspended housebound state until she broke through the barrier by a direct question to the visiting physician. Once she had received a straight answer, she called in all her friends and family for a great farewell party and died peacefully the next day (Higgs, 1982). This sort of request from the spouse may reflect not the patient's view but the spouse's own overwhelming anxiety, and it is this, once the patient's clear right to direct information about their condition has been established, that needs help in its own right. Moving relatives towards coming to terms with terribly painful reality is an undervalued skill in adult as well as paediatric practice. But the relatives' distress in such situations is a crucially important side effect, and to see it as not the physician's proper business is callousness in the extreme. A family that usually faces serious problems by denial has either to be allowed this as a (temporary) refuge or given proper help to change their ways. The hard-pressed or thoughtless physician who cracks open these defences and leaves the rest to chance could be as harmful a predator as a thrush with a snail. However, the insights in psychology of affective forecasting indicate that we usually overpredict the negative effects of our emotional reactions. With time and help, both patient and family will usually move on (Rhodes and Strain, 2006).

Medical ethics is full of examples of brave decisions being reached, either personally or as policy, but there has been much too little discussion of the *management of the process* as an ethical issue in its own right, or of the handling of *side effects* so as to minimize harm here too. Some writers have called these side effects *the residue*, others the moral *shadow* (Boyd et al., 1997). In terms of theory, choosing one principle or concept as the winner or trump still leaves the others less favoured in play, unless the argument has seriously discredited them. In practice, if one person or group has been identified with the way forward that is not chosen, satisfactory ways of handling this also have to be found. As an example, in Britain a laudable process of reporting back from hospital to general practitioner has recently been developed whereby the specialist writes her report to the patient and copies this to the GP. This brings the patient into the information loop, but in situations of uncertainty often excludes the GP from knowing about other issues that are not yet resolved and have not yet been told to the patient. The previous form of exchange would have dealt with these and allowed the GP to contribute to the debate or make plans to help prepare the patient for other news.

KINDNESS AND HOPE

Medicine is something of a victim of its own recent success. Patients and relatives have very high expectations. The doctor surely will know what to do. She will have something up her sleeve. In desperate situations, it is not at all uncommon for an arm to be grabbed and the terrible question asked: 'I will be all right, won't I doctor?' Something has to be said. The instinct of kindness is to provide an answer that does not present the bleak outlook in all its unpleasantness: but it is not necessarily the truth. A lot more might be broken in the ensuing seconds than just a reputation for honesty. What is behind the question is a desperate need for support and skilled companionship in a dark hour. The response needs to provide as much as the doctor can muster without making false promises or setting up trust to be broken. Fortune favours the prepared mind, as Pasteur said, and every clinician must be prepared with a reply that is kind and strong but not a lie. To be honest about what the clinician thought would happen at this stage might seem more like a curse than an objective assessment of the truth. If the question is repeated, then it becomes clear that a careful discussion is needed between two people who are giving each other their full attention. Time may need to be set aside, and perhaps other companions called in. It may have to be done gradually, in small stages, or repeated without irritation. Talking about the future and prognosis needs extreme care. Doctors may have a vague or a pretty good idea of how and when it will all end, but it can never be a certainty, and so putting it across as definite, with precise timing, is not only cruel but silly. Entering the patient's frame of mind and discussing what needs to be done, and how urgently, is a practice that creates an atmosphere of prudence, not panic. Doctors have seen or read about the worst, but whether this is relevant or not, in my view that is a burden to be borne by them and not by patients unless it is openly and explicitly requested.

CHALLENGES

How to deal wisely in context with problems such as the above cannot be specified or made a subject of routine. Likewise as a society we are only beginning to face the difficulties posed by talking openly about their illnesses with children or people with restricted minds, discussing the likelihood of genetic disorders or relatively certain diseases in later life with young people and families, or facing squarely how to speak out about poor professional performance. Corporate practice in health care and insurance advice to professionals often seem to be trying to muzzle conversation rather than open up communication, and the results often appear self-defeating or even to raise much higher costs than were trying to be saved. To some observers, lying in government in Britain has become an object of concern (Slessor, 2004), and as a very politicized area health care cannot help being affected by these issues.

Within clinical work, the modern practice of disclosure, to be as open as possible while being sensitive to a patient's overall needs, is not an easy road. For the professional it is a process of constant attention to detail, and being able to think through what should be done, with reasons made explicit (and if necessary made a note of), while proper time is given to this as much as to any vital process in medicine. Reflection about what happened and learning from it should continue, with help from other people when difficulties occur. Performing pianists must practise, actors need directing, yet doctors once trained strangely still try to work without recording or watching themselves and without supervision or mentorship. That we should be truthful to each other is based on respect, trust and keeping promises. That we should be so in practice needs a lifelong commitment of attention.

REFERENCES

Bok S. *Lying; Moral Choice in Public and Private Life*. London: Quartet, 1980.

Boyd KM, Higgs R, Pinching AJ. *The New Dictionary of Medical Ethics*. London: BMJ Publishing Group, 1997.

Higgs R. Truth at last – a case of obstructed death? *J Med Ethics* 1982 **8**: 48–50.

Oken D. What to tell cancer patients: a study of medical attitudes. *J Am Med Assoc* 1961; **175**: 1120–1128.

Radovsky SS. Bearing the news. *N Engl J Med* 1985; **313**: 586–588.

Rhodes R, Strain JJ. Ethical considerations. In: Blumenfield M, Strain JJ, eds. *Psychosomatic Medicine*. New York: Lippincott Williams & Wilkins, 2006.

Slessor T. *Lying in State*. London: Aurum Press, 2004.

Williams B. *Truth and Truthfulness*. Princeton, NJ: Princeton University Press, 2002.

45

Personal Beliefs and Patient Care[1]

JENNIFER JACKSON

The General Medical Council (GMC) to which all doctors practising in the United Kingdom must register, issues to medical students a handy, pocket-sized card summarizing briefly 'the essential duties of a doctor'. Most of the items which it lists are, as one would expect, plainly worded and unexceptionable (which is not to say unneeded); for example: 'Respect and protect confidential information' or 'Treat every patient politely and considerately' and 'Respect patients' dignity and privacy'. One item in the list, though, seems not so obvious in its meaning and maybe, were its meaning made obvious, it would not (or should not) seem unexceptionable. It does not correspond to anything in the Hippocratic Oath. Indeed, one suspects that were it possible to resurrect some medical sage of bygone times – Hippocrates himself or Galen or Thomas Percival or Sir William Osler – none of them would have a clue as to what it was about.

The 'duty' in question is expressed in the following terms: *'Make sure that your personal beliefs do not prejudice your patients' care'*. In this chapter, I want to explore what the GMC might have in mind by this injunction and discuss whether the GMC does right to include it in the list.

Naturally, anything we might say of the form 'Make sure that your Xs do not prejudice your patients' care' sounds like the sort of thing that a doctor should be signing up to – just as we expect clergymen to be against sin. The schema will have various appropriate fillings-in. Try replacing 'your Xs' by 'your dogs' or 'your drinking habits' or 'your absent-mindedness', for example. But if we substitute 'your personal beliefs', matters are not at all plain sailing.

Presumably 'patients' care' should be understood to cover whatever is available from the health care services, broadly speaking. I say 'broadly speaking' to include various procedures that are offered by health professionals that have nothing in particular to do with health care, with illness or injury: such as elective cosmetic surgery, vasectomies or the provision of contraceptive drugs. It is worth making this point because by sweeping various services under the description 'care', we lend a favourable glow to the injunction which it might not quite deserve. Everyone will agree – in broad terms – that doctors owe their patients the care they need. It is another matter whether doctors owe patients the services they want.

Making sense of what might be meant by 'personal beliefs' is more difficult. Is not *every* belief the belief of some person or other? The injunction with which we are concerned, unlike the other three mentioned above, seems to be written in a kind of code. Would it, perhaps, be too embarrassing to have made its meaning plain? I have a hunch that were the GMC to speak its mind on the matter more forthrightly, it would be saying: 'Do not let your nasty, illiberal and irrational, if not downright batty, beliefs stand in the way of patients having access to the services they want.' But they could hardly come out with that, could they? Let us see, however, whether there is a less provocative way of construing the alleged duty.

What, then, are we – in a more accommodating mood – to suppose that the GMC has in mind? There is clearly a difficulty. Doctors will sometimes knowingly deny things to their patients which would be of benefit to them. This could be entirely reasonable. Suppose, for example, a doctor routinely prescribes a drug that he believes is 'good enough' for his patients though he knows that there is another drug, considerably more expensive, that he could prescribe that

[1]For help in writing this chapter I want to thank Christopher Coope who has soldiered through its successive drafts, making many detailed and extensive criticisms and improvements.

would be somewhat better for them. This seems to be a clear case where a doctor's belief (here, a belief in the need to economise) would prejudice the patient's care. Yet the GMC might approve of this doctor's economizing policy, thinking it well judged. One of the essential duties it lists is, after all, 'pay due regard to efficacy and use of resources'.

There are, to be sure, ways in which patients' care might be compromised on account of their doctors' beliefs where the GMC would not approve: when these beliefs betray culpable ignorance. It would be entirely reasonable for the GMC to enjoin doctors to avoid that. And so it does. One of the duties on its list is: 'Keep your professional knowledge and skills up to date'. Although the duty we are trying to explain might be intended merely to add weight to this same duty by repeating it in different words, it is plausible to assume, given the space constraints of a small card, that the GMC has something distinctive in mind. What might it be?

Let us try the following: a doctor might have beliefs that cause him to discriminate unfairly against certain of his patients, prejudicing their care. It would be entirely reasonable for the GMC to enjoin doctors not to allow their patients' care to be prejudiced in this way. And so it does: 'you must never discriminate unfairly against your patients or colleagues'. But the inclusion of this rule shows once again that we have failed to come up with something distinctive.

Perhaps a clue to what the GMC has in mind may be gleaned from its use of the word 'personal'. Is the injunction meant to discourage doctors from allowing their *moral* judgements to prejudice their patients' care? People say, with quite uncertain import, that 'morality is personal'. Is this at last a plausible interpretation of the injunction?

Hardly so. Suppose a surgical team could provide the treatment a patient wants and needs but only by stealing something – perhaps by stealing an organ from someone else or some money from the bank. The patient says: 'Go ahead! That's all right by me.' The surgeons' reply: 'You must be joking! It is out of the question!' Are these surgeons deviating from the GMC guidance, allowing their personal – here understood as moral – beliefs to prejudice their patient's care? It would seem so. Seeing, though, that stealing is against the law, and it is reasonable to suppose that the GMC does not mean to encourage doctors to break the law, we may assume these surgeons are not after all deviating from the guidance intended. We need a different example.

Suppose, then, a family doctor could speed up the patient's access to needed surgery, but only by deliberately exaggerating to the consultant the acuteness of the patient's symptoms – that is, by lying. Again, the doctor might refuse saying: 'Are you seriously asking me to lie? I cannot possibly do that.' The doctor who says this might believe ('personally' believe, if you like) that it is always wrong to lie even when the motive is benevolent. Or he might believe that although lying is sometimes defensible it is not so here, where it means telling a bare-faced lie on a serious matter to a colleague. Either way, we may presume, the GMC injunction we are trying to understand is *not* meant to encourage doctors to overcome their personal reluctance to lie even if, as in this case, that is the only way of getting their patient the care that is needed. Among the basic duties on the GMC list, after all, is this one: 'be honest and trustworthy'.

Maybe, then, the injunction amounts to this: 'make sure that your moral beliefs *other than those to do with honesty* do not prejudice your patients' care'. Imagine, then, a doctor who is a firm advocate of the Beauchamp and Childress 'four principles'. He, however, attaches more weight to the principle of autonomy than is usual. He believes, let us suppose, that the principle of autonomy should always trump any other principle with which it conflicts. This is his personal belief in the sense that we are now giving to the phrase. It concerns what he takes to be his duty. And if he acts on it, his patients' care will sometimes be prejudiced as a result. Yet, it seems unlikely that the GMC would find fault with his conduct. He might after all defend his commitment to safeguarding patient autonomy by appealing to certain items in the GMC list of essential duties, such as: 'Listen to patients and respect their views' and 'Respect the rights of patients to be fully involved in decisions about their care'.

There is a broad lesson to be drawn from these examples. The moral law, or what we take to be its teachings, is apt to limit what we can do, not only by way of helping ourselves but also by way of helping others. And this applies, quite generally, to doctors as to everyone else. Think of promising. One might not be able to help patient Smith as one would like because one has promised to be elsewhere. It can be reasonable in the appropriate circumstances for a doctor, a *good* doctor, to respect such a promise – and this even though he cannot find, or does not propose to find, a locum. Of course, I am not saying that this would *always* be reasonable.

'Prejudicing the patients' care' is an intimidating phrase. One is supposed to tremble at the very thought. At the very least it may be supposed that an excuse is called for. But not so. We need to guard against this moralistic assumption. A doctor may do what will somewhat prejudice his patients' care for the lightest of reasons – yet need no excuse. He may take time off to go fishing, simply because he likes to do so and not just because he needs to refresh himself in order to keep fit for his patients' sake. Naturally, the doctor who takes time off has a duty to arrange suitable cover for his absence, in case of emergencies. But even so, there will be occasional non-emergency cases where patients will be somewhat disadvantaged because 'Doctor has gone fishing'. Similarly, some doctors may choose to practise on a part-time basis so as to allow more time for their hobbies. If they are particularly good doctors, their choice to go part-time – or take early retirement – is liable to prejudice patients' care. The patients may still get good care, but not as good (for more on this see Jackson, 2006, ch. 8).

We have so far tried out various ways of making sense of the alleged duty to make sure that personal beliefs do not prejudice patients' care, none of which seems satisfactory. Maybe we should approach the matter from a different angle. Instead of casting around for some interpretation of what principle the GMC might have had in mind, let us ask rather whether it might perhaps have been influenced by certain cases or paradigms. The GMC may have no complaint against doctors who prejudice a patient's care because they refuse to lie or steal for the patient. But it is another matter entirely – is it not? – if doctors are being obstructive to patients requesting abortions. Suppose a doctor refuses, saying: 'You are asking me to arrange for the killing of your baby. I cannot possibly do that.' Now is not this last kind of refusal exactly what the GMC would have had in mind as contrary to the principles of good medical practice? One wonders why they did not say so outright.

Yet is it not singularly inapposite to talk about 'prejudicing patients' care' when (a) it is a 'service' provided to a 'client' rather than provided to a patient, and (b) in so far as there are patients in the picture at all, the dispute in part turns on who is included as a patient and what counts as a prejudice to care? The decision to 'terminate' sounds mighty prejudicial to foetal care. True enough, one may want to *say* that the foetus is not a patient in the circumstances, and that is very understandable. For all that, is it not a matter of averting one's eyes? In the adjacent ward, where strenuous efforts are being made to maintain a pregnancy, no one will find it strange to think of the (wanted) baby as a patient. These familiar problems notwithstanding, I will assume that objection to abortion is very much, though perhaps not exclusively, what the GMC had in mind as the sort of 'personal belief' that should not be allowed to 'prejudice patients' care'.

Is it to be assumed, then, that doctors refusing to arrange abortions are acting from merely personal beliefs, unlike the doctors who refuse to steal or lie for their patients? What makes the conviction about abortion any more 'personal' than the conviction about lying or stealing? After all, as we noted in regard to lying, a doctor might have quite an individual view about the badness of lying in this or that circumstance, a view that other doctors might not share. There are some possible explanations. We will consider two.

First, it may be supposed that the objection to abortion is *religious*, whereas the objection to stealing or lying is moral. Out of respect for religious freedom the medical profession quite properly tries to accommodate members' religious beliefs – provided that they do not allow these to 'prejudice patients' care'. Thus, for example, Jewish doctors are entitled on their Sabbath day to refuse to see

their patients. But they are not entitled, and do not think that they should be, to obstruct patients from seeing other doctors on that day. They are perfectly willing to refer. So likewise, it might be said, if a religion forbids abortion, that is no justification for doctors who are members of that religion refusing to refer. Duties which are merely religious are for members only.

But plainly no one with religious beliefs sees the duty not to procure abortions as a matter of religious observance in this way. It is never thought of as a members-only matter. To be sure, it might suit those who defend abortion to portray things in this light, but wishing does not make it so. So we can lay this point aside.

Suppose, then, it is said that if the duty is not one of religious observance, it is at any rate religiously inspired, and this *of necessity*. The crucial thought here would be this: such a teaching about abortion must depend upon premises peculiar to one or more religions or denominations and that in consequence it would not be reasonable to deny others who do not share these assumptions access to what they want. Fortunately, we need not pursue this latter claim as to reasonableness unless the claim about dependence and necessity is true. But in real life hardly anyone ever supposes this. It is evident that both those who object to abortion and those who defend it against these objections proceed 'in a wholly secular way'. Revelation and tradition are not appealed to.

Let us allow, however, that some such appeal to religion might in fact be necessary to underwrite the objection to abortion, whatever the disputants assume in practice. We would be trying here to separate off certain 'non-religious' or universal moral claims, in order to say that beliefs in regard to these, and these only, *may* reasonably 'prejudice patients' care'. We would then hope to say something else in regard to abortion. It is thought safe to assume that beliefs about lying or stealing, or, say, the killing of adults and of born children are non-religious deep down, in the sense that they could be thoroughly understood and justified, given sufficient hard work and intelligence, without religious premises.

This assumption, however, remains a hope rather than a certainty. How do we know that some of our *shared* convictions about honesty, stealing and homicide are not (perhaps embarrassingly) religiously dependent – dependent on *some* religious presuppositions – in their rationale? Not just causally or historically, but, as we say, 'logically'? Philosophical understanding in these areas is plainly pretty limited. There seems to be some reason to suspect – I put it no more strongly – that the boundary line between the dependent and the independent might not run exactly where many of us would so like it to run. Without a resolution of this difficulty, the distinction which we have been trying to make between purely moral and religiously contaminated beliefs could not be made in a way suitable to the case in hand. The objection to abortion could not comfortably be put into quarantine all on its own.

The upshot would seem to be this. At a superficial level the objection to abortion seems quite non-religious, even though many of those who object obviously do have religious beliefs. More deeply considered, however, the objection could indeed be religiously dependent, but not in a way which allows us confidently to single it out as was hoped.

We have been asking what there might be about abortion which would enable the GMC to complain when a doctor allowed his conviction on *this* matter to prejudice his patients' care (or rather, their access to a service). We have now to consider a second possibility. The objection people have to abortion, it might be said, falls into quite a different moral category from the objection to lying, stealing, promise-breaking and so on. Some moral teachings concern obligations – perhaps called strict or minimal – whereas other teachings concern ideals or aspirations which reasonably differ from person to person. Might we be able to use this distinction to clarify the word 'personal' as it occurs in the GMC injunction? Perhaps it could read: 'Make sure that your enthusiasm for your personal ideals does not prejudice your patients' care'. That might seem a reasonable rule-of-thumb teaching.

And might not this enable us, after all, to single out abortion in the way desired? As everyone knows, people who are opposed to abortion call themselves 'pro-life'. This description seems exactly to indicate the sort of thing we have in mind. Those who are pro-life are committed to saving life – admirably, we might add. But not everyone need feel called upon to be committed in this way. After all, even as a doctor, there are many good things to do with one's life, which do not involve saving lives. We will be able to say then to every doctor: by all means have these personal enthusiasms, these moral ideals, but do not let them get in the way of the humble task of patient care required of you. This captures rather well how some people will interpret the word 'personal'. But of course it has been quite hard to write this last paragraph with a straight face, for it so conspicuously fails to engage with the topic in hand.

Let us try an entirely different tack. The injunction about prejudicing patient care can be seen in another light: as an instruction to doctors to be prepared to 'refer the patient to another doctor'. That there is some kind of duty on a doctor to 'refer' is evident. In its booklet *Good Medical Practice* (General Medical Council, 1998), the GMC offers guidance on how to apply the duties or principles summarized on its card. One of the items (item 14) there reads: 'If you feel that your beliefs might affect the treatment you provide, you must explain this to patients, and tell them of their right to see another doctor'. Seeing as your beliefs must *always* affect the treatment you provide (or refuse), we must assume that what the GMC has in mind here is something more

specific – like, maybe, your unusual or eccentric beliefs. Patients, it may be said, should not be disadvantaged, or denied the treatment they want, simply because they happen to be treated by a doctor whose views are out of line with the views of a majority of his colleagues.

But we need to consider just when and why this duty to refer arises. Sometimes a doctor, faced with a particularly difficult case, may be tentative or uncertain how to proceed. Assuming the difficulty is not that the problem lies quite outside his own field of competence, he need not refer the patient, but maybe he should, time permitting, seek a second opinion. If, however, a doctor is faced with a problem which is outwith his own clinical experience but where he knows (or should know) that it is within the experience of other colleagues, then surely he does have a duty to refer. But is the duty to refer in such circumstances grounded in the particular injunction we are examining? There is, I think, a more obvious grounding for it in another duty listed on the small card: 'Recognize the limits of your professional competence'.

Suppose a doctor is justifiably confident about the clinical judgement on which his advice is based – in so far as one can ever be confident about such things – but he realizes that his patient remains unconvinced. Here, too, it may be appropriate to refer the patient to another doctor, and this other doctor will naturally be selected with the expectation that his judgement will be the same.

Compare now the situation where a doctor is justifiably confident about a moral judgement on which his refusal to comply with a patient's request is based, and where the patient remains unconvinced. Does it make sense for a doctor in such a case to recognize a duty to refer – and moreover a duty to refer not just to another doctor whom he expects will confirm his opinion but rather to a colleague whom he knows will disagree with his moral view on the matter? If Dr Jones firmly believes that X-ing is wrong (unjust), he presumably believes too that arranging with Dr Smith to do X is wrong. Let us return to our earlier example of lying for one's patient in order to speed up the patient's access to needed surgery. Does anyone suppose it would be appropriate for the doctor to say the following: 'I cannot do that. Lying is out of the question. However, let me refer you to my colleague across the corridor, he is perfectly willing to lie for his patients in such cases'?

No doubt it is important for doctors to be ever mindful of their limitations and to pursue their work with a certain humility. That granted, there will be times when they are convinced, and rightly so, that complying with a request would be wrong, be the conviction medical or moral. Where there is a duty to refer, it could hardly be fulfilled simply by passing the patient on to any old colleague; only to a colleague whose judgement one trusts and respects.

Although the GMC might well allow that referral would not be appropriate in a case which involved lying, it might still hold that referral is appropriate, and it is indeed a duty, in the case of abortion. The morality of abortion, unlike the morality of lying, at least in such a context, is 'morally controversial'; that is to say, it involves beliefs which are held, and which are controverted, by people of apparent goodwill who are judged to be informed and thoughtful. While doctors, it may be said, like everyone else are 'entitled to their own views' on these matters (entitlement here comes very cheap), they must be scrupulously non-directive and promptly refer patients if they are unwilling themselves to provide a service, at least if the service is not illegal. It is actually quite usual for those who maintain this doctrine to represent it as a fair compromise, even-handed to both sides on the abortion debate (see, for example, Cantor and Baum, 2004).

It is natural to suppose that the GMC, in laying out its list of essential duties, is wanting to appear neutral, not wishing to take sides on such a contentious issue as abortion. But it is hard to avoid the suspicion that under the guise of being neutral, it is in fact adopting a permissive or liberal stance. Being neutral and being permissive are not one and the same thing. The permissive or liberal stance in regard to abortion is *protective* of 'a woman's right to choose'. Thus, it insists that doctors who object to abortion have a duty to refer, whereas if the stance were really neutral about abortion, it would have to be neutral with respect to referral. If the GMC were being neutral in its guidance it might express itself, quite gently, thus: If you are in difficulties about this matter you might find it *appropriate* to refer.

It is easy for this distinction (between the neutral and the permissive) to be overlooked. The British Medical Association (BMA), for example, seems to want to have it both ways: 'The Association makes no policy statement about the morality of abortion. Nevertheless, this implies that there are circumstances in which the BMA considers that abortion is acceptable . . .' (British Medical Association, 1993, p. 103). Besides saying it makes *no* policy statement and then apparently gainsaying this claim in the very next sentence, the BMA goes on to insist that doctors who object *must* refer (British Medical Association, 1993, pp. 108–109).

The BMA used not to adopt a neutral stance on abortion. Back in 1947, the Council of the BMA issued a statement affirming its continuing commitment to the Hippocratic Oath observing that: 'Although there have been many changes in Medicine, the spirit of the Hippocratic Oath cannot change and can be reaffirmed by the profession'. It went on to say that this oath 'enjoins' 'the duty of curing, the greatest crime being co-operation in the destruction of life by murder, suicide and abortion' (British Medical Association, 1947).

The distinction between a neutral and a permissive attitude is instructively illustrated in the different positions taken by the GMC and the BMA on the issue of non-therapeutic male circumcision of infants. And this will in fact tell us something revealing about attitudes to abortion.

According to some, circumcision is a mutilating procedure which can be painful and even harmful and which should not be inflicted on a child merely to accommodate the religious or cultural beliefs of its parents. According to others, the procedure, if competently performed, carries little risk, and refusal to provide this particular service fails to respect the religious or cultural beliefs of the families who seek it. The GMC reports that the consultation it conducted on this issue yielded 'widely conflicting views in society'. It says that these 'cannot' be resolved by the GMC. It notes that the legal position is untested; hence, unclear. In view of all this, it advises doctors who may happen to be opposed to the procedure where, as is usually the case, it is requested 'for non-therapeutic reasons' that they should explain their objection to the parents who ask for it and refer them to another doctor (General Medical Council, 1997) .

However, the BMA, as of 2003, has adopted a different position on this matter. It says: 'Clearly where patients or parents request a medical procedure, doctors have an obligation to refer on promptly if they themselves object to it (for example termination of pregnancy). Where the procedure is not therapeutic but a matter of patient or parental choice, there is arguably no ethical obligation to refer on.' The distinction made here is quite material. If male circumcision is not a medical procedure when performed for non-therapeutic purposes (though, of course it may be, for instance, to remedy an anatomical anomaly or a pathological condition like phimosis), one must wonder whether elective abortions are not medical procedures either – in which case the BMA should admit that it is equally arguable that doctors opposed to abortion are *not* obliged to refer. To be sure, as the law has developed in England the grounds for abortions are *supposedly* 'therapeutic', but it is common knowledge that in practice this grounding is nearly always a fiction.

Perhaps the GMC, after all, really does mean to be neutral on the abortion issue, not permissive. Perhaps its injunction is intended merely to remind doctors *to comply with the law* and not obstruct patients' access to any services to which it entitles them to lay claim. On this interpretation the injunction is targeting only personal beliefs that might lead a doctor to act contrary to the law. But this raises a problem.

If the GMC's list really does contain 'the essential duties of a doctor', these duties must surely apply wherever and whenever one is practising medicine. Although the GMC's jurisdiction is confined to the United Kingdom, students in UK medical schools come from all over, and many return, after qualifying, to pursue their careers in other continents and cultures. And besides, in its booklet *Good Medical Practice*, where the GMC explains the scope of its listed duties or principles, it says that 'They apply to all doctors involved in health care'. The other items in the list do seem straightforwardly applicable world-wide, just as we would expect. Consider, for example, those items that were cited earlier: 'Respect and protect confidential information', 'Treat every patient politely and considerately' and 'Respect each patient's dignity and privacy'. These duties are no less relevant and appropriate for doctors working in Somalia than for doctors working in the United Kingdom. Can the same be said of the alleged duty that we are considering?

Suppose a medical student is doing an elective abroad – in Somalia. He or she might be asked to assist in female circumcision, routinely available there (98% of women undergo it) but illegal in the United Kingdom (Prohibition of Female Circumcision Act 1985). Suppose, for the sake of argument, that in Somalia a law is passed that protects parents' entitlement to this customary service, imposing a duty on doctors to provide it on request. Should the GMC guidance to British medical students working abroad be that though they are entitled to refuse to assist, if they do refuse, they are morally obliged to refer to colleagues who are willing to take part? Otherwise, won't it be said, these students would be improperly 'imposing their values'? More generally, should the GMC instruct medical students always to comply with the law of the country where they happen to be working, or should it instruct them always to act as if English law were everywhere applicable? The former instruction would belie any notion of doctors' moral duties being prior to the law of this or that jurisdiction.[2] The latter would presuppose that the provisions of current home-grown English law cannot be morally defective.

Is it not possible that the law, not only abroad, but even on our own home ground, might in some important ways be deeply unjust? I do not need here to assert that it *is* so, merely that it *might be* so. This danger would hardly be diminished merely because the law happened to reflect faithfully the democratic will of a populace. The fact that a new statute, for example, the statute in the Netherlands permitting voluntary euthanasia, The Termination of Life on Request and Assisted Suicide (Review Procedures) Act, which came into effect as of 1 April 2002, has overwhelming popular support in that country, gives us scarcely any ground for thinking that the statute could not all the same be deeply contrary to the moral law.

Let us now briefly review our discussion. It might be thought very unfair to scrutinize as we have been doing the precise wording of an item in a list that has been designed to fit into a student's pocket or wallet. But the points raised in this chapter seem to have confirmed that the wording in this item is not unclear merely because its authors were having to compress a complex thought into a few words, but rather because its authors were unwilling to say frankly what was on their minds. It is to be expected that the GMC would like to avoid getting itself enmeshed in matters of moral controversy. No doubt it would hope to stand above the fray in setting forth what are supposed to be the essential duties. But, as we have remarked, where controversies involve issues of justice, of what we owe one another, the permissive or liberal stance that insists on protecting the patient's choice – or the parent's choice – by imposing on doctors a duty to comply or refer is not after all neutral.

And so, it seems, we have come full circle. We have come back to our original unfriendly interpretation of the injunction. It seems to be saying this: 'Make sure your *unreasonable* beliefs, which we just about put up with, do not prejudice your patients' care'. That guidance is unexceptionable, but is rather empty unless it is accompanied by some indication as to *which* beliefs are unreasonable. The GMC, being understandably reticent to add this, has to rely on doctors supplying the specifics, something like: unreasonable beliefs – such as hang-ups about the so-called 'sanctity of life'.

REFERENCES

British Medical Association. *Female Genital Mutilation Caring for Patients and Child Protection Guidance*. London: BMA, 1996 (Revised April 2001).

British Medical Association. *Medical Ethics Today: Its Practice and Philosophy*. London: BMA, 1993.

British Medical Association. Statement by the Council of the British Medical Association for submission to the World Medical Association, 1947; http://www.donoharm.org.uk/leaflets/war.htm.

British Medical Association. *The Law and Ethics of Male Circumcision: Guidance for Doctors*. London: BMA, 2003.

Cantor J, Baum K. The limits of conscientious objection – may pharmacists refuse to fill in prescriptions for emergency contraception? *N Engl J Med* 2004; **351**: 2008–2012.

General Medical Council. *Good Medical Practice*. London: GMC, 1998.

General Medical Council. *Guidance for Doctors who are Asked to Circumcise Male Children*. London: GMC, 1997.

Jackson J. *Ethics in Medicine*. Cambridge: Polity, 2006.

World Health Organization. *Information Pack on Female Genital Mutilation*, 1996; http://www.who.int/frh-whd/FGM/index.htm.

[2]Such a stance would be hard to square with the Female Genital Mutilation Act 2003, which makes it a criminal offence for any UK national or permanent UK resident to carry out this procedure abroad, *or to aid, abet, counsel or procure its being carried out abroad, even in countries where the practice is legal.* (My italics.) Admittedly, aiding, abetting, etc. is only an offence under this Act if the person on whom the procedure is carried out happens to be herself a UK national or permanent UK resident. But that merely reflects the limitations of the law's reach. The moral requirement of doctors implicit in such legislation presumably is not thought to apply in respect to the treatment of British women only. The World Health Organization maintains that health professionals should not carry out this procedure on anyone anywhere. The BMA appears to share this view (British Medical Association, 1996).

46

Conscience and Health Care Ethics

PIERS BENN

It is almost universally accepted that there is more to being a good doctor or nurse than the possession of clinical
skills. The health care professions are committed, explicitly
or implicitly, to certain basic ethical values. Medicine, for
example, is generally regarded as having certain ethical
goals and as bound by certain principles in the pursuit of
those goals. In addition, a widely shared assumption is that
in order to promote the values of medicine, practitioners
need personal virtues, such as honesty, benevolence and justice. In this, medicine is different from certain other types
of legitimate employment. For example, although the welfare of the consumer is not the main concern of a business
trying to sell a product at a profit, the welfare of the patient
is central to the good practice of medicine.

Accordingly, most health care professionals place considerable importance upon acting with integrity in their work.
This entails acting upon their moral principles and doing
what they consider to be right. Usually this coincides with
what their profession and patients expect from them. But
there are occasions when such expectations conflict with
the demands of professionals' personal conscience. Many
people believe that acting with integrity involves more than
doing things which merely happen to be right. It also means
following one's own conscience and not doing what one
believes to be wrong. Largely for that reason, doctors and
nurses often have the right to refuse participation in certain
procedures, on grounds of conscientious objection. One of
the purposes of this chapter is to examine the pros and cons
of 'conscience clauses' that permit such exemptions.

THE IDEA OF CONSCIENCE

But there are several problems that should be mentioned
first. What is it to follow one's conscience, and why might it
be important to do so? What authority does an individual's

conscience have? Is it wrong to require someone to act
against her conscience? And in general, do people's sincerely
held conscientious positions deserve 'respect'? Such questions are unavoidable in discussions of the supposed moral
right of health care professionals to refuse involvement in
certain procedures they object to, and we need to pause to
examine them before looking at the vexed and controversial
problem of conscientious objection.

There is one underlying issue we should mention, but
only to leave it on one side. This is to do with moral epistemology in general – of how, if at all, we can justifiably adopt
any moral convictions. This matter connects with a complex
problem in the realm of 'meta-ethics', namely whether moral
judgements are factual statements, or something else, such
as the expression of emotion or attitude. Those who take
the latter view are likely to say that, strictly speaking, there
are no moral facts, no objective moral truths 'out there', and
that therefore conscience does not yield awareness of any
such facts. One cannot know facts or truths that do not exist.
But people who do believe that morality really is objective
and 'out there' (whatever that may amount to) face the challenge of saying how, if at all, we can *know* what is good or
bad, right or wrong. Is there a special moral sense? Do we
know moral truths by a kind of intuition? If challenged to
say how we know the truths of morality, is it reasonable to
answer: 'by the exercise of conscience'?

This is an issue that has occupied much philosophical
thought about ethics, but in practice, almost everyone has
moral convictions and commitments, whatever their theory
of moral truth – or indeed, whether they have a theory at
all. Moral philosophers have often distinguished between
'first-order' and 'second-order' moral views, the former
being about practical moral issues, and the latter about the
nature of morality itself. Perhaps the two issues cannot be
entirely separated; one might wonder how someone can
reconcile her moral views with a radical scepticism about

Principles of Health Care Ethics, Second Edition   Edited by R.E. Ashcroft, A. Dawson, H. Draper and J.R. McMillan

the existence of moral truths or properties. But philosophers tend not to be bothered by this – not many people can sincerely think or act as if there were no moral obligations or values. So if morality is a kind of 'given', we can ask how we should go about forming our moral judgements. It is here that some people will answer that this requires the exercise of conscience. Conscience, on some such accounts, is the faculty for knowing what is required of us.

CONSCIENCE AS AN 'INNER VOICE'

If this is correct, how does it work? Historically, many people have thought of conscience as somewhat like an inner voice, telling us what is right and wrong and giving us a hard time if we go wrong. Thus, to have a 'guilty conscience' is to experience an uncomfortable feeling of having transgressed in some way, and perhaps deserving punishment. Socrates, as recorded by Plato, spoke of his internal 'voice', or inner guide which required obedience – forbidding him, for example, to break the laws of Athens by trying to escape from prison, even though he had been unjustly condemned (Plato, 1954). The rise of Protestantism after the Reformation produced an emphasis on the individual conscience, conceived as a source of knowledge that is binding upon us, even if it went against official authorities. Indeed, the emphasis on obedience to what you have worked out for yourself, as opposed to external authority (e.g. the Church) is a hallmark of early Protestant conceptions of conscience.

But how seriously should we take the idea of an authoritative inner guide or 'voice'? It is associated with an 'oracular' conception of conscience, in which 'consulting your conscience' is a bit like consulting an oracle or seer. You frame a moral question, consult your conscience and return with an answer almost as if it had been dictated. However, though useful as a metaphor, there are some serious difficulties with this idea.

One obvious problem is that people's consciences tell them very different things. Pacifists have a conscientious objection to fighting in wars, whereas other people think there are some wars one is obliged to fight in. Some health care professionals are absolutely opposed to abortion, whereas many others think it is a woman's right. There is an endless range of ethical issues on which sincere and reflective people profoundly disagree. If they disagree, then as a matter of logic they cannot all be right. Therefore many people have erring consciences. However authentic the deliverances of conscience may seem, it can and does mislead on some very important issues. If conscience were literally an oracle, it would be a dangerously fallible one.

Here, someone might interject that conscience is 'personal' or 'individual', perhaps adding that we do not have a right to judge the conscientious position of others, even if it apparently conflicts with our own. And in a very limited way, this is true. There are certain things that my conscience might forbid me to do, even though I would not condemn the behaviour of others who do it. But whenever this is the case, we can surely find differences in circumstances that can explain this. For example, a doctor who is an orthodox Jew will have a conscientious objection to working on the Sabbath or eating pork. But she does not in the least condemn non-Jews who do these things, since according to her, these obligations *apply only to Jews*, not Gentiles. She might admonish a fellow orthodox Jewish doctor for working on the Sabbath because as a Jew, he is supposed to observe the Sabbath. But she may be entirely happy to refer a patient needing treatment on the Sabbath to a Gentile colleague. Similarly, a 'recovering alcoholic' might think it very important for him not to drink alcohol, whilst not at all condemning others who drink. Because his situation is different from that of most other drinkers, he sees himself as subject to a requirement of abstinence that does not apply to most others. But neither of these examples shows that conscience is 'personal' in the way believed by many who make this claim. For the Jewish doctor, the fact that she is Jewish is relevant to whether or not she should work on the Sabbath. She does not have a conscientious view that applies only to her because she would presumably hold that no Jew should work on the Sabbath. And the recovering alcoholic would probably say that anyone else in his situation ought not to drink.

So the fallibility of conscience remains a problem, at least for anyone who takes its oracular nature too literally. When I make a moral judgement, I mean it to apply not just to me but also to anyone in a similar situation (what counts as a similar situation is a hotly debated issue that I shall not discuss here). Although I might tolerate the conscientious convictions of someone I disagree with – that is, although I might be polite, friendly and anxious to avoid nasty arguments – I cannot think his view is just as correct as my own.

However, a promising way to rescue the idea of conscience, in spite of moral disagreement, is to abandon the idea that it is like an oracle, still less an infallible one – something which few people really believe in any case – and see it instead as a fallible but perfectly respectable facility for reflecting on ethical issues and arriving at judgements.

The main difference between the oracular conception of conscience and the more reflective conception advocated here is that the first makes moral deliberation appear passive – a matter of somehow gleaning moral information from somewhere – whereas the second involves the agent in active and often difficult reflection. But how are we to reflect on ethical issues? The process is easily caricatured as looking inside your mind and discovering what moral views you have, in other words, doing no more than 'consulting yourself'. But this distorts how we ordinarily do make judgements, which surely involves many processes: testing our views for consistency; thinking of counter-examples to our initial opinions; honestly asking ourselves what our instinctive reactions are and then asking whether these reactions are tenable; examining how our existing principles apply to a particular situation; and especially, trying to imagine the situation of others who will be affected by our actions. If this is nothing but consulting ourselves, then this is an objection not only to moral reflection but pretty much to any enquiry we try to conduct.

'CONSCIENCE CLAUSES'

But if conscience is fallible and often misleads us, what is the importance of letting people follow their conscience? Many people, and especially health care professionals, think it very important that they should be allowed to act according to their conscience, even when doing so goes against what is normally expected of them. For this reason, 'conscience clauses' can exempt doctors and nurses from direct involvement in a range of acts they consider morally wrong (Dyer, 2003). Abortion is probably the most familiar and widely discussed example. But one can think of several other highly realistic, non-contrived examples of such refusal that can involve many practitioners. Consider the following possible examples of conscientious refusal by doctors and other health care professionals:

- Refusal to reach targets for childhood MMR vaccination, while being prohibited from using single disease vaccinations, on the part of a doctor who believes that the MMR single vaccine can cause autism in children.
- Refusal to prescribe post-coital contraception, on the ground that this really amounts to abortion. This of course is the position of most of those who describe themselves as 'pro-life'. In the United States, there have recently been a number of cases not only of doctors refusing to prescribe the 'morning after pill' but of pharmacists refusing to honour prescriptions for it (Hopkins, 2005).
- Perhaps more unusually, refusals by some Roman Catholic doctors to prescribe contraception to adults, on the basis of the Church's condemnation of all sexual acts that are not 'open to the transmission of life'. There is published guidance on how to avoid prescribing contraception in general practice (Catholics in Practice Committee of the Guild of Catholic Doctors, 1995).
- Refusal to treat a terminally ill person with possibly life-prolonging treatment, on the grounds that it is a misuse of resources and is unlikely to bring about net benefit for the patient.
- Conversely, refusal to stop providing life-prolonging treatment despite the patient's refusal to have it. This

was the background to the Miss B case in the United Kingdom in 2002, when a competent adult paralysed from the neck down won her case in the High Court to have her ventilator disconnected, contrary to the wishes of her doctors.
- Refusal to refer a patient for palliative care when, in the doctor's opinion, the curative options have not been exhausted, but the patient wishes for no more curative treatment.
- Refusal to refer a patient for sterilization, or refusal to refer for sterilization under particular circumstances (e.g. the patient requesting it is in her early twenties and has never had children).

It is widely believed that in at least some such cases doctors and nurses should have the right of conscientious refusal, if they harbour moral objections. However, in recent medical literature there is not a great deal of explicit *ethical* discussion of conscience clauses, or of the moral importance of acting according to one's conscience. Fundamental questions face us. What is conscience, and why, if at all, should it be obeyed? Are we obliged to 'respect' another person's conscience – whether that of medical colleagues, or indeed of patients? Can an action be morally wrong *just* because it goes against the agent's conscience?

To some extent, the concern with respecting doctors' conscientious objections has a similar basis to the contemporary concern to respect the autonomy of competent patients. The shift away from medical paternalism over the past two or three decades has given birth to increased awareness that patients may have individual or cultural perspectives that do not entirely square with the values of mainstream medicine. The GMC guidelines on the duties of a doctor require doctors to listen to their patients and respect their views. It is not always clear what this amounts to in practice. But given the emphasis on patient autonomy, which can entail respecting a competent patient's conscientious refusal of a life-saving treatment (e.g. the textbook example of a competent adult Jehovah's Witness's refusal of a blood transfusion) it seems reasonable that there should be a reciprocal duty to respect the conscientious positions of doctors.

But, as is familiar, there is potential for conflict between the conscientious stance of a doctor and what may be in the best interests of a patient – or at least, with what the patient desires. Of course, if a patient demands a treatment that is not clinically indicated, most doctors would feel under no obligation to supply it. But there are occasions when a doctor conscientiously refuses to be involved in a procedure, even though the procedure is legal and the patient satisfies the usual clinical criteria for it. In these cases there is a conflict between the medical consensus and the doctor's conscience. This generates a debate about the extent to which doctors should be allowed to resist involvement. Should doctors be required to provide such procedures or treatments, perhaps on pain of disciplinary action? Or should their conscientious position be given pride of place?

ARGUMENTS FOR RESPECTING CONSCIENTIOUS OBJECTION

There are various arguments in favour of respecting sincere conscientious positions. Some of these arguments are quite weak. For example, it might be said that conscience should be respected just because it is usually distressing to be required to do something you consider seriously wrong, and distressing to suffer guilt after having done it. However, if doctors were routinely spared involvement in procedures that caused them distress, the practice of medicine would virtually collapse. All kinds of things are distressing, such as watching a patient die in pain, breaking bad news, tending to accident victims – but we still expect doctors to do these things. Another relatively weak argument stresses that the mere legality of a procedure does not make it morally permissible; that there have been plenty of bad laws allowing wrong things and plenty of laws forbidding things which are morally permissible. Of course, this is true. But it is not a strong ground for permitting a doctor to refuse participation, just because he *thinks* a procedure is morally wrong. Just as there are morally bad laws or practice guidelines, so there are morally misguided views about the badness of laws and practice guidelines.

But there are stronger arguments. There is a tradition about the importance of following one's own conscience, which dates back at least to St Thomas Aquinas, though one need not be religious to hold to it (Kenny, 1987). This has two elements. First, it says that it is always wrong to act against one's conscience. Thus an 'erring conscience' binds (Jackson, 2006). Someone who deliberately does what he believes to be wrong, even though it is not, shows a general lack of concern with morality. It is as if he said to himself: 'This is wrong, but I don't care – I'm going to do it anyway.' In Aquinas's theological context, a man's conscience was his opinion, correct or not, about the law made by God. Deliberately acting against one's conscience was therefore acting against what one believed to be God's law and was therefore sinful. But second, someone who *obeys* his conscience may *still* be acting wrongly because his conscience may be misguided, badly educated or even plain evil. According to Aquinas, a person might do what he sincerely thinks is God's will, but be in error about God's will when he should know better. In short, obeying one's conscience is *necessary*, but not *sufficient*, for acting in a morally permissible way.

This idea has a theological origin but permits a secular reading – if you do something wrong when you should have known better, then merely having acted in accordance with

your conscience will not exonerate you from blame. Admittedly, it may not be your fault if you do not know the truth. If you had no means of knowing what was right and wrong in a particular situation – for example (in the religious context), if you had no way of knowing the Church's teaching, then although you may act in a way that is objectively wrong, you may not be blamed for it, or at least, not fully. But when your ignorance of the truth arises from negligence – you could have found it out, but you did not bother – then your erring conscience does not excuse you.

How can this be turned into an argument for respecting conscientious objection? The idea is that if acting against one's conscience is morally wrong, then no one should be required to do so because that amounts to being required to act wrongly. It is beside the point that one may be morally mistaken and one's conscience misguided. No one, on this argument, should be professionally required or pressurized into doing something they consider wrong, because to accede to such pressure would itself be wrong.

Note that this does not preclude attempts to persuade the objector that her stance, is mistaken. Conscience is not sacrosanct, in the sense of being properly immune to argument. We do and sometimes ought to express our moral disagreements with people. If we think someone's conscience is standing in the way of something important, it can be legitimate to try to reason with her. But there is an important, though fine line between rationally persuading someone to abandon a conscientious stance, and putting her under pressure to violate her principles while still retaining them. This can apply to patients too. It is well known that competent adults have a nearly absolute right to refuse any treatment, and treatment is sometimes refused on grounds of conscience. But it is usually hard for a doctor to stand by and watch a patient come to serious harm or death, through such refusal. If, say, a competent adult Jehovah's Witness is refusing a blood transfusion, then (subject of course to time constraints) it may be legitimate for an informed doctor to try to persuade the patient that the interpretation of the Bible that apparently forbids transfusions is irrational. This is unlikely to be feasible in practice for various reasons. But such attempts at persuasion do not amount to coercion. The patient can always refuse in spite of the doctor's arguments (Savulescu and Momeyer, 1995).

Other, perhaps more common arguments may also be brought in. A person's integrity may be violated if she is made to act against her conscience; the deepest values by which she defines her life are under assault. It is a cause of distress and anger that she should have to do what she thinks is wrong, and even if that alone is not decisive, it still counts. With these arguments in mind, we can say that there is very good, if not decisive reason to respect the conscience of health care professionals, just as there is good reason to respect the refusal, conscientious or otherwise, of competent patients.

RESPECT FOR REFUSAL VERSUS THE INTERESTS OF PATIENTS

To return to a familiar example: a doctor with strong moral objections to abortion. She feels bound not to violate her conscience by involving herself in this practice. At the same time, those who disagree with her might say that she has an overriding duty to her patients, including those who seek abortions that would be sanctioned by existing law. If she is mistaken in her views on abortion, then she does a disservice to those women whom she refuses to help. Yet it is widely accepted that a right of refusal should normally be granted. The right of refusal does not depend on that refusal being ethically reasonable.

However, can we find any coherent policy on how the right of refusal can be fairly balanced against the interest patients have in obtaining the services or treatments in question? Are the rights of doctors being given unfair priority over the rights and interests of patients? It may be that in large cities, where there are a number of doctors whom patients can choose to see, there is little cost to patients in allowing some doctors the right of refusal. The patient can probably find another doctor. But the situation may be very different in rural areas or small towns where the only doctor a patient can see has rigid views about abortion, the 'morning after pill' or even all contraception. In those cases, a patient may find herself at the mercy of the moral views of the doctor. Similarly, if a certain conscientious position becomes very common in the medical profession – let us say that a very large number of doctors become persuaded of some currently minority moral view – the patients may have understandable cause for complaint. They will feel that doctors are effectively imposing their moral views on them, maybe even in defiance of the GMC guidance that doctors should not allow their 'personal views' to prejudice their care of patients. Such arguments against doctors being allowed to refuse legal procedures on conscientious grounds have been vigorously put forward (Savulescu, 2006).

Doctors might reply that were they to yield to such requests, patients would be imposing their own values upon *them*, and this indeed is the view of the Guild of Catholic Doctors concerning contraception (Catholics in Practice Committee of the Guild of Catholic Doctors, 1995). But this manoeuvre is somewhat disingenuous; patients would not necessarily be forcing doctors to provide certain services, but rather asking them for those services, leaving it up to the doctors whether or not to agree. The issue of imposition does, however, arise if doctors are disciplined for sticking to their positions, or denied entry to their desired area of practice because of their views. However, if the legitimate interests of patients are to be protected, such measures may be necessary. The difficult question is how to strike the right balance.

We have seen how a relatively forceful argument for permitting conscientious objection is that it is wrong to do what you consider wrong (even if you are mistaken) and, because it is wrong to make someone do wrong, it is wrong to make someone do what he considers wrong. But this must be weighed up against an important consideration on the other side, namely that there is no *right*, in general, to be admitted into the medical or nursing profession or to a particular specialism within it. Just as a declared pacifist is unlikely to be admitted to the Army, so an aspiring doctor might not be admitted into a particular area within medicine if she declares herself unwilling to do what is normally required by the job. And whatever the merits of her conscientious position, her rights are not violated if she is denied entry to her preferred area because no such right existed in the first place. She might feel aggrieved, in effect made to choose between her principles and the career she had always wanted. It is no doubt but unfortunate to be in this situation, but being denied the right of conscientious refusal need not entail being made to act against conscience. There is always the option, however unappealing, of seeking another line of work, or another specialism within medicine.

CONSCIENTIOUS OBJECTION AND THE CORE VALUES OF MEDICINE

But granted that there is strictly no *right* to be admitted to one's preferred line of work, might it not be *unreasonable* to deny a well-qualified candidate her preferred post, on the grounds of her moral position? This, I suggest, depends, not so much on whether her position is morally defensible, but more on whether her moral position bears sufficient affinity to certain generally accepted core values of medicine (Wicclair, 2000).

To illustrate this, imagine two candidates for medical placements. One is an aspiring GP who will not prescribe the 'morning after pill' or refer for abortion. The other is an aspiring obstetrician who, it turns out, opposes the use of any pain relief during labour. His reason is that in the Book of Genesis, the pain of childbirth was Eve's punishment for her transgression in the Garden of Eden. Labour pains are a punishment for sin, and no attempt should be made to alleviate them. His position is conscientious and based on his fundamentalist understanding of the Bible.

Of course, the latter case is highly unrealistic. But it serves to focus the question of whether there are any conscientious positions that simply should not be accommodated, however sincerely held. I suggest this would be one such, whereas the matter is different with the pro-life woman who wants to be a GP. The reason, briefly stated, is that even if we disagree with the pro-life position, we can see that it relates intelligibly to generally accepted values. It is based on respect for human life, which is a core value of medicine; it bases itself on non-maleficence and regards abortion as maleficent because it is deliberate killing. We do not have to agree with this position to see how it is connected to positions we do accept. However, the views of the anti-epidural doctor do not connect with such core values of medicine. Relief of pain, when it conflicts with no other central value, is a core aim of medicine. Of course, he would perhaps argue that it should not be, but ultimately any profession has its first principles, and concern for human suffering should be one of them.

In summary, the challenge posed by conscientious objection in medicine is complex, and some balance must be struck between respect for objection and the legitimate interests of patients, who pay taxes for health care services in a democratic society and have some right to determine what kind of services they receive. There is no easy method for finding this balance, and conflict is inevitable. The most fruitful suggestion is that those conscientious positions that most accord with the basic values of medicine have the best claims to our respect.

There is another advantage of allowing limited conscientious refusal, and this is that the profession flourishes best if there are diverse ethical views to be found within it. A monolithic ethical culture tends to stagnate. Under pressure from dissenters, commonly accepted views about a variety of things have changed. One change frequently noted is that from a predominantly paternalistic conception of the doctor–patient relationship to one far more focused on patient autonomy. Another is in attitudes to impairment and the quality of life; it is less common now to 'let die' infants with impairments when they can be kept alive.

Certain issues, however, probably cannot be solved to everyone's satisfaction because people start from radically different premises. The issue of conscientious objection is essentially that of whether certain refusals should be allowed, *regardless* of whether the refusers are correct. This is important. For it is clear, for instance, that if one already opposes abortion on moral grounds, then one will support the right to refuse participation in abortion. And not only that, but also the right to refuse to refer the patient to someone else. For one difficulty with current practice is that a doctor who conscientiously refuses is obliged to refer the patient on to someone with no objections. Clearly this raises the issue of complicity, and it is hard to see how a doctor who seriously believes that abortion is murder can be happy to refer a patient to someone else who is prepared to commit murder. Doubtless, the granting of a right of refusal of direct participation, but with no right to refuse to refer, is a pragmatic compromise designed to give some leeway to all views. But it is not one that a clear-headed 'pro-life' doctor should be able to accept.

The main point, though, is that views about which practices one should be allowed to refuse participation in will largely, though not entirely, depend on one's prior views about the morality of those practices. If one does not believe that abortion is murder – if one believes, in fact, that it is any woman's right to have it on request – then it is not clear that one has any decisive reason to believe refusal should be allowed.

To sum up: ideally the issue of which refusals should be respected and which not, would be settled by coming up with an agreement among all parties, irrespective of their moral views. This is an ideal worth striving for and is indeed the basis of the theory of law in a liberal democracy: most people agree that certain practices they think immoral should be legally allowed, partly because they desire a similar tolerance from others. But with fundamental issues to do with life or death, some people consider certain actions to be so terrible that they will not agree that dissenters should be allowed to perform them. We have found good reason to accept certain conscientious refusals, provided they are not too out of kilter with the accepted core values of medicine. But views about what those core values are will remain, to some extent, irresolvably contentious. Thus, although we have argued in favour of conscience clauses, we should not expect our arguments to be found convincing by all parties. We can get closer to the necessary consensus, but never fully achieve it.

REFERENCES

Catholics in Practice Committee of the Guild of Catholic Doctors. *Contraception and the Catholic GP Trainee and Partner in a Group Practice*, 1995; http://www.catholicdoctors.org.uk/books/contraceptbook.htm

Dyer C. Health authorities cannot force doctors to act against conscience. *BMJ* 2003; **327**: 1187.

Hopkins TJ. Emergency contraception is under attack by US pharmacists. *BMJ* 2005; **330**: 983.

Jackson J. *Ethics in Medicine*. Cambridge: Polity Press, 2006; ch. 5.

Kenny A. The conscience of Sir Thomas More. In: Kenny A, ed. *The Heritage of Wisdom: Essays in the History of Philosophy*. Oxford: Blackwell, 1987.

Plato (Translated by Tredennick H). Crito, *The Last Days of Socrates*. Harmondsworth: Penguin Books, 1954.

Savulescu J, Momeyer RW. Rational non-interventional paternalism: why doctors ought to make judgements of what is best for their patients. *J Med Ethics* 1995; **21**(6): 327–331.

Savulescu J. Conscientious objection in medicine. *BMJ* 2006; **332**: 294–297.

Wicclair M. Conscientious objection in medicine. *Bioethics* 2000; **14**(3): 205–227.

47

Care in Families

HILDE LINDEMANN

Physicians, nurses, therapists and other professionals provide much of the care for those who suffer from disease or injury, but it is sometimes forgotten that there is another, far larger system of health care delivery: the family. Familial health care ranges from preventative care (teaching children how to brush and floss their teeth) to care of the bedridden (picking up prescriptions and providing soup and sympathy when someone is down with flu), to unremitting long-term care (looking after a son who suffers from schizophrenia)and to sacrificial care (live kidney or liver lobe donation to a loved one in need). The biomedical advances and socioeconomic forces that have given professional health care systems their current shape have put pressure on families to provide more care, of a more technical nature, than ever before. At the same time, changing social views as to how families may or must be configured, what the division of labour in the family is supposed to be and the extent to which families are expected to rely on professional health care all exert pressure in the opposite direction.

The demands the two systems put on one another can give rise to considerable friction between them, particularly when there is a danger of exceeding the capacity of either to provide the needed care. A further source of friction, however, is that although a great deal of attention has been devoted to the moral understandings that govern the conduct of health care professionals, the ethics of families has received short shrift. As a result, health professionals may treat families dismissively, view them with suspicion or hold them to their professions' own standard of conduct. And because families often cannot even articulate – let alone defend – the morality that governs them, they may experience frustration, fear or anger in their encounters with health professionals.

TWO SYSTEMS OF ETHICS

Until recently, moral philosophers have not been much interested in families, often perceiving them as natural entities outside the purview of morality, or, on the few occasions when they have taken notice of them, characterizing them uncritically in accordance with the social prejudices of their time (for example, Rousseau, 1993). Since roughly 1980, however, a handful of philosophers and bioethicists have produced a modest but growing literature on the ethics of families (Schoeman, 1980, 1985; Blustein, 1982; Rhoden, 1988; Okin, 1989; Hardwig, 1990, 2000; Arras, 1995; Nelson and Nelson, 1995; Nelson, 1997; Levine, 2000; Hardart and Truog, 2003). What this literature shows us goes some distance towards explaining why families are sometimes misunderstood in health care contexts. Consider the following contrasts between key ethical orthodoxies of the two systems of care.

ORTHODOXIES OF HEALTH CARE ETHICS

In health care ethics, as elsewhere, what confers orthodoxy on a belief or practice is not that it is never challenged, but that it is widely held and that it is recognized to be orthodox even by those who dissent from it. I have identified six such orthodoxies, though the list is hardly comprehensive:

1. *The focus of attention ought to be on the patient, not on the health care professionals.* The purpose of health care is to provide vulnerable patients with a safe and therapeutically effective clinical encounter; therefore, everything and everyone should revolve around the patient.
2. *The patient's autonomy must be respected.* Autonomy is understood to require two abilities: (1) the ability to make decisions and perform actions that originate from

Principles of Health Care Ethics, Second Edition   Edited by R.E. Ashcroft, A. Dawson, H. Draper and J.R. McMillan
© 2007 John Wiley & Sons, Ltd

oneself rather than being imposed from the outside; and (2) the ability to understand the facts of one's situation and to engage in practical reasoning on the basis of these facts. Autonomy is, therefore, a matter of individualism: to exercise autonomy is to move under one's own steam, free from external constraints.

3. *Nothing is supposed to be done to or for patients without their free and informed consent.* This orthodoxy follows from the orthodox understanding of autonomy as individualistic. Physicians and other health care workers may not lie to their patients as this impedes their ability to consent freely. Emergency treatment of patients who are in no condition to give consent is permitted, but only because such patients would presumably consent if they could. When patients are not mentally capable of giving consent, their proxies are supposed to use substituted judgement, deciding the way the patient would have decided. In the absence of any way of ascertaining what the patient would have wanted, the proxy should decide according to what is in the patient's best interests.

4. *The patient's best interests must be understood as self-interests.* This orthodoxy also follows from the orthodox understanding of autonomy as individualistic, and it entails, among other things, that proxies using the best interest standard may consider no one's interests but the patient's. If others' interests are considered, the proxy may be presumed not to understand his or her duties, and the health care professional has a responsibility to intervene.

5. *Patient confidentiality must be preserved except when the health, well-being or safety of others would be threatened by the failure to disclose information about the patient.* Confidentiality is necessary because patients must often entrust their most personal weaknesses and secrets to the health care professional; to break confidentiality is to abuse the trust at the heart of the patient-professional relationship.

6. *Advance planning is good and should always be encouraged.* Patients should have advance directives that appoint proxies to act for them if they ever become incompetent to make their own health care decisions. The directives should also stipulate the sort of life-sustaining treatments patients would want to have withdrawn or withheld were they to become irreversibly comatose or terminally ill.

Over the last 30 years or so (roughly since bioethics' inception as an interdisciplinary field), bioethicists have identified, developed and refined these tenets, conferring on them the stature they enjoy today.

ORTHODOXIES OF FAMILY ETHICS

Families, by contrast, tend to operate on a set of orthodoxies that are far less explicit. Many are unspoken, and although not all families embrace all of them, they are perfectly recognizable when they are articulated. In the list that follows, I confine myself to widely shared moral understanding governing families in contemporary, post-industrial European and English-speaking societies, acknowledging that even within those bounds, families exhibit many differences in their moral values and practices.

1. Where health care ethics is patient-centred, *in families, everyone counts.* Each member of the family is meant to be cherished by the others, singled out specially and shown loving concern. Although it is true that in many families the husband and father has counted for more than his wife, children and other dependants, all family members are nevertheless supposed to receive some special regard.

2. Where health care ethics understands autonomy as individualistic, *in families, autonomy is relational.* Jodi Halpern argues that even in health care settings, autonomy is 'an interpersonal process in which other people's recognition of a person's agency, or the lack thereof, is highly influential' (Halpern, 2001, p. 114). This interpersonal feature of autonomy is particularly visible in families, however. Family members are nested in a web of identity-constituting relationships, and because families shape and maintain the selves within those relationships, they both constrain and powerfully undergird their members' ability to be the authors of their own actions and choices.

3. Where health care ethics insists that nothing may be done to or for a patient without the patient's free and informed consent, *in families, trust is often more important than consent.* Touching in families is frequently unconsented because family members are supposed to be able to trust one another, to touch lovingly and not to touch when touching is wrong: marital rape and incest are particularly awful precisely because the perpetrators violate their victims' trust. When family members are needy and vulnerable, it is relationships of trust, not consent, that typically undergird their care.

4. Where health care ethics understands the patient's best interests as self-interests, *in families, interests extend beyond selves.* Because families are more than merely a collection of individuals, what happens inside one is often assessed in terms of its impact on the overall family, in a manner that is hard to reduce to the interests of individual family members. Family traditions are perhaps the clearest example of how family members participate in an ongoing process of group self-definition, but important decisions primarily affecting one family member are also usually made with due consideration for their impact on the family as a whole.

5. Where health care ethics emphasizes the importance of preserving patient confidentiality, *in families, many*

confidences are shared. Although family members surely have a right to privacy, parents are supposed to know where their children are and what sort of friends they have, whether they are unhappy in school, in the grip of an eating disorder or taking drugs. By the same token, a person in an intimate relationship is expected to tell her partner that her job has been terminated, that she has come into an inheritance or that she has a serious illness.

6. Where health care ethics extols advance planning, *in families, things don't always go according to plan.* Many families are too poor and their livelihoods too precarious for long-term plans to be feasible; other families move around too much or find themselves in circumstances where planning does not make sense. Still other families may plan for retirement or their children's higher education but do not try to control what sort of health care they would want under various hypothetical scenarios in the distant future.

THE FEATURES OF FAMILIES

To understand why the ethics of families differs in so many important respects from health care ethics, we need only to consider the differences between the two systems of care. The most striking difference, obviously, is that professional health care delivery systems have no purpose other than to provide health care to patients, whereas families have many functions: making and maintaining the homes where family life goes on, rearing children, fostering intimate relations, serving as a basic economic unit, transmitting cultural and religious values and so on. But unlike health care institutions, which are valuable only instrumentally, families are also *valuable as ends in themselves.* We prize them not only for what they can do for those inside them but also for what they are. The kinship relations that change but also endure over time, the network of ongoing connections that situate us in the world, the people we love just because they are *our* people – these are valuable quite apart from any goods or services the family might provide.

A second characteristic of families is their *gendered division of labour.* Beginning in the eighteenth century, the Industrial Revolution had a permanent impact on families because it forced increasing numbers of people to work outside their homes rather than on family farms or in cottage industries. For poor families, this meant that able-bodied women as well as men (and often children) had to work long hours in mills, coal mines or factories, but in middle-class families, women were excluded from the paid workforce and expected to devote themselves to domestic duties. They were responsible, with or without the help of servants, for the smooth running of the home and whatever caregiving was needed, whether for children, the ill or the elderly members of the family (Mintz and Kellogg, 1988). In the second half of the twentieth century, as middle-class wives and mothers took jobs outside the home to help support their families' higher standard of living, the gendered division of labour persisted; women still do a vastly greater amount of domestic work than men do, clocking in for the notorious 'second shift' after the paid workday is over.

A third feature of families is their *non-consensual relationships.* Some family ties are created voluntarily – for instance, when a man and woman marry or same-sex partners make a commitment to a long-term relationship – but many are not. None of us chose our parents, and while some of our parents might have chosen to procreate at a particular time, they did not choose the particular children who came into existence. Nor do we choose our siblings, grandparents, aunts, uncles or in-laws. Despite our not having agreed to these relationships, however, they often give rise to responsibilities: Aunt Marjorie must be invited to your wedding; Great-uncle Herbert must be taken for grocery shopping; your little brother must be helped with his homework.

Fourth, family members are *not fungible.* In a comedy classic, a distraught mother wails to W. C. Fields, 'You've killed my baby!' Fields looks doleful for a moment and then brightens up. 'Never mind, Madam,' he leers at her, 'I will gladly get you with another.' The exchange is funny not only because of its sexual innuendo, but also because family members are not replaceable in the way Fields seems to imagine. Family members are to be prized for who they are, not what they do, and for that reason they are not interchangeable. The person who sells you a halibut could just as easily be another fishmonger, but no one can take the place of your firstborn child.

Fifth, families are typically (as well as ideally) *sites of love.* Love, along with protection from harm, nurture and socialization, is required for children to grow normally, and because children grow in families, it is the families' responsibility to provide it. Love need not be expressed or felt as an emotion; it is perfectly possible to love a sister who irritates you beyond bearing. But familial love does not turn its back on its own, which is why, as Robert Frost puts it, 'home is where, if you have to go there, they have to take you in.'

And sixth, families play a central role in *constructing their members' identities.* If personal identities are a complicated interaction between our self-concepts and others' understandings of who we are, it is in our families of origin that we first come to have an identity at all. And just as families *shape* the identities of their youngest members, so too do they help *maintain* the identities of the older members. Many factors combine to hold each of us together as a particular 'who', including our experience of familiar places, activities, commitments and memories, but perhaps the most powerful source of identity maintenance is found in our intimate relationships, particularly those that have endured over time. Through many acts of recognition, large and small, the people who know us well mirror back to us who they think we are, and in so doing they help us stabilize our identities even as we change and grow.

What counts as a family? As the current struggles over gay marriage demonstrate, that is a contested question. There are single-parent families; gay and lesbian families; childless families; families where the adults are remarried and the children are stepchildren or half-siblings; divorced families extending over several households with children in joint physical custody; families in which the adults are roommates and serve as 'othermothers' (Collins, 1991) to each other's children; families in the sense of kinship relations whereby people are connected by blood, marriage or adoption but who do not live together. Because there is no one feature that is characteristic of all families, it is perhaps best to regard 'family' as what Ludwig Wittgenstein calls a family-resemblance notion, consisting of many overlapping features but with no features that are common to them all.

FAMILY CAREGIVING

The features that are characteristic of families give shape, naturally enough, to the ways in which families take care of their own. It is therefore convenient to take up in turn each of the six features enumerated above, to examine its contribution to families' practices of care.

FAMILIES AS ENDS IN THEMSELVES

Because families are valuable not only for the goods and services they provide but also intrinsically, in themselves, they too are objects of care. The relationships that constitute them must be fed and watered; family traditions must be observed; family members must have occasions on which to enjoy each others' company, air grievances and mend any rifts that arise among them. To ensure that this self-care is possible, families must see to it that they do not exceed their capacity for giving other sorts of care. Like ships, families have a Plimsoll line – the point at which, no matter how the load is distributed, any additional weight will cause the craft to sink. It is true that families that are suddenly burdened with previously unimaginable amounts of caregiving sometimes discover that their caring capacity is much greater than they suspected. But it is also true that heavy demands on a family's caregiving resources pose a threat to the family's integrity.

Health care providers would do well to keep this point firmly in mind, rather than simply assuming that family members will eagerly pick up all the slack where professional care leaves off. Carol Levine tells the story of how, after her husband was severely disabled in a car accident, she was initiated into the role of family caregiver. 'A nurse stuck my husband's soiled sweat pants under my nose and said, "Take these away. Laundry is your job." . . ., The nurse's underlying message, reinforced by many others, was that my life from now on would consist of performing an unrelieved series of nasty chores. The social worker assigned to my husband's case had one goal: discharge. I was labelled a "selfish wife," since I refused to take him home without home care. "Get real," the social worker said. "Nobody will pay for home care"' (Levine, 2000, pp. 73–74). Levine's plight is exacerbated because she lives in the United States, where access to professional care largely depends on how much health care insurance one can afford. The uncaring and judgemental attitude of the professional staff, however, would seem to have less to do with health care economics than with a deep misunderstanding of what families are for.

GENDERED DIVISION OF LABOUR

Families provide a range of care: infant care, child care, elder care, long-term care, care of the mildly ill, acute care on hospital discharge, care of the dying. And this care may be given by mothers, grandparents, young children, disabled family members, fathers, nieces, nephews, siblings or cousins. But under the gendered division of labour that governs most families, the vast preponderance of family care is given by women. According to the National Alliance for Caregiving (2003), for example, approximately one quarter of US households contain someone caring for an elderly relative or friend, and nearly 73% of these long-term caregivers are women. The reasons for this are complex, but it seems clear that gender, understood not as sexual difference but as an abusive power relation favouring men's interests over women, is heavily implicated. The social institutions, practices and accompanying ideology that systematically assign an overwhelming proportion of unpaid caring labour to women create a system that is inherently exploitative – a fact that must be kept firmly in mind in any ethical analysis of family caregiving.

Because the material and social forces that create this division of labour are not likely to wither away any time soon, it is all the more important that the other family members do what they can to take care of the primary caregiver (Nelson, 2003). They could, for example, provide respite care so that she can have a weekend away from caregiving. Or they could run errands for her, take on some of her other chores, offer moral support, pamper her with foot massages or whatever else she regards as a luxury. Nor should the care of the caregiver be the sole responsibility of other family members. Diemut Bubeck (1995) suggests that respite care is a duty of citizens. Her idea, modelled on military service, is that men and women alike would spend some period of their lives in a 'caring service' whose mission would be to provide back-up care for family caregivers.

NON-CONSENSUAL RELATIONSHIPS

Although the gendered division of caring labour puts family caregivers at special risk of exploitation, so does the non-consensual nature of many familial ties. Consider, for example, an elderly parent suffering from a moderate degree of Alzheimer's disease. He is divorced and has never remarried, so the responsibility for looking after him devolves on his two sons. Someone must see to it that he gets regular meals, that his bills are paid on time, that he keeps his doctor's appointments, that he remembers to shower and shave, that his clothes and house are clean, and so on. If one of the sons is reluctant to shoulder his half of these responsibilities, then the other, whether he likes it or not, must do double duty. The son who leaves it all to his brother is surely open to moral censure, but the exploited son cannot responsibly remedy the injustice by doing only his fair share. He did not ask to have such an unreliable brother, nor did he agree to assume the full burden of his father's care. His consent, however, is not what binds him morally. Here, the source of normativity is the father–son relationship.

Because family caregivers may not exit the relationship that gives rise to their caring responsibilities, the patients who are the recipients of care have a special duty to consider their caregivers in turn. This consideration can take many forms. The patient might, for example, opt for a slightly more painful form of treatment because it lightens the caregiver's burden of care. Or the patient might decline a treatment – even a life-sustaining treatment – so as not to deplete altogether the caregiver's physical and financial resources. The idea here is not that the caregiver's interests take precedence over the patient's, but rather that because the patient–caregiver relationship is non-consensual, decision-making must extend some consideration to the caregiver as well as to the patient.

NON-FUNGIBILITY OF FAMILY MEMBERS

When a patient is cared for by someone she loves, she receives more than the aspirin, the backrub or the tea and toast her caregiver provides – she receives the goods that inhere in this particular intimate relationship (Blum, 1982). Put more precisely, she receives the good of this particular known, loved and trusted person. That is why it matters within families, in a way that it does not at the fish market, just who is taking care of the customer.

It can also be important just who makes treatment decisions for an incompetent family member. Suppose a computer could be programmed with every conceivable bit of information about you such that it can predict, with 99% accuracy, precisely what you would want under any imaginable medical scenario. You could then arrange for the computer to be your proxy decision-maker in the event that you become too ill to make decisions for yourself. Here, we have the height of fungibility: any computer that could do this is perfectly replaceable by any other properly programmed computer. But for some of us, *who* will decide is more important than what will be decided. Even if they do not choose exactly as we would, we might prefer our children – simply because they *are* our children – to a smoothly functioning machine (Nelson 2003).

FAMILIES AS SITES OF LOVE

It is in our families of origin, unless we are very unlucky indeed, that we first experience love. But love, unlike most other things that children need for healthy growth, is incomplete unless it is given as well as received (the same is true of language: a conversation requires speaking as well as listening). So, typically, parents and other family members hold very young children in a one-sided loving relationship, anticipating the time when love is returned, first childishly and often imperfectly, and later maturely, adult to adult. Love encumbers us with duties, however, in that it sets up the expectation that it will eventually be returned. That is why it is a serious moral matter when, in the absence of a pressing reason, adult children walk away from familial love.

If this is right, there are implications for family caregiving here as well – specifically, for the care that adult children owe their frail elderly parents. On the account of love offered here, filial obligation is grounded in need: first, the young child's need for love, and later, the loving parents' need for care. The kind and extent of care given will depend on the grown child's resources and the kind and intensity of the parental need, but whether to respond at all is not open to discretion. The seed of the duty to care for one's elderly parents was planted long ago, when the young parents heeded their duty to love their infant child.

FAMILIAL IDENTITY MAINTENANCE

Serious injury or illness can, and frequently does, play havoc with one's identity. To be critically ill for more than a few days is to lose control over one's physical and mental processes. It puts a stop to one's professional and social activities and interferes with one's memories, hopes, plans for the future and ongoing projects. It usually involves hospitalization, which means that one is uprooted from one's customary surroundings; denied access to cherished people, pets and objects; and thrust into a milieu governed by insider understandings to which one is not privy. All of this contributes to a disintegration of one's sense of self. Eric Cassell (1982) conceptualizes this disintegration as *suffering;* to suffer is to feel oneself being undone. Suffering persists, writes Cassell, until the threat to the identity has passed or until the integrity of the identity can be re-established in some manner.

It is when we suffer in Cassell's sense of the word that we most need the help of others to preserve our identities. Torn out of the contexts and conditions in which we can maintain our own sense of ourselves, we run the risk of losing sight of who we are, at least temporarily, unless someone else can lend a hand. Because our intimates know us best and their lives are closely intertwined with ours, they are in the best position to hold on to the 'who' of us until such time as we can pull ourselves together. And they are in the best position to help us incorporate into our identities the changes wrought by the experience of deep illness.

The orthodoxies of health care ethics might easily give rise to the assumption that when a patient is ill enough to enter the health care delivery system, the role of the family is two-fold: first, to serve as the mop-up caregiver by providing all the necessary care that the system is not designed to provide; and second, to supply professional caregivers with expert knowledge of the patient's wishes when the patient cannot convey these herself. Fortunately, professional practice seems wiser than bioethical theory. In a recent survey of physicians affiliated with American medical schools, a majority of neonatologists and intensivists said that family interests should be considered in decisions for incompetent patients, even if those interests are not coextensive with those of the patients (Hardart and Truog, 2003). These data, limited though they may be, suggest that health care practitioners have their own views of the importance of their patients' family ties. Arguably in this respect, theory could benefit from closer attention to practice. Perhaps bioethicists could learn, from what professionals actually do, the moral value of taking patients' families seriously.

REFERENCES

Arras J, ed. *Bringing the Hospital Home: Ethical and Social Implications of High-Tech Home Care.* Baltimore, MD: Johns Hopkins University Press, 1995.

Blum L. *Friendship, Altruism, and Morality.* New York: Routledge, 1982.

Blustein J. *Parents and Children: The Ethics of the Family.* New York: Oxford University Press, 1982.

Bubeck DE. *Care, Gender, and Justice.* New York and Oxford: Clarendon Press, 1995.

Cassell E. The nature of suffering and the goals of medicine. *N Engl J Med* 1982; **306**(11): 639–645.

Collins PH. *Black Feminist Thought: Knowledge, Consciousness, and the Politics of Empowerment.* New York: Routledge, 1991.

Halpern J. *From Detached Concern to Empathy: Humanizing Medical Practice.* New York: Oxford University Press, 2001.

Hardart G, Truog R. Attitudes and preferences of intensivists regarding the role of family interests in medical decision-making for incompetent patients. *Critical Care Medicine* 2003; **31**(7): 1895–1900.

Hardwig J. What about the family? *Hastings Center Rep* 1990; **20**(2): 5–10.

Hardwig J. *Is There a Duty to Die? and Other Essays in Bioethics.* New York: Routledge, 2000.

Levine C. The loneliness of the long-term caregiver. In: Levine C, ed. *Always on Call.* New York: United Hospital Fund, 2000.

Mintz S, Kellogg S. *Domestic Revolutions: A Social History of American Family Life.* New York: Free Press, 1988.

National Alliance for Caregiving, 2003; http://aging.senate.gov/public/events/hr76gh.htm

Nelson HL, ed. *Feminism and Families.* New York: Routledge, 1997.

Nelson HL, Nelson JL. *The Patient in the Family: An Ethics of Medicine and Families.* New York: Routledge, 1995.

Nelson J. *Hippocrates' Maze: Ethical Explorations of the Medical Labyrinth.* Lanham, MD: Rowman & Littlefield, 2003.

Okin SM. *Justice, Gender, and the Family.* New York: Basic Books, 1989.

Rhoden NK. Litigating life and death. *Harvard Law Rev* 1988; **102**(2): 375–446.

Rousseau JJ. *Emile* (Translated by Barbara Foxley). London: J.M. Dent, 1993.

Schoeman F. Rights of children, rights of parents, and the moral basis of the family. *Ethics* 1980; **91**(1): 6–19.

Schoeman F. Parental discretion and children's rights: Background and implications for medical decision-making. *J Med Philos* 1985; **10**(1): 45–61.

48

The Ethics of Primary Health Care

ANNETTE J. BRAUNACK-MAYER

Primary health care has been a key concept in debate about health care systems throughout the last 30 years. Notwithstanding changes in patterns of disease, demographic profiles, and in socioeconomic environments, primary health care has retained a central place as the means through which a comprehensive, universal, equitable and affordable health care service can be provided for all countries (WHO-UNESCO, 1978).

The first challenge for any account of the ethics of primary health care is the term 'primary health care' itself. There are a number of definitions of primary health care currently in use, not all mutually exclusive, but each with slightly different implications for our understanding of its ethics. This chapter provides a general introduction to primary health care and then explores the ethics of primary health care by drawing a distinction between two approaches to primary health care ethics: the 'individual' account and the 'community' account. The individual account is built upon contributions from the general practice ethics literature; the community account draws mainly on writing within the ethics of health promotion and public health ethics. Taken together, they provide a balanced introduction to the ethics of primary health care.

THE DEFINITION OF PRIMARY HEALTH CARE

The term 'primary health care' came into widespread usage following the International Conference on Primary Health Care in Alma-Ata, USSR in 1978 (WHO-UNESCO, 1978). In the Alma Ata Declaration, primary health care is defined as:

> essential health care based on practical, scientifically sound and socially acceptable methods and technology, made universally available to individuals and families in the community through their full participation and at a cost that the community and the country can afford to maintain at every stage of their development in the spirit of self-reliance and self-determination. It forms an integral part both of the country's health system, of which it is the central function and main focus, and of the overall social and economic development of the community. It is the first level of contact of individuals, the family and community with the national health system bringing health care as close as possible to where people live and work, and constitutes the first element of a continuing health care process (WHO-UNESCO, 1978).

Integrated care, comprehensiveness and efficiency have been key themes in primary health care rhetoric (Welton et al., 1997). Primary health care has offered a vehicle for eliminating the vertical nature of isolated health care (Tarimo and Fowkes, 1989), reducing health inequalities and ensuring effective universal coverage, while simultaneously limiting the escalating costs of institutional care (OECD, 1990).

The Declaration of Alma-Ata defines primary health care in a number of different ways. Primary health care is, first, a set of value commitments – to community participation and empowerment, equity, accessibility and services and programmes that are culturally appropriate. Second, it is a set of *strategies* for the organization of health systems and the delivery of health care. Primary health care should:

- be based on relevant research and experience;
- provide the full range of health services – health promotion, prevention, cure and rehabilitation – to address community needs;
- be intersectoral, involving agricultural, housing, education, public works and communication programmes, as well as health programmes;
- promote community and individual self-reliance and participation in the planning and delivery of health care;

Principles of Health Care Ethics, Second Edition   Edited by R.E. Ashcroft, A. Dawson, H. Draper and J.R. McMillan

- be supported by appropriate referral systems; and
- be provided locally by health workers who are trained to work effectively as a team and to be responsive to community needs.

These principles are to be realized through a set of *core activities*, which should include, at least:

- health education;
- promotion of food supply and proper nutrition;
- an adequate supply of safe water and basic sanitation;
- maternal and child health care, including family planning;
- immunization;
- prevention and control of locally endemic diseases;
- appropriate treatment of common diseases and injuries; and
- provision of essential drugs.

Finally, primary health care can be defined in terms of its *goals*, or strategic imperatives. Primary health care is to deliver:

- decreases in excess mortality of poor, marginalized nations;
- decreases in major risk factors that increase morbidity and mortality;
- sustainable health systems; and
- an integrated approach to wider social policy and community development.

Countries around the world adopted the values, principles, core activities and strategic imperatives of primary health care after Alma-Ata. In low-resource countries, where access to care is still limited, primary health care has remained a system-wide strategy for health and social development (Kekki, 2003). In developed and middle-level countries, where access to basic services is generally less of an issue, primary health care has come to mean two things. The first is a level of care, essentially that type of care that is provided by a health care professional in the first contact of a patient with the health care system. This articulation of primary health care is controversial, as there is ample evidence in the literature that primary health care should not be regarded as a synonym for front-line primary care and basic health services (WHO-UNESCO, 1978).[1] Nonetheless, in practice, in developed and middle-level countries, general practice is considered the professional face of primary health care, and a sizeable component of primary health care is often subsumed under the heading of general practice.

The second view defines primary health care in terms of policymaking in health care, and regards it as a strategy to integrate all aspects of the health care system. So, for example, the New Zealand Health Strategy defines primary health care as

> essential health care based on practical, scientifically sound, culturally appropriate and socially acceptable methods. It is universally accessible to people in their communities, involves community participation, is integral to, and a central function of, the country's health system, and is the first level of contact with the health system (New Zealand Ministry of Health, 2001).

The first definition tends to focus attention on personal interactions between primary health care workers and the individuals for whom they care; the second places more emphasis on initiatives that occur at the level of communities.

This difference between primary health care as a level of care and as a system of health care is important. It circumscribes the context within which discussion of the ethics of primary health care takes place. In the two sections that follow, I give an account of the ethics of primary health care from each of these perspectives. The next section of the chapter considers the ethics of primary heath care from the perspective of the level-of-care definition. This account of primary health care ethics I label the 'individual' account. The final section of the chapter uses the system definition of primary health; this account I label the 'community' account.

PRIMARY HEALTH CARE ETHICS: THE 'INDIVIDUAL' ACCOUNT

The content of the individual account of primary health care ethics derives principally from the general practice ethics literature. This literature, in turn, has grown out of a discussion of the nature of general practice and the role of the general practitioner (GP), so I begin with that definition.

General practice defines itself principally through the doctor–patient relationship:

> GPs are personal doctors, primarily responsible for the provision of comprehensive and continuing medical care to patients irrespective of age, sex and illness...they take account of physical, psychological, social and cultural factors, using the knowledge and trust engendered by a familiarity with past care. They also recognize a professional responsibility to their community.

---

[1] In the health promotion literature, the distinction is reinforced by referring to this type of primary health care as *primary care*, to distinguish it from the system-oriented focus of *primary health* care.

GPs exercise their professional role by promoting health, preventing disease and providing cure, care or palliation. This is done either directly, or through the services of others according to health needs and the resources available within the community they serve (Royal College of General Practitioners, 2002).

Clearly, parts of this definition overlap with the definition of primary health care. General practice is the first point of contact for many people with health problems and the means through which they access specialist and hospital care. It is located in the community and is therefore locally accessible. General practice also provides comprehensive care services, including health promotion, disease prevention, curative services and rehabilitation. Finally, general practice has a broad understanding of health, acknowledging the role of broader social and economic factors in people's lives and the import for health status.

A range of ethical issues emerges from this definition (Rogers and Braunack-Mayer, 2004), and these issues apply equally to GPs and other primary health care professionals. First, the primary health care professional's role as first point of contact and provider of accessible, comprehensive care creates particular ethical demands. Once a person is 'through the door', the primary health care practitioner is committed to help, regardless of their familiarity with or distaste for the problem. They cannot shift a patient on to others, secure in the knowledge that this person will not return. As Pellegrino notes:

> The generalist cannot take refuge in the limitations of his specialty. For him the healing relationship must be entered in the fullest sense . . . He must help, care for, comfort and ease when the specialist has nothing to offer . . . The patient often has made the rounds of the specialties; he is still ill, still needing answers to the key clinical questions. Even if the patient's illness has been 'negotiated' out of medicine by other physicians, someone must remain who can help.
> The generalist, on this view, is the physician par excellence since he has the most intimate relationship with the healing and helping functions of medicine. A specialist, especially if his domain is a technique, might get away with only scientifically right decisions; but a generalist, never (Pellegrino, 1983, p. 679).

Pellegrino draws our attention to the importance of the professional–patient relationship for ethical practice. The centrality of this relationship means that primary health care workers are often closer to their patients and their patients' lives than health professionals in other specialities. Insights into patients' values that would be masked in other settings become clear within the context of primary health care. For example, in primary health care there is more opportunity to know the patient as a person above and beyond their illness, so that beneficence can come to mean

far more than doing what is in a patient's best medical interests (Christie and Hoffmaster, 1986).

Similarly, a more nuanced understanding of patients' circumstances can also shape views about patient autonomy. The traditional medical ethics view of respecting autonomy is that if patients are fully informed, have a good understanding of the information necessary to make a decision and are not coerced, then any decision they make is autonomous and should be respected by the doctor. For primary health care workers this is an unduly narrow view. Their unique position in relation to their patients allows them to build a wider range of factors into decisions about their patients' capacities (Doyal, 1999). So, for example, a primary health care worker may not immediately accept her patient's apparent decision to do without treatment if she knows that this patient generally requires a supportive environment and two or three consultations to really make up his mind. Her unique relationship with her patient provides a vehicle for the exploration of fears and concerns that otherwise might go unvoiced.

Although relationships with people can make the primary health care practitioner's role rewarding, it can also cause ethical difficulties. It can be demoralizing when, for example, a series of treatments yield little success and a patient returns again and again with no improvement. Primary health care workers can be confused and challenged by the need to set limits on relationships, particularly in small communities in which one regularly meets one's patients in the street.

The proximity of primary health care means that confidentiality is also a key issue. The ethical requirements are straightforward: information about patients cannot be divulged to anyone except in strictly regulated situations. For health workers removed from the communities in which their patients live, it is not difficult to maintain confidentiality. For the primary health care worker, embedded in a local community and perhaps caring for more than one family member, keeping information private can be very challenging.

Finally, the primary health care practitioner has a particularly demanding role to play as advocate for individuals and communities. Such advocacy is consistent with the primary health care practitioner's commitment to equity and social justice, not least because the connections between health status and powerlessness, inequality and poverty are well recognized in both developed and developing countries. Yet, the advocacy role, although central to primary health care practice, is not without difficulties. It can create an open-ended commitment – where should primary health care practitioners draw the line in advocating for their patients? There are no clear boundaries; health problems inevitably merge into social matters that the primary health care practitioner may be unable to address effectively.

In addition, the practitioner may recognize that such problems are often dealt with more effectively when they are treated as public issues rather than private troubles (Mills, 1970).

The individual account of primary health care ethics that I have sketched in this section is built on the foundation of the relationship between primary health care professionals and their clients. Although this approach has its strengths, it also has weaknesses. For example, the focus is inevitably on individual relationships, yet, as noted in the introduction, such an approach only provides a partial picture of the definition of primary health care. The primary health care worker's domain is considerably larger than these individual interactions; it encompasses working with families, community members and whole communities to prevent illness, maintain and promote health and change the environment. It is to this interpretation of primary health care that I now turn.

PRIMARY HEALTH CARE ETHICS: THE 'COMMUNITY' ACCOUNT

The 'community' account of primary health care ethics begins from an assumption that communities are more than just aggregates of individuals. Rather, they are dynamic entities with interactive links between individuals, families, friends, groups, organizations and structures. Sometimes these links are created by geography; just as often communities are built around shared cultures, values, interests or beliefs.

This broad view of the nature of community implies that ethical challenges for primary health care cannot be defined merely as the sum of challenges for individual participants or professionals. Instead, they reflect the interplay between the interests and values of individuals and those of communities. Not surprisingly, therefore, the community account of primary health care ethics is characterized by a range of tensions that intersect and cut across each other: tensions between compliance- and empowerment-oriented approaches to community participation, between individual and social responsibilities for health, between commitment to health status change and social change, and between private freedoms and public benefits.

COMPLIANCE- AND EMPOWERMENT-ORIENTED APPROACHES TO COMMUNITY PARTICIPATION

Community participation[2] is a key principle in primary health care; indeed it is often described as the 'heart of

primary health care' (Wass and Griffith, 1998). It is intended to apply at all stages of primary health care, from planning of policies and services, through to delivery and evaluation. Yet, it is also rather like motherhood: everyone is in favour of it, but there is often certain vagueness about the detail. The reasons for the vagueness become clear when one examines the ethical positions that underpin community participation. There are at least two positions: the first focuses on the role of participation in enhancing compliance; the second on participation in the interests of empowerment. These positions are often, but not inevitably, in conflict.

Community participation is sometimes promoted because it is believed to improve compliance with primary health care interventions. Encouraging community participation can provide the primary health care professional with a better understanding of a community's beliefs, values, knowledge skills and concerns; with this the professional can ensure that interventions are appropriately tailored to the local context. Participation can also foster understanding in the community of the likely impact of a health intervention, and this in turn can create a more satisfied community. All these things are helpful because they enhance the likelihood that communities will support and benefit from health interventions.

Much early primary health care practice subscribed to this justification for participation. However, primary health care delivered with this rationale in mind may not necessarily empower communities. In fact, compliance-oriented participation can actually disempower people because it retains control of health interventions, programmes and policies with health professionals rather than with communities themselves.

The second justification for community participation directly addresses this criticism by focusing not on the good outcomes, as defined by professionals, that might result from a better-informed and participating community, but rather on the moral obligation to respect the right of people to make decisions about things that concern them. It argues that if people are to gain control over their lives, primary health care needs to be a liberating and emancipating force in people's lives.

This rationale has its own problems: what about communities that are not willing or able to consider the issues at hand? What about people who, despite the primary health care worker's efforts at informing or educating in appropriate ways, cling to 'wrong' beliefs? How does one deal with communities that want programmes that, on the basis of evidence and experience, are unlikely to work?

[2] There is a range of overlapping terms used as alternatives to community participation; these include consumer participation and citizen advocacy.

Rogers' example of a public health intervention in Scotland provides an excellent example of these sorts of tensions (Rogers, 2006). This programme aimed to improve child health through a home visiting programme complemented by strategies to enhance community participation in decision-making. These strategies included a series of public meetings to ask community members what extra services for children and families they would like. One of the services the community requested was baby massage; there is, however, no evidence that baby massage actually enhances child health. Given that resources were limited, public health professionals decided not to provide a service that they thought would not work. Concerns such as these are often voiced by primary health care practitioners who want to be confident that their programmes will actually deliver health benefits, which takes us full circle to the compliance-oriented approach to community participation.

There is thus a fundamental ethical tension for primary health care in the way it conceptualizes community participation: 'Are we aiming to have people comply with the wishes of professionals, or are we aiming to empower people to make their own informed decisions?' (Wass and Griffith, 1998).

INDIVIDUAL AND SOCIAL RESPONSIBILITIES FOR HEALTH

The Declaration of Alma-Ata called for community participation in primary health care 'in the spirit of self-reliance and self-determination' (WHO-UNESCO, 1978). Thus, encouraging individuals and communities to take responsibility for their health is central to the primary health care approach.

The notion of *individual* responsibility has been an important part of primary health care programmes since the relationship between lifestyle and health status was recognized in the 1970s. Yet, primary health care also acknowledges that health is socially determined and that health is a *social* responsibility (Marmot, 2005). Social, economic and political structures constrain the choices that people are able to make; to 'blame the victims' for their health status when they do not have control over the factors that affect their health is neither fair nor likely to change the situation. Victim blaming is not just restricted to individuals; communities can equally be called to answer for their failure when they do not appear to improve after time, energy and money have been invested in them.

Balancing individual and social responsibilities for health is a key challenge in primary health care practice. On the one hand, the concepts of community participation, development and empowerment make no sense unless one accepts that individuals and communities are able to interpret their own circumstances, reflect on them, identify what needs to change and act on their decisions. On the other hand, the emphasis in primary health care on governmental responsibility for health, intersectoral collaboration and political action highlights the limitations of individualist responses to health problems.

A pertinent example of this dilemma can be found in tobacco control. Health promotion programmes that focus on individual responsibility tend to use warnings on cigarette packages, education programmes and behavioural modification strategies to encourage people to give up smoking. By contrast, programmes oriented towards social responsibility legislate to restrict cigarette advertising, increase taxation on cigarettes and ban smoking in workplaces. Finding the right balance between these two approaches in tobacco control can be difficult. For example, increasing taxation on cigarettes affects poorer smokers to a much greater degree than it does wealthier smokers. Unless primary health care practitioners are careful, here, as elsewhere, those who are least able to take control of their lives can be most disadvantaged by structural change.

Of course, primary health care is not the only place in which one encounters this tension: debates between structure and agency, freewill and determinism are hardly new. Yet, the robustness of the debate in other arenas has not seemed to spill over into primary health care and one is left with a sense that this is a domain in which good theoretical discussion is still required.

CHANGING HEALTH STATUS AND CHANGING SOCIETY

Related to the tension between individual and social responsibilities for health is a tension between the twin goals of decreasing excess mortality and morbidity and eliminating inequity. The commitment to equity is central to primary health care; it is implicit in the World Health Organization slogan 'health for all.' The reasons for this commitment are well known: in both developed and developing countries relative poverty is a risk factor for morbidity and mortality (Marmot, 2005). Thus, primary health care has a strong social justice focus, with a commitment to addressing the social and structural determinants of health status.

One dilemma for primary health care is that programmes that focus on eliminating poverty, disadvantage and oppression may have undesirable outcomes for health status. Consider, for example, a primary health care programme that seeks to increase employment opportunities for women in order to increase wealth in the community. In the long run, such changes will benefit not only the women but also the whole community. However, in the short run, shifting power from men to women may also lead to family and community disharmony, higher divorce rates and increases in physical or emotional violence.

A second dilemma is that a general commitment to equity does not always serve the health interests of all equally. Providing equal access to health services may not take account of the fact that not all people are equally able to exercise their right of access (Rogers, 2006). Similarly, in culturally diverse communities, the programme that works for one group may have no impact on another. For example, health promotion campaigns that encourage adults to give up smoking by emphasizing the negative impact of passive smoking on their children may completely miss the mark with gay men.

PRIVATE FREEDOMS AND PUBLIC BENEFITS

The tension between the interests of individuals in making their own decisions about their health and the collective interests of a society in the promotion of health, safety and security is crucial for many aspects of primary health care practice. For example, successful primary health care interventions often work best if they encourage people to make healthy choices by limiting the availability of unhealthy alternatives. Similarly, health education programmes that use complex social marketing campaigns often succeed precisely because they manipulate people's understanding of health issues. Initiatives such as these raise questions about how we can balance the sometimes intrusive and restricting nature of programmes that promote health and prevent disease with the need for individuals to take responsibility for their own health.

One classic example of this dilemma is the delivery of immunization programmes (Dare, 1998; Dawson, 2004). Immunization has been one of the core activities of primary health care, in both developed and developing countries. Vaccination programmes have eradicated or significantly reduced the incidence of a number of diseases associated with high levels of mortality and morbidity (for example, smallpox and polio). These benefits accrue to individuals, but they also accrue to whole populations in ways that extend beyond the benefits to those individuals who choose to be vaccinated. Mass vaccination programmes, if their coverage is extensive enough, can lead to herd immunity, which can protect not only those who are immunized but also those who are not. The dilemma for immunization programmes is that allowing individuals to choose *not* to be vaccinated can also harm people who have been vaccinated. If enough people choose not to be vaccinated, eventually the value of herd immunity is lost, potentially leading to outbreaks which will affect people who have been vaccinated (because vaccines do not have a 100% success rate), a version of the tragedy of the commons (Hardin, 1968).

The problem of the tragedy of the commons is often dealt with by enforcement (May, 2005). Because individuals cannot be trusted to act collectively for the common good, we may have to require people to be vaccinated to ensure that the common good is served. In the United States, for example, school entry is conditional upon proof of vaccination against a range of common childhood diseases. All states grant exemptions on medical grounds, but only some states allow exemptions on religious or philosophical grounds. In other countries, childhood vaccination is not mandatory, but there is a range of strategies in place that strongly encourage it.

The arguments against enforced immunization stem explicitly from the position that the state (or another benevolent authority) ought not to interfere with people's right to make their own decisions about their own lives. The classic defence of this position was offered by John Stuart Mill, who argued that limiting people's free action is a greater evil than any other good that might be done (Mill, 1874).

Of course, Mill did allow some exceptions to state paternalism. He was willing to limit people's liberty when he thought that they would act differently if they were better informed (so, for example, school attendance can be mandated); when people were likely to make decisions now that will limit their freedom in the long term (so, for example, injecting heroin can be illegal); and when what one chooses to do for oneself might harm others – what is usually called the harm principle.

Mill's harm principle is frequently used to support a range of regulatory strategies that enhance health by restricting individuals' freedoms. Yet, some scholars question whether the principle is actually capable of doing the ethical work required of it. Does the harm principle provide sufficient justification to compulsorily treat patients for tuberculosis or to prohibit all alcohol sales in isolated indigenous communities? Goodin, for example, has argued that trying to use the harm principle to justify intrusive primary health care interventions is merely a strategy to avoid being labelled as paternalistic. He thinks we would do better to openly acknowledge the paternalism inherent in many freedom-restricting primary care and public health interventions:

> We do not leave it to the discretion of consumers, however well-informed, whether or not to drink grossly polluted water, ingest grossly polluted foods or inject grossly dangerous drugs. We simply prohibit such things on the grounds of public health . . . to a very large extent . . . the justification of public health measures, in general, must be paternalistic, their fundamental point is to promote the well-being of people who might otherwise be inclined cavalierly to court certain sorts of diseases (Goodin, quoted in Bayer, 2003).

The debate about private freedoms versus public benefits in health has been developed mainly under the auspice of scholarship in public health ethics. If the dilemma is sig-

nificant for public health practice, it is even more important in primary health care, because of the key role primary
health care gives to self-determination and empowerment.
Yet, here, as elsewhere, there seem to be no straightforward
resolution in sight.

CONCLUSION

The field of primary health care is a complex and contested
domain. This complexity and confusion is reflected in the
ways in which the ethics of primary health care is defined
and the tensions inherent in articulating those definitions.
The result is a jumbled array of perspectives in which general practice ethics, public health ethics, ethics of health
promotion, human rights and justice and the ethics of resource allocation all seem to have something to offer.

I have provided an account of primary health care ethics that attempts to impose order by drawing primarily on
general practice, public health and health promotion ethics
and making a distinction between 'individual' and 'community' accounts of the ethics of primary health care. Such
an approach is essentially permissive. It allows a broad
range of issues, challenges, theories and perspectives to be
included under the umbrella of the ethics of primary health
care and it does not attempt to advocate for one or other
approach. As the field develops, it is likely that the tensions
highlighted in my account will be sharpened and theorized
more effectively.

ACKNOWLEDGEMENTS

Dr Afzal Mahmood and Mr James Smith, both of the Discipline of Public Health, University of Adelaide, provided
helpful comments on earlier drafts of this chapter.

REFERENCES

Bayer R. Ethics of health promotion and disease prevention. In:
    Jennings B, Kahn J, Mastroianni A, Parker LS, eds. *Ethics and
    Public Health: Model Curriculum*. Washington: Association
    of Schools of Public Health, 2003; http://www.asph.org/docu-
    ment.cfm?page=782.
Christie RJ, Hoffmaster BC. *Ethical Issues in Family Medicine*.
    New York: Oxford University Press, 1986.

Dare T. Mass immunization programmes: some philosophical
    issues. *Bioethics* 1998; **12**: 125–149.
Dawson A. Vaccination and the prevention problem. *Bioethics*
    2004; **18**: 514–530.
Doyal L. Ethico-legal dilemmas within general practice: moral
    indeterminacy and abstract morality. In: Dowrick C, Frith L,
    eds. *General Practice and Ethics*. London: Routledge, 1999; pp.
    45–61.
Hardin G. *The Tragedy of the Commons*, 1968; http://
    www.garretthardinsociety.org/articles/art_tragedy_of_the_
    commons.html.
Kekki P. *Primary Health Care and the Millennium Development
    Goals: Issues for Discussion*. Geneva: World Health Organiza-
    tion, 2003; http://www.who.int/chronic_conditions/primary_
    health_care/en/mdgs_final.pdf.
Marmot M. Social determinants of health inequalities. *Lancet*
    2005; **365**: 1099–2004.
May T. Public communication, risk perception, and the viability of
    preventive vaccination against communicable diseases. *Bioeth-
    ics* 2005; **19**: 407–421.
Mill JS. *On Liberty*. London: Longmans, 1874.
Mills CW. *The Sociological Imagination*. Harmondsworth: Pen-
    guin Books, 1970.
New Zealand Ministry of Health. *The Primary
    Health Care Strategy*, 2001; http://www.moh.govt.
    nz/moh.nsf/238fd5fb4fd051844c256669006aed57/
    7bafad2531e04d92cc2569e600013d04?OpenDocument.
OECD. Health care systems in transition: the search for efficiency.
    Social Policy Studies No. 7, 1990.
Pellegrino E. The healing relationship: the architronics of clinical
    medicine. In: Shelp EA, ed. *The clinical Encounters: the moral
    fabric of the patient-physician relationship*. D. Reidel Publish-
    ing Company, Dordrecht 1983, p. 679.
Rogers W. Feminism and public health ethics. *J Med Ethics* 2006;
    32: 351–354.
Rogers WA, Braunack-Mayer AJ. *Practical Ethics for General
    Practice*. Oxford: Oxford University Press, 2004.
Royal College of General Practitioners. *European Definition of
    General Practice/Family Medicine*, June 2002; http://www.
    rcgp.org.uk/default.aspx?page–3294.
Tarimo E, Fowkes F. Strengthening the backbone of primary
    health care. *World Health Forum* 1989; **10**: 74–79.
Wass A, Griffith P. Concepts and values in health promotion.
    In: Wass A, ed. *Promoting Health; The Primary Health Care
    Approach*. Sydney: Harcourt Saunders, 1998.
Welton W, Kantner T, Katz S. Developing tomorrow's integrated
    community health systems: a leadership challenge for public
    health and primary care. *Milbank Q* 1997; **75**: 261–288.
WHO-UNESCO. Declaration of Alma-Ata. In: International Con-
    ference on Primary Health Care, 6–12 September, 1978; http://
    www.euro.who.int/AboutWHO/Policy/20010827_1.

49

The Nurse–Patient Relationship: A 'Principles plus Care' Account

STEVEN D. EDWARDS

In what follows I will begin by providing a description of some common models of the nurse–patient relationship. These will be analysed in terms of Beauchamp and Childress's (B&C) four principles. The principles will also be employed as tools of analysis to aid criticism of some models of the nurse–patient relationship. Then, more positively, some necessary components of any credible model of the nurse–patient relationship will be proposed; these are care plus the four principles.

It should be added that the chapter focuses solely on 'level three' of B&C's approach and no discussion is attempted on moral judgement, rules or theories and the relationships between these and the principles in B&C's approach (see Beauchamp and Childress, 2001; Edwards, 1996).

MODELS OF THE NURSE–PATIENT RELATIONSHIP

In their text on nursing ethics, Thompson Melia and Boyd (TM&B) identify four models of 'carer–client relationships' (Thompson, Melia and Boyd, 2000, p. 70) – obviously these will include nurse–patient relationships. The four models are the code, contract, covenant and charter models (Thompson, Melia and Boyd, 2000; see also Callaghan, 1988, ch. 4).

The 'code' model is said to emphasize the importance of promoting the well-being of patients and of preventing them from coming to harm. TM&B are critical of this model because, they suggest, it emphasizes and fosters the dependence of patients on nurses. The reason is that, according to the model, nurses are best placed to determine both what count as harms and benefits and how these are best prevented or promoted. The 'paradigm case' behind this model is said to be that of response to crisis. Thus, the nurse responds to the crisis by preventing harm or promoting the well-being of the patient.

The 'contract' model, as TM&B envisage this, involves the patient voluntarily seeking help. The nurse offers the help if she considers it appropriate, and the patient can then decide whether or not to enter into an agreement with the nurse concerning the service to be provided. As may be anticipated, this model views the nurse–patient relationship as no different in principle from any other contractual relationship, such as one that may enter into with a plumber, solicitor or car mechanic, and so on.

The covenant model is said to be of particular relevance in situations in which a patient has a chronic or terminal condition. In a contractual relationship, the parties concerned may enter into it out of mutual self-interest. But in a covenantal model a kind of commitment which exceeds self-interest is said to be involved (May, 1988). The strength of the commitment is sometimes claimed to be 'unconditional', (Thompson, Melia and Boyd, 2000, p. 79) or less strongly, to involve commitments which are supererogatory (Thompson, Melia and Boyd, 2000).

The last model that TM&B identify is a 'charter model'. In this, a series of commitments are issued concerning standards and the kinds of actions which patients have a right to expect from nurses. For example 'You will be seen within 2 hours of admission to Accident and Emergency Unit'; 'Information will be kept confidential' and so on (The Patient's Charter, 1991). The suggestion here is that prospective patients can make choices about which health care institutions to engage with should they be in need of a health-related service. As TM&B point out these kinds of documents tend to emerge within certain systems of health care delivery, specifically those which involve tendering for services and which are motivated by a desire to enhance consumer/patient choice. In addition

Principles of Health Care Ethics, Second Edition Edited by R.E. Ashcroft, A. Dawson, H. Draper and J.R. McMillan

to the four models suggested by TM&B, other models of the nurse–patient relationship to be found in nursing literature include the following.

Chadwick and Tadd (1992) identify four models. The first is that of 'parent surrogate' in which the nurse acts towards the patient, as a parent would to a child. The second is that of nurse as a 'technician'. In this, the nurse does not engage with the patient in any deep moral sense, she simply performs technical tasks as needed and provides information as requested by the patient. The third model is that of the 'contracted clinician'. As with the contractual model described by TM&B, what is envisaged here is a contractual agreement voluntarily entered into in which the terms of the contract are agreed on both sides before the approval of the contract. The fourth model Chadwick and Tadd identify is that of 'patient advocate' of which they identify several varieties, and which will be returned to below as it is a commonly expressed view.

Looking further back, in a classic text on nursing, Henderson (1966) identified three models of the nurse–patient relationship each of which is appropriate according to the differing stages of the patient's health condition: (a) the nurse as patient substitute, (b) the nurse as patient helper, and (c) the nurse as patient partner. To explain, consider a situation in which a patient is completely unable to feed himself due to poor motor co-ordination, but can take food orally if he is spoon-fed – perhaps the patient is recovering from a stroke. In feeding such a patient, the nurse as patient substitute adopts the role the patient would were he well enough to do so. Suppose that now the patient's condition is gradually improving. The nurse as helper does not feed the patient, but, say, guides the spoon which is being grasped unsteadily by the patient, and so helps the patient to feed himself. As the patient continues to recover, the nurse as partner engages with the patient in discussion of his plan of care, to ensure this is a plan the patient agrees with and is happy to embrace.

As mentioned, the idea of nurse as patient advocate – an advocacy model of the nurse–patient relationship – is one which many have favoured in the last 30 years or so (International Council of Nurses, 1973; UKCC, 1989, 1996). The standard dictionary definition of an advocate is 'one who pleads for another' (Concise Oxford Dictionary). It is easy to appreciate that this is unhelpfully broad when placed in the nursing context. Who decides the nature of the relevant cause to be pleaded? Is it to be the nurse, the patient, the doctor, Trust managers or other parties?

The UKCC (predecessor to the current NMC) discuss advocacy in their *Guidelines for Professional Practice* (1996). According to the *Guidelines*:

> Advocacy is concerned with promoting and protecting the interests of patients or clients, many of whom may be vulnerable

and incapable of protecting their own interests . . . You can do this by providing information and making the patient or client feel confident that he or she can make their own decisions ... (UKCC, 1996, p. 13).

Unfortunately, this seems vulnerable to an ambiguity similar to that which besets the dictionary definition. The first sentence concerns the protection and promotion of the interests of patients/clients. So the nurse as advocate, it seems, can determine what precisely the interests of patients/clients consist of, and then seek to promote or protect them as appropriate. The second sentence, though, emphasizes much less the interests of the patient. Instead, the prime concerns are information-giving and providing a kind of psychological support for the patient so they will feel empowered to make their own decisions – be these about what is in their best interests, or the kind of regime of care they would prefer to receive.

So in this construal of the nurse–patient relationship, nurse-as-advocate involves one or both of two things. Seeking to promote the patient's best interests and/or enhancing their autonomy by providing them with relevant information whilst at the same time reinforcing their confidence in themselves so they feel capable of making their own decisions.

An obvious difficulty with this understanding of advocacy is of course that the two components of it may conflict. Notoriously, what if promoting the patient's view conflicts with promoting their best interests? Suppose a patient refuses a plainly therapeutic intervention, or wants to discharge himself against medical advice, or wants to revert to taking hard drugs after a period of abstinence, or wants to commit suicide and so on. The idea of nurse as advocate as construed by the UKCC appears problematic.

Further general difficulties arise in the determination of best interests, such as might arise in the care of an incompetent patient (e.g. enforced dental care, or bad dental hygiene); or when there is disagreement about what is in the patient's best interests, say between nursing staff themselves or between them and a patient's relatives.

Other conceptions of the nurse as advocate seem problematic too. For example here is Gates' definition:

> [Advocacy is] the process of befriending and, where necessary, representing a patient . . . in all matters where the nurse's help is needed, in order to protect the rights or promote the interests of that person. The practice of advocacy must be taken in a true partnership, where the nurses see these partners as friends and therefore afford them the same care and love as they would to any of their own friends or relatives (Gates, 1994, p. 2).

In fairness to Gates, he expresses this definition in the context of nursing people with intellectual disabilities. But even there it seems problematic. The latter part seems far too demanding. It is reasonable to expect some degree of distance to obtain between nurses and patients/clients, and it is very implausible to expect a nurse to display the same level of moral commitment to her patients that she might have to her close relatives.

Let us turn to yet another conception of the nurse as advocate role, this time proposed by Gadow. She writes,

[existential advocacy requires] that individuals be assisted by nurses to authentically exercise their freedom of self-determination. By authentic is meant a way of reaching decisions which are truly one's own . . . (Gadow, 1980, p. 85).

For present purposes we can set aside the nuances involved which lead Gadow to coin the term 'existential advocacy' to characterize her particular brand of advocacy. As is evident from the quote, the core of advocacy as Gadow sees it is helping people make the decisions which are truly their own and which stem from consideration of their values and plans for the future.

It may be said that this too seems vulnerable in the same way in which one interpretation of the UKCC conception seemed vulnerable. Specifically, it can seem as though Gadow's line completely severs respect for autonomy from all considerations relating to the patient's well-being or harm. So in principle if a patient decides the best option for them is suicide or reverting to a life of hard drug abuse, this is fine. The nurse's proper realm of concern is confined to the means by which the eventual decision is made regardless of any assessment of the content of the decision reached by the patient from a moral perspective.

The last conception of advocacy to be mentioned here is that provided by Kohnke. According to her, 'The role of advocate is to inform the client and then to support him in whatever decision he makes' (Kohnke, 1982, p. 2).

As with the conceptions offered by UKCC and Gadow, this is again vulnerable to the charge of focusing exclusively on means and neglecting consideration of the moral content of the end of the decision-making process. In this and other conceptions, the nurse plays the role of facilitator to safeguard and create the conditions under which the autonomous patient can decide how they want to act.

Before moving on to look at a further key model of the nurse–patient relationship – a care-based model – it is appropriate to make explicit what we have been doing so far in describing and offering occasional evaluations of the models set out.

First, the four principles have provided a useful analytical tool in elucidation of the models. Each model can be interpreted in terms of the emphasis placed upon respect for autonomy, beneficence, non-maleficence and justice. Hence, we saw that several conceptions of advocacy stress obligations to cultivate, foster and respect patient autonomy and place much less emphasis upon obligations of beneficence, non-maleficence or even justice.

Second, the principles can also provide a means for critical assessment of the models of the nurse–patient relationship. For example, if it is true that some models really do neglect obligations of beneficence, non-maleficence and justice, then that seems a credible starting point for a critical assessment of the relevant model. To give a couple of examples of how this might work, return first to consider Gadow's conception of advocacy. As we have seen, considerations of beneficence and non-maleficence seem neglected. But so too, importantly, do obligations of justice. It is as if the nurse as existential advocate has one patient only at the forefront of her concern. What of the rest of her caseload, or the workloads of her colleagues? Surely, a credible account of the nurse–patient relationship must be one that recognizes these wider obligations of justice. Also, consider Gates' conception of advocacy once more. He does clearly take into account obligations of beneficence, non-maleficence and autonomy. But it seems that he attaches far too much weight to obligations of beneficence and non-maleficence. For he expects the nurse to be as committed to promoting the well-being of her patients as she is to promoting the well-being of her family members. As mentioned above, this weighting of obligations seems very implausible and appears incompatible with the demands of professional practice – at least insofar as these require the maintenance of some professional distance between patient and nurse.

So, it is clear that the principles provide some useful analytical tools which can be employed both to understand claims concerning the nature of the nurse–patient relationship and also to critically appraise such claims. Still further, the kind of critical analysis of models of the nurse–patient relationship just employed also exposes something fundamental about models of that relationship. This is that a credible model of the nurse–patient relationship must involve some place for the kinds of moral obligations set out in the four principles. There must be a place for obligations to respect autonomy, promote beneficence, prevent harm and strive for fairness. As mentioned, some of the models described above are vulnerable to criticism for failing to include one or more of these kinds of obligations.

To put the claim being made here slightly more technically, the proposal is that any credible model of the nurse–patient relationship must recognize a key place for the kinds of obligations specified in the four principles. Of course there will be occasions when this is not possible due to the condition of the patient; it will not be possible to respect the autonomy of a neonate for instance. But the claim that an adequate model of the nurse–patient relationship should include a place for the four principles seems a sound one. In situations in which a principle has no application, it will still in all likelihood be possible to apply the other three.

CARE VERSUS PRINCIPLES?

The proposal that the obligations specified in the four principles amount to conditions of adequacy in models of the nurse–patient relationship will not go down well in some quarters. This is because many nurse theorists and commentators have argued in favour of the idea that care is fundamental to the nurse–patient relationship and that an ethics of care should underpin nursing practice. Moreover, such commentators are often severely critical of a principle-based approach to nursing ethics, and it is reasonable to infer that their criticisms would extend to the suggestion that models of the nurse–patient relationship should embody the four principles.

The proposals that care is the key feature of the nurse–patient relationship and that nursing practice should be informed by an ethics of care have been advanced fairly widely over the last 20 years or so (Watson, 1988; Benner and Wrubel, 1989; Fry and Johnstone, 2002). Moreover, some commentators have advanced the claim that care comprises the 'essence of nursing' (e.g. Benner and Wrubel, 1989), And generally, commentators who champion an ethics of care are hostile to principle-based ethics. The hostility has its origins in the work of Gilligan (1982), who claimed to identify two differing ways of thinking about moral problems. She coined the terms 'ethics of care' and 'ethics of justice' to label the distinct approaches (principle-based ethics would be said to comprise an ethics of justice within Gilligan's taxonomy).

The claimed distinction between them can be drawn, rather crudely, in the following way. First, in an ethics of care personal involvement in moral problems is viewed as a good thing; such involvement certainly does not constitute an obstacle to proper moral judgement. Also, and relatedly, viewing moral problems as 'concrete', as actually situated in real-life contexts, does justice to their real natures. Further, viewing moral problems in terms of ongoing personal relationships also does justice to their real natures. Lastly, emotional involvement is recognized as a central component of the moral life, and so an adequate account of ethics should again do justice to this aspect of it – of moral phenomenology so to speak.

In contrast to the features of morality just described, the so-called ethics of justice is said to embrace rival claims about the nature of morality. Hence, in an ethics of justice personal involvement is viewed as an impediment to moral judgement and not an advantage. The ideal moral vantage point is one of detachment as opposed to involvement (see, Singer, 1993 and his 'principle of equal consideration of interests'). This is illustrated in the structure of the judicial system in the United Kingdom and elsewhere in which an 'impartial' judge or jury offers decisions on the culpability of alleged offenders on the basis of cool deliberation over presented evidence. Emotional responses to situations are

considered flawed moral judgements rather than reliable sources of moral judgement. Given that the principle-based line is best regarded as falling within an ethics of justice, it can be seen that there is this fundamental difference between it and an ethics of care.

Further, as mentioned, in the ethics of care the focus is on 'concrete' moral problems, anchored in a context and arising from networks of relationships which have evolved over time. But the principle-based approach involves abstracting out features common to many moral problems, such as conflicts between autonomy and non-maleficence. Care-based theorists see this as failing to do justice to the real nature of moral problems as proper attention to them involves focusing 'further in' on them so to speak as opposed to 'abstracting out' moral properties common to classes of moral problems.

Relatedly, the principle-based approach appears to foster an approach to moral judgement which stems from a 'snapshot' analysis of a situation – see Gilligan's (1982) discussion of Amy and Jake. So, for example, a problem may be presented as involving a clash between principles and an answer to the problem sought. But in the care-based approach the problem is not viewed as a 'snapshot' but as an ongoing narrative; the problem arises from historically grounded relationships and has ramifications for the futures of those relationships.

To recap. A review of some standard models of the nurse–patient relationship led us to analyse and assess these in terms of the four principles. This motivated the proposal that any credible model of the nurse–patient relationship must find a place for the obligations referred to in the four principles. But a challenge to this proposal was anticipated. The anticipated challenge is likely to emerge from proponents of a care-based model of the nurse–patient relationship. Such proponents typically embrace an ethics of care, and this is standardly taken to be incompatible with principle-based ethics. A description of the differences between the two approaches has just been offered.

CARE PLUS PRINCIPLES

Instead of responding to each of the criticisms of principle-based ethics as this is viewed from the perspective of an ethics of care, what I propose to do is to borrow a definition of care and show how it can be plausible to hold both that the nurse–patient relationship should be grounded in care *and* at the same time subscribe to the view that any credible model of that relationship should include a place for the obligations specified in the four principles.

I'll begin with a couple of quotes. 'Cure cannot be understood or accomplished without a background of care and caring practices' (Benner and Wrubel, 1989, p. 8).

What I take Benner and Wrubel to be claiming here is roughly this. The very intelligibility of health care practices presupposes care. The reason is that nursing and medicine are most credibly conceived of as responses to human suffering and such responses presuppose care on the part of those who respond to the suffering. But what is meant by 'care' in such claims? One helpful place to begin to answer this is provided by Noddings (1984). She writes, 'Caring involves stepping out of one's personal frame of reference into the other's. When we care we consider the other's point of view, [and] . . . his objective needs' (Noddings, 1984, p. 24).

Although this proposal is not without its problems, it can help to cast light on what is meant by 'caring' and 'care'. When read sympathetically, Noddings' claim can be understood as follows. In caring for others one tries to view the situation from the other person's perspective. We also try to make some assessment of the other person's 'objective needs'. Hence, what distinguishes caring in the health care context from caring for inanimate objects is that the latter have no perspective to try to grasp. So it is not possible to care for inanimate objects in the same way in which it is possible to care for human beings. The latter do typically have a perspective on the world; inanimate objects do not, of course.

So exploiting this understanding of caring it can be seen that nursing necessarily involves caring. It follows that the nurse–patient relationship is grounded in care. The nurse has a responsibility to try to view the situation as the patient sees it and also to be aware of the patient's needs.

It is in the sense just described, then, that care forms the foundation of the nurse–patient relationship. Recall the earlier claim that the obligations referred to in the four principles are also fundamental to an adequate model of the nurse–patient relationship. Given the understanding of 'care' that has just been offered, it can be seen that there need, in fact, be no incompatibility between (a) endorsing the view that the nurse–patient relationship is grounded in care; and (b) endorsing the proposal that the obligations referred to in the principles are fundamental to an adequate model of the nurse–patient relationship. To see this, consider an example of an encounter between nurse and patient.

Mrs M is an elderly, frail patient with poor mobility. She is currently in hospital recovering from a nasty fall in which she broke an arm and badly bruised her leg. Nurse N is caring for M. N is concerned that M begins to become active again after a period of bed rest. This is because it is important that M retains her mobility as much as possible, as this will be in her interests once discharged – at least as N views the situation. Also, N believes it is important for M to begin to try to recover her mobility so that her tissue does not start to break down causing pressure sores to develop. In the light of these concerns N suggests to M that she starts to make more of an effort to recover her mobility as much as possible,

for example, by taking some short walks on the ward with the eventual aim of walking to the ward bathroom instead of relying on being wheeled there in a wheelchair. M is very reluctant to take any steps apart from the one from her bed to the chair immediately adjacent to it, this is in spite of N's encouragement and gentle exhortations to do so.

Consider this situation, then, in the light of the crude model of the nurse–patient relationship suggested above. With regard to the 'care' component, it is plausible to suppose that the strategies initiated by N to foster M's mobility are motivated by care. N considers M's plight and makes a reasonable judgement concerning what is in her best interests and what kinds of interventions will best promote her 'objective needs'. It is in this way, then, that 'care' is central to the nurse–patient relationship in the present example.

(Of course the idea of 'objective needs' is not unproblematic, but I take it to be fairly easy to apply, for example, in a situation of the kind described here. Given M's situation, it does seem in her best interests to maintain her mobility and derivately her independence.)

With regard to the other components of the nurse–patient relationship, those concerning the obligations referred to in the principles, it seems straightforward, again, to apply them in the case of N and M. As seen, N's strategy is motivated by care. In the implementation of N's strategy, the obligations stated in the principles arise as follows. N's actions have to take into account the principle of respect for autonomy. The obligations generated by this principle oblige N to inform M of the reasoning behind her regime of care. Put simply, this is of course to try to ensure that M's mobility is restored to its former level. Also, respect for the obligations of this principle oblige N to listen to M's view of the strategy: Is she happy with it? Does she agree with it? Will she go along with it or does she object? With regard to the principle of beneficence, N's implementation of the strategy appears motivated by that, as it should be. N has made a reasonable and defensible judgement to the effect that M's interests are best promoted by the restoration of her mobility. With regard to the principle of non-maleficence, implementation of this obliges N to act in a way that does not harm M. Again, it is credible to conclude that the regime of care planned by N respects these obligations. Lastly, with regard to justice, this obliges N to act fairly. This principle is normally taken to apply to issues of distributive justice. In our case, N's time and efforts count as a 'good' to be distributed fairly. N has other patients to care for, so obligations of justice require N to take these into account and not to jeopardize the health of other patients by spending an unfairly large proportion of her time with M.

So this example has illustrated the way in which the four principles, plus a care component, can provide a credible, minimal model of the nurse–patient relationship. No doubt a fully adequate model would need to supplement these bare bones, but 'care plus principles' seems a reasonable foundation for a model of the nurse–patient relationship, or so it has been argued here.

REFERENCES

Beauchamp T, Childress JF. *Principles of Biomedical Ethics*, 5th edition. Oxford: Oxford University Press, 2001.

Benner P, Wrubel J. *The Primacy of Caring, Stress and Coping in Health and Illness*. Menlo Park: Addison-Wesley, 1989.

Callahan JC, ed. *Ethical Issues in Professional Life*. Oxford: Oxford University Press, 1988.

Chadwick R, Tadd W. *Ethics and Nursing Practice*. London: Macmillan, 1992.

Edwards SD. *Nursing Ethics, a Principle Based Approach*, Macmillan, Basingstoke, 1996.

Fry S, Johnstone MJ. *Ethics in Nursing Practice*, 2nd edition. Oxford: Blackwell, 2002.

Gadow S. Existential advocacy, philosophical foundations of nursing. In: Spicker S, Gadow S, eds. *Nursing, Images and Ideals*. NY: Springer, 1980; pp. 79–101.

Gates B. *Advocacy, A Nurses' Guide*. London: Scutari, 1994.

Gilligan C. *In a Different Voice*. Cambridge, MA: Harvard University Press, 1982.

Henderson V. *The Nature of Nursing, A Definition and its Implications for Practice, Research and Education*. New York: Macmillan, 1966.

International Council of Nurses. *Code of Nursing Ethics*. Geneva: ICN, 1973.

Kohnke MF. *Advocacy, Risk and Reality*. London: Mosby, 1982.

Liaschenko J, Davis AJ. Nurses and physicians on nutritional support, a comparison. *J Med Philos* 1991; **16**: 259–283.

May WF. Contract or covenant? In: Callahan JC, ed. *Ethical Issues in Professional Life*. Oxford: Oxford University Press, 1988; pp. 92–95.

Noddings N. *Caring, A Feminine Approach to Ethics and Moral Education*. Los Angeles: University of California Press, 1984.

Singer P. *Practical Ethics*, 2nd edition Cambridge: Cambridge University Press, 1993.

The Patient's Charter. London: Department of Health, 1991.

Thompson IE, Melia KM, Boyd KM. *Nursing Ethics*, 4th edition. London: Churchill Livingstone, 2000.

UKCC. *Guidelines for Professional Practice*. London: UKCC, 1996.

Watson J. *Nursing, Human Science and Human Care*. Boulder, CO: University Press of Colorado, 1988.

50

Dual Responsibilities: Do They Raise Any Different Ethical Issues from 'Normal' Therapeutic Relationships?

ANN SOMMERVILLE AND VERONICA ENGLISH

Dual responsibilities occur in a wide range of settings. Indeed, in this chapter, we argue that they occur to some degree in every branch of medicine. All health professionals sometimes find themselves owing a simultaneous moral, legal or contractual duty to several parties whose aims do not coincide. Nevertheless, duties to people other than the patient are likely to weigh persistently and considerably more in some branches of health care, such as prison medicine, than they usually do for doctors in normal therapeutic settings. The latter generally – but not invariably – experience conflicting loyalties on a lesser scale. Here we look to both extreme and mundane examples, in an attempt to capture the common elements of the issues that arise for the doctors and patients involved.

In practice there is no such thing as a doctor–patient relationship that occurs in total isolation and so all doctors have dual loyalties to some extent. In everyday medical practice, in both primary care and hospital medicine, doctors must be mindful of their broader responsibilities, towards other patients – for example, in terms of the use of scarce resources – and to society generally, such as to take action when their patients represent a serious risk of harm to others. In addition, many doctors enter into contractual arrangements with third parties such as insurance companies or employers where they are paid to provide medical examinations or reports. These doctors have more clearly articulated dual loyalties – to their patient and to their paymaster. Although in many circumstances the interests of their patient and the third party will coincide, this is not always the case. Where dual loyalties are most acute, however, and where there is the greatest potential for conflict, is where doctors

are contracted to an organization or institution to provide care for patients who may be in a particularly vulnerable position or for patients whose freedom is restricted in some way by their circumstances. Examples include prison doctors, forensic physicians and those working with asylum seekers or in the armed forces. So to some extent all doctors have dual loyalties, but there are varying degrees to which these affect doctors' practices and the extent to which the circumstances present ethical dilemmas.

It should be said at the outset, however, that in many instances where a duality of obligation comes into play, there is no ethical dilemma. This is because it would be abundantly clear to any detached observer whose interests should take precedence and which moral principle carries more weight in the particular context. If a patient asks for the concealment from an employer of information about an infection or impairment which could endanger others in the workplace, all other things being equal it is clear that the rights of the group not to be put at risk weigh more than the privacy rights of the individual. If a nurse sees that colleagues are performing badly or that lack of cleaning staff means a service is unsafe, it is clear that whistle-blowing action is needed. If an individual asks a doctor to provide false information to support an insurance claim, it is clear that, however much the doctor may wish to support the patient, he or she cannot become complicit in fraud. There is no moral conflict in such situations because in all their activities health professionals should be impartial in advice and decision-making, not unjustly biased by their loyalties to individual patients, employers or colleagues or heedless of the needs of the community at large.

Principles of Health Care Ethics, Second Edition   Edited by R.E. Ashcroft, A. Dawson, H. Draper and J.R. McMillan
© 2007 John Wiley & Sons, Ltd

The question, therefore, arises as to why we perceive dual responsibilities as so potentially problematic in ethics terms. There are several factors to explain this. Health professionals approaching such ethical dilemmas may be less attuned to them, given that medical ethics throughout its history has focused primarily on aspects of relationships between doctors and individual patients. Traditionally, far less attention has been given in ethical debate to those situations where doctors have duties primarily to populations rather than individuals or where their loyalty to the individual routinely has to be balanced against other bigger pressing concerns. Public health ethics and the norms governing medicine in the armed forces, prison or immigration services, for example, are emerging areas of ethical debate, but are significantly underdeveloped in comparison with the plethora of ethical guidance for other areas of medical activity. Also some spheres of medical practice, such as prison medicine or that related to police work or the judicial system, are also subject to laws, regulations or contractual rules aimed at promoting efficiency, but that do not necessarily echo best ethical practice. In the United Kingdom, for example, it is legal for detainees in a police station to be subjected to intimate body searches by doctors against their wishes if authorized by a senior police officer (British Medical Association and Association of Police Surgeons, 2004). Ethically, doctors carrying out such searches should still attempt to seek consent and weigh up whether the risks of proceeding without it in a particular case are justified. Frequently, the fact that highly detailed prison or immigration rules specify how detainees' medical care is managed may leave little opportunity for discussion of rather vaguer ethical duties. Respect for patient autonomy is difficult to achieve if all one's patients are routinely shackled, and respect for confidentiality is also a challenge if prison officers and police colleagues are present during examination, or have access to medical files, in order to exercise their duties of keeping control.

Although an independent observer in many cases might think it self-evident whose interests should predominate in the case of a conflict, human frailties, the desire to avoid disturbing the status quo and employment loyalties mean that the judgements are not made by completely independent observers but rather by health professionals embedded in the values of a particular setting. They can sometime come to identify more with the goals and standards of their co-workers than with their patients. In a prison setting, both prisoners and other staff tend to see doctors as part of the management team rather than the prisoners' advocate. In large enterprises, occupational health services can also be seen by employees as part of management even though doctors providing such services have a moral responsibility to individuals as well as to the workforce as a whole.

HOW DIFFERENT ARE THE ISSUES RAISED BY DUAL LOYALTY CONFLICTS?

In their medical careers, all doctors face increasingly complex ethical challenges and need to be vigilant about the potential for real or perceived conflicts of interest. Nevertheless, most who work in a straightforwardly therapeutic setting can unambiguously sign up to the traditional Hippocratic dictum that, all things being equal, their patients are their first concern (World Medical Association, 1947). This is clearly not true for health professionals with more pronounced dual responsibilities. By definition, the individual in front of them is never their sole concern nor necessarily the subject of their most important ethical obligations. Nevertheless, this is not completely divorced from the dilemmas encountered in other settings. As mentioned above, occasions arise for all health workers, including those in normal therapeutic settings, when the duty to individual patients is subordinated to greater over-arching concerns. Classic examples for general practitioners arise when visually impaired patients continue to drive contrary to medical advice or when a firearms licence is sought by someone with incipient mental illness. Any health professional involved in the provision of fertility treatment must not only consider the wishes of the patient but also bear in mind society's desire for the welfare of future children so that those who have abused or neglected children may not receive such treatment. Whenever an individual patient represents a risk to others, all practitioners have to consider the bigger picture as well as their patients' interests. On a more routine level, whenever questions arise about equitable allocation of scarce resources and management of waiting lists for care, doctors must be seen to act fairly on behalf of all in the community rather than prioritize particular patients.

In such cases, even though they are partners in a therapeutic relationship, the potential harm of supporting the patients' wishes outweighs doctors' duty to them and a concern for others in the community takes precedence. So, in some respects, it can be argued that there are no such things as dual loyalty dilemmas as a separate category of ethical concern because circumstances arise in which the pull of dual responsibilities is experienced by all health professionals regardless of their sphere of work. The need to put community safety above individuals' goals is precisely the same for the above-mentioned GPs as it is for police, prison or army doctors whose dual loyalty is more precisely articulated. Also, even when the welfare of individual patients is not their main focus, all doctors have some moral responsibility for the people they see or advise professionally. Independent doctors paid to carry out insurance examinations, for example, have some duty to ensure that symptoms they identify in insurance applicants are made known to that individual's usual doctor, if there is any doubt about them having been missed. Prison doctors not only contribute to the maintenance of order and the smooth running of the institution but also have clear ethical duties to their patients. Thus, all doctors have multiple loyalties. They all have duties to the group as well as to the individual before them, although they may be less clearly spelled out in most ordinary therapeutic partnerships compared with the potential for conflict for doctors concerned with public health or the welfare of prison populations. The difference then is one of degree rather than one of principle.

HOW DUAL RESPONSIBILITIES ARISE

Hard-wired into all medical training is a concern for the individuals that doctors encounter professionally, regardless of whether the latter are actual 'patients' receiving treatment or are more like clients needing independent medical examination for insurance, employment or immigration purposes or inmates of an institution to which the doctor is contracted to provide services. Dual obligations arise whenever doctors have strong moral, legal or contractual obligations to another party whose interests or priorities might conflict with those of these individuals. Such split loyalties are particularly acute in prisons, police stations and facilities for the dangerously mentally ill where care for individuals is provided within a framework of strict supervision and heightened awareness of the needs of the community at large. Conflicting loyalties can arise in courts where a medical interpretation of a situation might effectively exonerate or incarcerate a defendant. Doctors examining people claiming political asylum on grounds of maltreatment in their country of origin have duties both to the individual and to the state. Medical officers in the armed forces have to try to achieve a balance between the needs of recruits and the welfare of the unit in which they serve. Contrasted with such stark conflicts, doctors completing insurance or employment reports for their patients reflect the more routine face of dual responsibilities.

WHAT ETHICAL PROBLEMS DO DUAL RESPONSIBILITIES CREATE?

The ethical dilemmas raised by dual responsibilities are generally a more acute version of the ordinary dilemmas experienced by all doctors. When there is a strong obligation to another party or a wider population, such as to the courts or the police, this can conflict with the patient's usual rights, particularly the right to consent freely and to confidentiality. When individuals are compulsorily detained, the usual emphasis on autonomy and consent to medical care can be

blunted. Medical responsibilities towards the patient may be ill-defined in comparison with the way that doctors' duties to the other party are expressed in very clear rules. There are also risks of health professionals employed, for example, in the prison or immigration services assimilating the norms and values of their employer or the non-medical staff around them rather than acting in accordance with their professional standards. Clearly, however, although doctors may be employed outside the normal therapeutic relationship, the usual ethical standards still apply. Professional norms must still be respected, and doctors have a duty to inform those they come into contact with about their role and the nature of their obligations to other agencies.

There is a controversy, however, as to whether it is the fact of having medical skills that gives certain workers extra moral duties or whether the moral duties that often feature in arguments about dual responsibilities belong to the job being done. An example of the problems that can arise was illustrated by media coverage in 2004–5 (Lewis, 2004; Slevin and Stephens, 2004; Bloche and Marks, 2005) of the alleged involvement of health personnel in interrogation of detainees held by US forces in Cuba. Health professionals employed by the military shared detainees' health information with interrogators which allowed prisoners' physical and psychological weaknesses to be exploited. The US Defense Department published guidance (Assistant Secretary of Defense, 2005) saying that 'health care personnel charged with the medical care of detainees' had clear duties to protect those patients and act in their interests. Other 'health care personnel engaged in non-treatment activities, such as forensic psychology or psychiatry, behavioral science consultation, forensic pathology or similar disciplines' were not deemed to be employed in a therapeutic capacity. They had other job titles – such as interrogation adviser – and although medically qualified, they were not perceived as being bound by conventional medical ethical standards. In other words, no dual responsibility was involved if a medically qualified person was not actually engaged in providing therapeutic services even though the prisoner was unaware of the distinction. This view contravenes most widely accepted perceptions of the binding nature of doctors' ethical duties which see medical skills as invariably entailing special moral obligations (British Medical Association, 2001). A core facet of medical ethics dating back to Hippocratic values is that doctors should not use their medical skills in a way designed to bring harm to individuals in their care. British military guidance, for example, does not accept that doctors can have a separation of roles between clinical caregivers and physicians with intelligence-gathering responsibilities. This specifies that health personnel 'are only to be involved in professional relationships with prisoners or detainees for the purposes of evaluation, protecting or improving their physical and mental health' (Defence Medical Services Department, 2005).

WHAT ETHICAL PRINCIPLES APPLY TO DUAL RESPONSIBILITIES?

It is generally accepted that the same ethical principles that apply to doctors with explicit dual responsibilities apply to other practitioners, although the former may be constrained by the context in which the doctor works. Like other areas of care, having divided professional loyalties can involve doctors in ethical problems that range from the very dramatic to the extremely mundane. Ethical methodologies for dealing with such problems can also vary. As in other areas of medicine, in resolving ethical dilemmas practitioners may resort to concepts such as that of the four principles or frameworks that balance rights and duties, but where the dual loyalties are particularly acute – such as where doctors are working in institutions – a human rights approach may be considered.

In recent years split loyalties and dual responsibilities have particularly become the focus for medical human rights groups who see them as part of the key to preventing abuse of vulnerable groups such as detainees and asylum seekers (Physicians for Human Rights, 2002). Their approach is to apply national and international human rights norms to some of the most pressing dilemmas of dual responsibilities, where repressive, abusive or unfairly discriminative practices are most likely to occur. They begin from the principle that 'the most basic and fundamental purpose of human rights is to respect and protect individual persons' by applying a universally applicable set of moral principles expressed through international conventions, treaties and instruments. Dual obligations are increasingly seen as a particularly relevant debating ground for human rights organizations because it is generally assumed that doctors with pronounced dual obligations are at risk of subordinating the rights of patients to other interests. Those generally considered to be most likely to do so are doctors working in custodial settings, the armed forces, police and immigration services.

COMMON PRINCIPLES IN ALL SETTINGS

Some general points apply to all situations in which doctors examine individuals or write reports for purposes other than treatment, whether they be for insurance, court hearings, benefits applications or asylum proceedings.

EXERCISING PROFESSIONAL INDEPENDENCE

We have identified that one of the potential problems with having dual responsibilities is that health professionals can be constrained, influenced or misled by the prevailing rules and ethos among those they work with in a way that

downgrades the rights of patients/clients. If doctors absorb the perspective of the state or the employer, they may lose sight of the ethical obligations owed to the individuals they examine or treat. On the contrary, there is also a risk of sympathizing too much with the individual being examined. A key principle, therefore, is that of maintaining independence. This principle can be expressed in various terms. In a four-principle framework, it might be labelled attention to justice. In a human rights framework, it might be seen as the duty to uphold international norms by maintaining full technical and moral independence from the state and those in authority. Relevant related principles are the duty of fairness, equity and impartiality.

In practice it can be hard to implement with vulnerable populations like detainees or asylum seekers, especially if health professionals with dual responsibilities develop relationships with vulnerable people and see part of their role as being the patient's advocate. Similarly in collecting evidence in relation to court hearings of child protection cases, remaining detached and unbiased can be a challenge. Independence is skewed, however, if doctors' sympathy for their patients who may have suffered maltreatment in any way influences their objectivity. This can be an emotive area, and doctors must ensure both the impartiality of their report and that each individual application is subject to careful and disinterested scrutiny. The doctor's role is to discover and report on any relevant material features, even if they may adversely affect the case of the instructing party. As with all medical reports – including more mundane requirements for an insurance claim or for compensation for workplace injury – doctors must be impartial and should indicate where there is more than one possible cause of the individual's symptoms. Doctors who examine victims of abuse invariably build up expertise in prevalent patterns of maltreatment or abuse or injury in different settings. They can offer an opinion as to the most likely aetiology of the individual's condition, based upon observed facts, but should not speculate more widely. In court cases or asylum appeals tribunals, medical witnesses' primary duty is to assist the court and to speak with detached objectivity rather than support the case of an individual patient or that of the side paying the fee. Doctors acting in this capacity are not advocates and must have no interest in the outcome of the case.

Maintaining independence can also be an ethical issue in various situations where the outcome of the case is likely to affect many people seriously. Doctors serving in the armed forces need to ensure that the unit is fit for tasks assigned to it, but some soldiers may seek to be declared unfit if notified that they are to be sent to a war zone. Clearly, doctors should make a dispassionate and independent evaluation, swayed neither by the commanders' need to maximize numbers nor the individual's reasons if exclusion is not medically indicated. In less constraining settings, doctors employed by sports teams and by sports clubs can equally find themselves subject to the tension of conflicting loyalties. They owe duties to the team or club for whom they have the contractual obligations of an employee but, as doctors, they must also consider the needs of the athletes or players. The latter may come under pressure from managers to continue to play, even if they have sustained injuries and where continuing to play could exacerbate risks of long-term damage. In professional football, for example, there appears to be a presumption that players should continue to play with pain and injury. Maintaining independence and upholding their duty to minimize harm requires doctors to avoid this happening by informing both player and manager of the risks.

Occupational medicine deals with the effects of work on health and the impact of employees' health on their own performance and that of colleagues in the workforce. The objectives of an occupational health service include promoting the health and safety of all employees and to advise on rehabilitation and suitable placement of employees who are temporarily or permanently disabled by illness or injury. Consent to disclosure of employees' information to employers is still a prerequisite and managers should not have access to their employees' medical records. Occupational health professionals must act as impartial professional advisers, concerned with the health of all those employed. Such responsibilities can, however, lead to dilemmas such as when the doctor believes that the working environment may exacerbate health problems for certain employees or applicants for employment. It is vital that such situations be handled with complete impartiality so that information about risks to employees' health is not concealed and people who have already suffered injury can gain appropriate compensation.

RESPECTING AUTONOMY: THE DUTY TO ENSURE THAT APPROPRIATE CONSENT IS OBTAINED

Listening to individuals and demonstrating an appropriate respect for autonomy is an ethical requirement in all settings, even though individuals' own wishes may not be determinative or even acknowledged as important by others in authority. Convicted prisoners, for example, may have little choice about who examines them or the range of treatment on offer, but their consent to examination and treatment should still be sought. Their informed refusal of medical interventions can only be overridden in cases comparable to where valid refusal would be superseded in the community, such as when the patient's condition represents a serious threat to others. Like detainees, individuals joining the

armed forces lose some of their autonomy and are expected to follow orders issued for the benefit of the unit, platoon, ship or squadron of which they are part. Discipline is an essential part of the effective functioning of the services and it inevitably limits the exercise of autonomy. This extends to consent for certain medical procedures. Where there may be a doubt, for example, about soldiers' fitness for combat, or where their mental or physical health presents a threat to others, they may be ordered to submit to appropriate medical testing, or to certain forms of treatment such as vaccination. A refusal to obey a direct order in this context may well be dealt with by means of the ordinary disciplinary procedures that would apply to any refusal to obey an order. Doctors as well as their patients must obey any lawful command. Disobedience is punishable, including sanctions determined by court martial. Like all other doctors, however, those serving in the forces must behave in accordance with professional ethics. They are responsible for their professional actions to the same extent as any other doctor and are expected to work to the same ethical standards. Deciding whether to disobey a clear order so as to uphold good ethical principles requires a careful analysis of the balance of benefits and harms in each individual circumstance.

ENSURING APPROPRIATE CONFIDENTIALITY

All health information about identifiable individuals which doctors learn in a professional capacity is subject to the professional duty of confidentiality. In all situations, however, confidentiality can be breached if individuals consent to that happening or if there are strong arguments for subordinating the individual's wish to the needs of others. Where information might avert a miscarriage of justice or foreseeable serious harm to others, disclosure is likely to be justified.

Doctors writing medical reports for purposes such as insurance, employment, housing applications or compensation for injury may consider that patients' apparent co-operation in examination or volunteering of health information means that disclosure to others of that information can be assumed. In a straightforward therapeutic setting, information is routinely put onto the patient's record and shared with others providing care to that person, but this is not the case when dual medical responsibilities come into play. Police surgeons, for example, may examine individuals who have been victims or perpetrators of assaults and record the data they find. Particular effort needs to be taken to ensure that individuals understand the basis on which they are being examined and what will happen with the data obtained from it. If they are medically examined in connection with a prosecution, for a court report or in connection with an immigration appeal, doctors need to check that the individual knows the exact reason for the examination. They need to reiterate the fact that it is not a therapeutic exchange and indicate how information will be disclosed in the doctor's subsequent report.

Joining the armed forces also means that individuals relinquish some rights, including that of confidentiality. The interests of the individual have to be balanced against the interests of the unit. Medical officers may need to discuss the personal health information of their patients – who include not only soldiers but also their families – with commanding officers. Although prevailing military rules may not require consent for disclosure of medical information, it is nonetheless good practice for doctors in the armed forces to seek the individual's consent, whilst recognizing that any consent obtained may not be entirely free from pressure and is likely to be given in the context of a contractual obligation on the patient to agree to disclosure of certain information. As the ill-health of service personnel can put others at risk and jeopardize military goals, cases arise where even if the patient refuses, the 'public interest' in disclosure overrides confidentiality. In such instances, only information necessary to the issue at hand should be released. Information without any bearing on the individual's health, such as his or her sexual orientation, should not be released.

In sports medicine, problems can also arise regarding confidentiality, especially in the case of high-profile athletes, where considerable pressure from officials, from the media or even from sponsors can be exerted on doctors to release confidential information (Waddington and Roderick, 2002). Players may have contractual obligations to disclose relevant information to their managers and there is no commonly held code of ethics governing the way in which football clubs handle confidential information (Waddington and Roderick, 2002). Ethically, sports doctors need to be aware that contractual issues notwithstanding, the duty of medical confidentiality remains unchanged. Unless expressly indicated in the terms of the player's or athlete's contract, confidential information can only be released with the express consent of the patient, and breaches of confidentiality can only be justified where there is a risk of serious self-harm or harm to a third party.

For GPs providing routine employment or insurance reports, there may be no evidence of a dramatic harm if the subject asks for some potentially relevant information to be fudged or kept hidden but professional integrity is sacrificed if doctors agree to what is basically a fraudulent report. Clearly, doctors must avoid being influenced by either the requirements of a third party commissioning a report or by sympathies they may have for the individual being examined.

In an occupational health care setting, statutory and other periodic medical examinations can affect individuals' continued employment. Examples include pilots, workers in the atomic energy industry and medical staff who may develop potentially infectious conditions. If pre-employment testing is carried out, the consent of the individual must be obtained. Individuals should be informed of the nature of the tests and to whom the results may be disclosed. In some occupations, drug or alcohol testing may also be a facet of employment. Employees and prospective employees should be told of any circumstances in which testing in the workplace is carried out for illicit substances (Faculty of Occupational Medicine, 2006). Where employers wish to use pre-employment testing, a clear explanation must be given to potential employees so that they can make an informed choice as to whether or not to undergo that test. Where individuals are found to be a risk to others, either because of their health or due to addictive behaviour, occupational physicians must be careful not to take over the role of the line manager in deciding whether such an individual should be offered employment or dismissed. The patient must be reminded of the doctor's role as the agent of a third party and that the doctor's role in such cases is to advise the employer, with the individual's consent, of possible health problems which could arise.

CONCLUSION

To an extent, all doctors have dual loyalties, but in some specialities these play a greater role in the doctor's day-to-day practice and there is more scope for conflict and ethical dilemmas. Although on a less dramatic scale, precisely the same divided loyalties arise for occupational health doctors, whose responsibilities include protecting individual workers' health and advising management on all aspects of workforce welfare, as they do for those working in prisons or the immigration services. In all of the situations mentioned throughout this chapter, there are common elements and some common principles. They can be summarized by saying that even when health professionals are appointed and paid by another party, they still have a duty of care to the patients whom they advise, examine or treat. In all situations, doctors must abide by professional guidelines on ethics even if these are not reiterated in law. All health professionals in any sphere of work have a duty to monitor and speak out when services with which they are concerned are inadequate, hazardous or otherwise pose a potential threat to health or human rights. Respecting the autonomy of others by seeking their voluntary consent and co-operation is as important as it is in other areas of medical practice. Also the ethical duty of confidentiality remains, even though contractual terms may inhibit how much freedom patients have to exercise it. Nevertheless, information should normally not be disclosed without the patient's knowledge and consent. Doctors with clearly articulated dual responsibilities – like all other health professionals – must ensure that they remain objective and impartial even though the situations in which they work can make this difficult to achieve. Above all, it is essential that they are open and transparent about their dual loyalties and that their patients are aware of how the doctor–patient relationship differs from the usual therapeutic encounter and the practical implications of this in terms of consent and confidentiality.

REFERENCES

Assistant Secretary of Defense, Washington DC. *Medical Program Principles and Procedures for the Protection and Treatment of Detainees in the Custody of the Armed Forces of the United States*, 3 June, 2005.

Bloche MG, Marks JH. When doctors go to war. *N Engl J Med* 2005; **352**(1): 3–6.

British Medical Association and Association of Police Surgeons. *Guidelines for Doctors Asked to Perform Intimate Body Searches*. London: British Medical Association, 2004.

British Medical Association. *Medical Ethics and Human Rights*. London: Zed Books, 2001.

Defence Medical Services Department. *Surgeon General's Policy Letter: Medical Support to Persons Detained by UK Forces Whilst on Operations*. Ref DMSD/29/3/5, 6 January, 2005.

Faculty of Occupational Medicine. *Guidance on Alcohol and Drug Misuse the Workplace*. London: Faculty of Occupational Medicine of the Royal College of Physicians, 2006.

Lewis N. Red Cross finds detainee abuse in Guantanamo. *The New York Times*, 30 November 2004; p. 1.

Physicians for Human Rights. *Dual Loyalty & Human Rights in Health Professional Practice*. Physicians for Human Rights and University of Cape Town, 2002.

Slevin P, Stephens J. Detainees' medical files shared: Guantanamo interrogators' access critized. *The Washington Post*, 10 June 2004; p. A01.

Waddington I, Roderick M. Management of medical confidentiality in English professional football clubs: some ethical problems and issues. *Br J Sports Med* 2002; **36**: 118–123.

World Medical Association. *Declaration of Geneva*, 1947.

51

Violent and Abusive Patients:
An Ethically Informed Response

G.M. BEHR, J.S. EMMANUEL, J.P. RUDDOCK

Like many in vocational professions, those working in the field of health care will often be asked what prompted their career choice. Whilst eschewing the hackneyed response, 'To help people', the response of many will reflect an instinctive desire to 'do good'. Underpinning this is the assumption, dating from innocent student days, that the recipients of your care will bestow upon you their gratitude. Less persuasive in this choice of career will be the contrasting reality of not just a lack of gratitude, but also, on occasion, being subject to frank abuse. Consider the following example:

A female receptionist in an inner city general practice is wary when a well-known patient, Mr A, approaches the counter. Recalling previous hostile encounters, she is unsurprised when he demands, 'I want to see a doctor NOW. Don't ask me why, you stupid bitch, it's private and urgent'.

Take the response of one general practitioner, Dr Millpond (the middle-aged 'elder statesman' of the practice) to the above scenario. Although sympathetic to the feelings of his long-suffering colleague who is in the front line, his instinct is to focus on providing care to the patient. The feelings of his staff can be managed as a lower priority compared to fulfilling his duty of care to the patient and the need to avoid further confrontation. At what point, however, does his threshold for tolerance get breached – when the receptionist complains of being undermined? When she threatens to resign? Maybe only when she is physically assaulted on a later occasion?

The opinion of his younger colleague, Dr Hastie, is in stark contrast, having been influenced by her years as a registrar in a busy Casualty department. Impressed by seeing the results of the hospital's 'zero tolerance' approach, she is minded to be extremely firm and have Mr A escorted from the premises. Dr Millpond questions whether her feelings are so strong that she would be prepared to call the police.

Would she remove Mr A from the practice list? Would her mind be altered if she noticed that the patient was flushed and showed signs of ill-health?

Dealing with violent and abusive patients challenges all working in health care. How do we reconcile our duty of care with our rights as a citizen not to be subject to abuse? If the above scenario was played out in a different setting, perhaps Mr A confronting a shop assistant with demands to see her manager, the decision to remove him from the premises and call the police would be much more intuitive. One could envisage an attempt to calm the situation, hear Mr A out under the 'customer knows best' mantra, but few would defend Mr A's behaviour. Why, then, is our instinct so different in the health care setting? We would suggest that there are two fundamental assumptions underpinning this relative tolerance of abusive behaviour. First, the concern that the behaviour is itself a manifestation of a medical condition or at the very least that their illness renders the individual vulnerable such that their antisocial behaviour is excused. The second assumption is that there exists an unconditional right to health care for all. There are countless examples of illnesses presenting with a change in behaviour: the hypoglycaemic diabetic, the early presentation of a frontal brain tumour, the relapsing manic-depressive to name but a few. It is unquestionably our duty to provide care for these patients, with the hope that appropriate treatment will ameliorate the behaviour. There is a fear that focusing on 'managing' the behaviour alone and failing to diagnose and treat any underlying condition causing the behaviour would at best show a lack of empathy, a core attribute of those in caring professions, at worst leave us open to charges of negligence. However, the reality in the clinical world is far less clear-cut than this dichotomous response, and we spend much of the chapter exploring the ethical principles

Principles of Health Care Ethics, Second Edition Edited by R.E. Ashcroft, A. Dawson, H. Draper and J.R. McMillan
© 2007 John Wiley & Sons, Ltd

that can help guide us in individual clinical situations. First though we dwell on the assumption that all citizens should have unfettered rights to health care.

IS HEALTH CARE A RIGHT?

Paying taxes for a service does not create an inalienable right to that service. For instance, children can be excluded from school if they repeatedly misbehave, and social services are not obliged to re-house someone if they are thought to have been responsible for their own homelessness. In other words, if the duties of the recipients of a public service are not fulfilled, this may compromise their right to receive those services (Behr et al., 2005).

The American Medical Association Code of Ethics (Council on Ethical and Judical Affairs, 2002) has a chapter on 'Patients' responsibilities' which states, 'Like patients' rights, patients' responsibilities are derived from the principle of autonomy … autonomous, competent patients assert some control over the decisions which direct their health care. With that exercise of self-governance and free choice comes a number of responsibilities.'

Eleven items are listed as patients' responsibilities, which include, among others, being cognizant of the effects of their conduct on others. Draper and Sorell (2002) describe how, in terms of medical ethics, duties have come to be focused purely on service providers and not on service users – possibly because of the perception of their being less powerful and more vulnerable. In a transaction between the powerful and the vulnerable in the course of which the latter suffer, they point out that there is a (flawed) presumption that the vulnerable are innocent and the powerful guilty (or at least that the powerful have a responsibility to ameliorate the suffering of the vulnerable). They go on to argue forcefully that patients should observe their duties, and Richardson (1993) has suggested that patients should be informed, as precisely as possible, of what these duties are and what the consequences of transgression will be.

Failure of patients to observe their responsibilities is not necessarily sufficient for withholding health care (e.g. smokers are generally provided with treatments for illnesses associated with smoking). However, we subscribe to the view that health care is *not* an inviolable right, but based on a relationship of good faith (Behr et al., 2005), in which there is no obligation for professionals to provide a service in certain circumstances. So, what aspects of a patient's presentation should we consider to guide our management of abusive and violent patients in a proportionate way along the spectrum of zero to infinite tolerance? We begin with a discussion of moral responsibility – a useful starting point when considering cases challenging the boundaries of acceptable behaviour.

MORAL RESPONSIBILITY

Mr Pain has a diagnosis of schizophrenia although the acute symptoms of this illness have been controlled by depot medication for many years. He also often displays aggression and racial abuse against black people. He will only interact with white staff.

In considering an approach to dealing with Mr Pain, instinctively we form a view as to how responsible he was for his actions. We do this because one's moral responsibility for an action determines our response, namely whether to blame and punish or whether to care for or even pity the perpetrator. There is an alternative (utilitarian) view that it is not responsibility that should determine our response but, rather, the likely effectiveness/benefit of the particular response (this is considered in more depth later in the chapter). However, most philosophical and legal approaches (to punishment) do consider blameworthiness. Health professionals and managers do face the question of whether to prosecute offenders but, more often, have to decide such things as whether to assume responsibility for a patient's actions (e.g. detain under mental health legislation), what treatment would best serve their interests and whether to continue offering a service at all. An understanding of Mr Pain's ability to direct his actions as an autonomous agent will have an important bearing on these questions.

To some it may seem clear that Mr Pain is an unpleasant person who ought to be held responsible for his actions. To others it may be equally clear that he suffers from a major mental illness with an unstable mental state which will influence his actions and that he therefore cannot be held responsible for his behaviour, repugnant as it is.

There is no clear agreement as to what the requisite mental capacities are for one to be deemed responsible for one's (criminal) actions (Wilson and Adshead, 2004). Furthermore, one might argue that this capacity is not an all- or-nothing phenomenon but rather exists on a continuum and shifts in time and circumstance (Mele, 2004). However, dichotomous judgements of responsibility are taken by clinicians and courts every day, for example whether people can consent to treatment, be allowed to take the consequences of self-harm or drug addiction and whether they go to jail or hospital for crimes they commit. So, we would argue that whilst the 'threshold' of such decision-making is inevitably subjective, violent and abusive patients demand a response which forces us to make a judgement about responsibility, for example, to deny treatment/remove from a health care setting and so on. Although these judgements are made intuitively most of the time, it may be helpful to consider the factors that impinge on an individual's ability to understand his actions and ability to refrain from these actions.

Examples do exist of attempts to define explicit criteria in this regard. The US President's Commission report (President's Commission for the Study of Ethical Problems, 1996) suggested that the threshold of morally responsible agency should encompass the following attributes:

(1) Possess a set of values and goals.
(2) Be able to communicate and understand information.
(3) Be able to reason and deliberate about choices.

Elliott (1996) suggests that the requirements might be: having rational beliefs and actions, moral values and emotions roughly like those that most persons possess as well as the ability to communicate, deliberate, manipulate information and have some degree of knowledge about one's actions.

A CLINICAL APPROACH TO MORAL RESPONSIBILITY

It is difficult to attribute moral responsibility to an individual uniformly across time and circumstances. Thus it may be helpful to consider what features of a person's current mental state contribute to their volitional abilities (ability to control their actions) at a specified point in time. If one views actions as the end point of a chain of events resulting from one's perceptions, thoughts and feelings it is helpful to consider the impact of each of these.

SENSORY PERCEPTIONS AND THOUGHTS

Sensory stimuli are often the first events in the chain. On the face of it there is no abnormality of the sensory perceptions experienced by Mr Pain. If, however, he experienced auditory hallucinations of voices with African accents making derogatory comments about him that may impair his 'knowledge of his actions'.

Mr Pain's interpretation of the hallucination may be that he is either experiencing some awful abnormal phenomenon, which he recognizes as not being real, or that there are genuinely black people insulting him. The differences in these cognitive responses clearly have significance in that in the latter scenario he would be considered less blameworthy if he acted on that belief. Other questions could further elucidate his 'knowledge/ignorance' of his violent/ abusive response to black people such as 'Were there other ways of achieving your objective?' and 'What would have been the consequences for you if you didn't do it?' That is, does he truly believe he would have come to some harm if he did not 'defend' himself aggressively? Understanding of one's actions involves both factual knowledge as well as moral knowledge. Thus an action could not be justified if based only on factual ignorance, for example, he believed

blacks were insulting him but knew that assaulting them would be hurtful, unacceptable as a general practice and frowned upon by society ('Would they be hurt by what you did or said?' 'Would you be punished if caught?' and 'What would others say about the deed?'). Contemporary moral practices may not be the best judge in all circumstances, but *his knowing society's views of his actions* would increase his imperative to act in a morally responsible way.

EMOTIONAL/AFFECTIVE RESPONSES

Philosophers have long grappled with the difficulty of distinguishing an *inability* to refrain from acting (compulsion) from weakness of will or an *unwillingness* to refrain (Mele, 2004). The kinds of feelings and the strength of the feelings associated with an action have a bearing on this moral attribute of an action. So, for example, if Mr Pain was motivated by fear (i.e. prevention of harm to himself) in his aggressive behaviour we would instinctively be more forgiving than if he were motivated by anger or vengefulness and certainly more so than if he was motivated by the wish to gratify himself by violence. We would judge him differently if his response to his own action was remorse and a wish to address his problem as opposed to feelings of indifference or of pleasure. These intuitive responses are quite well captured by the notion of duress (Elliott, 1996). He has defined this as 'acting on a choice between two undesirables'. A man might *either* perform an act despite finding it morally repellent *or* refrain from acting even though this would cause considerable distress (psychological harm). Consider the following example.

> Mr Waters is 45-year-old and has chronic renal failure receiving haemodialysis three times a week. He has a lifelong history of interpersonal problems as a consequence of his hostile feelings towards the world and frequently attends the dialysis unit in a state of anger (often drunk) culminating occasionally in his throwing books and equipment around and exposing himself publicly. This causes both staff and other patients to feel very threatened. He behaves the same way when visiting his renal unit counsellor and social worker.

If the episodes of 'bad behaviour' were experienced by Mr Waters as being the only alternative to his enduring intolerable feelings (anger, anxiety, tension) and he felt ashamed and repelled by what he did each time, we might consider that he acted under duress (i.e. was compelled) and exonerate him or, at least, lessen the blame. Similarly, if Mr Pain felt that his not acting aggressively would force him to endure intolerable fear (in this case perceived persecution by black people) *and* he felt shame and remorse for the suffering he caused that would further heighten our sympathy for his case.

We may not have the same expectations of people who have emotional responses outside the range of that considered normal for most people. For example, if Mr Waters had had a frontal lobe injury and was prone to outbursts of extreme anger after relatively slight provocation, he would be less blameworthy than if he had 'normal' emotional responses. But we would still exonerate him further if he showed remorse and sought help to address his problem (assuming he had the insight to do so). He may or may not be acting out of character when under the influence of alcohol. However, his ability to foresee the consequences of his having a drink would mean he is no less blameworthy (and possibly more so if his intention was to diminish his inhibitions by drinking).

IDENTITY

Thus far we have said that there are aberrations of *perception and thought* that may lead people to be violent or abusive out of 'ignorance' and that people may experience *emotions* that compel them to act despite their knowing the wrongfulness of their action. Sometimes, however, these 'unusual' experiences are so much a part of a person's usual character that they cannot be considered exculpatory (Elliott, 1996). For example, Mr Waters may have a paranoid outlook that leads him to believe that he has received a 'raw deal' from society, which now 'owes him'. If this view was acquired recently and was a significant departure from his usual view of life we might regard his beliefs (and associated aggression) as *not being his own* and therefore excuse him from blame (or at least seek to understand this radical change). If, however, that view had always been held, regardless of whether it was an aberrant thought or resulted in extremes of emotional response, this reflects *who he is* – he owns those thoughts and feelings and owns the consequences of the actions resulting. Elliott's rationale for this is primarily that really radical changes in a person's thoughts and emotional life usually occur for reasons *outside of one's control* (e.g. psychosis, head injury, severe trauma). One might say the same of a childhood of abuse, but Elliott (1996) qualifies this further by pointing out that recently acquired changes in mental life have not afforded one the same *time for rational scrutiny* as lifelong-held views.

GLOBAL IMPRESSION

We have teased apart some of the factors that may influence our judgements about a person's moral responsibility for his/her behaviour in clinical situations. However, Elliott points out that intuitive global judgements are valid in and of themselves, 'We simply recognize that this person is impaired in enough ways to render him insufficiently *like other persons* to be included with them in a scheme of moral responsibility'. Clearly, there are inherent dangers in relying purely on our intuition yet we would contend that by

exploring the factors giving rise to our intuition, as detailed above, we can be more confident that we are making a more informed assessment.

CONCLUSION

In practice, clinicians and managers in health care are faced with decisions about what to do about a violent or abusive act committed (e.g. criminal prosecution) as well as planning management strategies for these individuals in anticipation of future similar acts. The capacity to be regarded as morally responsible informs these judgements. Further guidance may be achieved by assessing the relative benefit and harm from any proposed course of action.

BENEFICENCE AND NON-MALEFICENCE (DOING GOOD AND NOT DOING HARM)

Health care professionals and organizations have a duty to 'do good' to our patients and, arguably, an even more compelling duty to do no harm. Of course, if we never risked any harm we could do very little good and so most decision-making is based on what utilitarians would call the 'hedonic calculus' – that which would yield the most good and the least harm. These duties, however, apply not just to individual patients but to the wider group of patients we are responsible for, the community and society we are located in. The 'hedonic calculus' needs to be cognizant of this scope of application. Let us consider this in respect of Mr Waters.

A number of possible options exist with respect to the management of Mr Waters, and it is worth considering a few to see how we might weigh up the benefit and harm. For the purpose of this discussion, let us assume that he is deemed morally responsible for his violent and offensive acts.

TOLERATE THE ABUSE

The obvious benefit is that Mr Waters continues to receive treatment and will remain in a stable state physically. Perhaps treatment will relieve some symptomatology which could otherwise be contributing to his irritability. However, choosing this option could be seen as rewarding Mr Waters for his (bad) behaviour, as one might give a child the sweet he has been screaming for, reinforcing the behavioural problem to his own detriment. Widening the scope of this debate, we might consider the message such an action sends out. On one hand it may advertise the compassionate nature of the service. On the other it may undermine morale of staff in the unit and affect recruitment and retention of staff, thus impacting on the welfare of the wider patient group. At a societal level it may create the impression that abuse is tolerable within the health service and that patients have little ability or responsibility to refrain from such behaviour. This could potentially result in increasing prevalence of such problems (Mele, 2004), to the detriment of patients and staff alike.

WITHHOLDING TREATMENT

All the negative consequences of tolerating the abuse, as set out above, might be overcome by withholding treatment. Proportionality with respect to the gravity and immediacy of risk is obviously central to weighing the benefit and harm of any proposed course of action. If we withheld his renal unit counsellor and social worker visits only, we might consider that as a more proportionate response than 'condemning him to death' by withdrawing dialysis altogether. If Mr Waters came into A&E one night intoxicated, kicking and lashing out and demanding attention for his superficially lacerated wrists, one might cheerfully show him the door. If, however, he was bleeding from his ear and demanding immediate attention for his headache we ought to respond differently as the potential consequences are much more serious. Although proportionality is helpful when weighing the infringement of others' rights against the benefits of his treatment, most clinical scenarios are complex and arouse a range of clinical opinions. The responsibility of judging proportionality should be a shared one.

The corollary of this argument is that in some situations all options for treatment are regarded as clinically futile which might also be grounds for withholding of treatment. If, for example, Mr Waters was considered for the renal transplant programme, his ability to collaborate might be so impaired as to make successful transplant very unlikely and withholding this treatment could be deemed justifiable.

TRANSFERRING CARE TO ANOTHER SERVICE

This option would circumvent the problems mentioned above for the service concerned, though it may replicate the problems elsewhere. It would be sensible to anticipate the likelihood of the latter and, once again, weigh the infringement of others' rights and the collective welfare against the likely benefit to the individual.

PROVIDE TREATMENT WITH SAFETY

Specific, high-security treatment centres are sometimes made available to such challenging patients or it may be that providing security guards at each visit would contain the risk and allow for the benefits of treatment. Pursuing these options demands careful consideration of the message it sends to both patients and the public about responsibility.

This will also have implications for allocation of finite resources, which we consider later in the chapter.

PUNISHMENT

Health care workers' primary concern is to act in their patients' best interests. It is therefore not surprising that there is an inherent reluctance to consider overt punishment as an avenue of management, often despite powerful intuitions to do so. However, decisions *are* made to prosecute patients who commit offences. Clearly, there are benefits in asserting health workers' rights as citizens to enjoy the protection of the law and furthermore in justice being seen to be done. Punishment can be viewed though, not simply as delivering justice but as a way of positively influencing future behaviour, in other words as a beneficent act. However, in the context of health care settings the decision to, for example, withdraw treatment can be perceived as punitive. When we, as practitioners, are violated or abused in any way, it arouses strong feelings and, not uncommonly, the desire for retributive justice. Decisions about a person's treatment or withholding of that treatment can be easily influenced by these feelings and we should guard against that lest we allow our own gratification to be the focal point of a decision. So, if we sought to 'punish' Mr Waters for his behaviour we should do so exercising our citizen's right to prosecute him, creating a precedent that might deter others and in the hope that we might modify his views of what constitutes acceptable behaviour. Any decision to withdraw treatment, however, should not be motivated by a wish to punish.

In summary, the duties of beneficence and non-maleficence are perhaps more complex than they appear at first glance. Benefit and harm may occur not only directly by treatment or non-treatment but also more subtly through the messages one gives by one or other course of action. Further, both of these types of consequence need to be evaluated for the individual, the wider patient and provider group and for society. One specific aspect of the debate about individual versus collective welfare, which merits further thought, is resource allocation or distributive justice.

DISTRIBUTIVE JUSTICE

Aristotle's early argument that there should be equal treatment for those of equal need (so-called horizontal equity) remains at the heart of a consideration of issues of distributive justice today. Focusing on Mr Waters' situation, it could be argued that he merits the same access to treatment of his chronic renal failure as any other person with the same level of disorder. However, to enable delivery of the requisite treatment, he requires a higher level of care (extra nursing staff, security guards, repair of equipment, etc.). Aristotle also argued that unequal needs should be treated unequally (so-called vertical equity) – resources should be proportionate to need. As such should Mr Waters' extra requirements be justified in that he has two separate problems – not just his renal impairment but the additional issue of alcohol misuse? His needs *are* greater and therefore, he merits 'unequal', in this case increased, care.

This would not present a problem if the size of the resource pie was infinite, but it is not. If a physician were responsible *only* for Mr Waters' care, concerns about the use of extra resources would perhaps be peripheral to the physician's central priority of delivering optimum treatment for his patient. Indeed, it has been argued that doctors should not be simultaneously providers and rationers of care, that is, their focus should be on the individual's care without concern for the wider societal and cost issues. In our example, this perception would be challenged perhaps if we recognized that other patients were being denied dialysis who would, by virtue of their greater collaboration with care, get greater benefit than Mr Waters. So, we are always faced with a dilemma about how to ration care. The utilitarian concept of welfare maximization can help us to decide how to divide the resource pie, namely delivering the greatest benefit for the greatest number. Another approach to rationing has been to consider whether the *worthiness* of an individual should be a determining factor for receipt of a service. Does Mr Waters' aggressive and demanding behaviour, or his conscious decision to use alcohol despite the negative effect it has on him, make him less deserving of a scarce resource? This is exemplified more starkly by the choice of giving one life-saving treatment to Alexander Fleming instead of Adolf Hitler, as Mr Fleming 'deserves' it more. The main objection to this approach is the way in which it legitimizes the prejudices and values of the decision-makers. If we deny Mr Waters dialysis because of his lifestyle choices, does it pave the way for denying a pensioner their dialysis purely because of their age?

It is hard to avoid the conclusion that providers of care have a wider duty to apportion resources responsibly. In the context of resource decision-making, Mr Waters should be given (or denied) treatment on the basis of his need and the likely effectiveness of the proposed treatment, compared to the need and effectiveness of the treatment of others competing for the same resource, *not* because we find his behaviour morally repugnant.

CONCLUSION

We conclude that, in responding appropriately to patients who are abusive or violent, neither zero tolerance nor infinite tolerance is appropriate. Infinite tolerance seems to imply unfettered rights to access health care – a notion we reject – and has negative consequences for society and the individual patient. Zero tolerance seems to require people who may have diminished ability to be morally responsible, to take the full consequences of their actions. This is unjust in our view and an act of maleficence. We argue that our response should be informed by a number of different considerations, which can at times be conflicting: a patient's ability to act in a morally responsible way, what benefit and harm may arise from any course of action and also what implication that has on the equitable distribution of resources. In assessing moral responsibility, it is a common error to take a determinist view, for example, one acts because one is 'ill' or because one had a 'bad childhood', and we have proposed a more sophisticated approach to its determination. We believe that this is a critical concept in our response to violence and abuse, not simply to decide on a person's blameworthiness, but because it is central to the respect for autonomy of individuals. Henderson (2005) suggests that removing responsibility for behaviour may not only be unhelpful but can also be demeaning because it implies that the person is 'in some way incomplete, being deficient in self-control'. It may seem intuitive for doctors, nurses and other health and social workers to lean towards infinite tolerance because of the perception of patients as vulnerable and powerless. It has been suggested (Komrad, 1983) that the aim of any medical intervention ought to be an attempt to maximize the autonomy of the patient, meaning perhaps the restoration of physical or mental well-being. Equally though, this may mean fostering a person's emotional growth and the 'power of choice in action' (Henderson, 2005) through thoughtful and compassionate, yet firm, responses to their behaviour.

REFERENCES

Behr GM, Ruddock JP, Benn P, Crawford MJ. Zero tolerance of violence by users of mental health services: the need for an ethical framework. *Br J Psychiatry* 2005; **187**: 7–8.

Council on Ethical and Judicial Affairs, American Medical Association. Opinion 10.02, Patient Responsibilities. *Council on Ethical and Judicial Affairs, American Medical Association. The Code of Medical Ethics: Current Opinions.* Chicago: American Medical Association, 2002; pp. 140–142.

Draper H, Sorell T. Patients' responsibilities in medical ethics. *Bioethics* 2002; **16**(4): 335–352.

Elliott C. *The Rules of Insanity: Moral Responsibility and the Mentally Ill Offender.* Albany, NY: State University of New York Press, 1996.

Henderson AS. Free will and volition. *Br J Psychiatry* 2005; **187**(3): 290.

Komrad MS. A defence of medical paternalism: maximising patients' autonomy. *Journal of Medical Ethics* 1983; **9**: 38–44.

Mele A. Action: volitional disorder and addiction. In: Radden J, ed. *The Philosophy of Psychiatry: A Companion* (*International Perspectives in Philosophy and Psychiatry*). New York: Oxford University Press, 2004; pp. 78–88.

President's Commission for the Study of Ethical Problems in Medicine and Biomedical and Behavioral Research. *Making Health Care Decisions*, vol. 1, 1982; pp. 57–60 (in Elliott C. *The Rules of Insanity: Moral Responsibility and the Mentally Ill Offender.* Albany, NY: State University of New York Press, 1996; p. 122).

Richardson G. *Law, Process and Custody: Prisoners and Patients.* London: Weidenfeld and Nicolson, 1993.

Wilson S, Adshead G. Criminal responsibility. In: Radden J, ed. *The Philosophy of Psychiatry: A Companion* (*International Perspectives in Philosophy and Psychiatry*). New York: Oxford University Press, 2004; pp. 296–311.

The Moral Significance
of the Human Foetus

NORMAN FORD

The term 'foetus' is generally used after the first eight weeks of human development following conception. Believers in the Bible as God's word support absolute respect for the human foetus, while most contemporary secular philosophers hold that a human foetus has no right to life and is not a person. This chapter explores these two positions and argues that the human foetus is a person.

BIBLICAL APPRECIATION OF LIFE BEFORE BIRTH

Biblical language has engendered profound respect for the life of the human foetus in western culture, literature and law (Frye, 1993). From its beginning the Bible shows that God is the creator of human life in a distinct way. We read in Genesis 1: 27:

Reprodurt created man in the image of himself,
In the image of God he created him,
Male and female he created them (Wansbrough, 1985).

Men and women are called by God to procreate children in Genesis 1: 28:

Be fruitful, multiply, fill the earth and subdue it (Wansbrough, 1985).

God is portrayed as actively involved in the formation of human beings from conception. Job 10: 8–12 eloquently testifies to this belief:

Your hands having shaped and created me,
Did you not pour me out like milk,
and then let me thicken like curds,

clothe me with skin and flesh,
and weave me of bone and sinew? (Wansbrough, 1985)

Jeremiah 1:4 says:

Before I formed you in the womb I knew you (Wansbrough, 1985).

Psalm 139: 13–16 adds:

You created my inmost self
knit me together in my mother's womb. …
Your eyes could see my embryo (Wansbrough, 1985).

Finally in Luke's Gospel we read what Elizabeth said to Mary: 'Look, the moment your greeting reached my ears, the child in my womb leapt for joy' (Wansbrough, 1985). Luke indicates that Elizabeth receives the revelation of Mary as the mother of the Messiah through the prophetic leaping of John the Baptist, her unborn child of six months. This implies the unborn children miraculously communicate in this unique encounter (Brown, 1993; John Paul II, 1995).

CHRISTIAN TRADITION AND CATHOLIC TEACHING

Inspired by the Bible, the early Christian tradition held that it was gravely immoral to destroy life in the womb; to do so was seen as an offence against God. This was a powerful *culture favouring prenatal life*, contrary to the practice in the Mediterranean world where abortifacients were used to destroy the fruit of conception (Leone, 1998). The early Christian book, the *Didache*, contains a moral instruction for Christians, which reads: 'You shall not murder a child, whether by abortion or by killing it once it is born' (Niederwimmer, 1998). Germain Grisez gives a good summary of early Christian writings on the respect due to the human foetus (Grisez, 1970). At the end of the second century, Tertullian, aware that the foetus is a human being, wrote: 'For us, murder is once for all forbidden; so even the child (*conceptum*) in the womb, while yet the mother's blood is still being drawn on to form the human being, it is not lawful for us to destroy' (Tertullian, 1931). Boethius (d. 524) understood a human being is philosophically a natural person, defined as an 'individual substance of a rational nature' (Boethius, 1953). St Thomas Aquinas (d. 1274), not wishing to restrict person to the process of reasoning, said: 'Person means ... what subsists in rational (intelligent) nature' (Aquinas, 1965).

Witness to the continuing Christian tradition of support for the intrinsic value and moral respect due to foetal life was given by over 2000 Catholic bishops gathered at the Second Vatican Council in 1965: 'Life must be protected with the utmost care from the moment of conception: abortion and infanticide are abominable crimes' (Flannery, 1975). Pope John Paul II went further in his *Gospel of Life*: 'The human being is to be respected and treated as a person from the moment of conception; and therefore from that same moment his rights as a person must be recognized, among which in the first place is the inviolable right of every innocent human being to life' (John Paul II, 1995).

CONTEMPORARY SECULAR CONCEPTS OF THE HUMAN PERSON

Since the time of the English philosopher John Locke (d. 1704), a shift began in the understanding of the human person. Locke held that although a human being's identity is determined by biological criteria, a person must be able to exercise rational faculties and acts:

> We must consider what *person* stands for; – which I think is a thinking intelligent being, that has reason and reflection, and can consider itself as itself, the same thinking thing, in different times and places; ... It is a forensic term, appropriating actions and their merit; and so belongs only to intelligent agents, capable of a law, and happiness, and misery (Locke, 1924).

Michael Tooley developed Locke's insight and put it on the ethical and philosophical agenda in his seminal article (Tooley, 1972). He acknowledges that in ordinary discourse the term 'person' is used to refer to living beings whose mental life and language is similar to that of normal adult human individuals. But when Tooley critically analyses the rationale for the respect due to persons, he finds that there are certain similar characteristics that are usually employed to describe what makes someone a 'person'. If one were to ask what property on its own would suffice to make a living

being a person, he suggests that 'the capacity for rational thought is sufficient, that being a moral agent is sufficient, that being a subject of nonmomentary interests is sufficient, that having a mental life that involves an adequate amount of continuity and connectedness via memory is sufficient and that simple consciousness is sufficient' (Tooley, 1998).

Tooley admits it is logical to expect that if the relevant property that makes personhood could be present in individuals in varying degrees, then personhood itself could likewise be present in humans in corresponding degrees. This implies different persons would each have a different moral status. He says: 'the acquisition of personhood may very well be a gradual process, and similarly for the loss of it, in at least some cases – such as, for example, Alzheimer's disease, which ultimately results in a permanent, degenerative, vegetative state' (Tooley, 1998). Tooley goes on to consider the claim whether a fertilized ovum might be a potential person on a par with the moral status of a person. He dismisses the claim because the isolated fertilized ovum is unable to actualize itself without environmental support for warmth and nutrients (Tooley, 1998). Incidentally, adult persons cannot survive without the support of the earth's environment.

Tooley likewise dismisses as grounds for personhood being members of the species *Homo sapiens* whose adult members usually have the moral status of persons. The presupposition here is that such members would have the intrinsic property of having interests in need of protection. Tooley points out that the morally relevant and significant concept of interest is 'one that connects up with being a conscious being, and being capable of having desires' (Tooley, 1998). Tooley says that 'species membership is not itself morally significant' (Tooley, 1998). He concludes that many of the above-mentioned criteria for personhood

> entail that something is not a person unless it possesses, or has possessed, the capacity for thought, and this means that if any of the criteria mentioned above is even roughly correct, then human fetuses and newborn infants cannot be persons unless the capacity for thought is something that develops at some point prior to birth – a possibility that does not seem very likely (Tooley, 1998).

In short, the absence of self-consciousness means there can be no desires and hence neither rights nor personhood. Tooley effectively repeats what he first published in 1972:

> In my usage the sentence 'X is a person' will be synonymous with the sentence 'X has a (serious) moral right to life' .... An organism possesses a serious right to life only if it possesses the concept of a self as a continuing subject of experiences and other mental states, and believes that it is itself such a continuing entity' (Tooley, 1972; 1983).

Peter Singer popularized the views of both Locke and Tooley and emphasized the significance of the concept of the person for ethical decision-making at the beginning and end of human life. In his opinion, a human person is understood 'in the sense of a rational and self-conscious being'; thus he excludes members of the species *Homo sapiens* who lack this characteristic (Singer, 1993). Singer holds that 'we accord the life of a fetus no greater value than the life of a nonhuman animal at a similar level of rationality, self-consciousness, awareness, capacity to feel, etc. Since no fetus is a person, no fetus has the same claim to life as a person' (Singer, 1993).

Singer's definition of person is used to determine what beings have rights to live, based on their interests and desires. Human foetuses could neither count as persons nor have the interests of persons: 'The fact that a being is human, and alive, does not in itself tell us whether it is wrong to take that being's life' (Singer, 1994). Singer and Helga Kuhse agree that 'when we kill a new-born infant there is no *person* whose life has begun. When I think of myself as the person I now am, I realise that I did not come into existence until sometime after my birth' (Kuhse and Singer, 1985).

Michael Lockwood's concept of person is similar and could only apply to human beings after birth: 'A person is a being that is conscious, in the sense of having the capacity for conscious thought and experiences, but not only that: It must have the capacity for reflective consciousness and self-consciousness. It must have, or at any rate have the ability to acquire, a concept of itself, as a being with a past and a future. Mere sentience is not enough to qualify a being as a person' (Lockwood, 1985). He admits the foetus is a human being, but not a person, and holds that once the human foetus becomes a person, he or she remains the same human being as before. What he or she requires is some discernible common substratum between the human being and the human person. He believes this could not occur before the formation of the brain with its ongoing physical organization over time. As Lockwood puts it:

> I came into existence only when the appropriate part or parts of my brain came into existence, or more precisely, reached the appropriate stage of development to sustain my identity as a human being, with the capacity for consciousness. When I came into existence is a matter of how far back the relevant neurophysiological continuity can be traced. Presumably, then, my life began somewhere between conception and birth' (Lockwood, 1985).

[He would in theory allow an immaterial soul to supply the required substratum, but finding no empirical evidence for this, opts for the organized physical structures of the brain].

Mary Anne Warren denies that a foetus is a person: 'Prior to the latter part of the second trimester, and probably somewhat later, a fetus almost certainly lacks the neurophysiological structures and functions which are necessary for the occurrence of conscious experience, as well as for thought, self-awareness and other more complex mental capacities' (Warren, 1998).

Walter Glannon thinks much the same but allows for a person's existence once sentience is reached: 'A person begins to exist when the fetal stage of the organism develops the structure and function of the brain necessary to generate and support consciousness and mental life. This is when the fetus becomes sentient, at around 23–24 weeks of gestation' (Glannon, 1998). For these philosophers, foetuses cannot be persons until they have the capacity to exercise some minimal degree of rationally self-conscious acts by expressing interests or desires.

PHILOSOPHICAL RESPONSE TO SECULAR CONCEPTS OF THE HUMAN PERSON

The views of most contemporary secular philosophers on the moral significance of human foetuses give little comfort to foetuses. Denying that foetuses are persons does not ring true, thereby suggesting that the underlying empiricist philosophical premises are flawed, especially when two-thirds of foetuses born prematurely at 24 weeks' gestation survive (Ford, 2002). Such a restricted meaning of 'person' needs to be critically examined in the light of its serious implications for human foetuses. The views of these secular philosophers may be consistent with their philosophical presuppositions, but this does not discount the validity of the traditional view that unborn children are natural, if not legal, persons. I will argue that it suffices to be a subject of a rational nature to be a person and that a spiritual soul is required to render human nature rational. Further, I argue that because the foetus is a living being with a rational human nature, we must conclude that a spiritual soul is created within the embryo when each human being begins.

HUMAN SUBJECT WITH A RATIONAL NATURE IS A PERSON

Secular philosophers are right on many aspects of the human person viewed *subjectively*. Great importance should be given to the interests of persons and their autonomy. Many people, however, differ significantly from secular philosophers on what is required to constitute a human person. It is necessary to ask why it is that only human beings, who are rationally self-conscious and have interests, are deemed to be persons. Can this secular criterion for 'personhood' be rationally justified? Must there not be a foundation that accounts for the human person's subjective perception of his or her interests and desires?

Reflection on the human person from an *objective* viewpoint complements a subjective approach. These approaches do not represent mutually exclusive polarities in our self-understanding. Rationally self-conscious acts and choices do not exist in themselves. They are expressions of the human individual who is their subject. Their existence is made possible by the intrinsic capacity of the human subject's nature (Ford, 2002). Rational self-conscious desires, interests and acts of knowledge owe their existence to the rational nature of the human subject to whom they belong, of whom they are an expression and for whom they are meaningful. Whenever we see a horse and admire its beauty, we are aware of it and of ourselves as the subject who admires the horse. Likewise, known interests are good for their subject: indeed the person as a subject of a rational human nature is the primordial good for whom all goods are good and without whom goods could not be experienced (Ford, 2002). As Charles Taylor says, all kinds of rational self-conscious acts are 'properties which can only exist in a world in which there are subjects of experience, because they concern in some way the life of the subject *qua* subject' (Taylor, 1985).

We have a rational (intellectual) nature that enables us to be aware of the self as the same subject of knowledge of present and past objects of thought and events in our environment. This natural dynamism spans the mental and bodily dimensions of our rationally self-conscious activities. The dimensions of body and mind apparent in these activities indicate each person is a living subject, a body–mind unity. It is preferable, with Chappell, to view the self as a subsisting substance in an Aristotelian sense which 'allows us to be aware of the substance itself, directly, in our immediate experience – and not just the properties of the substance' (Chappell, 2004).

We may conclude that the intellectual nature of a human subject suffices to constitute a human individual as a person. Jenny Teichman understands this when she says: 'In ordinary life *person* and *human being* refer to the same things. For this reason the *ordinary* sense of the word *person* does not, indeed cannot, detach moral import from the concept of the human' (Teichman, 1992). Again she says: 'Human beings are paradigm persons.... for many centuries now it has been the case that "a person" signifies a natural person, i.e. a human being, in all human discourse' (Teichman, 1985). As such, human persons realize they are subjects of inherent dignity and intrinsic value and rightly claim moral and legal inviolability. Patrick Lee agrees: 'From conception on, the unborn human being is a developing entity with the basic, natural capacities to reason and make free choices. She *right now* is that type of thing or substantial entity' (Lee, 2004a).

IMMATERIAL SOUL

Our conscious acts are not merely acts of the brain, as though it was the organ for thinking as the eye is the organ for seeing. Though a functioning brain is needed to think, it is not itself conscious. The intellect together with the senses and the brain enables us to think. The person is one with its rational nature and cannot be separated from it. We need to explain what enables humans to have a rational nature, including the intellect (Ford, 2002). There is no denying a sense-polarity in our knowledge, which focuses on concrete bodies. Human knowledge, however, goes well beyond sense knowledge, which is limited to a perceptual field and images of the imagination and memory within space–time parameters. A cow sees the green grass. A human individual likewise sees the green grass but also knows the truth 'that the grass is green'. Aquinas says this could not be known unless the intellect knows its own self, 'to whose nature it belongs to be conformed to things. Consequently, it is because the intellect reflects upon itself that it knows truth' (Aquinas, 1952). We furthermore understand concepts such as 'square root', 'virtue', 'immaterial soul' or 'God'. We make predications about abstract truths with certainty, for example 'the square root of 49 is 7'. This predication is made by our intellect, not by a sense organ. We know this objective truth and we are aware that we are the subject of this knowledge.

Sense knowledge does not know its own essence because it 'knows nothing except through a bodily organ, and a bodily organ cannot be a medium between a sensing power and itself' (Aquinas, 1952). Aquinas adds that unlike sense knowledge, in intellectual knowledge, 'the act of cognition mediates between the knower and the thing known' in as much as it knows its own essence (Aquinas, 1952). This sort of awareness implies a turning back on itself, like *total self-presence* which transcends the capacity of material senses and requires an intellect of an *immaterial* or *spiritual* nature (Ford, 1991). Each part of a body is only present where it is, not elsewhere. Aristotle (d. 322 BCE) knew that a body could not know truth as such 'for no bodily activity has any connection with the activity of reason' (Aristotle, 1963).

Aristotle and Aquinas rightly understood that intellectual acts require an immaterial soul to perform what a bodily organ alone cannot do. Traditionally, it has been said that this type of knowledge is made possible by a human spiritual soul or life-principle, which Aristotle aptly defined as 'the first actuality of a natural body possessed of organs' (Aristotle, 1957). It actuates matter into an organized living body – an animated body or an incarnate spirit – and constitutes each person into a single entity and an enduring subject. Each one of us experiences this unity: it shows that the soul must be one with the body to constitute one living human individual – a human person (Ford, 2003).

DEFINITION OF A HUMAN PERSON

In the light of what has been discussed, it seems that there is no rational necessity to restrict the concept of person to those who are actually able to exercise intellectually self-conscious acts. What is it that enables a child to first have intellectually self-conscious acts like knowing the truth or expressing desires? This would not be possible unless a rational human nature was already present to enable self-conscious acts of the intellect to be exercised. Lee rightly comments that secular philosophers who admit that people who are asleep or in reversible comas are persons do so 'because they have the potentiality or capacity for higher mental functions' (Lee, 2004b). It seems that a human person may be defined as 'a living individual with a rational [intellectual] human nature' (Ford, 2002).

THE HUMAN FOETUS AS PERSON

Human foetuses are human beings and members of the species *Homo sapiens*. It seems they should be classed as persons because they are human individuals who, through development and growth alone, normally acquire the actual ability to use their natural capacity to perform intellectual acts. Time alone is needed for the requisite brain development to occur before these acts can be expressed. Each human being is chromosomally male or female from conception, even though typical sexual activities can only be exercised after puberty. Human nature usually enables foetuses to develop to the stage where, without ceasing to be the same living human individuals, they can exercise intellectually self-conscious, free and moral acts. They are persons with potential, not potential persons (Ford, 2002). As Beckwith says: 'One can only develop certain functions because of the sort of being one *is*' (Beckwith, 2005).

Lockwood admits an immaterial soul could explain a person's enduring identity, but finding no empirical evidence for it, he favours the human brain as a material substratum (Lockwood, 1985). Because an immaterial soul could not be derived from matter, it must be created when the individual is formed to constitute a human person (Ford, 1991). Hence, it is philosophically credible to hold that the human person begins once an individual with a rational human nature is formed.

These antithetical views on the moral significance of the human foetus are due to two fundamentally different philosophies: one that admits the existence and meaningfulness of non-material reality and the other that practically denies both.

Empirical theories of knowledge are sufficient for ordinary experience and scientific knowledge, but they are inadequate for considering realities which transcend the range of matter and material energy, such as God and the immaterial soul. Simply because our knowledge begins with sense knowledge, it does not mean it is justified to limit human knowledge to the empirical domain. For the human intellect 'reality as such' cannot be reduced to 'empirical reality'. To do so is to disregard how we successfully engage in meaningful discourse about realities which transcend experience (Ford, 2002). This seems to be the epistemological foundation of positions which unwarrantedly deny personhood to human foetuses and embryos.

IMPLICATIONS OF THE MORAL SIGNIFICANCE OF THE FOETUS AS A PERSON

Unborn children are quite significant to their mothers, especially after the first movements are felt and bonding increases. Some pregnant women who undergo a prenatal diagnostic test are reluctant to bond with their unborn children and regard the pregnancy as *tentative* until after they find out their children are free of the abnormality for which tests were done (Ford, 2002). People who believe human foetuses are persons are morally opposed to any acts which are inconsistent with foetuses' personal status. On the other hand, those who do not accept that human foetuses are persons deny them a right to life and hold induced abortion is morally permissible. The legal protection that should be provided for human foetuses is split along the same lines.

Respect for the human foetus, however, would not morally forbid the performing of medically indicated procedures which save the life of a pregnant woman or safeguard her health from a serious pathological condition, provided there is no direct assault on the life of the foetus. The death of the foetus may be foreseen as a side effect of the intervention, but it should not be intended. Such a situation arises, for instance, if a pregnant woman has a cancerous uterus that needs to be removed. There is a significant moral difference between directly choosing to terminate a pregnancy and permitting the unwanted loss of human life as a side effect of a life-saving act. Furthermore, the foetus should not be treated as a commodity. This implies that foetal tissue legitimately obtained from a deceased foetus may be donated for transplantation – but not sold like products at the market.

Warren regards 'both sentient foetuses and infants as having significant moral status based upon their capacity for sentience' (Warren, 2000). There is, however, no agreement on when a human foetus begins to experience pain – ranging from 30 weeks' gestation to 10 weeks (Ford, 2002). Aristotle himself opposes abortion after the foetus 'has developed sensation and life' (Aristotle, 1967). There is now universal agreement among philosophers that human foetuses should not be subjected to unnecessary pain, regardless of whether the actions are, or are not, therapeutic. In cases of medical procedures which could potentially cause human foetuses to suffer pain, some clinicians may well need to learn a lesson from the following Australian guideline for researchers using animals: 'Unless there is specific evidence to the contrary investigators must assume fetuses have the same requirements for anaesthesia and analgesia as adult animals of the species' (NHMRC, 1997).

CONCLUSION

We have been discussing two concepts of the human person. The traditional concept is based on the ontological constitution of a person, who is a subject of moral inviolability. It focuses on the kind of being a person is in itself, from the beginning of the person to death, regardless of the person's stages or conditions of life. The contemporary secular concept, instead, focuses on the ability of the human being to have rationally self-conscious acts and interests. This is very much akin to considering a person as a moral agent as suggested by Locke's above-mentioned reference to the person being 'a forensic term' (Locke, 1924). Only human beings with the requisite properties are considered to be persons with a right to life. The former concept of person is compatible with the second, but the second concept of person is not compatible with the former.

Consequently, the moral significance of the human foetus varies according to people's fundamental religious and/or philosophical beliefs on what constitutes a human person. At the same time it also depends in practice on the value people attribute to the human foetus, especially pregnant women. Wanted unborn children are cherished: but, it needs to be asked, whether depriving unwanted unborn children of life is justified.

REFERENCES

Aquinas T. In: Mulligan RW (Translator). *Truth*. Chicago: Henry Regnery Company, 1952.

Aristotle. In: Hett WS (Translator). *On the Soul* (De Anima). London and Cambridge, MA: Heinemann, 1957.

Aquinas T. In: Velecky C (Translator). *Summa Theologiae*, vol. 6. London and New York: Blackfriars, 1965.

Aristotle. In: Peck AL (Translator). *Generation of Animals*. London: W. Heinemann; Cambridge, MA: Harvard University Press, 1963.

Aristotle. In: Rackham H, ed. (Translator). *Politics*. London: W. Heinemann; Cambridge, MA: Harvard University Press, 1967.

Beckwith FJ. Of souls, selves and cerebrums: a reply to Himma. *J Med Ethics* 2005; 31: 56–60.

Boethius. *A Treatise against Eutyches and Nestorius, Also commonly known as De persona et duabus naturis*. In: Stewart HF, Rand EK (Translators). *Boethius. The Theological Tractates and The Consolation of Philosophy*. London: W. Heinemann Ltd; Cambridge, MA: Harvard University Press, 1953.

Brown RE. *The Birth of the Messiah*. New York: Doubleday, 1993.

Chappell TDJ. Persons as goods: response to Patrick Lee. *Christian Bioethics* 2004; 10: 69–77.

Flannery A. Pastoral constitution of the church in the modern word. In: Flannery A, ed. *Vatican Council II The Conciliar and Post-Conciliar Documents*. Dublin: Dominican Publications, 1975; pp. 903–1014.

Ford NM. *When Did I Begin? Conception of the Human Individual in History, Philosophy and Science*. Cambridge: Cambridge University Press, 1991.

Ford NM. *The Prenatal Person: Ethics from Conception to Birth*. Oxford: Blackwell, 2002.

Ford NM. Stem cell research and ethics. In Ford NM, Herbert M, ed. *Stem Cells. Science, Medicine, Law and Ethics*. Strathfield, NSW, Australia: St Paul's Publications, 2003; pp. 71–83.

Frye N. *The Great Code*: The Bible and Literature. London: ARC Paperbacks, 1993.

Glannon W. Genes, embryos, and future people. *Bioethics* 1998; 12: 187–211.

Grisez G. *Abortion: the Myths, the Realities and the Arguments*. New York: Corpus Books, 1970.

John Paul II. Gospel of Life. Homebush, Australia: St Paul's, 1995.

Kuhse H, Singer P. *Should the Baby Live? The Problem of Handicapped Infants*. Oxford: Oxford University Press, 1985.

Lee P. Abortion and Christian bioethics: the continuing ethical importance of abortion. *Christian Bioethics* 2004b; 10: 7–31.

Lee P. The pro-life argument from substantial identity: a defence. *Bioethics* 2004a; 18: 249–263.

Leone S. The ancient roots of a recent debate. In: *Identity and Statute of the Human Embryo*. Vatican City: Juan de Dios Vial Correa and Elio Sgreccia, Liberia Editrice Vaticana, 1998; pp. 28–47.

Locke J. In: Pringle-Pattison AS, ed. *Essay Concerning Human Understanding, Book II*. Oxford: Clarendon Press, 1924.

Lockwood M. When does a life begin? In: Lockwood M, ed. *Moral Dilemmas in Modern Medicine*. Oxford: Oxford University Press, 1985; pp. 9–31.

National Health & Medical Research Council. *Australian Code of Practice for the Care and Use of Animals for Scientific Purposes*, 6th edition. Canberra: Commonwealth Department of Health and Family Services, 1997.

Niederwimmer K. In: Attridge HW, ed. *The Didache. A Commentary*. Minneapolis: Fortress Press, 1998.

Singer P. *Practical Ethics*, 2nd edition. Cambridge: University Press, 1993.

Singer P. *Rethinking Life & Death: The Collapse of Our Traditional Ethics*. Melbourne: The Text Publishing Company, 1994.

Taylor C. *Human Agency and Language, Philosophical Papers I*. Cambridge: Cambridge University Press, 1985.

Teichman J. The definition of person. *Philosophy* 1985; 60: 175–185.

Teichman J. Humanism and personism. *Quadrant* 1992; 36: 26–29.

Tertullian. In: Glover TR (Translator). *Apology*. London: William Heinemann, 1931.

Tooley M. Abortion and infanticide. *Philos Public Affairs* 1972; 2: 37–65.

Tooley M. *Abortion and Infanticide*. Oxford: Clarendon Press, 1983.

Tooley M. Personhood. In: Kuhse H, Singer P, eds. *A Companion to Bioethics*. Oxford: Blackwell, 1998; pp. 117–126.

Wansbrough H, ed. *The New Jerusalem Bible*. New York: New York, Doubleday, 1985.

Warren MA. Abortion. In: Kuhse H, Singer P, eds. *A Companion to Bioethics*. Malden, MA: Blackwell, 1998; pp. 127–134.

Warren MA. The moral difference between infanticide and abortion: a response to Robert Card. *Bioethics* 2000; 14: 352–359.

53

Will We Need Abortion in Utopia?

ADRIENNE ASCH

Philosophical literature on abortion has examined the moral status of unborn human life and comes to no consensus. As Gillon (2001) discusses in his summary of the abortion debate, views range from equating embryos and foetuses with born individuals as soon as conception occurs to views that accord with the foetus's increasing moral status as it develops. Supporters and opponents of abortion might agree that a foetus implanted in a woman's body is a genetically different entity from the woman who gestates it and has the potential for separate biological and social life. There is no harm done to pro-choice arguments by acknowledging that a foetus is both a part of a woman's body and a genetically different being.

In nations that permit abortion, courts and legislatures recognize the absence of consensus on the moral status of unborn life. They accept abortion based on the circumstances of adults and children already born. Arguments for abortion often focus on societal factors that both advocates and opponents of abortion would change. Discussions emphasize the 'distressful life and future' that attends a woman's unchosen social motherhood (*Roe v Wade*, 1973). Others emphasize that women's childbearing role has been used to justify affording them inferior educational, employment and civic opportunities (Ginsburg, 1985, 1994; Siegel 1995). But abortion is not merely a remedy for socially constructed gender inequalities; it allows people to maintain deeply felt attitudes towards sexual relationships, parenthood and familial obligations. For that reason, it would be needed even in a world without sex discrimination and with vastly improved societal arrangements for children and adults.

US scholars and courts generally have supported women's need for abortion using concepts such as 'privacy' and 'gender equality', but this chapter proposes that legal, social and technological developments should lead us to justify access to abortion on different grounds. These developments also compel us to struggle with some hitherto under-addressed topics if we are to continue arguing for abortion in a better world than one we may ever inhabit. Even in a world where coerced sex was rare, where women did not face economic discrimination, where employers structured their expectations in line with family responsibilities, and where women and men took on an equal share of those responsibilities, we would need birth control and abortion. To justify society's need for abortion – not merely women's – I would make three claims:

1. Women and men benefit from expressing themselves in sexual relationships, and the personal and interpersonal value of such expression does not reside solely in sexual acts having procreative potential;
2. Coerced parenthood, even if only biological and not social, is likely to have profound, negative psychological and social ramifications and should therefore be discouraged;
3. Even when an adult consents to become a parent, there are moral and legal limits to what we expect parents to do for their already born children; we should not demand that members of one sex make a sacrifice of their bodies to gestate new life, if we do not demand that members of both sexes make comparable sacrifices (donating blood, for example) to meet the needs of the children with whom they are already connected.

ABORTION AND SEX

Rather than grounding views about abortion on the question of the moral status of the foetus, let us examine the moral status of sexual relationships. Without heterosexual sex there would be no intended or unintended pregnancies, no foetuses in women's bodies, and no question about the appropriate handling of those pregnancies. Some major world religions do not endorse sex when it is deliberately separated from openness to procreation, but they accept sexual relations between people who cannot reproduce because of infertility or menopause. Such religious acceptance comes from understanding what others writing from a secular tradition also recognize: sexual relationships can be a powerful way to create and express deep, enduring human connections. Such relationships serve to demonstrate and renew companionship, caring, commitment and love (Karst, 1980). For anyone who believes that sexual intimacy can be legitimate, worthwhile and morally acceptable apart from its procreative potential, one must follow McDonagh (1996) in arguing that consent to sexual expression says nothing about consent to creating a new human being. We should acknowledge the psychological and interpersonal value of sexual relationships in human life and agree that their worth and goodness need not derive from their link to reproduction.

In the United States and many other nations, the law now gives some legitimacy to consensual non-procreative sexual relations, regardless of the marital status or sexual orientation of the participants. Beginning with cases supporting the rights of the married and unmarried to use contraception (*Griswold v Connecticut*, 1965; *Eisenstadt v Baird*, 1972) and now extending to protection for homosexual relationships (*Lawrence v Texas*, 2003), a body of US law affirms that consenting parties should be able to conduct their sexual lives without fear of government censure or intervention. The law implicitly acknowledges and protects the human need for closeness, love and self-expression that can characterize such relationships.

Like contraception, abortion permits women as well as men to participate in the goodness of sexual relationships without facing an automatic link between sexual expression and potential parenthood. Along with seeking equality of opportunity in the public sphere, women seek and benefit from the goods to be found in sexual intimacy; what women achieve through access to contraception and abortion is the opportunity to discover their potential for giving and receiving passion, joy, tenderness, comfort and all the other emotions and experiences that can be found in sexual intimacy. Birth control and abortion change the playing field for women not merely in public life, but also in the private world of interpersonal relationships and psychological development. Whether or not they countenance the way in which many men view their sexual lives as free from the consequences of parenthood, abortion opponents need to examine why men, but not women, can often participate in sexual relationships that are not intended to lead to parent–child relationships. I would be surprised if people could support a double standard of sexual life for women and men. If in fact they could not account for such different standards and social consequences, we might have a more honest conversation about how views on abortion depend upon views about the proper role of sex in human relationships.

VOLUNTARY AND COERCED PARENTHOOD

Women and men eagerly anticipating a new child will attest that becoming a mother or father is a momentous, life-changing event. Writing about the difference between chosen and unchosen pregnancy, Daphne de Marneffe said: 'The reality of pregnancy is that having a baby one does not inwardly consent to is a traumatic offence to one's integrity as a person; having a baby that one desires is an ultimate fulfilment of oneself as a person' (2004, p. 241). De Marneffe is speaking here not merely about the physiological facets of pregnancy, but about pregnancy as the prelude to a chosen parenting relationship. For a host of religious, social and psychological reasons (Hoffmann and Hoffmann, 1973; Alpern, 1992), the vast majority of people treasure the opportunity to raise a child, and thwarted fulfilment drives the practices of adoption, assisted reproduction and the world of infertility clinics. The cultural significance of parenthood is the very thing that makes the prospect of having a child that one does not desire so psychologically distressing and socially offensive.

As law professor Kenneth Karst has written, 'The decision to have a child, whether within or outside marriage, strongly implicates the values of intimate association, particularly the values of caring and commitment, intimacy and self-identification. The decision ranks in importance with any other a person may make in a lifetime . . .' (1980, p. 640).

Thirty years before addressing pregnancy termination, the US Supreme Court affirmed the significance of chosen parenthood when it forbade governments from sterilizing prisoners (*Skinner v Oklahoma*, 1942). Along with Anita Allen (1995), I argue that to preserve the special, intimate, self-defining qualities of parent–child relationships, governments must neither prevent people from forming such ties nor compel them to do so.

Much of the writing on abortion portrays the adverse social and economic circumstances in which many women raise children, with male partners or alone. The decision in *Roe v Wade* described the difficulties many mothers face:

> Maternity, or additional offspring, may force upon the woman a distressful life and future. Psychological harm may be imminent. Mental and physical health may be taxed by child care. There is also the distress, for all concerned, associated with the unwanted child, and there is the problem of bringing a child into a family already unable, psychologically and otherwise, to care for it.

The *Roe* court paints a vivid picture of the many complications that can make childraising very difficult. Implicit in this description is the recognition that whether women are raising children with partners or alone, in poverty or material comfort, they continue to do most of the day-to-day work of feeding, clothing, protecting, educating and socializing children. If a mother is not living with her child's father, she often raises their child without the financial or social support she might have expected when the child was conceived. In nations without state-supported health care or daycare, many parents may fear that they cannot provide their children with basic safety, security and protection. In this social context, the desire to avoid parenthood is understandable. Conceivably, with affordable childcare and health care, jobs with wages and hours that fit the needs of families, paid childrearing leave routinely used by men as well as women, and men's equal responsibility for the children they father, some of today's reluctant or unwilling prospective parents might change their minds.

However, others would probably still demur. The psychological and social requirements of adult partnership and childraising are not identical. Some people are far better suited to being loving companions to another adult than they are to meeting the needs of a growing child. Men and women may feel that they lack the patience, imagination, generosity or empathy to change their lives in ways that will nurture a child from infancy to adulthood. Others may be confident that they are most fulfilled as human beings and best able to contribute to their societies by devoting their entire lives to art, public service, social causes, scientific discovery or national security. The capacities and virtues associated with good parenting may be those towards which everyone might aspire, but it is hard to imagine a world in which all adults will attain them. A society that validates many different kinds of lives cannot insist that all women or men should find parenthood rewarding.

So far I have been discussing voluntary or coerced social parenthood, where pregnancy would lead to raising the resulting child. Interestingly, so did the Supreme Court in *Roe v Wade*; other legal theorists who have revisited this decision have followed suit (Balkin, 1995). They did not address the implications of carrying a pregnancy to term if the child was to be raised by others. Today, however, litigation over implanting frozen embryos, and the acceptance of adoption and 'donor'-assisted reproduction, all underscore that parenthood is biological as well as social. In a society that permits separating the biological from the social components of parenthood, the meaning of parenthood is rapidly evolving, and abortion must be re-examined as well.

Biological motherhood or fatherhood – even when separated from the day-to-day life of the child – has significant psychological and social implications. The cherished social norm underlying all discussions of reproduction and parent–child relationships is that those who cause the existence of a new human life should take some responsibility to care for that life (Nelson, 1989). In the United States, the English-speaking world and many other nations, the norm is that biological parentage should lead to social parentage unless there is a good reason to do otherwise. Causal responsibility should entail social responsibility for a child.

The assumed connection between genetic causation and social parenthood has been changing as practices of gamete 'donation' have increased. In other writing, (Asch, 1995). I have argued that pre-birth intention to parent and post-birth rearing should be recognized as more important than genetic or gestational connection to a child. People may transfer the responsibility that genetic causation typically confers when they provide gametes to those who will raise a child of their eggs and sperm; they may choose to gestate a child for other people, as in 'surrogate' or 'contract' motherhood; or two genetic parents may decide that they should not raise a child they have conceived and may have the child adopted by others. In all these instances, the biological contributors to the new human being have chosen this arrangement and have thus assumed responsibility for the new life. By intentionally separating biological from social parenting, their actions indicate both to themselves and others that while acting outside the norm, they have still made conscientious decisions about the fate of their genetic offspring. They have accepted both the idea of becoming parents only in the biological sense, and the emotional significance of creating a child.

In disputed embryo cases, one genetic parent would compel the other to become a genetic parent against their will. Only state courts have confronted disputes about the fate of unimplanted frozen embryos, but several decisions in the last 15 years apparently adhere to the view that parenthood should not be forced upon an unwilling person (Pachman 2003). Although Pachman herself argues that a woman's greater role in the IVF process – analogous to her unique role in pregnancy – should give her the final say in any dispute about unimplanted embryos, the courts have concentrated on the psychological and social ramifications of parenthood and have found any compelled parenthood to be offensive (*Davis v Davis*, 1992). They have done so regardless of whether the unwilling prospective parent was male or female. Pachman cites a New Jersey case (J.B. V M.B., 2001) where the woman did not wish to have embryos she created with her former husband implanted in his new wife or used by infertile couples. Commenting on the negative consequences of unwanted genetic motherhood, the court stated that '[i]mplantation, if successful, would result in the birth of her biological child and could have life-long emotional and psychological repercussions

. . . Her fundamental right not to procreate is irrevocably extinguished if a surrogate mother bears J.B.'s child.'

One wishes the New Jersey court had articulated more precisely why purely biological parenthood is so invested with emotional and psychological weight. Even as some men and women choose to separate biological from social parenthood, the status of each type of parental relationship persists as culturally and religiously significant. Knowing that your genetic material has been used by others to create a new life against your will differs markedly from deciding to give or even sell eggs, sperm, embryos or gestation. Whether or not she will ever see or hear about the child after its birth, a woman lives with the knowledge that a child with her genes exists in the world. The child may look like her or her relatives. If the behaviour geneticists are accurate (a deeply contested question, as discussed in Parens et al., 2006), the child may manifest some of her aptitudes and personality even if they never interact.

In the era before widely available abortion, some women and some male partners went through pregnancy and found themselves either the coerced social parents discussed earlier, or coerced by families and social agencies into making adoption plans for children. After a stigmatized out-of-wedlock pregnancy and childbirth, they would sign papers terminating parental rights, contact and usually all knowledge about where the child was, how the child was faring and who was raising the child (Solinger, 1992). Before access to birth control and abortion, adoption resembled the unchosen genetic parenthood that courts today would discourage in the disputes over unimplanted embryos.

The ineradicable differences in the biology of reproduction inevitably lead to differences between woman and man when it comes to continuing or ending pregnancies. As long as foetuses can grow only in women's bodies, and as long as women are permitted to decide whether they will continue or end a pregnancy, some men will be denied fatherhood even if they would happily assume responsibility for a child they helped create. Other men will become genetic and social parents against their will and may find themselves with financial obligations to children they never intended to exist.

Could or should any imaginable social changes affect men's and women's relationship to pregnancy, abortion and parental roles and obligations? If pregnancy and involuntary motherhood were once seen as the inevitable consequences of sexual relationships, perhaps compelled financial support for undesired children has been accepted as a way to impose some check on men's sexual behaviour. If we accept birth control and abortion as legitimate decisions for women to make, we may want to rethink our expectations of men and of the society as a whole. In order for women to imagine raising a child without the participation of the man who fathered the child, she must believe that she has adequate emotional and financial resources in herself, her social network and the community. The trend in the disputed embryo cases that opposes coerced parenthood should influence the social and legal response in the abortion context. Fairness, decency and concern for greater equality and mutuality between women and men leads me to oppose the automatic presumption that men should pay support for children they never intended or expected. The state that wants women to have genuine choice in matters of parenting should help women who want to raise children even without the co-operation of the men who engendered them.

Of course, in today's very imperfect world, many divorced men stop supporting children despite years of being recognized as their genetic and social father. However men rationalize such behaviour, it harms children by depriving them of material and emotional resources. Such acts give men and fathers a bad reputation, and nothing else I say in favour of change should be taken to excuse paternal neglect.

Many unintended pregnancies now carried to term would not occur in a society where men respected women's views and interests. Outright male violence forces sex and pregnancies; men often refuse to use condoms or to accept women's use of birth control. When women decide to carry these unintended pregnancies to term and to raise the resulting children, they may also decide that the men should give financial support to the child, even if they provide nothing else. A woman could understandably feel betrayed and abandoned by the child's father and might deeply regret the relationship that engendered the child she nonetheless decides to raise. The courts could uphold a woman's and her child's claim for support on the grounds that the man did nothing to forestall impregnation and instead behaved in ways that made it more likely to occur.

In some cases where men have been required to pay support for children they never wanted, however, fact is stranger than fiction. In a law review article, Donald Hubin recounts stories of women who lied to men about using birth control, of a woman who inseminated herself with sperm from the condom her partner wore, and of another woman who obtained sperm from a man who was unconscious during the act from which she became pregnant (Hubin, 2003). The men who pay child support for children brought into existence through deception may be a small minority of the men supporting children, but they certainly exemplify unsought parenthood. Perhaps they have no other contact with the child or the mother than sending a monthly, quarterly or yearly sum; perhaps they grudgingly, awkwardly or curiously spend time with the child they never wanted. These men live with the resentment of having been deceived, assaulted or robbed of their genetic material; they have obligations towards children they did not want and towards whom they may feel at best distance, at worst dislike.

In most instances of unintended pregnancy, however, both the woman and the man do not expect a pregnancy to result from a particular sexual encounter. Human beings make mistakes and there is no foolproof contraception. A man may have no idea why his partner decided to maintain the pregnancy and raise the child; he may be deeply distressed about having to take on a parenting role he never intended. If the partners are going to maintain an ongoing relationship, he may feel that he must embrace her decision and the child. If her decision to continue the pregnancy strains and breaks their emotional connection, it is worth asking whether he should be required to assume a financial tie to the woman and a child whose existence he sought to avoid.

If women change their minds and decide to continue a pregnancy when their sexual partner had reason to believe they would not, they should not demand their partner's financial or emotional involvement with the child. The biological father will have to face an unsought genetic tie to a child, and he may decide that he has obligations to the child he helped create. If he voluntarily comes to such a decision, rather than being compelled by a court or government agency, there is a good chance that his child, his partner and he will derive psychological and social benefits from chosen rather than coerced connection. If his partner, the law and social practice do not compel his financial involvement, and if he genuinely feels that the unexpected parental status is well beyond what he understood his sexual relationship to entail, a complete exit may ultimately be fairer and more helpful to the child and to his former partner than their awareness of a cheque that arrives with no interest, no love and none of the commitment, caring and identification that ideally accompany parenting responsibility.

I have been arguing that in order to realize the virtues that can make sexual intimacy and parenthood among the most special parts of human life, they each should be undertaken voluntarily. Birth control and abortion permit women to avoid involuntary genetic and social motherhood, and the trend in disputed embryo cases endorses the approach I have taken here. The biology of pregnancy will not prevent some men from being involuntary genetic fathers, but we could change our law and practice to free men from the financial consequences of unchosen parenthood. Such a proposal could only be fair to children and women if society acted to ensure that women's educational and economic opportunities were not diminished under such circumstances.

Until now, I have been discussing abortion as a response to undesired genetic or social parenthood of any child that might be born, having nothing to do regardless of the characteristics of the particular foetus or the number of foetuses a woman may be carrying. It is important to comment on what some people have described as a new facet of the abortion debate (Gillon, 2001), the matter of selective abortion. Tests can now determine the number of foetuses being carried, their sex and whether or not they have such disabling traits as Down syndrome, spina bifida, cystic fibrosis or Tay Sachs disease. For many reasons, women (and their partners) may believe that it is emotionally, financially or socially difficult or unacceptable to raise a child of 'the wrong sex' (usually a girl), or a child who would have a disabling condition. They may conclude that they live in a group or a society that will not treat a girl or a child with a disability well and may fear that the child's life will be hard, physically and emotionally painful, and ultimately unrewarding. They may decide that the psychological, time and financial demands of bringing triplets into their lives or of raising a child with a disabling condition would jeopardize their work lives, their other children or their own relationship. Even if they recognize that any childraising is likely to be demanding and life-changing, they may suspect that the distresses and hardships of parenting children with certain characteristics are ultimately incompatible with their parenting and life goals.

As I have said in other writing, (Asch, 2000; Asch and Wasserman, 2005) I believe that selectivity is counter to the virtues of parenting that strike me as ideal: the openness to welcoming, appreciating and nurturing new life and the flexibility to understand that any one characteristic such as disability will not obscure all the other qualities present in the new child. I recognize that others disagree with my view on parental selectivity (Ruddick, 2000) and that some of those who generally object to futuristic 'designing' of children do not object to selecting against those who would have disabilities (Sandel, 2004). I, however, maintain that a disability is almost never incompatible with a rewarding life for the child, or with a rich, positive parenting experience (Asch, 1999; Ferguson, 2001). Along with such scholars as Newell (1999) I have extended to all selective abortions the arguments made by abortion supporters who nonetheless object to sex-selective abortions: that they undermine the societal goals of women's equality and reinforce restrictive sex stereotypes (Wertz and Fletcher, 1992; Holmes, 1995). Professional and public expectations that prenatally diagnosed disability automatically should lead to abortion can undermine the barely won recognition that people with disabilities can contribute to family and society (Asch, 1999). Although these remain minority positions, I am not alone in viewing most of the existing difficulties of disability as remediable by changes in societal attitudes and institutions, much like the changes that have improved life for women. However, I recognize that although many thoughtful people can envisage social changes that would improve conditions for girls in India, or for all non-disabled children everywhere, many fewer are ready to extend this analysis to life with disability, and they therefore maintain that selective abortion on grounds of foetal health is among the strongest reasons to support available abortion (Harris, 2001; Glover 2006).

Despite my opposition to parental selectivity, my objections to any unchosen parenthood lead me to believe that no woman should continue her pregnancy if she cannot face becoming the rearing or even the genetic non-rearing parent of a child of 'the wrong sex', of triplets rather than twins, or of a child who will have a disabling condition. If society accepts selectivity against foetuses with disabling traits, it should accept selectivity based on other characteristics that can be determined before birth such as sex. Societies that try to halt parental selectivity by banning sex-selective abortions while encouraging abortions based on disability will endanger the willingness to accept and include people who are born with or who acquire socially unacceptable conditions. Emily Jackson's response to sex-selective abortion captures my position on all selective abortions:

> Sex-selective abortion represents a powerful example of the implausibility of separating reproductive choices from the web of social networks within which decisions must be taken. But recognizing that a preference may be socially constructed does not necessarily mean that it should be ignored. The decision to abort a fetus because it is female may only be comprehensible in the light of a deeply embedded cultural and economic preference for sons, but that does not make an individual woman's choice less real or compelling . . .[W]here a competent adult woman has made her own decision that she wishes to terminate a particular pregnancy, restricting her access to abortion may be incompatible with a strong commitment to the principle of self-determination (Jackson, 2000, p. 485).

In my utopia there might be no selection because all prospective parents would feel that they had the social, psychological and material resources to care for any child that was born to them. Moreover, they would live in a society that legitimated their choices with institutions equally committed to the well-being of each new child. But the goal of only chosen parenthood leads me to accept that others will reach different conclusions from those I advance; those choices must be respected.

BODILY INTEGRITY AND PARENTAL OBLIGATION

I strive for a world in which social parenting would be valued more than genetic ties, and a world in which men and women were equally committed to raising children. Could I imagine a world in which women with unintended pregnancies accepted the pregnancy as a prelude to transferring the child to the child's father if he sought to take responsibility for it, or to a would-be adoptive parent? Yes, but many pre-

vailing attitudes would have to change. Thinking about possible changes requires discussing pregnancy itself: how it affects women's bodies, creates a new relationship between woman and foetus, and entails obligations.

As the *Roe* court and others note, (Mackenzie, 1992; McDonagh, 1996) pregnancy is anything but a physically trivial event in a woman's life; rather, most women report it to be intense, physically demanding, sometimes exhausting, health-threatening and even life-threatening. A woman goes through morning sickness, fatigue, substantial weight gain; her bodily changes affect her way of moving, what food and how often she eats, how she feels awake or asleep. Her body and her day-to-day life are influenced by the presence of the new being growing within her. She will not be able to ignore the pregnancy, just as no one can ignore the realities of hunger, fatigue or pain. This awareness constitutes some form of psychological relationship to the foetus. Once the pregnancy becomes apparent to others, the woman's life also changes socially, because they respond to her as a pregnant person, a mother-to-be. These physiological and social changes accompany any gestation, irrespective of whether the gestational relationship to the foetus will lead to a social, rearing relationship with the child.

A great deal of legal and philosophical writing centres on the idea that human beings, as possessed of physical bodies, cannot psychologically detach themselves from their bodies (Rao, 2000). We experience the world with and through our bodies, and our body is an essential aspect of our personhood. The law in the United States affirms that the human mind and self are not separable from the human body, and protects the individual's bodily privacy. Ninety years ago, the US Supreme Court established the notion of bodily integrity and asserted that no one could be touched or medically treated without his or her consent (*Schloendorff v Society of New York Hospital*, 1915). Bodily integrity is also violated if our bodies are used by others without our consent. Courts have applied the idea that individuals must consent to uses of their bodies to the instance of life-threatening situations of family members. In the case of *McFall v Shimp* (1978), for example, one cousin could not be required to save his cousin's life by providing bone marrow, and the cousin died for lack of another suitable donor.

When Judith Jarvis Thomson (1971) wrote her classic article justifying abortion, she did so on grounds of bodily integrity. She likened the bodily and life changes of pregnancy to those that would occur to a woman suddenly attached for nine months to another human being (a violinist using her kidney). Several courts had already determined that no familial relationship entitled one person to the blood, bone marrow or organs of another when Thomson offered her defence of abortion. Thomson highlights that pregnancy – as a process that uses a woman's body to sustain potential human life – requires sacrifice and involvement analogous to the sacrifice and involvement of someone who provides her kidney to an ailing person. Bodily use without such consent violates not only one's physical integrity but also one's sense of self. The foetus has the same properties regardless of whether the woman gestating it desired to be pregnant, psychologically accepted it when she learned she was pregnant, or resented, feared and disliked being pregnant; McDonagh (1996) and de Marneffe (2004) expanding on Thomson's powerful analysis when they insist that pregnancy, gestational relationship and gestational parenthood should offend our understanding of bodily integrity, selfhood and self-determination if they become compelled and if childbirth becomes literally forced labour.

As West (1995) has argued in her justification for abortion, we do not require either women or men to use their bodies to aid their own children, much less strangers with whom they have no relationship. Parents of 5-year-old children may be prosecuted for child abuse if they do not feed their children enough to keep them alive; but the same father or mother is not required to provide blood, bone marrow or a kidney to their dying 5-year-old child if they do not want to do so. They may be admired for doing so and perhaps even morally censured for failing to make this sacrifice to save their child's life, but they cannot be compelled to have their body used to aid even that child. If law and custom accept limits to parental obligation to children with whom they have entered into a relationship of daily care, it is difficult to understand why women should use their bodies to create new life if they do not wish to do so. Abortion opponents should require men to promise their kidneys to their children in case of need. If we asked comparable sacrifices of women and men to their existing children, we might be better positioned to suggest that women make a 9-month physical sacrifice of their health and comfort to give life to a new human being.

Should a woman be willing to let her body be used to create new life even if she does not wish to become the child's social mother? If the child's father asks her to maintain the pregnancy and be absolved of any obligation to the baby after it is born, should she do so? I think it would be desirable for men and women to aid their children, their friends and possibly strangers much more than is expected today. It could be praiseworthy for a woman who found herself pregnant to agree with the child's biological father that she will gestate the baby and give it to him, free of any stigma or involvement if she does not want to raise the child. I can also imagine women saying that they could use their bodies to create new life that friends or strangers would care for if they themselves did not want a parenting role. If we valued primarily the social work of parenthood and not the ties of genetics or gestation, we might see our way to donating pregnancies to others without detachment from the experience of gestating, and without developing unexpected attachment to the baby after birth.

For those who cannot embrace raising children and cannot accept that other people are unwilling to raise a child or have others raise a genetic child they had gestated, the reality of unintended pregnancies probably means the reality of abortion. In 1990, legal scholar Lawrence Tribe asked whether we would need abortion if foetuses could be transferred from the body of one woman to the body of another, or to an artificial womb, or even possibly to a man (Tribe, 1990). He concluded that the economics of substitute gestation would make it unrealistic. I am more concerned with its moral or social desirability and its effect on human psychology and social life. Even if we could safely remove a foetus from a woman and implant it elsewhere, ending her pregnancy and freeing her physical body might not free her from the knowledge of a life to which she could not consent, of a status of genetic mother that implicated her in a connection she did not want. To protect chosen genetic, gestational and social parenthood, I must remain committed to a world where abortion and foetal death – not simply foetal removal and transfer – are possible.

Under changed psychological conditions, we might not need abortion in utopia. But I stop short of such a claim or wish because I believe that people will and should make their own evaluations about how they want to use their bodies to sustain life; about whether they must raise a child of their genes or whether they should see the child as available to others; about whether to select the characteristics of the children they will raise. Creating a new life is such a momentous event that it should ideally be chosen, and my utopia ultimately must make way for a range of choices to fit the diverse psychological needs of different women and men.

I hope that these reflections will stimulate pro-choice theorists to better articulate their justifications for a procedure that still troubles many people. We need more conversation about the different weights to put on genetic, gestational and social ties to children; on the separation of sexual from reproductive relationships; on the obligations of fathers; about what limits, if any, to place on parental selectivity; on whether we should change our account of bodily integrity and parental obligation to include entitlements of others to the use of our bodies; and whether we would like to replace abortion with a reformed society that included foetal transfers and unstigmatized adoption. Proponents of abortion should acknowledge that foetal life is indeed a form of human life; however, they should ground their acceptance of this procedure on the claim that human life must be wanted and accepted in order to have a chance at flourishing. Abortion permits women – alone or with their   decide that only those children with whom they accept some type of relationship, and for whom they accept some responsibility, will come into being.

ACKNOWLEDGEMENTS

This chapter benefited from wonderful conversations with Leslie Francis, Betty Wolder Levin, Bruce Levin, Vivian Lindermayer and Carmel Shachar. Despite philosophical disagreements on some points, Ari Schick provided excellent research and many suggestions for phrasing and organization that clarified and sharpened my argument. John Fousek's editing tightened the writing. Finally, my thanks to Heather Draper for inviting me to contribute this chapter and for patient support and encouragement that kept me from giving up on it.

REFERENCES

Allen A. In: Balkin JM, ed. *What Roe v. Wade Should Have Said: The Nation's Top Legal Experts Rewrite America's Most Controversial Decision*. New York: New York University Press, 1995 (concurring in the judgment); pp. 92–108.

Alpern KD. Genetic puzzles and stork stories: on the meaning and significance of having children. In: Alpern KD, ed. *The Ethics of Reproductive Technology*. New York: Oxford University Press, 1992; pp. 147–169.

Asch A. Parenthood and embodiment: Reflections on biology, intentionality, and autonomy. *Graven Images* 1995; **2**: 229–236.

Asch A. Prenatal diagnosis and selective abortion: a challenge to practice and policy. *Am J Public Health* 1999; 89(11): 1649–1657.

Asch A. Why I haven't changed my mind about prenatal diagnosis: reflections and refinements. In: Parens E, Asch A, eds. *Prenatal testing and Disability Rights*. Washington, DC: Georgetown University Press, 2000; pp. 234–258.

Asch A, Wasserman D. Where is the sin in synecdoche: prenatal testing and the parent–child relationship. In: Wasserman D, Wachbroit R, Bickenbach J, eds. *Quality of Life and Human Difference: Genetic Testing, Health Care, and Disability*. New York: Cambridge University Press; 2005; pp. 172–216.

Balkin JM. In: Balkin JM, ed. *What Roe v. Wade Should Have Said: The Nation's Top Legal Experts Rewrite America's Most Controversial Decision*. New York: New York University Press, 1995 (opinion of the court); pp. 31–62.

Davis v. Davis, 842 S.W.2d 588, Tenn., 1992.

de Marneffe D. *Maternal Desire: On Childhood, Love and the Inner Life*. Boston, MA: Back Bay Books, 2004.

Eisenstadt v. Baird. 405 U.S. 438, 1972.

Ferguson PM. Mapping the family: disability studies and the parental response to disability. In: Albrecht GL, Seelman KD, Bury M, eds. *Handbook of Disability Studies*. Thousand Oaks, CA: Sage Publications, 2001; pp. 373–395.

Gillon R. Is there a 'new ethics of abortion'? *J Med Ethics* 2001; **27**: ii5–ii9.

Ginsburg RB. Some thoughts on autonomy and equality in relation to *Roe v. Wade. Univ North Carolina Law Rev* 1985; **63**(2): 375–386. (Reprinted in Pojman LP, Beckwith FJ, eds. *The Abortion Controversy: A Reader*. Boston, MA: Jones and Bartlett Publishers, 1994; pp. 119–28).

Glover J. *Choosing Children: The Ethical Dilemmas of Genetic Intervention*. New York: Oxford University Press, 2006.

Griswold v. Connecticut. 381 U.S. 479, 1965.

Harris J. One principle and three fallacies of disability studies. *J Med Ethics* 2001; **27**: 383–387.

Hoffmann LW, Hoffmann ML. The value of children to parents. In: Fawcett JT, ed. *Psychological Perspectives on Population*, New York: Basic Books, 1973; pp. 19–76.

Holmes HB. Choosing children's sex: challenges to feminist ethics. In: Callahan J, ed. *Reproduction, Ethics, and the Law: Feminist Perspective*. University of Indiana Press: Indianapolis, 1995; pp. 148–177.

Hubin DC. Daddy dilemmas: untangling the puzzles of paternity. *Cornell J Law Public Policy* 2003; **13**: 29–80.

J.B. v. M.B., 783 A.2d 707, NJ, 2001.

Jackson E. Abortion, autonomy and prenatal diagnosis. *Social Legal Stud* 2000; **9**(4): 467–494.

Karst KL. The freedom of intimate association. *Yale Law J* 1980; **89**: 624–692.

Lawrence v. Texas. 539 U.S. 558, 2003.

Mackenzie C. Abortion and embodiment. *Austr J Philos* 1992; **70**(2): 136–155.

McDonagh EL. *Breaking the Abortion Deadlock: From Choice to Consent*. New York: Oxford University Press, 1996.

McFall v. Shimp. 10 Pa.D. & C. 3d 90, 1978.

Nelson HL, Nelson JL. Cutting motherhood in two: Some suspicions concerning surrogacy. *Hypatia* 1989; **4**(3): 85–94.

Newell CJ. The social nature of disability, disease and genetics: a response to Gillam, Persson, Holtug, Draper and Chadwick. *Journal of Medical Ethics* 1999; **25**(2): 172–175.

Pachman TS. Disputes over frozen preembryos and the 'right not to be a parent'. *Columb J Gender Law* 2003; **12**: 128–153.

Parens E, Chapman A, Press N, eds. *Wrestling with Behavioral Genetics: Science, Ethics, and Public Conversation*. Baltimore, MD: Johns Hopkins University Press, 2006.

Rao R. Property, privacy, and the human body. *Boston Univer Law Rev* 2000; **80**: 359–460.

Roe v. Wade. 410 U.S. 113, 1973.

Ruddick W. Ways to limit prenatal testing. In: Parens E, Asch A, eds. *Prenatal Testing and Disability Rights*. Washington, DC: Georgetown University Press, 2000; pp. 95–108.

Sandel MJ. The case against perfection: what's wrong with designer children, bionic athletes, and genetic engineering. *Atlant Month* 2004; **293**(3): 50–62.

Schloendorff v. Society of New York Hospital. 211 NY. 125, 105 N.E. 92, 1915.

Siegel RB. In: Balkin JM, ed. *What Roe v. Wade Should Have Said: The Nation's Top Legal Experts Rewrite America's Most Controversial Decision*. New York: New York University Press, 1995 (concurring); pp. 63–85.

Skinner v. Oklahoma ex rel. Williamson. 316 U.S. 535, 1942.

Solinger R. *Wake up Little Susie: Single Pregnancy and Race Before Roe v. Wade*. New York: Routledge, 1992.

Thomson JJ. A defense of abortion. *Philos Public Affairs* 1971; **1**(1), 47–66.

Tribe LH. *Abortion: The Clash of Absolutes*. New York: Norton, 1990.

Wertz DC, Fletcher JC. Sex selection through prenatal diagnosis. In: Holmes HB, Purdy LM, eds. *Feminist Perspectives in Medical Ethics*. Bloomington, IN: Indiana University Press, 1992; pp. 240–253.

West R. In: Balkin JM, ed. *What Roe v. Wade Should Have Said: The Nation's Top Legal Experts Rewrite America's Most Controversial Decision*. New York: New York University Press, 1995 (concurring in the judgment); pp. 121–147.

54

Maternal–Foetal Conflict

ROSAMUND SCOTT

INTRODUCTION

The term 'maternal–foetal conflict' is troubling. When pregnant, a woman typically worries hugely about the impact of her choices and actions on the foetus she carries and the child it will become. Pregnant women are generally renowned for accepting considerable burdens and facing significant risks for the sake of their unborn child. Sometimes, however, the needs of the foetus may conflict with the wishes of the woman who has, in fact, chosen to carry it to term. For instance, she may have a difficulty of some kind about accepting a caesarean section recommended for her foetus, herself or both. The difficulty may be of a religious nature (*Re S*, 1992); or a previous experience of a caesarean may have seriously traumatized her (*Rochdale*, 1997); or she may be very ill, even terminally so, so that a caesarean may compromise her health (*Re A.C.*, 1990). Alternatively, some aspect of a pregnant woman's daily life may negatively affect the foetus, such as the way she drives her car (*Dobson v Dobson*, 1999). These may be instances of maternal–foetal conflict.

The most obvious case of maternal–foetal conflict arises when a woman wishes to terminate a pregnancy. Although some of the arguments relevant to this discussion originate in the abortion debate, this chapter is not about abortion. Instead, the focus is on a woman who, whether or not originally voluntarily pregnant, has decided to continue with a pregnancy. At first glance, this seems to simplify the analysis of a pregnant woman's moral obligations. However, unless we say that in accepting a pregnancy, a woman undertakes to have any treatment apparently needed by the foetus or refrain from doing anything which may negatively impact on it, regardless of the importance of what may be at stake for her – and it is worth considering whether we *should* say this – the moral picture may be even more complex than that inherent in the issue of abortion.

Should moral analysis of the maternal–foetal relationship begin with the foetus or the woman? At one level, either of the starting points is problematic because we are concerned with the maternal–foetal *relationship* and instances where this results in conflict. Some analyses, often associated with the abortion debate, start and effectively finish with either one of these (Finnis, 1973). Others go further and, more satisfactorily, relate the claims of the foetus to the interests of the pregnant woman (Feinberg, 1979; Dworkin, 1993); I shall start with the foetus and, while still considering the foetus, move to explore the situation and interests of the pregnant woman. But is it necessarily the foetus that we are concerned with?

Indeed, although sometimes a woman's choice or action may risk the death of the foetus, at other times it may risk harm to the 'future child'. In yet other cases, either of these outcomes could occur: the result of the refusal of a caesarean could be that the foetus is fine, that it dies or that it is born as a child who has been harmed. Does the possibility of a damaged child mean that the term 'maternal–*foetal* conflict' is a misnomer and the conflict is sometimes the one between a pregnant woman and a future child? John Robertson has criticized the use of the term 'foetus', arguing that it is only where the foetus is at risk of death that the term is apt. In other cases, where harm rather than death is at issue, the real focus should be on the future child the foetus will become (Robertson, 1994). He thinks the term 'foetus' confuses and biases the issue in favour of the woman because the future child is a moral person with interests and rights and therefore has a much stronger moral (and legal) status than that, particularly, of a relatively early foetus.

It is appropriate to draw attention to the ultimate 'identity', if you like, of the future child the foetus will become. However, if we focus on the future child in the sense of the 'subsequently born child', we lose sight of the fact that, for the purposes of the current discussion, we are in fact concerned

Principles of Health Care Ethics, Second Edition   Edited by R.E. Ashcroft, A. Dawson, H. Draper and J.R. McMillan
© 2007 John Wiley & Sons, Ltd

with choices made or actions taken when that child is still *in utero*. Indeed, there is another sense of future child, namely the 'child who will be but is not yet born'. The benefit of this sense is that it forces us to confront the real difficulty, which is to determine the *weight* of its moral claims compared with those of the woman in whose body it resides: at the moment of the conflict, the future child is not yet born. Within the treatment context, when harm to the future child could result from the refusal, say, of a caesarean, the degree to which that surgery impinges on her body is a significant consideration. By contrast, and importantly, the physical situation of the future child may well be less relevant beyond the treatment context, where a woman's actions do not implicate her moral interest, particularly in bodily integrity, such as the manner in which she drives her car or crosses a road. In these cases, to some degree her moral relationship with the future child may be more akin to the relationship between a third party and a foetus inside a pregnant woman, which he may harm by his conduct.

Because the future child as I have defined it is the one who will be but is not yet born, we need to consider the moral claims of the foetus. In any event, these are also at issue in the case of foetal death.

THE MORAL CLAIMS OF THE FOETUS

The foetus is human. Does this give it full moral status? On the human species argument, at conception the human genetic code attaches to the new being, and '[a] being with a human genetic code is man' (Noonan, 1970). This sounds somewhat tautologous, but the point is to attribute to the zygote, embryo or foetus the full moral status and so full rights of a born human being. So the morally relevant quality must be humanity itself; or, put another way, the criterion of moral status *is* humanity. A problem, however, is that this immediately rules out the claims of other beings, such as the higher apes, to serious moral concern.

Perhaps being a person gives moral status. On this argument, the moral community consists of all and only persons (Warren, 1973). The criteria of descriptive personhood are primarily consciousness, rationality and agency, and also the ability to communicate and self-consciousness. Possession of only some of these criteria may be sufficient for personhood, and it may not be necessary to possess any one criterion, but because a being with *none* of these characteristics is not a person, a pre-sentient foetus (who thereby lacks even consciousness) is not a person. A post-sentient foetus still lacks most of these characteristics, so it is not a person either. Further, because only persons have rights, foetuses have none. The personhood argument shifts the moral frame of reference from humanity to personhood, but why should this be a constructive move? What is the

normative significance of personhood? Warren considers it would be as absurd to grant full moral rights to a being which is not a person as it would be to consider that such a being has 'moral obligations and responsibilities'. So the implied link may be the idea of moral agency.

The personhood argument is a serious one, particularly because it may let beings which are not human into our range of moral focus, but it has notable weaknesses. As regards the foetus, the argument has no space for the fact that the foetus, unlike a fish, is on the way to becoming a person. Nor does it have anything to say about a foetus's place inside a pregnant woman. The narrow and rather technical nature of the argument is revealed by its implications for infanticide: because very small infants lack most of the characteristics of descriptive personhood, they are not persons and so have no rights. To tidy up a conclusion which is unfortunate when viewed from a wider moral perspective, the personhood approach must look elsewhere, to consequentialist arguments about the effects of destroying unwanted children. Similarly, the answer that the foetus has no moral claims because it is not a person and therefore lacks rights is ultimately unsatisfactory.

Although it does not have rights, perhaps the foetus has interests of some kind, of which we should take account. To have an interest is to have a stake in something and conscious awareness is a 'prerequisite' for the possession of interests (Feinberg, 1984a). If consciousness is sufficient for the possession of interests and hence minimal moral status, then a sentient foetus is such a being (Steinbock, 1992). There are two senses of 'interest': first, those things which promote the good of a being are *in* its interests; second, there are those things one seeks, in which one *takes* an interest. A sentient foetus cannot *take* an interest in its welfare, but arguably it has an interest in its welfare because it may feel both pleasure and pain. Scientific work on foetal pain gives weight to this view (Glover and Fisk, 1999). However, although helpful in relation to the sentient foetus, the interest approach has no way of granting any moral claims to the pre-sentient foetus. Does the latter have none?

An argument which gives space to the potential of beings may be helpful here. On the argument from potential, because a zygote is potentially a fully-fledged human being, so it has full human rights (Finnis, 1973). The classic objection is that it is illogical to deduce actual rights from potential qualification for those rights (Benn, 1973). The response is that the argument stands for the normative proposition that those who are potential persons *ought* to have the same rights as actual persons, which requires justification but does not itself depend on a logical mistake (Steinbock, 1992). However, many people, particularly if not religious, find it difficult to accept that the zygote has the same moral status as a born person. Further, we have returned to the language of rights. If we then bring the pregnant woman into focus, we may find we have two sets of at least *prima facie* rights in direct conflict with one another, unless we think she has none.

Significantly, the moral frame of reference of the argument from potential can be shifted away from the constraints of the language of rights (Feinberg, 1979). On this approach, we can say that the fact that the foetus is potentially a person could be a basis, not for ascribing rights to it, but for owing it certain duties, the kind which do not have to correlate with rights. This is worth further thought.

It is trite to say that the foetus is developing, but one way to think about its moral claims is to focus on this aspect. An embryo of 8 weeks is less developed than a foetus of 16 weeks. We can say that it has 'invested' less in life (Dworkin, 1993) or that it has less of a 'claim' (Feinberg, 1979). Both Ronald Dworkin and Joel Feinberg have argued, in different ways, for gradualist approaches to the moral claims of the foetus, as has Ian Kennedy (Kennedy, 1991). On a gradualist approach, the longer a pregnancy has been allowed to develop, the greater must be the justification on the woman's part for in any way compromising it. Another way of expressing this is to say that the strength of the moral duties owed in pregnancy become progressively stronger. If one does not think that the foetus has full moral status from the moment of conception (as a zygote) or that only personhood and rights are prerequisites to moral consideration, morally and intuitively a gradualist approach has much to commend it.

My own view is that the foetus's moral status increases gradually throughout pregnancy and that there is also an increase in the strength of its moral claims with the acquisition of interests at sentience, but that it never acquires rights. Roughly speaking, the development of sentience may coincide with the point of viability. An attractive feature of this gradualist approach is that it allows for an interplay of maternal and foetal interests: by definition it looks both to the foetus and to the pregnant woman who carries it. This is highly appropriate to the maternal–foetal relationship. Because it is not concerned with whether the foetus has rights but instead with the duties that may be owed it, it has a moral sensitivity to the developmental and physically dependent story which is the foetus's journey into the world; and because it acknowledges the possibility that a woman's serious reason may justify compromising the foetus's position, it recognizes the physical, emotional and other burdens of pregnancy for her. This approach can be refined to apply to the future child who may in due course be born with damage suffered *in utero*: in this case, a woman's reasons for refusing treatment must relate particularly to her body (which will likely be the case especially where invasive treatment is in issue), given that the most important distinguishing feature between a born child and a future child is that the latter is *in utero* until birth. Of course, a gradualist approach will not

be helpful if one thinks a woman's duties in pregnancy must be absolute, because the claims (or rights) of the foetus are similarly absolute.

Shortly, I turn to consider the maternal–foetal relationship directly from the woman's viewpoint. What we can already see is that a gradualist approach looks to her reasons for possibly compromising the foetus's position, for instance through the refusal of certain medical treatment, so that where she has serious reasons these may displace her *prima facie* duties to the foetus (Kennedy, 1991). In this way, the approach requires that we think closely about what is asked of her and what her response might be. In line with this, the approach can be developed to take on board the key moral interests which may be implicated for her in pregnancy, particularly when medical treatment or surgery is apparently needed by the foetus, namely her interests in bodily integrity and self-determination (in essence, in making important choices) (Scott, 2002). These interests also underpin her moral right to refuse medical treatment for herself when not pregnant.

When we are considering whether she also has the right to refuse medical treatment when pregnant, when it seems reasonable to suppose that what was an absolute right becomes a *prima facie* right, we need to think about whether her reasons for refusal are serious. Here, it is helpful to consider whether her reasons have a sufficiently strong connection with the moral interests which underlie her *prima facie* right. Where they do, we might say that she retains her right to refuse medical treatment despite the harm to the foetus. Here, there is a 'coincidence' between the serious reason and the right. But where her reasons have no real connection with the interests underpinning her right to refuse treatment, we might say that her *prima facie* right 'gives way' to a duty to the foetus to accept the treatment it apparently needs. Further, if she does still 'claim' that right by exercising it, we could say that she does so *unjustifiably*.

For example, consider the purely hypothetical case of a woman who refuses to swallow a pill which would significantly benefit the foetus/future child. In fact, foetal arrhythmias and vitamin deficiencies can be treated in this way (Ouellette, 1994). Most unlike major surgery, a pill impinges on the body very minimally, in that it simply has to be swallowed. Further, and importantly, if we assume that the pill has no possible adverse effects on the woman, then it will be very hard to think of a reason, let alone a serious one, why she should refuse it. The implication is that she would clearly have a moral duty to take it. We can see, then, that the link between the serious reason and the right can be broken, so that a right can be 'claimed' and, in effect, exercised without good reason. In effect, to refuse the beneficial pill seems an entirely arbitrary choice. Indeed, this analysis implicitly rejects the Choice theory of rights (Hart, 1955) in favour of a hybrid approach which combines the ideas of interest and autonomy as discussed generally by Jeremy Waldron (1984).

On my account so far, a gradualist approach to the maternal–foetal relationship can be related to ideas both about a woman's rights and the moral interests underpinning these, and her duties in pregnancy. More importantly, the approach opens up scope for reflection on the moral quality of her decision to exercise her *prima facie* rights on any given occasion. Where her reasons for refusing treatment are sufficiently strong and thereby seriously implicate her interests in self-determination or bodily integrity or both, she may be justified in doing so; where they are not, in effect she has the duty to accept the treatment. In practice, however, how can we say whether or not her reasons are sufficiently strong?

THE MORAL INTERESTS OF THE PREGNANT WOMAN

We need to explore further the link between a woman's reasons for refusing treatment and her interests in self-determination and bodily integrity. Because we are effectively concerned with when a *prima facie* right 'gives way' to a duty and when it does not, we also need to look at the problem in terms of a woman's rights and duties. I will use a woman's interest in self-determination to explore the extent of her *prima facie* rights and her interest in bodily integrity to explore the extent of her *prima facie* duties by considering the idea of a duty which might be owed through the body.

SELF-DETERMINATION – EXPLORING THE EXTENT OF A PREGNANT WOMAN'S RIGHTS

If we were concerned with harm to the foetus occurring in the course of a woman's general daily conduct, such as the way she crosses the street or drives her car, we would not have to consider her interest in self-determination to decide whether she has a duty, in those activities, to avoid harm to the foetus. Such activities do not seriously invoke her interest in making important personal choices. We can easily say, therefore, that she has a duty to do these things carefully because this would only be reasonable. But where a woman refuses a caesarean section, for instance for religious reasons, we have in part to look at the nature and strength of her interest in self-determination.

We must now address the question of how to determine the seriousness or strength of a woman's reasons for refusing treatment where those are not trivial, given that we do not share her religious beliefs and that it is her body, not ours, which will be the subject of surgery. Can the belief of a

Born Again Christian that it would be a serious sin to accept surgery be so important as to justify foetal death or harm to the future child? (In fact, this person believes surgery is unnecessary.)

The problem raised here is how to take account, in our moral reasoning, of the reasons of others. One obvious way we do this is by according rights. By granting people the right to refuse medical treatment, for instance, we are partly saying that we recognize the individual's interest in making deeply personal choices which affect his or her body. Yet where we are contemplating whether a *prima facie* right should not 'give way' to a duty – whether the pregnant woman's interest in self-determination which underlies (in part) her right to refuse a caesarean should not give way to the foetus – we have to go 'behind' the right and think about her reasons for refusing the surgery.

When we do this we realize that a religious faith amounts, in some sense, to an internal system (rational or otherwise) which makes it hard to criticize from outside. This means that we cannot both step inside the religious belief and retain the external perspective from which we need to weigh the belief against the interests of the foetus. Instead, we must reflect on the significance of the belief for the pregnant woman and so the place of religion in her life. One way to understand religion in this context is as a 'construct which gives meaning to people's lives' (Savulescu, 1994). By recognizing the important role religion plays in a woman's deliberations about how to live, we can accord significant weight to the question of religion in moral argument without ourselves being religious or sharing the same religious faith. It follows that unless we are to disrupt the place of religion in her life, we must accept the seriousness of her religious beliefs. So, by means of a sincerely held religious faith which partly consists in beliefs about the body, she justifiably asserts the right to refuse the surgery or, put another way, does not have the moral duty to submit to it. If we do not respect her reasons (as we would not in the case of a parent refusing treatment for religious reasons for a separate born child), we contemplate operating on her without her consent, which is highly morally problematic. In effect, the strength of her religious reasons in the treatment context can best be seen in their relationship to her body. In turn, this brings the significance of the body and a woman's interest in bodily integrity firmly into view.

BODILY INTEGRITY – EXPLORING THE EXTENT OF A PREGNANT WOMAN'S DUTIES

I now turn to a pregnant woman's interest in bodily integrity to explore the idea of a duty which might be owed through the body. Judith Jarvis Thomson first approached the maternal–foetal relationship in this way, focusing on the issue of abortion and asking whether a woman has a duty to be a 'Good Samaritan' to the foetus (Thomson, 1971). I am concerned with the idea of duties to avoid physical harm or death to others and whether such a duty can be owed to the foetus through a woman's body, such that she has a duty to accept medical (including surgical) treatment for it.

Strikingly, unintentional or negligent physical harm to others typically occurs in the course of general day-to-day conduct and is a breach of an individual's *negative* duty not to harm others. By contrast, a pregnant woman's duty to accept treatment for the foetus (to avert physical harm to it) would be a duty *positively* to assist it. The significance of this is that it is generally easier to determine the reasonableness of negative duties not to cause physical harm to others than of positive duties to aid them. This means it is easier to determine when a negative duty not to harm another exists and when it has been breached, such as when a cyclist accidentally knocks a child into a river. By contrast, when we consider whether someone has a positive duty to rescue that child, particularly where the river is fast-flowing and he cannot swim, we see that questions about the abilities and nature – physical or psychological – of the would-be rescuer become relevant, eventually to the extent that we may question whether a duty to rescue actually lies.

This is acutely accentuated when we move beyond the idea of a rescue in the sphere of 'general conduct', which may at most carry physical risks (the swimming case) to the idea of rescuing others quite literally through one's body, as in the case of a relative who 'rescues' another relative by the donation of a bodily organ or tissue, or the pregnant woman who 'rescues' the foetus by means of the caesarean. In other words, the determination of reasonableness – and hence, crucially, of the existence and extent of the duty – becomes more complex and uncertain in the latter scenarios. Given the intensely personal and physical nature of such rescues, it will be very understandable (in one sense, one might even say rational) that someone may have intense concerns about such a rescue. In the case of the pregnant woman, for instance, previous experience of a caesarean may have seriously traumatized her. Ultimately, this reveals the limitations of attempts to analyse a pregnant woman's duties to the foetus in terms of Good Samaritan arguments because these typically concern duties in the course of daily conduct. Similarly, the idea of a pregnant woman's duty to accept a caesarean for her foetus's sake is wrongly characterized as an instance of an 'ordinary neighbourly duty' to help another person, as John Finnis would likely describe it (Finnis, 1973), because by definition such duties do not involve extraordinary bodily invasions.

Nevertheless, the women who are typically the subject of the maternal–foetal conflict cases are essentially voluntarily pregnant or at least did not abort (though the availability of abortion should not be assumed), and therefore intended to carry their foetuses to term. So it might be said that they necessarily took on certain particular or special responsibilities towards their foetuses/future children. How can this not include the duty to submit to a caesarean the moment before the birth? This objection relies on the idea that assumed responsibilities give rise to stringent positive duties. Feinberg has argued that where certain individuals, such as firemen, have accepted special duties to assist others and thereby run exceptionally high – what passers-by would regard as unreasonably high – risks for others, then the (positive) duties of passers by are reduced (Feinberg 1984b). He argues that voluntarily pregnant women are analogous to firemen. Pregnant women are, in fact, the only people able to help foetuses directly. This means that there is no question of chaos or confusion arising about who should be doing the rescuing which might arise (as Feinberg's argument implies) were we not to appoint firemen. Does pregnant women's peculiarly essential role heighten the degree of positive duty to which they are subject?

THE 'SOCIAL CONTEXT OF PREGNANCY'

At this point, I think we must attend to what I shall call the 'social context' of pregnancy. A woman who undertakes a pregnancy is not simply analogous to a fireman with special and stringent positive duties to aid others. Beginning a pregnancy is not just the assumption of a social role with concomitant social duties, but rather is a choice to reproduce – to create – another human being. Individuals such as firemen who undertake strict positive duties to aid others can choose other ways of helping others (although those roles will then need to be filled by others who do not have qualms about the burdens or risks involved). But pregnant women (and their partners) cannot choose another way to have a child (subject to irrelevant exceptions). Given the acute personal importance to the woman (and partner) of reproduction, it is unfair and unjust to say that either a pregnant woman must accept any treatment required by the foetus, in particular the seriously invasive and potentially religiously problematic caesarean section, or not reproduce. The possible objection that such a woman should adopt, rather than reproduce, is highly unsympathetic to the reality of a woman's (or a couple's) emotional involvement in reproduction. Hence, rather than insisting that voluntarily pregnant women owe a duty to the foetus entailing large sacrifices (and that women should not become pregnant unless they are prepared to make such sacrifices), biological facts at the heart of our social life may here lessen, rather than intensify, the positive duties to promote foetal welfare imposed upon pregnant women in this regard, so that these are indeed less stringent than the negative ones.

Curiously, the extraordinary nature of the invasiveness of surgery to benefit the foetus such as a caesarean – by comparison with the way we typically avoid physical harm to others – is belied by the very ordinary, indeed fundamental nature of pregnancy in human life. It is this ordinariness which may incline some (Finnis, 1973) to consider that the incidents and burdens of pregnancy must surely be accepted 'as a matter of course', to use a phrase from the US Supreme Court abortion decision of *Planned Parenthood of Southeastern Pennsylvania v Casey* (1992), in which this view was criticized, effectively giving legal expression to my 'social context' argument.

Moving briefly beyond the treatment context, the difficulties of determining the reasonableness of a duty not to harm the foetus by accepting medical treatment for it are not present when we turn to consider possible instances of maternal conduct which may, particularly, harm the future child, such as smoking, alcohol consumption (which is more than minimal) or solvent abuse. In the light of the severe harm to the future child which may result from these activities on the one hand and the lack of value to the pregnant woman in engaging in such conduct on the other, the judgement can here be made that a pregnant woman is breaching a negative moral duty she owes to her future child. Social problems of addiction, however, may cloud the duty issue in relation to maternal use of drugs, smoking and alcohol. Further, beyond such obviously harmful activities as smoking or solvent abuse, we would at some point encounter difficulties in determining the extent of a woman's moral duties, particularly in relation to activities of value to the pregnant woman, such as those relating to her work, family or other important commitments. Unfortunately, there is even medical evidence that maternal stress affects the foetus to some degree (Teixeira, Fisk and Glover, 1999). As the Supreme Court of Illinois recognized in the case of *Stallman v Youngquist* (1988), unlike the detached third party whose conduct may harm the foetus, it is a pregnant woman's 'every waking and sleeping moment which, for better or worse, shapes the prenatal environment which forms the world for the developing fetus'. Further, this is not a 'pregnant woman's fault' but 'a fact of life'. Again, this gives (legal) expression to my 'social context' argument.

CONCLUDING THOUGHTS

I have briefly discussed some of my ideas developed elsewhere (Scott, 2002), concentrating on the medical treatment context. I have suggested that a pregnant woman cannot fairly be said to have the duty, in becoming pregnant, to make extraordinary sacrifices on the foetus's behalf. This is not to say that she does not have a duty to 'do all she can'. This much is only reasonable. Yet doing all she can will involve doing all those things which she does not have serious reason to refuse to do (including serious doubts grounding

such reasons). In other words, to say that she must 'do all she can' is at the same time to allow for the constraints of her religious faith or her concerns and fears in relation, for instance, to invasive surgery.

The unique sense in which, physically at least, a pregnancy is something which, in a very real sense, 'happens' to a pregnant woman, coupled with the fact that the reproduction of the species is always a task falling principally upon women, suggests that justice is broadly served by recognizing how important it is for women to have as much control as possible over medical treatment issues in this process. In the unlikely event that a woman lacks serious reasons for her treatment choice, there should be a place for discussion and, very rarely, persuasion in relation to treatment decisions. In such a case, her *prima facie* moral right has 'given way' to the claims of the fetus, and she would unjustifiably claim and exercise a moral and legal right to refuse the treatment. However, compelled – especially surgical – treatment is unwise for a range of moral, legal and policy reasons. It is therefore appropriate that English law and the law of some US states protect her right to refuse treatment such as a caesarean (*Re M.B.*, 1997; *Baby Boy Doe*, 1994). Ultimately, society's interests lie in recognizing a pregnant woman's moral and legal right responsibly to decide treatment issues herself. This approach values pregnant women and, overall, will be in the best interests of unborn children.

REFERENCES

Baby Boy Doe. 632 N.E.2d 326. Ill. App. 1 Dist., 1994.

Benn S. Abortion, infanticide and respect for persons. In: Feinberg J, ed. *The Problem of Abortion.* Belmont, CA: Wadsworth, 1973; pp. 135–144.

Dobson v Dobson. 2 Can. S.C.R. 753, 1999

Dworkin R. *Life's Dominion: An Argument about Abortion and Euthanasia.* London: Harper Collins, 1993.

Feinberg J. Abortion (1979). In: Feinberg J ed. *Freedom and Fulfillment.* Princeton, NJ: Princeton University Press, 1992; pp. 37–75.

Feinberg J. *Harm to Others.* New York: Oxford University Press, 1984a.

Feinberg J. The moral and legal responsibility of the Bad Samaritan (1984b). In: Feinberg J, ed. *Freedom and Fulfillment.* Princeton, NJ: Princeton University Press, 1992; pp. 175–196.

Finnis J. The rights and wrongs of abortion: a reply to Judith Thomson. *Philos Public Affairs* 1973; **2**: 117–145.

Glover V, Fisk NM. Fetal pain: Implications for research and practice. *Br J Obstet Gynaecol* 1999; **106**: 881–886.

Hart HLA. Are there any natural rights? *Philos Rev* 1955; **64**: 175–191.

Kennedy I. A woman and her unborn child. In: Kennedy I, *Treat Me Right.* Oxford: Oxford University Press, 1991; pp. 364–384.

Noonan JT Jr. An almost absolute value in history. In: Noonan JT Jr, ed. *The Morality of Abortion: Legal and Historical Perspectives*. Cambridge, MA: Harvard University Press, 1970, pp. 51–59.

Ouellette A. New medical technology: a chance to reexamine court-ordered medical procedures during pregnancy. *Albany Law Rev* 1994; **57**: 927–960.

Planned Parenthood of Southeastern Pennsylvania v Casey. 120 L.Ed. 674, 1992.

Re A.C. 573 A.2d 1235, D.C. App. 1990.

Re M.B. (Caesarean Section). 8 Med. L.R. 217, 1997.

Re S (Adult: Refusal of Treatment). 4 All E.R. 671, 1992.

Rochdale (N.H.S.) Trust v C. 1 F.C.R. 274, 1997.

Robertson J. *Children of Choice: Freedom and the New Reproductive Technologies*. Princeton, NJ: Princeton University Press, 1994.

Savulescu J. Rational desires and the limitation of life-sustaining treatment. *Bioethics* 1994; **8**: 191–222.

Scott R. *Rights, Duties and the Body: Law and Ethics of the Maternal–Fetal Conflict*. Oxford: Hart Publishing, 2002.

Stallman v Youngquist. 531 N.E.2d 355. Ill., 1988.

Steinbock B. *Life Before Birth: the Moral and Legal Status of Embryos and Fetuses*. New York: Oxford University Press, 1992.

Teixeira JMA, Fisk NM, Glover V. Association between maternal anxiety in pregnancy and increased uterine artery resistance index: cohort based study. *Br Med J* 1999; **318**: 153–157.

Thomson JJ. A defence of abortion. *Philos Public Affairs* 1971; **1**: 47–66.

Waldron J. Introduction. In: Waldron J, ed. *Theories of Rights*. Oxford: Oxford University Press, 1984.

Warren MA. On the moral and legal status of abortion. *Monist* 1973; **57**: 43–61.

55

Limits to Reproductive Liberty

THOMAS H. MURRAY

The phrase 'reproductive liberty' is a battle cry in the political and legal fight over abortion. Supporters of women's access to abortion frame the issue as a matter of women's freedom and welfare. Abortion opponents retort that the woman's desires and interests must take second place to the life of the foetus; for them, 'reproductive liberty' must seem a profoundly suspect idea.

In any event it is a simple phrase which conceals a more complex and interesting terrain. Liberty is generally understood to have two aspects: the freedom *from* and the freedom *to*. Abortion is about the freedom *from*: freedom from an unwanted pregnancy, freedom from the life-altering responsibilities of raising a child. Abortion and contraception as well are better described as means of supporting the right to non-reproductive liberty, that is, the liberty not to reproduce when one does not want to reproduce. Of course, some people would describe it differently: as access *to* abortion. But abortion is a means, not an end in itself; it is a means to terminate a pregnancy which is unwanted for whatever reason. The end which is sought is not to be pregnant, not to have this child at this time.

Conflicts over access to abortion roil the political landscape in some countries. But I will not deal further with abortion in this chapter. There is little new to be said about it for one thing; but most of all, I want to examine critically what happens when the battle cry of reproductive liberty is used to understand the freedom *to* reproduce: to have a child, whether it be any child at all, or a child with some particular qualities (Parens and Knowles, 2003). How well does it encompass and illuminate what is important about becoming a parent?

When in vitro fertilization (IVF) was first introduced, it was seen as an aid for couples who could not conceive a child through normal sexual intercourse. The typical story might look like this: couples who desperately wanted to have a child, who had been infertile for years, were now being given an opportunity to create the family they so urgently sought. There were critics of IVF from the beginning, but the critics' objections were not to the couple's ultimate goal – to become parents, to have and raise a child. Indeed, the critics of IVF then, as much as the critics of certain uses of assisted reproductive technologies (ARTs) now, tended to be strong supporters of parenthood, children and families. The disagreements were over what were seen as potential misuses of the new reproductive options, over erosions in long-held social understandings and practices these new alternatives might cause and over the creation, use and destruction of embryos. But these disagreements over means and ancillary consequences should not distract us from the deep core of moral agreement between the early advocates and users of IVF and their critics: that having children and becoming parents were a profoundly good thing. It is useful to keep that in mind as we explore the ethical complexities wrought by new ARTs and new uses for old ARTs.

At the heart of the debate over the limits of reproductive liberty lies a conundrum wrapped in a confusion. First, the confusion: the liberty to have a child, to reproduce, is not merely the flipside of the liberty to choose *not* to have a child. The great battles over reproductive liberty have been fought mainly on the grounds of the rights to contraception and access to abortion, the principal means women have to prevent or end unwanted pregnancies. Contraception and abortion are aspects of the reproductive liberty to choose not to have a child, at least not at this time, not in this manner. Some commentators want to apply precisely the same analytical framework to decisions, technologies and laws aimed at creating and raising children. But that move leaves something, or more properly someone, out: the child.

Whatever one's views about abortion and contraception, the result of the effective application of both of these is the same: no child; no child to carry through pregnancy, no child to give birth to, no child to care for, raise and prepare

Principles of Health Care Ethics, Second Edition   Edited by R.E. Ashcroft, A. Dawson, H. Draper and J.R. McMillan

for adult life. There are many good reasons to think that reproductive liberty is important, especially for women whose fate depends in many ways on whether, when and in what circumstances they have children. Having a child is a life-altering event. A child can be a long-sought blessing; but there are times when bearing and rearing a child come as great, unwanted burdens – and this can be so even when the child is loved and cared for. Life does not arrive in neatly wrapped packages of all-chosen-and-good and unwanted-and-all-bad.

Once there is a child, so much in one's life changes. From the moral point of view, the interests and well-being of the child are now entitled to the same consideration as the interests of the other members of the family. From the point of view of living one's life, accepting the responsibility of caring for a child is a profoundly significant event. I used to frequently err in describing someone as single when he or she was, in fact, married, but there was a core of truth in my mistake: marriage changes a person's legal status, to be sure, but life for a married couple without children is not all that different from life together without marriage. Having a child, though, changes everything.

Here is the conundrum: if unfettered liberty is what you seek, then the very last thing you should do is have a child – unless your idea of liberty is being awakened multiple times in the night by crying and returning to bed with spit on your shoulder. I will not even mention the terrors parents endure as their daughter or son navigates the shoals of adolescence.

So something seems askew in the effort to lump all of reproductive liberty into one big ball which emphasizes the liberty rights of reproducing – or not – adults. That may be a suitable framework for thinking about contraception. It is the framework generally adopted by supporters of access to abortion and vilified as leaving the foetus out by abortion opponents. But once a child is born, whatever one's views on abortion, there is a creature whose interests are every bit as valuable and worthy of respect as the adults who participated in bringing it into the world. A thoughtful ethical analysis of ARTs, then, must take into account the well-being of the children who will be created, who are, after all, the fundamental goal of ARTs. It is simply not enough to focus exclusively on the interests and wishes of the adults involved.

How should we evaluate a moral framework like reproductive liberty as it is applied to the creation of a child? For a good many philosophers, the theoretical framework comes first. Consequentialists such as utilitarians have an exceptionally encompassing conceptual framework (Harris, 1992). A talented utilitarian moral theorist can stuff just about every conceivable problem into the theory's great maw, chew on it a bit and spit out some sort of answer. Nevertheless, some problems seem to be more easily digested by utilitarianism than others. Utilitarians have notable

difficulty dealing with so-called special relationships. If everyone should be accorded precisely the same moral weight in the utilitarian calculus, what are we to say about our most special, intimate relationships? Should our child be counted exactly the same as our neighbour's child or a child in some distant village? There is a certain appeal to this sort of moral levelling, as a counterweight against our propensity towards ignoring the welfare of strangers, hardening our hearts towards those who are distant and different from ourselves. So, a utilitarian framework has some appeal in thinking about justice on national and international scales. But it seems particularly ill-equipped to say anything insightful about our relationships, not with *any* child or all the world's children, but with this, *our very own* child, the one who has lived with us since birth, whose illnesses have inspired fear, concern and devoted care, whose first steps were greeted with joy, whose first words named us, who is beloved to us, whose life is intertwined with ours until death. Even after our death, we will live on in our child's memories, and should our child die before us, the memory of our life with our child pervades what remains of our own lives (Murray, 2002).

My point here is not that a moral theory like utilitarianism can say nothing about the relationship of parent and child; utilitarian philosophers can and do offer their observations about ARTs and the like. Rather, my point is that utilitarianism's insistence on moral levelling can render it insensitive to the most central, intimate and important relationships in our lives, none more important than the relationship between parent and child. Perhaps it is like asking a tone-deaf person to become a music critic. This critic could describe certain aspects of the concert experience, perhaps do a sophisticated mathematical analysis of the score. But this poor critic cannot hear or describe the *music* as it soars, moves us or disturbs us. Now, I am certainly not claiming that any philosophers or legal scholars, by virtue of their theoretical commitments, are incapable of having deep and authentic relationships. That is clearly false. But I do think it worth considering the difficulty such commentators face in reconciling what they experience in those vital relationships with their preferred moral or legal theories which are ill designed to be sensitive to those relationships. And I suggest that one way of assessing the adequacy of some ethical account of a problem is to begin by asking how well it comes to grips with what is centrally important to that problem. A conceptual or theoretical framework which does not, in some deep sense, 'get' what is most important in the situation is unlikely, I believe, to offer either insightful analysis or helpful advice.

Consider another, very prominent theoretical account of the ethics of reproduction: procreative liberty as developed by its leading exponent, Robertson (1994). Procreative liberty is rooted in a legal analysis of the rights of adults to choose not to have a child through contraception or abortion, and extended to the rights of adults to use alternative means to create a child, including a child with a particular set of traits desired by the procreating adults. The theory's proponents are aware that a completely unrestrained version of procreative liberty may become impossible to defend. They acknowledge that the interests of the children created by ARTs deserve some sort of consideration. The standard they have typically employed was that the child so created should not be worse off than if it had never been born at all.

A little reflection reveals that this standard prohibits very little if it prohibits anything at all. For one thing, it requires developing and defending an account of a life worse than no life at all – for an infant or child. We are accustomed to the idea that an adult may feel, as death from some implacable disease grows near, that death may be preferable to a continuation of a life shrouded by pain, indignity and the loss of all one has cared for in life. But procreative liberty requires that we make similar judgements for infants and children, who may never have known a different sort of life than the one they now live. Attending to the voices of people with disabilities should alert us to the distinction between a life we may have preferred for ourselves without disability, and the insight and testimony of uncountable persons with disabilities who live rich and fulfilling lives and who object fiercely to any attempt to devalue them and the lives they lead (Parens and Asch, 2000).

I regret having to use the following hypothetical case, but it sharpens the point: imagine a couple that wishes to use pre-implantation genetic diagnosis (PGD). They explain that they wish to select only those embryos which have profound but not lethal genetic or chromosomal defects so that a child will be born, but with profound impairments and a shortened life expectancy. Or if this hypothetical case is not clear enough, imagine parents who ask that the developing spinal cord of their foetus be surgically damaged to ensure that the infant will be paraplegic. What possible reasons could parents have for such requests? Perhaps their marriage is endangered, and they believe that caring for a severely impaired child might become the glue which keeps them together. Perhaps they wish to make a statement about the value of persons with disability. Perhaps they have a seriously impaired child and want that child to have company. Perhaps their reasons are unfathomable. The point of the hypothetical is this: procreative liberty disallows any inquiry into or critique of the procreating adults' reasons. As long as the child is not worse off than never having been born, the principle of procreative liberty grants adults complete discretion as to what they do and why, in their pursuit of a child.

I have virtually no doubt that defenders of procreative liberty would be appalled to see their principles used to defend decisions such as the ones I have just laid out. Nor would they approve of such actions by parents or health professionals. But the test of a principle is not merely its application to cases for which we applaud the outcome; we must also explore what it permits or prohibits when applying the theory yields troubling results. The heart of procreative liberty's shortcomings is its almost complete failure to take the child into account. In practice, the standard of a life worse than non-existence is likely to be useless, devoid of clear, uncontroversial applications. I have described it as analogous to dividing by zero in arithmetic: it is an operation we can describe, but it is incapable of yielding a meaningful answer.

The theory may be a prisoner of its own birth in law and in response to cases in which autonomous adults were making decisions not to have children. When ARTs are being used to create a child, but before an embryo is created or implanted, or a foetus brought to term, why should adults give any moral consideration to the interests of this not-yet-existing child? In earlier research I explored the concept of our moral responsibilities to a not-yet-born child, by which I meant a child that will ultimately be born (Murray, 1996). This should not be confused with the rhetorical use of the notion of an 'unborn child' to refer to a foetus that has been aborted. In the cases I want to consider, the adults responsible for the creation, gestation and birth of the child intend for it to be brought to term and born alive and viable. The question is, what moral responsibilities towards this not-yet-born child do the adults who have some influence over its fate have?

The first stumbling block in assessing the usefulness of the concept of the not-yet-born child is the problem of timing: how can I have a responsibility at time 1 towards a child who does not even exist until time $(1 + n)$? What if n equals 9 months and the not-yet-born child was a newly formed embryo at the moment my decision must be taken? What if n equals one hour? And what could my moral obligations possibly be if n equalled 3 years, long before the child was even conceived?

It may be helpful to point out that the obligations to not-yet-born children can fall on people other than those directly involved in the child's procreation. Suppose that someone is the manager of a chemical plant that is secretly releasing toxic materials into a community's water supply. These chemicals do not affect children or adults, but they cause serious damage to developing embryos because they disrupt the delicate balance of endocrine hormones and result in infants born with physical abnormalities and brain dysfunction. Or perhaps they do not affect embryos but rather gametogenesis, so that men's sperm is abnormal – still capable of creating a viable embryo, but one that will result in a severely damaged infant. The plant manager argues that he should not be held responsible in any way for the damage done to these children because the harm was not to persons but to cells, to gametes; any harm therefore occurred before any embryo was formed, and besides, the plant stopped discharging these toxins years ago. Would we regard these as cogent and persuasive excuses? Or would we say to the plant manager that he knew that future children would be damaged by his actions and that he should be held responsible? If the facts of the case are sound and the chemicals damaged gametes resulting in the births of seriously affected children, and if we agree that the plant manager's arguments do not exculpate him, then we have accepted the idea that people can have moral obligations to not-yet-born children, even not-yet-conceived children. (This last point underscores the difference between the rhetoric of 'unborn children' in the abortion debate and the concept of the not-yet-born child as a helpful means for thinking about our moral responsibilities prior to the conception or birth of a child.) Timing, in the end, may figure in our analysis of the nature and extent of moral responsibility. (The effects of our actions on outcomes in the far future are typically much less certain; our ability, and therefore duty, to foresee such outcomes likewise can be attenuated by time.) But time itself does not excuse us from responsibility. A terrorist planting a bomb in a nursery school, which is intended to kill and maim a dozen children, is morally culpable for his evil actions whatever the length of the timer – 1 hour, 1 month, 1 year or 5 years – even if in this last case the children had been neither born nor conceived when the bomb was placed.

In place of the rather feckless constraint which proponents of procreative liberty suggest, when we consider the ethics of ARTs we should employ a robust standard, focused on our moral obligations to the not-yet-born children whose very existence is the point of pursuing ARTs in the first place. Using such a standard would mean that the welfare of the children so created deserves full consideration, not merely the preferences of the adults participating in that child's creation.

There is another fundamental point to be made here: purchasing reproductive services is not like purchasing a new car or a relaxing massage. The point of ARTs is not to acquire or consume something, but to create a child with whom we hope to have a life-long relationship. Now, there are people who become very attached to their cars, but short of heroic anthropomorphizing, they cannot expect their cars to love them back, to grow in wisdom and maturity, or to flourish the way people can. If someone wrecks, neglects or junks an expensive car, we may think he or she is foolish or imprudent, but we do not regard this as a terrible moral offence. If someone neglects or harms a child, on the other hand, we see this as a great moral failing and a tragedy.

Children differ from mere objects. Imagine a man who covets his neighbour's television. It is the latest model: huge, brilliant, with stunning clarity. Desires of this sort may be ultimately destructive of one's happiness in the long run. But then again it may be just a run-of-the-mill sort of covetousness, shallow perhaps, but not completely foolish. Suppose his neighbour offers to trade his marvellous new TV for his old, small one. After getting over his astonishment, the man could rejoice in his good fortune. His neighbour may be generous, manipulative or crazy – but now he can have a state-of-the-art TV set!

Suppose that instead of offering to trade TV sets, the man's neighbour offered to trade 5-year-old children. He thinks yours is more talented and attractive; you have noticed that his seems considerably brighter than yours. And let us imagine that both judgements are correct: your child is the more talented and attractive, and his is the more intelligent of the two. Economists might even describe such an exchange as Pareto-optimal, in that both men are increasing the satisfaction of their preferences. Would such a trade be morally acceptable?

I assume that most readers would not approve. For one thing, the children's interests were not mentioned at all. But suppose that the two men were equally competent parents, who provided roughly comparable levels of financial support to their families. These considerations, however, seem to miss the fundamental point: children are not fungible objects who can become the subject of voluntary exchanges in the same way we exchange items of furniture, appliances or books. The oddest thing in this hypothetical case is the complete absence of any mention of anything to do with relationships, with the histories of giving and receiving care in each family, with the love which grows between parent and child. The more likely response to a request to trade children, once it became clear that the offer was not a joke, would be astonishment and outrage. This child is *my* child, not in a sense of ownership the way I would describe my bicycle, but *my child* as the child who lives with me, whom I love, for whom I have made uncountable sacrifices, whose smile unfailingly cheers me, whose sadness penetrates my heart, whose happiness and flourishing are central to my own life. Relationships between parents and children sometimes begin with an explicit choice, sometimes not; choice, so important for much of our moral lives, fades into insignificance once we have taken on the responsibilities and joys of raising a child.

I was once asked about using PGD to have a child who was both free of a lethal genetic disease *and* also a prospective source of healthy umbilical cord stem cells and bone marrow for an afflicted older sibling. I responded that people seemed to have children for three sorts of reasons: good reasons, bad reasons and no reason at all. I added that in my experience, the last accounted for the great majority of children, although falling birth rates in many countries in Europe and elsewhere suggest that fewer children are coming into those parts of the world without at least some reason on the part of their parents.

But the reasons, or lack of them, under which children are conceived and born should matter less to an ethics of ARTs than may first appear. The fundamental purpose of having a child is not merely to produce a child, but rather to create a life-long relationship within the circle of people who will love and nurture that child. And so we should look to those relationships and the goods we seek in and through them, for moral guidance on ARTs.

One of the first things to note is the inability of the usual categories of moral motivation used by philosophers to apprehend what is most important about relationships between parents and children. Moral philosophers most often divide moral motivation into two types: selfishness and altruism. The arguments are frequently over such questions as whether altruism is possible or wise, given our fallible perceptions of others' preferences and interests. But parenthood does not fit neatly into either category. Take selfishness. We cannot and should not expect parents to surrender all their needs and desires to their child's interests. Parenthood is a complex balancing act among many factors, for example, when the child's desires or needs should take first place and when the parent may reasonably pursue his or her own interests. So a certain dose of selfishness can exist within a healthy parent–child relationship. But often parents are called upon to set aside their own preferences in order to attend to their children. This looks like altruism, but with an odd twist to our usual understanding of the concept. The twist is this: one of the great revelations of parenthood is that by being caring and loving parents who sacrifice their own comfort at times for the betterment of their child, they also further their own flourishing. Through caring for others, as in parenthood, we can become better, more mature, loving and wise people. Parenthood is also one way, though not the only way, to meet what the psychologist and psychoanalyst Erik Erikson called the challenge of generativity – learning to care for people and ideas beyond ourselves. Theory aside, the practical experience of parenthood confirms the inadequacy of the usual understandings of selfishness and altruism to describe what goes on between parents and children. When we care for our child, we also flourish – but only if we aim at our child's flourishing, not in the first place at our own interests. Erikson's term for this is *mutuality* (Erikson, 1964).

If the point of having a child is to create a vitally important type of relationship, a relationship of profound significance for the child and for the adults whose lives become intertwined with that child, then it makes sense to frame our thinking about the flipside of reproductive liberty – ARTs and the arrangements people make to create children – in terms of what makes those relationships fulfilling for both parents and children. Unconstrained wilfulness and the unconditional satisfaction of procreative whims are not likely to be to the benefit of children. It is worth contemplating whether they would serve the deeper and long-term interests of parents either. ARTs are neither inherently suspect nor utterly beyond moral scrutiny. Each application of an ART invites consideration of its impact on the people directly affected – the procreating adults and the children created – as well as its broader, long-term impact on the social institutions and practices that shape the possibilities of flourishing for both parents and children. These assessments will not be simple or easy, or without controversy. But we cannot escape them through a glib and vacuous invocation of procreative liberty without real limits.

REFERENCES

Harris J. Wonderwoman and superman: the ethics of human biotechnology. New York: Oxford University Press, 1992.

Murray TH. *The Worth of a Child.* Berkeley, CA: University of California Press, 1996.

Murray TH. What are families for? Getting to an ethics of reproductive technology. *Hastings Center Rep* 2002; **32**: 41–45.

Parens E, Adrienne A. In: Parens E, Asch A, ed. *The Disability Rights Critique of Prenatal Genetic Testing: Reflections and Recommendations.* Washington, DC: Georgetown University Press, 2000.

Parens E, Knowles LP. "Reprogenetics and public policy: Reflections and recommendations". *Hastings Center Rep* 2003; **33**(4): Special Supplement.

Robertson JA. *Children of Choice: Freedom and the New Reproductive Technologies.* Princeton, NJ: Princeton University Press, 1994.

56

Disability without Denial

TOM SORELL

Much medical treatment is aimed at restoring human states and capacities to a range that is normal for patients of a certain general type in a population. Thus, someone in their teens who is unable to walk for 60 seconds without becoming breathless might be said to need treatment because their capacities fall (well) below the relevant local threshold for tolerable physical exertion in teenagers. But someone of roughly the same age who huffs and puffs after half an hour of quick walking might not be suffering from any disorder at all. Perhaps he is not in excellent physical condition, but he is not necessarily ill either, or in need of treatment. On the contrary, he might set an attainable standard of normal functioning for the person who, before treatment, gets breathless after only a minute of walking.

On this view, functioning that falls below the lower threshold of a normal range calls for treatment, other things being equal; but functioning or states above the threshold do not necessarily call for treatment, and medical interventions merely to fine-tune or enhance functioning or states so that they exceed the threshold as far as possible may be a waste of medical resources, or a perversion of medical practice. Thus, administering performance-enhancing drugs to sports stars might be claimed to be (at best) medically unnecessary. In the same way, cosmetic surgery might be said to be medically unnecessary if it only assists an ageing beauty king or queen to satisfy a vain wish to look a little younger. Or the injection of growth hormone into someone whose adult height is predicted to be at the low end of, but not outside, the normal range, might be said to be unnecessary.

Call this a 'medical model' of cosmetic surgery or sporting performance or human growth – one that calls for treatment *only* below a certain medically defined threshold.[1] The model tells against the enormous quantities of time, energy and admiration commonly invested in stereotypical good looks on the one hand and success in sporting competition on the other. The medical model implies that there is nothing medically wrong with people who do not fit these stereotypes, and, therefore, that there is no need for some of the medical skills and resources that might be directed, and that are in fact routinely directed in the West, at helping people to fit these stereotypes. The medical model even implies that medical skills and resources that could otherwise be directed at improving functioning well *below* the threshold for normal functioning are *wrongly* used or wasted if directed at improving functioning far above it.

Some disability activists refer very critically to a 'medical model of disability'. This is an approach that defines a given disability as a medical disorder, often a genetically based disorder, or one connected with a certain sort of bodily injury. Disorders amounting to disabilities are usually characterized by functioning well below the normal range that can only exceptionally be brought up to the normal range. The medical model gives indications of treatment, if any is available, and, where the disorder is genetically based, an indication of the genetic markers that enable it to be diagnosed before birth. According to disability activists, this sort of model works quite differently from the 'medical model' outlined in the preceding paragraph. Instead of going against questionable stereotypes, the 'medical model of disability' is said to reinforce them. For example, because many impairments resist treatment, even the lower threshold for relevant normal functioning can be made to seem unattainable. This fact can seem to set people with

---

[1]Of course, there are conditions where some function *above* the normal range might also justify medical intervention, for instance an over-functioning thyroid gland or higher than normal blood pressure. I have been referring to cases where functioning above the normal range is *enhanced* functioning.

Principles of Health Care Ethics, Second Edition   Edited by R.E. Ashcroft, A. Dawson, H. Draper and J.R. McMillan
© 2007 John Wiley & Sons, Ltd

such impairments apart from, and a cut below, the medically normal. On the other hand, because capacities above the threshold for the normal range sometimes turn out to be unnecessary for an acceptable standard of work or life, the location of the medically defined threshold can itself look arbitrary, or look as if it is influenced by questionable stereotypes. Finally, because changes in social policies can, without any medical breakthrough at all, seem to people with impairments to improve their lives significantly, what is bad about impairment cannot only be to do with bodily injury, genetic abnormality, or with thresholds of functioning. This is what disability activists mean when they say that what is disabling is not the impairment itself, but the ways in which able-bodied society refuses to accommodate it.

As we shall see later on, disability activists' criticism of the medical model sometimes suffers from exaggeration. The medical model does not tell us everything about disability, admittedly, but it does not tell us nothing either. And although the medical model may lend itself to reinforcing questionable stereotypes, its implication that impairments are disorders does not by itself reinforce those stereotypes. Or so I shall argue. I shall consider cases of both mental and physical impairment, and cases where impairment is both life-long and where its onset is a considerable time after birth. The testimony of those who have experienced life-changing impairment has to be considered alongside the testimony of those who have experienced life-long impairment. When it is, the idea that serious impairment is always a disaster can be questioned, but so, too, can the claim on the part of some disability activists that impairment is never something that makes people objectively worse off, only different. This claim can sound as if it is made by people in denial. As will emerge, the claim that those with impairments are only 'differently abled' is helped along by a questionable philosophy of science, just as the belief that those with impairments should be socially and economically sidelined is helped along by paternalism, prejudice or both.

DOES IMPAIRMENT LEAVE PEOPLE WORSE OFF?

An interesting source of testimony about the effects of at least one impairment comes from an edition in December 2005 of the BBC radio programme *In Touch*. *In Touch* deals with the whole range of issues raised by disability. The presenter, Peter White, who has been blind from birth, interviewed a retired academic, John Hull, whose book about losing his sight (Hull, 1991) impressed White for its power of teaching even him something about blindness. In the interview, Hull looks back on nearly two decades of being blind. His wife also reflects on the difference that her

husband's blindness made to their marriage, to the routine tasks of running a household, and to the experience of bringing up children.

The testimony is striking for more than its effect on Peter White. For one thing, it is not influenced at all by a medical model of disability. For another, it is provided by people who have experience of being sighted and of being blind, or having a partner who has been both sighted and blind. The effects of the blindness on others who might not have been fully prepared for it are addressed. Finally, although it is clearly the testimony of people who have coped quite successfully with blindness and who are looking back on a long period after its onset, the testimony treats blindness as a significant misfortune, all things considered.

An exchange from the beginning of the programme (BBC, 2005) introduces the issue in relation to how it was for John Hull at the time his blindness came on:

> WHITE: I suppose the point is, John, it does become an issue, though doesn't it, because there is inevitably in any relationship, however self-sufficient the blind person is, there is an element of reliance, and of course if you're newly blind, that's all the more so. I mean how much did you feel you had to rely on Marilyn in those early days?

> JOHN HULL: Oh well, of course the actual onset of blindness was crushing, really, it was just a total change of life. I was swept away, wasn't I sweetheart?

> MARILYN HULL: Well yeah, I mean of course you had access to your notes at the beginning of the summer and when you went back you couldn't see them. So as you were a lecturer it was a bit difficult, really. But I suppose one thing, Peter, was it was such a strange time coincidence because I was expecting our first baby. So you know, I mean it literally coincided. And so I think my attention was strangely diverted, well obviously diverted...

> WHITE: I just wonder, Marilyn, just going back to this question of how sanguine you were about it, I mean yes I can understand why the birth of a first child would divert you slightly. Do you think youth also may have had something to do with it?

> MARILYN HULL: Yes certainly, obviously, I think it did, I can't imagine what it would be like to lose your sight much later in life, as many people do, and the impact that would have on a partner then who perhaps was old themselves. I think that must be a colossal challenge. I'm not saying it wasn't a colossal challenge for us, I mean it's a huge loss, and of course I was devastated. I mean, who wants to become invisible?

> WHITE: And that's a recurring theme in John's writing, his awareness that if he can't see you, that makes you, feel invisible to him. And you did feel like that did you?

> MARILYN HULL: Yes, I mean who wants to lose the person they love, who wants to lose eye contact, eye contact – I mean that's just a whole chapter isn't it about how I felt then, I feel

it now, that never goes away: you've lost a whole register of relationship.

JOHN HULL: Indeed, I remember, people often used to talk to me about this, of course, and people assume the problems were in the university, but the problems in the university were soluble. Where you encountered the absolutely utter irretrievable face of loss was at home because of eye contact, both with Marilyn and with the children, your children's faces. I mean it goes, that's all, you can't do anything about it, you can't.

MARILYN HULL: Yes, I mean the awareness – my awareness of John not being able to see our new baby, well you had a sort of outline of his shape didn't you, but in all intents and purposes you couldn't get an impression of what he was really like. And then, of course, we went on to have three more children, so I mean basically anybody walking into our house today can know one of my children...and somebody who is sighted can know Tom or any of the others in a way that John – in one way that John never has and never can. And that's in just a moment and that is, of course, if you think about it, still painful.

Both John and Marilyn Hull speak here unequivocally about great loss, loss that has not been compensated for. A 'whole register' of marital and family communication is lost when eye contact is lost. Not being able to see one's notes as a lecturer was a setback, but it was relatively easily overcome.

Peter White comments on how the Hulls' point about eye-contact chimed in with something in his own experience:

WHITE: It's interesting, in some ways, you see, you still continue to show me in a way how insensitive people who are born blind are about this, because I can remember a girlfriend of mine . . . saying to me how difficult it was not to be able to make that eye contact and she said at a party or in a crowded room not to be able to look across, she could see me but I couldn't see her. And it has never occurred to me because . . . I know that if I'm at a party and I want to do that reassuring thing that people who go to parties together do, like, aren't these people awful, or how the hell do we get out of here, I know I've got to go and look for her. But of course what sighted people do is, they look at each other. I've discussed lots of issues like this with Jo, my wife, but never the idea that it might make her feel invisible. I suppose I'm curious to know whether the fact that I couldn't see her when I met her . . . makes a difference.

White does not say that, because he was born blind, the loss of eye contact makes no difference. He agrees that not having it is a dimension of loss in a relationship with a sighted partner.

John Hull goes on in this interview to speak of further factors that both aggravated and partly eased the loss, and of the deep depression he went through that was only broken by writing about his blindness. He came to think that

blindness is an intact world of its own with its own characteristics. And at the time when we began to realize that,

it was very profoundly difficult. I don't think it was a crisis of love but it was a crisis of worlds because we felt that we were being washed away on to opposite shores with a great dark river flowing between us (BBC, 2005)

Among the factors that aggravated John Hull's feeling of separation was a sense that the normal burdens of running the household and raising the children fell disproportionately on his wife. Another was a sense that he had broken faith with Marilyn's family, who did not think, when she was entering into the marriage, that it would be to a blind man. John Hull thought things would have been worse if he had been a blind man without money. He was able to keep his job as a lecturer and to retain a good income, though many other blind people were unable to remain economically self-sufficient. Marilyn Hull thought that her husband's blindness would have been more difficult to cope with if it had come on when they were not young and robust.

Evidence of a different kind for the claim that impairment is a misfortune comes from someone who is autistic, and who is a disability activist. Wendy Lawson[2] is a campaigner in Australia for a non-medicalized understanding of autism. In an interview for a BBC series on psychology and psychiatry (BBC, 2005), she admits that autism is a 'developmental disorder, if you like' in which people develop more slowly than normal, but not to the exclusion of high-level cognitive capacities, as in her own case. (She has five academic degrees.) She admits that people with autism have difficulty dividing their attention in comparison to other people, but she points out that if allowed to break up tasks and follow them through one at a time, they can function quite successfully. Autism can even be seen to afford a 'superior' degree of functioning, she says, as it enables people not to be as preoccupied as non-autistic people are by the trivialities of how they look or sound (BBC, 2005). But Lawson agrees that autism is a spectrum disorder affecting many whose functioning does not come close to hers, including people who are unable to speak at all. Although she says that some of those at the lower-functioning end of the spectrum communicate quite well in their own way, she does not claim that they function just as well as any other autistic person. Again, while she dislikes medical definitions of autism, she points out that autism, though not a medical disorder itself, is associated with medical disorders, such as epilepsy.

A more radical approach to autism is adopted by Jim Sinclair, an American autism campaigner. 'Autism is not something a person has or a "shell" that a person is trapped inside,' he says. 'Autism is a way of being. It is pervasive. It colours every experience, every sensation, perception, thought.' So when parents say, 'I wish my child did not have autism', what they are really saying is, 'I wish the autistic child I have did not exist'. It is true that if autism *defines* someone

[2]Wendy Lawson's website: http://www.mugsy.org/wendy/index2.htm

or is essential to someone, as Sinclair is claiming, wishing it away is in effect wishing away the person. But what is the ground for the essentialist claim? Consider the parallel claim that when one is suffering from cancer it pervades one's whole life: does it follow that in wishing that a certain person did not have cancer one is wishing *them* out of existence? If the reply is that autism, unlike cancer, is a life-long condition whenever it occurs, and that its pervasive character is connected with its being life-long and ineliminable, then that seems to be false in view of the changes to the condition that different kinds of therapy are known to bring about. On the essentialist view, children with autism who are placed in special schools and gradually change behaviourally might have to be regarded as denatured rather than helped, even if they themselves are glad of the change!

An autism campaigning website called 'Getting the Truth Out'[3] takes images of the autistic that it says are exploited for fund-raising based on revulsion, and reinterprets them in ways that are more accepting. The curled-up postures, motionless sitting and hand-flapping of some adults with autism are reinterpreted as ways of relaxing, playing or simply coping with sensory input that is hard to organize and sometimes overwhelming. These reinterpretations are plausible, and they often succeed in showing that the lives of those with autism do not in the least justify revulsion. They do not show, however, that people whose lives are mostly spent curled up, sitting motionless or engaged in hand-flapping are as good as the lives of people who are not autistic. Nor do they seem to discredit, as they seem intended to discredit, the efforts of mainstream autistic charities to find treatments.

The radical autism campaigners often argue as if anything short of accepting and supporting autism without trying to change it were a kind of expression of support for a new eugenics. A magazine article sympathetic to autism campaigners and the points they are trying to make Brune (2005) says:

> But there seems an air of special pleading about all this. In fact, everyone knows that some autistic people can have remarkable abilities and, fascinating as the differences between autistic and non-autistic brains may be, the bottom line is that many people with autism seem not to function well at all, to be deeply unhappy and disturbed and to need a lifetime of special care. How can it be wrong to try to help them?

How indeed?

IMPAIRMENTS AND LIVES WORTH LIVING

On the essentialist view we have seen being expressed by Jim Sinclair, a person with autism who ceased to be autistic

would cease to be. Again according to Sinclair, someone who wishes that a person with autism were not autistic really wishes that person had never been born or were dead. Still according to Sinclair, a parent who wants autism cured in a child is involved in some sort of conceptual mistake, perhaps the mistake of thinking that autism traps a normal person in an autistically behaving body-shell. These claims seem to me to be highly contentious if not obviously false. Nor does their being put forward by someone who has *been there* make them authoritative. Being autistic no more makes Jim Sinclair an expert on the *concept* of autism than cancer makes a cancer sufferer an expert on the concept of cancer. In the cancer case, there is, in addition to the experience of suffering the disease, the physical basis of it. There is no reason to think that autism is different. It, too, has a physical basis as well as an experiential side, and the concepts of autism and of cancer must encompass both. But being autistic or having cancer gives one no special insight into its physical basis. Indeed, because autism is a spectrum disorder, and possibly even more than one disorder, it is not even true that one person's *experience* of autism is entirely representative. Nor does the wish to express solidarity with the most friendless of those with autism mean that essentialist claims are true. At best, it makes them well-intentioned.

The essentialist thesis does not *argue* down the natural thought that those with impairments are worse off. It simply rules it out by stipulation. But why should it be so important to block the possibility that impairments make people who have them worse off?

It might be thought that *not* blocking this possibility opens the way to eugenics. Consider abortion policy. In the United Kingdom, abnormality of the foetus is a ground for a termination. If abortion is permissible for foetuses that will develop into, for example, babies with Down Syndrome, does not that policy on abortion express the thought that anyone who has been born with Down Syndrome is better off dead, and that society is better off without such people? And does not this show a profound disrespect for those with Down Syndrome who have already been born? If so, then it may seem that the only way *not* to show disrespect to people with Down Syndrome is to deny that their impairment makes them more than different. This pulls the rug out from under the abortion policy, it might be thought, because no one would claim that anyone who is simply different – who simply belongs to a minority – is better off dead, or that the prospect of a foetus developing into a member of a minority is a ground for abortion.

But this line of thought overstates the message of the abortion policy. The most the abortion policy expresses

---

[3]www.gettingoutthetruth.org

is the thought that babies with Down syndrome typically have significantly worse life-chances than babies without abnormalities, and impose much greater life-long demands on their carers (and perhaps the state) than people without Down syndrome. This thought can be true without it being denied that, were particular people with Down Syndrome to come into existence, they might (atypically) have entirely fulfilling lives that imposed no burdens. This thought can also be true without implying that existing people with Down Syndrome should be killed off, or that they and their lives are worthless. At most, it implies that no one is obliged to add to the number of those with Down Syndrome if they have a pregnancy affected by it. After all, couples who want to go ahead with such a pregnancy are not prevented from doing so by a policy that merely permits abortion for Down Syndrome.

The essentialist line against the Down Syndrome abortion policy is also questionable in the way it connects respect with creating or prolonging life. The fact that someone's life deserves respect does not mean that they should stay alive by all means or have their lives prolonged by others by all means possible. Someone who very heroically survives 40 years of pain and relative loneliness may have had a very unpleasant life, notwithstanding the heroism, and notwithstanding the fact that heroic lives rightly command great respect. The unpleasantness is a reason for thinking that an earlier death might have been a deliverance, or that the prospect of bringing into existence another sufferer of the same condition was better avoided than not.

Both of the following can be true together:

(1) Impairments make people worse off, adding to the difficulties of making a life go well; and
(2) people who have impairments deserve respect.

Not only are these claims consistent, but it is also natural to connect them; it is natural to say that (2) is true *because* (1) is true. People who need to overcome great obstacles to succeed deserve respect for trying to overcome them, let alone for succeeding. The essentialist thesis denies (1) and takes away a *special* reason for respecting those with impairments, leaving only the personhood they share with everyone else.

The following are also consistent with (1) and (2), and are, in my view, true:

(3) Some impairments leave people less badly off than the able-bodied or minded think;
(4) those with impairments are worse off than they would be if social policies were different; and
(5) the basis for many if not all impairments is physical.

(3) contains the main truth in the otherwise exaggerated-seeming positions of the disability activists. The disability activists are right to claim that many of us are too quick to write off the possibilities of life as a person with autism or Down Syndrome. Not only are we too seduced by a very narrow range of stereotypes of what children should be like, and of what it is to be a successful adult; we exaggerate the drawbacks of lives that depart markedly from these stereotypes. Even within the normal range, many of us probably *overvalue* academic success, conventional good looks and wealth as signs of excellence or flourishing. These valuations probably denigrate average performance in the normal range, and probably undercut the possibility of positive valuations outside the range. They condescend to the *merely* normal, and perhaps show contempt for those who do not reach the threshold of normal performance. Against *this* background, without the essentialism, Sinclair seems right to say:

> Non-autistic people see autism as a great tragedy, and parents experience continuing disappointment and grief at all stages of the child's and family's life cycle.
> But this grief does not stem from the child's autism in itself. It is grief over the loss of the normal child the parents had hoped and expected to have. Parents' attitudes and expectations, and the discrepancies between what parents expect of children at a particular age and their own child's actual development, cause more stress and anguish than the practical complexities of life with an autistic person (Sinclair, 1993).

Without denying that those with impairments are worse off, we can also agree that, as (4) says, a range of social policies makes those with impairments worse off still. The Getting the Truth Out website speaks of the way institutions for the autistic sometimes enforce a brutal regime to make them responsive. Then there is the isolation of institutional life, and the routine economic marginalization of those with impairments who are not institutionalized, to say nothing of the marginalization of people with physical impairments by thoughtless architecture, town planning and so on. Hardly anyone denies that, in this area of non-medical ways of improving life for those with impairments, there is much still to do.

It does not follow from the truth of (4), or from the fact that many doctors have sometimes shared the stereotypes that have blinded the public in general to the truth of (3), that impairment is entirely a 'social construct' and that (5) is false. If repudiating the 'medical model' of disability means denying that there is a physical basis to autism or blindness, then the baby is being thrown out with the bathwater. Although it is sometimes unclear in campaigning material, opposition to the medical model from disability academics does not in fact involve a denial of (5). The 'social model of disability', pioneered in Britain, distinguishes between impairment (a biological phenomenon) and the oppression of those with impairments consisting of social attitudes and practices, which is social and is disabling. Impairment is the phenomenon that the medical model and the social model both recognize – albeit in different ways – but the social model takes account of other things as well. Lately, even disability theorists who are in sympathy with the consciousness-raising and political power of the social model have begun to complain that the social model does not make enough of impairment, or the experience that arises specifically from impairment (Thomas, 1998).

Once impairment is in the picture, it is hard to see that the social model of disability must be at war with a medical model, so long as a medical model does not come with the claim that it tells us everything about impairment. Some disability theorists, however, taking their cue from certain feminist theorists, and *their* philosophical predilections, dislike deep and fundamental dichotomies, including the dichotomy between a physical or biological notion of impairment, and a social notion of disability. According to them, impairment is not one thing and a social phenomenon of disability another. Instead, impairment, too, is a (thoroughly) social notion, partly because it is inevitably characterized linguistically, and language is social (Shakespeare and Watson, 2002). The same 'argument' would show that geology, intended to characterize processes that occur in our planet long before the advent of human beings, is 'social', or that the physical processes that came a moment after the Big Bang are social!

In analytic philosophy, it is customary to suppose that social facts depend upon but are not reducible to psychological facts, that psychological facts depend upon but are not reducible to physical facts, and that physical facts are basic: ontologically basic. This way of thinking about ontology does not deny that the social sciences, psychology and the brain sciences and physics all have a linguistic medium; but this medium is not to be confused with content. Whatever makes it *true* that there was for a long time

no life or intelligence on earth, it has nothing to do with language. Language may make it *thinkable* or *expressible* that there was once no life or intelligence on earth, but it does not make it true. Nor can it be coherently claimed that the existence of society makes it true that once life or intelligence did not exist on earth. In a related sense, a particular impairment, understood as an expression of a genetic disorder, is not inherently social. It is inherently biological, and because the biological depends on the physical, inherently physical, but not inherently social.

Considerations like these support the *maintenance* of the distinction between impairment and the social aspects of disability for theoretical purposes. As impairment is the focal point of the medical model, it is hard to remove all vestiges of it from thinking about disability. It is hard *and* unnecessary. Insisting – even in theory – that it is all social is another kind of denial.

REFERENCES

BBC (British Broadcasting Corporation). *Radio 4 In Touch*, 2005; http://www.bbc.co.uk/radio4/factual/intouch_20051227.shtml#transcript

BBC. *Radio 4. All in the Mind*, 2005a; http://www.bbc.co.uk/radio4/science/allinthemind.shtml

Brune J. *Say it Loud, Autistic, and Proud*. London: Observer Magazine, 13 November 2005; http://observer.guardian.co.uk/magazine/story/0,11913,1639392,00.html

Hull J. *Touching the Rock: An Experience of Blindness*. New York: Vintage, 1991.

Oliver M. *Understanding Disability: From Theory to Practice*. Basingstoke: Macmillan, 1996.

Shakespeare T, Watson N. The social model of disability: an outdated ideology? *Res Soc Sci Disab* 2002; **2**: 9–28.

Sinclair J. Don't mourn for us. *Our Voice, the Newsletter of Autism Network International* 1993; **1**(3): http://web.syr.edu/jisincla/dontmourn.htm

Thomas C. The body and society: impairment and disability. In: Paper Presented at BSA Annual Conference on Making Sense of the Body. Edinburgh, 1998.

Disability and Equity: Should Difference Be Welcomed?

TOM SHAKESPEARE

CHANGING ACCOUNTS OF DISABILITY

Disability is a word with strong cultural associations. In the minds of many professionals, patients and members of the public, the term evokes ideas of medicine, invalidity, tragedy, failure and lack of competence. In modern western societies, the dominant ways of thinking about disability have been individualist: disabilities are unfortunate medical problems which we are morally compelled to prevent or failing that, to cure. Society may have progressed beyond pre-modern ideas about disability being punishment for former sins, or karma, but it generally regards disabled people as defined by their deficits (Oliver, 1990).

This powerful tradition of thinking has been challenged by disabled people themselves, who have self-organized in political movements in many countries of the world since the 1960s, and particularly since the formation of Disabled People's International in 1981 (Dreidger, 1989). This challenge has involved political action to promote civil rights and independent living; it has included cultural initiatives to promote disability pride and alternative images of disability; and it has been closely related to the growth of disability studies, a cross-disciplinary endeavour to understand disability as an issue of equal opportunities and human rights, not predominantly of medicine and rehabilitation (Shakespeare, 2001).

Disability studies has been based on the work of disabled people themselves, both activists and scholars, and often activist-scholars. It has followed the precedents of other subaltern studies: Marxism, feminism, lesbian and gay studies, post-colonialism. To use C. Wright Mill's formulation, disabled people have used their sociological imagination, turning private problems into public issues (Wright Mills,

2000). The research agenda has included efforts to redefine disability, to trace patterns of exclusion and domination through history and culture, to bring disabled people's own perspectives, experiences and voices into the mainstream and to develop alternative ways of supporting and including disabled people in areas such as employment, education, personal care and community living.

The redefinition of disability which has been central to disability politics and disability studies has taken slightly different forms in different countries. For example, in many countries normalization or social role valorization concepts (Wolfensburger, 1992) have been influential in promoting deinstitutionalization and social inclusion, particularly for people with learning difficulties. American activists and writers have developed minority group conceptions of disability (Hahn, 1988), following civil rights traditions. The Nordic countries have relied on a relational model of disability in developing a research agenda: This emphasizes the complex and situated interaction between individual factors and the environment (Gustavsson, 2004). The strongest version of the social account of disability derives from Britain, where the Union of Physically Impaired Against Segregation invented the social model in the 1970s (Campbell, 1996). Whereas other social approaches focus on the social and political consequences of having a disability, the social model redefines disability itself, producing what Michael Oliver (1990) termed a 'social creationist' understanding. For the mainstream of UK disability studies, disability refers not to any physical or mental limitation, but to the failure of society to include those who have physical or mental differences. People are disabled by society, not by their bodies. This sets up a distinction between

Principles of Health Care Ethics, Second Edition   Edited by R.E. Ashcroft, A. Dawson, H. Draper and J.R. McMillan
© 2007 John Wiley & Sons, Ltd

impairment (individual medical difference) and disability (social barriers or social discrimination).

The family of social approaches to disability have been important in different ways. First, these different models have focused attention and political action on removing environmental and social barriers. This instrumental effect has enabled greater participation of disabled people in the mainstream. Second, these approaches have relocated the disability problem away from individuals and onto society, and hence enabled the person with impairment to move from a position of self-pity and failure, to a position of anger and pride. Rather than feeling sorry for herself, a disabled person can now blame society for her difficulties. The problem is not her incapacity or invalidity, but social barriers and social neglect. She can now join up with other disabled people – regardless of impairment – to form a collective response to discrimination. In other words, this psychological effect has created the conditions for an identity politics of disability. Of the family of social approaches to disability, the most powerful tools for the promotion of barrier removal and identity politics have been the minority group and social model versions of the social conception of disability, because they have been the basis for vigorous, disabled-led campaigns of direct action and civil rights based on strong collective identity as disabled people.

In summary, the social approach to disability shifts the emphasis from individual or medical responses to collective and structural responses. The implication is that disabled people are to be welcomed and accommodated, not prevented or cured. Disability becomes an issue of citizenship. Impairment is to be accepted, whereas action should be taken against the unfair discrimination which makes impairment a problem or leads to social exclusion and disadvantage. The following sections unpack and develop these points, before concluding with a critical assessment of disability politics.

IMPAIRMENT IS PART OF THE HUMAN CONDITION

The political challenge of disability rights and disability studies highlights an important existential truth about the inescapability of impairment. Although biomedicine seeks to eliminate suffering and ill-health, in practice impairment and mortality are inextricable elements of embodiment. Rather than society dividing into two different groups – a majority of able-bodied people and a minority of people with disabilities – in practice it may be more useful to think in terms of a continuum (Zola, 1989). It is obvious that able-bodied people have limitations, and disabled people have capabilities. Equally, everyone shares a vulnerability to

accident and disease. For example, the Human Genome Project has demonstrated that every genome contains mutations, at least 100 spelling mistakes that could predict vulnerability or cause ill-health. As people age, they collect injuries and chronic illnesses. Disability disproportionately affects people in the later stages of life.

Many medical initiatives to remedy disability may ironically contribute to the increase in the number of disabled people. This is because the effect of interventions is often to reduce mortality, but at the cost of increased morbidity. For example, good health care enables people to live longer lives: however, in later life they may be prone to diseases of ageing such as macular degeneration and dementia. Orthopaedic surgery, nursing care and rehabilitation enable people to survive spinal cord injury, where once they would have died within a few years of trauma. Protease inhibitors have converted HIV/AIDS from an acute incurable illness to a chronic illness, for those who can access the drug treatments. Foetal medicine and neonatology enables more babies who are born prematurely to survive, but half of these children will have life-long impairments as a consequence (Wood, et al., 2000). The argument is not that these interventions should be abandoned, but instead that the concept of eliminating disability is misguided, perhaps impossible.

A more balanced understanding of disability would disavow the perfectionist ambitions often found in biomedical or bioethical writing. For example, some have seen antenatal genetic screening as the route to eliminate disability. This overlooks the fact that although only 2% of births are affected by congenital abnormalities, some 10–20% of the population are disabled: in other words, the vast majority of impairment is caused by poverty, ageing, injury or disease, not by genetic factors. The ambition to minimize illness and impairment is important, but so too is the acceptance of the frailty and limitations of the human condition. More realism about the reality of embodiment might mitigate some of the hostility and prejudice which is directed towards disabled people, who serve as uncomfortable reminders of vulnerability and dependency. Adopting the principle of universal human rights means extending respect and recognition to disabled people, rather than devaluing and oppressing people who are physically or mentally different. Awareness that disabled people will always be part of society leads to the realization that society has to change to support and include disabled people, now and in the future.

PEOPLE ADAPT WELL TO DISABILITY

Although there has been an assumption in biomedicine and bioethics that disability is an individual tragedy – in John Harris's terms (Harris, 2000,) a harmed condition which people have a strong subjective preference not to be in – the reality of many disabled people's lives is rather different.

Those who are born with their impairments do not have anything with which to compare their situation. They have no need to 'come to terms' because they have never known anything different. Because they have only experienced life with impairment, they usually feel comfortable with their situation. For this reason, they do not generally feel deficient or in need of medical attention, unless they have a degenerative condition. It is common for people born impaired to reject attempts to cure them or correct their abnormalities: often they reply that they are happy the way they are. Disability has become part of their identity, and they can no more conceive of being non-disabled than a man can conceive of being a woman. Those people who develop impairment through injury or disease may have more difficulties coming to terms with their situation because they have usually lost function or suffered reduction in health. Nevertheless, here too there is evidence that people can adapt very well to changed circumstances. Some disabled people have even said that their accident was the best thing ever to happen to them.

These findings are counter-intuitive. Disabled people, whom the mainstream regard as suffering, or being in a state of ill-health, claim to feel healthy and happy. The 'disability paradox' (Albrecht, 1999) is that many disabled people report a high quality of life. Indeed, in some surveys disabled people actually report a higher quality of life than non-disabled people. Whereas non-disabled people may express sentiments such as 'I'd rather be dead than disabled' or 'disability is the worst thing that could happen to a person', those who actually experience disability first hand have a very different view.

One implication of this disparity is that it is dangerous to conflate or confuse objective accounts of quality of life with subjective accounts of quality of life. Disabled people can experience pleasure and happiness; they can have their preferences satisfied; they can lead flourishing lives (Edwards, 2005). Aspects of impairment and disability – for example, pain and fatigue, or poverty and loneliness – should not be glossed over or ignored. Yet there may not be an easily drawn qualitative difference between disabled and non-disabled people, all of whom are also vulnerable to these diswelfares. A second implication of these findings is that non-disabled people often do not understand the reality of disability, and that their attempts to imagine what it may be like to be disabled, or to empathize with disabled people, can be prejudiced and misleading (Young, 1997). Non-disabled people often project their own assumptions onto the disabled other, and they assume that they know what it must be like or what must be best for the disabled person.

DISABILITY IS A RELATIONAL ISSUE

Understanding disability as socially created (Oliver, 1990) or at least socially mediated, switches attention from prevention or cure of impairment, to removal of barriers in society. Disability movements have claimed that the priority for investment and action should not be a biomedical research seeking to correct impairment, but a social change in order to enable people with impairment to participate. Building a more inclusive society can promote independence, by providing access to employment and ensuring disabled people access mainstream education, transport, housing and other services. This reduces the costs of maintaining disabled people on welfare and of providing segregated services.

A relational approach to disability shows that disability is not an unchanging and static condition, but that it is influenced by cultural values, assumptions and arrangements. For example, Nora Groce (1988) demonstrates how Martha's Vineyard, an isolated New England community with a high proportion of deaf members, was accepting of the impairment to the extent that this difference was not a salient feature which marked out the sub-population: everyone there spoke sign language. Equally, dyslexia, an obstacle in an information society for which reading and writing are requisites for employment, was no barrier in pre-literate societies based on agrarian skills which were learned through demonstration and example.

In the contemporary world, those societies which have mandated Universal Design and barrier removal – for example the United States, and increasingly the United Kingdom – are far more accessible to people with mobility or sensory impairments. Educating all children in the mainstream increases familiarity with disability and challenges the stigma and poor educational achievement historically associated with those who experience 'special' or segregated schooling. Removing discriminations – the unfair burdens placed on people who communicate, travel or behave differently from the norm – enables participation by those who are otherwise qualified to perform mainstream roles.

Attention to the environments and relationships which generate disability and disadvantage highlights the extent to which professionals and other non-disabled people, often unwittingly, create problems for disabled people. This can be a challenging realization for non-disabled people. It is easy to oppose overt prejudice, hostility and violence towards disabled people. It is harder to accept that one's own well-intentioned behaviour is inappropriate. For example, often the parents, assistants or helpers of disabled people are asked questions, rather than the disabled persons themselves. It is often assumed that the health issue is always associated with the impairment, as if disabled people do not have the usual range of medical problems. Those who provide assistance sometimes do so in patronizing ways, which imply that the individual is childlike or intellectually deficient. The basic rights of privacy and respect are not always accorded to disabled people in the same way as to non-disabled people: Curiosity or embarrassment leads to inappropriate questioning or handling. In summary, it is common for disability to be treated as a master status, which overwhelms other aspects of the individual's identity and dominates the interaction. Those who set out to help can sometimes end up hindering.

RESPONDING TO THE DISABILITY CHALLENGE

The claims outlined above represent an orthodox reading of the disability rights argument. However, it is important to test and challenge some of the claims of the disability rights community which may be based more on rhetoric and political correctness than on logic or evidence. The demands of disability identity politics may sometimes conflict with best practice. Moreover, disabled people are an extremely diverse group, not only in the experience of impairment, but also in attitudes to it. A nuanced approach to disability and a deeper debate about some of the complexities are needed.

Disability politics has explicitly followed precedents established by civil rights, feminist and lesbian and gay liberation thinking, and some leading thinkers have argued on marxist principles. Despite the value in such analogies, there are limitations to the parallel. Other social experiences – such as those of race, gender and sexuality – can be explained in terms of unfair discrimination or restriction of negative freedom (Bickenbach et al., 1999). An individual or group who could otherwise participate equally or compete fairly is denied the opportunity due to barriers or burdens placed in their way. Although this certainly applies to disabled people, in the ways demonstrated above, the removal of discrimination may not equalize outcomes in the same way. This is because disabled people experience intrinsic limitations, to varying degrees, by virtue of the impairments of body or mind which are an inextricable part of being disabled. In the case of gender, race or sexuality, there is no pathology associated with that form of embodiment and no inferiority of functioning which restricts independence and participation.

For the emancipation of disabled people, it is not sufficient to remove social barriers. It is also important to provide additional support and investment. For example, many disabled people cannot work as hard or as effectively as people who do not have impairments. A person with serious mental illness may sometimes be unable to work at all, perhaps for weeks or months at a time. A person with a condition which causes pain or fatigue may not be able to work for a full day or a five day week. And some people with intellectual impairments may not be able to work at all, in any capacity. Although there are certainly many more disabled people able to work than do so currently – in Britain, up to one million people, who could otherwise participate, are excluded from employment – there are others whose intrinsic physical or mental limitations prevent them being productive.

The problem of impairment limitations challenges the claims of those disability activists who have argued in terms of difference and the value of diversity. Although all individuals are worthy of respect and equal in human rights, people are not equal in terms of capacities or contribution. Respect for diversity appeals to rhetoric, but in practice it might be good, where possible, for fewer people to be affected by life-limiting conditions. For example, supplementing food with folic acid reduces the incidence of births affected by spina bifida: this seems intuitively desirable.

Rightly, disability activists have challenged the notion of disability as tragedy. The evidence is that most disabled people's lives are not tragic or unhappy. However, it would be wrong to claim that impairment was irrelevant or even a positive concept. Rather, impairment and disability might be seen as a predicament: not neutral, not awful, but something to be coped with and overcome.

The implication of seeing impairment as a predicament is that it is good to prevent or cure conditions which cause impairment and disability, wherever possible. Although acknowledging that some of the biomedical rhetoric about cure raises expectations of rapid benefits which are unlikely to be realized, or overlooks the side effects of interventions, or disrespects those who are living successfully with their conditions, it would be misguided if radical disability activists rejected completely investment in medical research and the development of therapies and regimes which improve functioning.

Some disability scholars and activists have developed an 'expressivist' challenge to prenatal diagnosis or other attempts to reduce the incidence of impairment (Parens and Asch, 2000). This claims that because preventative measures express the view that it would be better for disabled people not to be born, they are therefore discriminatory to disabled people. In my view, this confuses the requirement to respect, accept and include existing disabled people, with the imperative to reduce the chance of existing or future people becoming impaired.

It is not inconsistent to support disability rights and work to prevent more disabled people existing. Undoubtedly, some of the current language, imagery and arguments about disability prevention is offensive, unbalanced and discriminatory to disabled people. Those who offer screening or other measures have an obligation to do so in ways which do not denigrate disabled people or represent their lives inaccurately or unfairly.

DISABILITY AND HEALTH CARE

In conclusion, the development of disability rights has issued a challenge to all sections of society, including health care. Professionals and carers alike need to examine their assumptions, and develop reflexive practice, rather than unconsciously perpetuating oppressive or discriminatory ways of thinking. The way forward is to listen to disabled people themselves and to understand that disability is a multidimensional problem, not just of physical or mental functioning but also of environmental access, employment discrimination, social support, equality and justice. When encountering a disabled person, the professional should ask 'need to know' not 'want to know' questions, according the disabled individual the same privacy and respect as any other patient. Disabled people are the experts on their own lives, but need to work in partnership with the professionals and carers who can facilitate their inclusion and independence. When disabled people face problems, they are often the same problems as those which non-disabled people encounter, just as their needs are normal needs, not abnormal ones: education, information, employment, friendship and support.

In the words of the title of a Canadian academic collection (Rioux, 1994), *Disability is not Measles*: unlike illness, impairment often becomes part of identity (Edwards, 2005) and paradoxically may even be welcomed and celebrated, as the example of Deafness indicates. Biomedicine aims at the elimination of illness and impairment, and the continuing existence of disabled people may be challenging to many who practise or research medicine. However, disability is not simply an unwanted medical problem, it is a complex social reality, and humane and egalitarian medical responses have to take their place alongside social change and political equality if disabled people are to be truly emancipated.

REFERENCES

Albrecht GL, Devlieger PJ. The disability paradox: high quality of life against all odds. *Soc Sci Med* 1999; **48**: 947–988.

Bickenbach JE, Chatterji S, Badley EM, Ustun TB. Models of disablement, universalism and the international classification of impairments, disabilities and handicaps. *Soc Sci Med* 1999; **48**: 1173–1187.

Campbell J, Oliver M. *Disability Politics: Understanding Our Past, Changing Our Future.* London: Routledge, 1996.

Dreidger D. *The Last Civil Rights Movement.* London: Hurst, 1989.

Edwards S. *Disability: Definitions, Value and Identity.* Oxford: Radcliffe, 2005.

Groce N. *Everyone Hear Spoke Sign Language: Hereditary Deafness in Martha's Vinyard.* Harvard, MA: Harvard University Press, 1988.

Gustavsson A. The role of theory in disability research – springboard or straitjacket? *Scand J Disab Res* 2004; **6**: 55–70.

Hahn H. The politics of physical differences: disability and discrimination. *J Soc Issues* 1988; **44**(1): 39–47.

Harris J. Is there a coherent social conception of disability? *J Med Ethics* 2000; **26**: 95–100.

Oliver M. *The Politics of Disablement.* London: Macmillan, 1990.

Parens E, Asch A. *Prenatal Testing and Disability Rights.* Washington, DC: Georgetown University Press, 2000.

Rioux M, Bach M, eds. *Disability is not Measles: New Research Paradigms in Disability.* North York: L'Institut Roeher, 1994.

Shakespeare T, Watson N. Making the difference: disability, politics and recognition. In: Albrecht G et al., eds. *Handbook of Disability Studies.* Thousand Oaks, CA: Sage, 2001; pp. 546–564.

Wolfensburger W. *A Brief Introduction to Social Role Valorization as a High-Order Concept for Structuring Human Services.* Syracuse, NY: Syracuse University, 1992.

Wood N, Marlow N, Costeloe K, Gibson AT, Wilkinson AR. Neurologic and developmental disability following extremely preterm birth. *N Engl J Med* 2000; **343**(6): 378–384.

Wright Mills C. *The Sociological Imagination.* Oxford: Oxford University Press, 2000.

Young, IM. Asymmetrical reciprocity: on moral respect, wonder and enlarged thought. *Constellations* 1997; **3**(3): 340–363.

Zola IK. Towards the necessary universalizing of a disability policy. *Milbank Q* 1989; **67**(2, Pt. 2): 401–428.

58

Genetic Counselling

ANGUS CLARKE

'Genetic counselling' applies to both an activity and a profession. This chapter will identify and address many of the issues that arise for those who 'do' genetic counselling as part of clinical genetic services, whether as a genetic counsellor or clinical geneticist. No attempt is made to resolve all these issues.

The use of the knowledge and technologies collectively referred to as 'human genetics' in health care raises a number of difficult and sensitive issues. The very existence of genetic counselling as a distinct clinical activity acknowledges the potential for problems to arise for individual clients and their families. As cytogenetic, biochemical and molecular genetic techniques have developed over the last 40 and 50 years, it has become possible not only to provide diagnostic assessments and to give prognoses but also to detect genetic alterations that are clinically silent and that may not manifest as disease until later in the individual's life or even not until a future generation. This can raise social or ethical difficulties within families and between clients and professionals as the individual's previously concealed identity is revealed (Armstrong et al., 1998). Testing that gives an indication of risk to future generations but not to the health of the individual tested is referred to as carrier testing. A test that reveals information that is likely to be relevant to the future health of the individual is referred to as a predictive test.

ETHOS, GOALS AND OUTCOMES

NON-DIRECTIVENESS IN GENETIC COUNSELLING

It is impossible to consider modern genetics without reference to the movement that linked knowledge about genetics to the improvement of society. Eugenics, as it was termed by Galton, became a social movement associated with the loss of reproductive liberties for anyone found to be unfit, whether by reason of social class, mental condition or racial origin. Eugenics-inspired concepts developed variably across Europe and North America, reinforcing racist immigration policies in the USA, attitudes to social class in Britain and notions of Aryan racial superiority in National Socialist Germany. The defeat of Nazi Germany in the second world war led to the recognition that the German medical profession had colluded heavily with eugenic ideas and, in the name of 'race hygiene', had played an active role in the forced sterilization, incarceration and even the killing of many patients (whatever their 'race') with diseases attributed to inherited weakness (Müller-Hill, 1988). This resulted in a reassessment of Galton's eugenic ideals as deeply flawed.

The scientists, clinicians and 'counsellors' (often social workers) who set up the first genetics clinics were committed to avoiding the sin of eugenics, principally by enabling their patients to make decisions for themselves and based on their own values. Non-directiveness, as it has become known, is seen not only as the opposite of eugenics, enabling counsellors to distance themselves from the abuses of the past, but also as a professional commitment to respect for client autonomy and an openness to consider the wider family impact of genetic information and choices. But it may also enable professionals to keep an emotional distance from their clients, especially those with whose actions or values we are out of sympathy; the full moral and legal responsibility for clients' decisions rests with them alone (Clarke, 1997a).

Fraser's (1974) formulation of the goals of genetic counselling emphasizes the need for professionals to help families understand their situation correctly, support them as they make their own decisions and help them make the best possible adjustment to the disorder in question. While

Principles of Health Care Ethics, Second Edition   Edited by R.E. Ashcroft, A. Dawson, H. Draper and J.R. McMillan
© 2007 John Wiley & Sons, Ltd

this may have minimized the problems of families feeling pressured by professionals, being told what to do or even being coerced to act against their own wishes and judgements, an excessive focus on avoiding 'directiveness' has resulted in other problems. In particular, continual reference to an unexamined ideal of 'non-directiveness' may have misled professionals into providing clients with information but then backing away from supporting them in their decision-making, in case this is interpreted as an attempt to influence their decision. This approach fails to recognize that there is no clear separation between giving information on one hand and giving advice or influencing a client on the other. It assumes that any influence is bad, whereas the client may be looking both for information and for some interpretation of it, which may well amount to influence. This misunderstanding of non-directiveness may block emotional engagement with clients, risking the charge of over-distancing or abandonment (Quill and Cassel, 1995), and may discourage professionals from challenging clients constructively (Wolff and Jung, 1995) or speaking plainly and directly (Benkendorf et al., 2001), when to do so would help clients to arrive at the their own (autonomous) decisions. There is scope within genetic counselling for professionals to make frank recommendations as to what decisions they think their clients should make within a framework of shared decision-making (Elwyn et al., 2000). This would be entirely appropriate – as a form of beneficence – not only in the context of medical management intended to limit the harm caused by genetic disorders but also in the moral sphere; for example, making recommendations intended to promote open communication within a family or promoting the future autonomy of young children by deferring predictive testing for a late-onset disorder. In response to these appropriate criticisms of non-directiveness, other verbal formulae have been proposed, such as 'shared decision-making' (Elwyn et al., 2000) or 'psychosocial genetic counselling' (Weil, 2003).

CLINICAL GENETICS CONTRASTED WITH POPULATION GENETIC SCREENING PROGRAMMES

The most serious challenge to autonomy arises in population screening programmes, where the institutional context of screening serves to promote the uptake of screening despite the intentions of the individual health professionals involved. The screening of newborn infants for treatable genetic disorders or malformations, such as phenylketonuria (PKU) or congenital hypothyroidism, has such clear benefits to the infant (because early treatment makes such a difference to the outcome) that screening is mandatory

in some jurisdictions. *Not* to screen for such disorders would be reprehensible, so the routinization of screening without a requirement for informed parental choice may be entirely defensible. Indeed, a professional would be failing in their duty of care to an infant if they failed to challenge a parent who declined the 'offer' of newborn screening. This approach would not be appropriate, however, with other disorders where the benefits from early diagnosis are not as clear, or where the potential benefits are for the family as a whole rather than the affected child. Screening for these disorders, such as some inborn errors of metabolism and also Duchenne muscular dystrophy, should not, therefore, be routinized but should only be performed where properly informed parents judge that it would be helpful. This brings us up against a tension present in many population screening programmes.

Most clinical genetic services are made available to individuals concerned about a disorder in their family; for example, parents may wish to know the cause of a developmental disorder affecting their child or someone may wish to know if they will develop a condition that has affected other family members. The genetic service attempts to answer these questions, while ensuring that the client understands the implications of their situation as fully as is feasible. This may entail the professionals listening to the client's questions or concerns, perhaps probing or challenging them, and gathering information so as to establish the genetic facts. These facts are then used to answer the client's questions. In the context of population screening programmes, however, the context is very different.

In population screening, the health care system makes a proactive offer of testing instead of waiting passively for interested clients to seek out information. This proactive role can be justified where the health benefits of testing are clear. It is less straightforward to justify the population screening of pregnant women for cases of genetic disorders or structural malformations in the foetus, however, when the principal intervention available, where some anomaly has been detected, is the termination of the pregnancy. Although it may be reasonable to make such tests available to those who want them, the active promotion of testing by the health care system as a part of routine antenatal care can be seen as an implicit but strong recommendation that pregnant women *should* have antenatal screening, and that a pregnancy in which the foetus is affected by Down syndrome or spina bifida *should* be terminated. If the offer of antenatal screening is made in such a way that women experience it as a 'considered choice', then there is no problem; those who wish to have screening can do so, those who do not want it do not have it, and those who do not know much about it can be given information and arrive at their own decision. If screening is routinized, however, so that women have the tests by simply complying with normal clinic procedures, then the individual women may have made no considered decision; the screening has *happened to* them rather than having been *chosen by* them. When staff explicitly direct women to have screening tests, or when they treat those who opt not to have screening as in some way deviant, then the operation of the screening programme has clearly been directive or coercive. This institutional directiveness can be avoided in a population screening programme only when the professionals involved actively ensure that the women in clinic understand that this test is different from the other tests being performed on the basis of a clear medical recommendation. There may also be institutional decisions about the way in which the programme is structured that can usefully modify the experience of choice in a screening programme (Parsons et al., 2000).

The ethos of an antenatal screening programme, all-important to avoid institutional pressure on pregnant women, may be influenced by the goals of screening and the outcome measures used to evaluate its performance. Programmes that justify their existence through reducing the birth incidence of Down syndrome or neural tube defects will want to maximize the uptake of the test and the proportion of identified foetal anomalies that lead to a termination of the pregnancy. Programmes that claim to justify their existence by offering choice may find it difficult to put this into practice if the outcome measures they use are, in practice, those relating to uptake of screening, terminations of pregnancy and the birth incidence of affected infants (those that could have been detected prenatally and thereby terminated). It is now less common for such calculations to be the explicit force driving antenatal screening programmes, but this may owe more to the expectation that health services should adopt the rhetoric of informed patient choice and not appear to discriminate against, or to treat disrespectfully, those with disabilities than to a change of justification. It is only in the day-to-day operation of such programmes, and the experiences of the women going through the antenatal clinics, that the values-in-action of a programme can be assessed (Clarke, 1997; Williams et al., 2002).

Justifying antenatal screening by preventing the birth of infants with disorders that are expensive to look after seems very close to the 'race hygiene' of National Socialist Germany (Duster, 1990; Asch, 1999). A coercive programme that routinized antenatal screening could of course be avoided by not offering screening at all, leaving those who actively want it to seek it out. But this threatens the autonomy of those who would choose screening if only they knew about it (and perhaps if they could afford to pay for it). Emphasizing the importance of the personal views of pregnant women and avoiding institutional pressures to maximize the uptake of screening could in principle resolve

this tension. Other pressures would however remain. Pregnant women and their partners may regard the way in which society treats those with genetic disorders and other disabilities as a reason for not bringing an affected child into the world.

Those with family experience of a specific genetic disease often have first-hand experience of the life lived by an affected person and their family. Their views are likely to be grounded in lived reality, and the pregnant woman may decide to terminate an affected pregnancy so as to spare her child the suffering that she fears would be his or her lot or to spare her family the effects of life with an affected child. Others will not usually be so well informed, and may base their decisions on a fantasy image of a range of disorders. They will be influenced by their impressions of the behaviour of others towards those with mental and physical impairments in their local communities. Anticipation of the stigma experienced by affected individuals, the social discrimination encountered by many with disabilities and the unsatisfactory provision of health, social and educational support made available to individuals and families with genetic conditions inevitably influence individual decisions, whatever be the person's own values and the ethos of the institutional process.

UNANTICIPATED ANOMALIES

One important additional consequence of prenatal diagnosis generally, and especially prenatal screening programmes using foetal ultrasound anomaly scanning or chromosome analysis, is the detection or recognition of unanticipated anomalies (e.g. Turner syndrome or XYY syndrome). Such a finding – even if relatively minor or of little significance – must be disclosed, but it may cause much heartache, especially if there is real uncertainty about what it will mean for the future welfare of the child. The manner of disclosure may greatly influence the parents' response. The possibility of unanticipated findings should be explained in advance, so that the unanticipated result is less likely to induce an immediate, visceral response that forces a decision to terminate the pregnancy that will be regretted later, especially when the likely favourable outlook for an affected child subsequently comes to be appreciated. Some couples seek genetic counselling after a termination. How honest should the counsellor be when the condition would most likely have resulted in a generally healthy child requiring only modest medical intervention? Should the counsellor's compassion towards the grieving couple lead them to restrict or modify the information they give about the condition, in the hope that it will generate less guilt and remorse?

RESPECT FOR PEOPLE AND SELECTION AMONG EMBRYOS

One challenge to prenatal genetic screening programmes is that at least some people with genetic conditions are distressed by the very existence of prenatal screening programmes that intend to detect and then terminate pregnancies with *their* condition; they, and sometimes their families or carers, feel that they are being devalued. Another is that they aggravate the existing stigmatization and social discrimination through seeming to legitimize it, thereby making the lives of affected individuals even more difficult. These considerations should be taken into account when societies or health services consider what types of screening programme to introduce or maintain. Further, we need to reflect upon the differences between prenatal screening programmes 'for' Down syndrome and foetal sex selection. Our society's apparent wish to eradicate Down syndrome could be compared to the collective decision in some communities to value sons so much more highly than daughters.

These issues take on a somewhat different shape in the context of pre-implantation (or pre-gestational) genetic diagnosis, when they are uncomplicated by the issues around the termination of an established pregnancy and are considered elsewhere in this volume.

PREDICTIVE GENETIC TESTING

When a competent adult requests predictive genetic testing for a serious inherited disorder, genetic services would, in general, proceed to arrange the appropriate investigation as long as the diagnosis in the family could be confirmed, and the client and counsellor had together considered the range of possible consequences of a favourable result, an unfavourable result, an unclear result or a decision not to proceed with testing. To permit adequate time for counselling, it would usually be regarded as good professional practice to impose some delay before carrying out a genetic test, unless there are clear medical benefits to be gained from immediate testing. Even when testing has these clear benefits, for instance surveillance for tumours in adults at risk of an inherited form of cancer, it is usual to discuss the possible disadvantages of testing as well as explaining the anticipated benefits of testing. With an effectively untreatable disorder, such as Huntington's disease (HD) and other familial neurodegenerative conditions, there is usually a more detailed and extended counselling process with perhaps three or four appointments before the person at risk receives the test results. Professionals expect to cover a number of topics before going ahead with the testing, including an explanation of the range of possible test results, the likely impact of testing on the client and others, and issues of insurance and employment.

'Favourable' results can be difficult to live with, for instance, if other family members are given unfavourable results, or remain at high risk, because the client can feel that she or he does not deserve the good result or may now feel emotionally isolated from the rest of the family. Surveillance for tumours is often reassuring if the disorder in the family is a predisposition to cancer. Clients may be unwilling to discontinue surveillance even when it is no longer regarded by professionals as appropriate (Michie et al., 2003). Some effort must be made by counsellors to help the client to engage with their risk and to reflect upon how they (and those around them) might respond to a range of possible results – especially a favourable or an unfavourable test result, or the decision not to proceed with testing (Evers-Kiebooms et al., 2000; Sobel and Cowan, 2000). Some clients readily participate in such reflection at the suggestion of counsellors, others resist (McAllister, 2002; Sarangi et al., 2005). Experience shows that some of those initially most resistant to engagement in reflection are helped by it nonetheless – either deciding not to proceed with testing after all, or finding it a surprisingly useful preparation for their test results.

Some clients are helped by the courteous firmness with which the professionals resist their impatient insistence that a test be performed at once. Nevertheless, it is paternalistic for a professional not to comply with a request if a client makes it clear that they would prefer to go ahead without any of the associated counselling. There is a professional consensus that predictive genetic tests should be available only as part of a package along with the counselling, but not all agree. Others claim that genetics professionals are seeking to stake out a professional territory at the expense of the excessive medicalization and mystification of genetic knowledge.

It may be necessary to use samples or information from other family members in order to test the individual concerned. If the particular gene involved is unknown or is very difficult to test, linkage-based methods may be required that compare the at-risk individual's pattern of genetic markers to those of their family members. If the gene is known but the mutation present in the family is unknown, then it may help to identify the mutation in someone who definitely has (or had) the disorder. If this can be found, it becomes possible to look specifically for that in the at-risk person. Without access to such samples or such knowledge, the interpretation of test results in the at-risk person may be hampered. The person seeking testing has then to obtain consent for the professionals involved to access that person's medical records. The affected relative may have to undergo mutation testing, as is regularly the case in familial breast and ovarian cancer. Affected individuals, however, can be distressed by such a request because there may be important prognostic or emotional implications for them, which they would prefer to avoid (France et al., 1999). A woman with breast cancer, and in whom a BRCA1 gene mutation is found, is thereby identified as being at high risk of a second breast cancer and also perhaps of ovarian cancer. She may prefer not to be tested, while feeling an obligation to comply with the request for the sake of her family. This could be regarded as an unfair pressure to apply to a sick patient. Some think that the moral obligations a person feels to their kin is an unfair restriction on their autonomy; others that, because we live within a network of reciprocal relationships and mutual obligations, a person's autonomy cannot sensibly be considered as though they live in a social vacuum. However we resolve this, any request to perform genetic testing on a client's affected, and possibly sick, relative must be made gently and with respect, so that they are not too distressed by the process (Hallowell et al., 2003).

Sometimes, testing one willing family member almost inevitably affects other family members who are unwilling to be tested. For instance, if HD affected one's grandparent, one's own *a priori* chance of being affected is 1 in 4, but one's parent's is 1 in 2. If one is found to have the mutation that causes HD, then one's parent does too, something that they may prefer not to know. Is it justified to perform testing of those at 1 in 4 risk against the wishes of those with a 1 in 2 risk? Practice varies on this issue. Although all professionals should attempt to initiate a discussion within the family to resolve the difference, some would permit their client's interest in being tested to outweigh the contrary wishes of their parent if the differences were not resolved, especially if the client wanted to use the test result to make important reproductive decisions. In some circumstances, it might be helpful to use a linkage-based molecular exclusion test before performing a direct mutation test, as a way of involving the intervening parent and slowing the pace of testing to promote a more constructive, consensual resolution (Lindblad, 2001).

PRIVACY, CONFIDENTIALITY, DISCLOSURE

Respect for confidentiality in genetic services is as important as it is in any other health service. There are occasions, however, when professionals encourage clients to pass on information about their genetic constitution to members of their family. When a client fails to do so but the professionals think that the information is important and relevant to the relatives, then what sort of obligation does the professional have to the client's family? When might this override their obligation to respect the privacy of the original client?

In support of forcing disclosure, several commentators have suggested that genetic information does not belong to just one individual but to the whole family (Somerville and English, 1999; Parker and Lucassen, 2004). Such arguments can appear rather contrived, however, because information generated about one person may or may not be relevant to

any particular relative. We would be unlikely to know this in advance of testing the relative, and so the account begs the question of whether the information is in fact shared. Furthermore, to insist on the disclosure of genetic information within families may appear to be recommending a clear course of action, but we know from empirical data that it can be very difficult to track the flow of information within family networks, and that individuals may give much careful thought to whether they should pass information to specific relatives and sometimes conclude that they should not do so, at least at that time (Forrest et al., 2003; Featherstone et al., 2006). It can be difficult for professionals to challenge the reasoning employed by clients as they do not know the family members. Forcing disclosure can have unintended and unwelcome consequences and may not deliver the hoped-for benefits of an early diagnosis. In addition, there will be an impact on medical services in general and genetic services in particular as members of society – our fellow citizens – reassess their willingness to entrust sensitive personal information to their medical practitioners, once it becomes common knowledge that practitioners regularly do force the disclosure of personal information to other members of the family. The consequences of that shift in trust in the discretion of health professionals may be difficult to define and impossible to measure but need to be taken into account in setting a policy of forced disclosure.

Concern for genetic privacy also arises in relation to third parties, especially insurance companies and employers. This is not such an issue within the clinic, or between the individual practitioner and client, because confidentiality would almost always be respected in relation to third parties unless the clinician or counsellor had a clear legal duty to disclose information. In the United Kingdom, genetic counsellors would not pass on any personal information about a client to a third party without the client's (usually written) permission – except in the case of incapacity to drive – so the issues arise more at a general, societal level rather than within the clinic.

GENETIC TESTING OF CHILDREN AND ADOLESCENTS

Diagnostic genetic tests performed to establish the cause of a child's current health problems do not raise any very serious ethical issues, although the familial dimension of a genetic diagnosis may require great tact and sensitivity to avoid causing distress to a child and their parents. Equally, predictive genetic tests that will be useful in the medical management of a child are not especially problematic. Timing is more of an issue than whether or not to test. This is something to be settled between family and professionals in close co-operation and may differ substantially depending upon individual family circumstances.

The ethical issues that do arise in relation to the genetic testing of legal minors centre on predictive testing for late-onset genetic disease and testing to determine carrier status – of importance to children's future reproductive decisions but not usually their own health. These issues often arise in two quite different contexts. First, where parents, or those with parental responsibility, see testing as a means to help them discharge their duty of care towards the child, and perhaps to settle their own anxieties. Second, where older children wish to discover their genetic constitution, especially if this has implications for their future health or decisions about reproduction. Only the first set of issues will be considered further here; issues arising in the second context relate primarily to deciding when a young person is sufficiently mature to make important and irreversible decisions about genetic testing.

Many parents agree that testing for late-onset disorders should be left until the child can decide for him/herself. The issue then is when and how to introduce to the child the fact of their being at risk or, for carrier testing, the fact that they might be healthy carriers of the disorder present in the family. The grounds for deferring these decisions are three-fold: respecting the future autonomy of the child, preserving their future right to genetic privacy, and avoiding the potentially difficult or damaging emotional consequences of parents (or others) treating children differently because of their genetic test results. In effect, these three principles are weighed against the parental rights to make decisions for and about their children. There is no parental right to order genetic tests on a child, and in UK law, the best interests of the child have primacy. In many circumstances, genetic counsellors aim to persuade the parents to defer testing (Clinical Genetics Society Working Party, 1994); the child is not a property to be treated as the parent/owner thinks best. In the last resort, differences between parents and professionals could be decided in courts of law, but legal rulings have not yet clarified how professionals should approach disagreements in this area.

Where parents persist in requesting that a non-therapeutic predictive or genetic carrier test is performed, the professional's concern is to protect the child's future autonomy and privacy and to avoid any emotional problems from testing. This does not mean that parents do not have their child's interests at heart; they may intend to rear the child to cope better with the genetic issues that will face them in the future, or to be in a position to inform the child gently, in an age-appropriate fashion, or they may simply want to know so as to relieve their own anxiety and uncertainty. These concerns can be addressed by asking them to reflect upon how the knowledge will actually affect the child's rearing, to consider that *preparing* a child could actually be counter-productive – how do you *prepare* a child

to be ready to face the inevitable onset of HD considering that a clear majority of at-risk adults do not choose to have such tests?

In relation to carrier testing, the situation may differ between the two types of carrier status, autosomal recessive carriers, where a carrier will have affected children only if their partner is also a carrier, and sex-linked disorders and chromosomal rearrangements, where a carrier can have affected children irrespective of the genetic constitution of their partner. In the former case, the genetic constitution of the child's future partner is relevant, not in the latter. In either case, parents might wish to influence the child's whole attitude to the possibility of having genetically related children. This is an activity fraught with problems; indeed, parents' attempts to influence their children's decisions about partners and reproduction litter mythology, history and fiction and seem generally to be doomed to failure. Explicitly handing responsibility for such matters to an adolescent seems more likely to promote autonomy than trying to force a particular pattern of conduct. Moreover, a decision not to test a young child does not in any way prevent parents from talking about the situation with the child from a young age and in such a way as to help them make their own decisions about testing. The principal problem in these circumstances appears to be the reluctance of some parents to discuss the possibility of genetic disease with their children (e.g. Jarvinen et al., 1999).

Where parents persist in their desire for testing, a counselling-based approach may allow professionals to keep the relationship open with parents and to avoid taking an unhelpfully rigid, predetermined position (McConkie-Rosell and Spiridigliozzi, 2004).

Disorders in one child may provoke the decision to have diagnostic testing in future pregnancies. This may reveal the genetic carrier status of an unaffected foetus, and – if generated – this information would usually be passed to the parents. The parents, then, may know the carrier status of subsequent children but not of older children. They may request testing to clarify the situation for any older children, in part so as to ensure that the children are all treated in a similar fashion.

Similar anomalies in genetic services provision may be experienced by parents when newborn screening for cystic fibrosis (CF) or sickle cell disease (SCD) identifies a newborn infant as an unaffected carrier. Genetic counsellors will usually aim to defer such testing until the teenage years, but newborn screening (in the United Kingdom) sets out a programme of testing that will identify a small proportion of carriers for cystic fibrosis and effectively all carriers of sickle cell disease. The few CF carriers identified in this way can be regarded as an unintended but inevitable consequence of seeking to identify affected infants because, so far, the molecular genetic testing for affected infants is not sufficiently accurate to distinguish between a small number of affected and carrier infants without a physiological test (measurement of sweat electrolytes), so these few carriers are tested in case they might have been affected. For SCD, the situation is different: the technology used to screen infants is protein-based, looking to see if the HbS (sickle haemoglobin) molecule is present. Screening, therefore, identifies every carrier infant, who will have one copy of the HbS gene. If the health consequences of being a carrier are significant in the UK context, this may be justified – but if not, then the reasoning behind the active and universal disclosure to parents of HbS carrier status is flawed.

DYSMORPHOLOGY ASSESSMENT AND DIAGNOSTIC LABELS

The diagnostic assessment of patients with unusual physical features can cause profound disquiet or even humiliation in patients and their families. It must therefore always be conducted with great sensitivity and respect. To study a person's facial features for evidence of a genetic disorder can threaten identity and self-esteem.

There is an extensive literature about the social consequences of diagnostic labelling for disorders affecting physical or cognitive development, especially about the stigma that can be associated with genetic disease. The complex interplay between labelling and stigma can be appreciated if one considers the position of the parent of a child, whose disruptive behaviour attracts censure, drawing attention to his age and to how he ought to know better. If the child has dysmorphic features – that is, looks clearly 'different' so that he is readily recognized as having a medical condition – then the criticism may be reduced. Having a diagnostic label may also ward off criticism when the child has no dysmorphic features; it can also assist in gaining access to appropriate educational and social support, even though such services should be made available on the basis of need rather than label, and may facilitate membership of a support group.

A related matter is the coining of diagnostic labels for the new clinical entities. There have been a number of disorders where the name itself or an acronym can lead to social or emotional difficulties, such as LEOPARD syndrome, CATCH22 and DEFECT syndrome (Schrander-Stumpel, 1998). Given that affected patients and their families will have to live with these syndrome labels for decades, and will perhaps gain a good part of their sense of identity from them, they need to be chosen with care, consideration and respect. Furthermore, eponyms can also be inappropriate labels if the physicians so honoured in fact behaved in a profoundly unethical way (Harper, 1997).

CURRENT INSTITUTIONAL ISSUES

There are several ethical issues under active consideration by genetics professionals, and these can be outlined here in brief. One is the extent to which professionals are obliged to maintain contact with clients so as to provide updated information or to revisit diagnostic issues as new knowledge becomes available. Given the pace of advance within human and clinical genetics, this obligation – if it is regarded as an enforceable obligation – could make clinical work in genetics quite impractical (Hunter, 2001). Another approach to the continuing involvement of genetic services with specific families is the operation of genetic registers through a contract drawn up between the families involved and the services, with obligations on both sides including the requirement that families notify the services of important changes of circumstance and any change of address.

Genetic services do sometimes become involved in the provision of continuing care to their clients. In the United Kingdom, for example, some genetic services coordinate the provision of screening for tumours in those found to be at risk of complex, multi-organ cancer syndromes (e.g. von Hippel–Lindau disease). What is appropriate will depend upon local and historical factors – including what other health services are available – but it would clearly be impossible for specialist genetic services to take on the general medical care of all those with any inherited or genetic condition. The issue is one of where to draw lines within a given institutional framework.

CONCLUSION

We can see that genetic services operate within a socially and ethically complex set of tensions. There are competing demands on the professional – duties to the individual client, to whole categories of patients affected by genetic disorders, and to the institutional framework within which the genetic services are provided. This is always true of health services, but is true in a stronger sense in the context of genetics because there is so often a wider family dimension to be considered – the professional may feel obliged to other members of the family who are not present in the consultation (Parker and Lucassen, 2003). In addition, reproduction is involved, and this raises the issues of the termination of pregnancy and of selection (discrimination) between categories of person. As genetic knowledge and technology develop, the issues faced by families and professionals are continually changing. Furthermore, the intrusion of commerce into the client–professional relationship is also changing that relationship as families learn to gain access to services they want outwith the traditional pathways of clinical referral. Because of these continual changes, a stable, workable resolution of the various tensions has not been reached. This is an area to keep under frequent review: we anticipate that further challenges will arise as the knowledge base of human genetics develops over the coming decades.

REFERENCES

Armstrong D, Michie S, Marteau TM. Revealed identity: a study of the process of genetic counselling. *Soc Sci Med* 1998; **47**: 1653–1658.

Asch A. Prenatal diagnosis and selective abortion: a challenge to practice and policy. *Am J Public Health* 1999; **89**: 1649–1657.

Benkendorf JL, Prince MB, Rose MA, de Fina A, Hamilton HE. Does indirect speech promote nondirective genetic counselling? *Am J Med Genet* 2001; **106**: 199–207.

Clarke A. The process of genetic counselling: beyond nondirectiveness. In: Harper P, Clarke AJ, eds. *Genetics, Society and Clinical Practice*. Oxford: Bios Scientific Publishers, 1997a; pp. 179–200 (Chapter 13).

Clarke A. Prenatal genetic screening: paradigms and perspectives. In: Harper P, Clarke AJ, eds. *Genetics, Society and Clinical Practice*. Oxford: Bios Scientific Publishers, 1997b; pp. 119–140 (Chapter 9).

Clinical Genetics Society Working Party. Report on the genetic testing of children. *J Med Genet* 1994; **31**: 785–797 (and BSHG and CGS websites).

Duster T. *Backdoor to Eugenics*. London: Routledge, Chapman and Hall, 1990.

Elwyn G, Gray J, Clarke A. Shared decision making and non-directiveness in genetic counselling. *J Med Genet* 2000; **37**: 135–138.

Evers-Kiebooms G, Welkenhuysen M, Claes E, Decruyenaere M, Denayer L. The psychological complexity of predictive testing for late onset neurogenetic diseases and hereditary cancers: implications for multidisciplinary counselling and genetic education. *Soc Sci Med* 2000; **51**: 831–841.

Featherstone K, Bharadwaj A, Clarke A, Atkinson P. *Risky relations. Family and Kinship in the Era of New Genetics*. Oxford: Berg Publishers, 2006.

Forrest K, Simpson SA, Wilson BJ, van Teijlingen ER, McKee L, Haites N, Matthews E. To tell or not to tell: barriers and facilitators in family communication about genetic risk. *Clin Genet* 2003; **64**: 317–326.

France E, Gray J, Elwyn G, Tischkowitz M, Brain K, Sampson J, Anglim C, Clarke A, Parsons E, Sweetland H, Mansel R, Barrett-Lee P, Harper PS. Genetic testing considerations in breast cancer patients. *J Genet Counsel* 1999; **8**: 289–299.

Fraser FC. Genetic counselling. *Am J Hum Genet* 1974; **26**: 636–659.

Hallowell N, Foster C, Eeles R, Ardern-Jones A, Murday V, Watson M. Balancing autonomy and responsibility: the ethics of generating and disclosing genetic information. *J Med Ethics* 2003; **29**: 74–83.

Harper PS. Naming of syndromes and unethical activities: the case of Hallervordern and Spatz. *Lancet* 1996; **348**: 1224–1225. (See also Harper P, Clarke AJ. *Genetics, Society and Clinical Practice*. Oxford: Bios Scientific Publishers, 1997; pp. 221–5).

Hunter A, et al. Ethical, legal and practical concerns about recontacting patients to inform them of new information: the case in medical genetics. *Am J Med Genet* 2001; **103**: 265–276.

Jarvinen O, Aalto A-M, Lehesjoki A-E, Lindlof M, Soderling I, Uutela A, Kaariainen H. Carrier testing of children for two X-linked diseases in a family based setting: a retrospective long term psychosocial evaluation. *J Med Genet* 1999; **36**: 615–620.

Lindblad AN. To test or not to test: an ethical conflict with presymptomatic testing of individuals at 25% risk for Huntington's disorder. *Clin Genet* 2001; **60**: 442–446.

McAllister M. Predictive genetic testing and beyond: a theory of engagement. *J Health Psychol* 2002; **7**: 491–508.

McConkie-Rosell A, Spiridigliozzi GA. 'Family matters': a conceptual framework for genetic testing in children. *J Genet Counsel* 2004; **13**: 9–29.

Michie S, Smith JA, Senior V, Mareau TM. Understanding why negative genetic test results sometimes fail to reassure. *Am J Med Genet* 2003; **119A**: 340–347.

Müller-Hill B. *Murderous Science*. Oxford: Oxford University Press, 1988.

Parker M, Lucassen A. Concern for families and individuals in clinical genetics. *J Med Ethics* 2003; **29**: 70–73.

Parker M, Lucassen A. Genetic information: a joint account? *Brit Med J* 2004; **329**: 165–173.

Parsons EP, Clarke AJ, Hood K, Bradley DM, Feasibility of a change in service delivery: the case of optional newborn screening for Duchenne muscular dystrophy. *Community Genet* 2000; **3**(1): 17–23.

Quill TE, Cassel CK. Nonabandonment: a central obligation for physicians. *Ann Int Med* 1995; **122**: 368–374.

Sarangi S, Bennert K, Howell L, Clarke A, Harper P, Gray J. (Mis)alignments in counselling for Huntington's disease predictive testing: clients' responses to reflective frames. *J Genet Counsel* 2005; **14**: 29–42.

Schrander-Stumpel C. What's in a name? *Am J Med Genet* 1998; **79**: 228.

Sobel S, Cowan DB. Impact of genetic testing for Huntington disease on the family system. *Am J Med Genet* 2000; **90**: 49–59.

Somerville A, English V. Genetic privacy: orthodoxy or oxymoron? *J Med Ethics* 1999; 25: 144–150.

Weil J. Psychosocial genetic counselling in the post-nondirective era: a point of view. *J Genet Counsel* 2003; **12**: 199–211.

Williams C, Alderson P, Farsides B. Is non-directiveness possible within the context of antenatal screening and testing? *Soc Sci Med* 2002; **54**: 339–347.

Wolff G, Jung C. Nondirectiveness and genetic counseling. *J Genet Counsel* 1995; **4**: 3–25.

59

Ethics and Psychotherapy:
An Issue of Trust

TIM BOND

I have long been interested in how clients and therapists appear to approach the ethical basis of their work in different discourses. In my experience, clients tend to think of ethics as rooted in the character of the therapist as this character is communicated through the therapeutic relationship. If you ask clients what are the ethical factors they take into consideration in deciding whether or not to enter or continue therapy, they are most likely to raise the issue of trust and whether or not they perceive the therapist as trustworthy or untrustworthy. 'I want a therapist I can trust' is a typical response. Other characteristics such as competence, compassion and respectfulness are also frequently mentioned, but trust appears to be a critical issue and, where it is present, any deficiencies in other desirable ethical criteria may be ameliorated or overcome.

However, our clients' concern over trust is not matched by the degree of attention given to trust and being trustworthy in professional ethics written to support the practice of therapists, such as counsellors, psychotherapists, counselling psychologists and psychoanalysts. Trust is either completely omitted or considered too insignificant to be indexed (Francis, 1999; Gordon, 1999; Tjeltveit, 1999; McFarland and Twyman, 2003b). Where trust is considered only briefly, it is either as an ethical background against which to consider confidentiality and breach of sexual boundaries with clients (Corey et al., 2003) or is translated into a principle of fidelity, as a commitment to honour each other's promises (Thompson, 1990 ; Bond, 2000).

I have felt increasingly challenged by this neglect of trust as a potential point of ethical reference. It seems inconsistent with professional roles which justify their contribution to society on the basis of listening attentively to the communications of their clients and responding appropriately in terms which are meaningful and therapeutically productive for the client. What does this discrepancy in the ethical aspirations of clients and therapists indicate about the integrity of professions founded on listening and creating relationships based on mutual understanding?

For several years, the potential discrepancy between a client's instinctive approach to ethics and the rapidly developing professional ethics, to which I was a contributor, sat in the background as a low-grade but persistent irritant, soothed by cognitive dissonance. It nearly ignited into a point of active interest when I realized that it might provide a key to finding a seemingly elusive professional ethic across the cultural diversity of Europe (Bond, 1999), but was quelled by another project: the challenge of reviewing the ethical framework of one of the biggest professional bodies concerned with counselling and psychotherapy and the complexity of developing ethics to encompass the practice of over 20 000 practitioners in the increasingly diverse moral and cultural context of the United Kingdom (BACP, 2000). It was in the bicultural context of New Zealand that the potential of a relational ethic of trust became clearer to me.

I was to work with a distinguished Maori woman, an experienced counsellor and tribal elder. It was to be my first time working across the deeply bifurcated cultural divide between Maori and pakeha, and from the unfamiliar position of being pakeha. In my preparation I expected to be working across traditional and modern culture, tribally and individually focused ethics, different relationships to land and the historical struggles over that land, and completely different approaches to the purpose of life and the role of our respective ancestors. My familiar points of reference were stripped away, and all we had between us was the human relationship as a platform

Principles of Health Care Ethics, Second Edition   Edited by R.E. Ashcroft, A. Dawson, H. Draper and J.R. McMillan
© 2007 John Wiley & Sons, Ltd

on which we could build some mutual understanding and appreciation of what each of us brought to the relationship. Only trust seemed a common point of contact. I learnt so much from this experience as I observed my struggle to be trustworthy and moments when I became untrustworthy, largely through ignorance. Every aspect of my ethical landscape looked unfamiliar as I began my first steps in biculturalism.

When I returned to my more familiar English context, I realized that I had been deeply affected by the experience. The ethical potential for relational trust to bridge differences was at the forefront of my thinking and experience. I had also realized experientially for the first time a distinction between ethics which operated primarily unilaterally and bilaterally. When I had started my work as a counsellor and therapist in mental health services in the 1970s, the dominant ethic was paternalistic, a unilateral expectation that client's would trust you to use your power and expertise to their benefit. As paternalism fell into disrepute as an abuse of power, it was replaced with respect for client autonomy, which I embraced enthusiastically and worked on its application in counselling ethics in some detail: first as the only principle (Bond, 1993) and later as first amongst a set of equal principles (Bond, 2000). The unilateral flow of trust substantially switched to the other way round with the introduction of an ethic of respect for autonomy. The professional was increasingly expected to facilitate and trust clients to make decisions on their own behalf within an ethic of respect for client autonomy. As I reflected on the best and worst of my experiences in New Zealand with both Maori and pakeha colleagues, I began to appreciate the potential of bilateral trust as a bridge which could span substantial human differences.

I began to wonder if I had experienced an extreme example of how many clients might experience their encounter with an unfamiliar therapeutic culture and ethics. I started to glimpse how a relational ethic of trust might be highly relevant to therapy. I was encouraged by the Reith and Gifford Lectures by Onora O'Neill published in 2002 and her use of trust as a credible position from which to criticize an ethic of autonomy. My gloss on her detailed and tightly argued points was that mistrust is fundamentally a relational problem which requires a relational remedy. No amount of elaborating consent procedures, transparency, audit and extending bureaucracy could be a satisfactory substitute for attending to trust in the relationship between people (O'Neill, 2002a, 2002b).

AN ETHIC OF RELATIONAL TRUST

What is so daunting about trying to develop any ethic of trust is the loose and ill-defined way in which 'trust' is used in everyday speech. It can mean little more than a vague sense of a good feeling about someone or something. At the other end of the spectrum, it can represent a major commitment on which someone is prepared to risk his or her well-being or even life. As I listened to clients and therapists in many different circumstances talk about their experiences, I began to appreciate afresh that the major dangers in therapy arose from the sense of psychological intimacy and exposure between client and therapist in close-up relationship. The quality of the relationship had to be sufficient to withstand more than just bridging difference, which had been my preoccupation in New Zealand. Through a process of trial and error, which involved creating categories inductively and testing them abductively in practice, a definition of the key features of relational trust was constructed. *Trust is a relationship of sufficient quality and resilience to withstand the challenges arising from difference, inequality, risk and uncertainty.*

Trust is envisaged as a dynamic counterbalance between quality and resilience of relationship and potential threats to that relationship and, thus, to the individuals concerned. Difference and inequality are envisaged as primarily relational challenges. Risk and uncertainty are primarily existential but may be manifested relationally in therapy. I will elaborate each element of the definition in turn.

A RELATIONSHIP OF SUFFICIENT QUALITY . . .

There is currently a resurgence of interest in the contribution of relationship to therapy. Some of these are scientifically and empirically based (Norcross, 2002). Others have been inspired by the possibilities opened up by the development of post modern epistemologies in social sciences (Reason and Rowan, 1981; McLeod, 2001; Denzin and Lincoln, 2005) to enrich and challenge the prevailing realist approaches to therapy, which present the therapist as a technician making adjustments to the client's self-contained psychological system (Cornell and Hargaden, 2005). Yet others have drawn on the interplay between science and the humanities, particularly philosophy and literature, to examine the implications of relationship from fresh perspectives (Gordon, 1999).

One of the consequences of these new social science paradigms is that ethical issues are no longer necessarily the residues of issues for which there are no technical solutions. Instead, from a paradigmatically interpretivist view of knowledge and rationality, values inform all aspects of the therapy. Nothing is value-neutral. Ethics pervade all aspects of the therapeutic work and are therefore central to any consideration of what constitutes a relationship of sufficient quality. Thus, creating a relationship of sufficient quality to undertake the therapy becomes more than just a practical requirement to enable therapy to take place. It becomes an ethical aim for both therapist and client, which affirms the ethical significance of relationship for any vision of a good life. Attention to the relationship and its struggles with trust and mistrust in all its variations become an affirmation of what is meaningful in life.

. . . AND RESILIENCE . . .

One of the essential qualities of the relationship is its sustainability over time, at least for the duration of the therapy, and that it is of sufficient strength to withstand any turbulence and difficulty. It is conventional to represent therapy as heavily reliant on the person and personal resourcefulness of the therapist; however, this can be exaggerated as a form of heroic altruism to support the client's autonomy or healing. Instead, trust focuses attention on a two-way dynamics in which both contribute to the resilience.

With an inexperienced or troubled client, the greater responsibility rests with the therapist. The therapist's resilience acts like a metaphorical storm anchor to protect a boat which would otherwise drift into greater danger with the turbulence. By protecting the boat, the anchor protects both passengers: therapist and client. These observations tend to reinforce the widespread, but by no means universally accepted, requirement that trainee therapists are required to undergo therapy. An ethic of trust would not only support the existing justifications for trainees receiving therapy in order to develop insight into the client's experience and promote personal awareness to improve competence, but it would also extend the task of therapy for trainees to include a focused opportunity to examine and promote the resilience of the trainee to identify areas of vulnerability, consider any implications for becoming a therapist and promote strategies to promote a compassionate resilience. For example, many people who become therapists do so initially out of an interest stimulated by their own struggles in life. This can be a great source of insight and empathy, but unless it is examined it may lead to over-identification with clients facing similar difficulties. Over-identification may diminish the quality of listening as differences between the client's and therapist's experience are overlooked, or may create sufficient additional stress for the therapist so that there is heightened risk of burnout.

Resilience also directs attention to the types of support required to undertake this type of work. The significance of this has long been recognized with the almost universal requirement of regular and ongoing supervision or therapeutic consultation throughout the therapist's working life. Supervision is a form of non-managerial support, which addresses ethical dilemmas, provides informal training to extend competence and offers personal support. However, resilience is also enhanced by mobilizing other available sources of support in the working environment, such as belonging to a network of colleagues and being adequately resourced for the type of work undertaken. A great deal has been done in conventional ethics about the vulnerability of the client to the therapist, but the therapist is also vulnerable to secondary traumatization as a result of exposure in a psychologically intimate way to other people's distress and difficulties. It is one of the unavoidable personal costs of this area of work which can be greatly ameliorated and sometimes prevented by collegial support within relationships of sufficient strength and resilience to withstand the challenges associated with the type of work.

However, relational resilience does not just depend on the resourcefulness of the therapist. The reciprocal nature of trust also directs attention to the conditions the client require to sustain the relationship. For both, a dialogue may be the most trust-enhancing way of resolving ethical dilemmas which arise in the work. This is not a new idea. Thompson (1990) suggested a principle of fidelity in order to focus attention on the implicit and explicit promises involved in offering and receiving therapy. What is distinctive, from his approach, is the shift in focus towards the implications for trust in the therapeutic relationship and away from a quasi-contractual task of explicating the mutual promises offered to each other. An examination of the implied and explicit exchange of promises can all too easily become a means of apportioning risks and responsibilities to each other like a typical business contract. Instead, an ethic of relational trust would support considering how risks and responsibilities could be shared to the advantage of the relationship.

One of the unexpected findings from an abductive analysis of these ideas is the extent to which responsibility and energy for sustaining the relationship is shared between client and therapist: in particular, the number of times clients experience a sense of taking responsibility for sustaining the relationship. The energy to perpetuate the relationship flows back and forth between the client and therapist, much more than the conventional therapist-centred ethics would suggest. In some instances, the client has also taken the lead in re-establishing the ethical basis of the work when the therapist has acted unethically by, for example, breaching confidentiality or falling asleep. An ethic of trust values the client's contribution to the ethical dynamics much more than most therapist-centred approaches to ethics.

. . . TO WITHSTAND THE CHALLENGES . . .

The quality of the relationship needs to be disproportionately weighted in favour of 'sufficient quality and resilience' in order to withstand the challenges which will be encountered both from within the therapeutic relationship and externally, for example arising from adverse changes in the circumstances of either person. The obvious threats are events which arise outside the immediate relationship, for example one or other becoming ill, bereaved or other adverse circumstances. However, the less obvious threats are those which arise from within.

. . . ARISING FROM DIFFERENCE . . .

Difference between people poses significant challenges in human relationships in general. Gender, race, culture, ethnicity, sexuality, style of dress, physical size and hair colour are all examples of the myriad of differences which frequently carry significance in social settings and therefore may also become significant in the therapeutic relationship. Belonging and shared identity as a social unit are strongly associated with sameness. Differences set people apart from the group, especially in times of collective stress unless the group has the wisdom to recognize the ways in which differences can enrich and strengthen the resourcefulness of the group. Differences may elicit forceful responses to enforce conformity. Differences create the risk of prejudice and unfair treatment, bullying, rejection, or exclusion and abandonment. Differences are such a frequent cause of hurt that clients feel vulnerable and are justifiably fearful of revealing differences from the perceived social norm or from the norms communicated by the therapist. The psychological intimacy of the encounter increases the potential vulnerability to a negative reaction by the therapist.

The therapist also faces distinctive challenges to listen beyond his or her own life experience. These challenges are substantial when listening across obvious differences in experience, such as life stages, gender, ethnicity, culture or religion. It tests the therapist's knowledge, capacity to elicit relationship-forming information, curiosity and empathic imagination in order to form the basis for a therapeutic relationship in which the client feels sufficiently understood to want to undertake the challenges of change. Differences are a source of vulnerability for both client and therapist. Differences are capable of 'making a stranger' of others and hence creating a potential breakdown in trust and the viability of the relationship.

. . . INEQUALITY . . .

Within the therapeutic relationship, there are intrinsic and extrinsic sources of inequality. The extrinsic ones are unlikely to be resolved by therapy, certainly in the short term, or by therapy alone, but will be present as an influence on the dynamics of the relationship. These are inequalities arising from the social structure of society and the unequal distribution of power, status and personal achievement.

Class, wealth, education, occupation and other social factors are part of the daily realities for both the therapist and client outside the therapy room but are also likely to be present within it as part of the background against which the therapeutic relationship is formed. Sociological factors may pass unnoticed in a primarily psychological discourse, but they deserve attention because they carry the potential to support or undermine the relationship (Sennett, 2003), and may have complex and contradictory implications for trust. For example, a therapist may become so familiar with a power dynamic, which gives them the advantages of being a professional over their clients that they may be caught unawares when faced with a client from a more prestigious occupation or a public celebrity. Such unexpected encounters for most therapists may rekindle a conscious awareness of the challenges of creating a therapeutic relationship capable of overcoming differences in social standing with clients who are more or less powerful in society. A therapist's deference or over-assertiveness can be equally threatening to the development of a relationship of sufficient quality to support the work. A well-grounded respect is a much better basis for establishing the relationship.

Intrinsic to the therapeutic relationship are the inherent differences in status and power within the relationship between person seeking help and the person offering help. Typically, the therapist is credited with greater knowledge, expertise and being more 'healed' or psychologically healthier than the client who is disadvantaged by the vulnerability for which help is being sought. From the position of vulnerability the client may have a vested interest, at least initially, in amplifying and idealizing the characteristics of the therapist who carries power because the power differential carries with it the power to heal. Therapists work with these idealizations in many different ways. The popularity of the metaphor of the 'wounded healer' is partially inspired by some therapists' egalitarian instincts to redress the power imbalance by reducing the power differentials based on fantasies of what it means to be healthy.

One aspect of the therapeutic relationship leading to potential inequalities is the power of experience, *perezhivanie* (Mahn and John-Steiner, 2002). With all the power vectors usually favouring the therapist, a therapist's experience may tend to predominate and become the point of reference, although translated and subtly communicated. When experiential power flows from the therapist to the client, it carries the potential for healing and new learning. But the flow is not just one way. Experiential power, once engaged, is always reciprocal. The aims of therapy are that it should be beneficial, but one of the risks is that it can cause harm and traumatize the client or therapist.

. . . RISK . . .

The risks that are most frequently addressed in ethics are the breaches of boundaries concerning privacy, intimacy and restricted contact. The first two are particularly prominent in any approach to ethics because they are some of the most frequently raised issues in professional conduct or disciplinary proceedings. The third appears to be much more of an issue than may have been appreciated through the lens of other approaches to therapeutic ethics.

Confidentiality and privacy: A heightened concern over confidentiality and privacy is a distinctive preoccupation of therapists (Nash, 1996). We are aware that we are the recipients of personally sensitive information which could be deeply damaging to the social standing of our clients, if inappropriately disclosed. However, we are deeply divided in the approaches to confidentiality. For some, confidentiality is an essential and inviolable requirement for therapy to be possible. Others see it as secondary to primary ethical values of doing good and avoiding harm, which may justify overriding confidentiality in order to achieve a more pressing ethical commitment. These could include protecting the client from self-inflicted serious harm or preventing serious harm to others, such as a client intending to inflict abuse or assault and the protection of vulnerable others from harm by third parties such as child abuse by a client's relative. These variations in views about the boundaries between the private and public domains are also evident in the law, with different jurisdictions offering different levels of protection to confidences and imposing requirements to disclose confidences. Clients appear generally more sanguine about confidentiality and treat it as an issue of trust, which they can assume will be attended to by the therapist unless they have reason to believe otherwise. It may be that they are seduced into blind trust (a contradiction in terms) by the evident professional concern over confidentiality, but this has led some therapists to worry whether this trust is well placed (Bollas and Sundelson, 1995) and others to go to heroic lengths to protect confidentiality (Hayman, 2002).

Intimacy: Holmes and Lindley, in their contribution to the first edition of this volume, presented a systematic analysis of the perennial issue of psychological intimacy crossing over into sexual activity. The analysis was guided by the principle of autonomy, and on this issue there appears to be little to divide an ethic of autonomy from an ethic of trust. Trust has the merit of avoiding the paradoxical prohibition on consensual sex between adults by reference to their autonomy. It is much more straightforward to argue that sex with clients is wrong when considered against an ethic of trust. If someone enters therapy on the expectation that it will be psychologically intimate, but will be confined to this level of intimacy, it is a clear breach of trust to move the boundaries towards sexual activity. In addition, there is a reasonable expectation that the therapist ought to be able to withstand sexual advances and projections from clients. Whether approaching the issue of sex between clients and therapists from an ethic of autonomy, like Holmes and Lindley, or from an ethic of trust, the conclusions are much the same.

> There is a need therefore for a set of safeguards which are likely to ensure the ethical practice of psychotherapy. These include personal therapy for therapists, regular supervision for therapists at all levels and the organization of properly regulated psychotherapy profession. Such measures will not be watertight. Patients and therapists will occasionally fall in love, not always with disastrous results. No doubt, sexual and other forms of therapeutic exploitation will also continue despite all these measures, but at least they will ensure that an atmosphere of good practice prevails ... and that the public can have some legitimate confidence in a profession whose basis must always be that of a trusting and secure relationship (Holmes and Lindley, 1994, pp. 678–679).

Restricted contact: Most approaches to therapy are time-limited in terms of individual sessions and overall duration. Typically, there is an expectation that the therapeutic work will be confined to the sessions either by avoiding social contact outside the sessions or avoiding discussion of the work where social contact is permitted or unavoidable. This works well for most clients and therapists. However, I have heard anguished accounts from clients who hoped for lifelong friendship, which was not forthcoming from the therapist. I have also heard from therapists whose clients have resisted an appropriate containing or ending of the work and have been harassed or stalked by current and past clients. Some of these situations may be the result of poor practice by a therapist, but more often it appears to be the irrational and unconscious needs if one party has rendered them unable to remain trustworthy to the other. An analysis of the limitations on contact within therapy and its implications for trust reveals that this is ethically a much more complex issue than simply the therapist's responsibility to manage boundaries and to accomplish endings well.

Exposure to relational traits of the other: A major source of risk arising from the psychological intimacy is the exposure of one person to the relational traits of the other. These are often presented as unconscious transferences and countertransferences or as projective identification in the more psychodynamically oriented approaches to therapy. Some of the more optimistically inclined therapies encourage positive transferences, without necessarily using this terminology; for example, the core conditions of person-centred therapy or the relational background to a primary focus on problemsolving in solution-focused and cognitive therapies. No matter how the relationship is conceptualized, negative interactions will inevitably occur. The act of offering therapy creates an expectation that the therapist will be able to withstand a reasonable degree of negative relational dynamics from the client, perhaps evoked by a refusal to act in accordance with a client's projective identification (Cashdan, 1988), or the hostility evoked by a therapist's congruence (Mearns and Cooper, 2005). However, both people are vulnerable to each other's unconscious sadism (perhaps evoked by an alarm at the psychological threat posed by the other), narcissism (the need to elicit positive self-affirmation through the good opinion of the other) and the potential to over-identify with the other so that subjective identities homogenize unhelpfully or to under-identify with the other so that there is no imaginative reaching out to understand the other's subjective experience (McFarland and Twyman, 2003). Therapists are humans and most of us will have caught ourselves in counterproductive psychological relationships with clients: if not in the moment that it occurs in therapy, then later in the opportunity for self-reflection provided by supervision. The ethic of relational trust accepts that there will be moments of counterproductive dynamics, but invites us to redress the relationship in order to bring it back within its therapeutic purpose.

Paradoxically, after pointing out many dangers associated with risk, an ethic of trust also requires appropriate risk-taking. The alternative would be to offer false reassurance or to collude with a client's problematic patterns from which the client wants relief. Risk-taking by both therapist and client is an essential aspect of personal change. Over-anxious risk avoidance can be as damaging to the therapy as excessive risk-taking. This is a different approach to risk from that usually adopted in clinical governance, where risks are invariably negative and only justifiable if they are minimized and outweighed by the sufficiently probable benefits. An ethic of trust challenges us to consider how compatible the risk-taking is with the relationship which has formed in dialogue with the client, as an alternative to being over-reliant on formal consent procedures. An ethic or trust requires the following:

- engaging in dialogue and evaluation, openly and non-defensively, with the client and probably a supervisor, which strives for mutual agreement over risk-taking;
- being aware that a risk has been taken;
- carefully observing the consequences, evocatively phrased as 'exquisite curiosity' (Eusden, 2005) or 'respectful attentiveness' (Gordon, 1999);
- offering a relational remedy for any unwanted effects and substituting or reframing the intervention according to the therapeutic circumstances;
- avoiding becoming defensive or switching to a shame-based response by asserting authority over the client or making accusations about the client's complicity or inadequacy;
- sustaining the therapeutic flow in dialogue with the client;

- maintaining heightened ethical awareness and engagement throughout.

Risks do not become unethical merely because they produced unwanted results. They become unethical because of a lack of awareness that they have been experienced as counterproductive, persistently reinforced or even compounded by further mistakes. It is persisting with a mistake regardless of the therapeutic and relational consequences which creates the conditions for a breakdown of trust.

. . . AND UNCERTAINTY . . .

Therapy is both science and art. An overemphasis on the scientific dimensions may be good for professional status and may comfort the therapist's omnipotence or the client's idealization of the therapist's powers. Science is the discourse of high status and control. But over-reliance on science alone is at the price of underestimating the opportunities which arise from unpredictable nature of a creatively unfolding process which involves two (or more) people reflexively responding to one another in a flow of communications, each in turn adjusting to the preceding communication. Current therapeutic knowledge exists in both scientific and creative domains. Perhaps, the greatest challenge for any therapist is finding knowledge which is applicable to a particular client. An ethic of trust challenges the automatic application of well-validated scientific knowledge or a highly persuasive creative insight from the humanities to a particular person without critically evaluating its applicability. Good therapists are well versed in generalizable insights and are skilled in the use of appropriate rationality (Habermas, 1986) and in the conversions required to meet the needs of a particular person.

Excessive uncertainty avoidance can be just as damaging to trust as exaggerating the levels of uncertainty. One form of uncertainty avoidance reported by both therapists and clients is the way in which the therapist's excessive fear of an external authority, whether in the abstract form of the law or the authority of a specific person, perhaps a trainer, supervisor or manager, can frustrate the development of trust or destroy the trust which is already established. The client senses the switch of attention to an external authority, and the therapist's fear creates a corresponding fear of being betrayed because of the therapist's apparent powerlessness. The therapy room is not hermetically sealed from all external forces, but how these are managed can be critical to trust. One of the unresolved puzzles from this work so far is why does one therapist make a successful referral to an outside agency and sustain the client's trust whilst another loses it, in seemingly similar circumstances and responding to similar constraints on confidentiality, concerning child protection?

AN ETHIC OF TRUST: STRENGTHS AND LIMITATIONS

The distinctive strength of an ethic of relational trust is the way it directs attention to the embodied and reciprocal relationship between two people. It is a situational ethic which sits closer to the client's concerns and language than some other approaches to ethics. This increases the potential for resolving ethical dilemmas bilaterally and dialogically and in ways that are more congruent with a professional role which is so dependent on listening attentively.

Like utilitarian and deontological ethics, an ethic of trust has limitations in its application.

An ethic of trust is a form of virtue ethic but with a relational twist so that the point of reference is not an individual's character considered in isolation, but lies in the relationship between the characters of two or more people. The philosophical roots are primarily Buber and Levinas, although not exactly mapping onto either.

The aim of this exploration of the application of an ethic of trust in psychotherapy is to expand the range of ethical perspectives and awareness available to the therapist, which supplements the talionic rules of professional bodies as part of their disciplinary procedures and looks beyond the unilateral application of principles, currently characteristic of westernized professional ethics. Each of these discourses serves important functions but, even in combination, fails to give sufficient weight to the ethical significance of the relational context and dynamics of therapy. An ethic of trust provides a distinctive lens through which to view the bilateral dynamics of therapy in which being in relationship is both the source of ethical meaning and the context from which the evaluative function of ethics arises. In this sense it is an intrinsic ethic. Although inspired in circumstances where there appeared to be an absence of extrinsic points of reference because of the depth of cultural difference, thus leaving only relationship as a point of contact, an ethic of trust is enriched in counterpoint to other ethical discourses:

'A meaning only reveals its depths once it has encountered and come into contact with another, foreign meaning . . . such a dialogic encounter of two cultures does not result in merging or mixing. Each retains it own unity and open totality, but they are mutually enriched' (Bakhtin, 1986, p. 7).

This is work in progress. One of the next stages in the development of this ethic will be to pay more attention to the double dynamics of trust than I have been able to here. The intrinsic dynamics between balancing the quality of relationship and danger is becoming clearer. There are comparable limitations to deontological and utilitarian ethics, where respecting an ethic of trust would lead to serious harm to another or significant disruption of their entitlement to trusting relationships, for example where a client is using therapy to gain the courage to exact physical revenge on a former partner in an acrimonious separation. The failure to offer to others what clients expect for themselves undermines the integrity of the relationship, and as a consequence, the protection of a vulnerable other from an identified substantial risk may take priority over keeping trust with a client, if the threat cannot be resolved in any other way. A more equivocal situation arises where the client is contemplating an action which will cause significant unhappiness to others, perhaps by leaving an established relationship. This is just the sort of issue which may be ethically deepened by a dialogue in which both client and therapist examine the implications for their individual and relational integrity. Although the primary focus is likely to be on the client's sense of integrity, there may be implications for the therapeutic relationship and the therapist's integrity. Listening is seldom neutral and there is much more to be said about the ethics of listening (Todd, 2003). However, there is a second dynamic, which also deserves attention. O'Neill identifies this dynamic as the Cassandra Problem (O'Neill, 2002a). Merely being attentive to issues of trust and being trustworthy does not guarantee that someone will be trusted. It is possible to be trustworthy and not trusted or more dangerously to be untrustworthy and trusted. Not only is this relevant to therapy but the relational insights of therapy may also help to cast new light on a long-standing ethical conundrum.

REFERENCES

BACP. *Ethical Framework for Good Practice in Counselling and Psychotherapy.* Rugby: British Association for Counselling and Psychotherapy, 2000.

Bakhtin MM. Response to a question from *Novy Mir* editorial staff. In: Emerson C, Holquist M, eds. *Speech Genres and Other Late Essays* (Translated by McGee VW). Austin, TX: University of Texas Press, 1986; pp. 1–7.

Bollas C, Sundelson D. *The New Informants: Betrayal of Confidentiality in Psychoanalysis and Psychotherapy.* London: Karnac Books, 1995.

Bond T. One size fits all? The quest for a European ethic for counselling and psychotherapy. *Eur J Psychother Counsel Health* 1999; **2**(3): 375–388.

Bond T. *Standards and Ethics for Counselling in Action.* London: Sage, 1993.

Bond T. *Standards and Ethics for Counselling in Action*, 2nd edition. London: Sage, 2000.

Cashdan S. *Object Relations Therapy: Using the Relationship.* New York: Norton, 1988.

Corey G, Corey MS, Callanan P. *Issues and Ethics in the Helping Professions*, 6th edition. Pacific Grove, CA: Brooks/Cole, 2003.

Cornell WF, Hargaden H, eds. *From Transactions to Relations: The Emergence of a Relational Tradition in Transactional Analysis.* Chadlington: Haddon Press, 2005.

Denzin NK, Lincoln YS. *Handbook of Qualitative Research*, 3rd edition. Thousand Oaks, CA: Sage, 2005.

Eusden S. *When Does a Mistake Become Unethical?* Personal communication, 2 July, 2005.

Francis R D. *Ethics for Psychologists: a Handbook*, Lerusters British Psychological Society, 1999.

Gordon P. *Face to Face: Therapy as Ethics.* London: Constable, 1999.

Habermas J. *Knowledge and Human Interest* (Translated by Shapiro JJ). Oxford: Polity Press, 1986.

Hayman A. Psychoanalyst subpoenaed. In: Jenkins P, ed. *Legal Issues in Counselling and Psychotherapy.* London: Sage, 2002; pp. 21–23.

Holmes J, Lindley R. Ethics and psychotherapy. In: Gillon R, ed. *Principles of Health Care Ethics.* Chichester: John Wiley & Sons, Ltd, 1994; pp. 671–680.

Mahn H, John-Steiner V. The gift of confidence: a Vygotskian view of emotions. In: Wells G, Claxton G, eds. *Learning for Life in the 21st Century.* Oxford : Blackwell, 2002; pp. 46–58.

McFarland Solomon H, Twyman M. Introduction: the ethical attitude in analytic practice. In: McFarland Solomon H, Twyman M, eds. *The Ethical Attitude in Analytic Practice.* London: Free Association Press, 2003a; pp. 3–12.

McFarland Solomon H, Twyman M, eds. *The Ethical Attitude in Analytic Practice.* London: Free Association Books, 2003b.

McLeod J. *Qualitative Research in Counselling and Psychotherapy.* London: Sage, 2001.

Mearns D, Cooper M. *Working at Relational Depth in Counselling and Psychotherapy.* London: Sage, 2005.

Nash RJ. *'Real World' Ethics: Frameworks for Educators and Human Services Professionals.* New York: Teachers College Press, 2002.

Norcross JC, ed. *Psychotherapy Relationships which Work: Therapist Contributions and Responsiveness to Patients.* New York: Oxford University Press, 2002.

O'Neill O. *Autonomy and Trust in Bioethics.* Cambridge: Cambridge University Press, 2002a.

O'Neill O. *A Question of Trust.* Cambridge: Cambridge University Press, 2002b.

Reason P, Rowan J, eds. *Human Inquiry: a Sourcebook of New Paradigm Research.* Chichester: John Wiley & Sons, Ltd, 1981.

Sennett R. *Respect: the Formation of Character in a World of Inequality.* London: Allen Lane, 2003.

Thompson A. *Guide to Ethical Practice in Psychotherapy.* New York: John Wiley & Sons, Ltd. 1990.

Tjeltveit AC. *Ethics and Values in Psychotherapy.* London: Routledge, 1999.

Todd S. *Learning from the Other: Levinas, Psychoanalysis and Ethical Possibilities in Education.* Albany, NY: State University of New York Press, 2003.

60

Mental Illness and Compulsory Treatment

JOHN R. MCMILLAN

In Chapter 61, Matt Matravers discusses the arguments surrounding compulsory detention for those with personality disorders. Attempts to justify preventative detention emphasize the importance of preventing risk to the public. Although 'harm to self' is not particularly relevant to whether or not preventative detention can be justified, it is the most important and keenly debated justification for the compulsory treatment of those with mental illness. There are a number of possible positions, ranging from those who think that the possibility of somebody benefiting is usually sufficient for coercive treatment to 'abolitionists' or those who think that compulsory treatment can never be justified. The first half of this chapter will outline these positions, and the second half will show how both of them neglect the appropriate justification of compulsory treatment. This chapter will argue that the significant degree of non-voluntariness that mental illness can cause, coupled with the risk of a serious harm (for example, attempting suicide), provide a justification for compulsory treatment in some cases.

MENTAL HEALTH LEGISLATION

In most liberal democracies adults are legally permitted to refuse medical treatment even when a physician believes that treatment is clearly in that person's interests. This principle applies even in cases where a refusal of treatment might risk the death of that patient. In effect, mental health legislation provides the means by which people who are mentally unwell might lose this right to refuse treatment.

Although there are some important differences between mental health acts in different jurisdictions, they tend to have some common features. In general, they all attempt to define a reference class for 'mental disorder', 'mental illness' or some other equivalent concept. There are a number of legislative options when doing this and they can have

important implications for whether a person can be treated against their will (see Dawson, 1996).

Mental illness itself is rarely thought to be a sufficient condition for compulsory treatment. Legislation usually also requires that in addition to fitting one of the prescribed classes of mental illness, this person must also be at a serious danger to themselves or other people (Bartlett and Sandland, 2003).

There are a number of other common legislative conditions that are likely to make a moral difference to the acceptability of compulsory treatment. In England and Wales, it is a requirement that a viable therapy is available before someone is compulsorily detained and treated (Bartlett and Sandland, 2003). The rationale for this is sensible and fairly clear: unless a person can actually be provided with a clinical benefit, compulsory treatment ceases to be treatment at all and compulsory treatment becomes another form of preventative detention.

Even though there is a significant amount of legislative concordance about the preconditions for compulsory treatment, there is still a significant disagreement about whether the law is justified or whether it is restrictive enough.

Matravers mentions some of the ways in which definitions of mental disorder have been used and manipulated to achieve other social or political ends. There are clear-cut examples of the political abuse of 'mental illness' such as the 'treatment' of political dissidents in the USSR. However, according to antipsychiatrists this abuse is much more widespread, and the concept of 'mental illness' is necessarily linked to political or social ends in a much more general way.

ANTIPSYCHIATRY

For some time now I have maintained that commitment – that is, the detention of persons in mental institutions against their will – is a form of imprisonment; that such deprivation of liberty is contrary to the moral principles embodied in the Declaration of Independence and the Constitution of the United States; and that it is a crass violation of contemporary concepts of fundamental human rights. The practice of 'sane' men incarcerating their 'insane' fellow men in 'mental hospitals' can be compared to that of white men enslaving black men. In short, I consider commitment a crime against humanity (Szasz, 1998, p. 299).

Thomas Szasz is probably the most ardent and consistent critic of compulsory treatment for mental illness. In his view the wrongness of compulsorily treating the mentally ill is on a par with slavery, a serious criticism indeed if true. Peter Singer's (1995) comparison of our treatment of animals to our past treatment of people with different coloured skin demands that we consider whether we are in fact justified in eating animals and using them in research. Szasz is making a similar analogy: there is nothing morally different between slavery and compulsory treatment; everyone believes the former to be wrong so the latter must be too. Eating animals and using them in research is easy for us and, according to Singer, the ease with which we use them has blinded us to the fact that we are acting wrongly. Likewise, the social function that compulsory treatment serves, according Szasz, blinds us to the absence of a sound justification.

One obvious response is to insist that slavery and compulsory treatment are disanalogous because slavery necessarily involves the exploitation of slaves for the benefit of their masters whereas compulsory treatment can aim at benefiting or avoiding harm to the mentally unwell person. The paradigmatic example of this is the compulsory treatment and hospitalization of those who are at risk of self-harm. Arguably the worst form of self-harm, and one which is all too common amongst those with mental illness, is suicide. However, Szasz thinks that compulsory treatment cannot be justified even when it aims at preventing suicide.

ANTIPSYCHIATRY AND SUICIDE

There are interesting arguments for and against the permissibility of suicide. Hume argued that suicide should be permissible and even praiseworthy in some instances (Hume, 1985). Hume considers whether suicide might violate a duty to God, neighbour or self and denies the existence of any such duty. Although Szasz does not consider the question of whether suicide is wrong or a duty, he does believe that there is a fundamental right to commit suicide and that psychiatrists violate it.

The right to kill oneself is the supreme symbol of personal autonomy . . . Now, psychiatry, as an arm of the state, prohibits the act and 'treats' it as if it were a symptom of an underlying disease (typically, depression or schizophrenia). The deprivation of liberty intrinsic to such an intervention is viewed not as human rights violation but as a human rights protection (Szasz, 2003, p. 228).

Szasz appears to derive the right to commit suicide from respect for autonomy. More needs to be said about this: does not intervening when a person is about to commit suicide respect that person's autonomy? According to Kant, suicide necessarily involves a failure to respect autonomy. He famously argued that

someone who has suicide in mind will ask himself whether his action can be consistent with the idea of humanity as an end in itself. If he destroys himself in order to escape from a trying condition, he makes use of a person merely as a means to maintain a tolerable condition up to the end of life. A human being, however, is not a thing and hence not something that that can be used merely as a means, but must in all his actions always be regarded as an end in itself (Kant, 1997, p. 38).

For Kant, suicide not only involves an agent failing to respect themselves as an agent but is also an intrinsically irrational act. We might consider Kant's views on the matter to be slightly out of step with what most people believe about suicide now. Nonetheless, it is important to bear in mind that for Kant's classic defence for autonomy, the rationality of a rational will is what grounds the importance of respect for autonomy. Although we might not agree with Kant's claim that suicide is always irrational, the claim that an irrational suicide fails to respect autonomy is very plausible. One influential study showed that 90% of those attempting suicide were suffering from some form of mental illness at that time (Beautrais et al., 1996). It does not follow from the fact the person has a mental illness that he or she is irrational, nor does it follow from the fact that a person has a mental illness that a suicide attempt is irrational. However, mental illnesses frequently impair or alter the rationality of the person afflicted. Although we might disagree with Kant that suicide is intrinsically irrational, we might agree with him that significantly irrational actions that lead to great harm should not be considered as supreme expressions of autonomy (McMillan, 2003).

This worry is perhaps even more significant when we consider what a Millian should say about suicide prevention and mental illness. Mill claimed that the only kind of case where it is acceptable to limit the liberty of an individual is when harm might be caused to another person by that liberty being exercised. Mill goes on to state that the welfare of that individual is not a sufficient warrant for limiting liberty (Mill, 1998). So far so good, this sounds like a strong argument in favour of a right to commit suicide. The problem is that Mill goes on to say that a full set of liberties should only be granted to

human beings in the maturity of their faculties. We are not speaking of children, or of young persons below the age which the law may fix as that of manhood or womanhood. Those who are still in a state to require being taken care of by others must be protected against their own actions as well as against external injury (Mill, 1998, p. 14).

Of course, many suicidal, mentally unwell people are adults and ordinarily possess 'mature faculties': Mill is primarily referring to children. Nonetheless, Mill's point is a deeper one; the reason why children should not be extended a full set of liberties is because they have not developed the capacity to judge what is likely to be in their interests. In the case of a person who has temporarily lost the ability to make sound decisions about their own interests, there is a Millian justification for not extending a full system of liberties. Szasz might respond that there is a difference between children, who have not yet developed the capacity to make important decisions about their interests and mentally unwell adults who may have this capacity, yet are unable to exercise it because of mental illness. This would not be an adequate response. In the case of those who are temporarily unable to judge their interests, we might be warranted in temporarily restricting their right of self-determination. If a child is particularly mature and is in fact a very good judge of their interests, failing to respect their wishes might be legally permissible but is, from a moral point of view, on a much shakier footing.

This is significant for Szasz because he cites Mill's *On the Subjection of Women* with enthusiasm (Szasz, 2003). He suggests that the mentally unwell are discriminated against in much the same way as women. Moreover, Szasz is a libertarian and seems to take Mill's version of this doctrine as his motivation.

THE MYTH OF MENTAL ILLNESS

Although Szasz is a political libertarian (someone who believes in the minimal state), this is not an essential feature of antipsychiatry. Although many of the other people described as antipsychiatrists, such as Cooper (1970) and Laing (1960) do argue for freedom from traditional psychiatry, they should not be described as libertarians in the same sense as Szasz. The feature common to all of these versions of antipsychiatry is the belief that mental illness is not a real disease entity and serves other social functions:

> Mental illness, of course, is not literally a 'thing' – or physical object – and hence it can 'exist' only in the same sort of way in which other theoretical concepts exist. Yet, familiar theories are in the habit of posing, sooner or later – at least to those who come to believe in them – as 'objective truths' ('or facts'). During certain historical periods, explanatory conceptions such as deities, witches and micro organisms appeared not only as theories but as self evident causes of a vast number of events. I submit that today mental illness is widely regarded in a somewhat similar fashion, that is, as the cause of innumerable diverse happenings (Szasz, 1961, p. 104).

The claim here is simply that mental illness is an explanatory concept in much the same way as 'electron' or 'phlogiston' are. Although we have a number of reasons for continuing to believe in the electron, at least as a theoretical concept, the theory, predictions and assumptions that are essential to phlogiston mean that we should ditch this explanatory concept. Szasz is saying that 'mental illness' also has an important explanatory role, but that instead of looking for a disease entity we discover this role by looking at how it actually functions as an explanation. This move is common to most forms of antipsychiatry: they tend to believe that we need to examine the assumptions and social functions that 'mental illness' serves.

> In actual contemporary social usage, the finding of a mental illness is made by establishing a deviance in behaviour from certain psychosocial, ethical or legal norms. The judgment may be made, as in medicine, by the patient, the physician (psychiatrist) or others. Remedial action, finally, tends to be sought in a therapeutic – or covertly medical – framework, thus creating a situation in which psychosocial, ethical and/or legal deviations are claimed to be correctible by (so-called) medical action (Szasz, 1961, p. 105).

It is important to bear in mind that Szasz and the other antipsychiatrists do not deny that mental illness exists, in the way that phlogiston does not exist. Instead, they claim that 'mental illness' masquerades as a natural kind or scientific concept when it is not. At the heart of antipsychiatry is the view that psychiatry is not concerned with genuine disease entities but rather concerns itself with what can be called 'problems in living'. Essentially, 'mental illness' is a concept that attempts to legitimize 'treatment' aimed at correcting what are behavioural deviations.

There are a number of positions on the concept of mental illness. There are connections between the debate about 'mental illness' and the broader debate about the concept of disease (for more on the concept of disease see Lennart Nordenfelt in Chapter 73 of this volume). If there is no viable account of 'disease' that puts it on a par with other natural kind terms, then there is not much hope for a scientifically robust account of mental illness.

The debate about compulsory treatment has given a significant amount of weight in the debate about whether or not mental illness demarcates genuine disease entities, but, as will be argued, the relevance of this debate is not as obvious as it might first appear.

Abolitionists, like Szasz, think that compulsory treatment for mental illness can never be justified so compulsory treatment should be abolished.

It is important to distinguish abolitionism from antipsychiatry. Although it is the case that antipsychiatrists are the most important antagonists in the debate about compulsory treatment, it is possible to believe in abolitionism but not antipsychiatry, that is you might not only think that there is never an adequate defence for forcing treatment upon someone but also believe that mental illnesses are real disease entities (see Morse, 1982).

It is also possible to think that antipsychiatry is true and that abolitionism is false. It might be that you think that mental illness is not a real disease entity and does tend to function as a way of correcting deviancy, while also arguing that there are some cases where it is still justified to treat a person against their will. The truth or falsity of antipsychiatry might be interestingly independent of the truth of abolitionism.

The abolitionists can be contrasted with what Chodoff calls the 'medical model psychiatrists' (Chodoff, 1998; Peele and Chodoff, 1999).

THE MEDICAL MODEL PSYCHIATRISTS

Although most mental health acts will set a fairly high standard of risk to self before permitting compulsory treatment, there are some interesting arguments in favour of a more permissive view. Chodoff gives the following case by way of illustration:

> A man with a history of alcoholism has been on a binge for several weeks. He remains at home doing little else than drinking. He eats very little. He becomes tremulous and misinterprets spots on the wall as animals about to attack him, and he complains of 'creeping' sensations in his body, which he attributes to infestation by insects. He does not seek help voluntarily, insists there is nothing wrong with him, and despite his wife's entreaties he continues to drink (Chodoff, 1998, p. 288).

Although it seems likely that this man is mentally unwell, there is nothing in this story to suggest that he is about to cause himself serious harm or to attempt suicide. It is likely that for many mental health acts his excessive drinking and poor eating are not sufficiently serious for him to be treated against his will. A 'Medical Model Psychiatrist' is likely to think that in this case there are good reasons for forcing treatment upon him, if this is necessary to treat him. Chodoff believes that

> mental illness is a meaningful concept and that under certain conditions its existence justifies the state's exercise, under the doctrine of parens patriae, of its right and obligation to arrange for the hospitalization of the sick individual even though coercion is involved and he is deprived of his liberty' (Chodoff, 1998, p. 290)

Like Szasz, Chodoff thinks that the status of mental illness as a disease plays an important role in the justification of compulsory treatment. He thinks that the concept of disease should not be restricted to organic disease but should also include

being negatively valued by society, by 'nonvoluntariness,' thus exempting its exemplars from blame, and by the understanding that physicians are the technically competent experts to deal with its effects (Chodoff, 1998, p. 291).

This seems like rather a lot to pack into a concept of disease and cannot be an adequate account of 'mental illness'. One problem is that it is possible for people to be mentally unwell yet still be deemed capable of voluntary action. An important English legal case is in *Re C*, in which a man was judged competent to refuse the amputation of his leg even though he suffered from chronic paranoid schizophrenia and believed that he was a world famous surgeon (*Re C*, 1994). Furthermore, it is hard to see why being 'negatively valued by society' should be a part of the concept. Although having a mental illness is, in general, a bad thing for the person concerned, in some cases, mental illness can provide the impetus for creative expression. Many famous artists and musicians have suffered from mental illness and in some cases, Van Gogh being a particularly good example, their art is inextricably linked to their mental illness. In these cases perhaps mental illness should not be negatively valued.

Even though Chodoff is wrong to identify mental illness with responsibility and being negatively valued by society, he is right that there is an important connection between the justification for compulsory treatment and the moral responsibility of the mentally unwell. Chodoff suggests that one necessary condition for involuntary hospitalization is that there is an 'impairment of the patient's judgment to such a degree that he is unable to consider his condition and make decisions about it in his own interests' (Chodoff, 1998, p. 292). It might be that this condition is sufficient for compulsory treatment when there is a good reason for supposing that it will be in that patient's interests.

COMPULSORY TREATMENT: JUSTIFIED PATERNALISM?

As was mentioned earlier in this chapter, Mill thinks that we are justified in not extending a full set of liberties to those who are at risk of compromising their own good when there is a question mark over the 'maturity of their faculties'. However, more needs to be said about how this can provide a defence of compulsory treatment for mental illness.

If there is an adequate justification of compulsory treatment for the purpose of preventing harm to self then this is a justification for a kind of paternalism: paternalism necessarily involves acting on behalf of another person to further the good of that person or others. There are many forms of paternalism (for an excellent overview see James Childress' Chapter 29 in this volume). The most important distinction is between hard and soft paternalism. Hard paternalism usually 'involves interventions intended to benefit a person despite the fact that the person's risky choices and actions are informed, voluntary, and autonomous' (Beauchamp and Childress, 1994, p. 277). Clearly, paternalism of this kind is likely to be morally problematic given the way that it runs roughshod over the autonomous wishes of an agent. This is clearly in contrast with soft paternalism where

> an agent intervenes on grounds of beneficence or nonmaleficence only to prevent substantially nonvoluntary conduct – that is, to protect persons against their own substantially nonautonomous action(s) (Beauchamp and Childress, 1994, p. 277).

This version of paternalism is much less problematic, if it is problematic at all. In cases where a person is acting in a substantially non-voluntary way, it is arguable whether they are performing their own actions at all. If mental illness causes non-voluntary conduct, then there might be a soft paternalist justification for compulsory treatment. Note that this justification does not rely upon the presence of a 'mental illness' and *a fortiori* nor does it rely upon the reality of 'mental illness' as a disease entity. The relevant moral and jurisprudential category is non-voluntariness, and mental illness is only relevant insofar as it is one of a number of possible causes of this.

Although this might appear to provide an adequate justification, it still remains to be shown that the right degree and kind of non-voluntariness is present in those who are likely to be compulsorily treated. Feinberg distinguishes actions that are 'fully voluntary, involuntary and nonvoluntary' (Feinberg, 1986, p. 104). Fully voluntary actions are those performed by adults in 'full control of their deliberative faculties'. Involuntary actions are those which are clearly not causally related to the agency of that person, or as Feinberg says those that do not involve

> choice at all, properly speaking – when one lacks all muscular control, or when one is knocked down, or pushed, or sent reeling by a blow or an explosion – or when through ignorance one chooses something other than what one means to choose, for instance thinking arsenic powder is table salt and thus choosing put it on one's scrambled eggs (Feinberg, 1986).

Voluntariness admits of degrees: There is a broad array of pressures, deficiencies of reason and so on that creates a spectrum of actions from those that are clearly and obviously involuntary and those which are fully voluntary. Non-voluntary actions are those that fall on the spectrum of voluntariness between the fully voluntary and the involuntary. In cases where mental illness causes a person's actions to become involuntary there is a sound justification for acting paternalistically and treating compulsorily if this is necessary to prevent self-harm. If mental illness

causes a person's actions to become non-voluntary or even 'substantially nonvoluntary', it is less clear that compulsory treatment has a sound moral justification. Our choices and actions are often less than 'fully voluntary', and it would be highly inappropriate in many of these cases to interfere with our liberty. For example, someone might have an irrational fear of all medications and refuse antidepressants on this basis. In this kind of case, we might consider their choice and action nonvoluntary, to some extent, but it would still be inappropriate to force treatment upon them. However, as Beauchamp and Childress suggest, there are likely to be some cases where a persons actions are 'substantially non-voluntary' without being involuntary, where it is appropriate to be paternalistic. Determining when this is the case creates a hard moral question: how non-voluntary does a person's behaviour have to be before we are justified in overriding their autonomy?

Feinberg suggests that we should weigh the degree of nonvoluntariness against the risk of harm in order to determine whether paternalism is justified:

> Most harmful choices, like most choices generally, fall somewhere in between the extremes of full voluntariness and complete involuntariness. It follows that we may formulate relatively strict (high) standards of voluntariness or relatively low standards of voluntariness in deciding, in a given context and for a given purposes, whether a dangerous choice is voluntary enough to be immune from interference. In some contexts, we may even want to permit choices that are quite substantially less than 'fully voluntary' to qualify as voluntary enough (Feinberg, 1986, pp. 104–5).

Feinberg is in effect saying that we must weigh the extent to which a person's autonomy is compromised against the risk to that person's welfare if they follow through with that risky choice or action. (This approach to the justification of paternalism and surrogate decision-making is also defended by Buchanan and Brock (1990), McMillan and Gillett (2005) and Eastman and Hope (1988)). Compulsory treatment is always a serious and significant imposition, so it is important that it only occurs when the risks are quite high and the degree of involuntariness quite severe. Mental health acts tend to require a significant degree of risk before permitting compulsory treatment, so perhaps they often succeed in balancing risk and 'non-voluntariness' in the right way. In any case, there is a good case for at least some instances of compulsory treatment being justified on soft paternalist grounds that do not rely upon mental illness being a real disease entity.

CONCLUSIONS

This chapter began by outlining Szasz's abolitionist and antipsychiatric critique of compulsory treatment. This was contrasted with what Chodoff calls 'the medical model' approach. Both of these positions focus upon the status of 'mental illness' as a disease entity and attempt to use their conclusions about this to justify or reject compulsory treatment. This chapter has shown that the debate about whether mental illnesses are genuinely diseases is not obviously relevant to the debate about whether or not compulsory treatment can be justified. Of course, the existence of at least some form of treatment that can aid those with mental illness is necessary for a paternalist justification to work. If it could be shown that compulsory treatment can not benefit people (which seems very unlikely) then there really are no good grounds for forcing treatment upon people.

REFERENCES

Bartlett P, Sandland R. *Mental Health Law and Practice*, 2nd edition. Oxford: Oxford University Press, 2003.

Beauchamp T, Childress J. *Principles of Biomedical Ethics*. Oxford: Oxford University Press, 1994.

Beautrais A, Joyce P, Mulder R, Fergusson D, Deavoll B, Nightingale S. Prevalence and comorbidity of mental disorders in persons making serious suicide attempts: a case-control study. *Am J Psychiatry* 1996; **153**: 1009–1014.

Buchanan A, Brock D. *Deciding for Others: The Ethics of Surrogate Decision Making*. Cambridge: Cambridge University Press, 1990.

Chodoff P. The case for involuntary hospitalization of the mentally ill. In: Pence G, ed. *Classic Works in Medical Ethics*. Boston, MA: McGraw Hill, 1998.

Cooper D. *Psychiatry and Antipsychiatry*. St Albans: Paladin, 1970.

Dawson J. Psychopathology and civil commitment criteria. *Med Law Rev* 1996 (Spring).

Eastman N, Hope T. The ethics of enforced medical treatment: the balance model. *J Appl Philos* 1988; **5**: 49–59.

Feinberg J. *Harm to Self: The Moral Limits of the Criminal Law*. New York: Oxford University Press, 1986.

Hume D. Of Suicide. In: Miller E, ed. *Essays, Moral Political and Literary*. Indianapolis: Liberty Fund, 1985 [1777].

Kant I. In: Gregor M, ed. *Groundwork of the Metaphysics of Morals*. Cambridge: Cambridge University Press, 1997 [1785].

Laing R. *The Divided Self: A Study of Sanity and Madness*. London: Tavistock, 1960.

McMillan J. Dangerousness, mental disorder and responsibility. *J Med Ethics* 2003; **29**: 232–235.

McMillan J, Gillett G. Moral responsibility, consciousness and psychiatry. *Austr NZ J Psychiatry* 2005; **39**: 1018–1021.

Mill J. On liberty. *John Stuart Mill on Liberty and Other Essay*. Oxford: Oxford University Press, 1998 [1859].

Mill J. On the subjection of women. *John Stuart Mill on Liberty and Other Essay*. Oxford: Oxford University Press, 1998 [1869].

Morse S. A preference for liberty: the case against involuntary commitment of the mentally disordered. *California Law Rev* 1982; **70**: 54–106.

Peele R, Chodoff P. The ethics of involuntary treatment and deinstitutionalization. In: Bloch, Chodoff, Green, eds. *Psychiatric Ethics*. London: Oxford University Press, 1999.

Re C. (adult refusal of treatment). ER 819 1 WLR 290, 1994.

Singer P. *Animal Liberation*. London: Pimlico, 1995.

Szasz T. *The Myth of Mental Illness: Foundations of a Theory of Personal Conduct*. New York: Dell Publishing, 1961.

Szasz T. Involuntary mental hospitalization: A crime against humanity. In: Pence G, ed. *Classic Works in Medical Ethics*. Boston, MA: McGraw-Hill, 1998.

Szasz T. Psychiatry and the control of dangerousness: on the apotropaic function of the term 'mental illness'. *J Med Ethics* 2003; **29**: 227–230.

Szasz T. Response to comments on psychiatry and the control of dangerousness: on the apotropaic function of the term 'mental illness'. *J Med Ethics* 2003; **29**: 237.

61

Personality Disorders and Compulsory Detention[1]

MATT MATRAVERS

INTRODUCTION

Consider the following three cases from England, the USA and Australia, respectively:

Michael Stone: Stone was convicted (twice, because of a successful appeal against his first conviction) for the 1996 murders of Lin and Megan Russell and the attempted murder of Josie Russell. They were attacked, and the mother and one daughter bludgeoned to death with a hammer. Josie was similarly attacked, but survived. Stone had a police record dating back to the age of 12 and a fairly prolific adult criminal career. He was gaoled in 1981 for robbery and grievous bodily harm; in 1983 for wounding, assault and dishonesty; and in 1987 for armed robbery. He was released in 1994 and, in the same year, sectioned under the Mental Health Act at De La Pole Hospital in Hull. Doctors there decided he was not mentally ill and discharged him. Defending this decision, the chief executive, Ruth Carnall, pointed out that Stone's release was quite proper for, although he had a severe personality disorder and was considered dangerous, his condition was untreatable so he could not be detained under the Mental Health Act. Carnall described Stone as a classic 'psychopath' who was incapable of feeling guilt or empathy and was resistant to treatment (Summers, 2001).

Leroy Hendricks: Leroy Hendricks spent a large part of his life in custody. At his trial to determine whether he should be civilly committed, he admitted to a long history of sexual offences with children. He had five convictions, for indecent exposure, lewdness, and molestation of children. In addition, he confessed to forcing his two stepchildren to engage in sex with him while on parole. Hendricks claimed that the only

way to ensure that he did not sexually molest another child was for him 'to die' (Kansas v. Hendricks, 1997).

Garry David: David had a long history of violent offending, of self-mutilation, and of making threats of violence to others. Shortly after being released from prison for a serious violent offence, he attempted to murder a woman and two police officers. During his fourteen year sentence for those offences, he assaulted fifteen other inmates and prison guards. He was also hospitalized more than 80 times 'for a range of self-inflicted injuries, including cutting off his nipples and parts of his penis' (McCallum, 2001). Coming up for release, he threatened, once free, to murder several people and to poison the local water supply. The Mental Health Board found that he suffered from Antisocial Personality Disorder, but that he was not mentally ill and so could not be certified under the Mental Health Act. For a discussion of the case see Williams (1990).

These three cases have a number of things in common. In each case, we are presented with an individual who is apparently a dangerous risk to others. None is mentally ill. Rather, each is said to suffer from a disorder of personality that predisposes him to activities harmful to others. Yet, despite the danger they present, in all three cases, they are not – or at least, not at the relevant time – liable to criminal punishment because all three had served their most recent sentences and, in that sense, had wiped the slate clean. The risk is that they might do something in the future, and criminal liability and punishment is for acts already attempted or committed. However, because they had personality disorder and were not mentally ill, they do not fit the usual model for civil confinement. Finally, and perhaps most remarkably,

[1] I am grateful to the British Academy for the award of the Thank-Offering to Britain Fellowship, which made research on this paper possible.

all three of these individuals can lay claim to some kind of legal or legislative notoriety: Stone's murders prompted the British Government to propose legislation to deal with what it calls 'dangerous severely personality disordered people' (Great Britain, 1999, 2000); Hendricks was the first man to be committed under the Kansas statute, later tested in the US Supreme Court, allowing for the civil confinement of 'sexually violent predators'; and David's case led to the euphemistically called 'Community Protection Act' enacted in 1990 by the district of Victoria solely to ensure that he was not released into the community.

Although these three cases are particular, the legislation (or legislative proposals) with which they are associated is of a kind that is becoming common. The idea is to plug a perceived gap that arises when someone is thought to be 'dangerous', but (i) has not committed a (fresh) criminal offence – and so cannot be dealt with by the criminal justice system – and (ii) is not mentally ill, and in need of treatment – and so cannot be dealt with by the mental health system. Politicians declare that something must be done, because the public, it is said, will not tolerate sexually violent predators, paedophiles, and psychopaths living among them simply because the experts cannot agree amongst themselves about how to classify such people and what to do with them.

Precisely because these issues are politically sensitive, hotly contested, and (at the moment at least) of great public interest, it is critical that the difficult ethical questions that surround them are given careful consideration. On the one hand, it is easy to feel the force of the thought that 'something must be done' when confronted by the possibility of dangerous, antisocial, people with personality disorder living unsupervised in the community, or when having read of the latest victim of a person with personality disorder recently released from a criminal or health care institution. On the other hand, it is equally easy to fear the 'risk society' that threatens to lock people up for what they might do and to worry about the use of mental health legislation being used as a means of social control. However, neither response is helpful.

The ethical issues surrounding personality disorders and compulsory detention are many, various, and controversial. One reason for this is that personality disorders are perhaps the most controversial of all psychiatric conditions. Another is that the *compulsory* element of compulsory detention makes it particularly ethically problematic. Rather than beginning with personality disorders, I want to start by asking whether, and if so under what kinds of conditions,

compulsory detention can ever be justified. Having identified those conditions, the question then is does an individual with a personality disorder (or with some particular personality disorder) meet these conditions.

COMPULSORY PREVENTIVE DETENTION

When a liberal state acts to detain an individual, it manifests an awesome and defining power. To deprive someone of his or her liberty is, after all, normally a serious violation of that person's rights. Yet, the state claims the (monopoly of) legitimate power to do so under certain circumstances. Sometimes, these circumstances are relatively uncontroversial (even if the details and justifications are disputed). So, the state routinely uses deprivation of liberty as a criminal punishment and, for the most part, its right to do so (at least in some cases) is widely recognized. On most accounts of just punishment, the state's right to punish depends on the past offence committed by the agent. Indeed, some people argue that punishment is, by definition, something that can only be done to an offender for an offence.[2] However, it is not the case that the state only detains people for what they have done. It may also detain people to prevent future harm and, again, in some cases this power is largely uncontroversial.

Consider three instances of the state's use of preventive detention. First, a mentally ill person who is judged by competent professionals to pose a serious risk to himself or others. Such a person may well be detained for treatment and in order to prevent future harm to himself or others. Second, a state may preventively detain a person who has a major communicable disease such as smallpox or cholera. Third, in the criminal law, the state may detain pretrial defendants when, and because, they are judged to be dangerous or likely to abscond. Although this will generally be accompanied by regulations or guidelines concerning how quickly trial should follow, it can nevertheless mean that legally innocent persons are detained for several months because of what they might do.

These three instances of compulsory preventive detention are relatively uncontroversial, and these powers are commonly held by democratic states across the world. What makes them uncontroversial? One answer to this emerges if we compare them with Stephen Morse's criteria for justifiable 'pure preventive action'. Such action would be justified, Morse claims: '(1) if the potential harm were sufficiently grave; (2) if the prediction

---

[2]This argument by definitional fiat is not very satisfactory. Purely consequentialist theories of punishment appeal to the future consequences of punishing (or not punishing) the offender rather than the past act. However, and in part for that reason, purely consequentialist theories of punishment are widely thought to be unsatisfactory (for a review of the different justifications of punishment (Matravers, 2000; Duff, 2001). Thus, the phrase 'preventive detention' will be used here to describe (only) non-criminal detention justified by the claim that it aims to prevent a future harm.

technology were sufficiently accurate; (3) if the preventive response were maximally humane and minimally intrusive under the circumstances; and (4) if the preventive action was preceded by adequate due process' (Morse, 1999).

The three examples meet these criteria. The severely mentally ill person must pose a grave threat to himself or others; the disease in cases of quarantine must be a 'major' one; and the criminal defendant must be thought to pose a serious risk. Similarly for the other criteria: it is important that we are confident about the threat, that there are proper procedures, and that the intervention is as humane as possible; the conditions in quarantine and while on remand should not be the same as the conditions in prison.

Morse's criteria, sensible as they are, cannot of course be used in any straightforward way to settle disputes about when some particular instance of preventive detention is justified. The criteria require interpretation: when is a potential harm 'sufficiently grave'? how accurate need the 'predictive technology' be? and what counts as 'maximally humane' and 'minimally intrusive'? It is against this background that I want now to consider personality disorders, and in particular, proposals to detain people regarded as dangerous in virtue of their having a (or some combination of) personality disorder(s).

PERSONALITY DISORDERS

People may well have been wondering about personality, and differences of personalities, for as long as they have been able to communicate. Hippocrates (around 460–380 BC) famously proposed that individuals' personalities depended on the relative quantities of four 'humours' found within them: yellow and black bile, phlegm, and blood. His categories, of course, remain in everyday use when we call someone 'phlegmatic', 'sanguine', or describe someone's melancholy disposition as 'black'. The modern idea of personality disorder first arises in the eighteenth century in contradistinction to mental illness (Ferguson & Tyrer, 1988). Remarkably, the distinction between mental illness and personality disorder has been controversial ever since. Psychiatrists – and perhaps as Kendell speculates – 'British psychiatrists more than most' – have remained 'ambivalent' about whether personality disorders are mental illnesses or even medical conditions at all (Kendell, 2002; Moran, 1999). As Ferguson and Tyrer comment, this issue was of little medical importance given the very limited treatments available for any and all abnormal mental states (Ferguson & Tyrer, 1988). Although this has changed with the advance of treatments for some mental abnormalities, it is in the legal domain that the distinction has always mattered most.

Moreover, the kinds of legislation described in the first section above have now made the issue urgent.

Given that what is proposed is to detain people, against their will, for reasons of prevention, it is important to start with the most radical challenge: the claim that 'personality disorder' is merely an evaluative label that is used to justify the use of medical power to manage those of whom society disapproves (see, for famous versions of this argument; Foucault, 1965, 1978; Szasz, 1972). Two features of personality disorders seem to support the radical challenge.

The first is the indisputable fact that the history of psychiatry contains numerous examples of the abuse of the idea of disorder. To give just two examples: in 1851, in a paper in the *New Orleans Medical and Surgical Journal*, Dr Samuel Cartwright proposed that runaway slaves suffered from 'drapetomania', identified by an irresistible desire to run away (to be cured, apparently, by whipping or amputation of the toes). In the twentieth century, in China and the Soviet Union, psychiatric conditions such as 'political monomania' justified the detention of those opposed to the state. These examples are, according to radical critics, the forerunners of disputes over homosexuality, alcoholism, and hyperactivity.

The second is that personality disorders, unlike (it is claimed) other illnesses, are diagnosed on the basis of the patient's behaviour rather than, for example, on the basis of the identification of some underlying organic abnormality. The result, the critics claim, is a vicious circularity. For example, the *DSM-IV-TR* states that 'the essential feature of Antisocial Personality Disorder is a pervasive pattern of disregard for, and violation of, the rights of others that begins in childhood or early adolescence and continues into adulthood' (American Psychiatric Association, 2000). Or, to put it another way, what defines someone with Antisocial Personality Disorder is that they are persistently antisocial.

These two difficulties are exacerbated by continuing disputes over the reliability and validity of current diagnoses of personality disorders and controversy over their categorization. To the lay person, all of this might seem to add up to a simple question with a simple answer: are personality disorders illnesses (to be treated by the medical profession) or are they not (in which case if there is problematic behaviour then it ought to fall to criminal justice or social work professionals)? Clearly, 'drapetomania' is not an illness, so (given the time) the 'problem' of runaway slaves should have been a matter for the police.

The trouble with that, seemingly so sensible, approach is that the problems of definition that afflict 'personality disorder' are present, too, in the identification of 'illness'. Thus, in defining illness, there are radical critics who claim that illness is nothing other than a social construction.

As one writer puts it, 'the attribution of illness always proceeds from the computation of a gap between presented behaviour (or feeling) and some social norm' (Sedgwick, 1982). Others regard this as far too extreme and argue that illness is purely biomedical and spell this out in terms of something like biologically disadvantageous statistical deviation from what is normal (Scadding, 1967, 1990; Cohen, 1981). This is not the place to discuss the concepts of disease and illness; the point is just to emphasize that whatever difficulties are associated with the concept of personality disorder, they are not likely to be resolved by asking whether such disorders are, or are not, 'really' illnesses (Kendell, 2002).

That said, there is one way in which the debate over illness may help. No matter how much difficulty we have in defining illness, only the most radical sceptic would argue that we should discard the concept. The fact is that having the concept serves useful medical and social purposes. Moreover, among non-sceptics, few would deny that the way to characterize illness (disorder or dysfunction) is to accept that it involves *both* biomedical facts and socio-political judgements. That is, to be ill (disordered or dysfunctional) is to suffer from some biological abnormality (which can be understood in a number of ways) that is *harmful* or that gives one a *handicap* (which is a judgement relative to social norms). Such an account fits well with our intuitions and practices. As Kendell pointed out in 1975, both a 'child with spina bifida' and one with 'fused second and third toes' suffer from an 'anatomical defect acquired early in embryonic development' yet we do not tend to regard the latter as ill (Kendell, 1975). It also fits well with the *DSM-IV* definition of personality *disorders* as against personality *traits*. The latter are 'enduring patterns of perceiving, relating to, and thinking about the environment and oneself that are exhibited in a wide range of social and personal contexts'. Whereas, such traits only become disorders when they 'are inflexible and maladaptive and cause significant functional impairment or subjective distress' (American Psychiatric Association, 2000).

Arguing that the concept of personality disorder may be a useful one and is one that is not categorically distinct from other illnesses or dysfunctions, however, is not the same as arguing for the current list, and categorization, of personality disorders in either the *ICD-10* or the *DSM-IV*. We should expect continuing controversy over, and revision to, both the lists of disorders and the ways in which they are categorized and diagnosed. Nevertheless, for the purposes of considering personality disorders and compulsory detention, the above analysis at least allows us to ask the question of whether the compulsory detention of people with personality disorder could be justified.

PERSONALITY DISORDERS AND COMPULSORY DETENTION

Why might a society detain people with personality disorder in a health care institution against their will? One answer is in order to prevent harm to the patient and/or to others. In addition, in the case of the mentally ill, society may detain someone in order to ensure that they receive proper care and treatment.

The issue of treatment goes to the heart of much of the controversy around personality disorders. *If*, as many psychiatrists think, personality disorders are not treatable, then to detain sufferers from such disorders in health care institutions turns such institutions into, at best, warehouses and, at worst, gaols. Psychiatrists have understandably resisted both of these roles. However, there is a great deal of controversy over whether personality disorders can be treated and over what constitutes 'treatment'. So, for example, the UK Government has recently agreed that 'it would be inappropriate to use the Mental Health Bill to detain (or otherwise apply compulsion to) people who are not in need of specialist mental health care', but has gone on to argue that it does *not* believe 'that compulsion should be limited to those cases where the benefit of treatment will be expressed by an improvement to the patient's condition, or by preventing deterioration' (Great Britain, 2005, pp. 14–5). This issue is considered further below in the discussion of 'maximally humane' preventive interventions.

Of course, the purposes of compulsory detention are not limited to treatment and the sites of such detention are not limited to health care institutions. We need, then, to turn to the core issue of preventive detention.

Consider again the four criteria for justifiable preventive detention identified in the second section above: detention is justified '(1) if the potential harm were sufficiently grave; (2) if the prediction technology were sufficiently accurate; (3) if the preventive response were maximally humane and minimally intrusive under the circumstances; and (4) if the preventive action was preceded by adequate due process'. Condition (4), although not always met in practice, ought to be beyond dispute in theory in a liberal democratic society governed by the rule of law and so can be put to one side. What of the other three?

Rape, homicide and self-mutilation are serious harms. Put self-harm to one side, so as to concentrate on preventive detention to avoid harm to others. If we grant that there are some people – people like those identified at the start of this paper – who, because of their disordered personalities, will rape and kill, then we cannot dispute that condition (1) can be met. Of course, a critic might say that there is nothing particular about people with personality disorder in this context. If we knew that a person, who did not suffer from a personality disorder, would kill someone in the future then whatever applies to the person with personality disorder applies to him, too. Many people would agree and would allow that both can be detained, if and only if condition (2) could also be met.[3] Putting that to one side, it seems at least plausible that the threat, if it can be predicted, posed by someone like Garry David is a grave one and so that condition (1) is met by some people.

The degree to which condition (2) can be met is a matter of dispute, and even as it stands, we would need to decide what degree of accuracy was 'sufficient'. In a 2001 paper, Buchanan and Leese estimated that, under the UK Government's proposals, six people would have to be detained in order to prevent one person acting violently (Buchanan & Leese, 2001), which led the *Lancet* to comment that 'the forecasting of dangerousness remains like that of the weather – accurate over a few days, but impotent to state longer-term outcome with any certainty' (Farnham & James, 2001). Such scepticism is widespread (see, for example, Morse, 1999; White, 2002). Given this, one might wonder why this issue is still of philosophical or ethical interest. For surely, if the rate of false positives is above some very small proportion, then there can be no morally justified practice of preventive detention. (Even a straightforward consequentialist would be likely to agree that the disutility of detaining multiple false positives would outweigh the utility of preventing some one grave harm.)

Given the existing predictive tools, that answer seems right. There can be no morally justified general rule allowing people (whatever their personality) to be picked from the general population to be detained against their wills because of the prediction that they might be dangerous in the future. Our predictions are simply not accurate enough and were they ever to become so, we would probably need to rethink many of our ethical categories and much of our criminal justice system. However, in practice (and sometimes in principle) that is not what is proposed. What drives the legislators is not some vision of 'dangerousness tribunals' picking likely offenders from the general population before they have offended, but the problem of existing offenders – like Stone, Hendricks and David – who may reach the end of the criminal sanction and be released. In the past, many such offenders were held on indeterminate sentences and so could be detained in the criminal justice system until deemed to be no longer dangerous. However, since the mid-seventies, the criminal justice systems of the USA and UK have increasingly turned to determinate (and sometimes mandatory) sentencing (sometimes in response to the abuse of indeterminate sentencing) so this option is no longer available.

As one might expect, restricting the population assessed to existing violent or sexual offenders increases the predictive accuracy of the existing tools, and it is a plausible conjecture that one reason that legislators have felt confident enough to intervene in this area is the rise of actuarial assessments such as the Violence Risk Appraisal Guide (VRAG) and the revised Psychopathy Check List. Even these, however, produce sufficient false positives for their use to be morally problematic (for an overview, and further references, see Dolan & Doyle, 2000).

If we grant that the careful use of clinical and actuarial measures, applied to a population of serious offenders, could generate sufficiently accurate predictions of future grave harm, then for this small group, it would seem that both conditions (1) and (2) for justified preventive detention could be met. That leaves condition (3): that the intervention be maximally humane and minimally intrusive. Discussing this condition inevitably means revisiting the issue of treatment mentioned above.

If treatment is not available for the kinds of personality disorders from which those identified as potentially violent suffer, then psychiatrists are likely to continue to maintain that detention in medical health institutions is inappropriate. Should society wish to warehouse its dangerous members, it will be claimed that the job should be done by the criminal justice, or some other system. Of course, if treatments are developed (or if existing treatments can be shown to work), then the situation would be different. However, it should be remembered that, as Moran puts it, 'offenders with abnormal personalities do not adapt to the penal system any better than they do to health care' (Moran, 1999). If such people are to be detained in conditions that are maximally humane, then, it seems just as wrong to warehouse them in an inappropriate criminal justice institution (particularly if they have completed their sentence) as in a hospital. The solution, if condition (3) is to be met probably lies with properly resourced specialist centres that combine the security of the prison system with the therapeutic environment of the hospital (for a proposal of this type see Fallon et al. (1999).

CONCLUSION AND THOUGHTS FOR THE FUTURE

The argument above attempts to show that the compulsory detention of people with personality disorder could be morally justified if, and only if, certain stringent conditions are met. However, it also demonstrates the difficulty

---

[3]Kantians might think that the extra control available to the 'normal' person means that we should always allow that he might autonomously choose to act differently at the crucial moment and so should not intervene. In so far as this is found plausible, I think it is because people doubt that condition (2) could be met. If we were certain that an aggressor was about to attack his victim, we would surely be entitled to intervene even if this thwarted the autonomous choice of the aggressor.

of meeting these conditions. Personality disorders are controversial; if they exist they are difficult both to diagnose and to treat. Finally, the predictive technologies that we have are insufficiently accurate to be relied on for general legislation.

Predicting the future is, as we have seen, a risky business. However, there are some signs of progress in many of the difficult areas identified above. Neurobiological findings may lead both to a better understanding of certain kinds of personality disorder (particularly those associated with violence) and of how early intervention in childhood might help divert the person from a life of persistent antisocial behaviour. In risk assessment, we have a better understanding of the epidemiology of violence and more sophisticated risk assessment tools based on a clearer identification of risk factors. Nevertheless, there is a long way to go in all these areas. Finally, no matter how great the technological and biomedical advances, one must never forget that the right of the state to detain people against their will is a moral and political matter and that the balance of power between the state and its citizens – particularly its marginalized and non-conforming citizens – is not even. For these reasons, it will always be important that proposals of the kind discussed in this chapter be subject to rigorous, critical, moral argument and appraisal.

REFERENCES

American Psychiatric Association. *Diagnostic and Statistical Manual of Mental Disorders: DSM-IV-TR.* Washington, DC: American Psychiatric Association; 2000. 686, pp. 701.

Buchanan A, Leese M. Detention of people with severe personality disorders: a systematic review. *Lancet* 2001; **358**: 1955–9.

Cohen H. The evolution of the concept of disease. In: Caplan AL, Engelhardt HT, McCartney JJ, eds. *Concepts of Health and Disease: Interdisciplinary Perspectives.* Reading, MA: Addison-Wesley, 1981; pp. 209–20.

Dolan M, Doyle M. Violence risk prediction: clinical and actuarial measures and the role of the psychopathy checklist. *Br J Psychiatry* 2000; **177**: 303–11.

Duff RA. *Punishment, Communication, and Community.* Oxford; New York: Oxford University Press, 2001.

Fallon P, Bluglass R, *et al. Report of the Committee of Inquiry into the Personality Disorder Unit at Ashworth Hospital.* London: HMSO, 1999.

Farnham F, James D. Editorial. *Lancet* 2001; **358**: 1926.

Ferguson B, Tyrer P. History of the concept of personality disorder. In: Tyrer P, ed. *Personality Disorder: Diagnosis, Management and Course.* London: Wright, 1988; p. 1

Foucault M. *Madness and Civilization: A History of Insanity in the Age of Reason.* New York: Vintage Books, 1965.

Foucault M. *The History of Sexuality: Volume 1. An Introduction.* New York: Pantheon Books, 1978.

Great Britain, Department of Health. *Reforming the Mental Health Act Part II: High Risk Patients,* 2000.

Great Britain, Department of Health. *Government Response to the Report of the Joint Committee on the Draft Mental Health Bill 2004.* London: HMSO, 2005; pp. 14–15.

Great Britain, Home Office. *Managing Dangerous People with Severe Personality Disorder: Proposals for Policy Development.* London: Home Office 1999, 1999.

Kansas v. Hendricks, 521 U.S. **346**: 1997.

Kendell R. The concept of disease and its implications for psychiatry. *Br J Psychiatry* 1975; **127**: 305–15.

Kendell R. The distinction between personality disorder and mental illness. *Br J Psychiatry* 2002; **180**: 110–5.

Matravers M. *Justice and Punishment: The Rationale of Coercion.* Oxford: Oxford University Press, 2000.

McCallum D. *Personality and Dangerousness: Genealogies of antisocial personality disorder.* Cambridge: Cambridge University Press, 2001; p. 16.

Moran P. Should psychiatrists treat personality disorders? *Maudsley Discussion Paper 7.* London: Institute of Psychiatry, 1999; p.17.

Morse SJ. Neither desert nor disease. *Legal Theory* 1999; **5**: 265–309.

Scadding J. Diagnosis: the clinician and the computer. *Lancet* 1967; **2**: 877–82.

Scadding J. The semantic problem of psychiatry. *Psychol Med* 1990; **20**: 243–8.

Sedgwick P. *Psycho Politics.* London: Pluto, 1982; p. 34.

Summers C. *Stone Case Could Prompt Law Change.* London: (BBC News 2005), 2001.

Szasz TS. *The Myth of Mental Illness: Foundations of a Theory of Personal Conduct.* New York: Harper & Row, 1972.

White S. Preventive detention must be resisted by the medical profession. *J Med Ethics* 2002; **28**: 95–8.

Williams CR. Psychopathy, mental illness and preventive detention: issues arising from the David case. *Monash Univer Law Rev* 1990; **16**(2): 161–83.

62

Labia mea, Domine[*]: Media, Morality and Eating Disorders

SIMONA GIORDANO

INTRODUCTION

La donna e` mobile; qual piuma al vento; muta d'accento; e di pensiero; Sempre un'amabile; leggiadro viso; in pianto e in riso; La donna e` mobile; qual piuma al vento; muta d'accento; e di pensier; e di pensier; e di pensier . . .
(Giuseppe Verdi, *La Donna è Mobile/The Duke's Aria, Rigoletto*)
(The woman is mobile, such a feather in the wind, mute in the word and in thought. Always an amiable graceful face, in tears and laughter . . . The woman is mobile, such a feather in the wind, mute in the word and in thought, and in thought, and in thought)

I do not care for the body, I love the timid soul, the blushing, shrinking soul; it hides, for it is afraid, and the bold obtrusive body...
Emily Dickinson, Letter No. 39 (Johnson, 1958)

Giuseppe Verdi's *Rigoletto* contains one of the many celebrations of female grace in arts. Verdi's *Rigoletto* praises traits such as lightness ('feather in the wind') and capacity to control words and thoughts, which should characterize the woman (Giordano, 2002). Similarly, Emily Dickinson's letters and poems are replete with celebrations to spirituality and references to the body as '*mouldering casket*' (Johnson, 1958, note 2, p. 140), which ought to be transcended.

Many people believe that anorexia results from pressure by the media to be thin. (I will mainly refer to anorexia, as anorexia is the most striking form of food control, but the arguments of this chapter extend to any form of suffering which relates to dissatisfaction with the body, including bulimia, bulimic-anorexia and subclinical abnormal eating behaviours. The arguments articulated here should give us a better understanding of the relationship which we all might have with food and our body, and the way this relationship is shaped by our moral values.) Considering anorexics as victims of fashion, however, is a misanalysis of the problem. Anorexia is not the result of *aesthetic pressure*. Anorexia has its foundation in moral principles and beliefs.

Studies on anorexia show that many of those who develop anorexia are indeed influenced by TV and magazine models (Eating Disorders Association). However, even when the sufferer apparently diets for aesthetic reasons or in response to an alleged social imperative to be thin, the deeper reasons for anorexia are to be found in the idea that the person should be able to control the 'lower' desires emanating from the body with her/his 'higher faculties' (intellect, rationality or spirituality), that there is something moral and admirable in the capacity to exert will power over the body and something immoral in the incapacity or, worse, unwillingness to do so. The body becomes the arena of a moral fight.

This chapter looks back into the history of philosophy, to identify the values which, across the centuries, have shaped our way of thinking about goodness and rightness and how

---

[*]The title of this chapter, 'Labia mea, domine', is the moaning of those condemned for the sin of gluttony, in the VI Canto of the *Divine Comedy* by Dante Alighieri. An English translation is available online at http://dante.ilt.columbia.edu/comedy/. An earlier version of this chapter was presented at the FAB/IAB, World Congress of Bioethics, Sidney, 9 November 2004. The title was: 'How Morality Shapes Our Bodies, Anorexia and Socio-cultural Values'. Some of the arguments of this chapter have been previously published in Giordano's *Understanding Eating Disorders, Conceptual and Ethical Issues in the Treatment of Anorexia and Bulimia Nervosa*, Oxford: Oxford University Press.

Principles of Health Care Ethics, Second Edition Edited by R.E. Ashcroft, A. Dawson, H. Draper and J.R. McMillan
© 2007 John Wiley & Sons, Ltd

should we act. We shall see that anorexia is the consistent implementation of ordinary moral principles and values.

The arguments of this chapter do not pretend to be a comprehensive explanation of anorexia. It seems likely that many factors (psychological, social, familial, biological and genetic) contribute to the genesis of the disorder and to the conceptualization of food refusal as psychiatric disease. This chapter will consider the claim that anorexia is the result of the fashion of thin women. It will argue that the preference for thinness is not primarily *aesthetic*. In order to understand why many people value thinness and are prepared to make many sacrifices for the sake of thinness (up to the point of dying), we need to look at a certain conception of the human being and at moral values related to that conception. In the light of this argument, anorexia no longer strikes as either a 'caprice' of vain women or as 'irrational' behaviour, symptomatic of a mental illness, but appears to be an understandable and coherent behaviour.

ANOREXIA AND THE MEDIA

Anorexia is one of the most widespread and threatening conditions affecting young people. It is the most lethal of psychiatric disorders. The mortality associated with the disorder is up to 20% (Griffiths & Russel, 1998).

In common discourse, anorexia is said to be caused by pressure by the mass media to be thin. The illness, the argument goes, is an inevitable effect of an indiscriminate fashion, which, by using unnaturally thin models, spreads the pernicious and overwhelming idea that thinness is a necessary attribute of beauty and imposes an unhealthy model of beauty on innocent young women.

A similar argument has even persuaded serious medical organizations. The British Medical Association (2000) and The Institute of Psychiatry (London), for example, agree, that fashion and the media may play a role in the causation of eating disorders (debate available at http://www.edauk.com/).

However, publishers of women's magazines have objected that people tend to buy magazines where skeleton-like bodies are pictured, and this is why super-thin models are used (*Guardian*, 30 May 2000, 31 May 2000). Supply, they say, satisfies demand. What is more likely to be the case, that people like thinness *because magazines are replete with thin models*? Or is it (also) the other way round – magazines are full of thin models *because this is what people like*? It is not just that *what we see, we want*. Instead, in an important sense, *what we want, we see*. The question, therefore, is why do we like *these very thin women?* Or what is attractive in thinness?

Some studies reveal that, historically, thinness has been valued at times when women were expected to demonstrate their intellectual skills. The more numerous are the women who aspire to 'male' positions, the more numerous

are those who pursue a cylindrical or tubular (androgynous) body (Gordon, 1991). From this perspective, thinness is valued not *in itself* – simply because *it is beautiful* – but for what it signifies.

As we shall see, thinness corporealizes a cluster of moral values with a long history, which have been embodied in western morality across the centuries and which remain dominant in western societies. These values rest on a particular metaphysic of the person, according to which we are composed of two ontologically distinguishable 'parts': mind and body.

THE BODY/MIND SCHISM: ITS ORIGINS

In the western thought the mind has often been juxtaposed to the body (Krugovoy, 2003; Giordano, 2005a). The philosopher Gilbert Ryle has defined this idea as 'The Official Doctrine', given that most people seem to take it for granted.

> The official doctrine, which hails chiefly from Descartes, is something like this. With the doubtful exceptions of idiots and infants in arms every human being has both a body and a mind[...] In consciousness, self-consciousness and introspection he [the man] is directly and authentically apprised of the present states and operations of his mind[...] It is customary to express this bifurcation of his two lives and his two worlds [...]It is assumed that there are two different kinds of existence or status. What exists or happens may have the status of physical existence, or it may have the status of mental existence (Ryle, 1978).

This metaphysics is influential in contemporary bioethics although it is still debated in philosophy. Many bioethicists, for example Singer (1995), Harris (1992), Parfit (1976) and Engelhardt (1996) argue that persons, in their 'complete' or 'higher' form, possess certain mental capacities – self-awareness, for example, as the capacity to consider itself as the same being over time. Beings that do not possess the requisite mental capacities are not persons. The assumption here is that human beings have a mind and a body, as two conceptually distinguishable entities, and that the mind is the entity which gives us our special and unique status among all living beings.

Usually, contemporary philosophers do not provide an elaborate gnoseology (a theory of human faculties) as for example Locke, Berkeley or Kant did. That *we have* rationality or a mind seems so self-evident that it does not require any justification. If *we have* a mind, then we *also have a body* – as something ontologically different from the mind. This idea has had important implications in bioethical debates on abortion and euthanasia, relating to the moral status of humans. But these arguments go beyond the scope of this chapter.

The dichotomy of mind and body probably originated in Orphism (Reale & Antiseri, 1984, Vol. 1; Giordano, 2005b).

Orpheus was a Greek (probably legendary) poet. Orphism understands the human being as composed of soul and body. The soul is a *demon* (δαίμων), a divine principle which fell into the body because of an original sin. The soul is immortal and reincarnates in different bodies, until the rituals and practices of the 'Orphic life' put an end to the cycle of reincarnations (metempsychosis) and the soul is set free.

This schema of thought had an irreversible effect on original Greek naturalism. For the first time the human being was presented as composed of two sides in contrast with each other, and physical impulses were presented *as something which needed to be transcended*. Orphism had a major impact on Greek culture, including philosophy and science.

For example, the mathematical studies of the School of Pythagoras were all informed by the conception of the soul as *trapped or incarcerated* in the body. Pythagoras and his scholars considered Science as a means of purification. A similar idea is found in Empedocles. In his poem *Katharmoi* (purifications), he developed the Orphic teachings: Empedocles believed, in a similar way to Pythagoras, that the soul (*psyche*) was a demon expelled from the *Olympus* (a paradise) and destined to reincarnate itself in different bodies.

Plato also included in his philosophy the concepts of Orphism. In the *Gorgias,* he argued that 'the body is for us a grave' (Reale & Antiseri, 1984, note 21, p. 112). It is by dying that the soul is set free and that we come to life. In his later thought, Plato softened this mysterifical conception, but always preserved the metaphysical distinction between *psyche* (entity similar to the intelligible) and body (sensitive entity). The theme of the soul recurs in virtually all his writings: *Meno, Phaedo, Republic, Phaedrus Timaeus.*

Aristotle talked about the human being as a compound of form and matter. The material is the body, the animal part, and the form is the mind (the *nous*): 'the part of the soul by which it knows and understands'(Aristotle, 1986). The *nous* expresses our very nature (Aristotle, 1998). There is no human being without *nous*.

The metaphysical distinction was accepted in the Latin world. Christianity presented the body and physical life as secondary and non-important, even as a source of sin. Suffering in the body and suffering in our 'physical' life is irrelevant provided that the soul is pure and not ill, and if suffering helps purify the soul, then it is a good thing. In Puritan New England, Emily Dickinson wrote:

[W]ho cares for a body whose tenant is ill at ease? Give me the aching body, and the spirit glad and serene, for if the gem shines on, forget the mouldering casket
Emily Dickinson, Letter No 54 (Johnson, note 2, 1958, p. 140).

The body–mind split remained unquestioned in the various interpretations of the Christian thought (Patristic doctrines and Scholastic philosophy), in the whole medieval western philosophy and theology, in the various denominations of Christianity and in Renaissance humanism.

Many modern philosophers have incorporated the metaphysics of body and mind (or soul or spirit) into their theories. Probably Decartes (with his partition of *res cogitans and res extensa* – literally the 'thinking thing' and the 'extended thing') and Kant (with his division of *phenomenal* – or physical – dimension and *noumenal* – or supernatural dimension) provide some of the most remarkable systematizations of the dichotomous conception of the human nature in philosophy.

KANT AND THE MORTIFICATION OF THE FLESH

According to Kant, there are two ontological dimensions: one is phenomenal and the other is noumenal. Animals belong to the phenomenal dimension. Human beings with their animal nature also belong to the phenomenal dimension. However, there is also a noumenal, transcendent dimension, and the human being also participates in this dimension, with its *reason*.

From his ontology and theory of human faculties, Kant drew his moral doctrine. For Kant, a person behaves morally if (and to the extent that) she or he submits the 'phenomenal' side (which is the physical side, with its impulses and desires) to the 'rational' or 'noumenal' side. In order to be moral, human beings need to sacrifice their physical nature and to act according to the precepts of the reason.

Kantian moral philosophy, whose basic lines have only been summarized here, represents one of the clearest and most consistent expressions of the idea that morality is achieved by the submission of the 'physical' to the 'rational' (Kant, 1948).

This does not mean that if one reads Kant or Plato, he or she will become anorexic or is more likely to develop anorexia. What I am suggesting is that the doctrines of many philosophers and theologians express principles and values which are crystallized in the western culture, and these principles and values become one of the determinants of eating disorders. Viewing physical life as something which can and should be controlled and submitted to the will, may in fact have an obvious impact on the way people perceive their physical impulses, including *hunger*.

MORAL INTEGRITY AND *HUNGER*

Within an ethic which demands the submission of the 'physical' to the 'rational', it is obvious that control over one of the most pressing physiological impulses, hunger, is praised. Fasting has historically been and is still associated with ideas of *control* over the chaotic passions of the body, and the person who is able to exert control over hunger, such a powerful physiological impulse, has often been presented as an example of moral integrity (Bruch, 1974).

Moreover, fasting has been and is currently often associated with the idea of *purity*. In the Christian tradition, gluttony is a sin. In 1996, Papa Giovanni Paolo II suggested fasting as a 'therapy for the soul. [...] It facilitates [...] contact with God. [...] Penitential fasting, among other meanings, helps us recuperate our interiority [...] and is of a great support to the life of the spirit' (Christus Rex Information Service, 1996).

The idea that fasting is *good for you* has over time been divested of the original religious significance and has taken a pseudomedical connotation. Anyone who can make a simple search through the internet will verify that hundreds of health farms offer fasting as a form of 'detox', of purification. Fasting 'cleans up' the organism. This implies that eating is a form of pollution. Invariably, the suggestion is that there is a connection between emptiness (freedom from food) and purity (spiritual catharsis, freedom from stress and disease). Control of the body is physical–spiritual catharsis, demonstration of will power, virtue and moral character.

This is the cultural background which generates anorexia (among other types of abuses of the body). The anorexic does not need to be religious or a regular custumer of health farms. Anorexia, however, should be understood in the light of this cultural and moral substrate. Control of food intake, self-induced vomiting, abuse of laxatives, diuretics and exercise, which interestingly are called 'cathartic practices', are central to anorexia. Anorexics do not only want to be thin: they want to be empty and clean of food. Food is experienced not only as fattening but it is also a pollutant, an undesirable intruder which makes you bloated, dirty and heavy.

One anorexic said:

> Before I eat (or ate) I felt afraid that I had held out too long; while eating my main idea was how I could get rid of the food in one way or another – and this thought filled my head until I felt empty again (MacSween, 1995).

Through control of hunger and body shape, people affirm their *purity:* a purity which is not only physical but also mental and moral. They are able to control their body with their will: they win over their body.

EATING DISORDERS AND MORALITY

It may be objected that to connect anorexia and contemporary fashion with ancient values professed by Orpheus, Plato, the Christian Fathers or Kant is too speculative because no one, nowadays, believes in reincarnation or would sacrifice his or her life in the name of a Christian ethic.

However, sociological studies show that this ethic is still dominant in contemporary society (Weber 1976; Turner, 1984). The body–mind split is part of the way most people ordinarily think about persons. The moral values which follow, related to the idea that the body is inferior to the mind and ought to be controlled, remain unquestioned in the history of western thought for over 3 000 years. It seems likely that they persist in contemporary societies, and it is possible that such moral substrate explains permeability to elements of other cultures, which seem congruent with that substrate.

Moreover, experts on eating disorders agree that moral values such as self-control, perfectionism, responsibility, intellectual achievement, hard work and values which traditionally are a part of Christian ethics are invariably internalized by people with eating disorders, (Bruch, 1974, note 27, p. 25; Duker, 2003, pp. 121–22; Vandereycken & Van Deth, 1994; Lawrence, 1984, pp. 32–35).

Duker and Slade, for example, point out that an intense morality is one of the underlying characteristics of any sufferer of an eating disorder. People with eating disorders

> [...]are completely rule-bound[...] They apply their moral rules to food, to eating, to exercising as to everything else in their life [...] sufferers typically adhere very strongly to a cluster of values that centre on hard work, self control, personal responsibility, high standards of achievement, deferred gratification, not receiving rewards that have not been earned, not receiving where this is not deserved...these values and aspirations can be applied to food and body regulation as effectively as they can be applied to work, educational achievements, career success, personal relationships and of course sports, where encouragement for these values to be extended to body regulation is explicit [...] Anorexics, bulimics, all those striving to get their body "into shape" [...] are people who place very high value on control [...] it is the continuity between the sufferers' moral attitude and that of their social group or culture that again explains why the condition can be lethal (Duker & Slade, 2003, note 31, pp. 108–110).

Although anorexia is a complex condition and it is likely that many other factors contribute to its genesis, we can *make sense* of it, we can understand it better, by also looking at it in the light of a particular morality.

In the context in which the body is regarded as the 'lower grade' part of the human person, 'corpulence' (from the Latin *corpus* = body + *ulentus* = abounding in) is *unacceptable* and therefore *cannot* be considered beautiful. When not openly considered immoral, the judgement may be more subtle and severe: 'incontinence' (the vice of indulging in physical desires) will cause hilarity or disgust. Thinness is the demonstration of successful abnegation, whereas heaviness is the expression of the most repugnant vices: indolence, weakness and moral collapse (MacSween, 1995, note 28, pp. 249–50). It is not co-incidental that overeating which characterizes bulimia is the reason for *shame and guilt*, whereas rigid regimes of diet and exercise are reasons for *pride*, in people with eating disorders. Eating disorders are the consistent implementation of a moral-ity which places high status on self-control and will power, a morality which is widely accepted in the western world. *To be thin is to be good.* This is why the more the sufferer becomes emaciated, frail and vulnerable, the more powerful he or she feels. Kyle finds a similar psychological dynamics in other groups who commit self-harm (Kyle, 2004).

TWO UNRESOLVED ISSUES

WHY WOMEN?

It may be asked why, if eating disorders are the result of western morality, mainly women are affected. Would it mean that men are less sensitive to moral imperatives than women? It may also be asked whether the fact that anorexia is mainly a female problem invalidates the argument that the disorder is related to morality.

The fact that anorexia mainly affects women does not mean that morality does not play an important role in the develop-ment of the condition or that females are more sensitive than men to morality. What is more likely to be the case is that men and women can both be sensitive to the same moral impera-tives, but express their sensitivity in different ways. Men will fight for professional success or for a sculptured body, for ex-ample, whereas women will fight for a thin body. The differ-ent ways of responding to morality probably depend on gender stereotypes, which link the value of women to certain attributes (for example, frailty and thinness) and the value of men to other attributes (for example, physical strength and success).

This raises the further question as to why our society has these gender stereotypes. This would deserve a separate investigation. The metaphysics that I have outlined above, with its normative functions, can in part explain anorexia. Eating disorder behaviour expresses the way in which the person implements his or her conception of what being a person is and of what being a 'good or valid person' means, although it is necessary to look at other sociocultural and psychological determinants to explain why men and women articulate different patterns of behaviour in response to a common moral background.

WHY IS ANOREXIA NOT FOUND IN OTHER CULTURES?

The body–mind split is present in other cultures and religions, such as Hindu, Islam and others, which also place high status on the values of the spirit. Why is anorexia not found in those sociocultural contexts, if it is related to principles and values which seem to be also present in those contexts? Does the fact that similar values are found in other societies in which eating disorders are absent invali-date the theory that eating disorders are related to certain metaphysics and ethics?

In order to understand why anorexia is not found in some societies, it would be necessary to explore those other sociocultural contexts, to analyse the similarities and differences between the values accepted in cultures in which anorexia is found and those accepted in cultures in which anorexia is not found. Probably, it would also be necessary to study social and family settings in those societies. To my knowledge, such a comparative sociological study has not been yet made, and therefore an answer to the question as to why anorexia is not found in those sociocultural contexts can only be speculative.

What matters in this context, however, is that the fact that anorexia is not found in other societies does not mean that the moral values sketched above do not have a role in the causation of eating disorders. Anorexia and eating disorders in general are complex phenomena. A number of factors are likely to be involved in their development (psychological, genetic, biological, familial and social factors). The metaphysics and ethics discussed above seem to be necessary, but not sufficient to cause anorexia. They may improve our understanding of the meanings of anorexic behaviour. They are not bound to cause an-orexia. They may play a determinant role in our society because of the way they interact with other social factors (for example the structure of the family or the role of the woman in western societies). The fact that other cultures in which anorexia is not found share apparently similar metaphysics and ethics does not mean that those meta-physics and ethics do not play a role in the causation of eating disorders.

IS IT UNETHICAL TO BE NORMAL SHAPED?

Thomas Pogge raised an objection to these arguments (oral communication, Feminist Association of Bioeth-ics, Tuesday 9 November 2004). He said that instead of eliminating moral categories from judgements of people's shape, we should support positive moral judge-ment of 'normal' weight and shape. There is, he argued, something immoral in being obese, and probably there is something immoral in being extremely thin. It is morally right to be 'normal' – neither too fat nor too thin – to eat well and keep healthy, and this is what should be encouraged.

Of course it is preferable (especially for health) to have a 'normal' weight. So, there is something true in the statement: being too fat (or too thin) is 'bad for you'. But from this statement, it does not follow that being too fat (or too thin) is 'bad *of* you'. Although it is preferable to encourage people to appreciate the benefits of being healthy, it is unclear what can be gained by blaming or praising them if they are too fat or too thin. Moral condemnation has dubious benefits. And the exercise of moral police over eating can hardly produce any profit in terms of people's health, if this is what matters. Maybe you may convince some obese people to diet by claiming that it is morally bad of them to over-eat or by trying to make them feel guilty. However, moralization of eating behaviour is generally unsuccessful. Moral disapproval of fatness – which has been constant at least since the spread of Christianity – is not preventing increase in incidence of obesity in industrialized countries. Moreover, it is condemning many anorexics to suffering and premature death. How 'moral' can this be?

CONCLUSIONS

In common discourse, anorexia is viewed as a result of a contemporary mania for thinness, spread by magazines and the media. This chapter has shown the omnipresence of ultrathin models does not explain anorexia. Instead, both contemporary fashion and anorexia express a common phenomenon, the admiration of thinness, which is not a primarily aesthetic phenomenon, but is a moral phenomenon rooted in our conception of the human person. The preference for thinness symbolizes the idea that human beings are a composite of body and mind, and that there is something moral and admirable in the capacity to control the body. Emaciation displays, in the most direct way, the victory over one of the most pressing body needs, the need *to eat*.

Being thin is thus not merely beautiful: it is *valuable*. Thinness indicates the transcendence of the body. It is the emblem of the person's self-control and discipline. Concomitant denigration of fat reflects the conception that the body is potentially evil and corrupting, and needs to be contained, an idea which is invariably found in all eras of western culture.

The claim that anorexia is an effect of the negative influence operated by the media, therefore, hides the real causes of the disorders, which are found in ordinary ideas of what a person, a good person, should be. Blaming fashion or the media, or magazine directors, for using emaciated models is an easy way to avoid questioning our own moral values. It is to escape the fact that there is something potentially lethal in ordinary morality and in our conception of what is good and valuable.

REFERENCES

Aristotle. *De Anima (On the Soul)*. Harmondsworth: Penguin, 1986.

Aristotle. *Metaphysics*. London: Penguin, 1998.

British Medical Association. *Eating Disorders, Body Image & the Media. BMJ* (London) 2000.

Bruch H. *Eating Disorders: Obesity, Anorexia Nervosa and the Person Within*. London: Routledge & Kegan Paul, 1974; p. 25.

Christus Rex Information Service. Notizie dalla Santa Sede, 12 Marzo 1996; web: http://www.christusrex.org/www2/news-old/3-96/is3-12-96set.html.

Duker M, Slade R. *Anorexia Nervosa and Bulimia: How to Help.* Buckingham, Philadelphia: Open University Press, 2003; pp. 108–10, 121–2.

Eating Disorders Association; http://www.edauk.com/sub_effects_of_the_media.htm

Engelhardt HT Jr. *The Foundation of Bioethics*. New York; Oxford: Oxford University Press, 1996.

Giordano S. Qu'un souffle de vent . . . . *Med Human* 2002; **28**(1): 3–8.

Giordano S. Anorexia nervosa and its moral foundations. *Int J Child Health* 2005a; **13**: 145–56.

Giordano S. Is the body a republic? Ethics of organ and tissue post-mortem retention and use. *J Med Ethics* 2005b; **31**: 470–5.

Gordon R. *Anoressia e bulimia, anatomia di un'epidemia sociale* (Original English version Milano: Raffaello Cortina *Anorexia and bulimia, anatomy of a social epidemic*, 1990). Oxford: Blackwell, 1991; p. 92.

Griffiths R, Russel J. Compulsory treatment for anorexia nervosa patients. In: Beumont PJV, Vandereycken W, eds. *Treating Eating Disorders: Ethical, Legal and Personal Issues*. New York: New York University Press, 1998 (Chapter 6).

Guardian, 30 May 2000; web: http://www.guardian.co.uk/print/0%2C3858%2C4023718-103699%2C00.htm.

Guardian, 31 May 2000; web: www.guardian.co.uk/Archive/Article/0,4273,4023818,00.html

Harris J. *The Value of Life*. London: Routledge, 1992.

Johnson TH. *The Letters of Emily Dickinson*. Harvard University Press: Cambridge, 1958; pp. 103, 140.

Kant I. Critical examination of practical reason. In: Abbott TK, ed. *Critique of Practical Reason and Other Works on the Theory of Ethics*. London: Longmans, Green and Co, 1948; pp. 87–200.

Krugovoy SA. *Victorian Literature and the Anorexic Body*. Cambridge: Cambridge University Press, 2003; p. 9.

Kyle R. In: *Presentation at FAB Congress on Self Harming: The Body as Communication*. Sidney, November 2004.

Lawrence M. *The Anorexic Experience*. London: The Women's Press, 1984; pp 32–5.

MacSween M. *Anorexic Bodies: A Feminist and Social Perspective*. London: Routledge, 1995; pp 249–50.

Parfit D. Personal identity. In: Glover J, ed. *The Philosophy of Mind*. Oxford: Oxford University Press, 1976; pp. 143–63.

Reale G, Antiseri D. *Il pensiero occidentale dale origini a oggi*. Milano: La Scuola, 1984; p. 112.

Ryle G. *The Concept of Mind*. London: Penguin, 1978; pp 13–14.

Singer P. *Rethinking Life and Death*. Oxford: Oxford University Press, 1995.

Turner BS. *The Body and Society: Explorations in Social Theory*. London: Blackwell, 1984.

Vandereycken W, Van Deth R. *From Fasting Saints to Anorexic Girls, the History of Self-Starvation*. London: Athlone press, 1994.

Weber M. *The Protestant Ethic and the Spirit of Capitalism*. London: George Allen & Unwin, 1976; p. 180.

Intellectual Disability[1]

PEKKA LOUHIALA

Approximately 1% of people are intellectually disabled (learning disabled, mentally retarded). The cause of intellectual disability (ID) can be prenatal, perinatal or postnatal, but it often remains unknown. The commonest particular condition leading to ID is Down's syndrome.

Various terms referring to ID have been used, and they reflect both the times and the context of their use. The terms 'moron', 'imbecile' and 'idiot', for example, were originally introduced in the early twentieth century as technical terms to describe levels of ID. Later terms describing the phenomenon were, for example, 'feebleminded' and 'mentally handicapped'. Currently, there are three common terms. 'Mental retardation' is used in many American contexts (American Association for Mental Retardation), 'learning disability' is common in the United Kingdom (*British Journal of Learning Disabilities)*, and 'intellectual disability' is used in several international contexts (International Association for the Scientific Study of Intellectual Disabilities).

The terminologies reflect political correctness and the activities of interest groups, but basically all three terms refer to the same group of people. I prefer *ID* for the following reasons: *mental* refers to a broader set of functions than *intellectual*, and most of these people have no disability in many mental functions. Typically, they are fully capable of loving. In addition, no actual retardation takes place with many individuals who have ID. If *mental retardation* is too broad, then *learning disability* is perhaps too narrow a concept. These individuals have problems not only in learning but also in a wider set of intellectual functions.

Intellectually disabled people are often considered *not healthy*. Although it is obvious that many diseases and congenital conditions may lead to ID, there is no necessary association between ID and health. In fact, the statistical definition implies that there will *always* be a group of people at the lower end of the intelligence quotient (IQ) curve.

The group of people with ID is very heterogeneous, and the difference between mild and profound ID is huge. Even within one clearly defined category (like Down's syndrome) individual differences can be great.

DEFINITION

There are many possible definitions of ID, all of which are at least partly based on the concept of *intelligence*. The nature of intelligence is, of course, a controversial topic, but the following characterization by Robert Sternberg is useful for the purpose of understanding ID: '. . . I define intelligence as consisting of those mental functions purposively employed for purposes of adaptation to, and shaping and selection of, real-world environments' (Sternberg, 1990).

The tradition of *measuring* intelligence dates back to 1905, when Binet and Simon published the first test of intelligence (Binet and Simon, 1905, reprinted by Rosen *et al.*) (Rosen Clark, & Kivitz, 1976). Binet and Simon introduced IQ, which became a central concept in measuring intelligence.

A comprehensive definition of ID which would cover every individual and would be suitable for all purposes does not exist, and it may not even be worth aiming at. For the purposes of statistics and epidemiology, the following narrow definition is useful: *A person is intellectually disabled if he or she falls*

---

[1]This chapter draws upon material from the author's book *Preventing Intellectual Disability – Ethical and Clinical Issues*, © Cambridge University Press, 2004, extracts reproduced with permission.

Principles of Health Care Ethics, Second Edition   Edited by R.E. Ashcroft, A. Dawson, H. Draper and J.R. McMillan
© 2007 John Wiley & Sons, Ltd

below two standard deviations in a standardized intelligence test.

However, from the point of view of an individual, adaptation to the environment may be much more important than a test result. The definition of ID used by the American Association for Mental Retardation is broader: *Mental retardation is a disability characterized by significant limitations both in intellectual functioning and in adaptive behaviour as expressed in conceptual, social and practical adaptive skills.* In addition, the definition mentions five assumptions which are essential to the definition. These assumptions emphasize the context of community environments, cultural diversity, coexisting strengths and the need for support.

ID is clearly a normative concept, and to a large extent it has been socially constructed. Boddington and Podpadec (1991) even argue that 'what holds the class together is the assumption that they are excluded absolutely or in degree from certain valuable aspects of life'.

MORAL STATUS

Adult human beings with normal intelligence are usually considered to have full moral status. This is, however, a generalization which is obviously not valid even in contemporary Western society. In our time, race or sexual orientation are examples of traits used to deny full moral status. Intelligence has also been used as a criterion for full moral status. Thus, in addition to racism and sexism, there is something which might be called *intelligism.* (Vehmas, 1999a).

The moral status of a being or a thing can be based on its *intrinsic* or *relational* properties (Warren, 1997). Intrinsic properties which have been proposed as single criteria for moral status are life, sentience and personhood. Being 'alive' or 'sentient' is at least to some degree a *scientific* question. But whether one is a person is not a scientific question, but a philosophical one.

Evans (1996) argues that at the root of the conceptual disagreement (of the definition of 'person') is a moral disagreement about how, in fact, different individuals ought to be treated. Hallamaa (1994) ended up with very similar conclusions: '"Person" is not a theoretically "innocent" concept . . . it includes an implicit normative aspect in the sense that it states what is morally important and relevant and what can be left to one side . . . Person as a moral term implies our central normative commitments, it does not offer a neutral ground for solving moral disagreements.'

Steven Edwards (1997) has argued that the low moral status often accorded to people with ID derives from individualism. According to the *ontological* component of individualism, the existence of the self and the identity of the self do not depend upon the existence of anything beyond the self. The *normative* component of individualism states that the ideal moral agent is fully autonomous, thus being able to make his or her own decisions about a good life.

Both of these aspects of individualism refer to *independence* in their own ways. The self is an independent entity if its existence does not depend on the existence of other selves (Edwards, 1997). One is *socially* independent if one does not need the concern and care of others. This has obvious implications for the status of the disabled who are in many ways dependent on other people in their daily lives.

The issue of dependence can, however, be seen in a totally different light. Instead of the disabled being considered a marginal group, they can be seen as *distinctively human* because of their dependence on other people (Vehmas, 1999b).

The concept of ID cannot be applied to young infants. However, these children sometimes have conditions which lead to ID later in childhood. This development can often be predicted with high probability, but the degree of disability remains uncertain. According to some philosophers, (future) ID as such means lower moral status (e.g. Kuhse & Singer, 1985). Letting such a child die is more justifiable than letting a child with (future) normal intelligence die.

Such a view is, however, problematic for many reasons. First, the assumption that the quality of life related to ID per se must be lower than the quality of life with normal intelligence is clearly wrong. For example, the commonly held view that Down's syndrome is associated with a joyful and positive character may well be true. If it is true, a utilitarian should *prefer* the life of an individual with Down's syndrome to the life of someone without this syndrome.

Secondly, the reasoning of Kuhse and Singer seems to imply that the value of life decreases gradually with decreasing intelligence. What then would be the lower limit of intelligence which would guarantee full moral status? What about the individual with subnormal intelligence but no ID (according to current definitions)? What about extremely intelligent individuals and their quality of life?

Thirdly, the context in which one is born and lives is very important for one's happiness. Vehmas (1999b) has presented the following clarifying example (for which he acknowledged John Lizza):

> Suppose A is a boy without intellectual disabilities who grows up in an impoverished environment with bad familial and social relationships, whereas B has Down's syndrome but grows up in an excellent environment with good social and familial support. Which one has the prospects for a more satisfactory life? Probably the child with Down's syndrome, especially if the other child grew up in a neighbourhood where statistics showed that a high percentage of the young males end up in prison or dead. Would Kuhse, Singer and Rachels think it permissible to kill infants born in impoverished environments because the prospects for their lives would be much worse than for those born in a more affluent environment?

Young infants are not moral agents. During late infancy or early childhood the individual gains moral agency, and it also becomes possible to test his or her intelligence. *Possible* future ID is not relevant to the moral status of a foetus, a newborn or a young infant. What is the situation for older children and adults with *actual* ID? Does the degree of disability affect the moral status of an individual?

In practice, intellectually disabled people are often accorded a moral status which is lower than that accorded to intellectually able individuals (Edwards, 1997). Prenatal screening does not *necessarily* imply a lower moral status of affected individuals, but adult disabled people easily interpret screening as a message saying: 'They don't want people like us.'

Notions of personhood popular among some utilitarian philosophers may also be thought of as supporting the lower status of individuals with ID. However, even if the extreme views on personhood were adopted, there would be implications only for the status of the profoundly intellectually disabled, who form a small minority of the population with ID. Only in that group may intelligence as such be relevant to one's moral status. Although the great majority of intellectually disabled persons can be said to be moral agents in the full sense of the term, some individuals with profound ID obviously lack the qualities necessary for moral agency. In a possible conflict situation, the moral status of a full moral agent would be stronger.

PREVENTION OF INTELLECTUAL DISABILITY

It has been taken for granted that the prevention of disabilities, including ID, is per se a good thing. However, because there is no necessary association between ID and suffering, we have to ask the question *why* should it be prevented? Five arguments are briefly considered here: (1) the eugenic argument, (2) the foetal-wastage argument, (3) the family burden argument, (4) the societal burden argument and (5) the quality of life argument.

According to the *eugenic argument*, there is something bad or undesirable in certain genetic conditions which deviate from a norm that can be defined by statistical and scientific methods. The elimination of these conditions, defined as 'genetic diseases', can be considered a legitimate goal. It is thus assumed that 'genetically normal' or 'genetically healthy' can be defined.

The concepts of 'normal' and 'healthy' are, however, highly ambiguous. We all have unique genotypes, and it is a matter of convention which of them is considered normal and which abnormal or undesirable. In fact, virtually everyone carries a small number of harmful recessive genes. In addition, the interaction between one's genotype and the environment is, in many cases, a crucial determinant of health and well being.

It is also worth noting that the application of selective abortion is *dysgenic*, not *eugenic*, when the total effect on the human gene pool is considered. The fact that it is dysgenic is due to the possibility that the relative number of carriers of recessive genes leading to certain diseases may increase, while the homozygotes are selectively aborted. The magnitude of this dysgenic effect is, however, very small and slow (Jackson, 1990). Whether we want to utilize prenatal diagnosis or not has to be judged on other grounds.

It has been estimated that more than half of pregnant women lose their embryos during the first trimester and some miscarry during the latter two trimesters. According to the *foetal-wastage argument*, selective abortion is a continuation of this natural process (Boss, 1993). The argument seems to assume two things: first, that nature is able to differentiate between embryos or foetuses which have the possibility for full human life after birth and those which do not, and secondly, that nature or natural can be considered the standard from which we can infer how things should be.

The first assumption is partly true. It is not true, however, that the more serious a condition is, the more frequently spontaneous abortions occur. The second assumption seems to assume that nature is good, at least with respect to the particular issue of spontaneous abortions. This general idea of nature being good would, however, lead to odd implications, and the particular idea of certain spontaneous abortions being good leads us to ask why this and not some other natural process should be considered good. It may be that the supporters of the argument also base their view on a value judgement about the lives of individuals with a certain genotype or phenotype.

The *family burden argument* can be presented as a more general version referring to the rights of the parents or as a narrower utilitarian version comparing the family consequences of accepting a handicapped child or aborting it as a foetus. Discussion on the general version leads to questions about the ethics of abortion. Instead, I shall concentrate on the narrower formulation which has special relevance for the prevention of ID.

The burden on the family can be expressed in several ways. First, having an intellectually disabled child is an obvious risk for both marriage and the relationship between the parents and the other children in the family. Secondly, whatever the arrangements of care, the parents often experience feelings of guilt. Thirdly, the burden on the family can be expressed materially as the extra economic costs caused by the special care arrangements needed for the child.

Depending on the degree of the disability and the number of additional handicaps, the burden an intellectually disabled child places on a family can be anything from minor to major. The discovery of disability in a child of any age is always a shock, but a mildly intellectually disabled child with no additional handicaps may later bring only minor changes to

family life. On the contrary, the care of a severely intellectually disabled child with, for example, cerebral palsy and
epilepsy may be extremely time consuming and exhausting,
both physically and mentally.

The impact of an intellectually disabled child on a
family is not entirely and necessarily negative. There
are both families that have been weakened and families
that have been emotionally enriched by the presence of
a disabled child. It is important to note that the matter in
each case is *uncertain* and the experience may strengthen
as well as weaken the family. And, of course, as Bosk
(1992) has pointed out, 'chronic sorrow' and 'successful normalisation' are only analytically distinct. Empirically, it is possible to imagine the same person having
each feeling closely connected in time.

The political and economical structure of society and
the supportive service available highly influence the psychological and economic burden experienced by families
with an intellectually disabled child. According to Boss
(1993), 70% of families with a chronically disabled child
in the United States have significant financial problems
as a result of the child's disorder. In countries with subsidized medical care, the economic burden on families is
far less important.

Thus, the utilitarian family burden argument is not
generally true. It may be a good argument only in *particular* cases, in which the burden of a handicapped child
on the family can reasonably be expected to exceed the
burden caused by abortion.

According to the *societal burden argument*, the
intellectually disabled never become productive or benefit
society. Instead, they are a burden, and therefore, preventing ID is justified, if that prevention does not bring about
a greater burden in some form. The unit of measurement
in the discussions on social burdens is, in general, money,
because other social burdens or goods are more difficult
to quantify.

Cost–benefit analyses concerning the prevention of ID
have been carried out, and screening for disorders such as
Down's syndrome and fragile X syndrome has been shown
to be cost effective. The analyses are, however, problematic
in many ways. First, the accuracy and validity of the calculations are questionable because many assumptions must be
made about, for example, the uptake of tests and the proportion of women willing to abort after a positive diagnosis. In
a district in Wales, as a result of a quality-improvement
project, the uptake of serum screening *fell* from around
95% to 75%. In addition, the number of amniocenteses decreased as women were able to think more clearly about
their options and the limitations of the tests (Al-Jader,
1999). Secondly, political changes like deinstitutionalization, obviously reduce the costs remarkably. Thirdly, other
costs and benefits, like those related to the unavoidable

miscarriages related to amniocenteses, have not been considered. Fourthly, the hidden premise that prevention is justified if it can be shown to save money, however little, cannot be taken for granted.

The *quality of life argument* goes like this: individuals
with ID often have a low quality of life. Especially those who
have associated physical handicaps may have an extremely
low quality of life, in some cases even to the extent that life
can be considered worse than death. These kinds of lives
are not worth living; therefore, preventing states leading to
such lives is justified.

The concept of happiness is not equal to the concept of
quality of life, but the discourse on the latter has its roots in
the earlier discourse on the former. Classical utilitarianism
was interested in the maximization of happiness, roughly
the same as *subjective* quality of life, and, for it, how happiness was distributed in society was irrelevant.

The quality of life issue can also be approached from perspectives other than strictly utilitarian ones. Amartya Sen,
for example, has suggested the *capability* approach, which
is concerned with people's actual abilities to achieve various valuable functionings as a part of living (Sen, 1993). In
empirical sociology, Allardt (1993) has presented the *basic
needs* approach, which combines both subjective and objective aspects of well-being. This approach is categorized
by the catchwords having, loving and being. *Having* refers
to the material conditions necessary for survival and for
avoiding misery, *loving* stands for the need to relate to other
people and to form social identities and *being* stands for the
need to integrate into society and to live in harmony with
nature. With respect to having and loving, the position of
people with ID does, in most cases, not differ from those
without ID.

No obvious reason can be found as to why ID per se would
decrease the quality of life of the individual. The mildly intellectually disabled or so-called borderline people may be
the only ones who suffer from their inferior intelligence, not
being able to manage in the open labour market and feeling
rejected by their peers. On the other hand, they do not feel
that they belong to the world of the intellectually disabled
either. The suffering these persons experience is, however,
more a reflection of the attitudes of the environment and it
does not originate from low intelligence as such. It is easy
to imagine, for example, a rural community in which such
a person could find his or her place and would not suffer.
We can also imagine some suffering at the other extreme of
the IQ distribution: a highly intelligent child or youngster
might also suffer from rejection by peers.

We should ask the question whether those who are
unhappy feel so because they are intellectually disabled or
because they have been poorly cared for (Rose-Ackerman,
1982). In addition, it can be questioned whether burdens
external to the individual should be counted in calculations

of one's quality of life at all (Boss, 1993). These burdens can be considerable in the form of a lack of socioeconomic or familial support to establish a minimally satisfactory life. Counting these external burdens would, however, lead to problematic conclusions because it would then be logical to consider selective abortion also in cases in which the prospect of the foetus without a diagnosed condition leading to disability would be miserable due to unfavourable social conditions.

The quality of life of the intellectually disabled has been studied extensively, but very rarely has it been compared with the quality of life of the general population. In one study, the author concluded that, in general, the intellectually disabled are as satisfied with their lives as the rest of the population. The former, however, do experience physical violence and stress more often than the latter (Matikka, 2000).

Severe ID is almost always accompanied by physical handicaps, which may cause considerable suffering. The suggested justification for selective abortion in these cases refers to survivability or the possibility of a pain-free existence. The former issue poses the question of the length of 'normal' life which is considered worth while. Is it 6 months, as in Tay-Sachs disease, or 40 years, as in Huntington's disease? Or should we perhaps consider the ratio of 'normal' to 'abnormal' years? And, in the end, there always remains the question of whether the individual actually suffers in such a way that it would overcome the desire to continue life.

When trying to imagine what an intellectually disabled person feels, we may too easily think what *we* would feel if we suddenly developed similar mental and physical characteristics. The result, of course, does not tell anything about the feelings of the actual person, who, in most cases, has had the qualities for a lifetime.

We have seen that very different arguments have been presented to support the prevention of ID. Some of them focus on the individual, some on the family and some on society. Some arguments consider suffering, some economic good. In the medical context they are often presented superficially, ignoring the complexity of some more-or-less hidden assumptions behind each argument.

The family burden argument may be more successful than the other ones, but only if two conditions are met. First, reproductive autonomy of the families is given high value, and secondly, a psychological or economic burden is accepted as a justification for abortion. It is important, however, to separate two issues: the *general* justification for the prevention of ID (e.g. in the form of introducing nationwide programmes) and justification in *particular* cases. At the general level, the argument is not strong because of the substantial variation in the psychological and economic burdens. In particular, the economic burden is highly determined by the nature of the health and social services available in a particular society. In the case of an individual family, if obvious burden can be anticipated, the argument is strong. If a society accepts abortion on request, there are no convincing arguments to deny it from parents willing to prevent ID in their offspring. Health care providers do not, however, have a duty to perform prenatal diagnosis on any kind of request, and the other side of respecting parental autonomy is supporting parents' right to give birth to children who will be intellectually or physically handicapped.

REFERENCES

Al-Jader L. The achievements of antenatal screening programme for congenital abnormalities and lessons learned for clinical governance. *J Med Genet* 1999; **36**(Suppl. 1): S70.

Allardt E. Having, loving, being: an alternative to the Swedish model of welfare research. In: Nussbaum MC, Sen A, eds. *The Quality of Life*. Oxford: Clarendon Press, 1993; pp. 88–94.

Boddington P, Podpadec T. Who are the mentally handicapped? *J Appl Philos* 1991; **8**: 177–90.

Bosk CL. *All God's Mistakes. Genetic Counseling in a Pediatric Hospital*. Chicago/London: The University of Chicago Press, 1992.

Boss JA. *The Birth Lottery. Prenatal Diagnosis and Selective Abortion*. Chicago: Loyola University Press, 1993.

Edwards S. The moral status of intellectually disabled individuals. *J Med Philos* 1997; **22**: 29–42.

Evans M. Some ideas of the person. In: Greaves D, Upton H, eds. *Philosophical Problems in Health Care*. Avebury: Aldershot, 1996; pp. 23–35.

Hallamaa J. *The Prisms of Moral Personhood*. Helsinki: Luther-Agricola-Society, 1994.

Jackson LG. Commentary: Prenatal diagnosis: the magnitude of dysgenic effects is small, the human benefits, great. *Birth* 1990; **17**: 80.

Kuhse H, Singer P. *Should the Baby Live?* Oxford: OUP, 1985.

Matikka LM. Comparability of quality-of-life studies of the general population and people with intellectual disabilities. *Scand J Disability Res* 2000; **2**: 83–102.

Rose-Ackerman S. Mental retardation and society: the ethics and politics of normalization. *Ethics* 1982; **93**: 81–101.

Rosen M, Clark GL, Kivitz MS. *The History of Mental Retardation, Collected Papers*. Baltimore: University Park Press, 1976.

Sen A. Capability and well-being. In: Nussbaum MC, Sen A, eds. *The Quality of Life*. Oxford: Clarendon Press, 1993; pp. 30–53.

Sternberg RJ. *Metaphors of Mind – Conceptions on the Nature of Intelligence*. Cambridge: Cambridge University Press, 1990.

Vehmas S. Discriminative assumptions of utilitarian bioethics regarding individuals with intellectual disabilities. *Disability Soc* 1999a; **14**: 37–52.

Vehmas S. Newborn infants and the moral significance of intellectual disabilities. *J Assoc Persons Severe Handicaps* 1999b; **24**: 111–21.

Warren MA. Moral status. *Obligations to Persons and Other Living Things*. Oxford: Clarendon Press, 1997.

64

Ethical Issues and Health Care for Older People

JULIAN C. HUGHES

INTRODUCTION

There is a saying that old age does not come alone: it 'breeds aches'. The requirement for health care increases as we age and this, in turn, raises the possibility of ethical issues. But this is already to have indulged in preconceptions about ageing. I shall start this chapter by briefly considering general issues about being old and ageism. This will raise what could be regarded as the central ethical issue in old age, which is the problem of autonomy. I shall outline why it is an ethical problem. In my view the problem is resolved by taking a broader view of what it is to be a person. Having gestured at this view, the remaining parts of the chapter will show the difference it makes to discussions of a variety of ethical issues that arise in old age.

WHO ARE OLDER PERSONS?

The potential injustice to elderly people contained in the assumptions that are made about them because they are seen as old rather than individual is an injustice built into social institutions (Oppenheimer, 1991, p. 366).

Like younger people, older people are very varied. The notion of diversity in old age immediately suggests that our approach to older people should be flexible, capable of accommodating difference. Similarly, *issues* in old age will be many and various too. While some of these issues will be shared with people of a younger age, some of them will reflect ageing itself. I have listed, incompletely, a mixture of these issues in Table 64.1.

Talking of 'ageing itself' raises further questions. For what is ageing? Well, a quick glance at Table 64.1 should show that it is a complicated concept. It involves a biological

component; but there are also psychosocial factors stemming, for instance, from isolation and relative poverty. There are spiritual issues too. This is a time in people's lives when they might be able to focus on living authentically, focusing on what is deeply meaningful to them. And the nearness of death encourages this focus.

The issues for an individual older person will be unique, although shaped by a shared human nature. The concepts of human nature and ageing are not fixed (Bavidge, 2006); they change with time and place and so too will the ethical issues. Table 64.1 contains elements that are ambiguous concerning whether or not they represent a good thing for the ageing individual. Quality of life, for example, is a complicated notion (Bond and Corner, 2004) and one that is impossible to pin down – despite the numerous attempts to measure it objectively – except in so far as we can sketch what might be the good life for an individual person (Hughes, 2003). So, there is no simple paradigm for what it is to be an older person.

In approaching older people we approach a range of potential issues reflecting shared and idiosyncratic life experiences. Older people are themselves embedded in contexts or narratives that have their own character:

The elderly have been around the block, seen it all before, and developed habitual ways of responding. Their interests and behaviour are motivated by different ambitions, concerns, and anxieties from those of the young . . . there are also distinctive and valuable qualities in the experience and the attitudes of the elderly who have been in similar situations many times before (Bavidge, 2006, p. 49).

This experience should encourage us to engage with older people in finding ways to negotiate difficulties. But there may be, as Oppenheimer suggested, injustices built into our

Table 64.1. Some Issues in old age

Authentic existence	Autonomy	Cognitive impairment
Communication	Death	Dependence
Depression	Disadvantage	Diversity
Existential realization	Family	Frailty
Freedom	Fulfilment	Immobility
Independence	Isolation	Loss
Relationships	Religion	Sensory impairment
Social participation	Spirituality	Stigma
Time	Voluntary work	Vulnerability

social systems. It may be that the route the older person would be inclined to take – to remain at home, for instance, with appropriate home care – is simply not open. In care homes, the problem is sometimes that the person's 'needs can no longer be met', with the result that the older person – who has had to sell a *home* to afford the *care* of the *care home* – has to be moved willy-nilly.

There is much that goes on, therefore, to ensure the *true needs* of older people (especially those who are poor) are ignored because of political decisions and social structures. This reflects an incipient ageism that tends to direct energy and resources away from fairly basic levels of care for older people. Indeed, there is evidence that the standards of health and social care in many parts of even an affluent society like Britain are poor (e.g. Ballard et al., 2001; Eaton, 2006; Fisken, 2006).

AGEISM

There have been arguments for some time about whether rationing on the basis of age is ethically acceptable. Williams (1997) stated: 'In each of our lives there has to come a time when we accept the inevitability of death, and when we also accept that a reasonable limit has to be set on the demands we can properly make on our fellow citizens in order to keep us going a bit longer.'

The inevitability of death cannot be contradicted. But the second part of the sentence is motivated by a more arguable political view, which is asserted more starkly a little later by Williams (Williams, 1997): 'So the values of the citizenry as a whole must override the values of a particular interest group within it.'

Such a view would cause more consternation if it were uttered in connection with race, religion or sexual orientation. It seems to go against the values highlighted by Grimley Evans (Grimley Evans, 1997) in the same debate, where he emphasized 'the equality of citizens in their relation to the institutions of the state' and 'the uniqueness of individuals regardless of their physical or mental

attributes'. Yet many of us might feel a natural sympathy for the 'fair innings' argument, according to which there comes a point (perhaps after three score years and ten) when it would seem better to spend money on preserving the lives of younger people rather than of older people, who should instead only receive palliative measures. This natural sympathy, however, itself indicates a type of ageism inasmuch as it partly depends on the perception that all 'the elderly' are the same. This is what Grimley Evans (Grimley Evans, 1997) was objecting to: '. . . the exclusion from treatment on the basis of a patient's age without reference to his or her physiological condition'.

Individuals need to be treated individually. Groups of older people should not be excluded just because, like groups of poorer people, they are statistically (as a group) not such a good bet. In any case, the 'fair innings' argument requires a qualitative component – because an individual innings can be quite different depending on all sorts of factors – and cannot be judged 'fair' merely on the basis of length.

Thinking about who 'the elderly' are, therefore, as well as thinking about ageism, leads us to one point: older people are a very varied group and, if we are to do the right thing for them, we need to treat them individually. This leads us to the central ethical issue in old age: the problem of autonomy.

FROM AUTONOMY TO THE SITUATED PERSON

The pre-eminence of autonomy as an ethical principle in liberal thought is well established. If we are concerned about the individuality of older people, it is easy enough to see why respect for autonomy should be given a high priority. And yet it is a problem. For, if age breeds aches, it also breeds at least a degree of dependency. The ethical problem concerns how we can be both autonomous *and* dependent. It quickly becomes apparent that this is unavoidable. Most of us could not function without the help of other people. This is true even when we are in 'our prime', which is just when we like to think of ourselves as fully autonomous; in this respect old age is no different to other stages of our lives.

Thought about autonomy should help us to see, too, that we do not merely exercise our autonomy when we are faced by the big dilemmas. As Agich states:

> Autonomy fundamentally importantly involves the way individuals live their daily lives; it is found in the nooks and crannies of everyday experience; it is found in the way that individuals interact and not exclusively in the idealized paradigms of choice or decision making that dominate ethical analysis' (Agich, 2003, p. 165).

He goes on to argue persuasively that,

> The concept of autonomy properly understood requires that individuals be seen in essential interrelationship with others and the world (Agich, 2003, p. 174).

Hence, the notion of autonomy is itself complex (Collopy, 1988). For many older people, their autonomy is increasingly predicated on their dependency; but not because their autonomy is faulty, rather because this is the nature of being in the world as an older person. Moreover, it also emerges that autonomy as a concept, in relation to any age, must be circumscribed.

Now, one of the reasons that autonomy is circumscribed is because of the nature of personhood. One way to characterize this notion is to describe the person as a situated embodied agent (Hughes, 2001). It is because of the multifarious ways in which we are situated as human beings that autonomy *must* be circumscribed. It is entirely open to me to make a particular decision, but I remain historically and culturally embedded so that my decisions cannot be blind to laws and norms of ethical action. My autonomous decision-making is limited by the autonomous decisions of others. Although I am an agent, I am a *situated* agent, ineluctably bound by my nature as a human being in the world. While that nature entails the possibility of openness to new experiences and endeavours even in old age, it also entails a degree of dependency. Because, for one thing, as *embodied* agents, we are subject to the natural processes of ageing. As Agich went on to say in his seminal discussion of autonomy in connection with long-term care:

> The agent in the everyday world is thus an essentially dependent entity, . . . A theory of autonomy that provides a concrete view of persons must be one that is sensitive to the social nature of personhood and to the complex conditions that actually support the unique identity of those individuals needing long-term care (Agich, 2003, p. 134).

The problem of autonomy, therefore, is solved by taking a broad view of personhood so that autonomy itself is seen, *inherently*, as a notion that has to be worked out in the context of a world shared with others on whom we are, perhaps, increasingly dependent as we get older.

CONSENT, CAPACITY AND BEST INTERESTS

The issues of autonomy and dependency are seen clearly when the older person is considered to lack the capacity to make important decisions. However, we should not overlook the possibility that older people are sometimes denied their wishes, not because of any form of incompetence on their part, but rather because they are dependent upon inadequate social support. When a person's decision-making capacity is called into question, his or her autonomy is placed under considerable threat. The paradigm case is that of decisions to do with treatment, where valid consent – entailing that the person is informed, competent and uncoerced – is required. But while this might seem straightforward, it is fraught with difficulty because of the evaluative judgements that have to be made. When it comes to consent to research, where we might have anticipated that things would be more rigorous, there is evidence of older people being involved in research projects although they do not pass the tests of capacity (Pucci et al., 2001). On the face of it this looks like a bad thing. However, it might be that the legal standards for capacity are in danger of being too narrowly defined. Current law in England and Wales suggests that to have capacity, the person must be able to understand, recall, weigh up the material information and communicate his or her decision. All of this is rather cognitive, whereas some have argued that emotional and volitional aspects also come into the assessment of capacity (Charland, 1998; Culver and Gert, 2004). It is certainly the case that decisions about capacity can be problematic.

Case vignette: Mrs B and going home

Mrs B is a 93-year-old widow who has been admitted to a medical ward slightly confused following a fall. She has lived for some years with her 84-year-old younger sister who is known to have a mild dementia. The younger sister is, however, physically fit. She is looked after by a neighbour whilst Mrs B is in hospital. Mrs B remains unsteady on her feet. A question is raised concerning whether Mrs B has the capacity to make a decision about returning home.

Mrs B is able to recall why she had to come into hospital. She remembers the fall. She readily agrees that she is unsteady, but says that she will be able to manage at home by avoiding those activities that have in the past led her to fall over. She seems, therefore, to understand at least some of the material information. It is not so clear, however, that she is able to weigh the information in making her decision. Or, at least, she appears to the medical staff to give little weight to the concerns about falling. Instead, she emphasizes her desire to return home to look after her younger sister. She is able to talk about the ways in which her younger sister helps to look after her and the ways in which she looks after her younger sister.

The need to assess a person's capacity to make a decision about going home from hospital is commonplace. As the case of Mrs B demonstrates, the idea of *weighing up* the material information is difficult to conceive without bringing in some form of value judgement. Such judgements need to give weight to the emotional content of what Mrs B is saying, as well as to whether or not she will be able to pursue the care of her sister adequately. In this case, it might seem very reasonable to argue that not giving enough weight to the risk of falls amounts to a failure to weigh up the relevant information properly. Contrariwise, the importance of continuing to live with her sister with a degree of independence could (it might reasonably be argued) be regarded as enough to outweigh the (mere) possibility of a fall.

If it were determined that Mrs B lacks capacity, a decision would have to be made in her best interests. It should become immediately apparent that the notion of 'best interests' cannot be considered in an atomistic fashion (Hughes et al., 2002). Mrs B's best interests inevitably involve other people. A careful negotiation would have to be entered into, which would be about values and would involve taking the values of all concerned seriously. Such values-based practice accepts that, especially in moral dilemmas, there will be values diversity. It is fundamental to this type of practice that it encourages a process designed to support a balance of legitimately different perspectives, a balance that is usually achieved through sensitive communication (Fulford, 2004). It is, of course, perfectly possible that this sort of sensitive communication and negotiation might not occur.

In any event, the need for a broad assessment of capacity and of best interests is underpinned by a broad conception of personhood. In a similar way, the other means of supporting the person's autonomy (whether by surrogate decision-making, by the use of advance directives, or by appeal to the courts) must also be aware of the context and of the particular circumstances that obtain. Again, this will mean that there are inevitable limits to the exercise of autonomy because of the dependency that follows from our situatedness as human agents.

FAMILIES AND CARE

Older people can often become dependent upon their families. Most families will keep the older person's best interests firmly in view. However, there can be tensions and, sometimes, particular family members can be abusive. Health care professionals will need to communicate with families but keep the interests of the older person in mind. This can lead to dilemmas concerning confidentiality. Our dependency, especially where the person has dementia, means that some information must inevitability be shared. However, the particularities of the case will help to determine the extent to which confidentiality is maintained in accordance with professional guidance (Hughes and Louw, 2002a). The aim and intention behind the sharing of information will obviously be crucial to whether or not breaking confidentiality is morally justified.

A particular issue for some families of people with dementia is that of truth-telling (Baldwin et al., 2005, pp. 64–73). Disclosure of a diagnosis such as cancer can be different in different cultures (Akabayashi, 1999), although the strong trend has been towards more openness (Buckman, 1996). In dementia care, we see a significant variety of attitudes towards disclosure even among professionals with a similar sociocultural background (Bamford et al., 2004). These differences will reflect the different emphases placed on principles, such as respect for autonomy and the need for beneficence, as well as on the exercise of the virtue of honesty.

Once again, the balancing of autonomy against the realities of the person's situatedness in a (more or less) caring family is the key to ethical decision-making. If the person's dependency is a brute fact – something that cannot be got around – if it is not induced by the malignancy of the physical or psycho-social environment (Kitwood, 1997; Sabat, 2006), then it would seem perverse to act as if the person had full autonomy. Nevertheless, to override the person's autonomy because of a slothful disregard for his or her remaining capacities and agency would be to undermine his or her standing as a person and for this reason would be morally culpable.

TAKING RISKS

The case of Mrs B also raises the issue of risk. Sometimes, through frailty and vulnerability, the older person may place himself or herself at risk. This might include the risk of physical harm from falling or misusing appliances such as gas ovens, or the risk of financial (or other forms of) abuse. In the circumstances of dementia, there may also be risks attendant upon wandering. The dilemma here is to decide the extent to which a person's liberty and autonomy should be curtailed for the sake of their safety (Hughes and Louw, 2002b).

In general, respect for autonomy favours the preservation of liberty. However, for some people being free poses risks. In particular cases, once again, the question will concern the extent to which we have truly tried to aim at what is good for the individual. Institutional responses, where the system requires that people be restrained in one way or another, are likely to offend societal norms. But this is not to deny that in individual cases some restrictions of liberty might have to be tolerated, especially where the issue of safety is paramount. Here is an example of a husband caring for his wife with dementia where he felt the restriction of her liberty was warranted:

> I felt bad about locking the doors. But, on the other hand, I realised that it was for her protection. I couldn't let her out. Once she knew that I'd locked the door, she'd start to thump the door and thump me and scream and call for the police, and all sorts of things. I had a terrible job trying to calm her down (Baldwin et al., 2005, p. 20).

Alternatively, here is an example of a husband who took a different view:

> I used to say to the carers who came in, 'Don't stop my wife going out at all – just go with her.' It's quite simple really: stop them getting into danger, yes, by whatever means you have to, but certainly do not restrict their freedom. Definitely not (Baldwin et al. 2005 p. 21).

The juxtaposition of these two quotations raises an interesting challenge. Are we to say that one husband was wrong and the other right? My inclination is to say no such thing, but is this illogical? Is it to try to hold that both *p* and *not-p* are simultaneously true? One response would be to seek clarification from the two husbands. What were the resources (physical, financial, social) of the first husband that meant he had no option but to lock his wife in? What does the second husband intend by saying that danger must be avoided 'by whatever means', and why might this not extend to locking the door? The point of the clarification would be to understand the specific situations of the two husbands and their wives. Their inter-relations and circumstances are unique, so we are not comparing *p* and *not-p*, but *p* and *q*. They are situated differently, they have different narratives, and they must be judged accordingly. Nevertheless, complete incarceration (*deprivation* of liberty as opposed to *restriction* of liberty perhaps) is not something we would tolerate without significant justification and legal safeguards. This distinction between 'deprivation' and 'restriction' of liberty in a person who is compliant but who lacks capacity is to be found at the heart of the now famous Bournewood judgement in the ruling of the European Court (Bournewood, 2004).

The need to look at risk and individual circumstances is becoming increasingly, but slowly, recognized in connection with driving and dementia. It is clear that ageism exists in connection with older people driving generally, but when it comes to people with dementia, it is often presumed that they will be unsafe. The issue of autonomy is readily ignored. Yet, the evidence is that people with dementia are able to drive safely while the disease is in the milder stages. Therefore, if someone wishes to continue to drive, he or she should be offered a specialized assessment of driving (Snyder, 2005). This is a way of recognizing the person's continuing agentive abilities even in the midst of increasing dependency in other aspects of life.

TREATMENT DECISIONS

Arguments about when to treat and when not to treat are epitomized by the dilemmas as to when to use artificial nutrition and hydration. The use of percutaneous endoscopic gastrostomy (PEG) feeding following stroke seems unobjectionable when swallowing is only temporarily dysfunctional and where the prospects of a good recovery are high. In the case of the person with severe dementia, however, where the swallowing has gradually been worsening, the use of PEG feeding is highly suspect given the poor evidence of its efficacy (Gillick, 2000). But there are many cases between the extremes where the dilemma remains real.

A broad view of nutrition will tend to stress the role of food and feeding in our lives. However, the broad view must also take into account the values and inclinations that guided the person whose ability to feed is now compromised. This may require some form of interpretation of the person's prior wishes, requiring practical wisdom (Widdershoven and Berghmans, 2006) or it may require judgements about quality of life (Bond and Corner, 2004). In a casuistic way, the interpretation in a particular case will tend to make comparisons with precedent cases where the moral dilemma has already been determined (Louw and Hughes, 2005). However, the interpretation will need to relate to the particular person situated within his or her own life history and nexus of beliefs and values.

DEATH

The tendency to care for people who are physically and mentally disadvantaged seems to be a deeply ingrained pattern of behaviour. It underpins the need for good quality palliative care, not only for cancer patients, but also in other chronic illnesses that have a terminal course, such as dementia (Hughes, 2006). Nevertheless, there are increasing demands for the legalization of assisted dying. On the one hand, the prohibition against intentional killing is a strong restraint; while, on the other hand, claims about dignity and humane treatment exert a definite pull. To allow that a carer might aim at the destruction of human life would be to undermine the essence of caring. But the strongest argument in favour of euthanasia or physician assisted suicide is the one that stresses its voluntary nature. This plays on the notion of autonomy, but it ignores the extent to which we are situated, so that the nature of an action must be judged in a context. In a particular case, even if it were voluntary, the intention and aim would always be to kill a human life. To allow this type of action to become established as a norm would be to take away a prohibition that has supported health care practice in civilized society. It would be to allow a breach in the principled objection to non-voluntary or involuntary killing (Keown, 2002).

CONCLUSION

Older people require and deserve our respect. This means that we must respect their autonomy, because this will always involve respecting the person's selfhood. But autonomy is limited by dependency just as our situated agency coalesces with our situated embodiment. Thus, old age shows what is true at other times of our lives too, that as human beings in the world our narratives have a unique meaning. Clinical judgements, which are, at one and the same time, judgements about both facts and values, must be coherent with the broader fields that characterize our human concerns. Our responses to old age and older people must cohere with our responses to being-in-the-world generally.

REFERENCES

Agich GJ. *Dependence and Autonomy in Old Age: An Ethical Framework for Long-Term Care*. Cambridge: Cambridge University Press, 2003.

Akabayashi A, Fetters MD, Elwyn TS. Family consent, communication, and advance directives for cancer disclosure: a Japanese case and discussion. *J Med Ethics* 1999; **25**: 296–301.

Baldwin C, Hope T, Hughes J, Jacoby R, Ziebland S. *Making Difficult Decisions: The Experience of Caring for Someone with Dementia*. London: Alzheimer's Society, 2005.

Ballard C, Fossey J, Chithramohan R, Howard R, Burns A, Thompson P, Tadros G, Fairbairn A. Quality of care in private sector and NHS facilities for people with dementia: cross sectional survey. *Br Med J* 2001; **323**: 426–7.

Bamford C, Lamont S, Eccles M, Robinson L, May C, Bond J. Disclosing a diagnosis of dementia: a systematic review. *Int J Geriatr Psychiatry* 2004; **19**: 151–69.

Bavidge M. Ageing and human nature. In: Hughes JC, Louw SJ, Sabat SR, eds. *Dementia: Mind, Meaning, and the Person*. Oxford: Oxford University Press, 2006; pp. 41–53.

Bond J, Corner L. *Quality of Life and Older People*. Buckingham: Open University Press, 2004.

Bournewood Judgement in the ruling of the European Court. *HL* v. *The United Kingdom*. (Application No. 45508/99). Judgement 5 October 2004.

Buckman R. Talking to patients about cancer. *Br Med J* 1996; **313**: 699–700.

Charland LC. Is Mr Spock mentally competent? Competence to consent and emotion. *Philos Psychiatry Psychol* 1998; **5**: 67–81.

Collopy BJ. Autonomy in long term care: some crucial distinctions. *Gerontologist* 1988; **28**(supplement): 10–7.

Culver CM, Gert B. Competence. In: Radden J, ed. *The Philosophy of Psychiatry: A Companion*. Oxford: Oxford University Press, 2004; pp. 258–70.

Eaton L. Care of England's older people still "unacceptably poor". *Br Med J* 2006; **332**: 746.

Fisken RA. Elder abuse, 21st century style. *Br Med J* 2006; **332**: 801.

Fulford KWM. Facts/values. Ten principles of values-based medicine. In: Radden J, ed. *The Philosophy of Psychiatry: A Companion*. Oxford: Oxford University Press, 2004; pp. 205–34.

Gillick M. Rethinking the role of tube feeding in patients with advanced dementia. *N Engl J Med* 2000; **342**: 206–10.

Grimley Evans EJ. The rationing debate: rationing health care by age: the case against. *Br Med J* 1997; **314**: 822–5.

Hughes JC, ed. *Palliative Care in Severe Dementia*. London: Quay Books, 2006.

Hughes JC, Hope T, Reader S, Rice D. Dementia and ethics: a pilot study of the views of informal carers. *J R Soc Med* 2002; **95**: 242–6.

Hughes JC, Louw SJ. Confidentiality and cognitive impairment: professional and philosophical ethics. *Age Ageing* 2002a; **31**: 147–50.

Hughes JC, Louw SJ. Electronic tagging of people with dementia who wander. *Br Med J* 2002b; **325**: 847–8.

Hughes JC. Quality of life in dementia: an ethical and philosophical perspective. *Expert Rev Pharmacoecon Outcomes Res* 2003; **3**: 525–34.

Hughes JC. Views of the person with dementia. *J Med Ethics* 2001; **27**: 86–91.

Keown J. *Euthanasia, Ethics and Public Policy: An Argument Against Legalisation*. Cambridge: Cambridge University Press, 2002.

Kitwood T. *Dementia Reconsidered. The Person Comes First*. Buckingham: Open University Press, 1997.

Louw SJ, Hughes JC. Moral reasoning – the unrealized place of casuistry in medical ethics. *Int Psychogeriatr* 2005; **17**: 149–54.

Oppenheimer C. Ethics and psychogeriatrics. In: Bloch S, Chodoff P, eds. *Psychiatric Ethics*, 2nd edition. Oxford: Oxford University Press, 1991; pp. 365–89.

Pucci E, Belardinelli N, Borsetti G, Rodriguez D, Signorino M. Information and competency for consent to pharmacologic clinical trials in Alzheimer disease: an empirical analysis in patients and family caregivers. *Alzheimer Disease Assoc Disorders* 2001; **15**: 146–54.

Sabat SR. Mind, meaning, and personhood in dementia: the effects of positioning. In: Hughes JC, Louw SJ, Sabat SR, eds. *Dementia: Mind, Meaning, and the Person*. Oxford: Oxford University Press, 2006; pp. 287–302.

Snyder CH. Dementia and driving: autonomy versus safety. *J Am Acad Nurse Pract* 2005; **17**: 393–402.

Widdershoven GAM, Berghmans RLP. Meaning-making in dementia: a hermeneutic perspective. In: Hughes JC, Louw SJ, Sabat SR, eds. *Dementia: Mind, Meaning, and the Person*. Oxford: Oxford University Press, 2006; pp. 179–91.

Williams A. The rationing debate: rationing health care by age: the case for. *Br Med J* 1997; **314**: 820–2.

65

Organs and Tissues for Transplantation and Research

DAVID P.T. PRICE

This chapter explores one or two central ethical and legal themes relating to the use of organs and tissues from both living and dead persons for therapy (transplantation) and research. The use of these materials for other purposes is mentioned in passing. These themes recently achieved prominence in the context of the passing of the Human Tissue Act 2004, legislated in the wake of the organ-retention scandals exposed most notably in the Bristol Royal Infirmary Inquiry (Interim), Alder Hey Children's Hospital Inquiry and Isaacs Reports (Bristol, 2000; Royal Liverpool, 2001; Isaacs, 2003). The fallout from those events, which constituted one of the biggest public relations setbacks for the medical profession in contemporary times, has lingered on although partial closure was achieved with the recent settlements (one for Alder Hey, and another for all other, relatives) made to the affected families (*Guardian*, 22 November, 2005). The resulting legislation applies across a broad range of medical uses, including transplantation, and for the first time establishes a comprehensive regulatory regime governing the storage and use of tissue (the generic term 'tissue' is utilized here despite the difficulties it has generated, in contrast to the expression 'relevant material' employed in the 2004 Act), overseen by the Human Tissue Authority (HTA) (it is anticipated that the HTA will soon merge with the Human Fertilization and Embryology Authority to form the Regulatory Authority for Tissue and Embryos (RATE)). This is crucial as the volume and range of human tissue use expand exponentially. The autonomy of the tissue source, or at least that of the 'giver' of the tissue, is of growing and central significance in ethical and legal decision-making. It expresses itself in the requirement for consent.

CONSENT

Consent has become the central ethical and legal concept at the heart of recent debates and reforms (Price, 2003; Weir, Olick, 2004). However, 'consent' vis-à-vis the removal, storage and use of tissue from the dead is not straightforwardly and patently apposite. John Harris has observed that posthumous interests are not necessarily like those interests which consent standardly protects (Harris, 2002). As regards postmortem examinations and the subsequent use of tissue for research, the Scottish Independent Review Group shunned the term 'consent' altogether, principally because parental powers are typically constrained by the best interests of the child, a concept regarded as inept in this context (Independent Review Group on Retention of Organs, 2002). The term 'authorization' was preferred, and the Human Tissue (Scotland) Act 2006 recently legislated by the Scottish Parliament adopts this alternative terminology. Indeed, the language of consent was conspicuously absent from the legislative context in this sphere in the United Kingdom prior to the 2004 Act. Reference was made, instead, to 'an absence of objection' in the Human Tissue Act 1961, and the Anatomy Act 1984, in instances where there was no 'request' by the deceased person that the body, or tissue removed therefrom, be used.

Moreover, even as regards the living, consent is typically applicable to *treatment* interventions, legitimating intrusions upon the body, having weighed the benefits and risks. The use of residual tissues (removed for diagnostic or therapeutic reasons, e.g. removal of a tumour by resection) for research or other purposes is a separate matter from the treatment/removal of tissue itself, and necessitates discrete consent despite their close juxtaposition (MRC, 2005).

Principles of Health Care Ethics, Second Edition   Edited by R.E. Ashcroft, A. Dawson, H. Draper and J.R. McMillan

Indeed, it was previously uncertain whether consent for the *storage* or *use* of such materials was legally mandatory at all – by contrast, with tissue removed for research or transplantation in the first place. It was the view of the Nuffield Council on Bioethics that no consent for their use for research was necessary as regards residual tissue (Nuffield Council, 1995). Indeed, a common perception is that the only donor interests implicated relate to *informational* privacy. The Human Tissue Bill initially required consent to the storage and use of nonarchived human tissue for research in all circumstances. It was amended to eventually allow the storage and use of (pseudo)anonymized ('where the person carrying out the research is not in possession, and not likely to come into possession, of information from which the person whose body the material has come can be identified') tissue, where it is ethically approved by a recognized research ethics committee (REC). It might, however, be perceived that this exemption detracts from the interest which people have in controlling the use of 'their' tissue per se (see below).

The key Inquiry Reports in England, nevertheless, embraced the concept of consent wholeheartedly and considered it to be ethically and legally indispensable for postmortem examination and subsequent storage and use of tissue. This view was endorsed by the preponderance of respondents to the Department of Health Consultation Report *Human Bodies, Human Choices* published in 2002 (Department of Health, 2003). In Parliament, consent was perceived as being explicit and necessitating a proactive approach.

The 2004 Act constituted a resounding and unequivocal rejection of the notion of *presumed* consent despite it being characteristic of laws in nations having the highest rates of organ donation for transplantation (although in Spain, consent is routinely sought from relatives of deceased persons despite the law) in Europe (Gimbel et al., 2003). The 'presumed consent' law incorporated in the Human Tissue Act 1961 was never applied in transplantation practice; unlike most other nations with such laws, there was no mechanism (e.g. a register) available to record one's objections to donation prior to death, apart from informing family. Not only was reliance on evidence of 'objection' regarded as being at the heart of many of the problems surrounding organ and tissue retention following postmortem examination, primarily on account of uncertainty as to the efforts necessary to communicate with relatives and to solicit opposition, but also many regard a failure to object as no kind of real 'consent' at all. To some, it smacks of a 'taking' by the state for the benefit of others and no more (Erin & Harris, 1999). It is, however, conceivably viewed as a form of 'tacit' consent, where a knowing withholding of an objection occurs. It is the substance rather than the form of consent which is crucial, that is consen(sus). The vogue

for explicit consent will ensure that, by dint of the fact that most people have not formally recorded their wishes prior to death, the decision is made by relatives rather than deceased 'persons' themselves. In addition to symbolically expressing a communitarian sentiment, presumed consent arguably locates the wishes of the latter more centrally and decisively at the present time.

The rhetoric in the parliamentary debates, the majority of responses to the Consultation Report and the Scottish Independent Review Group, all supported the notion that the wishes of the deceased person should be accorded predominance. Under the 2004 Act, however, a relative can give or refuse consent, provided the deceased person made no 'decision' to give or refuse consent and had not appointed a nominated representative (a novel concept introduced by the Act). In such an event the weight which the relative accords to the known or presumed wishes of the deceased is uncertain and innately variable (by contrast, in Germany, by law surviving relatives must make the decision based on the assumed wishes of the now deceased person). Section 7(4) of the Human Tissue (Scotland) Act, by contrast, stipulates that the nearest relative would not be permitted to authorize the use of the part of the body for the requisite purpose where the relative had 'actual knowledge that the adult was unwilling' for this to occur.

Currently, there is an asymmetry between a request by the deceased to donate and an objection to the same. Although the 2004 Act does not allow the removal, storage or use of body parts for scheduled purposes where the deceased made a decision to refuse to do so, and permits the use, removal or storage of such tissue where the deceased consented to it, there is no *obligation* to take or use the material in the latter circumstances. Clinicians could not be considered duty bound to remove organs or tissue for transplantation, or research. Thus, account may be taken of the objections of close relatives, for example, even where there is no legal obligation to do so, which is already the general practice in this country in respect of transplantation. Similarly, although the 2004 Act establishes a hierarchical scheme, or pecking order, for relatives, a valid consent need not necessarily be acted upon where there are objections lodged by other (equally or lower ranked) relatives. However, it is probable that a consent will be acted upon and objections from others ignored, where the results of the research (e.g. genetic) have greater potential relevance to the consentor. The Act consequently encourages case-by-case assessment.

Thus, although consent may be seen as a reflection of respect for autonomy, this is very often the autonomy of relatives rather than deceased persons. This is partly a function of the prevailing infrastructure and partly because of the perceived potential public relations impact of ignoring the views of relatives. However, the moral decision-making authority of relatives of deceased adults remains elusive. Indeed, it might be thought that to merely defer to the *objections* of relatives, rather than to their decision-making authority per se, would better reflect an approach based on non-maleficence. The policy of the British Medical Association to permit organ donation for transplantation, where the deceased did not object and no severe distress was caused to relatives, may be seen to reflect such a stance (British Medical Association, 2004).

With regard to the living, the notion of non-maleficence (or *primum non nocere*) has held particular sway in the sphere of transplantation (Price, 2000). However, the very meaning of *primum non nocere* in this context requires sustained analysis, in so far as donation is intrinsically clinically non-therapeutic from the point of view of donors, in addition to which living donors run substantial peri- and post-operative surgical risks, as well as risks relating to subsequent tissue deficit. However, to focus solely on the physical risks is to ignore the positive and negative psychological and emotional dimensions of the procedure. Harms and benefits need to be viewed and weighed in the round. Moreover, although commentators such as Carl Elliott have doubted whether it is necessarily always ethical to endorse the 'sacrifice' of living organ donors by clinicians and society, it may be appropriate to view the process *holistically,* that is the donation 'to' another individual and the ensuing transplantation into the recipient, conceived as a composite (Elliott, 1995). The danger, of course, is that a utilitarian rationale may ostensibly emerge, although this arguably ignores the weight properly afforded to donor autonomy. Motivated by protection of donor interests, certain commentators, for instance Aaron Spital, however regard *donor* benefit per se as an independent criterion for legitimate donation (Spital, 2004).

An enhanced emphasis upon donor autonomy as regards living organ donation for transplantation can be perceived in terms of both regulation and practice, mediating and constraining the duty of non-maleficence. Although the ceiling of legitimate risk taking remains vague, donors are being permitted to take increased risks, albeit in many situations the potential benefits to recipients are also enhanced. Although developments are cautious, the first living-related liver transplants are shortly to be undertaken in adults in the NHS in Scotland, for instance (they are presently performed privately in London only) (Neuberger & Price, 2003).[1] They have already become quite common in many parts of the world, and lung lobe transplants are also regularly performed in the United States. An increasingly liberal attitude is also being taken everywhere towards emotionally, rather than genetically, related (typically renal) donation. The lack of decisiveness of relationship from an intrinsic moral and legal perspective is highlighted by the

growth of renal donation by strangers in North America, and its gradual acceptance in principle, although not yet in practice [the Unrelated Live Transplants Regulatory Authority (ULTRA) was not asked to approve a specific case] in this country. Ignoring issues relating to commercialism and recognizing that clinical outcomes using genetically unrelated living donors approximate those from cadavers, and indeed many living related donors, acceptance of risk has come to be seen to be primarily a matter for assessment by such prospective donors themselves where clinicians have ruled out any psychopathology. However, regulations now passed under the Human Tissue Act 2004 will for the first time bring oversight of *all* such potential transplants, and even bone marrow donation, within the regulatory purview of the HTA. Apart from the imperative to exclude commercial dealings, this will assist in ensuring that consents are properly informed and voluntary.

The extent to which patients (or relatives) should be informed about the intended procedures and uses has inevitably remained contentious. While on the one hand, communication failures (for instance, a lack of appreciation by parents that the term 'tissue' could be taken to extend to whole organs) were at the epicentre of some of the scandals exposed by the inquiries, on the other hand the different informational needs of patients or relatives, especially in the context of postmortems (alluded to in particular in the Scottish Independent Review Group Report, and which bolstered support for the notion of 'authorization' rather than 'consent'), suggest the possibility of information overload and its capacity not only to obfuscate clear decision-making but also to generate distress. In many situations, broad knowledge would satisfy the decision-maker's informational needs (O'Neill, 2003). Further, in many instances precise information regarding subsequent uses of tissue (e.g. for research) may simply not be available at the time.

In the event, the 2004 Act adopted the expression 'appropriate consent', which served to identify the *locus* of decision-making but not the informational content of the process. The substantive issue was left to be determined flexibly and contextually by reference to the Codes of Practice to be issued by the HTA, and the general law. However, it was made abundantly clear during the parliamentary debates that *generic* consent would generally suffice for research, subject to any requirements added by RECs. Although many will consider that a donor is entitled to specific rather than general information about subsequent uses and storage for such purposes, and indeed Article 22 of the Council of Europe Biomedicine Convention seemingly envisages a need for specific information about each intended use as part of a discrete consent given

[1]See The Guardian, November 8, 2005.

for each subsequent usage, the Government ultimately wished to appease the research community and to avoid deleterious practical effects on research (avoiding, inter alia, the need to typically recontact donors or their relatives). This will impact research tissue banks in particular. The Nuffield Council on Bioethics has stressed that in any event consent is always to action which is incompletely described (Nuffield Council, 2004). Moreover, RECs will undoubtedly continue to insist upon detailed information to be given about specific intended research uses, and indeed it would typically be a condition under the general common law to provide broad information about the nature and purpose of the research whenever the tissue is taken from living persons for research in the first place, as part of the consent to the *removal*. However, there may be difficulties and ethical tension where broad consent is given, yet the person has reservations about specific forms of research but is unaware that such types of research are envisaged. In such cases, protection through RECs might not always suffice.

Where comprehensive regulation is envisaged, it is necessary to decide not only the forms of material which are to be regulated [the 2004 Act applies to (virtually) all cellular material] and in what fashion but also the purposes (and storage for that end) for which consent should be required. It is here that the weighing of collective and individual considerations can be seen most overtly. There are exemptions under the 2004 Act for storage and use of tissue taken from *living* persons, relating to clinical audit, quality assurance, education or training relating to human health, performance assessment and public health monitoring. All, apart from the last, were sought to be justified on the basis that they are implicitly connected to the medical treatment itself, whereas the latter is grounded in the general public interest. This is not only where conceptual fuzziness creeps in, due to the indistinct boundaries of, say, clinical audit and research or public health monitoring and (epidemiological) research, but also where seemingly arbitrary judgements about the scope of legitimate exemptions and the duty to contribute to the public good arise. The original version of the Bill required consent unless the use of the tissue for education and training was 'incidental to medical diagnosis or treatment', but such purposes were eventually exempted entirely from the consent requirement, thus shifting the rationale to the general public interest (Price, 2005). But is research not as equally in the public interest as education and training? The true justification for the exemptions are ostensibly to be found as much in pragmatic as in ethical concerns.

Although consent and autonomy are, rhetorically at least, given pride of place in the new legislative scheme, the question arises as to what the role of consent is here, and what interest(s) it is designed to protect? Storage and use of tissue per se involve no infringement of personal physical integrity, and protection of personal data arising therefrom is broadly catered for under laws relating to data protection and medical confidentiality.

PROPERTY IN HUMAN TISSUE

Ambivalence and disagreement have characterized the legal response and ethical debate surrounding 'property' in human tissue, by which one means the (bundle of) rights relating to 'it' rather than the material per se (although the character of the latter substantially drives the former). The notion of ownership of human tissue is contentious by virtue of the typically open-ended and extensive rights generated thereby, notably relating to alienation and control of use. The tissue here may still, or subsequently (as in the case of a transplant), form part of the human corpus or have become severed from it, whether as a function of medical treatment or of its intended use (e.g. removal for transplantation). In the former circumstances the prevailing legal and philosophical view is that the tissue is part of the 'being' or 'self', rather than any form of property. Laws governing personal freedom and integrity undoubtedly appear more apposite in this context. In any event, it is only after severance that human tissue is usable for research or transplantation [although whole (dead) bodies may be used for anatomical examination or public display].

Laws generally deny property rights to the tissue source. A property-based claim was rejected by the California Supreme Court in *Moore* v *Regents of the University of California* (1990) 793 P 2d 479 (Cal. Sup. Ct.), although it was heavily influenced by consequentialist considerations relating to the utility of using residual human tissue (in this instance cells from the patient's spleen were developed into a commercial cell line) for research (it may be noted that the 2004 Act excludes cell lines from its regulatory purview altogether, implying that it is not to be regarded as human material). The Nuffield Council on Bioethics Report *Human Tissue: Ethical and Legal Issues* published in 1995 adopted a similar stance regarding the use of residual tissue from living persons for research, suggesting that patients 'abandon' such tissue. This view would now seem to be contrary to most contemporary ethical opinion and to the philosophy underpinning the 2004 Act, in so far as consent is required vis-à-vis identifiable tissue. This Act, however, fails to explicitly adopt a property framework, albeit that it was broadly accepted that the statute was underpinned by the proposition that a patient has a broad general right to *control* the use of his or her tissue(s). This merely translates into the typical necessity for consent to be obtained for the relevant storage and/or use, as already discussed.

By contrast, the law concedes the property-based rights of *others* over human tissue. The right to control over the deceased's corpse for the purpose of disposal (burial or cremation) is vested in either the next of kin or the executors/administrators depending upon the jurisdiction. The police have a right to possess and retain body samples taken for criminal justice purposes (e.g. under the Police and Criminal Evidence Act 1984, as amended by the Criminal Justice and Police Act 2001), and to exclude others (even the source). Similarly, a coroner or pathologist has a right to possess the corpse for the purpose of performing a legitimate postmortem examination. Such rights are both logical and essential (see *AB and Others* v *Leeds Teaching Hospital NHS Trust and Another* (2004) 77 B.M.L.R. 145 (QBD)).

Thus, although the conventional legal view is that there is no property in the human body, including a corpse, this is generally a statement concerning proprietary rather than possessory rights. However, apparently founded upon a Lockean notion of 'property' being generated by the investment of labour in it, courts have recognized proprietary rights as vesting in an individual who has applied work and skill to human tissue, thereby changing its inherent nature. It has been held that 'fixing' human material removed at postmortem and creating slides constitute such work and skill, besides dissecting and preserving limbs and other substantial body parts severed at anatomical examination (see *AB and Others* v *Leeds Teaching Hospital NHS Trust and Another* (2004) 77 B.M.L.R. 145 and *R* versus *Kelly* [1998] 3 All E.R. 741 (CA)). This concept is extremely important, partly because this may be regarded as generating rights to sell such tissue as well as exclusively control its use. Indeed, the 2004 Act apparently assumes that if human body parts are property by virtue of the application of work and skill, they are legitimately subject to commerce, as the prohibitions on trading in the Act relating to transplantation do not apply to 'property' (this also reveals the implicit legislative view that human tissue is *not inherently* to be conceived of as property). But not only need it not simply be assumed that if human tissue is property it may be legitimately traded, such rights which are created as a consequence will reside in third parties, generating potential tension with the tissue source or relatives of deceased persons from whom such tissue 'derives'.

With regard to the living it is submitted that it is indeed appropriate and desirable for property rights to vest in the tissue source, to permit such uses of tissue as are deemed acceptable and to alienate such tissue as necessary. This dispositional right to control any uses by third parties, what Beyleveld and Brownsword describe as the rule preclusionary conception of property, is necessary to properly protect the tissue source's interest in it (Beyleveld & Brownsword, 2001). Consent would create a right to use and a property

right to possess (retain) the tissue for that purpose. But if property rights are not the foundation of the right to control the storage and use of a person's tissue, what is the proper rationale?

HARMING THE DEAD

Property rights in dead persons or tissue deriving therefrom raise greater difficulties in so far as the tissue source has ceased to exist and the idea of ownership over another's body is typically regarded as unpalatable and inappropriate. But if consent is required for the medical use of tissue after death, what wrong is done when the same thing is done without such consent? Failing to obtain consent is not wrong in itself, ethically speaking.

It is common to perceive someone as having been 'used', even after his or her death, when organs are taken, retained and/or used for research or other purposes, without consent. This is perceived to be wrong to the person whose corpse it is. However, and paradoxically, that person has now ceased to exist. Can one 'harm' a dead person? In general, legal duties and entitlements cease upon the death of the individual. The deceased individual is 'unaware' of any wrong, but this is a far deeper matter than a lack of awareness, and in any event it is perfectly possible for a person to be harmed in the absence of an appreciation of this occurring (as when, for instance, one is relieved unknowingly of the contents of one's bank account). Harris contends that the role of consent in posthumous organ retention is highly problematic (Harris, 2002). He draws a major distinction between living and dead persons. Respect for persons in his view is essentially a duty owed only to the former, reflecting respect for autonomy and concern for welfare. He states that any interests which exist posthumously are, however, of a different character, and he comments

> Autonomy involves the capacity to make choices, it involves acts of the will, and the dead have no capacities – they have no will, no preferences, wants nor desires, the dead cannot be autonomous and so cannot have their autonomy violated. Equally, the dead cannot have their bodily integrity violated, for violation consists not simply in a breach of bodily integrity, but in a breach of bodily integrity that is not consented to (Harris, 2002).

This issue has been recently highlighted in a practical context. One method of preserving organs, principally kidneys, following death outside the intensive care unit environment, is by cooling and perfusing the organs, usually facilitated by way of a cut in the groin. In particular, this allows time to contact relatives not at the scene, in order to seek permission for organ donation. A number of transplant centres have implemented such protocols for uncontrolled non-heart-beating donors, the clinical results of which have proven very positive. In general, these practices have provoked no controversy, even when aired in the local press, despite the absence of specific legal authorization and, in many instances, a lack of prospective consent. Such authorization is now to be found in the Human Tissue Act 2004, yet the Health Minister, Rosie Winterton, even doubted during the parliamentary debates whether this was strictly necessary. But if there is no legal wrong done here in the absence of consent, then arguably no wrong would be done by the *removal* of organs or tissues for transplantation or research (or even anatomical or postmortem examination) either. The King's Fund Institute Report 'A Question of Give and Take' aired the possibility that presumed consent could be taken to have been given for such procedures in any event (King's Fund Institute, 1994). But could one have a presumed consent rationale for organ-preservation methods and an explicit consent rationale for organ removal? (The position would, of course, be different in a jurisdiction having a presumed consent regime, as in the absence of the deceased having objected, there would be authorization for organ removal quite apart from organ preservation). If so, on what basis? Merely the degree of intrusion into the body? Further, one would surely have to ensure common knowledge of these procedures across the community, and a straightforward and accessible method of registering disapproval. Truthfully, there appears to be no consent process here at all. Not that it is to say that it cannot be justified; which returns us to the central issue. There is clearly no assault and battery committed by invading the integrity of a corpse, as this concept is only applicable to the living. Moreover, all kinds of procedures are performed upon a cadaver to prepare and preserve it for burial or cremation without either general knowledge or consent.

Veatch, however, argues that prospective justification, typically consent, is necessary for any intrusion or invasion of a cadaver. He suggests that attempting to justify cooling and perfusion procedures on the basis of an appeal to autonomy to subsequently decide whether to donate (facilitating acquisition of knowledge regarding the deceased's and/or relatives' wishes) misses the point (Veatch, 1995). Certainly, with regard to the living, autonomy is usually respected as a negative right to control intrusions upon one's integrity, but can this view be simply extrapolated to the corpse? Harris argues that it cannot. Moreover, if autonomy has any content in the context of the deceased, it must presumably relate to that of the *former* person and his or her wishes. Harris even concedes the existence of enduring interests which survive death, including one's wishes as to the medical uses of one's corpse, but suggests they are 'relatively weak', and easily overridden by the interests of the living, especially those requiring transplants. He endorses the legitimate removal of organs from corpses for

transplantation without any consent. Indeed, other imperatives, such as the needs of the criminal justice system, are already catered for. Forensic coroners' postmortems for instance legally require no consent at all.

Margot Brazier alludes to the potential for practices to conflict with the religious views and beliefs of the now deceased person, sometimes relating to the afterlife (Brazier, 2002). Indeed, Article 9 of the European Convention on Human Rights creates a prima facie right to religion and freedom of conscience and to manifest one's religion in worship, teaching practice and observance. She then considers the wishes of deceased persons more broadly and observes that most of us consider that to fail to take account of the explicit objection of a person to the retention or use of his or her tissue after death, as *wronging* them (Brazier, 2003). Indeed, it is an almost universal feature of transplant laws that there is an obligation to respect an explicit objection by the deceased to donation. The once living person's interests are infringed by such treatment, and it is thus seemingly a 'person-affecting harm', even though that person is no longer in existence at the time.

By contrast, any harm resulting from activity undertaken without consent is frequently focused only upon surviving relatives. But what interests of relatives are infringed by such action? It is here that the concept of *profound offence*, developed by the late Joel Feinberg, comes into view. He notes that such offence is caused by the belief that such conduct is wrong, not simply *believed* wrong because it causes offence.

Feinberg observes that in such instances the offended party does not think of himself or herself as the victim (a feature reinforced by the experience gained by the Retained Organs Commission) and cannot avoid such offence by averting his or her eyes (Feinberg, 1985; Retained Organs Commission, 2004). He argues that it is reasonable to use the criminal law to protect persons from wrongful offence, where deep *personal* affronts are concerned. This is because 'the offending conduct is somehow addressed to them in an unmistakably direct way, even when not observed by them' (Feinberg, 1985). The relationship is crucial and this explains, coupled with the natural inclination of parents or spouses, in particular, to feel they have failed in their duty if they have not properly 'protected' their children/spouses after death, the deep wounds inflicted on many relatives by some of the organ retention practices recently revealed. It also helps to explain why, even from a liberal perspective, when the deceased's wishes are not known, partners or close relatives of deceased adults should be given powers to decide upon donation subject to criminal penalties for transgression, as they are in the scheme generated by the 2004 Act; although arguably they should generally decide according to the supposed wishes of the now deceased person.

CONCLUDING REMARKS

The plethora of uses of human tissue, contexts for the acquisition and storage of tissue, and various types of tissue themselves, demand flexible, sensitive and balanced regulation. But such proportionality can only be properly realized when the interests of tissue providers and their relations are fully understood. It is this sensitivity which will realize the better alignment of donor and recipient interests alluded to in the previous volume (Sells, 1994).

REFERENCES

Beyleveld D, Brownsword R. *Human Dignity in Bioethics and Biolaw.* Oxford: Oxford University Press, 2001.

Brazier M. Retained organs: ethics and humanity. *Legal Stud* 2002; **22**(4): 550–69.

Brazier M. Organ retention and return: problems of consent. *J Med Ethics* 2003; **29**: 30–3.

Bristol Royal Infirmary Inquiry Interim Report. *Removal and Retention of Human Material*, 2000; http://www.bristol-inquiry. org.uk/interim.report/report.htm.

British Medical Association. Organ donation in the 21st century: time for a consolidated approach. BMA 2004.

Department of Health. *Human Bodies, Human Choices.* Summary of responses to the consultation report. Department of Health Publications, 2003.

Elliott C. Doing harm: living organ donors, clinical research and *The Tenth Man. J Med Ethics* 1995; **21**: 91–6.

Erin C, Harris J. Presumed consent or contracting out. *J Med Ethics* 1999; **25**: 365–6.

Feinberg J. *Offense to Others.* Oxford: Oxford University Press, 1985.

Gimbel R, et al. Presumed consent and other predictors of cadaveric organ donation in Europe. *Prog Transplant* 2003; **13**(1): 17–23.

Harris J. Law and regulation of retained organs: the ethical issues. *Legal Stud* 2002; **22**(4): 527–49.

Independent Review Group on Retention of Organs at Post-Mortem. Scottish Executive, 2002.

Isaacs Report. *The Investigation of events which followed the death of Cyril Mark Isaacs*, 2003; http://www.dh.gov. uk/cmo/isaacsreport/

King's Fund Institute. *A Question of Give and Take.* London: King's Fund Institute, 1994.

MRC. MRC operational and ethical guidelines. *Human Tissue and Biological Samples for Use in Research*, 2005.

Neuberger J, Price D. The role of living liver donation in the United Kingdom. *Br Med J* 2003; **327**: 676–9.

Nuffield Council on Bioethics Report. *Human Tissue: Ethical and Legal Issues.* London: Nuffield Council on Bioethics, 1995.

Nuffield Council on Bioethics. *Response from the Nuffield Council on Bioethics to the Human Tissue Bill.* London: Nuffield Council, 2004.

O'Neill O. Some limits of informed consent. *J Med Ethics* 2003; **29**: 4–7.

Price D. *Legal and Ethical Aspects of Organ Transplantation.* Cambridge: Cambridge University Press, 2000.

Price D. From Cosmos and Damien to van Velzen: The human tissue saga continues. *Med Law Rev* 2003; **11**(1): 1–47.

Price D. Human Tissue Act 2004. *Modern Law Rev* 2005; **68**: 798–821.

Retained Organs Commission. *Remembering the Past, Looking to the Future.* NHS, 2004.

Royal Liverpool Children's Inquiry Report, 2001; http://www. rlcinquiry.org.uk/download/index/htm.

Sells R. Transplants. In: Gillon R, ed. *Principles of Health Care Ethics.* Chichester: John Wiley & Sons, Inc, 1994; pp. 1003–27.

Spital A. Donor benefit is the key to justified living organ donation. *Cambridge Q Healthcare Ethics* 2004; 13: 105–9.

Veatch R. Consent for perfusion and other dilemmas with organ procurement from non-heart-beating cadavers. In: Arnold R, Youngner S, Schapiro R, Mason-Spicer C, eds. *Procuring Organs for Transplant: The Debate Over Non-Heart-Beating Cadaver Protocols.* Baltimore: Johns Hopkins University Press, 1995; pp.195–206.

Weir R, Olick R. *The Stored Tissue Issue.* Oxford: Oxford University Press, 2004.

66

Living Donor Organ Transplantation

TIMOTHY M. WILKINSON

The first successful kidney transplant was performed on 23-year-old Richard Herrick in Massachusetts in 1954, using a kidney from his living identical twin, Ronald (Munson, 2002). After the development of powerful and sophisticated immunosuppressive drugs, it became possible to transplant organs from related living donors apart from identical twins, from unrelated living donors and from people who were dead (Le Fanu, 1999). The obvious ethical advantage of using organs from dead people is that they would not be physically harmed by having organs removed. The well-known drawback is that there are not enough organs to meet the growing demand. There are various strategies to increase supply, such as changing the arrangements for consent, or increasing awareness of donation in intensive care units, but it is commonly thought that, even if organs were transplanted from all potential dead sources, supply would still fall short of demand. As one recent editorial put it, 'Alternative sources of donors, especially live donors, must be sought in order to address the unremediable disparity between the number of available cadaveric organs and the number of potential recipients' (Langone & Helderman, 2003).

The numerically most significant organ that is transplanted from living donors is the kidney. Renal transplantation is where there is the greatest disparity between demand and the supply of kidneys from the dead, and it is not only the safest but also reasonably safe for the donor. Focusing just on mortality, the risks are estimated at less than 1 in 3000. Since the late 1980s, living donors have also been used to acquire livers. The liver, unlike the kidney, is capable of regenerating in the donor. Liver donation is none the less riskier than kidney donation, with an estimated mortality risk of 0.2–0.5% for donation from adult to adult and 0.06–0.18% for donation from adult to child (ASERNIP-S, 2004). Although riskier, recipients of livers

often stand to gain more than recipients of kidneys because, for those with acute liver failure, there is no equivalent of kidney dialysis to keep them alive. On a smaller scale, there have also been live donations of segments of the lung and, on a much smaller scale, the pancreas and the small intestine. There have even been living donations of hearts, but not with the fatal consequences one might expect; donations have occurred in domino fashion, when patients who receive heart-lung transplants donate their original hearts. (For references and further discussion of the facts of living donor transplantation, see Price, 2001; Veatch, 2000).

Transplanting organs from living people raises many ethical questions, some of which will be mentioned now and then excluded, and the rest will be mentioned in detail. One set of excluded questions is about the boundaries of the living. While some people, like you and I (while I write this) are uncontroversially living, and others, like William the Conqueror, are uncontroversially dead, there are some, relevant to organ transplantation, whose status is controversial. Deceased donor organs are almost always taken from people declared whole-brain dead, but some writers say that whole-brain death is not genuinely death (Singer, 1994; McMahan, 2002). Anencephalics, who are born with most of their brains missing but their organs often intact, are considered alive both according to law and according to prevailing medical views, yet considered dead, or at least not alive, on some conceptions of death (Singer, 1994). Some non-heart-beating cadaver donors have organs removed following withdrawal of life support, but it is not clear how long the heart must stop for a person to be really dead (Veatch, 2000, ch. 13). I shall set the problem of boundaries aside and consider only the uncontroversially living.

I shall also take seriously the idea of donation and focus only on those who can reasonably accurately be said to be

Principles of Health Care Ethics, Second Edition   Edited by R.E. Ashcroft, A. Dawson, H. Draper and J.R. McMillan
© 2007 John Wiley & Sons, Ltd

offering a gift of an organ. Thus the chapter ignores the question of whether people may be paid for their organs because, whatever the correct answer, people who sell are not donors. The chapter also ignores the conscription of organs from the living, which is taken seriously by at least some philosophers (Rakoswki, 1991; Fabre, 2003) because the conscripted are not donors.

The topics we shall focus on here are the legitimacy of risking the health of living consenting competent potential donors; the grounds, if any, which justify taking organs from non-competent people; and the justice or injustice of living donors stipulating who is to receive their organs.

DO NO HARM AND AUTONOMY

The duty not to harm patients, or non-maleficence, is to be found in various forms in codes of medical ethics from the oldest times to now. On the face of it, such a duty prohibits surgeons from removing organs even from consenting people and transplanting them into others. Unlike standard surgery, organ removal for transplantation is not done for the therapeutic benefit of the patient. The removal of an organ puts the donor at risk from the operation, from post-operative infection and, in the case of non-regenerative organs, from the drawbacks of losing one. However, surely if competent people are willing and know what they are doing, it would be permissible to subject them to risks that may not otherwise be imposed on them. Do doctors not have a duty to respect people's autonomous wishes to run risks? But how much risk? And could people's consent be truly free in cases where their organs are needed to save the lives of relatives? As it happens, these thoughts occurred to the very team that transplanted the kidney from one Herrick twin to another (Munson, 2002), and the issues raised are still not fully resolved.

It is sometimes thought that living donor transplantation involves a clash between the duty not to do harm and the duty to respect autonomy. This is somewhat misleading, however, because of plausible developments of the underlying principles, doing no harm need not speak against live donation and respecting autonomy need not speak in its favour.

A duty not to do harm obviously needs to be filled in with some account of what harm is. Any view of harm will include physical harm and, if that is all there is to harm, the duty would prohibit transplants from live donors. However, there are attempts in medical ethics and law to justify living donor transplants by broadening medical harm to include psychological or social harms (which I shall somewhat inaccurately call 'mental harms'). Parents might suffer greatly if their children die, and still more so if they could have saved their children by donating an organ. Although

proceeding with the operations would put the parents at risk of physical harm, not proceeding would put them at risk of mental harm. If the mental harm outweighs the physical, then performing the operations would not violate the rule to do no harm. It is a nice question whether refusing to proceed would.

From a philosophical point of view, widening the conception of harm from just the physical to include the mental still does not go far enough. On a fairly standard view of harm, a harm is a setback to an interest (Feinberg, 1984), and most philosophical views of well being do not take interests to be limited to the physical and mental (Parfit, 1984, Appendix I). Indeed, people can have vicarious interests. Thus a loving parent has an interest in the welfare of her child; a harm to the child is a setback to that interest; and so a harm to the child is a harm to the parent too. In standard cases, a parent whose child is harmed would suffer mentally, but the harm to the parent is not limited to that. The parent would be harmed even if she did not know what had happened to the child.

The duty not to harm requires assessing whether, in a given case of a potential donor, the physical risks of the operation to the donor outweigh or are outweighed by the costs *to the donor* of not proceeding. Except on an implausibly narrow view of harm as only physical, the do no harm rule need not condemn and may support proceeding, when the benefits to the potential donor outweigh the risks. But if benefits and risks to the potential donor are to be weighed, who is to do the weighing? Once it is accepted that physical risk is not all that is relevant, the answer is not obvious. The transplant team might be authorities on the physical risks to the donor of an operation, but they are not authorities on how significant these risks are to the well being of the donor, and how they compare with the potential benefits. Transplant teams that include psychiatrists, social workers and so on might have a better sense of the non-physical harms and benefits than teams that include only medical and surgical staff, but the question remains of how expert they can be on such personal matters. One might thus be tempted to claim that the rule against doing harm actually requires transplant teams to go along with the wishes of potential donors. The most promising argument is based on the best judge view, familiar in discussions of paternalism.

According to the best judge view, if the person whose life it is disagrees with others (doctor, family, the state) about where her interests lie, it is that person who is most likely to be right (Archard, 1994; Wilkinson, 1996). In the case of living donor transplantation, the best judge argument says that the potential donor faces a menu of risks and benefits, and her own choice about what to do is more likely to be correct than anyone else's. Consequently, if the aim is to avoid harming her, she should be the one who chooses.

The best judge view has its problems, and one such is whether it can properly be applied to living donor transplantation. It would work only if the potential donors were making a judgement entirely about their own interests, but they typically are not. They are deciding in large part about the interests of potential recipients who need the organs, interests that potential donors care about because of love, a sense of duty, a desire to help, or some such. The decision to donate or not is in large part about others. One could try to redescribe the decision in terms of self-interest: 'I don't want to run the risk of post-operative infection or organ failure, but on the other hand I would get a psychic benefit from donating, so I think I'll donate.' This redescription is ludicrous, in part because the relevant psychic benefits are a by-product of decisions taken on other grounds such as love or duty (Elster, 1983). Because the best judge view does not claim that donors are the best judges of their moral duties, or how to help others, but only of their own interests and because the decision whether to donate is not about only their own interests, the best judge view does not give a reason to think donors are best placed to decide.

Even if the best judge view does not show that the donor is the one to decide, it does not follow that anyone else is better placed. Although matters might be clear in particular instances, the very nature of the comparison of the various types of harms and benefits makes it tricky to assess the net effects on a donor. How are feelings of guilt to be weighed against post-operative infection, for instance? The conclusion at this stage, though, is that the duty not to do harm does not prohibit all living donor transplantation. However, then why have the duty at all? Why not just let competent people make choices for themselves? Some see the rule against doing harm as an outmoded relic of medicine's paternalistic days (Veatch, 2000, p. 202). Neither doctors nor the law should decide whether an operation is too risky. That should be up to the person who wants to donate. It is a matter of autonomy.

Autonomy is literally 'self-rule'. Autonomy rights include the right to decide what happens to one's own body. Autonomy rights thus include the right to refuse to donate. But do they give the right to donate? To be sure, one would have the right to try to remove one's own organs, but this would be atypical living donor transplantation. Transplantation is typically not a one party case but at least a three party case: donor, recipient and transplant team. Autonomy does not give a right over the other parties, so people do not have a right that others help with the donation. However, a classic liberal view says that autonomy extends beyond one party when there is proper consent (Feinberg, 1984). If A consents to sex with B and B consents to sex with A, then, so long as they are acting privately, it is a wrongful interference with the autonomy of both A and B if they are stopped. Similarly, if the recipient donor, and transplant team all consent to a risky operation, then they should not be interfered with by others.

How far should respect for autonomy go? If kidneys may be taken, if livers may be taken, are there any limits? May a second kidney be taken from a person who has already donated one? May a parent, who will thereby die, donate a heart to save her child? Or anyone's child? It is entirely possible, and by no means absurd, to stick with the idea of autonomy and accept that, with the proper consents, people may be killed for the sake of others (Harris, 1998). But many will want to try to find some middle position in between interfering whenever potential donors choose against their best interests and going along with their decisions, however misguided or even genuinely heroic they are. Where such a middle position should be and whether it could be successfully defended are difficult questions.

The middle position need not be a compromise between avoiding harm and autonomy. Although the duty not to do harm did not rule out living donor transplantation, nor does autonomy clearly justify it even when all parties say they are willing to go ahead. This is because of difficulties in ensuring proper consent (Price, 2001, ch. 7). How much must potential donors be informed? How far must they understand what they have been told? If donors are under pressure from within their families, does this render the consent invalid? Some believe that even competent living donors should never be used because their consent can never be determined to be free. This goes too far, but one might defend limits on what organ removal can be consented to as a protection for autonomy. That way, some people would not be bamboozled or pushed into doing what they do not really want to do. (Compare the abuse argument against voluntary euthanasia: that some people will be killed even though they would not really want to be.) This shows at least that the argument from autonomy to permitting living donor transplantation is not straightforward.

The law in most countries does not permit the removal of organs necessary for life, or anything approaching that level of risk, even when all parties consent (Price, 2001). As we have seen, whether this is justified is one area of genuine and hard to resolve controversy. While we are on the subject of what actually happens, note that many countries, either in medical practice or law, have regarded it as wrong or at least undesirable to use unrelated living donors. Clinical reasons aside, the objection seems to be that unrelated living donors must either be being paid secretly, or else they must be crazy. These grounds for preventing donation from the unrelated are quite rightly criticized by several writers (Price, 2001, ch. 8).

There is also the question of whether transplant teams ought to perform operations whenever there are willing recipients and donors. Even if recipients and donors have a right to consent, they do not have a right to insist on donation. The members of the transplant team have their autonomy too, and it would be unreasonable to insist that they perform a lethal or very risky operation even on a willing person. Arguably, and resembling the compromise over abortion that exists in some countries, they might have a right to refuse but have a duty to refer a person to another transplant team, if any, who would be willing to perform.

We have just been considering what ethically may be legally or professionally required of transplant teams. It is likely that teams should be left with considerable discretion. But from the perspective of a transplant team, having the discretion does not tell them how to exercise it. If potential donor and recipient are keen and competent, would it be wrong for the transplant team to refuse, even if it had a legal freedom to decide either way? The answer might well depend on why the team refuses and, in particular, on whether it is motivated by reasons that are not its affair. Consider three arguments for refusing to perform the operation when potential donor and recipient consent validly. One is that to go ahead in this case would bring transplantation into disrepute and reduce the number of organs from other sources. This reason is no insult to the autonomy of potential donors. Another is that the transplant team do not want to be causally responsible for killing or severely harming a healthy donor in the event that the operation goes wrong. This reason is at least understandable and also, I think, no insult to the autonomy of potential donors because it is a reason based on how the team expect to feel rather than on a judgement of the interests of the donor. A third reason is that potential donors should not run such risks because of the bad effects on them or their family (Elliott, 1995). Arguably, this would insult the potential donors' autonomy. These risks should be their affair and so should the decisions about their duties to others (Shiffrin, 2000).

INCOMPETENT DONORS

The previous section was concerned with donation from competent people. Consider now incompetent people, that is some but not all members of these groups: children, the intellectually disabled and the mentally ill. These incompetents are in some sense able to donate, but are not capable of giving valid consent, and so the questions of weighing consent against harm do not arise. I here consider two major arguments that try to justify some living donor transplantation from incompetents. One allows donation from the incompetent when it would not harm them; the other claims that the incompetent have obligations to donate.

As we saw in the last section, the idea of harm should be taken in a sense broader than just the physical and, once it is, it becomes an open question whether performing the operation would be in or against the overall interests of the donor. Two American court cases illustrate this reasoning.

In one, a Kentucky court ordered a kidney donation from Jerry Strunk, a 27-year-old man said to have a mental age of 6, to his brother, Tommy. The brothers were very close to each other, and the court held that the donation was in the interests of Jerry. In the second case, a Wisconsin court declined to order a transplant of a kidney from Richard Pescinski, a catatonic schizophrenic who had been institutionalized for many years, to his sister. Richard Pescinski had no concern for anyone, and so not for his sister, and the court was given no evidence that it would be in his interests to have a kidney transplanted (Munson, 2002). (For the inconclusive state of British law, see Price, 2001, ch. 8). The sensible conclusion is that the argument for harm to living donor transplantation on the incompetent has scope limitations. To be properly applied, there have to be good grounds for thinking that the person really would be worse off if the donation did not go ahead.

The argument for avoiding harm taken broadly is somewhat controversial, although mainly on the grounds of potential for abuse rather than that it is incorrect. Some writers, however, argue for other justifications. Robert Veatch draws a parallel between organ retrieval from living incompetent people and their use in research. He claims that it is permissible to use the incompetent in research on certain conditions, notably that risk is no greater than some minimum, on the grounds that the incompetent have moral obligations to the wider community. He accepts that organ removal is significantly riskier than any research that should be permitted on the incompetent, but argues that extra risk may be justified within families. This is because the bonds between donor – or 'donor' – and family are stronger than those between research subject and community at large, and that more may be expected of the incompetent in the family sphere. However, on Veatch's view, there is a limit to what risk may be imposed on the incompetent and, given their current risk profiles, the limit is reached with the kidney and exceeded by lung lobe and liver transplantation (Veatch, 2000, pp. 196–8). A supplementary argument can be found in the case of Pescinski, where a minority opinion held that doing the decent thing by his sister is probably what Pescinski would have wanted had he been competent (Munson, 2002, p. 136).This is an attempt to connect the idea of moral obligation to the idea of substituted judgement, familiar in deciding for the incompetent (Buchanan & Brock, 1990). There are many problems with these views, some of which I shall now mention.

Any argument that relies on the alleged moral obligations of incompetent people is, at best, likely to apply only to certain subsets of the incompetent. Consider the argument about the bonds of family. This is likely to work only where there are indeed tight bonds, and so would not work in a case like Pescinski's.

The argument from moral obligation faces more fundamental objections. It is conventionally held that, to be a subject of a moral obligation, one must be an agent, that is, able to understand the obligation and perform it. We do not think, for instance, that it makes any sense to attribute a moral failing to a male trout for neglecting its offspring because trout clearly do not have the necessary conceptual apparatus to understand an obligation to nurture one's young. Certain typically incompetent people, such as 12-year-olds, clearly can have the capacity for agency, but others, such as all 1-year-olds, do not. For this reason, organ retrieval from people below some intellectual and moral capacity could not be justified by citing an obligation that they could not have. This is also why it makes no sense to claim that people like Richard Pescinski would have wanted to donate. He never had the capacity for those kinds of judgement (Buchanan & Brock, 1990, p. 115).

The lack of agency shows up the argument for moral obligation as an odd one. The language switches from the active – that the incompetent should donate – to the passive – the organs of the incompetent may be removed. There is a parallel in Bertie Wooster's description of a man over whom a bucket is emptied: 'In one second, without any previous training or upbringing, he had become the wettest man in Worcestershire' (Wodehouse, 1981). Training and upbringing are relevant for doing something, but irrelevant to being made the wettest; agency and obligation are relevant to doing (including permitting) something, but irrelevant to removing the organs of the incompetent. Perhaps a different argument should be made: the very lack of agency that precludes small children, say, from having obligations also precludes them from having a full set of rights, and, in particular, no right against the removal of their organs. I only mention this line of argument, rather than endorse it. I note that it fits better with the practice the argument from moral obligation purported to justify, namely, doing things to incompetent people rather than having them do things.

JUSTICE AND CONDITIONAL ALLOCATION

Historically, the field of transplantation has shown great concern for the just allocation of scarce resources. Scarce organs may not be bought or sold, in part to prevent unfair access by those with money, and they are not allocated according to any criteria of desert or merit. Although details vary, organs tend to be allocated according to a queue, and people's places on the queue depend on a mix of capacity to benefit, urgency and time spent waiting.

Living donation has been an exception to the rule of allocating according to place in the queue. A family member who wants to help a relative has not had to donate to the general pool, but has been able to stipulate that the relative receive the organ. This practice is not very controversial, but accepting conditions from other live donors is. Some people

who have been waiting for organs have taken to advertising on billboards or the internet, or asking in their churches for living unrelated donors (Robertson, 2005). Sometimes strangers want to donate only to a named celebrity. Sometimes potential donors attach racist conditions. A common term for accepting donor stipulations is 'directed donation', but a better one is 'conditional allocation' because the controversy is not primarily over the donor's attaching a condition to an offer, but over the transplant service's accepting it and allocating according to the condition (Wilkinson, 2007).

Should a potential donor's offer be accepted even though the organ would not go into the general pool? Some say conditional allocation should be allowed within families, or between friends, but not when the result of solicitation from a stranger (American Society of Transplant Surgeons, 2005). Is it defensible to distinguish, or is the choice between permitting all conditional allocation or none? One line of argument points to the alleged bad side effects of conditional allocation. Perhaps public knowledge of racist allocation would affect other people's willingness to donate, whereas conditional allocation within families would not (Spital, 2003). Different side effects could justify the distinctions. But another major line of argument claims that conditional allocation would be unjust, and there are good reasons to think that this argument could not justify the distinctions.

Why think conditional allocation unjust? The argument goes that when an organ is allocated conditionally, it bypasses the queue in the general pool. The queue is ordered justly and for some people to bypass it simply because they are lucky enough or famous enough to attract a donor is unjust (Kluge, 1989). Conditional allocation is still more unjust if it gives expression to the donor's discrimination. This argument is supposed to rule out conditional allocation even if it would provide organs that would not otherwise be available and would not reduce anyone else's access to organs.

Who is supposed to have duties of justice? There seem to be three relevant people or groups: the recipient, the donor and the transplant team and the wider framework of procurement and allocation they are embedded in. If we take these in order, we can first ask: is it unjust and thereby wrong for someone who needs an organ but is not top of the queue to accept one from a living person? Some high-minded writers (Kluge, 1989) think so, although it seems hard to see why, given that, by hypothesis, no one in the general pool loses. Should the person stranded on the rock as the waters rise refuse the offer of a boat ride on the grounds that another person on a different rock was not offered? As for live donors, it is hard to see that it is in general wrong if they make offers that bypass the queue in the general pool. To condemn such donors seems as unattractively rigoristic as condemning people who sponsor a child in a developing country, that being a less efficient and just method than other forms of charitable contribution.

This leaves the transplant team, and it is much more plausible that they have relevant obligations of justice. But whether these condemn conditional allocation depends on what justice requires. The claim might be that justice requires some form of equality of opportunity for access that supports the ranking system of the usual queue and that to allocate conditionally would conflict with this requirement. This is a very controversial claim about justice. As mentioned, the argument is supposed to rule out conditional allocation even if it would reduce access to organs. Under these circumstances, to refuse the offer would be to insist on levelling down – making some worse off and perhaps die for no gain to anyone else (Parfit, 2000). Whether levelling down principles are justified in this or any case is too large a topic to go into. Veatch (2000) claims that conditional allocation from dead donors should not be allowed and endorses levelling down; Wilkinson (2007) argues that levelling down is not justified in this case.

Even some of those who endorse levelling down egalitarian principles of justice are willing to make exceptions for donations within families (Kluge, 1989). However, once one distinguishes the roles of recipient and donor, on the one hand, and transplant team, on the other, it is not clear whether they are entitled to make this exception. There is, of course, nothing wrong and indeed a lot that is right with family members wishing to make sacrifices for each other and there is nothing wrong in principle with one family member wanting to donate an organ to another, or with that other accepting it. However, the members of the transplant team are not usually members of the same family as donor and recipient, and it is not clear how in a case of within-family donation they would become exempt from the requirements of justice in the allocation of organs. Egalitarian principles do not say: to each who is lucky enough to have a family member able and willing to donate (Robertson, 2005). (Even if the transplant team were family members, giving priority to relatives would be unjust nepotism.)

The thought here is not that it is wrong of transplant teams to perform living donor transplantation outside the general pool. It is that the attempt to justify this in the case of families, but no one else, on the basis of principles of justice looks incoherent. Other cases of conditional allocation might be unjust for special reasons, for instance, to avoid condoning racism. Otherwise, if on reflection we are not prepared to condemn as unjust conditional allocation within families, we should not condemn it in other cases either.

ACKNOWLEDGEMENTS

My thanks to John McCall and Debbie Tseung for their helpful comments.

REFERENCES

Archard D. For our own good. *Austr J Philos* 1994; **72**: 283–93.

ASERNIP-S (Australian Safety and Efficacy Register of New Interventional Procedures – Surgical). Live Donor Liver Transplantation – Adult Outcomes: A Systematic Review, 2004.

ASTS (American Society of Transplant Surgeons). Statement on Solicitation of Organ Donors, 2005; http://www.asts.org/donor-solication.cfm.

Buchanan AE, Brock D. *Deciding for Others*. Cambridge: Cambridge University Press, 1990.

Elliott C. Doing harm: living organ donors, clinical research and The Tenth Man. *J Med Ethics* 1995; **21**: 91–6.

Elster J. *Sour Grapes*. Cambridge: Cambridge University Press, 1983.

Fabre C. Justice and the compulsory taking of live body parts. *Utilitas* 2003; **15**: 127–50.

Feinberg J. *Harm to Others*. New York: Oxford University Press, 1984.

Harris J. *Clones, Genes, and Immortality*. Oxford: Oxford University Press, 1998; p. 137.

Kluge E-H. Designated organ donation: private choice in social context. *Hastings Center Rep* 1989; **19**: 10–6.

Langone AJ, Helderman JH. Disparity between solid-organ supply and demand. *N Engl J Med* 2003; **349**: 704–6.

Le Fanu J. *The Rise and Fall of Modern Medicine*. London: Little, Brown and Company, 1999.

McMahan J. *The Ethics of Killing*. Oxford: Clarendon Press, 2002.

Munson R. *Raising the Dead*. New York: Oxford University Press, 2002.

Parfit D. *Reasons and Persons*. Oxford: Oxford University Press, 1984.

Parfit D. Equality or priority? In: Clayton M, Williams A, eds. *The Ideal of Equality*. Basingstoke: Macmillan, 2000; pp. 81–125.

Price D. *Legal and Ethical Aspects of Organ Transplantation*. Cambridge: Cambridge University Press, 2001.

Rakoswki E. *Equal Justice*. Oxford: Clarendon Press, 1991.

Robertson C. Desperate patients solicit volunteers. *J Law Med Ethics* 2005; **33**: 170–4.

Shiffrin S. Paternalism, unconscionability doctrine and accommodation. *Philos Public Affairs* 2000; **29**: 205–50.

Singer P. *Rethinking Life and Death*. Melbourne: The Text Publishing Company, 1994.

Spital A. Should people who donate a kidney to a stranger be permitted to choose their recipients? *Transplantation* 2003; **76**: 1252–6.

Veatch R. *Transplantation Ethics*. Washington, DC: Georgetown University Press, 2000.

Wilkinson TM. Judging our own good. *Austr J Philos* 1996; **74**: 488–94.

Wilkinson TM. Racist organ donors and saving lives. *Bioethics* 2007; **21**: 63–74.

Wodehouse PG. *Life with Jeeves*. Harmondsworth: Penguin, 1981; p. 501.

Euthanasia and Principled Health Care Ethics: From Conflict to Compromise?

RICHARD HUXTABLE

INTRODUCTION

No one is likely to have the last word in the euthanasia debate. The arguments for and against may seem increasingly sophisticated, but the fundamental claims have changed little. Appeals to principles and the like seem to get the disputants no closer to agreement and yet some form of resolution appears warranted, in view of the importance of the issues at stake. In this chapter, I argue that it is time to consider adopting a compromise on euthanasia. Using the hypothetical case of Patrick, a patient who wishes to be helped to die, I sketch the key features of the debate and suggest that there are strengths and weaknesses in both the cases for and against such assistance. Against that backdrop, I further reinforce the case for compromise and make some – admittedly tentative – steps towards identifying the possible processes for securing this and, perhaps more controversially, the possible substance of such a compromise.

PATRICK'S REQUEST

Two senior doctors, Dr A and Dr F, have each been called to see Patrick, a 30-year-old former teacher and amateur athlete, who is an in-patient in the hospital at which they both work. Patrick is paralysed from the neck down following a road accident and is largely ventilator-dependent and has been for several months. He has informed the team caring for him, on numerous occasions, that he no longer recognizes this as his life and that he wishes to be helped to die. Patrick understands that without the ventilator his likelihood of dying is high. He has discussed the possibility of the ventilation being withdrawn but, despite assurances that any pain or suffering can be addressed through the use of sedative drugs and analgesics, Patrick declines this option. For one thing, he fears that there is a small chance he might still be able to breathe unaided and would therefore remain alive in his current state. Moreover, he feels that this is a fudge, designed to make the team feel better; what he wants is active and immediate help to die, either through a lethal concoction being prepared for him to ingest or through a lethal injection being administered by a doctor.

Although both of them are sympathetic to Patrick's plea, Drs A and F radically disagree on whether Patrick's request ought to be honoured. In a meeting subsequent to each of them seeing Patrick, Dr A states that he is against acceding to the request. Dr A is partly mindful of the fact that the actions Patrick proposes are contrary to the laws of homicide prevailing in the jurisdiction, as they amount either to a crime of assisting suicide or to one of murder. Dr A has campaigned against recent proposals to relax the law, which would afford voluntary euthanasia and assisted suicide a legal justification, at least where particular criteria are satisfied. Dr F, however, has been a vocal campaigner for such changes and she believes that Patrick would indeed be eligible if the law were to be changed. Although she too is concerned about the spectre of criminality, Dr F would be happy, in principle, to grant Patrick his wish. Neither doctor is willing to budge from their position; they agree, however, that no action should be taken yet and they decide to research the issue further so that they may present their respective cases more comprehensively at their next meeting.

Principles of Health Care Ethics, Second Edition   Edited by R.E. Ashcroft, A. Dawson, H. Draper and J.R. McMillan
© 2007 John Wiley & Sons, Ltd

THE SEARCH FOR A SOLUTION I: PRINCIPLED HEALTH CARE ETHICS

The first port of call for many health professionals faced with an ethical dilemma, at least in the developed world, will be the four principles approach (Beauchamp and Childress, 2001). Beauchamp and Childress's theory crops up in many medical curricula, and personal experience suggests that even those health professionals less well versed in ethics theory are familiar with the mantra of respecting autonomy, beneficence, non-maleficence and justice. Spurred on by Gillon's insistence that the principles can be of help in resolving virtually any dilemma confronted in health care, both Dr A and Dr F begin here (e.g. Gillon, 2003).

Unfortunately, at their next meeting, the two doctors are no closer to a solution. Dr F emphasizes the notion of respecting patient autonomy. Both doctors agree that Patrick satisfies criteria for deeming an individual autonomous because he appears appropriately well informed, free from outside pressure and is able to understand and reason through his decision in a competent manner. However, although he believes that individual choice must be respected in many situations, Dr A feels that this is not always so and that respect for individual choice certainly does not exhaust morality. Referring to the principles of beneficence and non-maleficence, he argues that to kill or be involved in the killing of a patient constitutes the most serious harm which anyone can inflict, particularly a doctor; to his mind, protecting life is the most beneficial course. Furthermore, to act otherwise would be to violate important principles of justice, in signalling that a disabled life is not due the same protection as an able life (Gormally, 1994). Legal endorsement of euthanasia would therefore unjustly undermine the rights of, and protection due to, the vulnerable in society (Campbell, 1998).

Dr F thinks Dr A is misinterpreting the principles. She maintains that life is only really worth while or beneficial when the individual living that life judges it so and asks, where is the harm in helping, if Patrick does not see death as harmful, but rather sees life in this condition as such (Nowell-Smith, 1994)? Dr F is also willing to go further, although she confesses that she has found less support for her next opinion. To her mind, justice is not only served by valuing every life equally (although she still insists that the value is to be determined by the individual). Despite confessing to some discomfort with the idea, she feels that justice might occasionally require the shortening of life, in order that the skills and materials currently devoted to a patient (particularly a patient like Patrick who does not want them) are redirected to the needs of other patients (Battin, 1987). However, given her disquiet, she confirms that this is not a key feature of her case, and she agrees to leave such considerations aside. (She nevertheless resolves to ask the hospital ethicists to devote more attention to the issue in the future.)

On one point the doctors are agreed: the four principles have not suggested a single answer or at least one on which they can agree. Furthermore, they are both willing to concede that the other's reading of the principles is *prima facie* plausible. They decide to postpone the issue again and to go deeper into the ethics literature in the hope of identifying a way forward.

THE SEARCH FOR A SOLUTION II: THE INTRINSIC VALUE OF LIFE

Dr A takes the lead at the next meeting. He now develops his argument that the best way of interpreting the injunctions to 'confer a benefit' and 'not do harm' involves recognizing that life has intrinsic value, such that its continuance is generally beneficial, whereas its intentional, premature ending is harmful.

Such an account is prevalent in the literature on euthanasia (Keown, 2002). The central ideas are most common in Judaeo-Christian and particularly Catholic thought, although they may be articulated in various ways, whether drawing upon a theistic heritage (the 'sanctity of life' doctrine) or not (the 'right to life'). Dr A's attention centres upon the Catholic account, not only because it commands much support (and, indeed, serves as a major focus of the criticism levelled by those in favour of euthanasia) but also because its terminology and distinctions (futility, acts and omissions) are familiar in both ethical and clinical circles.

The central idea is that life ought not to be brought to an end intentionally. This holds whether the killing is effected by active means (for example, a lethal injection) or passive means (an omission, such as deliberately declining to ventilate in order that the patient may die). Dr A recognizes, however, that he needs to do more work, for example, in relation to the notion of 'intention' and the distinction between acts and omissions. Fortunately, Dr A has recourse to two subordinate concepts, which give further specification and which serve also to mitigate against the potential severity of a strict, 'vitalistic' insistence on the intrinsic value of life.

The first subordinate concept is the doctrine of double effect. Application of this doctrine suggests that some activities which will pose a risk of death can be permitted, provided that death is not aimed at but is only an incidental side effect of the individual's otherwise worthwhile aim. Four conditions must be satisfied. First, the action itself must not be inherently morally wrong. Seeking to relieve a patient's pain, contends Dr A, is worth while, although he accepts that the use of strong opioids can curtail a patient's life, if only in the *rare* case (Huxtable and Forbes, 2004). Second, the intention must be to produce the good effect. So, says Dr A, the doctor using such drugs must intend only to relieve pain. Third, the good effect must not be brought about by the bad effect. It would be wrong therefore, claims Dr A, for the doctor to seek to achieve palliation through administering a demonstrably lethal dose. Finally, the good effect must outweigh the bad. The risk of death posed by drugs like morphine and some sedatives is, says Dr A, outweighed by the obligation to afford the patient relief, particularly in their final days or hours.

The second subordinate concept clarifies the distinction between actions and omissions. Deliberate fatal actions, Dr A postulates, will always violate the primary injunction. Yet, although it is also impermissible to intend (and secure) death through inaction, this does not mean that everything that can be done to prolong life must be done; sometimes withdrawing or withholding life-sustaining treatment (both of which are omissions) can be permissible. Here, Dr A invokes a distinction between 'ordinary' (or 'proportionate') means and 'extraordinary' (or 'disproportionate') means. In this context, he cautions Dr F not to think in terms of everyday treatments as opposed to unusual or 'high-tech' interventions. Rather, the point is that an extraordinary treatment is one that is futile or otherwise involves such high burdens for the patient that its benefits are disproportionately outweighed. Such a treatment or response is not morally obligatory. In contrast, where the benefits outweigh the burdens or the treatment is not likely to be futile, it is ordinary and thus morally obligatory.

Dr A, therefore, draws the following conclusions. To actively assist Patrick to die, whether through an action at his request or some form of joint enterprise, is morally impermissible. However, it is morally necessary to respond to Patrick's suffering. Although he has some difficulty with the conclusion, Dr A also tentatively concedes that it may even be acceptable to withdraw Patrick's ventilation, at least provided that this is not done with the intention of causing Patrick's death but rather with the intention of relieving his burden. If withdrawal were to occur, Dr A would seek to ensure that Patrick is kept comfortable through palliation and/or sedation, even if the drugs used might cause respiratory repression and thus entail a risk of Patrick, who is already experiencing respiratory difficulties, dying sooner than he would otherwise.

Dr F is unimpressed with this thinking. She identifies three particularly problematic areas, concerning its meaning, scope and appeal. First, asking what these related doctrines are to mean, Dr F complains that the terms invoked by Dr A all require further interpretation before they can be applied in practice. Thus, she says, there is nothing in this account to persuade her that she and Dr A are using terms like 'intention', 'futility', 'omission' and 'burden' in the same way. They are, she feels, morally loaded from the outset and, therefore, seem to beg the question as to what is the right thing to do.

Dr F also dismisses Dr A's account for being either too narrow in scope or else so wide that it defeats itself. It is at least too narrow in the sense that the focus on the moral sensibilities, intentions and so on of the doctor means losing sight of Patrick, who should, she claims, properly be the focal point of their thinking (Price, 2001). But even aside from this, the doctrine founders when it introduces notions like 'futility'. Such terms are unavoidably value-laden (Halliday, 1997). For them to make any sense some account must be taken of the condition of the patient and, indeed, the patient's own opinion thereof: how else are we to know whether a particular treatment will achieve a purpose for this patient? Moreover, to insist that the focus is on the quality of the treatment is to draw an illusory veil over what is really being judged: whether or not, in view of his condition, the patient is worth expending such effort on. She has similar points to make about the doctrine of double effect, which she also feels smuggles in assessments of the quality of the patient's life (Singer, 1993, p. 210). However, she concludes this point by arguing that Dr A can only avoid this charge of inconsistency by defining the relevant terms so narrowly that the doctrine ultimately entails a 'vitalistic' commitment to preserving all lives at all costs, which he claims he wishes to avoid (Kuhse, 1987).

Dr F also finds Dr A's approach to Patrick's plight unappealing. For one thing, Dr F claims that the doctrine is unlikely to persuade unless some underlying reason is offered for maintaining that life is intrinsically worth while; mere assertion alone will not suffice. If the reason lies in some appeal to a higher power like God then she, like many others in her pluralistic society, feels at liberty to reject this basis and all that ensues from it. Dr F concedes that nontheistic arguments can be offered in support of the principle, but she counters that even the most robust of these seem to allow the individual the right to determine when their life can be brought to an end (e.g. Beyleveld and Brownsword, 2001). If, then, the fates of Patrick and other patients, who may or may not have faith in a higher power, are to be determined by a primarily religious account of the value of life, then the doctrine is not only incoherent but also tyrannical, in holding the majority hostage to the views of an arguably dwindling minority (Dworkin, 1993, p. 217).

THE SEARCH FOR A SOLUTION III: THE INSTRUMENTAL VALUE OF LIFE

Dr F prefers the view that life is of instrumental value and only has value for the individual when he himself judges it as such. This, she says, gives a better way of judging when continued life is beneficial and when killing might not actually be harmful. She wants the matter to be determined by individual choice, although she is willing to make some small steps towards recognizing that outsiders too can judge the value of another individual's life.

Dr F does acknowledge Dr A's right to cleave to the sanctity of human life because this is perfectly consistent with respect for individual choice, but she resists the idea that his view can be imposed on her, let alone patients like Patrick who do not share it (e.g. Dworkin, 1993, p. 217). After all, she argues, many people do in fact support the case for allowing voluntary euthanasia (e.g. Voluntary Euthanasia Society, 2003). She feels she also has an advantage over Dr A in so far as her case for respecting autonomy is grounded in what she considers to be a rational conception of human agency or 'personhood'. A person is a creature capable of valuing one's own existence; where the person no longer so values existence, it may be brought to an end (Harris, 1985, 1997a).

She is willing to go a little further, however. She recognizes that the case for voluntary euthanasia also partially rests on regard for the condition of the patient. In keeping with her first argument, the autonomous individual (or 'person') must be the one who concludes that their quality of life is sufficiently low to trigger a request for assisted dying. Involuntary euthanasia can never be countenanced, even if some outsider thinks this would be kindest. Non-voluntary euthanasia, however, might be another matter. Dr F finds the idea that it can be merciful to end the suffering of a non-autonomous individual, such as a seriously disabled young child or a permanently incapacitated adult persuasive. She knows, however, that such a claim is highly contentious, even if it is limited to those cases where the patient's loved ones agree that this would be for the best (Singer, 1993, pp. 182–91). She, therefore, chooses to leave this argument to one side and returns to Patrick: given that he is autonomous, she thinks he has a right to be assisted in a manner of his choosing.

Dr A is unwilling to leave that argument aside and nor is he persuaded by her other claims. Like Dr F, he starts with problems of meaning. He is particularly troubled by the highly individualistic stance which Dr F is taking. People are not isolated in the way which Dr F seems to assume, but rather exist within a web of social relations (Donchin, 2000). To his mind, 'I want' should not automatically translate into 'I get', even if someone is willing to 'give it'. Moreover, he feels that a fuller appreciation of autonomy would help Dr F to see that autonomy is not merely concerned with empowerment but also involves constraint because – at the very least – one person's autonomy must end where another's begins. He is even less impressed with her recourse to quality of life considerations. Who is to judge when the 'quality' is sufficiently low to warrant killing? It is all very well for her to say that this is a matter for the autonomous individual, but what about non-autonomous patients? Who should decide then and according to what criteria?

This leads Dr A to identify some problems with the scope of Dr F's claims. To start with, he worries that the logic of the 'I want, I get' mentality can be taken to extremes. Once Dr F invokes a right to assisted dying, she must agree that someone else is under a duty to assist (Hohfeld, 1964). But what if no one is willing to assist; or must they do so? Aside from this concern, the logic of Dr F's argument suggests that euthanasia need not be restricted to the classic cases of 'terminal' or 'incurable' illness, assuming we can even define such concepts. It rather seems that if perfectly autonomous and, indeed, physically able individuals decided that they wanted help in dying, then provided they found someone willing to so assist (who was equally autonomous), Dr F could have no objection in terms of respecting autonomy as she understands the concept (see Möller and Huxtable, 2001). Dr F's only possible objection would be to point to the need for the patient to be, in some sense, suffering. But that returns her to the previous problem of meaning and then introduces a new problem of scope: any restriction to, for example, terminal illness will be susceptible to a charge of arbitrariness. Dr A notes that suffering can take many forms; would Dr F be content to allow euthanasia for any suffering whatsoever?

Indeed, Dr A feels that Dr F was deceptively coy in saying that she *might* be prepared to judge the value of another's life. This is, in his opinion, a necessary step in her argument: the case for euthanasia cannot rest on an appeal to autonomy alone because the compliant doctor must be willing to at least share the patient's judgement on the worth of his life or else she has no reason for acting (De Haan, 2002). It is, claims Dr A, but a small step from this thinking to thinking that one can judge the value of life for those unable to voice an opinion. Although she preferred to, Dr F simply cannot leave the issue of non-voluntary euthanasia to one side; indeed, she may even have to reconsider her opposition to involuntary euthanasia. Then the problems of scope stack up because Dr F's proclaimed logic slides her into the murky territory of eugenics. However, Dr A resists levelling a charge of Nazism against Dr F because he accepts that her motivation, although mistaken, is benign (Finnis, 1997, p. 53; Harris, 1997b p. 53).

Dr A then finishes by challenging the perceived appeal of Dr F's arguments. He confidently asserts that only a very small minority would support any move towards legitimizing non-voluntary euthanasia. He also believes that people would be less swayed by the case for voluntary euthanasia if they were better informed about the potential dangers of abuse and the benefits of palliative care (Keown, 2002). He is also wary of opinion polls indicating substantial support for the practice, as they can be partial and emotive.

At this point the conversation falters. Although each sees some merit in the other's arguments and counter-arguments, neither doctor is inclined to abandon their initial view. They think they see a way forward, however. They resolve to refer the case, as a matter of urgency, to the hospital's clinical ethics committee. They notify the committee that they are prepared to make submissions and will accept the committee's decision as final and binding. The committee, as they know, is composed of a diverse group of health professionals and lay members; previous encounters also suggest that the committee is split on the issue of voluntary euthanasia, with a third in favour, a third against and a third holding no strong views either way. Dr A, Dr F and, most importantly, Patrick now await the committee's decision.

THE SOLUTION: TIME TO COMPROMISE?

Although no amount of fresh thinking is likely to do away entirely with the arguments just sketched, it is sobering to note that the debate between these doctors was dubbed 'jaded' as long ago as 1958 (Williams, 1958, p. 143). How then do we move beyond 'the present impasse where we heatedly debate "right-to-die" legislation' (Fraser, 2000, p. 122)?

Although he does not focus on euthanasia, Martin Benjamin's (1990) work suggests that the way forward lies in compromising. This is certainly borne out by the ways in which the debate slots into Benjamin's four conditions of compromise: uncertainty, moral complexity, an ongoing relationship and the need for a decision. With regard to the first condition, there is undeniably a dearth of factual certainty in the end of life context. It is, for example, not always obvious how a particular intervention will affect a patient's life or quality of life; medicine is not as exact a science as it is sometimes depicted. Equally, although such claims are themselves slippery (e.g. Williams, 1985), to say that a particular policy involves stepping onto a 'slippery slope' cannot easily be (dis)proven prior to taking the relevant step. Predictions that legitimizing voluntary euthanasia will in fact lead to a more general devaluing of life cannot be tested in a rigorous fashion, save for some consideration of the evidence from other jurisdictions where the step has been taken. However, not only do variations between jurisdictions preclude conclusive inferences from being drawn as to the likely impact of a particular measure, (Battin, 2005, pp. 47–68) but the results of comparative analyses are themselves disputed. For example, although some argue that the Dutch system shows the (empirical) slippery slope in action (Keown, 2002), others believe that the converse is true (Otlowski, 1997). There is further empirical uncertainty surrounding the possible future development of medical science. So, should lives be prolonged in the hope of finding cures or effective treatments? And if these are developed, will the case for euthanasia be rendered moribund?

There is also philosophical uncertainty. Opinions remain split on the value of life and the related dilemmas which this question poses regarding, for example, the provision or cessation of life support. Indeed, we cannot even agree on how to define and categorize the types of conduct usually in issue. Is withdrawing life support a form of euthanasia, and if so is it active or passive in nature? What is assisted suicide and (how) does it differ from euthanasia?

Such uncertainty can only impact adversely upon our discussions about the rights and wrongs of ending life. Indeed, the moral complexity of the issues is a second reason for viewing this as an area where compromise ought to be considered: each of the arguments offered by Drs A and F has at least some intuitive merit. A third condition identified by Benjamin is that the disputants are locked in an ongoing relationship. In Patrick's case, and assuming no one resigns in disgust, Drs A and F are colleagues; the members of the local ethics committee too must work together through these issues to find a broadly acceptable solution. We can raise this to the societal level, for everyone in society surely has a stake in how this debate is settled, even if the answer remains open to revision.

The final condition to which Benjamin refers is that the issue in question cannot be ducked: a policy is needed. This is easy to construct in a hypothetical case like the one presented here because we have a committee which has been asked to make a decision. (Again, leaving aside the fact that support for Dr F's position would likely mean the committee has broken the law. It should also be noted that such committees typically only provide advice, rather than a (binding) decision. If the arguments sketched here are worth taking forward, then the role and remit of bioethical committees (whether local, national or international) may need reconsideration.) But even where no individual decision is required, there is an increasing need to clarify our policies (whichever jurisdiction we happen to occupy). Medical science continues to progress, the situations and settings in which we die alter and the arguments for and against euthanasia constantly ebb and flow, but metaphysical or moral closure appears a will o' the wisp. And this issue – where lives are at stake – is scarcely one on which we should lack a clear policy.

However, even if there is a *prima facie* case for securing a compromise, there will be resistance on the basis that this threatens moral integrity. Yet Benjamin, coming from a morally pluralistic perspective, does not think that this has to be the case. He recognizes that at least some important values will be incapable of reconciliation, such that an individual may feel bound by conflicting duties. Drs A and F have the right to present their respective cases and they retain this right even if the committee decision, to which they ultimately defer, is at odds with their view. The same holds for those who sit on such committees. If the individual accepts that her values are in conflict with someone else's but that there must be some decision, that individual also owes it to herself and to those others to accommodate a decision which somehow splits the difference. After all, committees called on to make decisions or issue policies cannot easily shirk those responsibilities. As Benjamin says, '[c]ompromise is not, strictly speaking, resolution. It makes the best of what appears to be a bad situation . . . The resulting ambivalence is part of the price we must pay to avoid the dehumanization of simple consistency in an unavoidably complex situation' (Benjamin, 1994, pp. 274, 277).

Benjamin is evidently concentrating on the ethicist who serves on ethics committees and it may be that this is the best place (whether locally or nationally) for deciding on the way forward with regard to euthanasia. Bioethics committees are already familiar, but what is less familiar is the argument that we should be using this process precisely in order to achieve a *compromise* on the ancient questions of euthanasia. Some scholars are beginning to move in that direction, (Battin, 2005, pp. 35–38; McCall Smith, 1999) but more work can certainly be done on, for example, the appropriate composition and remit of such committees, in order to ensure that every argument is given a fair hearing (that Drs A and F were both senior colleagues and that the ethics committee was already split on the issues were two deliberate features of the earlier scenario).

CONCLUSION: GIVING CONTENT TO THE COMPROMISE?

Having said all this, the precise contours of the compromise will be hard to specify in advance, and understandably so, for the conditions outlined here prioritize procedure over product. We can, however, say a little about what splitting the difference could mean in practice.

To start with, there will be points of consensus: for example, a patient like Patrick ought to be provided with adequate palliative care and ought not to be forced to receive unwanted life-sustaining therapies. Exploration of these points of agreement remains worth while (Moreno, 1995, p. 34), but it still seems unlikely that consensus will be reached on the central ethical issues. Indeed, some will say, such options effectively amount to a victory for Dr A – they do not constitute the 'middle ground'. However, Dr A need not wholly win out. For example, he may still feel that the decision to withdraw or withhold life-support challenges his belief that life is sacred.

Dr F, however, will still feel this falls short of granting the patient's wish. So what if she were to go ahead and assist Patrick? Here, we need to look beyond the case to the community and consider how the legislators, policymakers, prosecutors and, indeed, the professional bodies ought to respond to Dr F's actions. If we focus on the legal dimension, you will recall that Dr F has lobbied for a relaxation of the prohibitive laws on euthanasia, while Dr A has campaigned against. Which way should the lawyers jump? As was earlier noted, the best way to decide this would be through recourse to an appropriately composed committee. If compromise is worth while and, indeed, necessary, then the answer for the committee would appear to be: do not jump but do *step* into the middle ground, by recognizing the circumstances in which Dr F acted without losing sight of the force of Dr A's objections.

One way of giving shape to this policy would be to afford Dr F a partial defence to the crime of murder and provide for sentencing flexibility. The idea of a distinct defence of 'mercy killing', modelled on familiar categories like manslaughter, is not new, but is being revived precisely because it offers a middle way (e.g. Grubb, 2001). In a compromise, both sides must gain and lose: the policy will have to hurt both sides while also accommodating each to an extent. A partial defence achieves this as it affords an *excuse*, rather than justification or condemnation. As such, Dr F will have to accept that the policy is not – and will not be allowed to become – one of *de facto* decriminalization or even legalization: that life has been taken will still be marked by a criminal conviction and some form of penalty. However, in recognition of the features highlighted by Dr F (such as the victim's request and suffering), the penalty may be light in 'paradigm' cases (an example would be probation with some form of counselling). In deference to Dr A, however, taking life will remain criminal, and the judges will be afforded an appropriately wide discretion to deal with cases which in some way fall outside the paradigm (for example, due to questions over the sincerity of the accused's motive). Dr A will nevertheless have to accept that the penalties will not usually be punitive.

Much more needs to be done to give shape to such a policy and to the means for achieving it. For example, sentencing and prosecution guidelines would need to be developed in order to ensure that the demands of formal justice (treating like cases alike) are satisfied. Equally, revisions to the criminal justice system might be needed if we conclude that compromise is best secured through recourse to committees, rather than reliance on an individual adjudicator.

Leaving such details aside, I nevertheless hope to have demonstrated that we need to devote more attention to ways of resolving the euthanasia debate. The debate has trundled along on the same parallel tracks for some considerable time, and the tracks look unlikely to meet. There may continue to be victories and losses on both sides, sometimes within one and the same jurisdiction, as occurred in the Northern Territories of Australia which saw voluntary euthanasia permitted and then prohibited in the space of one year (Keown, 2002, pp. 153–166). Furthermore, an argument in favour of compromise is likely to be roundly criticized from all quarters, and might also risk descending into confusion and incoherence (Campbell, 2003). Nevertheless, exploration of the middle ground remains worth while, not least in 'the rough landscape of policy-making in which one may need to compromise, not in the sense of defecting from duty but honouring duties which are multiple'(May, 2003).

ACKNOWLEDGEMENTS

Work on this chapter, which is part of a larger project, began during a period of study leave in the Hastings Center, New York, in 2004. I am grateful to the University of Bristol for the financial support and to, in particular, Tom Murray, Bruce Jennings and Stacy Sanders for offering their time and expertise. Thanks are also due to Lois Bibbings and Alastair V Campbell, who provided invaluable comments on previous drafts.

REFERENCES

Battin MP. *Ending Life: Ethics and the Way We Die*. Oxford: Oxford University Press, 2005.

Battin MP. Age rationing and the just distribution of health care: is there a duty to die? *Ethics* 1987; **97**(2): 317–40.

Beauchamp TL, Childress JF. *Principles of Biomedical Ethics*, 5th edition. Oxford: Oxford University Press, 2001.

Benjamin M. *Splitting the Difference: Compromise and Integrity in Ethics and Politics*. Lawrence, Kansas: University Press of Kansas, 1990.

Benjamin M. Conflict, compromise, and moral integrity. In: Campbell CS, Lustig BA, eds. *Duties to Others*. Dordrecht: Kluwer Academic Publishers, 1994; pp. 261–78.

Beyleveld D, Brownsword R. *Human Dignity in Bioethics and Biolaw*. Oxford: Oxford University Press, 2001.

Campbell AV. Euthanasia and the principle of justice. In: Gill R, ed. *Euthanasia and the Churches*. London: Cassell, 1998; pp. 83–97.

Campbell AV, Huxtable R. The position statement and its commentators: consensus, compromise or confusion? *Palliat Med* 2003; **17**: 180–3.

De Haan J. The ethics of euthanasia: advocates perspectives. *Bioethics* 2002; **16**(2): 154–72.

Donchin A. Autonomy, interdependence, and assisted suicide: respecting boundaries/crossing lines. *Bioethics* 2000; **14**(3): 187–204.

Dworkin R. *Life's Dominion: An Argument about Abortion and Euthanasia*. London: Harper Collins, 1993.

Finnis J. The fragile case for euthanasia: a reply to John Harris. In: Keown J, ed. *Euthanasia Examined: Ethical, Clinical and Legal Perspectives*. Cambridge: Cambridge University Press, 1997; pp. 46–55.

Fraser SI, Walters JW. Death – whose decision? Euthanasia and the terminally ill. *J Med Ethics* 2000; **26**: 121–5.

Gillon R. Ethics Needs principles – four can encompass the rest – and respect for autonomy should be "first among equals". *J Med Ethics* 2003; **29**: 307–12.

Gormally L. Against voluntary euthanasia. In: Gillon R, ed. *Principles of Health Care Ethics*. Chichester: John Wiley & Sons, Inc, 1994; pp. 763–74.

Grubb A. Editorial: euthanasia in England – a law lacking compassion? *Eur J Health Law* 2001; **8**: 89–93.

Halliday R. Medical futility and the social context. *J Med Ethics* 1997; **23**: 148–53.

Harris J. *The Value of Life: An Introduction to Medical Ethics*. London: Routledge and Kegan Paul, 1985.

Harris J. Euthanasia and the value of life. In: Keown J, ed. *Euthanasia Examined: Ethical, Clinical and Legal Perspectives*. Cambridge: Cambridge University Press, 1997a; pp. 6–22.

Harris J. Final thoughts on final acts. In: Keown J, ed. *Euthanasia Examined: Ethical, Clinical and Legal Perspectives*. Cambridge: Cambridge University Press, 1997b; pp. 56–61.

Hohfeld WN. In: Cook WW, ed. *Fundamental Legal Conceptions as Applied in Judicial Reasoning*. New Haven; London: Yale University Press, 1964.

Huxtable R, Forbes K. Glass v UK: Maternal instinct vs. medical opinion. *Child Family Law Q* 2004; **16**(3): 339–54.

Keown J. *Euthanasia, Ethics and Public Policy: An Argument Against Legalisation*. Cambridge: Cambridge University Press, 2002.

Kuhse H. *The Sanctity of Life Doctrine in Medicine: A Critique*. Oxford: Clarendon Press, 1987.

Möller M, Huxtable R. Euthanasia in the Netherlands: the case of "Life Fatigue". *N Law J* 2001; **151**: 1600–1.

May WF. *Oral evidence to President's Council on Bioethics*, 17 October 2003; available on the World Wide Web: http://bioethics.gov/transcripts/oct03/oct17full.html.

McCall Smith A. Euthanasia: the strengths of the middle ground. *Med Law Rev* 1999; **7**: 194–207.

Moreno JD. *Deciding Together: Bioethics and Moral Consensus*. New York: Oxford University Press, 1995.

Nowell-Smith P. In favour of voluntary euthanasia. In: Gillon R, ed. *Principles of Health Care Ethics*. Chichester: John Wiley & Sons, Inc, 1994; pp. 753–62.

Otlowski MFA. *Voluntary Euthanasia and the Common Law*. Oxford: Clarendon Press, 1997.

Price D. Fairly bland: an alternative view of a supposed new "Death Ethic" and the BMA guidelines. *Legal Stud* 2001; **21**: 618–43.

Singer P. *Practical Ethics*, 2nd edition. Cambridge: Cambridge University Press, 1993.

Voluntary Euthanasia Society. *VES Briefing: Opinion Polls* 2003; available on the World Wide Web: http://www.ves.org.uk/pdf/PublicOpinion_Apr03.pdf.

Williams B. Which Slopes are Slippery? In: Lockwood M, ed. *Moral Dilemmas in Modern Medicine*. Oxford: Oxford University Press, 1985; p. 126.

Williams G. Euthanasia legislation: a rejoinder to the non-religious objections. In: Downing AB, ed. (1969). *Euthanasia and the Right to Death: The Case for Voluntary Euthanasia*. London: Peter Owen, 1958; pp. 134–47.

Understanding and Misunderstanding Death

DAVID LAMB

If I could bestow animation upon lifeless matter, I might in the process of time ... renew life where death had apparently devoted the body to corruption.

Mary Shelley, *Frankenstein*

INTRODUCTION

The determination of death continues to be a problematic issue and doctors are frequently accused of being out of step with public perceptions of death. Doubts concerning the medical profession's competency to accurately diagnose death have been expressed throughout the history of modern medicine. These doubts were evident in scores of pamphlets and tracts written in the eighteenth and nineteenth centuries (Arnold, Zimmerman & Martin, 1968). In 1740 it was suggested by Jean Jacques Winslow that putrefaction was the only sure sign of death. Such a proposal expressed great scepticism and ignorance concerning criteria for death and consequently reflected a total loss of public confidence in the medical profession. As a general rule doubts concerning the reliability of medical criteria and tests for death have emerged with the introduction of new medical techniques. Moral and philosophical problems have tended to be more acute during periods when neither the medical profession nor the public have fully understood the philosophical implications of certain developments in medical science. Following an examination of the sources of confusion over concepts of death it is concluded that an acceptable definition of death must acknowledge its medical, cultural and philosophical aspects.

MODERN SCIENCE, DEATH AND MEDICAL CONFUSION

The modern scientific era in medicine has its intellectual roots in the seventeenth century when pioneers such as Harvey, Gassendi and Descartes advanced mechanistic theories of life. Living beings were depicted as complicated mechanisms, and analogies were drawn between physical systems of that time and living organisms. Thus bodily functions were depicted in terms of mechanical devices; the most successful model being Harvey's mechanistic account of heartbeat and circulation of the blood. The Cartesian account of the living organism is, perhaps, the most familiar one. According to the Cartesians, the living being was a machine which was powered by a mind or soul.

From the seventeenth century onwards, the mechanistic view of life dominated scientific medicine and concepts of death have often rested on mechanistic analogies. The patient is dead when the machine packs up, when the cardiac pump no longer functions or when the central computer is irreversibly dysfunctional. Mechanistic ideas about life and death are compatible with religious notions of death as the separation of the immortal soul from the perishable body; death can be presented as the boundary between the extinction of physical life and the beginning of spiritual life. The physician is concerned with the former; the priest is concerned with the latter. Despite cultural and religious diversity throughout the world, people have placed tremendous moral importance on the boundary between life and death. Whenever science has appeared to encroach upon moral and religious notions of life and death this has given rise to public anxiety, as frequently expressed in art and literature. Consider Mary Shelley's account of attempts to reverse death in her tale of Frankenstein's monster and Edgar Allen Poe's fear of misdiagnosis of death as depicted in *The Tell Tale Heart*.

Anxieties concerning the reliability of medical criteria and tests for death have accompanied developments in scientific medicine. These have been strongly expressed in controversies over the transplantation of vital organs such as

Principles of Health Care Ethics, Second Edition   Edited by R.E. Ashcroft, A. Dawson, H. Draper and J.R. McMillan
© 2007 John Wiley & Sons, Ltd

the heart and lungs. Developments in resuscitative technology led to a spate of claims throughout the 1960s, concerning patients who had been allegedly 'brought back to life', and consequent discussions concerning the uncertainly of medical criteria for death. There are parallels between the uncertainty created by techniques of cardiac resuscitation in the mid-twentieth century and that which accompanied the development of artificial resuscitation in the eighteenth century.

During the 1760s, enlightened doctors and reformers began to organize 'humane societies' to teach the newly discovered technique of 'artificial respiration' for the purpose of resuscitating victims of drowning or suffocation. Artificial respiration had a dramatic effect on popular perceptions of death and the dying process. By 1796, the London Humane Society claimed to have resuscitated over 2000 people. The fact that so many 'apparent' deaths could be reversed prompted suspicions regarding the possible number of people who had been diagnosed as dead and were consequently buried, but nevertheless might have been resuscitated by means of the miraculous new techniques. Misunderstandings over the nature of resuscitation generated confusion and disenchantment with the medical approach to death.

Today we understand a great deal more about resuscitation and can measure, with some reliability, the extent of damage which will occur if a brain is starved of oxygen for a given period. During the eighteenth century, medical science was ignorant about anoxic insults to the brain and doctors knew very little about oxygen and its properties. We are also aware that resuscitation has limits and that it will not restore life to a person whose brain has been destroyed. In the eighteenth century, many of those who marvelled at the miracle of artificial respiration were unable to consider this fact. Thus sceptics appealed to artificial respiration when they argued that medical criteria and tests for death were unreliable. This was the background to demands that putrefaction should be considered as the only true sign of death.

As resuscitative techniques developed throughout the eighteenth century, other interventions in the dying process were employed, which included measures to restore motion to the blood, such as violent shaking of the patient and thumping victims of drowning accidents. The introduction of smelling salts in 1721 was seen as an aid to resuscitative techniques, and later electric shocks were administered to restore heart, nerve and muscle functions. In 1755, Giovanni Bianchi used electricity to resuscitate a dog. The first human to be electrically 'resuscitated' was in 1774, and by 1800 electrical resuscitation was beginning to raise doubts with regard to criteria for death. Although little was understood about electricity at the time, exponents of electrical resuscitation convinced many people that traditional methods of diagnosing death were inadequate. Giovanni Aldini, Professor of Physics at Bolognia, gave public demonstrations of electro-resuscitation, and in 1803 Londoners was thrilled by the twitching and wheezing Aldini evoked from the electrified corpse of an executed convict. With the mysterious, life-giving, force of electricity available, who could trust the doctor who diagnosed death without first passing an electric current through the deceased? The link between the force of electricity and life is one of the themes in Mary Shelley's, *Frankenstein,* which vividly portrays the ethical and emotional uncertainties posed by the new electro-resuscitative technology – not to mention organ transplantation a century later – and the doubts medical science had raised regarding the public's understanding of death.

Problems with the medical diagnosis of death were to persist throughout the nineteenth century. Efforts were directed to solve problems with patients in coma, suspended animation and related conditions such as catalepsy, asphyxia, ecstasy and trance – the latter of which was examined by the notorious Franz Mesmer, who argued that in trances, the soul was free to leave the body. Hence Mesmerism cast further doubts on the certainty of a medical diagnosis of death. Mesmerism, so it was claimed, not only brought about a state of apparent death, but its practitioners also claimed the ability to reverse death.

With further technical innovation came pressing concerns regarding the diagnosis of death. The introduction of inhalation anaesthesia in 1846 generated concern over the boundary between life and death. There were also reports of 'fasting girls' who allegedly spent long periods in death-like states without ingesting or excreting. By the late nineteenth century there was widespread panic across Europe and the United States of America concerning the indeterminacy of medical diagnosis and possible reversals of death-like states. In response to widely expressed fears of premature burial, governments passed laws to extend the interval between death and burial. Open caskets with around-the-clock guards often featured in nineteenth century European burials. Stories of 'revived' corpses being rescued by grave robbers whet the Victorian appetite for sensationalism and horror. This was the context in which laws requiring death certificates emerged.

A century later, in the 1950s and 1960s, developments in resuscitative technology and the ability to reverse cardiac arrest meant that thousands of pulse-less and apnoeic patients could be restored to fully conscious states. Although some at the time interpreted this as resurrection – thus repeating confusion displayed in the eighteenth century development of artificial respiration – the prevailing cultural view was that as the condition was reversible, temporary cardio-respiratory standstill was not equated with death. In the 1990s a subfield of research developed in which the experiences of patients undergoing temporary cardio-respiratory suspension were described as 'near death experiences'(Woodhouse, 1992) thus implicitly recognizing that death had not occurred.

Success in cardio-respiratory reversal generated a major scientific and ethical problem: the problem of the 'beating heart cadaver', where ventilation to asystole was becoming distressing to doctors and relatives as a clear boundary between life and death was no longer apparent. It later became obvious that the artificial continuation of cardiac and respiratory activity, in certain conditions where brain function had irreversibly ceased, was not equated with the maintenance of life, and was of no benefit to the patient. In such cases, conventional cardio-respiratory criteria had proven incapable of giving a clear and unambiguous answer to the question of the borderline between life and death, and a reassessment of traditional criteria was inevitable.

THE EMERGENCE OF BRAIN DEATH

The way forward lay in considering the importance of the brain. Notwithstanding the emotional significance of the heart, the significance of the brain as both the unit of consciousness and cognition, and as the organizing faculty of the body 'as a whole,' had long been recognized. For centuries human beings have decapitated and hung or beaten the heads of their unfortunate fellows in the knowledge that a brain sufficiently damaged or separated from its body was equivalent to death. The connection between brain function and the respiratory and circulatory organs is straightforward. First, spontaneous respiration is dependent upon brain function. Second, the brain is dependent upon a supply of oxygenated blood. With total brain infarction spontaneous respiration is ruled out, although in certain circumstances respiration can be artificially maintained. If the brain has been deprived of oxygen (for example due to cardiac arrest) for about 15–20 min, then its functions will be totally and irreversibly lost, never to be replaced by surgery, medication or technical aids. These elementary facts are not new, and were known long before criteria for brain death were proposed. But resuscitation technology led to a reassessment of the connection between brain function and the respiratory and circulatory organs. What did emerge from the 1950s was the awareness that intervention could make it possible to prevent the brain from succumbing to cardiac and respiratory arrest on one hand, and make it possible, on the other hand, artificially to maintain heartbeat and circulation of blood in a person's body whose brain had ceased to function as an integrated whole. In short: the natural link between the function of the brain and the heart and the lungs had been severed.

The earliest reference to a state approaching brain death was in 1902, when Harvey Cushing described a patient whose spontaneous respirations ceased as a result of an intracranial tumour, but whose heart was kept beating for 23 hours with artificial respiration (Black, 1978, p. 395). The contemporary discussion of brain death began in a paper by two French neuro-physiologists (Mollaret & Goulon, 1959), who described a condition of complete unresponsiveness, flaccidity, altered thermal regulation, absence of mesencephalic reflexes, lack of spontaneous respiration and progressive circulatory collapse. They called it *'coma depassé'* (literally, 'a state beyond coma'), but did not equate it with death. Throughout the 1950s and 1960s, developments in the technology of intensive care undermined confidence in the traditional cardio-respiratory concept and redirected attention towards neurological criteria. In 1968 the report by the Ad Hoc Committee of the Harvard Medical School was a landmark in the development of brain-related criteria for death (Harvard, 1968).

One fundamental point emerged from the history of confusion and uncertainty regarding the diagnosis of death: until the development of neurological criteria for death no one had seriously examined the concept of death in its medical context. Doctors had sought to diagnose death without explicitly addressing the philosophical problem of relating their (usually implicit) concept of death to the criteria and tests they employed when diagnosing the deaths of their patients. The idea of a definition of death, in medical guidelines and legal statutes, appears to have emerged simultaneously with brain-related definitions of death.

BRAIN DEATH AND FURTHER SOURCES OF MISUNDERSTANDING

Tremendous confusion has been created in both medical and philosophical literature over the terminology employed to describe the neurological syndromes that have emerged over the past thirty or so years. While the expressions 'brain death', 'whole brain death' and 'brainstem death' are now well established in medicine and law, a variety of philosophical positions became entrenched behind terms such as 'higher brain', 'lower brain', 'coma', 'chronic coma', 'irreversible coma', 'appallic syndrome', 'persistent vegetative state' (PVS), 'locked in syndrome', 'cerebral death', 'neocortical death', and the anencephaly spectrum. The capacity for confusion was increased when translating into other European languages. The term *'coma depassé'* survived in France until 1988 when it was rejected in favour of 'brain death' by the French Academy of Medicine who commented that the decision 'ends semantic ambiguity which leads to clinical ambiguity' (*Le Monde*, 27 May 1988). In Italy *'morte cerebrale'* translates equally as 'brain death' (including the brainstem) and 'cerebral death,' where damage is confined to the cerebral hemispheres, thus sparing the brainstem (Lamb, 1987, 1995).

Several terms in the above list emerged when medical scientists were first grappling with the new syndromes associated with neurological impairment. Thus terms like 'higher brain' and 'lower brain,' which have no precise anatomical meaning, crept into the language as a convenient way of distinguishing between cortical and sub-cortical structures. The term 'coma' refers to a sleep-like state due to damage to the brainstem but it has been erroneously used by philosophers to refer to impaired levels of awareness where damage is confined to the cerebral hemispheres. In a comatose patient, survival mechanisms, such as cough, gag and swallowing reflexes are absent, and accordingly comatose patients are generally regarded as terminally ill. Terms like 'chronic coma' and 'irreversible coma' – although frequently used in the media – are best avoided altogether as they have no physiological or neurological meaning.

In 1968, the Harvard Committee formulated a definition of death in which 'brain death' was equated with 'irreversible coma'. In the 1970s, irreversible coma became a catchphrase for all permanently unconscious patients. Strictly speaking, death is the ultimate irreversible coma as it implies that all survival mechanisms have shut down. The term 'irreversible coma' should not be applied to either the PVS or the anencephaly spectrum. The term 'appallic syndrome' is an anachronism which has been replaced by the expression PVS, where massive brain damage is largely confined to the cerebral hemispheres, sparing much of the brainstem and in particular the capacity to breathe spontaneously. Although some philosophers and ethicists (Gervais, 1987) have argued that patients in a PVS have lost any semblance of 'personal identity' this condition is clearly distinguishable from brain death. Patients in a PVS have usually been the victims of severe head injury or anoxic insults to the brain – lack of oxygen wrecks the cerebral hemispheres before it destroys the brainstem. Such patients may be found in institutions for the chronically sick all over the world. In cases where recovery from the PVS is considered to be impossible, several health authorities now sanction the withdrawal of nutrition and hydration so that the patient may die. It is important, both scientifically and ethically, to avoid confusing brain death with such non-cognitive states. The expression 'locked in syndrome' refers to a condition where the level and content of consciousness is fairly normal but the patient is paralysed and unable to speak (Levy, Sidtis & Rottenberg, 1987). This should not be confused with the PVS as clinical tests reveal purposeful eye movements and confirmatory Positron Emission Tomography (PET) scans reveal near normal levels of cerebral metabolism. The expressions 'cerebral death' and 'neocortical death' are best avoided as they have been used ambiguously by philosophers to refer to both whole brain death and the PVS. For neurologists 'neocortical death' refers to PVS patients with an isoelectric EEG, but philosophers have used it in a loose

way to refer to permanently unconscious patients, the PVS and brain death, thus attributing levels of certainty to electrical readings from the scalp that few, if any, physicians in the world would regard as valid indicators of life or death.

When physicians communicate with the media the capacity for misunderstanding is further emphasized. Expressions like 'he is brain-dead, but we have just performed successful cardiopulmonary resuscitation' or 'the brain dead patient has been put on a course of antibiotics', are suggestive that a patient (as opposed to the parts of a corpse) is being cared for. Remarks to the effect that a patient is brain dead and being maintained on a 'life support machine', which one 'chooses' to 'turn off' is probably the most common source of confusion. Further confusion is manifest when the brain dead are referred to as 'living cadavers' because of the extension of artificial nutrition and mechanical support.

A significant source of confusion, and hence public concern regarding the concept of brain death, can be traced to early attempts to reconcile brain death with the traditional cardio-respiratory concept. During the 1970s and 1980s, there were attempts to legitimize brain death on the grounds that a diagnosis of the irreversible loss of integrated brain function meant cardiac arrest was inevitable. But this merely describes a sequence of events and cannot be construed as an argument supporting the claim that brain death is death. It gave the impression that brain death was merely a prognosis that death (portrayed as irreversible loss of cardiac function) was imminent. Irreversibly dying is not actual death. This line of thought led to arguments concerning the length of time irreversible cardiac arrest could be artificially delayed after a diagnosis of brain death, as if the extent of the delay somehow inflicted damage on the credibility of brain related criteria for death.

During the 1970s, the normal maximum delay between the diagnosis of brain death and cardiac arrest in a ventilated cadaver was believed to be a few hours or at most a few days. But techniques for the management of brain dead cadavers improved, and when a middle aged man was reported to have been resuscitated for 68 days after brain death was diagnosed (Parisi et al., 1982) it generated criticism of the accuracy of brain death. Other similar reports followed. The source of scepticism generated by these reports lay in the fact that many arguments in support of brain-related criteria for death appealed to the inevitability of almost immediate cessation of cardiac activity despite attempts at aggressive management of the brain dead. The reason for this appeal lay in the deep-rooted desire to demonstrate that brain death is equivalent to traditional cardio-respiratory definitions of death. In fact, the entire discussion of the time lag between brain death and irreversible cardiac arrest was a non-issue: what had to be realized is that the accuracy of the diagnosis of brain death is independent of predictions concerning the survival of artificially supported cardio-respiratory activity.

This point was made by Pallis (1990) who insisted that the concept of brainstem death should be addressed with regard to its own philosophical merits. As Pallis (1990, pp. 12–13) pointed out, with new drugs the 'heart of the brain dead can be kept going much longer than was originally thought', and that 'with the artificial heart on the horizon it will soon no longer be possible to argue that brainstem death is death "because of its hopeless cardiac prognosis". The real philosophical issue will then have to be confronted, namely that brainstem death is death in its own right (death being defined as the "irreversible loss of the capacity for consciousness combined with the irreversible loss of the capacity to breathe spontaneously, and hence maintain a spontaneous heartbeat").' Pallis insisted that brainstem death was death in its own right and that arguments about its accuracy are independent of any predictions regarding cardio-respiratory function. The maintenance of organs within a body following brain death is dependent upon the level of technology available. There never was any need to support brain-related criteria with appeals to the inevitable cessation of cardiac activity.

PUBLIC ANXIETY CONCERNING BRAIN-RELATED CONCEPTS OF DEATH

Although the medical profession has generally accepted brain-related criteria for death, this move has encountered a degree of public anxiety, despite the undeniable fact that the record for reliable brain death diagnosis is far more reassuring than diagnosis based on cardiovascular criteria. Doubts are frequently raised concerning the link between criteria for brain death and the need for transplantable cadaver organs but there are ethical and philosophical arguments which are supportive of a separation principle whereby the interests of the dying patient are distinct from the interests of the transplant team and the potential recipient (Lamb, 2003).

The main objections to brain-related criteria for death are found in various cultural beliefs concerning the understanding of death. In an examination of objections raised in Denmark and Japan, Paul Gill (2000, p. 219) notes that for several cultures: 'different interpretations of personhood are usually important reasons for objecting to brain death as a single entity signifying death'. In this context, he cites the Japanese concept of a mutual connection between body and spirit, which is not to be understood in terms of the relationship between the body and the rational brain as it is in the West. There are cultural reasons for anxiety in the Japanese community over both brain death and organ transplants. In traditional Japanese thought, it is the belly or gut which

symbolically represents the major organ. Hence the Samurai warrior commits hara-kiri by plunging the sword into his belly, not his heart or brain. Just as Europeans speak of the heart as the seat of emotions and virtue, thus reinforcing the attractiveness of cardio-centric definitions of death, Japanese refer to the gut: hence, being 'good and honest' is having a 'clean gut'. While the English have a 'heart to heart' talk, the Japanese refer to 'opening one's gut'. To say one thing and mean something else can be expressed as 'the gut and the mouth speaking differently'. This does not mean that Japanese doctors and nurses believe that the gut is actually the major organ, but such symbolic beliefs stand as a barrier to the acceptance of a brain-related concept of death and the removal of organs after brainstem death. The acceptance of brain-related criteria in Japan has been very gradual, with legislation being finally endorsed in 1997, although public unease with brain-related criteria persists.

As Gill (2000) points out, opposition to brain-related criteria for death on cultural grounds may appear naive and unsophisticated, yet it does not mean that these views are without foundation. The social and cultural issues are as important as the physiological. Belief that brain death is at variance with cultural beliefs and traditions is said to underpin reluctance to accept brain-related concepts throughout the 1990s (Gill, 2000). It follows that an acceptable medical definition should be compatible with mainstream cultural and religious beliefs. The following guidelines for a definition of brain death specify both medical and cultural requirements.

A DEFINITION MUST REFER TO A RECOGNIZABLE AND IRREVERSIBLE PHYSICAL TRANSFORMATION

Any valid medical concept of death must be linked to an irreversible physical change in the status of the individual which can be clearly and unambiguously determined by empirical means. It follows that if a patient, declared dead, were to recover, it should not be said that he or she was dead but is now alive again, but rather that he or she was alive all the time but mistakenly diagnosed as dead. It is, however, important to stress that although irreversibility is essential to any medical concept of death, the fact that patients have not recovered from a certain state is not sufficient to uphold the conclusion that this state is death. Additional proof is required to support the diagnosis. It is therefore important to stress the distinction between a 'failure to recover' and 'already dead'.

A DEFINITION OF DEATH MUST BE SELECTIVE

In practice, and throughout history, doctors have not sought to diagnose the death of the whole organism; they have sought to identify a stage in the ongoing course of events when the individual organism no longer functions as an integrated whole. It has long been recognized that residual functions may persist after death, that muscles may respond to percussion for several hours, and that tissues such as skin, bone or arterial wall, may remain viable for transplantation purposes for a day or more. Newly developing techniques involving the management of corpses are being established that can maintain the viability of certain organs postmortem for almost indefinite periods. Random electrical activity may persist after death; spinal reflexes may persist beyond the death of a brain, and in fact do so when cardiac activity can no longer be demonstrated.

It is therefore essential, when considering concepts of death, that a sharp distinction is maintained between (a) death of the whole organism (total destruction of every cell) and (b) death of the organism as a whole (irreversible loss of integrated functioning), which is sought in the implementation of criteria for brain death. The former has never operated in practice. Failure to appreciate this distinction largely explains public unease with brain-related criteria for death in Germany during the 1990s (Hogle, 1999) and the panic unleashed in the British media when it was announced that brain dead preparations were being anaesthetized to overcome residual spinal reflexes prior to organ removal (Allison, 2000).

A DEFINITION MUST BE UNIVERSAL AND HOLISTIC

The requirement for universality implies that criteria must be unambiguous and the results of tests repeatable. It also implies that the mechanism of death be the same for all people whether in the backwoods or in the most sophisticated intensive care unit of a university hospital. The requirement for a holistic definition is recognition of cultural beliefs regarding the significance of both mental and physical attributes of the dying person. A definition of death which disregards continuous mental functioning is morally unacceptable; the same applies to a concept of death which disregards essential physical functions such as spontaneous respiration – although some proposed formulations of the definition of death (Gervais, 1987; Puccetti, 1988; Veatch, 2000) have questioned the significance of this function. A holistic definition, in keeping with most theological and secular beliefs, should recognize that among the important features of life are integration and organization (Lamb, 1988, 1996, 2000, 2001).Thus death is not strictly equated with the loss of the vital functions of one or more organs, but with the loss of the capacity to organize and integrate vital functions. In

practice tests for the death of the brainstem have never been conducted to ascertain the viability of a particular organ, equivalent to a liver or kidney; they are designed to ascertain whether the sub-systems which constitute the organism as a whole are capable of integrated functioning. The claim that elimination of certain functions – for example, those of the skin, liver, heart and kidneys – may lead to death is not the same as saying that the loss of these functions is death. An individual undergoing dialysis is not dead, although she may well die if she forgoes dialysis. But she will then die – directly or indirectly – of the cerebral consequences of renal failure. The functioning of the organism as a whole will have been irreversibly compromised.

CONCLUSION

It is essential to seek precision regarding the determination of death, as it marks a significant transition from duties we owe to the living and obligations to the dead. In the context of escalating health care costs, it is inevitable that there will be proposals to limit heroic and expensive methods of prolonging life. Persistent failure to present a clear-cut boundary between life and death may lend support to proposals for the termination of treatment according to cost – benefit criteria or on other extraneous grounds. But if the doctor is not to be seen as executioner, criteria for the pronouncement of death and the termination of treatment must be based on a clearly defined, widely publicised, culturally and philosophically acceptable, and practically meaningful concept of death, not on a prognosis that death is imminent or on an estimate that residual life would be worthless.

REFERENCES

Allison R. Brain death debate may deter organ donors. *The Guardian* 21 August, 2000.

Arnold JD, Zimmerman TF, Martin DC. Public attitudes and the diagnosis of death. *JAMA* 1968; **9**: 1949–54.

Black PMcl. Brain death. *N Engl J Med* 1978; **299**: 338–44; 393–401.

Gervais KG. *Redefining Death*. New Haven: Yale University Press, 1987.

Gill P. Brainstem death—an anthropological perspective. *Care Critic Ill* 2000; **6**: 217–20.

Harvard Medical School. A definition of irreversible coma. *JAMA* 1968; **205**(6): 85–8.

Hogle LF. *Recovering the Nation's Body*. New Brunswick: Rutgers University Press, 1999.

Lamb D. *Il Confine Della Vita: Morte Cerebrale ed Etica Dei Trapianti*. Il Mulino: Bologna, 1987.

Lamb D. Brain death and brainstem death: philosophical and ethical considerations. In: Evans JDG, ed. *Royal Institute of*

Philosophy Series. Cambridge: Cambridge University Press, 1988; pp. 231–49.

Lamb D. *Etica E Trapianto Degli Organi*. Bologna: Il Mulino, 1995.

Lamb D. *Death, Brain Death and Ethics*. Aldershot: Ashgate, 1996.

Lamb D. *Transplante de Órgãos Ética*. São Paulo: Editora Hucitec, 2000.

Lamb D. *Ética, Morte E Morte Encefálica*. São Paulo: Office Editora e Publicidade Ltda, 2001.

Lamb D. Brain death and the cadaver organ donor. In: Draper H, Scott W, eds. *Ethics in Anaesthesia and Intensive Care*. London: Elsevier Ltd, 2003; pp. 192–204.

Levy DE, Sidtis JJ, Rottenberg A. Differences in cerebral blood-flow and glucose utilization in vegetative versus locked-in patients. *Annals Neurol* 1987; **22**(6): 673–82.

Mollaret P, Goulon M. *Le coma depassé, Revue Neurologie* 1959; **101**: 3–15.

Pallis C. Return to Ellsinore. *J Med Ethics* 1990; **16**(1): 10–13.

Parisi JE, Kim RC, Collins GH, Hillinger MF. Brain death with prolonged somatic survival. *N Engl J Med* 1982; **306**: 14–6.

Puccetti R. Does anyone survive neocortical death? In: Zaner RM, ed. *Death: Beyond Whole Brain Criteria*. Dordrecht: Kluwer, 1988; pp. 75–90.

Veatch RM. *Transplantation Ethics*. Washington: Georgetown University Press, 2000.

Woodhouse M. Philosophy and frontier science: is there a new paradigm in the making? In: Lamb D, ed. *New Horizons in the Philosophy of Science*. Aldershot: Avebury, 1992; pp. 26–48.

69

Ethics without Boundaries: Medical Tourism

GUIDO PENNINGS

INTRODUCTION

Medical tourism indicates movements by persons from one country to another to obtain health care services. The term was originally used for people who went on vacation to exotic places to take advantage of healing or health beneficial natural resources like health spas, vacations at the sea shore or in the mountains and so on. The term has been extended to indicate people going abroad for health care services. The recreational aspect may still play a role but need no longer be present. In recent years, more and more people are willing to travel in search of the medical treatment they need but cannot get at home. The main reasons why people look for medical services abroad are that such care is not available at home for instance because of lack of expertise, the treatment is not covered by their health insurance and consequently too expensive, the service is available at a much lower cost elsewhere and the waiting lists are too long. The availability of information on the internet about the services offered by any clinic around the world and the increased democratization of airplane travelling contribute to the phenomenon. In the meantime, medical tourism became a multi-billion dollar industry. Some countries are actively attracting foreign patients by offering them package deals that include flights, transfers, hotels, personal assistance and translation, visas, treatment and post-operative vacation.

HEALTH CARE AS A PUBLIC SERVICE

The evolution is not carried solely by individuals looking for a solution. The European Court of Justice ruling in Decker and Kohll has made mainstream health services subject to two principles on which the European Union was founded: the freedom of movement of goods and the freedom of movement of services. Health care is now deemed to be tradable (Hermans, 2000). The Commission of the European Communities proposes to simplify the existing rule on the coordination of social security systems and the procedures of a European health insurance to facilitate patient mobility (Commission of the European Communities, 2004). Globally, the General Agreement on Trade in Services (GATS) negotiations try to liberalize all services. Consumption in other countries (the medical tourism considered in this chapter) is one of the four modes of trade in health services besides movements of the personnel providing services, foreign direct investment in health care and health insurance and direct cross-border trade (telemedicine). The key concern about the GATS is that it will lead to the privatization of essential public services like health care, education and drinking water (Labonte, 2004). The changing balance between the public and the private sector may endanger equity and access to services by the most needy groups in society (UNCTAD, 1998). The second objection concerns the specific status of certain services. Many people believe that health is a special good. One of the most popular views is that health care is special because disease and disability affect a person's range of opportunities. Health care in all its forms aims to keep people functioning as close to normal as possible (Daniels, 1998). There is discrimination when some people, for instance because of the inability to pay, are denied access to the basic tier of services needed to protect normal functioning. The proponents of this view argue that the medically necessary services should be covered and controlled by public health care systems. Elective interventions or technologies not directed at pathological conditions are excluded from the right to health care.

Access to high quality health care is considered a fundamental right. As a consequence, it is one of the basic tasks of the government to guarantee this right. Social security

Principles of Health Care Ethics, Second Edition   Edited by R.E. Ashcroft, A. Dawson, H. Draper and J.R. McMillan
© 2007 John Wiley & Sons, Ltd

systems are based on solidarity, collective responsibility and equal contributions in order to ensure accessibility of high quality care for all. Universal access also implies that health care should be provided on the basis of need rather than on the ability to pay. The increasing commercialization may clash with this fundamental principle. Therefore, the government should have extensive regulatory powers to redress market imperfections and to prevent discrimination on the basis of income. Two elements are responsible for the specific status of the health care market and explain why the provision of these services cannot be completely left open to free competition (Baeten, 2004). The first is the involvement of the 'third party' (the public financier) who pays the major part of the bill. Because of this, price mechanisms, based on the relationship of supply and demand, cannot function properly. The second is the information asymmetry between patient (consumer) and physician (provider). Patients lack the necessary knowledge to make an informed decision about the care they need. This makes it impossible to achieve an efficient market in health care. Both elements make overconsumption at the expense of society, mainly due to provider-induced demand, more than likely. Given the restricted budget for health care and rising costs because of ageing populations, the public health care providers should be able to control their expenditure by controlling prices and number of services and by encouraging the most effective use of funds.

CONDITIONS FOR ACCEPTABLE CROSS-BORDER HEALTH CARE

One question is whether the state has a duty to enable all citizens to obtain a decent level of health care or whether it has a duty to organize a health care system which can provide decent health care to all citizens at home. The former would very well be compatible with cross-border care if a number of measures are taken. One such measure which could have a huge impact is the portability of health care insurance. This means that the costs of the intervention abroad would be covered by the health insurance of the person's home country. However, the whole undertaking of medical travelling may also constitute a high non-financial barrier for some. Poorly educated people, who are not used to travelling and who only speak their mother tongue, will find travelling for medical reasons very burdensome. The duty of the state is not only to enable people to have treatment but to enable people to have treatment reasonably close to their home. This is not only a matter of comfort but also of quality. Quality of health care not only concerns the success rate of the intervention but also counselling, psychological support and follow-up. As long as it concerns elective medical services, these

elements may be negligible. For serious health problems, however, psychological support and security become increasingly important. These aspects depend on fluent communication with the staff which may be hampered by language problems and cultural differences. A clear indication of the importance of these aspects can be found in the fact that about half of the Canadian cancer patients who were offered treatment in the United States refused to go even though the treatment was paid for by their health insurance (Vellinga, 2001).

One conclusion implied by the government's duty to guarantee health care is that cross-border health care should be exceptional and cannot be the solution for a structural deficit of the health care system. Medical tourism can be seen as a symptom signalling the flaws of the system. When for instance lower income patients have to travel to obtain the treatment they cannot afford at home, the state fails in fulfilling its duty. One can see this trend increasing in countries like the United States with a limited public health insurance or in states where large parts of the population are simply uninsured. Not surprisingly, the sometimes enormous difference in cost between home and host country for the same surgical intervention or treatment is the main argument in the marketing strategy of the providing countries.

When long waiting lists for several treatments persist or when patients move on a large scale, vigorous measures need to be taken to remedy the problem. Sending patients to another country does not have to be problematic when it is a solution for a temporary shortage or when it concerns very specialized services. Some Canadian provinces have made temporary arrangements with nearby facilities in the United States to meet pressing health care needs of cancer patients (Vellinga, 2001). Cooperation across borders may enable better use of resources, sharing of potential spare capacity and improving access of patients to quality care. For tackling rare diseases or conditions requiring specialized care, expertise and practice could be concentrated in a limited number of clinics. European centres of excellence for such diseases would be justified by higher efficiency and quality of care. For these instances of cross-border health care, portability of health care insurance could easily be organized.

BENEFITS OF MEDICAL TOURISM FOR THE PROVIDING COUNTRY

The most important motive for developing countries to export health services by attracting foreign patients is generation of foreign exchange. These additional resources may be invested in public health care. It could lead to an upgrading of the health care infrastructure and technologies. It could also provide health professionals with advanced training and could introduce new and more efficient management techniques. However, all these advantages, even if realized, will not benefit the global population. The National Human Development Report 2001 in India stated that 'technological advances, though, widen the spectrum of possible interventions but are well beyond the financial reach of majority' (Planning Commission, 2002). In other words, there is a widening gap between what can be done and what can be afforded. Because the money put into treating foreign patients is an economic investment, motivated by profit, the only way this newly created system will spread out to the general population is by regulatory measures of the government. This cannot be left to the charity of the clinics. Moreover, it is not enough to have a law. Private hospitals in India have an obligation under the Public Trust Act to provide free health care to the extent of 20% of their resources, but no one checks whether they do so (Chinai & Goswani, 2005).

The medical tourism industry should not be blamed for all the deficits of the health care systems of the developing countries. The inequity, lack of access, low quality and so on existed before this development and are largely due to internal factors. India, Thailand and other countries actively promoting health tourism are spending approximately 1% of their gross national product on public health care. This is unlikely to change even if no corporate hospitals are started in the country. It could even be argued that the medical tourism industry at least offers the possibility, however small, of making a change for the good. The absolute minimum, however, is that everything is done to prevent the situation from aggravating for the local population.

DISADVANTAGES AND RISKS OF MEDICAL TOURISM

There is the possibility that the development of a separate health care system catering to foreign nationals stimulates or reinforces a dual system in which there is a high quality private segment for rich nationals and foreigners and a low quality public segment providing treatment to the poor masses. 'In Mumbai, as in New Delhi, Chennai and Hyderabad, private sector health care centres are gleaming "islands of excellence" as the industry calls them, all too often surrounded by seas of medical neglect' (Chinai & Goswami, 2005). The National Human Development Report 2001 from India diagnosed that there is 'a misplaced emphasis on development and maintenance of private health care services at the expense of a broadening and deepening of public health care system targeted, essentially, at controlling the incidence of communicable diseases in rural areas' (Planning Commission, 2002). In itself, a dual system does not have to be a problem. In fact, most countries

(both developed and developing) have a mixed system. Still, a supplementary tier would be problematic if its existence would undermine the basic tier either economically or politically (Daniels et al., 2000). An additional ethical problem is generated by the fact that the public health system does not cover the basic needs of all citizens. Because this is a fundamental right of every person, all efforts should be directed at reaching this goal instead of developing a higher level of health care for the more prosperous groups. According to Rawls (1971) fairness implies minimizing inequalities in the distribution of primary goods. An unequal distribution can only be justified if it benefits those who are worst off more than the others (the maximin principle). This can be seen as the most basic challenge to medical tourism: how to make sure that trade in health services not only benefits the local population in developing countries but also effectively improves the quality and equity of the health care for them.

A second danger is that, mainly due to constraints on resources and personnel, the local population is crowded out (Chanda, 2002). Investment in hospitals catering to foreign patients in developing countries would only be appropriate if the host country has a sufficient number of physicians per capita. Otherwise poor local people will suffer as physicians will be drawn to affluent patients (Gonzales et al., 2001). Another predicted evolution is 'cream-skimming' whereby foreign investors serve those who are able to pay and thus leave the public sector to those who cannot pay (UN, 1997).

The third risk is that the services provided to foreign patients overemphasize acute therapeutic services as opposed to preventive and public health measures, preventive medicine, vaccinations and so on. In terms of efficacy, much more might be obtained by spending money on public health measures. The services for foreign patients will be focused on very high-tech interventions for which the costs are completely out of proportion and do not address broader social needs. Although expensive high-technological interventions can be accepted when the basic health care needs are met, the same interventions are difficult to justify in a country where this is not the case.

The final danger is the brain drain. Developing countries have been wrestling with the outmigration of trained health service workers for many years. The availability of an adequate number of health personnel is indispensable for good public health care. Countries like Canada, the United States and the United Kingdom have been actively recruiting nurses and physicians from developing countries like the Philippines and Southern Africa. In fact, this phenomenon, also called the 'global health conveyor belt', occurs on the basis of several characteristics (Schrecker & Labonte, 2004). Personnel moves from poor to rich, from rural to urban, from public to private sector and from developing to developed country. The movements are not limited to developing countries. Bauer mentions the shortage of physicians in rural areas in the United States as a problem for distributive justice (Bauer, 2003). However, in developing countries, several movements come together: professionals will move both from the public health care segment to the private sector and from their own country to richer countries, thus causing a real exodus from the public health sector. It is unacceptable that developed countries recruit health care personnel from poor countries (Commission on the Future of Health Care in Canada, 2002). They should invest more in their own educational programmes for health care professionals. This increased capacity would also decrease cross-border travelling for health care services. The recruitment of foreign professionals is especially condemnable when some of the qualified professionals from developed countries are engaged in non-basic health care. In the United States, for instance, 4.6 million cosmetic procedures are executed per year (Castle et al., 2002). This industry has an impact on the availability of general health care, even when these services are paid for by private funds. If these people would switch to basic public health, there would probably be a sufficient number to handle this care for everyone. The same reasoning would apply to catering for foreign patients. So, one solution for the brain drain would be to discourage the waste of health care capacity in elective interventions.

HOW TO PREVENT THE EXISTING SYSTEM FROM DETERIORATING?

The main weapons to prevent the existing health care system from deteriorating are regulation and control. The local government should prevent the already very meagre flow of resources to the public health system from being diverted to the private hospitals. Due to extensive lobbying, this is already happening in some countries. Clinics, like any other type of business, try to obtain favourable conditions for investment. An investor-friendly climate can be provided by tax cuts, subsidies, concessional utilities and preferential land allotments (Chinai & Goswani, 2005). This form of cross-subsidizing will inevitably have adverse effects on the public sector. Moreover, the treatment of foreign patients is considered an export and thus deemed eligible for all fiscal incentives extended to export earnings. Secondly, not only the direct costs (who pays for the service) but also the indirect costs (who pays for the steps that make the service possible) should be taken into account. At present, education of different professionals is organized by the state in order to have qualified persons to perform the essential tasks of society. These tasks include provision and organization of health care, housing, education, public transport and so on. In states with a heavily subsidized

educational system, every profession has a social role to fulfil. It is a loss to society if a physician or a nurse whose education was largely paid for by the community leaves the country, works for foreign patients or invests most of his or her time in medical activities outside the public health care system. He or she profits from a service provided by society (because he or she uses skills acquired during training) without reciprocating by alleviating the needs of that society. This loss in health care capacity for society should be compensated. An obvious solution is a special tax on the services that are beyond socially recognized health care (like cosmetic procedures) or services provided to foreign nationals. This is similar to a migration tax by which emigrating professionals reimburse the government for training costs (Chanda, 2002). Such taxation on foreign systems could be used to create equity in access to services for local people (Janjaroen and Supakankunti, 2002). Other measures can be imagined. The government could demand that a physician and/or nurse works for a limited period (say 2 or 3 years) in a specific sector. Greek doctors, for instance, have to work for 1 year in a small village before they are allowed to practise in town. Others countries require a mandatory period of service in the home country. This solution has been applied for decades in the military. Physicians who received substantial or full funding for their studies and training must serve for a number of years (depending on the extent of the funding and the specialty) in the military. A similar obligatory service period could be demanded from all doctors graduating from publicly funded medical schools. Although these measures focus on the medical personnel, another way to approach the problem is by counting on the receiving state to reimburse for the services. Rich countries attracting physicians and nurses from developing countries should pay an amount to that country to compensate for the loss.

BENCHMARKS OF FAIRNESS

It is an understatement to say that it is difficult to decide whether a development like medical tourism has on balance an overall positive or negative effect. A large number of factors should be taken into account: the general level of development of the providing country, the kind of health service (elective, cosmetic, urgent) for which persons travel, the reasons for which people travel, the mode of financing the system (public or private), the extent of health insurance, the capacity of the health system of the host country and so on. There is far too little research done on the impact of international trade in health services to assess who wins or loses and under which set of conditions or regulations. The complexity of the ethical evaluation is also enormous not only for the calculation but also for the prediction of the consequences. Because the impact of a new system of health care for foreign patients is mediated by the specific characteristics of the country, the appreciation will be highly case-specific. Cuba's effort to attract foreign patients differs completely from the same effort by India because Cuba has a full coverage health insurance system and an overcapacity in health care.

One interesting tool for assessing health system reforms is proposed by Daniels and colleagues: the benchmarks of fairness (Daniels et al. 2000). This proposal is an extension of the set of three criteria used by the WHO to evaluate public health: equity in access to care, quality of care and efficient use of resources. In the benchmarks' proposal, fairness is a concept containing nine criteria: exposure to risk factors, financial barriers to equitable access to health care, non-financial barriers to access the comprehensiveness of benefits and tiering, equitable financing, efficacy, efficiency, quality of care, democratic accountability and finally patient and provider autonomy. These benchmarks can best be explained by referring to the questions they address: does the reform reduce barriers to access public health services? Does it provide services appropriate to the need of the population? Does the system promote efficiency? Does it make institutions publicly accountable for their decisions (Daniels et al., 2000)? This tool should enable a systematic evaluation of the impact of health care reforms (like the introduction of a system of cross-border health services) on the fairness of the resulting health care system. However, although each benchmark contains various criteria for evaluating specific aspects of fairness, it remains fairly general. Moreover, the evaluation should be made both in the home country of the patients and in the host country, and the reform could get different marks in the two countries. For example, the autonomy of the travelling patient may increase whereas that of the patients in the host country diminishes due to financial barriers. I believe there are strong indications that an unrestricted and purely market-regulated introduction of hospitals catering to foreign patients will negatively affect the fairness of the health care system of developing countries.

REPRODUCTIVE TOURISM, PERSONAL AUTONOMY AND LAW EVASION

One category of cross-border travelling for medical services should be distinguished from the others, namely travelling for reproductive services. The oldest service for which women crossed borders is abortion. Even at this moment, thousands of women from all over Europe are having an abortion in The Netherlands (Inspectie voor de Gezondheidszorg, 2002). More recently, there has been a huge increase of movements for the new reproductive technologies (Pennings, 2002). A number of reasons for travelling are overlapping with general medical tourism,

such as unavailability of services due to lack of expertise (for instance preimplantation genetic diagnosis), long waiting lists and strong cost reduction. However, reproductive tourism is also motivated by some specific reasons. The first reason is when a type of treatment is forbidden by law because the application is considered morally unacceptable. In Italy and Germany, for instance, no oocyte donation is allowed. Sex selection for social reasons is banned in almost all European countries. A second reason is when a technique is not considered sufficiently safe in one's home country. Especially in the starting phase of a new technique, the views may differ. Oocyte freezing, intracytoplasmic sperm injection with non-ejaculated sperm and ooplasma transfer are some examples. A final and fairly large group of travellers are categories of patients who are not eligible for assisted reproduction in their home country. This applies to single women, lesbian couples and postmenopausal women. Probably due to the element of law evasion, reproductive tourism has an overall negative connotation. Reproductive tourists are seen as disloyal to the regulation in their country; they shop for the legal or moral system that allows them to realize their plans (Millns, 2002). The phenomenon raises some difficult ethical questions like the following: has a person a moral obligation to obey the laws of his or her country, and to what extent has a government the right to regulate individuals' private lives by restricting ways of procreation?

In a modern society, different groups hold different positions on a number of ethical issues. Although the majority has the political right to impose rules that correspond to their view on the good life, this right should be balanced against important ethical values. Among these values, we count tolerance, autonomy and respect for others' opinion. Once this position is adopted, cross-border reproductive health care can be seen as a solution rather than a problem. The real problem which causes the movements, is the restrictive legislation that ignores the moral views of minority groups (Pennings, 2002). One of the clearest examples is Italy. This country adopted the most restrictive law on assisted reproduction in Europe and one year later patients (and fertility specialists) started leaving the country in their thousands (Fornasiero, 2005).

CONCLUSIONS

Medical tourism is a highly complex phenomenon. The moral evaluation depends on a large number of factors. When states guarantee equitable access of all citizens to a decent level of health care services, there will be little need for travelling. The movements that fall outside the level of basic care do not raise specific justice issues in the home country. The main problem at the moment is that citizens from developed countries are travelling to developing countries for interventions not covered by health insurance and for elective procedures. This equals export of medical services for the developing countries although they are already unable to meet basic health care needs of their own population. All efforts should be directed at preventing these movements from adversely affecting the current public health system in poor countries. In order to do this, the government must have adequate legal instruments to regulate the development.

REFERENCES

Baeten R. The proposal for a directive on services in the internal market applied to health care. Paper prepared for the public hearing in the European Parliament, 11 November 2004; http://www.ose.be

Bauer K. Distributive justice and rural healthcare: a case for e-health. *Int J Appl Philos* 2003; **17**: 241–52.

Castle DJ, Honigman RJ, Phillips KA. Does cosmetic surgery improve psychosocial well being? *Med J Austr* 2002; **176**: 601–4.

Chanda R. Trade in health services. *Bull World Health Organ* 2002; **80**: 158–63.

Chinai R, Goswani R. Are we ready for medical tourism? *The Hindu*, 17/04/2005; http://www.thehindu.com/thehindu/mag/2005/04/17/stories/2005041700060100.htm.

Commission of the European Communities. Follow-up to the high level reflection process on patient mobility and healthcare developments in the European Union. Brussels: Commission of the European Communities, 2004.

Commission on the Future of Health Care in Canada. *Globalization and Canada's Healthcare System*. Policy dialogue no. 11, 2002; http://www.hc-sc.gc.ca/english/pdf/romanow/pdfs/Dialogue_11_Globalization_E.pdf.

Daniels N, Bryant J, Castano RA, Dantes OG, Khan KS, Pannarunothai S. Benchmarks of fairness for health care reform: a policy tool for developing countries. *Bull World Health Organ* 2000; **78**: 740–50.

Daniels N. Is there a right to health care and, if so, what does it encompass? In: Kuhse H, Singer P, eds. *A Companion to Bioethics*. Oxford: Blackwell, 1998; pp. 41–8.

Fornasiero C. Turismo procreativo: fotografia di una realtà. In: CECOS Italy ed. *Conferenza stampa. Turismo procreativo:*

fotografia di una realtà. Rome, May 25 2005; http://www.cecos.it/conferenze/cf_250505.pdf.

Gonzales A, Brenzel L, Sancho J. Health tourism and related services: Caribbean development and international trade. Final report submitted to the Regional Negotiating Machinery (RNM), 2001 http://www.crnm.org/documents/studies/RNM%20Health%20Study%20Final.pdf.

Hermans HEGM. Cross-border health care in the European Union: recent legal implications of Decker and Kohll. *J Eval Clin Pract* 2000; **6**: 431–9.

Inspectie voor de Gezondheidszorg. Jaarrapportage 2002 van de Wet Afbreking Zwangerschap. Den Haag: Inspectie voor de Gezondheidszorg, 2003.

Janjaroen WS, Supakankunti S. International trade in health services in the millenium: the case of Thailand. In: World Health Organization, ed. *Trade in Health Services*, 2002; pp. 87–106.

Labonte R. Globalization, health, and the free trade regime: assessing the links. *Perspect Global Dev Technol* 2004; **3**: 47–72.

Millns S. Reproducing inequalities: assisted conception and the challenge of legal pluralism. *J Soc Welfare Family Law* 2002; **24**: 19–36.

Pennings G. Reproductive tourism as moral pluralism in motion. *J Med Ethics* 2002; **28**: 337–41.

Planning Commission. *National Human Development Report 2001.* Government of India, 2002.

Rawls J. *A Theory of Justice.* Cambridge, Massachusetts: Belknap Press of Harvard University Press, 1971.

Schrecker T, Labonte R. Taming the brain drain: a challenge for public health systems in Southern Africa. *Int J Occup Environ Health* 2004; **10**: 409–15.

UNCTAD Secretariat. International trade in health services: difficulties and opportunities for developing countries. In: UNCTAD-WHO, eds. *International Trade in Health Services: A Developmental Perspective.* Geneva: UNCTAD, 1998; pp. 3–28; http://www.ictsd.org/issarea/services/resources/Docs/WHO-UNCTAD1.pdf.

United Nations. United Nations Conference on Trade and Development. Report of the Expert Meeting on Strengthening the Capacity and Extending Exports of Developing Countries in the Services Sector: Health Services. Geneva: Trade and Development Board, 17–21 November 1997.

Vellinga J. International trade, health systems and services: a health policy perspective. In: Department of Foreign Affairs and International Trade Canada, ed. *Trade Policy Research 2001*, 2001; pp. 137–87; http://www.dfait-maeci.gc.ca/eet/pdf/07-en.pdf.

70

Ethics of Performance Enhancement in Sport: Drugs and Gene Doping

BENNETT FODDY, JULIAN SAVULESCU

Dick Pound is the head of the World Anti-Doping Agency, WADA. In an interview with CBC Sports Online (2003), he was asked, 'What drives you in the fight against drugs in sports? Why do you feel this is such an important issue?' His reply reveals much about the motivation of the anti-doping campaigners:

> Well, sports is so important to so many people, particularly young people, and it's a precursor to how you're going to behave in other aspects of social intercourse…[I]t's very important to have some kind of activity where you can say to people 'this is on the level'. You respect the rules, you respect your opponents, you respect yourself. You play fair.

> I don't want my grandchildren to have to become chemical stockpiles in order to be good at sports and to have fun at it…It's a completely antithetical view to what sport should have been in the first place. It's essentially a humanistic endeavour to see how far you can go on your own talent.

Current dogma is that performance enhancement in sport is wrong. As Pound's response shows, this dogma is predicated mainly on the view that performance enhancement violates this 'humanistic' conception of what sport should be.

In this chapter, we will argue that performance enhancement is inevitable and unpoliceable, that it is not against the spirit of sport and that we should remove anti-doping legislation to permit safe performance enhancement. We should focus more on testing athletes' health and fitness to compete.

CURRENT GUIDELINES AND POLICY ON DOPING IN SPORT

Whatever we think that sport should or should not be, there is one good reason why the world's sporting bodies are undertaking such a concerted effort to eliminate doping in elite sport. There is one good reason why there are no 'pro doping' movements and no legal challenges to the laws against doping in sport. The reason is simply this: doping is currently the most widespread method of cheating. Professional athletes are cheating, and worse, they are using methods which quite often put their health at risk, as Table 70.1 illustrates.

These health risks give us good reasons to ban performance enhancing drugs. But not all the harmful drugs are banned, and a number of banned drugs do not threaten athletes' health. Is it possible that the sporting bodies are not worried, or not at least primarily worried, about health?

The World Anti-Doping Agency, which defines which drugs will be banned in international athletics, bans a drug if it has at least two out of three of the following criteria. First, it must have the potential to increase sporting performance. Second, it must represent an actual or potential risk to the athlete's health, and third, its use must be contrary to the 'spirit of sport', which they define in the same document (World Anti-Doping Agency, 2003b).

According to the Anti-Doping Agency's definition, you are not doping if you are taking harmful drugs which do not enhance performance or violate the spirit of sport, such as tobacco (see Table 70.2). And you are not doping if you take performance-enhancing drugs which do not harm you or violate the spirit of sport. Under the current code, for example, caffeine is not illegal, even though it can strongly increase performance. In endurance sports, caffeine helps to mobilize the fat stores of an athlete (Costill, Dalsky & Fink, 1978). It can make as much as a 20% difference in the time to exhaustion among competitive athletes. That is a massive difference. Dietary supplements such as creatine are also legal on this 2-out-of-3 rule, and they also strongly

Table 70.1. Performance enhancers. Examples of prohibited performance enhancers for which athletes have been banned

Name	Effect	Unwanted effects
Anabolic androgenic steroids	Increased muscle growth; increased red blood cell production	Decrease in endogenous sex hormones; acne; temporary infertility; rarely, increased aggression; ventricular hypertrophy; liver damage; virilization in females; testicular atrophy and gynecomastia in males; increased risk of prostate cancer
Human recombinant erythropoietin (EPO), darbepoitin	Increased red blood cell production (increases performance in endurance sports)	Can increase blood viscosity to dangerous levels in very high doses, increasing risk of stroke or heart attack
Some stimulants (Mesocarb, Bromantan, Etilefrine, Ephedrine, Amphetamine, Cocaine, Adrenaline (new in 2006))	Improved alertness and reaction time; increased stamina; increased confidence	Cardiovascular stress, increased risk of psychosis (amphetamine); cardiac arrhythmia, insomnia, bradycardia, tachycardia, anorexia
Enhancement of oxygen transfer – blood doping, perfluorochemicals	Increased red blood cell count	Risks identical to EPO or hypoxic training
Cannabinoids such as THC	None known – likely to decrease performance	None known

influence performance. Creatine is similar to the banned drug EPO – in that it supplements an endogenous substance. Two different double-blind studies found that the time to exhaustion in anaerobic exercise could be increased by over 10% by the use of creatine (Bosco et al., 1997; Prevost et al., 1997). But creatine, like caffeine, is legal because it is not thought to harm athletes or violate the spirit of sport.

However, the Code goes on to say explicitly that *all* '[d]oping is fundamentally contrary to the spirit of sport'. In other words, if a drug is banned because it is both harmful and performance enhancing, it is necessarily considered to violate the spirit of sport as well. This statement contradicts the 2-out-of-3 rule because it adds this spirit-violating property to *every* banned group. Perhaps this is a mistake, but if it is not, then WADA and its supporters are not seriously worried about health risks. Neither are

they seriously worried about performance enhancement. If either of these concerns were important to WADA, it would sometimes consider banning a drug just because it was harmful, like tobacco, or just because it was performance-enhancing like creatine. In fact, the WADA code is functionally identical to a single-criterion code which defines doping as 'any substance or method which violates the spirit of sport'. This obsession with the spirit of sport is echoed in Pound's rationale, quoted above.

So what is WADA's conception of the spirit of sport?

WADA defines the 'spirit of sport' using a long list of words (World Anti-Doping Agency, 2003a):

(1) Ethics, fair play and honesty
(2) Health
(3) Excellence in performance

Table 70.2. Examples of legal performance-enhancers

Name	Effect	Unwanted effects
Creatine	Improves time to exhaustion in anaerobic exercise. Faster recovery from training	May lead to muscle cramping
Caffeine	Assists mobilization of fat stores, during exercise, improving time to exhaustion; assists alertness and concentration, especially on repetitive motor tasks	Insomnia, tachycardia, gastrointestinal complaints, increased blood pressure (high doses); withdrawal symptoms include headache and fatigue
Hypoxic/altitude training	Increases endogenous EPO, boosting the production of red blood cells	Excessive use can increase blood viscosity to dangerous levels in some individuals
Some stimulants – pseudoephedrine, nicotine, buproprion, pipradrol	Increase alertness and concentration	Carcinogenic (cigarettes); increased stroke risk, insomnia, tachycardia, anorexia (Pipradrol, pseudoephedrine)
LASIK eye surgery	Improves eyesight	Some risk of vision damage during surgery

(4) Character and education
(5) Fun and joy
(6) Teamwork
(7) Dedication and commitment
(8) Respect for rules and laws
(9) Respect for self and other participants
(10) Courage
(11) Community and solidarity.

This may be a good list of features that embody the aspirational 'spirit of sport'. But as a way to choose which drugs to ban, it is terrible.

Many of the terms on this list refer only to the amateur sport, not the elite sport where the anti-doping effort is focused. Fun and joy, for example, seem to be only a very weak requirement in elite sport. Similarly, elite athletes do not compete to improve their health or their education. Some of the terms on the list represent concepts that are not threatened by doping at all. For example, it is hard to see how teamwork is threatened by doping, especially when a whole team is doping. In one way, we might even think it courageous, dedicated or committed to take a harmful drug in the pursuit of sporting success, especially where that success also benefits one's team. Finally, some of the terms on the list are not threatened if every athlete is doping or if doping is legal. Excellence in performance is only threatened by doping when doping is against the rules. If a drug is legal there is no threat to an athlete's 'character'. And 'solidarity' is not threatened in cycling, where we assume that almost every athlete is taking EPO or blood doping.

The only terms on the list that are threatened by doping are those concerned with cheating. 'Respect for rules and laws' is at the heart of what motivates the crusade against doping. If we retain the WADA code, but cut away the irrelevant parts of their 'spirit of sport', doping is just using a substance or a method which is against the rules of the sport. That is, doping is just cheating by using drugs.

And that is probably as good a definition of doping as we will get, but it begs the question – why do we need rules against these drugs and training methods? Cheating is bad for sport because a sport is defined by its rules, but eradicating doping is not the only way to eradicate drug cheats. The other way is just to erase the anti-doping rules.

FAILURE OF CURRENT POLICY

It would be much easier to eliminate the anti-doping rules than to eliminate doping. The current policy against doping has proved expensive and difficult to police. In the near future it may become impossible to police.

It is difficult even to estimate how much illegal performance enhancement occurs at elite level. We are all familiar with the regular doping scandals at each major sporting event. In some sports, such as cycling, it is said to be endemic. In 1992, Vicky Rabinowicz interviewed small groups of athletes. She found that Olympic athletes, in general, believed that *most* successful athletes were using banned substances (Rabinowicz, 1992). Only about 10–15% of participating athletes are tested in each major competition (International Association of Athletics Federations, 2004). This testing costs WADA alone over $US 20 million.

Newer designer drugs are constantly being developed (see Table 70.3). Growth hormone is very difficult to detect. Myostatin is a growth factor which controls muscle growth. One family has been identified with a genetic mutation resulting in no myostatin production (Schuelke, et al., 2004). This resulted in extraordinarily strong and developed muscles in the child affected. Genetically modified mice which do not produce myostatin have enormous muscles and have been called Schwarzenegger mice (Lee, 2004). Administration of myostatin blockers cause significant increase in muscle mass in mice (Lee & McPherron, 2001). Genetic manipulation to stop myostatin production

Table 70.3. Examples of prohibited performance enhancements for which no athlete has tested positive, but believed to be in use

Name	Effect	Unwanted effects
Gene doping	Wide range of possible effects, including increased red blood cell count, localized increase in muscle growth or growth of fast-twitch muscle fibres, and so on	Depends on gene chosen and vector for genetic enhancement
Luteinizing hormone (LH)	Increases testosterone production in men, increasing muscle growth and stamina	None known other than risks stemming from increased testosterone
Growth hormone	Increased height if used in children or adolescents; increase in muscle mass; increased red blood cell production	None established – possible links to diabetes, acromegly, hypertension and so on
Beta blockers	Decrease natural tremor and reduce effects of 'stage fright'	Hypotension, heart failure, shortness of breath, depression, and so on

or administration of blockers would be expected to significantly increase strength in athletes and are likely to offer real potential for doping in the future. Insulin-like growth factor injected into the muscles of mice increases strength. Direct injection into the muscles of athletes would be simple and very difficult to detect as DNA would be taken into muscle DNA, requiring muscle biopsy to detect it. As gene doping becomes more efficient, it is likely to offer great opportunities for doping in sport and 'for all intents and purposes, gene doping will be undetectable' (Andersen, Schjerling & Saltin, 2000). Detection will likely require not blood or urine tests (as occurs now), but invasive, difficult and dangerous muscle biopsies. As gene therapy works in animals nowadays (for example inserting the EPO gene), there is no reason why it could not be attempted by athletes.

HEATH RISKS IN CURRENT POLICY

As we have shown, the WADA code is focused on cheating rather than harm. But the present system actually creates an environment of risk for the athlete. This gives us another reason to change it.

Because doping is illegal, the pressure is to make performance enhancers undetectable, rather than safe. Performance enhancers are produced or bought on the black market and administered in a clandestine, uncontrolled way with no monitoring of the athlete's health. Allowing the use of performance enhancers would make sport safer as there would be less pressure on athletes to take unsafe enhancers and would generate pressure to develop new safe performance enhancers and to make existing enhancers more effective at safe dosages.

Allowing performance enhancers would not eliminate risk to athletes' health but it would reduce it. Some would still seek an advantage through the use of unsafe, illegal enhancers. Some would still take safe enhancers in unsafe dosages. But it would narrow the performance gap between those athletes who wish to avoid health risks, and those who do not. This would also reduce the coercive force to take unsafe enhancers. If this were coupled with greater focus on evaluating fitness to compete and health, as suggested below, rather than drug detection, there would be an even greater improvement in athlete health.

A PROPOSAL

We should develop safer drug options that are as effective and as cheap as the harmful substances of today. There is a real practical difficulty with this because all drugs are harmful if taken in megadose quantities. Even nandrolone

is safe enough if taken in a small dose. Even water is lethal if taken in a very large dose. Ideally, we need drugs which are as effective as existing drugs at a safe dose, but which do not become significantly more effective at an unsafe dose.

But as we will discuss, elite athletes are always pushing the boundaries of personal risk. Safe alternatives will help those few elite athletes who are risk–averse, but we suspect that elite athletes can and will always find new boundaries to push and new risks to take, whether or not drugs are allowed. The point about doping is to take more of a substance than your competitors – if taking more does not work, then you take more of something else. The reason why athletes take risks is because they are strongly motivated to have the best performance.

With that in mind, we *could* try to lower the incentives for winning, by reducing prize money and limiting athletes' earnings. If we deliberately underpaid them, we would make winning less valuable to athletes, and this would in turn make their health relatively more valuable to them. But athletes' wages are not usually decreed by some governing body; they are a function of the money that the athletes can make for their sponsors and team owners. Thus, this solution would likely be impossible to enact.

If athletes will always be so strongly motivated to win that they will take severe risks, a better risk-reduction strategy would be to exclude athletes for health reasons, as we currently do in cycling. In cycling, if your haematocrit is too high (over 50%), you cannot compete because your blood viscosity puts you at risk, whatever the cause. Similarly, if athletes have left ventricle hypertrophy from steroid use or other cause or if their testosterone levels are above a certain limit, they should be informed of the risk. It would be possible to exclude them, even if the drug itself was legal, or even if they just had a naturally high level of testosterone. In Melbourne, boxers are excluded from competition if they have measurable brain damage on magnetic resonance imaging (Spriggs, 2004).

Exclusion would give athletes an incentive to look after their bodies. We could fund medical spot checks using the enormous funds we currently spend in a doomed attempt to find drugs in athletes' blood and urine. WADA alone costs around $22 million per year – just to test around 15% of the athletes (IAAF, 2004).

It is not as though these suggestions have never been made before. In 1998, the president of the International Olympic Committee, Juan-Antonio Samaranch, suggested that athletes be permitted to use safe performance-enhancing drugs (Downes, 1999). However, every time these suggestions are raised, they face a familiar list of objections. We could go through these objections one by one, but in our view they are all united in their dependency on a smaller number of misconceptions about sport and about what makes a sport good or bad.

The current doping controls also depend on these misconceived beliefs. We have compiled a list of seven. Once we recognize these misconceptions, the current doping controls begin to look much worse than our simple proposal to revise anti-doping controls.

SEVEN MISCONCEPTIONS ABOUT DRUGS IN SPORT

MISCONCEPTION 1

If every sportsperson takes legal safe drugs, sport will be decided by drugs, not human ability.

Jonathan Vaughters wrote this in *Cycling Weekly*:

> To argue that if everyone is doping and using the same dope, then it's fair, is bunk. Different drugs affect different metabolisms in different ways and some people will always benefit more from certain drugs than others. This is why doping must end, or we will not get to see who is truly the best (Vaughters, 2004).

This last sentence reveals a popular belief – that doping stops us from seeing who is truly the best.

Why should differences in metabolisms not decide who is best at a sport? Metabolisms are part of who is good and bad at sport, with or without doping. If I metabolize carbohydrates better than my opponent, it will give me an advantage, just as I will gain an advantage if I metabolize steroids more effectively. Athletes have genetic differences in their metabolic rates (Bogardus et al., 1986) and different gene–nutrition interactions (Heck et al., 2004) that already form part of what makes them 'truly the best'.

One part of the meaning of sport comes from this kind of comparison of athletes' biological potential. This was the old naturalistic Athenian vision of sport – to find the strongest, fastest or most skilled man. This is what Dick Pound appealed to when he said "[Sport is] essentially a humanistic endeavour to see how far you can go on your own talent" (CBC Sports Online, 2003).

Training aims to bring out this potential. Drugs which improve our natural potential are against the spirit of this model of sport. But sport is not just a test of biological potential. Central to human sport is the competitive spirit. Humans are not horses or dogs. We make choices and exercise our own judgement and other mental abilities. We choose the kind of training required and how to run our race. We can display courage, determination and wisdom. We are not flogged by a jockey on our back but drive ourselves. It is this judgement that competitors exercise when they choose diet, training and whether to take drugs.

Sport is not a test of biological potential when some competitors enhance their biology whereas others do not. This enables the biologically inferior cheaters to win. But that can only happen when enhancement is not permitted. If enhancement is permitted, competitors need no longer be drug discordant.

MISCONCEPTION 2

That clean sport is fair as in 'a level playing field'.

Obviously if we remove the bans on all doping, this levels the playing field in one way because every athlete can obtain the same drugs. But some will still claim that the best drugs will only be available to the richest athletes, that this would make sport unfair and that it would create an unlevel playing field.

There are a number of different kinds of inequality in elite sport. Differences in socioeconomic status from one country to the next, and from one individual to the next, limit access to top-class training and equipment. In this sense, drugs *level* the playing field – for example, illegal EPO is more affordable for third-world athletes than legal hypoxic training facilities (Savulescu, Foddy & Clayton, 2004).

But differences in genetic endowment can also make a huge difference in elite sport and cannot be redressed. Elite sport can be fair if 'fair' is interpreted to mean that 'the rules are applied equally'. It can never be fair if 'fair' is interpreted to mean 'level playing field'.

There is no genetic level playing field – sport is a test of genetic inequality.

People have different capabilities, genetic and financial. That is a fact that cannot be changed. We *could* create separate leagues for people with different amounts of money or different degrees of genetic talent. But we think it is better to accept variations in capability. We should worry more about sport being 'fair' in the sense that 'the rules are applied equally to everyone'.

MISCONCEPTION 3

Training and diet, unlike drugs, do not tend to be harmful. Clean elite sport is not harmful and tends to promote good health.

The WADA Copenhagen Declaration's preamble says that '. . . sport should play an important role in the protection of health' (World Anti-Doping Agency, 2003c). More broadly, any time the health risks of performance-enhancing drugs are mentioned, there is an assumption that these risks are significant in comparison to the baseline risks of 'clean sport'. But this assumption is not correct.

Elite sport can be extremely harmful. Even clean elite athletes have to accept serious harms to be competitive. These risks are usually reduced or absent in amateur competition, so just like drug risks, they are risks which are *extrinsic* to a sport – they are not a necessary part of the sport. There is nothing special about a drug-related risk which demands that we intervene, if we permit these unnecessary non-drug risks to exist.

One group has written that there is a limit to human cardiac adaptation to sports training, placing some athletes at risk of sudden cardiac death (Claessens et al., 1999). This risk is elevated if exotic training schemes are undertaken to increase an athlete's haematocrit, such as altitude or hypoxic tent training. Athletes who are stressed or over-trained also suffer a depletion in their immune systems (Gleeson, 2000; Nieman, 2000). Normal amounts of exercise increase the effectiveness of a person's immune system. But when we begin to over-train, the effect is reversed. In elite sports, athletes are at heightened risk of infection. One Norwegian study found 15% of gymnasts were anorexic (Sundot-Borgen, 1994). Christy Henrich is one example: she was an American gymnast who died of multiple organ failure from anorexia when she was 22. Some elite sports require an unhealthily large body shape. Many American footballers have bodyweights that correspond to a dramatically increased mortality (Harp & Hecht, 2005). Dysfunctional eating also seems to create a high incidence of menstrual dysfunction and stress fractures in female athletes. The rates are shockingly high – Beals studied a group of female college athletes and found that 37% had suffered some form of menstrual dysfunction and 37% had suffered a stress fracture (Beals, 2001). A number of sports have a high risk of mild traumatic brain injuries – boxing and football are predictable examples, also skiing, snowboarding, cycling and horse-riding (Freeman et al., 2005). One group found that the brains of athletes with these injuries could not be differentiated from the brains of people who were abusing recreational drugs (Iverson, Lange & Franzen, 2005).

Depending on the sport, at elite levels athletes are always at high risk of some sort of accidental injury. In American football, there is nearly one 'significant' injury per game – meaning it caused them to miss at least one game (Nicholas, Rosenthal & Gleim, 1998). In the Australian Football League from 1997 to 2000, teams of 40 players had around 40 *new* injuries per season (Orchard & Seward, 2005). Playing these sports at an elite level commits you to about one injury every year. If a drug were suspected of having this kind of risk, there would be a major witch-hunt. But these baseline risks are imposed on every athlete who accepts a place in one of these teams. Some sports have chronic health conditions in almost every elite participant – for example, top-tier trampolinists have an 80% incidence of stress urinary incontinence (Bo, 2004) which is no less serious a problem than the oft-cited gynaecomastia which can result from steroid use.

Injuries are not limited either to ankle sprains or concussion. From 1990 to 1999, 14 people died playing Australian Rules football, mostly from brain injury following collisions between players (McCrory, Berkovic & Cordner, 2000). None of the deaths were drug-related. Australian Rules is a comparatively dangerous sport, but it comprises only a tiny fraction of the total number of sportspeople worldwide who play high-impact, contact sports.

Playing sport at an elite level is not suicide, but neither is steroid use. To be sure, elite athletes are healthier on average than any morbidly obese person. But elite athletes in some sports can expect to have a serious medical problem every year or two. This is not true of EPO, taken at a reasonable dosage. Even at very high dosages, and even if we take into account the poorly-substantiated rumours of EPO-related deaths, EPO does not present any risks that cannot be found from just over-training or especially from hypoxic training. If you have a low haematocrit for genetic or dietary reasons, EPO could actually improve your health (Fairbanks & Tefferi, 2000).

Elite sport *without* performance-enhancing drugs is not safe. It will continue to get less safe as athlete wages go up and they push the limits of human performance.

It is not made significantly less safe through the use of existing performance-enhancing drugs, even if everyone uses them. It is inconsistent to crack down on drugs for health reasons when we are indifferent to the serious risks athletes are exposed to all the time.

If we – unlike WADA – are mostly concerned about athletes' health, we should test athletes for health indicators rather than for drugs. It is far easier to test haematocrit, or the red blood cell level in the blood, than it is to try to detect EPO or whether someone has been using a transfusion machine. We can set a safe limit, as we do in cycling, and ban anyone whose haematocrit is unsafe, whatever the cause. We can evaluate heart size and function, heart rhythm and other cardiac parameters and disqualify athletes who are at risk, whether the cause is natural variation, training or use of steroids or growth hormone. And we could consider the limits on damage that will have later effects – we could evaluate joint structure and function and disqualify athletes if they were likely to get arthritis in the future, if we thought that health was very important.

The question is – what risks should athletes be exposed to? It is not – what is the origin of that risk?

MISCONCEPTION 4

Widespread introductions of radical technology change sport for the worse.

The universal adoption of doping would represent a radical technology changing the performance of athletes across the board. To some, this is offensive in its own right.

The US Anti-Doping agency has a booklet that promotes '6 pillars of ethical decisionmaking'. Pillar 6 begins with the claim: 'Play by the rules. Sport is defined by the rules. Without the rules, it ceases to be the same sport.'

This statement is of course trivially true. But the implication here is that it is a deeply undesirable outcome for a sport to become a different sport – that we want sport to stay the same and not be changed by drug use. The implication is that, by allowing certain kinds of progress, the character of a sport is changed in a way that invalidates it or makes it worse. This argument stated slightly differently claims that we are on a 'slippery slope' towards a point where sportsmen are like robots – bizarre cyborgs. The French philosopher Robert Redeker (2002) said,

> Cycling is becoming a video game; the onetime 'prisoners of the road' have become virtual human beings... The type of man once promoted by the race, the people's man, born of hard toil, hardened to suffering and adept at surpassing himself, has been substituted by Robocop on wheels, someone no fan can relate to or identify with.

Of course, advances in equipment, clothing and training put us on this slope as well. In tennis, large head tennis racquets changed the game. This allowed players to hit the ball harder from a wider range of places on the court. Ultimately, this, together with other changes to the game, reduced the spectacle as male players were hitting – particularly serving – the ball so hard that there were no rallies. Subsequently, the pressure of the balls was reduced to slow them down. The increase in the size of the racquet head was allowed because it was thought to be in the spirit of tennis at the time. However, double strung tennis racquets were never permitted. They would have allowed too much spin and would have changed the game in a radical way that people could not accept.

Though we resist some changes, sport has changed drastically over the decades. Provided those changes are modest and gradual, they seem to be acceptable and indeed form a part of the evolution of sport. One radical change that has afflicted almost every sport is the current obsession with catching drug cheats. These controversies overshadow each Olympic games; our favourite athletes are removed from the field, and an enormous amount of airtime is given to these issues instead of to the coverage of sport. We are all made poorer when our favourite athletes are banned for drug use. Sometimes in our fight to maintain the status quo, we can make the status quo worse. This is an intangible but serious cost of doping controls.

MISCONCEPTION 5

Athletes should have a right to compete – and win – without taking risks they would prefer not to take.

One popular argument against legal doping is that it harms clean athletes by forcing them to take harmful drugs against their will, by coercion.

The President's Council on Bioethics (2003) wrote this:

> Should the use of an enhancing agent become normal and widespread, anyone who wished to excel in a given activity . . . might 'need' to use the same (or better) performance-enhancements in order to 'keep up'. Anecdotal evidence suggests that this 'soft coercion' may already be a problem.

Here is a quote from Laura Morgan, which gives a rationale for why this coercion is wrong.

> . . . not giving your best effort for any given game is wrong. This seems to require taking steroids if one's opponent is. But one who is morally committed to the ethics of competition and fair play should not be obligated to incur unnecessary health risks (Morgan, 2004).

We already outlined the extreme (and unnecessary) risks which elite athletes take to win. These risks are not there by chance. Partly these risks are due to the limitations of the human body. But mainly, they are defined by how badly athletes want to win. If they want to win very badly, they will inevitably be willing to take great risks. To play any athletic sport at its highest level, you therefore need to accept a certain degree of risk. If you find that level of risk unacceptable, you cannot succeed at the highest level. How much success can a sprinter achieve without risking stress fractures or leg injuries? How much success could a gymnast achieve without dieting to stay light?

The idea of 'soft coercion' could only have some sort of validity if it were true that the drugs were substantially more harmful than the sports themselves. As we have suggested, this is not clearly the case. We did say that health should be our first priority when considering doping. But if the health risks are relatively low, then perhaps they are just none of our business. For us to step in and say 'you may not take this risk' to a consenting, informed adult is the kind of strong medical paternalism which we have all but abandoned in every other sphere.

It may be that many athletes are only poorly informed about the side-effects of performance-enhancing drugs because their coaches administer them, and that their consent is thus limited. If this is true, there may be truth to the claim that athletes are coerced (or more accurately, deceived or *tricked*) into accepting these minor risks.

Allowing *safe* performance enhancement would reduce coercion in sport. *Safe* performance enhancement would encourage full disclosure to athletes. Athletes will still need to take drugs to remain competitive, but this will be no more coercive than their need to eat a special diet or to train in a certain way. Offering safe performance enhancement is no more coercive than offering prize money.

MISCONCEPTION 6

What is good and bad for amateur sport is what is good and bad for elite sport.

One of the most common arguments against legal doping is that children in amateur sport will be harmed if we legalize doping in professional sport. Another version of this argument claims that allowing doping will send the wrong 'message' to the public, and that sportspeople should set an example, telling us that winning should not be so highly prized, and that drug use should be reviled.

This idea is revealed in WADA's Copenhagen declaration:

> . . . sport should play an important role in the protection of health, in moral and physical education (World Anti-Doping Agency, 2003c)

Recall some terms from WADA's definition of the 'spirit of sport' (World Anti-Doping Agency, 2003a):

- Health
- Character and education
- Fun and joy
- Community and solidarity.

Even without drugs, elite sport does not promote these qualities. Is the 100 m lessened by the agony of the defeated or the seriousness with which they contest the race? Is professional boxing degraded by the competitive spirit with which it is played? And do professional gymnasts really compete for their health?

Amateur sport is relevantly different to professional sport. We do not perform drug testing in amateur Sunday-league sports. This is partly due to lack of resources. It is partly because amateur athletes have a relatively weak incentive to win. But they also have a stronger incentive *not to cheat* because the goals of amateur sport are different and are more strongly compromised by cheating.

In amateur sport, it is important that a good match is created. We try to match amateur tennis players to players of similar skill to ensure an interesting game. But this is never done in professional tennis – in fact, the seeding system ensures that most games are lopsided until the final rounds. In an amateur game, we have a concept of giving the opponent a 'sporting chance' – self-handicapping to increase enjoyment. Elite sport is not about the players' enjoyment. Elite sport is mainly about the spectators' enjoyment – after all, they foot the enormous bill. In amateur sports, what is interesting to the spectators is of no importance. Amateur sport is often about health. Elite sport is deleterious to health. Elite sport already sets some very bad examples, as well as some good ones.

MISCONCEPTION 7

People will lose interest in sport if every athlete takes drugs.

It is sometimes claimed that the prosecution of a war on doping preserves the public level of interest in a sport. As we have argued, enhancements occur already in sport to an extent that it is largely undetected and will soon become practically undetectable. What removes interest is cheating. An athlete is cheating whenever we declare a rule prohibiting some substance that the athlete is taking.

There is a kind of common misconception that there is a clear line which marks where legal supplements end and performance enhancing drugs begin. The use of caffeine and creatine is now extremely widespread, and both enhance performance. Why is this not boring? Hypoxic training tents have exactly the same effect as blood doping or EPO, and they are similarly widespread among wealthy teams. Yet these teams are never accused of being boring.

If legal performance enhancements do not make a sport boring, then we can stop doping from being boring by making it legal.

CONCLUSION

The removal of doping controls would have major benefits: less cheating, increased solidarity and respect between athletes, more focus on sport and not on rules.

Most of the 'costs' of abolishing doping controls depend on false beliefs.

There will still be a small number of arguments against abolishing doping controls which do not depend on any kind of misconception. But in order to justify the current doping controls, these arguments have to justify the ban's yearly multi-million dollar cost, *and* the intangible costs, and they must outweigh the benefits we would get if we abolished doping controls. We should focus on the health of athletes, not performance enhancement.

Rather than attempting to detect undetectable enhancers, we should spend our limited resources on evaluating health and fitness to compete. There are good reasons to allow performance enhancement, to make sport fairer (in the sense that the rules are equally applied) and to narrow the gap between the cheaters and the honest athletes. It would provide a better spectacle, be safer and less coercive.

We cannot prevent sport from evolving, but we can and should begin to direct its evolution for the better.

ACKNOWLEDGEMENTS

We would like to thank Miriam Wood for her assistance with the preparation of this article.

REFERENCES

Andersen JL, Schjerling P, Saltin B. Muscle, genes and athletic performance. *Sci Am* 2000; **283**: 48–55.

Beals K. Changes in the prevalence of risk factors for the female athletic triad among collegiate athletes over a two-year period. *Med Sci Sports Exerc* 2001; **33**(S5) (Abstract).

Bo K. Urinary incontinence, pelvic floor dysfunction, exercise and sport. *Sports Med* 2004; **34**(7): 451–64.

Bogardus C, Lillioja S, Ravussin E, Abbott W, Zawadzki JK, Young A, Knowler WC, Jacobowitz R, Moll PP. Familial dependence of the resting metabolic rate. *N Engl J Med* 1986; **315**: 96–100.

Bosco C, *et al.* Effect of oral creatine supplementation on jumping and running performance. *Int J Sports Med* 1997; **18**: 369–72.

CBC Sports Online. *The Enforcer* [online], 2003; available from http://www.cbc.ca/sports/indepth/drugs/stories/qa_dickpound.html.

Claessens P, *et al.* Ventricular premature beats in triathletes: still a physiological phenomenon? *Cardiology* 1999; **92**(1):28–38.

Costill D, Dalsky G, Fink W. Effects of caffeine ingestion on metabolism and exercise performance. *Med Sci Sports Exer* 1978; **10**: 155–8.

Downes S. Samaranch Move Stuns Critics. London: *The Sunday Times*, January 31, 1999.

Fairbanks VF, Tefferi A. Normal ranges for packed cell volume and hemoglobin concentration in adults: relevance to 'apparent polycythemia'. *Eur J Haematol* 2000; 65: 285–96.

Freeman JR, Barth JT, Broshek DK, Plehn K. Sports injuries. In: Silver JM, McAllister TW, Yudofsky SC, ed. *Textbook of Traumatic Brain Injury*. Washington, DC, US: American Psychiatric Publishing, Inc, 2005; pp. 453–476.

Gleeson M. The scientific basis of practical strategies to maintain immunocompetence in elite athletes. *Exerc Immunol Rev* 2000; **6**:75–101.

Harp JB, Hecht L. Obesity in the National Football League. *JAMA* 2005; **293**: 1061–2.

Heck AL, Barroso CS, Callie ME, Bray MS. Gene – nutrition interaction in human performance and exercise response. *Nutrition* 2004; **20**(7–8): 598–602.

IAAF. *International Association of Athletics Federations* [online], 2004; available from: http://www.iaaf.org/antidoping/index.html.

Iverson GL, Lange RT, Franzen MD. Effects of mild traumatic brain injury cannot be differentiated from substance abuse. *Brain Injury* 2005; **19**(1): pp. 15–25.

Lee SJ, McPherron AC. Regulation of myostatin activity and muscle growth. *Proc Natl Acad Sci USA* 2001; **98**: 9306–11.

Lee SJ. Regulation of muscle mass by myostatin. *Annu Rev Cell Dev Biol* 2004; **20**: 61–86.

McCrory PR, Berkovic SF, Cordner SM. Deaths due to brain injury among footballers in Victoria, 1968–1999. *MJA* 2000; **172**: 217–19.

Morgan L. Enhancing performance: morally permissible? In: Boxill J, ed. *Sports Ethics: An Anthology*, 2004; p.187.

Nicholas JA, Rosenthal PP, Gleim GW. A historical perspective of injuries in professional football. Twenty-six years of game-related events. *JAMA* 1998; **260**(7): 939–44.

Nieman DC. Special feature for the olympics: effects of exercise on the immune system: exercise effects on systemic immunity. *Immunol Cell Biol* 2000; **78**(5): 496–501.

Orchard J, Seward H. Epidemiology of injuries in the Australian Football League, seasons 1997–2000. *Br J Sports Med* 2005; **36**(1): 39–44.

President's Council on Bioethics. *Beyond Therapy: Biotechnology and the Pursuit of Happiness*. New York: Harper Collins, 2003; Chapter 3.

Prevost MC, Nelson AG, Morris GS. Creatine supplementation enhances intermittent work performance. *Res Q Exer Sport* 1997; **68**: 233–40.

Rabinowicz V. Athletes and drugs: a separate pace? *Psychol Today* 1992; **25**(4): 52–3.

Redeker R. Tour de France, où es-tu? *l'Humanite*, 29 July 2002.

Savulescu J, Foddy B, Clayton M. Why we should allow performance enhancing drugs in sport. *Br J Sports Med* 2004; **38**(6): 666–70.

Schuelke M, Wagner KR, Stolz LE, Hubner C, Riebel T, Komen W, Braun T, Tobin JF, Lee SJ. Myostatin mutation associated with gross muscle hypertrophy in a child. *N Engl J Med* 2004; **350**(26): 2682–8.

Spriggs M. Compulsory brain scans and genetic tests for boxers—or should boxing be banned? *J Med Ethics* 2004; **30**: 515–6.

Sundot-Borgen J. Risks and trigger factors for the development of eating disorders in female elite athletes. *Med Sci Sports Exerc* 1994; **26**(4): 414–9.

Vaughters J. What would you do? *Cycling Weekly*, October 30, 2004; pp. 32–33.

World Anti-Doping Agency. *World Anti-Doping Code*, 2003a; p. 3.

World Anti-Doping Agency. *World Anti-Doping Code*, 2003b; pp. 15–16.

World Anti Doping Agency. *Copenhagen Declaration on Anti-Doping in Sport*. WADA, 2003c; p. 2.

71

Training Good Professionals: Ethics and Health Care Education

NAFSIKA ATHANASSOULIS

Medical education has seen some radical changes in the 10 plus years since the first edition of the present volume. The General Medical Council's paper on medical education, 'Tomorrow's Doctors' (General Medical Council, 2003), first published in 1993 (revised in 2003) laid down new ideas for medical curricula. There has been a shift from the idea that medical students should gain as much knowledge as possible to the idea that becoming a doctor is a life-long learning process. Medical schools are now expected to provide their students with a variety of skills such as research skills and communication skills, as well as cultivate patient-centred approaches to teaching and learning. Discussions of values and ideals relevant to the medical profession now form part of the integrated curriculum. One of the most comprehensive changes has been the inclusion of ethics in the curriculum.

This chapter discusses some of the general thoughts behind the inclusion of ethics in medical curricula with specific reference to the teaching programme of the School of Medicine at the University of Leeds. This particular programme, set up in collaboration between the School of Medicine and the School of Philosophy at this institution, has attempted to bring Aristotelian ideas about education to bear on curriculum design in medicine. Much of Aristotle's work in ethics focuses on the importance of education and sets out ideas on how we should go about encouraging and training the young in the study of ethics. This emphasis on Aristotelian ideas is intended as a recommendation of the kinds of qualities education should seek to instil in students and suggestions on how we can achieve this. (Much of the emphasis in recent moral philosophy has been on a rather confrontational style of analysis, which pits one type of normative theory against another. The aim of this

chapter is not to convince the reader of the relative merits of Aristotelianism (or virtue ethics) as opposed to deontology or consequentialism, but to use ideas from Aristotle to talk about the shape of moral education. Such ideas concerning the development of moral character could plausibly be adopted by other theories and do not represent any commitment to a particular kind of answer to normative questions because the emphasis is on the development of moral judgement and independent thinking.)

ASKING THE QUESTION

Moral philosophy is one of the central subjects in any undergraduate philosophy degree; so it may strike academic colleagues in philosophy as odd that one of the very first steps in teaching medical students is to introduce them to the fundamental questions ethics seeks to answer. At the very beginning of the *Nicomachean Ethics*, Aristotle warns us that the purpose of his book is a very practical one. He is not seeking to increase our theoretical, abstract knowledge, but rather this is an inquiry into how one becomes good. Aristotle wants to examine actions and how they should be performed; his fundamental question is 'How should I live my life?', 'What kind of person should I be?' For Aristotle, answering this question should be a central project in any human being's life because the distinctive function of humans is reason. Reading the *Nicomachean Ethics* should have a profound effect on how one leads one's life. This is not merely an intellectual, abstract exercise, but a practical, life-altering, life-long project. This realization, that morality is a practical concern, was central in Aristotle's thought

Principles of Health Care Ethics, Second Edition   Edited by R.E. Ashcroft, A. Dawson, H. Draper and J.R. McMillan
© 2007 John Wiley & Sons, Ltd

and has been revived in the development of virtue ethics in
the last few decades (for modern developments on this topic
see Crisp, 1996).

Having said that, this very question, 'How should I live
my life?', is difficult for students to grasp. Moral considerations, questions about right and wrong behaviour, about
the quality of our actions and the development of our characters, seem strange for first-year medical students. This
may be because this is their first contact with moral education, or it may be because of a misconception which identifies moral education with religious conviction or with a set
of conservative views, mainly about one's sexual conduct.
Even students who can give thoughtful answers to the question 'Why do you want to become a doctor?' often fail to
appreciate the depth of the kind of answer they need to give.
For example 'Because I want to help people' is a plausible
answer to why one might want to become a doctor, but understanding what it means to be a kind person, to behave in
a consistently and dependably kind manner in all areas of
one's life and doing so with the right emotions, easily and
freely, is a really different and difficult topic. Understanding kindness requires moral maturity, which is a life-long
project and we cannot expect to find it as standard among
young people.

Whatever the cause then, it seems that young students
find the very questions of morality perplexing; they fail to
see the relevance of these questions to their lives. The very
first task in teaching medical ethics then is to convince the
students that these are valid, pressing questions which they
need to ask of themselves and then attempt to answer.

How does one deal with highly motivated, but also
very busy and highly stressed students, who wonder why
they should bother with ethics? One quick answer is telling students that they have no choice. The various bodies
governing medical education have recommended the inclusion of ethics in the curriculum, and we all have to fall in
line with these recommendations. However, this is a very
unsatisfactory answer, which underestimates the students'
sensibilities. Medicine as a profession brings professionals
into close contact with other people, others who may be in
especially vulnerable situations, contemplating the most
difficult decisions at the edge of human life. Questions of
right and wrong are simply inevitable for medical professionals. It is a mistake, however, to approach such issues as
matters of bureaucratic necessity, as obligations imposed by
governing bodies and professional organizations. Consent
forms should be filled in, but not because one fears censure
from one's superiors or litigation from one's patients. Our
moral obligations are not external burdens to be discharged
in the least onerous manner possible. Rather the needs and
interests of others should engage us, and responding appropriately to those needs should form part of our conception
of the good life.

Medical students should not be taught ethics and medical
professionals should not practise ethically because they have
to, but rather because they want to, because they appreciate
how one human being stands in relation to others and how
a variety of values, some self-interested some other-regarding, play a part in one's life (for more on these ideas, see
Dent, 1999). What this means is that medical students have
to come to see the importance of ethical questions for themselves and appreciate the relevance they have to their lives.
The relevance they have to their lives not only as medical
professionals who will need to deal with matters of life and
death every day, but also as thinking human beings who
will have to interact with other human beings and work out
some way of taking the well being and interests of other
people into account.

One related issue here is the relationship between ethics
and the law. The two topics seem to have a very reasonable
connection, and one could see some advantages in teaching
them together. However, this can be misleading. Although
legal discussion can involve sophisticated interpretation and
debate, at an introductory level, matters of law are matters
of fact. Ethics, on the other hand, involves a completely different way of learning. Rather than handing out factual answers, ethical education challenges students to ask the questions of their own selves. For this reason it can sometimes
be counterproductive to introduce law and ethics together.
Students who may be focusing on a clearly identifiable way
of obtaining high marks may latch onto factual, legal answers, avoiding the challenge of thinking for themselves.
It may be best then to side step legal questions at the very
start of medical education or avoid discussing them alongside ethics, simply as a means of requiring students to think
for themselves rather than relying on the law for a quick and
authoritative answer.

MORAL PERCEPTION

Appreciating the basic, big moral questions is then a
first step. The second step is coming to see how these
considerations affect us all in practice. Invariably, because
of its very nature, medicine will bring students into contact
with a large number of complex, diverse and demanding
ethical issues. However, oddly enough, it is not always easy
to notice these issues.

One way of accounting for this is by considering the Aristotelian notion of moral perception. Seeing the world as full
of moral situations involves coming to see the world differently and also involves a process of sensitization. Central to
Aristotelian theory is the idea that virtue has both cognitive
and affective elements. Kindness is not merely theoretical,
abstract knowledge of the virtue but '...a full-hearted appreciation of the importance of caring for others, of their

needs and well-being. The "full-heartedness" comprises the free and willing giving of attention to other people, a readiness to interpret situations in a way favourable to others' interests, a reluctance to give up on others' problems and so on' (Dent, 1999, p. 26). The world is a morally rich environment, full of opportunities for taking into account the interests and well being of others and reflecting on our own values and attitudes. However, becoming sensitized to the relevance of particulars is not an easy task. It requires emotional maturity, the opportunity to discuss what one observes with others, moral imagination and effort.

MORAL IMAGINATION, MORAL JUDGEMENT AND THE DEVELOPMENT OF MORAL CHARACTER

For Aristotle the proper emotions, cultivated and guided by reason, are a crucial part of virtue. So, one task of medical education must be to appropriately sensitize medical students to the situations they are likely to encounter; '[a]rguably much of the harm in the world is done by people who lack a sense of the less obvious consequences of their actions or of how some of the victims experience them. Simply being able to enter into the point of view of people different from oneself can make a major difference in one's humanity...' (Kupperman 1999, p. 207). So one is seeking partly to open the students' eyes to the possibility of moral problems within the world and partly to sensitize them to the demands these problems make on them and the impact their own actions will have.

Aristotelian moral education then is the education of reason and the emotions in accordance with virtue. This is a life-long, arduous project for the development of one's moral character and moral judgement. Students of virtue must come to see what virtue requires of them, that is, what is the kind, courageous, friendly thing to do, why virtue requires this, as well as be motivated to act accordingly, with kind, courageous and friendly emotions. Rules and principles can form part of this development, used either as training tools or as 'rules of thumb' (Nussbaum, 1990), but their usefulness is limited. Ultimately, what one needs is moral judgement, the ability to respond to the particulars of each situation and judge their relative importance. This may often require seeing beyond rules and understanding how principles should be sensitive to context. Judgement is required because the right answer will be sensitive to context and the person making the decision. This should not be taken to mean that Aristotle supported relativism. Relativism, the idea that truth is relative and determined by social conventions or individual opinions, is an entirely different idea. For Aristotle there is a right answer, but it is difficult to find, requires moral maturity and is dependent on the particular circumstances of the case and the agent.

One implication of this idea is that a map of ethical education in health care cannot read as a grid of specific topics, ideas or principles which are taught in a specific order and then applied in a rather mechanical way by the students to arrive at the right answer. Unfortunately, ethical matters are much more complicated than that. There is no formulaic answer to moral questions and no easy theory which can be learnt by heart and applied by rote. Clinical judgement does not take this form, so why should we expect ethics to do so? Much of clinical education is about learning facts and methods; however clinical proficiency is mainly about the development of judgement, the ability to take in information and subject it to critical thinking processes. It is these reflective qualities we admire in expert doctors, the ability to see beyond rules and reason outside common parameters. Similarly, ethical reasoning cannot be captured in an easy-to-memorize formula.

IN PRACTICE

How do all these ideas work in practice, and what difference should they make to the curriculum? The first thought is that like many other aspects of medical education, moral development does not cease with graduation. Students of virtue will continue to mature and develop throughout their lives: this is not the kind of project one completes. Again like other aspects of the curriculum, for example like communication skills, ethics should be taught in an integrated manner throughout all the years of study. What I mean by integration is easy to grasp in theory, even though it can be demanding to apply in practice. Each discipline has a set of aims and objectives, an understanding of what the discipline is about, of what students should have achieved in order to be able to say that they have a good understanding of the discipline and a good education in it. These aims and objectives and the means by which they are achieved can vary, and vary radically, from one discipline to another. Two disciplines can be taught alongside each other to the same group of students but without achieving any degree of integration if they are taught in ignorance of each other. What I mean by this is that the first step of integration must be to learn about the other discipline; what is it trying to achieve, how does it go about doing this? The next step is to ask what is the degree of overlap between the two disciplines? If there is similarity in aims and objectives, can they be taught together? If there is difference can we incorporate new ideas, effect change and add to the existing curriculum? Integration means that philosophy is taught within medicine, as a part of medicine, and the aims and objectives of the ethics curriculum are adjusted to reflect and incorporate those of the medical curriculum. At the same time the medical curriculum is also subject to change to incorporate these new ideas, so both disciplines emerge from the process changed.

One way of integrating the two curricula, is to think of ethical education as a theme which runs through all courses and is raised and discussed as appropriate rather than as an isolated session. This will encourage students to view ethical problems simply as one dimension of the many issues patients will bring to them and will alert them to the possibility that all sorts of situations they come across will have ethical dimensions. For an excellent example of a fully integrated course, raising patient-centred issues in basic science, pathology, law and ethics as well as social and cultural issues, see the *Lifecycle* course at the University of Leeds available online at http://www.histology.leeds.ac.uk/icu4/. *Lifecycle* uses realistic cases to bring awareness of issues in practice and reflects real cases in that the issues that are raised are not individuated, compartmentalized nuggets of information; rather they are complex, multidimensional problems which require students to examine them by bringing to bear knowledge from a number of disciplines.

Integration within the existing curriculum must go hand in hand with a sense of ethics teaching as a whole. Progression must be possible from one year to the next as students become more accustomed to identifying ethical problems, expressing their views, formulating arguments, defending their positions and developing objections against other views. An overview of the entire ethics theme is also important to ensure there is no significant overlap in the material taught from year to year and that topics considered central are covered at some point or other. I have said almost nothing about the actual topics one might want to teach because this is, in a sense, beside the point. Specific curricula can identify different topics they consider central, but differences at this stage are unimportant. This is because philosophical training is really training students how to think; this skill, thinking, producing consistent, convincing arguments, can be applied to any topic. Students may choose to pursue topics they have an interest in within courses which offer individual choice (Special Study Modules, also known as Student Selected Components). Generic philosophical skills, along with more general skills such as research skills, teamwork, information gathering and presentation skills, can then come into play to help approach any new topic.

Full integration in the curriculum should help students identify ethical issues, as these will be discussed as they occur within the teaching. In addition, the use of real and fictional cases, direct contact with patients and the opportunity to learn from professionals who have a direct grasp of the realities of medical practice can be crucial. Putting oneself in another person's place, thinking about the possible outcomes of one's action, contemplating the repercussions of one's behaviour are all ways of developing one's moral competence. Highly realistic, detailed case studies used in teaching, case studies which raise not only issues regarding basic science, pathology or clinical skills but also social, cultural and ethical issues, allow students to learn in an environment which most closely mimics the kinds of situations they will come across outside the medical school. This effectively involves developing one's moral imagination.

Contact with professionals who have experience of what the practice of medicine is really like is also very important. Aristotle places a great deal of emphasis on the importance of the moral exemplar, the person of experience who can advise and lead by example. Health care professionals can teach alongside philosophers, and many teachers now have backgrounds in both medicine and ethics. Learning from professionals one can identify with and attempt to emulate is crucial for learning well. Sherman writes that suitable exemplars can fulfil many roles: they bring along their relevant experience, bringing the topic to life and making learning more accessible; students find it easier to identify with their teachers and be motivated by what motivates them; they bring a practical dimension to theoretical topics; and they can demonstrate practical decision making based on a grasp of the particulars (Sherman, 1999).

Finally, a question asked often enough is how does one go about assessing ethical competence? Well, in a sense one does not. Some students, like some of us from all walks of life, will be more successful than others at sensitizing themselves to ethical issues and attempting to resolve them. Some will be less successful, and the judgement of this failure will come from their colleagues and patients as well as their family, friends and everyone they come into contact with in due course. In another sense, general critical thinking skills which form the backbone of philosophy can be assessed as they are in straightforward philosophy courses. Here, one is looking for the ability to understand and construct arguments, express oneself clearly and in a structured manner, make relevant and convincing points, consider other positions and show knowledge of the relevant literature, include original thoughts and demonstrate independent thinking. All these skills can be demonstrated in a variety of assessable activities, such as essays, presentations, portfolios, among others; the limit really is the imagination of the course designers.

CONCLUSION

The inclusion of ethics has brought about two revolutions in higher education. One is in the design and delivery of the medical curriculum which has had to change radically and adapt to new demands. The other comes from philosophy itself. Traditionally perceived as a rather obscure, abstract, academic topic, philosophy has had to adapt and develop teaching methods which will appeal to students outside its usual demography. Interdisciplinary teaching is taking philosophy as a topic to a wide variety of new students ranging from health care students to engineering students to computing and business students. The skills remain the same, how to reason well, and the project is fundamental to all human beings: how should I live my life?

ACKNOWLEDGEMENT

I am grateful to a number of my colleagues for helpful comments on an earlier draft of this chapter and in particular I would like to thank Jennifer Jackson, Gerald Lang, Rob Lawlor, Chris Megone and Georgia Testa.

REFERENCES

Aristotle. *Nicomachean Ethics* (Translated by Thomson JAK). England: Penguin Books, 1976.

Crisp R. *How Should One Live?* Oxford: Clarendon Press, 1996.

Dent N. Virtue, *eudaimonia* and teleologiccal ethics. In: Steutel J, Carr D, eds. *Virtue Ethics and Moral Education*. London: Routledge, 1999.

General Medical Council. Tomorrow's Doctors, 2003; available on: www.gmc-org.uk/med-ed/tomdoc.hta.

Kupperman JJ. Virtues, character and moral disposition. In: Steutel J, Carr D, eds. *Virtue Ethics and Moral Education*. London: Routledge, 1999.

Nussbaum M. *Love's Knowledge*. USA: Oxford University Press, 1990.

Sherman N. Character development and Aristotelian virtue. In: Steutel J, Carr D, eds. *Virtue Ethics and Moral Education*. London: Routledge, 1999.

72

Ethics Consultation and Ethics Committees

ANNE SLOWTHER

INTRODUCTION

As philosophical medical ethics has developed as an academic discipline over the past 40 years, there has been a concurrent, though somewhat slower, development of a service delivery component of the field. Clinical ethicists or ethics consultants and clinical ethics committees have had an increasing presence in hospitals and other health care settings in many countries throughout the world, providing on the ground support and advice to clinicians, patients and their families when ethical difficulties arise in patient care (Slowther et al., 2001a). This involvement in, rather than a commentary on, the ethics of everyday medicine owes its development to a variety of philosophical, legal and social influences. This has resulted in both differences and similarities in provision of ethics support across different cultures and health care systems. A key feature of the structure of clinical ethics support, whether ethics consultation or ethics committee, is its multidisciplinarity. Clinical ethics committees include in their membership health professionals, lay members, lawyers, ethicists, hospital managers and chaplains (McGee & Caplan, 2001); ethics consultants have backgrounds in philosophy, medicine, nursing, sociology and theology (Slowther et al., 2001a). This reflects in part the diverse skills and knowledge base required to provide good clinical ethics support. Ethics consultants and ethics committees are not simply 'philosophers at the bedside'. In recent years there has been an expansion in the focus of the work of ethics consultants and ethics committees, making them include organizational and resource allocation issues in addition to individual case consultation (Christensen & Tucker, 1997). There has also been an increasing debate about the nature of ethics consultation (La-Puma & Schiedermayer, 1991b; Zoloth-Dorfman & Rubin, 1997; Agich, 2003), the competencies required to provide ethics consultation (La-Puma

& Schiedermayer, 1991a; American Society for Bioethics and the Humanities, 1998; Aulisio, Arnold & Younger, 2000) and the need for robust evaluation of this work (Fox, 1996; Tulsky & Fox, 1996; Phillips, 1996). In this chapter, I will briefly trace the history of ethics consultation and ethics committees in the clinical setting, consider some key issues in the structure, process and methodology of ethics consultation, and look to the future development of clinical ethics support.

HISTORY

Clinical ethics committees, as distinct from Institutional Review Boards or Research Ethics Committees, have been a feature of hospitals in North America for many decades, and a requirement for a hospital to have a clinical ethics committee or some mechanism for addressing the ethical issues that arise in patient care is now part of the regulatory requirement for accreditation of hospitals in both the United States (Joint Commission for Accreditation of Health Care Organisations, 1996) and Canada (Canadian Council on Hospital Accreditation, 2006). In Europe, the Netherlands probably has the most well established history of clinical ethics committees, serving nursing homes as well as hospitals (van der Kloot Meijburg & ter Meulen, 2001), although originally these committees were combined committees of clinical and research ethics. Combined committees are a feature of other European countries, for example Belgium (Carbonelle & Schmitz, 2000) and France (Arnoux, 2000), and in some countries there is a legislative requirement for hospitals to have a committee that considers ethical issues relating to clinical and research practice. Other European countries, such as the United Kingdom (Slowther et al., 2004) and Norway (Ruyter, 2000), have developed clinical ethics committees independently from the research ethics infrastructure. Where clinical ethics committees are independent of research ethics committees, there is less likely to be a legislative or regulatory requirement governing their existence. However, the Norwegian government has recommended that all hospitals should have a clinical ethics committee (Ruyter, 2000) and the Royal College of Physicians in the United Kingdom has published recommendations on the provision of ethics support for clinicians which include clinical ethics committees as one model of delivery (RCP Working Party on Clinical Ethics, 2005). Clinical ethics committees are also developing in Australia (Kerridge, Pearson & Rolfe, 1998) Asia (Tan, 2002), the Middle East, (Wenger et al., 2002) and South America (Tealdi & Mainetti, 1990).

The impetus for the development of clinical ethics committees varies between countries. In the United States, a major factor was a group of legal judgements (In Re Quinlan, 1976) and federal legislation for withholding and withdrawing life prolonging treatment in adults and neonates. In addition to these legal pressures, in 1983 the President's Commission for the Study of Ethical Problems in Medicine and Biomedical and Behavioural Research recommended that hospitals should establish clinical ethics committees as a way of resolving ethical conflict in individual cases. This 'top-down' approach has been consolidated in recent years by the Joint Committee on Accreditation of Health Care Organizations (JACHO) requirements for accreditation of health care institutions and further legislation in individual States (Joint Commission for Accreditation of Health Care Organisations, 1996). In contrast, clinical ethics committees in some European countries have developed in a much more 'bottom-up' manner as a result of clinicians seeking support for ethical difficulties that they were experiencing in their daily practice, or individual hospitals identifying a need for ethical input into the institution's policies and practices (Slowther et al., 2004).

Clinical ethicists or ethics consultants have developed alongside clinical ethics committees, and their respective roles are often integrated in an institution (La-Puma & Toulmin, 1989; Smith et al., 2004). Like clinical ethics committees, ethics consultants are much more common in North America than elsewhere, but their number is increasing in other countries (Reiter-Theil, 2001a; Wray, 2002). One impetus for the development of clinical ethicists has come from the academic departments of medical ethics where ethics consultation has developed as a natural progression of the department''s research and teaching role (Agich, 2003). Some clinical ethicists are employed directly by hospitals and may hold joint clinical and ethics appointments (clinician ethicists). Ethicists are usually members of their institution's clinical ethics committee (CEC) and are often seen as providing the moral expertise for the committee, or at least providing the ethics education for committee members. Several academic centres in North America run ethics internships and fellowships to train

clinical ethicists (Chidwick et al., 2004), but elsewhere there is no specific training for this new professional role in health care. A common concern expressed in the clinical ethics literature internationally is the lack of recognized training, qualifications, or generally accepted competencies for either members of clinical ethics committees or individual ethicists (Fletcher & Hoffmann, 1994; Aulisio, 1999; Slowther et al., 2001b). The American Society for Bioethics and the Humanities have published a document setting out the recommended core competencies for ethics consultation, (American Society for Bioethics and the Humanities, 1998) but there has been a reluctance by many in clinical ethics to be prescriptive in setting standards for those working in the field.

The roots of clinical ethics are firmly embedded in clinical practice and, perhaps, more specifically in clinical medicine and the doctor/patient relationship (Singer, Pellegrino & Siegler, 2001). There was certainly an initial reluctance by clinical ethics committees to become involved in wider ethical issues relating to patient care, such as resource allocation and organizational ethics. If hospital policies were considered, they were policies closely related to individual patient care, such as Do Not Attempt Resuscitation (DNAR) orders and advance directives. However, in recent years clinical ethics (and thus the work of CECs and ethics consultants) has expanded its focus beyond the limits of the hospital ward to consider wider institutional concerns, developing along the way a subspecialty of 'organisational ethics' (Pentz, 1999; Goold et al., 2000). The domain within which CECs and ethics consultants operate is still by and large the acute care hospital, with no meaningful expansion into community care, such as family practice, community services, or nursing homes. (The Netherlands is a notable exception in this respect with regard to nursing homes.) However, this may change as clinical ethics committees become more common in countries where community care is a major part of the health care system. A perceived need for CECs and ethics consultation in both the primary care and community settings has been documented (Busby & Rauh, 1991; Slowther et al., 2001b; Hoy and Feigenbaum, 2005). Development in these areas may pose organizational, methodological and theoretical challenges for ethics consultation as it operates in a less familiar context.

FUNCTIONS AND SCOPE OF ETHICS CONSULTANTS AND ETHICS COMMITTEES

A cursory glance at the copious literature on ethics consultation and CECs will identify a common theme in describing the functions of ethicists and committees. The triad of education, policy development, and case consultation is seen as defining the role of consultant and committee. When the President's Commission advised the establishment of clinical ethics committees in the United States, the recommendation was that they offer advice in individual cases (President's Commission, 1983). However, initially committees focused mainly on policy and education, and their case consultation role was minimal (Blake, 1992). A similar situation was found in a study of clinical ethic committees in the United Kingdom in 2000 (Slowther et al., 2001a). Reasons for avoidance of case consultation include lack of confidence in the moral expertise of the committee (by both health professionals in the hospital and committee members themselves), concern that the committee would usurp the clinician's role of medical decision-maker, and lack of resources to allow timely and appropriate responses to urgent requests for consultation. In contrast, clinical ethicists see case consultation as a key function of their role and may be less involved in policy formation, if at all. In some institutions case consultation is carried out by ethicists, and broader policy issues are considered by the committee, (La-Puma & Toulmin, 1989) although this clear separation of roles is unusual, and in institutions without an ethics post the CEC will carry out whatever ethics functions occur. The diverse nature of clinical ethics services both between countries and within individual health care systems, together with a lack of formal regulatory frameworks, means that CECs and clinical ethicists are to a great extent free to choose which functions they will focus on (subject to the agreement of the institution). However, a narrow focus on either policy formation or bedside case consultation is open to criticism. Clinical ethics is about practising ethics in the day-to-day clinical setting, and its aim is to improve patient care. Policies developed without any practical knowledge of individual cases, their clinical and moral nuances, and how they are resolved in practice, are likely to be too abstract or lack relevance to the situation on the ground, and consequently less likely to be implemented. However, individual case consultation in isolation, without addressing wider institutional norms and practices, may not achieve improvement in patient care throughout the institution (Benatar et al., 2001).

SOME KEY ISSUES FOR DEBATE IN ETHICS CONSULTATION

STRUCTURAL ISSUES: WHO DOES IT?

As has been noted, ethics consultation or support is provided in diverse forms, both in the mechanism of support provision and the scope of the support. Within this diversity, there is still further variation in provision of individual ethics case consultation. At least four different structural models of case consultation have been identified.

(1) *Case consultation by committee*: In institutions with a CEC but no clinical ethicist, the committee may provide case consultation. CECs that provide case consultation will have a mechanism for calling meetings at short notice to respond to urgent requests. In some instances a subcommittee may convene if the full committee cannot be called. Referrals to the committee may come through the chair or another member of the committee, and there is often an initial screening process to identify cases that would be more appropriately dealt with in a different forum, for example risk management or complaints procedures.

(2) *Case consultation groups*: This model can take several forms including
   (a) A sub-group of the ethics committee, with review of cases by the full committee.
   (b) Individual committee members providing an 'on call' service with support from a local ethics centre or an ethicist within the institution.
   (c) An ethics consultation service, which may include health professionals in the institution and/or members of an academic ethics centre.

(3) *Hub and spoke model*: In this model, the 'spokes' are individuals taking the ethics lead within their clinical areas, providing initial advice and support at a unit level. If the issues are complex, a formal case consultation can be requested from the CEC, ethicist or ethics centre acting as the hub. The hub is responsible for providing training to the individual ethics leads and reviewing their work in a systematic manner.

(4) *Individual ethicist*: In many North American and some European hospitals, the case consultation is provided by individual ethicists (who may work in isolation or as part of a group of clinical ethicists comprising a comprehensive clinical ethics service).

The relative advantages and disadvantages of the different models is a subject for debate. A committee provides a wider range of perspectives on a case, reducing the risk of bias in identifying and analysing the issues. Lay membership makes it less likely that the process will become institutionalized. However, concerns have been expressed about moral decision-making by committee consensus (Moreno, 1988), and there are practical difficulties in ensuring a timely response to urgent problems. An individual ethicist is more flexible (although if acting alone cannot always be available) and will have the requisite training in the knowledge and skills required for ethics consultation. But an individual may be less accountable than a committee, and personal bias or conflict of interest may be more of a problem. In practice a combination of models is probably desirable, and some institutions are able to provide this (Smith et al., 2004). There is currently no empirical evidence to suggest which model is more effective.

PROCESS ISSUES: WHO SHOULD BE INVOLVED?

Depending on the model of case consultation, a variety of people may be involved as 'consultants', the whole CEC, including health professionals and lay members, a small group of mainly health professionals, or an individual ethicist. The person requesting the consultation is presumably essential, as without that person there would be no 'consultation'. However, there may be situations where an ethicist working in the hospital identifies an issue and initiates the consultation process. An initial default position would be that all those directly involved or affected by the decision should be involved in the consultation process. Patients' families think that family members and those who know the patient best should be involved (Day et al., 1994). The nature of the involvement may vary depending on the situation. Agich describes the consultation process at the Cleveland Clinic as being flexible to the situational context and preferences of those involved, sometimes taking the form of a case conference and at other times consisting of a series of dialogues between the ethicist and the relevant individuals including patients and clinicians (Agich, 2003). However, requests for ethics advice and support may not present in a formal consultation request but may take the form of a telephone or corridor conversation in which a clinician seeks the counsel of an ethicist or member of the CEC to talk through a concern that has not reached the stage of requiring a full blown case consultation. Too rigid a conformation to a consultation process protocol could deter clinicians from drawing informally on the knowledge and skills of their ethics colleagues, and opportunities to empower clinicians to identify and resolve ethical issues as part of their daily work could be lost.

If ethics consultation can legitimately take place without the involvement of patients and their families in some situations, should they always be informed that a consultation has taken place? Conversations about patients taking place without their knowledge suggest extreme medical paternalism. The role of ethics committees and ethics consultants has generally been seen as counteracting such practices by ensuring that the voice of the patient is heard. For a committee or consultant to discuss a particular case without informing the patient that this was occurring runs counter to this key aim of ethics consultation. However, is a requirement to always inform a patient when her case is discussed with the ethicist a moral absolute? Ethical guidelines for clinicians would generally allow sharing of patient information with other health professionals when the purpose

of disclosure was to provide optimum care for the patient (General Medical Council, 2004). A key question in the context of ethics consultation must therefore be, is the ethics consultant a member of the health care team? An ethicist employed by and working in the hospital may be seen as a member of the team, but it is less clear that a member of the ethics committee who does not work at that hospital would be considered as such. An important consideration is the patients' *perception* of an ethics consultant as part of the team. If patients are unaware of the existence of an ethics consultation service they will not expect information to be shared with an ethicist or CEC. In such circumstances disclosure of information will be seen as a breach of their autonomy as implied consent cannot be assumed (UK Clinical Ethics Network, 2006).

Even in the case of a formal ethics consultation process, there may be occasional, if rare, circumstances when a patient or family member may not be informed of the consultation.

Consider the following cases:

1. A physician has been asked by the mother of an adolescent patient not to tell her daughter that the medication she is receiving for behavioural problems is an antidepressant drug. She is fearful that if her daughter knows this she will stop the medication and her behaviour will deteriorate such that it will be impossible for the family to function and her daughter will need to be taken into care.
2. Following genetic testing of a child and her parents for a familial disorder, it becomes clear that that the man is not the genetic father of the child. The geneticist is unsure about whether to disclose this information to the parents.

In both of these cases, to inform the patients of the case consultation would be to pre-empt the ethical enquiry raised by the referral. Unless we take an absolutist view of patient autonomy, consideration of harms and benefits to the patient, and to others, may on occasion justify consultation without patient involvement or knowledge.

THEORETICAL AND METHODOLOGICAL ISSUES: HOW IS IT DONE?

The extensive literature on ethics case consultation is characterized by recurring themes of the legitimacy of ethics consultation and the nature of moral expertise, (Agich, 1990), competencies required by ethics consultants (American Society for Bioethics and the Humanities, 1998), and the model of consultation (committee or consultant) (La-Puma & Toulmin, 1989). There has been less debate about the methods used by ethics consultants and CECs in facilitating a resolution of the ethical difficulties that precipitated the request for consultation. The historical development of clinical ethics and ethics consultation lent itself to an abstract principlist or deductive approach to consultation. One reason for the development of ethics consultants and committees was that ethics was no longer seen as an integral part of the practice of medicine generating its own rules and norms but as the specification of more general, perhaps universal, moral rules and as such a topic for philosophical reflection and analysis, external to the practice of medicine. The ethics consultant was someone who brought knowledge of moral theories and principles and skills of analytical reasoning to bear on the ethical conflicts that modern medicine created. The most well documented and frequently used example of this deductive approach is that of the Four Principles of Biomedical Ethics developed by Beauchamp and Childress (Beauchamp, 2003). The strength of the principlist approach is that it provides a clear framework with which to consider the moral complexities of an individual case. It is a model frequently used by CECs, particularly in the early stages of their development. A criticism of a principlist approach is that it oversimplifies the analysis of the ethical issues by not taking account of the realities of the clinical context.

Other methodologies have been suggested as alternative or complementary approaches to ethics consultation, and are used in practice to varying degrees. Casuistry or case based reasoning has a long tradition in moral philosophy, and persuasive advocates in clinical ethics (Arras, 1991; Jonsen, 1991). It seeks to find the moral meaning and resolution of the problem from a detailed analysis of the facts of the case and comparison with paradigm cases from the literature or past experience. It is an exercise in practical reasoning, recognizing the relationship between principles, circumstances and forms of argument relevant to cases of a similar sort. Narrative ethics and feminist ethics theories have also been drawn on to develop a richer theoretical approach to ethics consultation (DeRenzo & Strauss, 1997); (Charon & Montello, 1999). These approaches emphasize the importance of acknowledging the experiences that shape how moral agents (patients, their families and clinicians) perceive their role in a given situation. Thus, effective consultation must include an exploration of the different perspectives and different conceptions of the currently assumed values and principles of those involved in the case. It must also include a consideration of the broader context in which a dilemma has arisen (for example institutional policies or practices and social circumstances of the patient). Other theoretical approaches to ethics consultation include hermeneutics (Thomasma, 1994; Ten-Have, 1994) and deliberative ethics (Gracia, 2003), both emphasizing the interpretive nature of the endeavour in different ways. A phenomenological reading of ethics consultation has also been offered, arguing that the ethics consultant is inevitably a part of the case and sometimes shapes 'the very circumstances that give meaning to the case' (Agich,

2005). This interpretation sees clinical ethics and ethics consultation as part of medical practice rather than as a neutral facilitator or commentator, a striking contrast to the principlist approach.

In addition to the theoretical underpinning of case analysis in ethics consultation, there has been debate about the role of the ethicist or ethics committee in the process of consultation and how consultation is enacted in daily practice. Ethics consultation is commonly seen in terms of conflict resolution and mediation, recognizing that many of the issues that are referred to a CEC or ethicist arise from seemingly irreconcilable differences either between different health professionals or between physicians and patients' families (Reiter-Theil, 2001b; DuVal et al., 2001). In this scenario the ethics consultant is a neutral facilitator, with mediation and counselling skills providing a common language of ethics which can be used to move towards a consensus solution. Another view of the ethics consultant is one of the clinician ethicist working in the medical model of consultation (La-Puma & Schiedermayer, 1991b). The ethics consultant in this scenario focuses on the diagnosis of the ethical problem, works through the therapeutic options and reaches a solution. In contrast to this medical model, others see the ethics consultant as a member of a multidisciplinary team, with skills drawn from a variety of backgrounds including philosophy, sociology, theology, law, and health care (Baylis, 1994). What these slightly different views of the role of ethics consultation have in common is the focus on the care of the individual patient, whether this is conceptualized in a narrow medical model or in a broader social and psychological context. A slightly different view of the role of ethics consultation is that where the goal of consultation is not resolution of conflict in individual cases but the creation and sustenance of a moral community (Zoloth-Dorfman & Rubin, 1997). This interpretation envisages ethics consultation as an activity necessarily involving an ethics committee rather than the domain of an individual ethicist. These varying interpretations of the role of ethics consultants and ethics committees reflect the continuing debate about what is the exact nature of ethics consultation.

ACCOUNTABILITY AND LEGITIMACY OF ETHICS CONSULTATION AND ETHICS COMMITTEES

The legitimacy of CECs and ethics consultation within an individual health care institution, or within society as a whole, depends on a number of things. First, there must be an accepted understanding of what ethics consultation is, both generically and within a specific institution, and what a CEC or ethicist does. To put it simply, a CEC or ethicist must be able to articulate their role and function within the institution, the aims of their work, and the methods by which they plan to achieve their aims, and to demonstrate that they have the necessary knowledge skills and experience to carry out their work. If they are unable to do this it is unlikely that the community of clinicians, patients and managers for whom they are providing the service will seek their advice or support. The ongoing debate about the role of ethics consultation and the competencies required to do it means that there are no objective standards or guidelines that can be used to demonstrate legitimacy. Instead, this must be a local negotiation between the CEC/ethicist and the community they serve. Gaining legitimacy will also require that CECs/ethicists accept responsibility for their work. Although most ethics consultation is seen as advisory or facilitative (Slowther et al., 2001b) the aim must be in some way to influence behaviour, choices, and viewpoints, and acknowledging that this is so means accepting responsibility for the CEC/ethicist's part in this process (Agich, 1990).

A different kind of legitimacy is that conveyed by legal and regulatory frameworks, and for CECs and ethicists this varies between jurisdictions. In some European countries and in some US states, health care institutions are legally required to have a CEC (Slowther et al., 2001a). However, legislation does not require clinicians to follow the advice of such committees. Very few legal cases have considered specifically the role of CECs or ethicists in the decision-making process of the case in question. Where this has happened (mainly in the United States) the courts have differed in their views. Although early cases appeared to support the idea of a CEC consultation removing the requirement for a case to come to court (In Re Quinlan, 1976), others carried clear messages that decision-making responsibility should not be usurped by a committee (Wolf, 1986). More recently, some US courts have been critical of the role that CECs or ethicists have played in cases brought before them (In the matter of baby K, 1993). In the United Kingdom, there are no laws or regulatory frameworks governing CECs. There is debate within the UK clinical ethics community about the legal liability of CECs, and whether they could be open to a charge of negligence in carrying out their advisory work to health professionals. Much will hinge on the ability of a CEC to demonstrate due process, appropriate skills and knowledge, and the reasonableness of their actions (Hendrick, 2001). Similar debates about the legal legitimacy of CECs have occurred in the United States, and in both the United Kingdom and North America it is recommended that CEC members (and clinical ethicists) are provided with legal indemnity by their employing organizations.

EVALUATION

A striking, though perhaps understandable, feature of the literature on CECs and ethics consultation is the paucity of evaluative studies in this area. In 1996 a conference on evaluation of ethics consultation considered key issues for evaluation, including the aims of ethics consultation, (Fletcher & Siegler, 1996; Tulsky & Fox, 1996), setting the research questions, (Tulsky & Fox, 1996) and developing outcome measures (Fox & Arnold, 1996). A difficulty for any evaluation of ethics committees or ethics consultation lies in the debate over the nature of ethics consultation discussed above. The choice of outcomes to evaluate will depend upon the stated aims of the service concerned. The aims of ethics consultation are often not clearly articulated beyond the very general one of 'improving patient care'. This begs the questions that what do we understand by improved patient care in the context of ethics consultation, and whose understanding are we using in our definition (patients, clinicians, ethicists). Several studies have shown that patients' views on 'ethical' issues such as advance care planning do not correspond with the standard position of the clinical or ethics community (Singer et al., 1998; Martin, Thiel & Singer, 1999; Drought & Koenig, 2002). Thus care needs to be taken in designing evaluative studies of ethics consultation to ensure that relevant and measurable outcomes are identified.

The number and quality of studies on CECs and ethics consultation has risen in the past ten years. Many studies have looked at the process measures rather than outcomes, and others have measured user satisfaction, usually limited to clinician users. More recently, there have been some studies measuring specific outcomes, for example a randomized controlled trial of ethics consultation in intensive care using time spent on a ventilator as an outcome measure (Schneiderman et al., 2003). Some findings from evaluation studies include the following:

1. The frequency of requests to CECs for formal case consultation is low (median 4 per year in one national survey) (McGee & Caplan, 2001).
2. The commonest issues brought to CECs or consultants are around the end of life issues, autonomy and competence (McGee & Caplan, 2001).
3. Ethics consultations are more likely to be requested by clinicians with some training in ethics (DuVal et al., 2001).
4. User satisfaction with ethics consultation is high among clinicians but less among patients and families (McClung et al., 1996).
5. Knowledge of the existence of a CEC and its role in the institution is low among health professionals working in the institution (Hoffmann, 1991).

FUTURE DEVELOPMENTS

The expansion of clinical ethics consultation and clinical ethics committees in recent years seems likely to continue as health care becomes increasingly complex and expectations increase for clinicians to be accountable for their decisions. The increasing focus on the field of clinical ethics will intensify the debate about professionalization, and it seems likely that formal regulation including codes of practice and standards of competency for CECs and ethicists will develop. As empirical ethics is increasingly recognized as a legitimate research paradigm, the opportunities for evaluation and research on the process and outcomes of ethics consultation will increase. Although it is important that clinical ethics demonstrates that it is making a useful contribution to patient care, those working in the field need to resist the assumption that easily measurable outcomes can be identified. A major contribution of ethics consultation may be in the development of a transparent and reflective process of engaging with the moral complexities of clinical care. Demonstration of an effective ethical process is a legitimate outcome for ethics consultation.

The interconnectedness of individuals, organizations and systems in the provision of ethical health care is now being recognized. CECs are becoming involved in organizational issues, and ethics networks are contributing to the systems change at organizational, regional and national levels (Slowther et al., 2004; MacRae et al., 2005). The development and maturation of these networks will provide a sound base for an expanding national and international dialogue on how to achieve ethical health care in the best way wherever it is delivered.

REFERENCES

Agich GJ. Clinical ethics: a role theoretic look. *Soc Sci Med* 1990; **30**(4): 389–99.

Agich GJ. Joining the team: ethics consultation at the Cleveland Clinic. *HEC Forum* 2003; **15**(4): 310–22.

Agich GJ. What kind of doing is clinical ethics? *Theor Med Bioethics* 2005; **26**(1): 7–24.

American Society for Bioethics and the Humanities. *Core competencies for health care ethics consultation.* Glenview, Illinois: American Society for Bioethics and the Humanities, 1998.

Arnoux I. Specificities of French ethics committees. In: Lebeeer G, Moulin M, eds. *Ethical Function in Hospital Ethics Committees: Biomed 2 Working Papers.* Brussels: Universite Libre de Bruxelles, 2000; pp. 59–73.

Arras JD. Getting down to cases: the revival of casuistry in bioethics. *J Med Philos* 1991; **16**: 1–51.

Aulisio MP. Ethics consultation: is it enough to mean well? *HEC Forum* 1999; **11**(3): 208–17.

Aulisio MP, Arnold RM, Younger SJ. Health care ethics consultation: nature, goals, and competencies. A position paper from the Society for Health and Human Values–Society for Bioethics Consultation Task Force on standards for bioethics consultation. *Ann Intern Med* 2000; **133**(1): 59–69.

Baylis F, ed. *The Health Care Ethics Consultant.* Totowa, New Jersey: Humana Press, 1994.

Beauchamp TL. Methods and principles in biomedical ethics. *J Med Ethics* 2003; **29**(5): 269–74.

Benatar SR, Bhutta ZA, Daar AS, Hope T, MacRae S, Roberts LW, Sharpe VA. Clinical ethics revisited: responses. *BMC Med Ethics* 2001; **2**: E2.

Blake DC. The hospital ethics committee. Health care's moral conscience or white elephant? *Hastings Center Rep* 1992; **22**(1): 6–11.

Busby A, Rauh JR. Implementing an ethics committee in rural institutions. *JONA* 1991.

Canadian Council on Hospital Accreditation. *Guide to Accreditation of Canadian Health Care Facilities.* Section 6.11. 2006. Ottawa: CCHA, 2006.

Carbonelle S, Schmitz P. Ethical function in Belgian Hospital Ethics Committees: Historical overview. In: Lebeer G, Moulin M, eds. *Ethical Function in Hospital Ethics Committees: Biomed 2 Working Papers.* Brussels: Universite Libre de Bruxelles, 2000; pp. 39–45.

Charon R, Montello M. Framing the case: narrative approaches for healthcare ethics committees. *HEC Forum* 1999; **11**(1): 6–15.

Chidwick P, Faith K, Godkin D, Hardingham L. Clinical education of ethicists: the role of a clinical ethics fellowship. *BMC Med Ethics* 2004; **5**: E6.

Christensen KT, Tucker R. Ethics without walls: the transformation of ethics committees in the new healthcare environment. *Camb Q Health Ethics* 1997; **6**: 3–301.

Day JR, Smith ML, Erenberg G, Collins RL. An assessment of a formal ethics committee consultation process. *HEC Forum* 1994.

DeRenzo EG, Strauss M. A feminist model for clinical ethics consultation: increasing attention to context and narrative. *HEC Forum* 1997; **9**(3): 212–27.

Drought TS, Koenig BA. "Choice" in end-of-life decision making: researching fact or fiction? *Gerontologist* 2002; **42**(Spec No 3): 114–28.

DuVal G, Sartorius L, Clarridge B, Gensler G, Danis M. What triggers requests for ethics consultations? *J Med Ethics* 2001; **27**(Suppl 1): i24–9.

Fletcher JC, Hoffmann DE. Ethics committees: time to experiment with standards. *Ann Intern Med* 1994; **120**(4): 335–8.

Fletcher JC, Siegler M. What are the goals of ethics consultation? A consensus statement. *J Clin Ethics* 1996; **7**(2): 122–6.

Fox E, Arnold RM. Evaluating outcomes in ethics consultation research. *J Clin Ethics* 1996; **7**: 2–38.

Fox E. Concepts in evaluation applied to ethics consultation research. *J Clin Ethics* 1996; **7**: 2–21.

General Medical Council. *Confidentiality: Protecting and Providing Information.* London: GMC, 2004.

Goold SD, Kamil LH, Cohan NS, Sefansky SL. Outline of a process for organizational ethics consultation. *HEC Forum* 2000; **12**(1): 69–77.

Gracia D. Ethical case deliberation and decision making. *Med Health Care Philos* 2003; **6**(3): 227–33.

Hendrick J. Legal aspects of clinical ethics committees. *J Med Ethics* 2001; **27**(Suppl 1) i50–3.

Hoffmann DE. Does legislating hospital ethics committees make a difference? A study of hospital ethics committees in Maryland, the District of Columbia, and Virginia. *Law Med Health Care* 1991; **19**(1–2): 105–19.

Hoy J, Feigenbaum E. Making the case for ethics consults in community mental health centers. *Community Ment Health J* 2005; **41**(3): 235–50.

In Re Quinlan. 70N.J. 10;335 A.2d 647, 1976; N.J. LEXIS 181; 79 A.L.R. 3d, 1976.

In the matter of baby K. (832 F. Supp. 1022; 1993 U.S. Dist. LEXIS 12574; 2 Am. Disabilities Cas. (BNA) 1244). United States District Court for the Eastern District of Virginia: Alexandria Division, 1993.

Joint Commission for Accreditation of Health Care Organisations. *Joint Commission for Accreditation of Health Care Organisations: Comprehensive Manual for Hospitals.* Chicago: JCAHO, 1996.

Jonsen AR. Casuistry as methodology in clinical ethics. *Theor Med* 1991; **12**(4): 295–307.

Kerridge IH, Pearson S, Rolfe IE. Determining the function of a hospital clinical ethics committee: making ethics work. *J Q Clin Pract* 1998; **18**: 2–24.

La-Puma J, Schiedermayer DL. Ethics consultation: skills, roles, and training. *Ann Intern Med* 1991a; **114**(2): 155–60.

La-Puma J, Schiedermayer DL. The clinical ethicist at the bedside. *Theor Med* 1991b; **12**: 2–9.

La-Puma J, Toulmin SE. Ethics consultants and ethics committees. *Arch Intern Med* 1989; **149**(2):1109–12.

MacRae S, Chidwick P, Berry S, Secker B, Hebert P, Shaul RZ, Faith K, Singer PA. Clinical bioethics integration, sustainability, and accountability: the Hub and Spokes Strategy. *J Med Ethics* 2005; **31**(5): 256–61.

Martin DK, Thiel EC, Singer PA. A new model of advance care planning: observations from people with HIV. *Arch Intern Med* 1999; **159**(1): 86–92.

McClung JA, Kamer RS, DeLuca M, Barber HJ. Evaluation of a medical ethics consultation service: opinions of patients and health care providers. *Am J Med* 1996; **100**(4): 456–60.

McGee G, Caplan A. A national study of ethics comittees. *Am J Bioethics* 2001; **1**(4): 60–4.

Moreno JD. Ethics by committee: the moral authority of consensus. *J Med Philos* 1988; **13**: 4–32.

Pentz RD. Beyond case consultation: an expanded model for organizational ethics. *J Clin Ethics* 1999; **10**(1): 34–41.

Phillips DF. Ethics consultation quality: is evaluation feasible? *JAMA* 1996; **275**(24): 1866–7.

President's Commission. President's Commission for the study of ethical problems in medicine and biomedical and behavioural research. *Decisions to Forego Life Sustaining Treatment: A Report on the Ethical, Medical and Legal Issues in Treatment Decisions.* Washington, DC: US GPO, 1983; pp. 155–70.

RCP Working Party on Clinical Ethics. *Ethics in Practice: Background and Recommendations for Enhanced Support.* London: Royal College of Physicians, 2005.

Reiter-Theil S. Ethics consultation in Germany: the present situation. *HEC Forum* 2001a; **13**(3): 265–80.

Reiter-Theil S. The Freiburg approach to ethics consultation: process, outcome and competencies. *J Med Ethics* 2001b; **27**(Suppl 1): i21–3.

Ruyter K. Ethics committees: The national situation in Norway. In: Lebeeer G, Moulin M, eds. *Ethical Function in Hospital Ethics Committees.* Brussels: Universite Libre de Bruxelles, 2000; pp. 91–105.

Schneiderman LJ, Gilmer T, Teetzel HD, Dugan DO, Blustein J, Cranford R et al. Briggs KB, Komatsu GI, Goodman-Crews P, Cohn F, Young EW. Effect of ethics consultations on nonbeneficial life-sustaining treatments in the intensive care setting: A randomized controlled trial. JAMA 2003 Sep 3; **290**(9): 1166–72.

Singer PA, Martin DK, Lavery JV, Thiel EC, Kelner M, Mendelssohn DC. Reconceptualizing advance care planning from the patient's perspective. *Arch Intern Med* 1998; **158**(8): 879–84.

Singer PA, Pellegrino ED, Siegler M. Clinical ethics revisited. *BMC Med Ethics* 2001; **2**: E1.

Slowther A, Bunch C, Woolnough B, Hope T. Clinical ethics support services in the UK: an investigation of the current provision of ethics support to health professionals in the UK. *J Med Ethics* 2001a; **27**(Suppl 1) i2–8.

Slowther A, Hope T, Bunc C, Woolnough B. Clinical ethics support in the UK. *Current Position and Likely Development.* London: The Nuffield Trust, 2001b.

Slowther A, Johnston C, Goodall J, Hope T. Development of clinical ethics committees. *BMJ* 2004; **328**(7445): 950–2.

Smith ML, Bisanz AK, Kempfer AJ, Adams B, Candelari TG, Blackburn RK. Criteria for determining the appropriate method for an ethics consultation. *HEC Forum* 2004; **16**(2): 95-113.

Tan SY. Hospital ethics committees: will America's model work in Asia? *Ann Acad Med Singapore* 2002; **31**(6): 808–12.

Tealdi JC, Mainetti JA. Hospital ethics committees. *Bull Pan Am Health Organ* 1990; **24**(4): 410–8.

Ten-Have H. The hyperreality of clinical ethics: a unitary theory and hermeneutics. *Theor Med* 1994; **15**(2): 113–31.

Thomasma DC. Clinical ethics as medical hermeneutics. *Theor Med* 1994; **15**(2): 93–111.

Tulsky JA, Fox E. Evaluating ethics consultation: framing the questions. *J Clin Ethics* 1996; **7**(2): 109–15.

UK Clinical Ethics Network, 2006; www.ethics-network.org.uk.

van der Kloot Meijburg HH, & ter Meulen, R.H. (2001). Developing standards for institutional ethics committees: lessons from The Netherlands. *J Med Ethics* 27(Suppl1): i36-i40.

Wenger NS, Golan O, Shalev C, Glick S. Hospital ethics committees in Israel: structure, function and heterogeneity in the setting of statutory ethics committees. *J Med Ethics* 2002; **28**(3): 177–82.

Wolf SM. Ethics committees in the courts. *Hastings Center Rep* 1986; **16**(3): 12–5.

Wray E. The Padua bioethics service: a model of excellence in clinical ethics? *Bull Med Ethics* 2002; **183**: 13–5.

Zoloth-Dorfman L, Rubin SB. Navigators and captains: expertise in clinical ethics consultation. *Theor Med* 1997; **18**(4): 421–32.

PART III

MEDICINE IN SOCIETY

This third section, 'Medicine in Society', outlines and explores a set of conceptual and ethical issues relating to medicine in a broader social and political contexts. The section begins with some analysis of key concepts relevant to such issues (e.g. health, community, health promotion and prevention), before moving on to a series of chapters focused on the use of key methods in decision making and priority setting in health care (e.g. cost-effectiveness analysis, public preferences, decision analysis) as well as issues related to social structures (e.g. inequities, organizational ethics). The central chapters of this section are focused on discussing ethical issues as they arise in relation to the core issues in public health policy (e.g. epidemiology, screening, vaccination, infectious disease control, bioterrorism, drugs policy and smoking). Finally, the section ends with a return to three issues exploring the nature and limits of moral obligations for professionals and society in relation to human rights, refugees and asylum seekers, and disaster relief.

Lennart Nordenfelt opens this section by exploring the concept of health as a means of thinking about the aims of medicine. He discusses what 'health' is, and what is it to be 'healthy'. He does this through an outline of the different competing theories of health and the underlying philosophical issues, such as the degree to which judgments about health can be value-free. Bruce Jennings focuses, in his chapter, on the meaning and implications of the concept of 'community' and related ethical issues such as solidarity. He argues that such a concept is vital to our discussions in many areas of public health, but that this is often forgotten. He focuses on the potential conflict between the interests of

the individual and the community by considering a US legal case about vaccination. He argues that ultimately we should not see the individual and community as being in conflict, as the individual can only become who they are within the context of a community. Alan Cribb explores the meaning of 'health promotion' and the distinctive ethical issues that arise in this area of health work. He also argues forcefully for a key role for social science in our practical and theoretical reflections upon these issues. For example, any answer to the question about the extent to which inequalities are the result of, say, social class or individual behaviours should be central to the formation of ethical policy. Marcel Verweij's chapter discusses a key issue in public health policy, given its focus on prevention. He outlines a series of difficulties and problems with the idea that prevention is always preferable to cure. For example, the analysis of benefits and harms is difficult in such cases due to the distribution of these factors between individuals and populations; there are important concerns about the increasing medicalization of life; as well as a general worry about the imposition of restrictions as to what counts as a good life.

Beginning the second group of chapters, Daniel Wikler *et al.* focus on the ethical issues in relation to priority setting in health, particularly the way that assumptions shape the methodology of cost-effectiveness analysis. These hidden values are often taken for granted by policy makers, despite their contentious nature. Jeff Richardson and John McKie continue the same theme, by exploring the theoretical assumptions of economists, though this time the focus is on the role of public preferences. The role of preferences in general has been central to welfare economics, due to the idea that individuals are held to know better than anyone else what is best for them. This chapter explores some of the problems with such a view. Jack Dowie explains and defends the use of decision analysis in clinical decision making: indeed, he goes as far as to argue that it is unethical not to use it. He argues that this methodology allows the best possible decision to be made, explicitly taking into account both medical evidence and values, rather than being based on the shakier ground of 'intuition' or 'experience'. Wendy Rogers explores the role of social determinants of health as a source of many of the inequities in health that arise from both injustice and failures to respond to relevant duties. Health care policy can be focused on the reduction of such inequities if the will is there, and such an approach can be justified by appeal to values such as justice and fairness. Jacob Kurlander and Marion Danis provide an introduction to the new field of organizational ethics and demonstrate how these issues are relevant to health care. They outline a series of ethical questions that require discussion. What responsibilities does a health care organization have? What should its priorities be? What organizational structures are ethical? The discussion draws upon literature from both business and professional ethics.

Steven Coughlin opens the third group of chapters focused on key issues in public health, by discussing a series of ethical issues related to epidemiology, the key methodology of public health. Epidemiology is focused on the distribution and causes of disease at the population level. This means that many of the ethical issues it raises are different from those discussed in traditional research ethics, as there is a tension between individuals and their rights and the need to include everyone in the relevant population for an accurate analysis of the problem. Niklas Juth and Christian Munthe begin their discussion of screening by focusing on the definition of 'screening'. They argue that screening is a population-level intervention, and that this is the source of many of the ethical problems associated with this issue. They explore how values are integrated into decisions about screening, particularly in relation to the aims of such programmes. In his chapter on vaccinations, Angus Dawson outlines a number of different arguments that can be developed in relation to the ethics of vaccination policies. He argues that vaccinations are a classic public health issue because the focus of policy should not only be upon the individual. The existence of herd protection in a population is an important public good, and so vaccination policy should aim to promote this good, not just focus on decision making in relation to individuals. Peggy Battin *et al.* focus on the ethical issues in relation to infectious disease. They argue that these issues have been neglected until relatively recently, but that their conceptual tool of thinking about patients with infectious disease as being both victim and vector allows us to see the complexity of the relevant ethical issues. They suggest that looking at infectious disease in this way will also then allow us to develop a new perspective upon bioethics in general. Michael Selgelid focuses on a number of ethical issues related to the topic of bioterrorism. Some of these relate to clinical decision making about who should be a priority for treatment (e.g. those most in need or those most needed by society). However, he also explores the extent to which health care professionals have a duty to treat patients even when their own lives might be in increased danger as a result. He ends by considering more general policy issues such as the importance of research in this area, and the responsibility of scientists to take care in their publications not to reveal information that might be used by potential bioterrorists. Wayne Hall and Adrian Carter discuss a series of issues relating to the use of drugs in society. Are addicts responsible for their actions? Is it ethical to restrict access to certain drugs? What are the societal costs of drug use, and what role should such costs play in policy formation? Is there any role for paternalism and coercion in drug treatment policy? Bob Goodin's chapter picks up the idea of free choice and its limits in relation to smoking policy. To what extent do smokers choose to smoke, and what follows from our answer to this question? He argues that in relation to smoking, the issue is not about lack of information about the dangers, but the extent of free choice in the light of addiction.

In the final groups of chapters in this section, Doris Schroeder outlines a series of theoretical issues about the nature of human rights before turning to the role of doctors in supporting and promoting (as well as transgressing) human rights. She argues that given the nature of medicine, it is natural to think of doctors as playing a role in the protection of human rights, although it should not be forgotten that they could also be involved in their violation. Pascale Allotey *et al.* discuss the role of health care workers in nontraditional roles, such as judgements about the legitimacy of the social and political grounds claimed by refugees and asylum seekers. Beyond these professional roles, what obligations do host countries have to these new arrivals? Is there a difference between the obligations arising, for example, from mental illness caused by torture and the consequences of being HIV positive upon arrival? Finally, Soren Holm discusses our obligations in the special case of disaster relief. He argues that virtually all ethical theories support the idea that we have such as obligation, and that this might even be used as a means of judging the reasonableness of such theories. He suggests the real debate is over the extent of such an obligation in relation to both individuals and governments. He also discusses the separate issue about the difficult but inevitable role of triage in medical responses to disasters.

Angus Dawson

The Concepts of Health and Illness

LENNART Y. NORDENFELT

INTRODUCTION

It is often maintained that health is one of the major goals of medicine or even *the* goal of medicine. This idea has been eloquently formulated by the American philosophers of medicine Edmund Pellegrino and David Thomasma in their book *Philosophy as the Basis of Medicine* (Pellegrino & Thomasma, 1981, p. 26):

> Medicine is an activity whose essence appears to lie in the clinical event, which demands that scientific and other knowledge be particularized in the lived reality of a particular human for the purpose of attaining health or curing illness, through the direct manipulation of the body and in a value-laden decision matrix.

Although some other goals of medicine exist, such as the basic goal of saving lives and the recently developed goal of quality of life, health is, indeed, the foremost goal of medicine and public health (Pellegrino & Thomasma, 1981; Callahan & Hanson, 1999). Health that also has a prominent position in many life contexts is a crucial condition for maintaining and executing a profession, for enjoying leisure activities and, indeed, for living a good life in general. Health is indeed a formal prerequisite for performing certain tasks or taking up certain occupations such as that of soldier, policeman or fire-fighter. More compelling is the place of mental health as a condition for moral and criminal culpability.

However, the formidable task of interpreting the nature of health remains to be pursued. What, more specifically, is health? To what more precise goal shall we direct our efforts in medicine and health care?

These questions are not simply academic. They are of great practical and thereby ethical concern. The consequences for health care diverge considerably, not least in economic but also in social and educational terms, depending on whether health is understood as people's happiness, or their fitness and ability to work or, instead, just the absence of obvious pathology in their bodies and minds. There are adherents of all these ideas in the modern theoretical discussion on health.

Etymologically, health is connected with the idea of wholeness. This is evident in the verb 'heal', with the sense of regaining wholeness. The healthy person is a person who is whole in the sense of having all the properties that should pertain to a human being. Health has thus traditionally been viewed as an ideal notion, a notion of perfection that very few people, if any, can completely attain. Today health also sometimes functions as an ideal notion. This is, indeed, the case with the formulation of health by the World Health Organization in its initial declaration, published in 1948: 'Health is a state of complete physical, mental and social well-being and not only the absence of disease or injury.'

The notion of health is the object of scientific study from several points of view and within several disciplines. Besides research by those in medicine, public health, nursing and other paramedical disciplines, other investigations are based in anthropology, psychology, sociology and philosophy. In some of these disciplines the focus is on a particular aspect of the notion: in psychology, the experience of health and illness, or, in anthropology and sociology, health and illness as factors of social importance. Philosophical analyses of health have often involved an attempt to formulate global definitions of the idea. Thus, in the following, many references will be taken from philosophical theories of health.

THE VARIETIES OF HEALTH

Health, thus, is a notion primarily applicable to a human being as a whole. On the contrary, there are more specific derivative notions. Ever since antiquity, and reinforced by the Cartesian

This chapter draws upon material from the author's work Health in Albrecht *et al World Encyclopedia of Disability*. Reproduced by permission of Sage Publications.

Principles of Health Care Ethics, Second Edition   Edited by R.E. Ashcroft, A. Dawson, H. Draper and J.R. McMillan

distinction between body and mind, it has been natural to separate somatic health from mental health. The interpretations of mental health have varied over time. The ancient notion of mental health was closely connected to morality, whereby the mentally healthy person was a person who lived a virtuous life, but this idea has lost most, though not all, of its significance today. The idea of spiritual health is also current in the health sciences though it is not systematically recognized. Bernhard Häring (1987) is a leading spokesman for a notion of health including a spiritual dimension: 'A comprehensive understanding of human health includes the greatest possible harmony of all of man's forces and energies, the greatest possible spiritualization of man's bodily aspect and the finest embodiment of the spiritual' (Häring, 1987)

The various categories of health have connections to each other. Sometimes bodily health has been given priority in the sense that it has been viewed as a prerequisite for mental health. Galen (ca. AD 129–216/7) in some of his writings attempted to explain mental properties of the person in terms of specific mixtures of the bodily parts (Galen, 1997). Consider also the ancient proverb: *mens sana in corpore sano* (a healthy mind in a healthy body). In the modern discussion about mental illness, one position, favoured in particular by medical doctors, is that all mental illness has a somatic background, that is, all mental illnesses – if they exist at all– are basically somatic diseases (Szasz, 1974). The customary view, however, also in Western medicine, is that a person can at the same time be somatically healthy and mentally ill, or vice versa.

THE LATITUDE OF HEALTH

Since antiquity theorists of health have emphasized that the health–ill health dichotomy is not represented by two opposite states. There is instead a dimension or latitude of health from optimal health to maximal ill health. According to this idea a person can be in a state that is far from optimal health, but still be healthy. Likewise, people's state of ill health can vary between mildly ill and seriously ill. Galen is perhaps the philosopher who has contributed most to the analysis of the latitude of health. He made more distinctions in this respect than are customary today. He not only distinguished between health and ill health but also acknowledged a state in between these called the neuter state. This means that, according to Galen, a person can be neither healthy nor ill, but instead be in a neuter state along the health–ill health dimension. This idea concerning a latitude of health was developed in several sophisticated ways in the medieval medical discussion. For a thorough analysis, see Ottosson (1982).

HEALTH, DISEASE AND ILLNESS

In many contributions to the theory of health a distinction is made between the concepts of disease and illness

(Boorse, 1975; Twaddle, 1993; Fulford, 1989). The general idea behind this distinction – although it has been made in different ways by different authors – is that a disease is a deranged process in the person's body whereas an illness is the person's negative experiences, for instance, pain or anguish, as a result of the disease. In addition, some theories include disability in illness, see below. The distinction between disease and illness has proved useful in several contexts, including the clinical one, (Hellström, 1993) for separating the disease as a pathological phenomenon from its impact on the person as a whole.

THE BASIC THEORIES OF HEALTH

HEALTH AS BALANCE

An extremely powerful idea in the history of medicine is the one that health is constituted by bodily and mental balance. The healthy person is a person in balance, normally meaning that different parts and different functions of the human body and mind interlock harmoniously and keep each other in check. The Hippocratic and Galenic schools (Hippocrates 460–380 BC and Galen AD 129–216/7) were the first Western schools to develop this idea in a systematic way. They stated that a healthy body is one where the primary properties (wet, dry, cold, hot) of the body balance each other. In the medieval schools, following Galen, this idea was popularized and formulated in terms of a balance between the four bodily humours: blood, phlegm, yellow bile and black bile.

The idea of balance is strong in several non-Western medical traditions. The Yahurveda tradition in India, for instance, declares that there are three humours acting in the body, the breath (*vata*), the bile (*pitta*), and the phlegm (*kapha*). The proportions of the three humours vary from person to person, and their actions vary according to the season, the environment, the lifestyle of the individual and his or her diet. In good health the humours are in equilibrium. Disease is the result of their imbalance (Singhal & Patterson, 1993).

Balance is a powerful idea also in modern Western thought, in particular, within physiology. The idea is then often to be recognized under the label of *homoeostasis* (the Greek word for balance). Walter Cannon's (1871–1945) classical work on homoeostasis (Cannon, 1932) describes in detail how the various physiological functions of the body control each other and interact in feedback loops in order to prevent major disturbances.

The idea of balance or *equilibrium* (the Latin word for balance) has a rather different interpretation in the writings of Pörn (1993). Here balance is a concept pertaining to the relationship between a person's abilities and his or her goals.

The healthy person, according to Pörn, is the person who can realize his or her goals and thus retain a balance between abilities and goals. (Campare health as ability, below.)

HEALTH AS ABSENCE OF DISEASE; THE IDEA OF A NATURAL FUNCTION

Although health is often described in non-medical terms and with reference to non-medical contexts, it has its primary place and function as a medical concept. Health in the medical arena is contrasted in particular with disease, but also with injury, defect and disability. Culver and Gert (1982) have coined the term 'malady' to cover the negative antipodes of health. In many medical contexts (Hesslow, 1993) and in some philosophical reconstructions of the notion of health (Boorse, 1977, 1997), health has been defined as the absence of diseases or the absence of maladies. The perfectly healthy person, therefore, is the person who does not have any diseases or maladies.

If one looks upon the relationship between the concepts in this way, the burden of definition lies on the negative notions. Christopher Boorse (1997) for instance, defines disease in the following terms: 'A disease is a type of internal state which is either an impairment of normal functional ability, i.e. a reduction of one or more functional abilities below typical efficiency, or a limitation on functional ability caused by environmental agents.' The notion of functional ability, in this theory, is in its turn related to the person's survival and reproduction, in other words, his or her fitness. From this analysis it follows that we need not use the notion of disease in order to define health. The same idea can be formulated in the following positive terms: a person is completely healthy if, and only if, all his or her organs function with at least typical efficiency (in relation to survival and reproduction.)

Boorse (1997) calls his concept of disease a pathologist's concept. It is not the clinician's. Boorse does not here analyse the state of affairs normally denoted by the term 'illness', which has a subjective component, the feeling of illness (see above). Nor does he analyse any social or legal category, sometimes referred to as 'sickness', in other words the social and legal role adopted by the person who is ill (Twaddle, 1993).

The idea of functional ability is similar to, but not identical with, the notion of natural function proposed by Wakefield (1992) where the platform for analysis is biological evolutionary theory. The natural function F of an organ is, according to this idea, the function for which it has been designed through evolution. This means that the species in question (for instance, the human being) has been able to reproduce through history with the genetic set-up for the function F. This idea has been criticized partly because it relates the idea of health in the present context to developments in the past (Nordenfelt, 2003).

HEALTH AS WELL-BEING

It is an important aspect of health that the body and mind are well, both in order and function. But we may ask for the criteria of such well-functioning. How do we know that the body and mind function well? When is a body in balance?

A traditional answer is that the person's subjective well-being is the ultimate criterion (Canguilhem, 1978). Simply put: when a person feels well, then he or she is healthy. This statement certainly entails problems because a person can feel well and still have a serious disease in its initial stage. The general idea can, however, be modified to cover this case too. The individual with a serious disease will sooner or later have negative experiences such as pain, fatigue or anguish. Thus, the ultimate criterion of a person's health is his or her present or future well-being. (For a different approach suggesting that complete health is compatible with the existence of disease, see Nordenfelt, 1995, 2001).

It is a difficult task to characterize the well-being constituting health. If one includes too much in the concept there is a risk of identifying health with happiness. It is, indeed, a common accusation directed against the WHO definition that it falls into this trap. Health cannot reasonably be identical with complete physical, mental and social well-being, many critics say. The absurd conclusion of this conception could be that all people who are not completely successful in life would be deemed unhealthy.

Some authors (Gadamer, 1993; Leder, 1990) have pointed out that phenomenological health (or health as experienced) tends to remain as a forgotten background. Health in daily life is hardly recognized at all by its subjects. People are reminded of their previous health first when it is being disrupted, when they experience the pain, nausea or anguish of illness. Health is 'felt' only under special circumstances, the major instance being after periods of illness when the person experiences relief in contrast to the previous suffering.

Thus, although well-being or absence of ill-being is an important trait in health, most modern positive characterizations of health have focused on other traits. One such trait is health as a condition for action, that is, ability.

HEALTH AS ABILITY

A number of authors in modern philosophy of health have emphasized the place of health as a foundation for achievement (Parsons, 1972; Whitbeck, 1981; Seedhouse, 1986; Fulford, 1989; Nordenfelt, 1995). In fact, they argue, in partly different ways, that the dimension ability/disability is the core dimension determining whether health or ill health is the case. A healthy person has the ability to do what he or she needs to do, and the unhealthy person is prevented from performing one or more of these actions. There is a connection between this conception and the one that illness entails suffering. Disability is often the result of feelings such as pain, fatigue or nausea.

The formidable task for these theorists is to characterize the set of actions that a healthy person should be able to perform. Parsons (1972) and Whitbeck (1981) refer to the subject's wants, that is, the healthy person's being able to do what he or she wants, Seedhouse (1986) to the person's conscious choices, and Fulford (1989) to such actions as could be classified as 'ordinary doings'. Nordenfelt settles for what he calls the subject's vital goals. These goals need not be consciously chosen (also babies and people with dementia have vital goals). The goals have the status as vital goals because they are states of being that are necessary conditions for the person's minimal happiness in the long run. Health in Nordenfelt's theory is thus conceptually related to, but indeed not identical with, happiness.

Although it is evident that health, as ordinarily understood, is connected with ability, and ill health with disability, one may still doubt whether the dimension ability/disability can remain the sole criterion of health/ill health. An important argument concerns those disabled people who are not ill, according to common understanding, and who do not consider themselves to be ill. These people are to be classified as unhealthy according to the ability theories of health.

One answer to this question (Nordenfelt, 2001) is that disabled people need not be unhealthy if their disability is established merely according to conventional measurements. There are several standardized instruments for the measurement of disability today. (See for instance the so-called DALY-instrument (Reidpath et al., 2003). People are unhealthy only if their disability is established in relation to their individual vital goals. Moreover, a disabled person of course need not have any diseases. Both disability and ill health in Nordenfelt's system are compatible with the absence of diseases. Health can be reduced by causes other than maladies. Another answer, proposed by Svenaeus (2001) is that there is a phenomenological difference between the disabled unhealthy person and the disabled healthy person. The unhealthy person has a feeling of not being 'at home', with regard to his or her present state of body or mind. This feeling is not present in the case of the disabled in general.

Observe also that the notion of disease (or malady) will have a slightly different connotation given an ability- or well-being-centred concept of health than it has according to the naturalistic account. For the naturalist Boorse, a disease is a dysfunction in relation to the survival of the individual and the species. For the ability- or well-being theorist, on the other hand, a disease is a dysfunction in relation to the individual's ability or well-being.

SOME ISSUES IN CONTEMPORARY PHILOSOPHY OF HEALTH

HEALTH AND VALUE. NATURALISTS AND NORMATIVISTS

A crucial theoretical problem in the characterization of health is whether this notion is a scientific one or not. One can ask whether health and its opposites can be given a neutral, rather than value-laden description, or whether it follows by necessity that health is to be characterized as a 'good' bodily or mental state. Proponents of the former view are often called naturalists, whereas proponents of the latter view are often called normativists.

Different theorists have arrived at different conclusions with respect to this issue. Boorse (1977, 1997) claims that there is a value-neutral definition of the basic notion of disease. Donald Broom (1993), who analyses the notions of animal health and welfare, comes to the same conclusion. Wakefield (1992) argues for the thesis that the notion of disease has two parts, one of which is value-neutral, that is, the one that refers to the natural function of organs. The other part of the concept, however, refers to the value-laden notion of harm. Most other theorists, however, think that the notion of health and its opposites are with necessity value-laden. Some argue that these values are universal (Pellegrino & Thomasma, 1981), others that the values determining the concepts of health and illness are connected to the background cultures (Engelhardt, 1996). The physician/philosopher Canguilhem (1978), who wrote one of the most significant treatises of human health and illness of the twentieth century, though he drew almost exclusively upon medical data, came to the conclusion that health is an evaluative concept in a strong sense. The healthy organism, says Canguilhem, is not an organism whose functions are normal in a statistical sense. The healthy organism is one that is 'normative', that is, one that is capable of adopting new norms in life.

One can discern further differences in the contention that the notion of health is value-laden. Some theorists (for instance Khushf, 2001) claim that the notion is value-laden in the strong sense that its descriptive content can vary over time. As a result of this, the only element common to an ancient and a modern concept of health is that health is a 'good' state of a person's body or mind. Others, like the ability theorists above, would claim that there is a common descriptive content, in other words, the fact that health has to do with a person's abilities, but that one needs to make an evaluation in order to specify what aspect or level of ability is required for health.

HEALTH AND CULTURE RELATIVISM

If health is a value-laden concept then, as we have seen, some would argue that there are differences in the interpretation of health between cultures both historically and geographically. It is important to note that these differences can be more or less profound.

The concepts of health can vary from culture to culture because there are fundamental differences in the basic philosophy of health and health care, as between Western medicine and traditional Chinese medicine or the traditional Indian *Ayurveda* medicine. Western medicine, which is to a great extent based on a naturalistic philosophy of man, arrives easily at a naturalistic understanding of health, whereas oriental schools with a holistic understanding of man in a religious context derive a notion of health which incorporates forces and developments that are partly supernatural.

The ways of and reasons for ascribing health to people may, however, vary even if there is a basic common theory of health and disease. Consider a particular physiological state, the state of lactase deficiency, which has the status of disease in a Western country but not in most North African countries. In combination with ordinary consumption of milk, lactase deficiency causes diarrhoea and abdominal pain. Thus, in Western countries where people usually drink milk, lactase deficiency will typically lead to illness. Therefore, this state ought to be included in a list of diseases in these countries. In North Africa, however, people rarely drink milk. Therefore, lactase deficiency seldom leads to illness. Consequently it would be misleading to consider lactase deficiency a disease in this part of the world.

What makes the difference between the Western and the African cultures in this example is not necessarily different concepts of disease. It could be a question of different lifestyles and different environments judged from the point of view of a single concept of disease.

HEALTH AND ILLNESS AS GENDER-DEPENDENT NOTIONS

Some theorists contend that the way we define and in general look upon health and health care is dependent on our gender (Oakley, 1993). This difference is well reflected in the traditional health professions. The traditional doctor is a man who is basically concerned with the physical condition of his patients. He sees his primary task as being to cure the diseases of the patient by the use of well-established treatments often in the form of surgery and drugs. The traditional nurse is a woman who is basically concerned with the general well-being of the patient. She sees her primary task as being to care for the person as a whole. Caring, for her, means above all 'relating to the ill person as a whole person

whose psyche is equally involved with her or his soma in the illness in question' (Oakley, 1993).

HEALTH OF HUMAN BEINGS VERSUS HEALTH OF ANIMALS AND PLANTS

Health, disease and the other central medical concepts are not used only in the human context. We usually ascribe health and disease also to animals and plants. Do we then apply the same concept of health?

In this case the answers differ. The naturalists, who relate health solely to survival and reproduction, can easily transpose their concept to the world of animals and plants. The same could hold for balance theorists. It is more problematic to use the idea of health as ability or, even more, the idea of health as well-being all over the world of animals and plants. This can serve as an argument in favour of the naturalistic account. On the contrary, it can be argued that there is an enormous difference between the human context and the context of other living entities. Human beings live in complex societies with complex demands and with a system of health care that is supposed to serve these demands. Health is important for a human being because it enables him or her to engage in crucial activities, such as work, political activities and leisure activities, and not least, to engage in close human relations such as friendship and love. Thus, the health concept that is of interest to most people is a holistic concept embracing all such relevant abilities. Therefore, it is no wonder that the concept of human health has evolved in directions quite different from the concepts of health concerning animals and plants.

REFERENCES

Boorse C. On the distinction between disease and illness. *Philos Public Affairs* 1975; 5: 49–68.

Boorse C. Health as a theoretical concept. *Philos Sci* 1977; **44**: 542–73.

Boorse C. A Rebuttal on health. In: Humber J, Almeder R, eds. *What is Disease? Biomedical Ethics Reviews*. Totowa, NJ: Humana Press, 1997.

Broom DM. A usable definition of animal welfare. *J Agric Environ Ethics* 1993; 15–25.

Callahan D, Hanson MJ. *The Goals of Medicine: The Forgotten Issues*. Washington, DC: Georgetown University Press, 1999.

Canguilhem G. *On the Normal and the Pathological*. Dordrecht: D. Reidel Publishing Company, 1978.

Cannon WB. *The Wisdom of the Body*. New York: Norton, 1932.

Culver CM, Gert E. *Philosophy in Medicine: Conceptual and Ethical Issues in Medicine and Psychiatry*. Oxford: Oxford University Press, 1982.

Engelhardt HT Jr. *The Foundations of Bioethics*, 2nd edition. Oxford: Oxford University Press, 1996.

Fulford KWM. *Moral Theory and Medical Practice*. Cambridge: Cambridge University Press, 1989.

Gadamer H-G. *Über die Verborgenheit der Gesundheit*. Frankfurt am Main: Suhrkamp Verlag, 1993.

Galen. *Selected Works* (Translated with an introduction and notes by P.N. Singer). Oxford: Oxford University Press, 1997.

Häring B. *Medical Ethics*. Middlegreen, Slough: St. Paul Publications, 1987; p. 154.

Hellström O. The importance of a holistic concept of health for health care: Examples from the clinic. *Theor Med* 1993; **14**: 325–42.

Hesslow G. Do we need a concept of disease? *Theor Med* 1993; **14**: 1–14.

Khushf G. What is at issue in the debate about concepts of health and disease? framing the problem of demarcation for a post-positivist era of medicine. In: Nordenfelt L, ed. *Health, Science, and Ordinary Language*. Amsterdam: Rodopi Publishers, 2001.

Leder D. Clinical Interpretation: The hermeneutics of medicine. *Theor Med* 1990; **11**: 9–24.

Nordenfelt L. *On the Nature of Health: An Action-Theoretic Approach*, 2nd revised edition. Dordrecht: Kluwer Academic Publishers, 1995.

Nordenfelt L. *Health, Science and Ordinary Language*. Amsterdam: Rodopi Publishers, 2001.

Nordenfelt L. Health as natural function. In: Nordenfelt L, Liss P-E, eds. *Dimensions of Health and Health Promotion*. Amsterdam: Rodopi Publishers, 2003; pp. 37–54.

Oakley A. *Essays on Women, Medicine and Health*. Edinburgh: Edinburgh University Press, 1993; p. 40.

Ottosson P-G. *Scholastic Medicine and Philosophy*. Naples: Bibliopolis, 1982.

Parsons T. Definitions of health and illness in the light of American values and social structure. In: Jaco EG, ed. *Patients, Physicians, and Illness*. New York: The Free Press, 1972.

Pellegrino ED, Thomasma DC. *A Philosophical Basis of Medical Practice*. Oxford: Oxford University Press, 1981.

Pörn I. Health and adaptedness. *Theor Med* 1993; **14**: 295–304.

Reidpath DD, Allotey PA, Kouame A, Cummins RA. Measuring health in a vacuum: examining the disability weight of the DALY. *Health Policy Plan* 2003; **18**: 351–6.

Seedhouse D. *Health: Foundations of Achievement*. Chichester: John Wiley & Sons, 1986.

Singhal GD, Patterson TJS. *Synopsis of Ayurveda*, based on a translation of the Treatise of Susruta. Delhi and Oxford: Oxford University Press, 1993.

Svenaeus F. *The Hermeneutics of Medicine and the Phenomenology of Health*. Dordrecht: Kluwer Academic Publishers, 2001.

Szasz T. *The Myth of Mental Illness*, revised edition. New York: Harper & Row, 1974.

Twaddle AR. Disease, illness and sickness revisited. In: Twaddle AR, Nordenfelt L, eds. *Disease, Illness and Sickness: Three Central Concepts in the Theory of Health*. Studies on Health and Society, vol. 18. Sweden: Linköping, 1993.

Wakefield JC. The concept of mental disorder: on the boundary between biological facts and social values. *Am Psychol* 1992; **47**, 373–88.

Whitbeck C. A theory of health. In: Caplan AL, Engelhardt HT Jr, McCartney JJ, eds. *Concepts of Health and Disease: Interdisciplinary Perspectives*. Reading, MA: Addison-Wesley Publishing Company, 1981.

74

Community in Public Health Ethics

BRUCE JENNINGS

Community can be understood both as a description of a certain type of human situation and as a normative standard used for the evaluation of human situations. The former is marked, for example, by a strong sense of togetherness and solidarity and low levels of impersonality and anonymity, and the latter by a strong sense of mutual obligation and a relatively weak sense of conflict between the interests of the self and others. A strong sense of community can induce persons to give up their lives for the sake of others with whom they identify. Ethically, a robust conception of community can motivate an argument that there is a duty to die in order to protect your community; and, of course, community induces and motivates lesser sacrifices as well, including those often required to protect the public health. The mirror image concept, both sociologically and normatively, where the valences of the concept of community are reversed can be called autonomy (in the sense of negative liberty or the right to be let alone) or individualism. The aim of this chapter is to explore the contribution that a carefully rendered concept of community can make to the ethical and political vision of public health.

COMMUNITY: THE LOST TRADITION OF PUBLIC HEALTH

In bioethics and medical ethics the predominant emphasis has been on the concept of individual patient autonomy or self-determination. In public health ethics one might naturally assume that the core value would be community. The reasons are many. For one thing, public health is focused on the external social determinants of health in populations. Unlike clinical medicine, public health is not a patient-centred professional practice; it deals in the realm of policies and programmes that cover large numbers of people at one time and rarely has the intimacy of the doctor–patient relationship. The main scientific orientation and knowledge base of public health is epidemiology, which is a probabilistic and statistical rather than biologically reductive and experiential body of knowledge. Finally, approaches that benefit the health of individuals may be at odds with programmes or practices that affect the health of populations, and the allocation of resources indicated by a clinical perspective may be quite different from that indicated by a public health perspective (Rose, 1999).

But today the normative orientation in public health (both, I would say, in public health ethics as an academic study and in public health practice) is more individualistic than communitarian. Dan Beauchamp, a leader in the recent revival of interest in public health ethics, once referred to the concept of community as part of a 'neglected tradition' in public heath. He writes:

> Community is one of the most important words in our democratic lexicon, perhaps second only to the idea of the individual. In its most basic meaning, community refers to our life together, and the attachments which sustain that life together. A community is not simply a group of people living in close proximity. A community has a life in common which stems from such things as a shared history, language, and values (Beauchamp & Steinbock, 1999, p. 53).

During recent decades, the individualistic turn in public health has to do with the nature of the AIDS epidemic and the new, almost unprecedented civil liberties challenges that it posed for the field (Bayer, 1989; Bayer & Fairchild, 2004). Effectively contesting traditional public health responses to spread epidemics and sexually transmitted disease, AIDS activists forced public health officials to think in new ways and with new scruple about matters such as privacy, surveillance, prevention and the relative weight of health values in comparison with other cultural and social values.

Principles of Health Care Ethics, Second Edition   Edited by R.E. Ashcroft, A. Dawson, H. Draper and J.R. McMillan
© 2007 John Wiley & Sons, Ltd

Another reason for a declining emphasis on the concept of community – particularly as that concept has been used to support state action and the public health exercise of police power – was the more gradual shift in the epidemiology and demographics of public health problems in the developed world, with chronic illness and behavioural-related risk factors coming to the fore. More authoritarian, top down public health measures, which had proven tremendously successful in the twentieth century in combating infectious and environmental disease, were giving way to health promotion, education and counselling efforts in which persuasion and individual cooperation were the main elements of the public health armamentarium. (I refer to what has been called the 'new public health' (La Londe, 1974). During the past several years, to be sure, the 'old' public health has returned with the advent of SARS, fears of bioterrorism and the concern about the possibility of a pandemic of avian influenza.)

However this may be, there is also an underlying conceptual reason for the relative neglect of the concept of community in public health and public health ethics. The 'tradition' to which Beauchamp refers has not only been neglected of late, it is also weak and philosophically underdeveloped in the understanding of community it conveys.

Public health has appealed to a conception of aggregative welfare to legitimate its moral authority and legal 'police power', and this utilitarian conception of community (for want of a better term) is not nearly robust or persuasive enough to stand up against strong libertarian (or even egalitarian) critiques. This can be seen when we examine the predominant role of what I shall refer to as the 'Millian paradigm' in analyses of the legal and ethical justification of public health authority.

Creating community when it is lacking and bolstering it where it already exists are themselves important tools of public health policy and practice, not simply considerations of ethical justification. Public health is interesting in large part because it is about what ethics and political philosophy have also always been about: what constitutes the human good – the good life in the good society. Public health is not just about biological functioning on the inside, but it is about psychosocial functioning on the outside, in lived relationships with others, in (here it comes naturally to our syntax, there is no other adequate word) community.

Community denotes relationships that are of intrinsic and not merely instrumental value to the participants; it denotes relationships that involve a depth of commitment greater than strategic rationality; and finally it contains a fascinating dynamic in which participants are both shaped as selves by their life in community with others and at the same time have the power to shape and reshape their community through their own agency. These concepts have an integral and substantive place in public health and public

health ethics. Community is not simply to be treated as an empirical fact about the psychological states or social perceptions of certain individuals. Are communities things that individuals construct in the beliefs they hold and the actions they undertake, or are communities things that constitute and shape individuals? As we must understand them in public health ethics, they are both.

THE MILLIAN PARADIGM

By and large, the liberal tradition of moral individualism was given cannonical formulation by John Stuart Mill in the mid-nineteenth century and is best exemplified in recent times by the important work of John Rawls. Rawls defines community narrowly as 'an association of society whose unity rests on a comprehensive conception of the good' (Rawls, 1993), and he adopts the view that community is reducible to an aggregation of individual preferences and beliefs. By defining community in terms of the function of beliefs about the good and the good life, Rawls goes on to argue that the concept of community has its proper place only in private life and should be excluded from the domain of politics, government, law and public policy (Mulhall & Adam, 1996). Public relationships should be instrumental and advantageous, not communal and closely knit. Communities are dangerous in public life in a way that alliances for mutual advantage are not because communities will impose their conception of the good on dissenting individuals (and other communities) if they obtain the authority and coercive power to do so. Public morality, in contrast to religion and private morality, must be deontological, not teleological. That is to say, public morality and public policy must be based on justice, rights, and duties that are justified independent of the fact that adherence to these norms may promote the good or human flourishing.

We should ask, however, whether this type of liberalism – which gives priority to individual liberty over community solidarity and priority to the right over the good – would not place restrictions on the practice of public health so stringent that it would preclude, at least as a matter of public policy, most of the positive, health promoting, well-being enhancing aspects of the field. It would seem most straightforward to say that health promotion and disease prevention are policies and practices that are justified in virtue of the fact that they promote the good of large numbers of people and because sometimes the good of the group takes precedence over the liberty of individuals. But that answer is permissible within the framework of individualistic liberalism only within rather narrow bounds. Disease prevention is to be justified in virtue of its protective and harm prevention functions; health promotion cannot be justified in this way, and it may indeed be a violation of the proper boundaries that should be set between the public and the private. If the liberal tradition, and even its most sophisticated contemporary exponents, like Rawls, does permit state action and does permit the curtailing of individual liberty on some grounds, as of course it does, it has none the less always been most wary and sceptical about public ethical justifications made on behalf of community and its related concepts. Will a more communitarian public health, one that does base its public ethical justification on a conception of community and the human good, lead towards a kind of health theocracy in which the main tenet of faith is: *Mens sana in corpore sano*? That, I take it, is a conclusion that liberal individualists always fear and that indeed no civic, progressive communitarian should want.

As we consider the shortcomings of its individualistic alternative, we should not forget that using the concept of community in public health ethics is subject to several serious conceptual pitfalls. For one thing, the meaning of community varies so significantly across several different dimensions that it may need to be broken down into a series of more basic categories (such as fidelity, reciprocity, self-esteem and empathy) before it can best be used in such an analysis. Moreover, if community is characterized in a strongly affective way, as a bonding sentiment that produces internal belonging at the price of external exclusion, then its moral force in balance with opposing values such as equality, respect, and rights would not seem to be very compelling. Or perhaps, at certain historical moments, all too dangerously compelling.

At this point it is necessary to examine in closer detail the presuppositions and implications of the predominant individualistic ethical framework in public health, which I shall refer to as the 'Millian paradigm', because it brings up to date both the moral concerns and the conceptual structure adumbrated by John Stuart Mill in *On Liberty* (Mill, 1958). This is the ethical problem setting individual liberty against the authority of the state and the interests of society. The ethical problem is typically framed in terms of expertise and the clash of interests. It pits the autonomy or liberty (Mill calls it 'self-sovereignty') of the individual against state (and professional) paternalism and against the pressure of social opinion. (The most important general work on the nature of this type of problem and its analysis is of Feinberg (Feinberg, 1984–1988). One of the best discussions of this framework in relation to public health is of Leichter (Leichter, 1991)).

Let us consider one important example that shows both how pervasive the Millian paradigm has been and how it can be articulated both in ethical/political theory and in constitutional law. The text in question is the important 1905 decision of the US Supreme Court in *Jacobson* versus *Massachusetts* (Jacobson, 2002). In this case Henning Jacobson refused to comply with a public health ordinance in Cambridge, Massachusetts, requiring smallpox vaccination. Having lost in state court, Jacobson appealed to the Supreme Court on the grounds that the public health policy of mandatory vaccination violated his right to freedom and equal protection of the law under the Fourteenth Amendment of the US Constitution. The court denied Jacobson's claim and ruled to uphold the Massachusetts public health law requiring him to submit to vaccination or to face a fine or imprisonment. (The fine in question that he refused to pay was $5.00.)

Since the mid-nineteenth century when the Fourteenth Amendment was enacted, it has been the textual focal point for the balancing of individual liberty and state authority in American constitutional law. The Jacobson decision set out the elements of Fourteenth Amendment jurisprudence that is still used by the federal courts today. This jurisprudence sets up a balancing test to weigh the individual's liberty interests against the legitimate duties and functions of the state and inquires whether or not the state policy in question is reasonable and whether the state or public interest in question is compelling. It is significant in public health law because it clearly sets forth the nature of the police powers granting the state, through its public health agencies, the authority to protect the community from threats to its health and safety. (For an interesting and broad ranging interpretation of Fourteenth Amendment jurisprudence, especially that portion of the text known as the Equal Protection Clause, see Fiss (1977). Beauchamp (1988, 1999) reads the *Jacobson* decision as a part of the republican and communitarian legal tradition of the United States that both stands at the origins of American public health law and embodies a way of thinking that has been eclipsed by narrower forms of liberalism and utilitarianism.)

At times the language of the court opinion (written by Justice Harlan) seems strongly communitarian:

> It is a fundamental principle of the social compact that the whole people covenants with each citizen, and each citizen with the whole people, that all shall be governed by certain laws for 'the common good', and that government is instituted 'for the common good, for the protection, safety, prosperity, and happiness of the people, and not for the profit, honour or private interests of any one man, family, or class of men'. The good and welfare of the commonwealth . . . is the basis on which the police power rests . . . (Jacobson, 2002, p. 208).

In summarizing Jacobson's claim, the opinion is eloquent in expressing both sides of the individualism/community tension:

> The defendant insists ... that a compulsory vaccination law is unreasonable, arbitrary, and oppressive, and, therefore, hostile to the inherent right of every freeman to care for this own body and health in such way as to him seems best; and that the

execution of such a law against one who objects to vaccination, no matter for what reason, is nothing short of an assault upon his person. But the liberty secured by the Constitution of the United States to every person within its jurisdiction does not import an absolute right in each person to be, at all times and in all circumstances, wholly freed from restraint. There are manifold restraints to which every person is necessarily subject for the common good (Jacobson, 2002, p. 208).

However, as if remembering the admonitions of John Stuart Mill, the Court goes on to qualify and narrow the implications of the state power founded on community covenant and the common good:

There is, of course, a sphere within which the individual may assert the supremacy of his own will, and rightfully dispute the authority of any human government ... to interfere with the exercise of that will. But it is equally true that in every well-ordered society charged with the duty of conserving the safety of its members the rights of the individual in respect of his liberty may at times, under the pressure of great dangers, be subjected to such restraint, to be enforced by reasonable regulations . . (Jacobson, 2002, pp. 209–10).

The language that Mill uses to present his main argument about the limits of state action and the harm principle is strikingly echoed in the *Jacobson* decision. Compare Mill:

. . . the only purpose for which power can be rightfully exercised over any member of a civilized community, against his will, is to prevent harm to others. His own good, either physical or moral, is not sufficient warrant. He cannot rightfully be compelled to do or forbear because it will be better for him to do so, because it will make him happier, because, in the opinions of others, to do so would be wise or even right. These are good reasons for remonstrating with him, or reasoning with him, or persuading him, or entreating him, but not for compelling him or visiting him with any evil in case he do otherwise. To justify that, the conduct from which it is desired to deter him must be calculated to produce evil to someone else. The only part of the conduct of anyone for which he is amenable to society is that which concerns others. In the part which merely concerns himself, his independence is, of right, absolute. Over himself, over his own body and mind, the individual is sovereign (Mill, 1958, p. 13).

The limitations set up in *Jacobson* are suggested by such phrases as 'great dangers' and 'reasonable regulations'. The Court is persuaded by the nature and consequences of a disease like smallpox that the necessary threshold of danger has been passed. Reasonableness has to do with how effective the public health policy is, and it has to do with whether vaccination is the only effective alternative or the least violative of individual rights and liberty. But reasonableness also has to do with the seriousness of the impact on the individuals to whom the policy applies. Accordingly, the opinion is also quite concerned with Jacobson's failure to show that he himself would be placed at undue medical

risk by receiving a vaccination. Apparently the Court is willing to balance his liberty against the protection of the community, but not necessarily his life or health. Indeed, it could very well be in this instance that his life and health are on the side of community and not on the side of individual liberty.

A similar tacking back and forth between conflicting values and extreme claims is evident in the way the Court understands the basis and application of the police power. It is inherent in the very notion of the state, which is established essentially for the self-preservation and defence of its citizens. But this conception alone does not go so far as to establish intrinsic value in the community itself. In fact, sufficient justification for the limitation of individual liberty by state authorities can be found within the logic of the concept of liberty alone, without recourse to community at all. This argument, familiar in the contractarian tradition of political theory at least since Hobbes, has to do with the self-contradictory nature of unlimited freedom. Writing for the Court, Justice Harlan expresses it this way: 'Real liberty for all could not exist under the operation of a principle which recognizes the right of each individual person to use his own, whether in respect of his person or his property, regardless of the injury that may be done to others' (Jacobson, 2002, p. 208).

And after affirming the public health authority against Jacobson's individual claims in the circumstances of this case, the Court goes out of its way to make clear that individual rights remain at the centre of its legal, constitutional – to say nothing of its political and ethical – vision. The Court 'should guard with firmness every right appertaining to life, liberty or property as secured to the individual by the supreme law of the land...' (Jacobson, 2002, p. 214). And there are certain types of state policies, even in the domain of public health, that cannot be justified by appeal to community interests alone:

Before closing this opinion we deem it appropriate, in order to prevent misapprehension as to our views, to observe . . . that the police power of a state . . . may be exercised in such circumstances, or by regulations so arbitrary and oppressive in particular cases, as to justify the interference of the courts to prevent wrong and oppression (Jacobson, 2002, pp. 214–5).

In the final analysis, this text is not a vindication of community over the individual. On the whole the concept of community it offers is an aggregative one, and it keeps public health within the confines of the Millian paradigm by making harm to others the dividing line between public and private, licit freedom and illicit freedom and liberty and licence.

I argue that taking the concept of community seriously in public health ethics means breaking in fundamental respects with the Millian paradigm. Community is neither an aggregation of individuals nor an abstraction away from individual difference to single out some common principle; it is the medium, what Bourdieu (1977) calls the habitus, in which common features of our humanity are lived and experienced as they are reflected through particular, localized modes of cultural and symbolic expression. Community is not a paternalistic entity that imposes its understanding of the individual's good or best interest on that individual against her own will and judgement. Community is instead a concept that leads us to broaden and deepen our understanding of what it means for individuals to have a will and to make judgments. The conflict, if there be one, is not between a 'higher will' and the individual's will but between two possibilities of willing and discernment that reside, at least potentially, within each person. And finally, community is not a super-individual or trans-individual thing that exists above and apart from the persons who comprise it and that has its own person-like characteristics that may be opposed to the interests or needs of individuals. The challenge of a communitarianism that rejects individualism is not to lose sight of the moral importance – indeed the moral existence – of the individual. *Individualism* as a mistaken theory of human ontology (being and becoming) should not be confused with *individuality* as a fundamental safeguard of human rights and dignity.

If the justification and legitimacy of public health authority is tied in these ways to the concept of community, so too perhaps is our basic understanding of the determinants and the phenomenon of health itself, which from the public health perspective cannot be completely understood by recourse to biological reductionism or the so-called 'medical model'. Consider the growing body of work in epidemiology indicating that the uneven distribution of health and morbidity in a population – the public health 'gradient' – is not simply a matter of poverty and the distribution of wealth but also 'social capital' networks of meaningful activity and social support (Wilkinson, 1996; Marmot & Wilkinson, 1999; Evans, Barer & Marmor, 1994; Putnam, 2000). Public health is coming to understand that even physical health – to say nothing of mental health or quality of life – is directly linked to matters that are social and institutional and not merely material and economic. These matters include social identity, self-esteem, social involvement and connectedness, social support and membership, the experience of social discrimination and injustice, the stress of social hierarchy, competition, and uncertainty, the behaviour-shaping power of peer-group influences and one's sense of one's own power and efficacy.

The list goes on. The point is that public health takes us inherently and not simply fortuitously into the design and redesign of personal relationships, institutional capacities and moral connections; in a word, community. The new epidemiology has less to do with the causal nexus than it does with a kind of moral ecology. Moreover, the study of public health is becoming *public* or *civic* in a way that does not reduce to an interest in the health of populations. If we take it seriously, the goal of enhancing the health of large numbers of people from preventable, premature, or risk behaviour-related disease is a goal that will require our fundamental reconsideration of what it means to have a community, to be individuals in a community and to share a common or public good.

The individualism that public health ethics inherits from the liberal tradition involves a conception of self that stresses the uniqueness of each person, and values precisely that which symbolizes difference and separation rather than sameness and commonality. Relational ties with others are certainly morally permissible, even essential, on this view but only in as much as they are instrumental to the achievement of individual ends and only when they are entered into voluntarily. Liberalism sees personhood in terms of interests that are both morally and ontologically prior to the relationships the person has and to the symbolic (cultural) and institutional forms and practices in which one lives (Sandel, 1982). The liberal self seeks expression and affirmation *through* but not *in* social relations, which are at best instrumentally useful for the satisfaction of subjectively defined interests, and at worst confining. This instrumentalism holds liberal individualism back from more radical versions of individualistic anarchism, but there remains a wariness in liberal individualism about claims asserting the intrinsic value of belonging, communal membership, or public life. Connection with others is primarily seen as a source of threats, limits or the effacement of the self, rather than as an enabling or empowering medium of self-realization.

By contrast, a philosophy of public health informed by communitarianism would see personhood in terms of those dimensions of human selfhood and experience, such as physical frailty or need and membership in a community of shared life and purpose, that highlight connection and commonality rather than difference. It would seek self-realization in – as well as through – relations of shared purpose with others. And, as the epidemiological evidence indicates, relationships and life with a functional network of symbolic and institutional forms can have a positive effect on health promotion and protection against certain risk factors that undermine health. It may even be the case, as the Whitehall study seems to suggest, that hierarchy – or at least arbitrary power and unequal status – can undermine health, perhaps through stress and the workings of hormonal mechanisms as yet not well understood. This points communitarianism in public health not only towards relational resources and social capital, but also towards community and relationships of a particularly just and egalitarian kind. Community for public health as a possible empirical connection may hold important implications for community in public health as a discourse of normative legitimation.

This suggests an important reason why an individualistic, aggregative notion of community (collective interests or maximizing notions of net benefit) is inferior to a more complex notion of community (the common good). With only an aggregative notion of the public interest at hand, when faced with the advent of a social transformation (such as sprawl that leads to air pollution and sedentary lifestyle) or a new development in biotechnology, public health can only ask whether the benefits to individuals outweigh the costs.

Now, there are some kinds of moral costs (and benefits) that are conceptually invisible to this way of seeing the problem. They have to do with notions of public life and communal relationships that are not defined by the aggregation of particularistic interests but rather by the nurturing and transformation of democratic or communal interests – interests that flow directly out of institutions, customs and practices that foster inclusiveness, solidarity and mutual respect, as well as opportunities for the new forms of individuality and self-expression. The introduction of new technologies or the exercise of certain kinds of elite, professional authority might disrupt or undermine the norms sustaining these communitarian values and practices. New forms of social discrimination based on stigmatizing information revealed by new technologies of genetic screening is an example (Nelkin & Tancredi, 1994). The eroding of traditions and institutions that sustain communitarian values is a significant social 'cost' that must somehow figure in the ethical analysis of public health policy and practice. And yet in the literature not only of bioethics but of the new public health ethics as well, it is precisely this element that is missing and would be advanced by a more adequate critical vocabulary of community and related concepts.

REFERENCES

Bayer R, Fairchild A. Genesis of public health ethics. *Bioethics* 2004; **18**(6): 473–92.

Bayer R. *Private Acts, Social Consequences: AIDS and the Politics of Public Health*. University Park: Penn State University Press, 1989.

Beauchamp DE, Steinbock B, eds. *New Ethics for the Public's Health*. New York: Oxford University Press, 1999.

Beauchamp DE. Community: The neglected tradition of public health. In: Beauchamp DE, Steinbock B, eds. *New Ethics for the Public's Health*. New York: Oxford University Press, 1999; pp 57–67.

Beauchamp DE. *The Health of the Republic*. Philadelphia: Temple University Press, 1988.

Bourdieu P. *Outline of a Theory of Practice*. London: Cambridge University Press, 1977.

Evans RG, Barer ML, Marmor TR, eds. *Why Are Some People Healthy and Others Not?* New York: Aldine de Gruyter, 1994.

Feinberg J. *The Moral Limits of the Criminal Law*, vols. 4. New York: Oxford University Press, 1984–1988.

Fiss O. Groups and the equal protection clause. In: Cohen M, Nagel T, Scanlon T, eds. *Equality and Preferential Treatment*. Princeton: Princeton University Press, 1977; pp. 84–154.

Jacobson v. Massachusetts. 197 US 11. In: Lawrence O. Gostin, ed. *Public Health Law and Ethics* (reprinted). Berkeley: University of California Press 2002, 1905, pp. 206–15.

La Londe M. *A New Perspective on the Health of Canadians*. Ottawa: Department of National Health and Welfare, 1974.

Leichter HM. *Free to Be Foolish: Politics and Health Promotion in the United States and Great Britain*. Princeton: Princeton University Press, 1991.

Marmot M, Wilkinson RG, eds. *Social Determinants of Health*. Oxford: Oxford University Press, 1999.

Mill JS. *On Liberty*. Indianapolis: Bobbs Merrill, 1958.

Mulhall S, Adam S. *Liberals and Communitarians*, 2nd edition. Oxford: Blackwell, 1996; pp. 191–222.

Nelkin D, Tancredi L. *Dangerous Diagnostics: The Social Power of Biological Information*. Chicago: University of Chicago Press, 1994.

Putnam RD. *Bowling Alone: the Collapse and Revival of American Community*. New York: Simon and Schuster, 2000.

Rawls J. *Political Liberalism*. New York: Columbia University Press, 1993; p. 146.

Rose G. Sick individuals and sick populations. In: Beauchamp DE, Steinbock B, eds. *New Ethics for the Public's Health*. New York: Oxford University Press, 1999; pp 28–38.

Sandel M. *Liberalism and the Limits of Justice*. Cambridge: Cambridge University Press, 1982.

Wilkinson RG. *Unhealthy Societies*. New York: Routledge, 1996.

75

Health Promotion, Society and Health Care Ethics

ALAN CRIBB

It is impossible to give a full account of the nature or ethics of health promotion in a short chapter. That being the case I will concentrate on two issues which seem to me to illustrate something of the distinctiveness of health promotion but which also have implications for health care ethics more generally. I will begin with a discussion of the nature of health promotion and, in particular, its comparative open-endedness or formlessness. This open-endedness, I will suggest, has a number of implications for approaching the ethics of health promotion. It raises questions and uncertainties about the locus of responsibility for health promotion, about the knowledge base of health promotion and about how the object of ethical investigation and analysis is framed and conceptualized. I will then go on to consider one facet of this open-endedness in a little more depth, namely the relevance of social science based knowledge claims for health promotion ethics, and the relationship between social sciences and health care ethics.

THE ILL DEFINITION OF HEALTH PROMOTION

There is no unambiguous or agreed referent for the term 'health promotion'. The spectrum of interpretations ranges from the very broad (indeed virtually all-encompassing) to the relatively specific, where only specific examples of occupational or policy action would qualify as health promotion. For example, starting at the most expansive end, should we think of health promotion as referring to only activities, or to both activities and processes? In other words, should we be thinking of 'the promotion of health' in a way that makes it analogous to 'the production of health'.

Thus – leaving aside the notoriously problematic question of what 'health' is – all manner of things may be 'health promoting' just as all manner of things may be 'oxygen using', independent of human activity or agency. But even if we decide that health promotion must refer to a set of activities (those which promote health in some sense), then which set of activities is this? For example, do these activities have to be conducted with the *aim* of promoting health, or is what matters that an activity has the *consequence* of promoting health? Is a well-intentioned GP who is making a substantial contribution to the over prescription of antibiotics in a community acting as a health promoter? Is a plumber who is doing a thorough job of fitting heating, bathing and toilet facilities in a new housing estate thereby a health promoter?

These concrete examples take us closer to the other – more restricted – end of the spectrum, because health promotion might be thought of as a particular kind of occupational activity. This is not just a thought experiment; there are people who work in the field of health promotion and think of it as an occupation. Some of these people have the term 'health promotion' in their title, and many more have it in their job description. None the less, it would be odd to restrict the application of the term according to the simple contingency of where it happens to have been adopted. For my purposes I will treat health promotion in a way that moves between the more expansive and the more restricted poles. I am using it to pick out an ill-defined cluster of reforming discourses which have become, to varying degrees, influential in health policy and which, broadly speaking, seek to reorient health policy and health care around disease prevention or community health improvement. But I am also using it as shorthand for a range of specific health-related interventions,

Principles of Health Care Ethics, Second Edition Edited by R.E. Ashcroft, A. Dawson, H. Draper and J.R. McMillan
© 2007 John Wiley & Sons, Ltd

sometimes linked to occupational roles, each of which, of course, deserves consideration on its own terms.

Having begun by underlining the vagueness and interpretative elasticity that attaches to the idea of health promotion, I will briefly mention two influential 'definitions' of health promotion that may provide some gentle anchorage for those who are unfamiliar with the domain. First, the World Health Organization in the famous 'Ottowa Charter' (World Health Organization, 1986) describes health promotion as 'the process of enabling individuals and communities to increase control over the determinants of health and thereby improve their health'. Second, Tones and Tilford (2001), in the pithiest formulation of the very helpful accounts of health promotion they offer, describe it in a mathematical form as 'health education x public policy for health'.

The very idea of health promotion is inherent in the opening up of the time–space continuum in health care. Once we see health in the context of the whole causal nexus of events and processes, we can 'zoom out' from health care interactions to all of the possible determinants of health and illness. And once we are in the habit of thinking about the 'outcomes' of health care interventions, we are enabled to start thinking about the potential 'health outcomes' of any and every kind of social intervention. This is the essence of health promotion. It is the idea that we might turn our knowledge of the determinants of health into action for health. The idea of health promotion is thus a kind of logically necessary development in the historical evolution of health care. The different historical faces of health promotion emerge in the space between established patterns of health care and the logical possibility of 'universal' health promotion.

This process relates to the universalization of the means of health promotion. But the history of health promotion includes another – distinct but overlapping – dimension of diffusion which completes a 'totalizing' process; namely the frequent elision of health with conceptions of welfare or well-being. I will not review the various narrow or broad definitions of health here, nor the different possible conceptions of welfare and well-being. (In brief I am assuming that welfare refers to something like 'the satisfaction of basic needs' which provides the conditions for people to aim to live the life they want, and that well-being refers to something like 'a life being lived in a way that is judged (from some standpoint, left unspecified here) to be worthwhile and fulfilling'. I review the relationships between health, welfare and well-being in Chapter 2 of Cribb (2005).) My aim is simply to note that in much of the policy rhetoric of health promotion, there has been a lack of differentiation concerning the ends of health promotion. (Sometimes this is for the understandable reason

that welfare and well-being are, in various respects, themselves part of the causal nexus underpinning health.) These elisions mean – in their most careless manifestations – that the promotion of health is simply fudged with the promotion of well-being. According to this absurdly stretched conception just about anything that might contribute to making someone's life worthwhile counts as an example of health promotion.

The distinctiveness of health promotion ethics relates in part to the apparent boundlessness and formlessness reviewed above. In addition to the question about the ends of health promotion there are many other basic uncertainties. For example, who are the agents responsible for health promotion and whose health are they supposed to be promoting? Is everyone responsible for promoting everyone's health? Apart from those people working in health promotion, or in posts with a named health promotion function, it is difficult to know who else to include in, or exclude from, the category of 'health promoters'. If we think about the range of potential opportunities for promoting health, then we might be inclined to include everyone. However, if we ask who has not only the relevant expertise but also the ethical legitimacy to promote other people's health, we may be inclined to exclude almost everyone, perhaps even many who are officially employed as 'health promoters'. The more we move away from one-to-one health promotion encounters (e.g. a doctor counselling a patient about dietary changes), the more these overlapping *problems of expertise and legitimacy* come to the fore for three very good reasons.

First, although health care practices are conducted within an elaborate professional ethic – including systems for recognizing appropriate forms of expertise, client 'permission giving' and professional role-specific obligations – there does not appear to be any equivalent process of 'ethical licensing' for population health promotion. This is significant, not least because health promotion is normally initiated by the would-be health promoters rather than by the intended beneficiaries. Second, more 'long distance' health promotion interventions will inevitably produce more complex systems of 'side-effects' which are not only difficult to predict but also difficult to evaluate. And given the complex causal and constitutive links between aspects of health, welfare and well-being already noted, such evaluations, as well as the predictions they rest upon, have to be multidimensional. Third, in so far as health promotion interventions involve changes to social or cultural systems as well as to physical systems, this problem of knowledge is compounded, because of the notorious problem of attaining reliable knowledge in the social sciences.

Hence, in addition to definitional problems, population health promotion gives rise to characteristic ethical problems and dilemmas. (Of course not all health promotion is – on the surface – society-wide or population-oriented. Indeed arguably the most widespread penetration of health promotion discourse has been in the contexts of clinical health care where it refers to the introduction of a longer term health maintenance, health enhancement or disease prevention orientation into professional–client encounters. There are some very interesting ethical problems generated by the reorientation of individual health care relationships by health promotion (e.g. issues about the implications for professional responsiveness, respect for patient autonomy and client trust when clinical encounters are mediated through professionals' health promotion intentions) but I will not focus upon them here.) These ethical problems often revolve around what I have labelled as *problems of ethical legitimacy*, that is the problems of justifying various kinds of uninvited 'social influence' on individuals. These include, among other things, the health promotion uses of education, persuasion (e.g. by dis/incentives), cultural or environmental 'engineering', and legally enforced compulsion. This ethical agenda entails seeking possible justifications for different kinds and degrees of interference over individuals' freedom to frame, make and enact choices and, in turn, this typically means a consideration of the following themes: (a) the possibility of negotiating 'social consent' or, using a different idiom, of establishing conditions for properly grounded trust in health promotion interventions; (b) the balance between population goods and individual goods; (c) the scope and limits of justified paternalism in the name of health; (d) the fair distribution of burdens and benefits; as well as (e) fair processes for determining and balancing these burdens and benefits in theory and in practice. These are all fundamental themes in social philosophy, and I will not even attempt to address them directly here. In what follows I will merely touch upon a few aspects of these questions while concentrating on a set of overlapping ethical complications – complications that largely relate to what I have called *problems of expertise*.

I have been pointing to the potential distinctiveness of health promotion ethics as arising, at least in part, from the open-ended nature of health promotion. To talk about open-endedness here is partly to acknowledge the conceptual vagueness of the term, but it is also to indicate the ways in which many examples of health promotion work are unlike treatment oriented doctor–patient encounters. Health promotion is frequently not initiated by the client; it often takes place in socially diffuse fields rather than in well-defined professional and institutional fields; and it is often critically dependent upon social science knowledge claims rather than on claims which reside largely in the natural sciences. In the remainder of the chapter I will explore these

questions further, concentrating mainly on the question of social science knowledge.

HEALTH PROMOTION, SOCIAL SCIENCE AND ETHICS

The social sciences are of particular relevance in the areas of health promotion and public health. Social sciences form a key part of the practical knowledge base of health promotion in a way that does not apply in clinical health care. (I do not want to draw a clear distinction here just to note that the centres of gravity of the knowledge base of health promotion policy and practice on the one hand and clinical health care on the other are very different and that social sciences (especially the more 'social' social sciences e.g. sociology, policy analysis, economics) are a core part of the *toolkit* of health promotion practice.) As I have already noted, this raises questions about whether the knowledge base of health promotion is reliable and, in turn, this feeds into concerns about the legitimacy of, and trust in, the work of health promoters. This is one reason to consider the nature of social scientific knowledge in a discussion of health promotion ethics, but, as I hope to show, there are other such reasons.

One way of talking about the contribution of the social sciences to health promotion ethics is simply to say that the empirical component of health promotion ethics depends on social scientific knowledge. So, for example, if we want to know what factors encourage or discourage binge alcohol drinking, we can investigate this empirically. If we then want to know whether we are justified in trying to prevent binge drinking by attempting to manipulate these factors, we need to be able to do some ethical thinking and in order to do this – in any practical sense – we need to have some way of guesstimating what the possible effects of the range of proposed measures might be. On this model the job of the social sciences, roughly speaking, is to discover and set out the facts (especially the fact that *a* tends to bring about *b*) that feed into the reasoning of applied philosophy or ethics. But to put it in these terms is to see at once some of the problems that are attached to this model. That is, there are well known problems of making knowledge claims in the social sciences – at least of producing the kinds of broadly generalizable descriptions, explanations and predictions that are needed if social policy judgements are to have an evidence base which is remotely comparable to that available, for example, in pharmacology. And these problems are not only technical ones about finding suitable methods and instruments but also more deep seated philosophical problems which can be seen as resulting from the nature of the object under study – that is, social life – independently of any accounts of the shortcomings of methods.

These problems can be briefly summarized under four headings. There is the *problem of culture* – social life is partly constituted by culture, that is by systems of meanings, traditions, and so on. And cultures are both diverse and constantly evolving – there is no obvious equivalent to being able to add 2 milligrams of chemical A to 4 milligrams of chemical B in the same set of conditions. There is the *problem of open systems* – that is, social life takes place within extremely complex and open-ended systems. The sheer number of factors that might be relevant to explaining some phenomenon, along with the different dimensions and facets of social life – the religious, the political, the economic etc. – not to mention the many ways in which these can be modelled and measured produces a countless number of possible interactions. This leads to a particular difficulty in attaining predictive validity in the social sciences, a difficulty which is also associated with the third set of problems, namely the *problem of reflexivity and agency*, that is social science knowledge is not independent of the objects – social life, people – being studied. People faced with the predictions built into policy models can, to varying extents, choose not to behave as the models predict. Finally, closely linked to these challenges – especially to the challenges of working with culture and reflexivity – is *the problem of values,* that is, given the contestability of descriptions of the social life and the ways in which these competing descriptions are bound up with cultural perspectives and particular vantage points, social sciences are arguably inherently normative. (Again it might be worth underlining the point that the more natural science related elements of clinical science are by no means immune to these four problems – for example those who subscribe to the strong programme in the sociology of scientific knowledge emphasize the cultural and evaluative construction of medical categories and are sceptical about the performance of authoritativeness and relative closure in medical knowledge – but there does at least seem to be a difference of degree between the natural and social sciences as regards the balances between generalizability, indeterminacy and contestability.)

Now of course these challenges are not specific to health promotion policy making but apply to all policy related social science, and before focusing on some health promotion related examples, I want to offer a broad-brush account of the ways in which these challenges are managed in policy related social science generally. To do so, I will borrow and make use of a distinction which is sometimes made between 'problem-solving' and 'critical' policy analysis. It should be stressed that this is an extremely crude distinction. I am using the idea of two traditions of policy analysis merely as ideal types for the purpose of my argument.

The two broad approaches represented by the problem solving and the critical traditions can be viewed as two contrasting responses to the problem of social science knowledge that I have just sketched out. The problem solving tra-

dition does not see these problems as insuperable and looks to methods similar to those in the natural science tradition, especially to certain quasi-experimental and statistical methods, to find ways around the challenges posed by culture, open systems, reflexivity, and so on. In particular it places great stress on the aspiration towards descriptive and explanatory validity and rigour; and this aspiration is typically accompanied by an interest in – as far as possible – the insulation of factual claims from the risks of partisanship. The critical tradition tends to take as a starting point the ways in which social science claims are made from particular vantage points and embody normative assumptions of one kind or another. It is more comfortable with the idea that social science is partisan, and indeed sometimes advocates explicit partisanship. It tends to be hostile to the idea that the models of validity and rigour that apply in the natural sciences are applicable in the social sciences. Instead of treating the cultural and reflexive nature of social life as problems that can be managed by clever methods, the critical tradition takes the uncovering and unpacking of the cultural construction of social life as a core activity. (It should be noted in passing that the cultural constitution of the social world provides a further rationale for the important place of empirical work in health care ethics – it is impossible to get a sense of what many health-related goods amount to, or of what kinds of policy initiatives are feasible without a grounded account of the specific histories, climates and policy traditions that constitute the specific contexts under investigation.)

Now just to quickly illustrate some of these differences, I will return to the example I mentioned above, namely the study of binge alcohol drinking and how to reduce it. A problem solving approach to this question might, for example, seek to design and measure the effectiveness of some pilot intervention – local education campaigns, labelling strategies, experiments with the use of licensing laws or the social marketing of alternative drinks or recreations. A critical approach would ask who has identified binge drinking as a problem and why; whose interests are served by the various suggested strategies for dealing with it, and might ask, for example, 'Why are certain people's habits labelled as being about bingeing or indulgence? Are there not other parties with responsibilities in this area for whom the ascription of greed or excessiveness might not fit better?'.

My own position (in brief) is that aspects of these two approaches need combining and that the best social science often strives to work across the two approaches. It needs to be prepared to move back and forth between putting normative questions on one side and focusing explicitly upon them. Clearly, the balance we strike between them depends in large part upon our aims, that is, on what kinds of questions we are interested in asking and answering and why we are interested. Some questions lend themselves more to problem solving treatment than others, and the problems of drawing sufficiently well grounded and rigorous causal inferences to inform policy formation bite more deeply in some areas than others. Some matters are intrinsically more socially circumscribed and well defined. A project in which primary care nurses experiment with different models of smoking cessation classes and nicotine substitutes, comparing them for success rate, cost effectiveness and client satisfaction, is not very different from any evaluation of treatment alternatives. In this kind of case, there is a degree of insulation between the object of investigation and wider cultural and social-economic processes. This example can be contrasted with a case like research on conceptions of responsible alcohol use which does not depend on a clinical intervention, and which often takes place outside a specific and medicalized institutional framework. Other examples – such as action on housing or income taxation – are even more diffuse.

What is the relevance of the above debates about social science for health promotion ethics? The broad answer can be quickly summarized. The social sciences help to determine what counts as knowledge in health promotion and are thereby implicated in the construction of what counts as a 'problem' and a 'solution'. The fundamental point is that the categories and frameworks that we use to interpret the social world have value judgements embedded in them which feed into policies and practices that have effects. This process takes place when the social science activity is primarily descriptive, explanatory or evaluative, and it has a range of different kinds of potential effects – for example the ways in which health promotion problems and solutions are constructed may reinforce certain moralizing discourses; it may alter the distribution of health experiences whether narrowly or broadly conceived, or it may produce or reproduce patterns of discrimination or stigmatization. Social science and social research does not somehow 'float above' social action; they are a form of social action. Hence, health care ethicists need to have a dual relationship with empirical research claims about the social world. Ethics does depend upon empirical accounts, and hence, ethicists must be interested in these accounts being as rigorous and defensible as possible. At the same time – or as part of this concern with rigour – ethicists must be ready to see these empirical accounts as part of their problematic. I will mention a few examples to illustrate what I mean.

I will start with an example which is well known in health promotion and public health circles and which shows that the concern that I have raised about the construction of health promotion knowledge is not merely an academic worry. It arises from what has become a very familiar controversy in the United Kingdom ever since the publication of the Black Report in 1980 on class related health inequalities. The Black Report stated:

> At the most fundamental level, theoretical explanations of the relationship between health and inequality might be roughly divided into 4 categories:
>
> i. artefact explanations; ii. theories of natural or social selection; iii. materialist explanations; and iv. cultural/behavioural explanations (Whitehead, 1992).

The first explanation – the artefact explanation – essentially explains away the correlation between social class and health status as a product of models and measures. The second explanation suggests that any such correlation might best be understood as ill health causing downward social mobility, rather than relative disadvantage somehow causing poor health. But if we put these two explanations on one side – as is the mainstream position in health promotion and public health – as at best only explaining part of the social class health gradient, we are left with the well known debate about the explanatory power of lifestyle versus structure (and of course the interactions between them). When seeking to explain health inequalities, how far should we look to factors such as class related patterns of smoking, alcohol use, nutrition and recreation? Or how far should we look to the distribution of environmental and occupational hazards and to the distribution of fundamental resources, not just income and wealth but housing, education and so on?

The reason for the controversial nature of these interpretations is plain. It is because of the different ways in which agency, especially the agency of the disadvantaged, can be implicated in these models of explanation. The lifestyle model places the actions, and hence to some degree the agency of the disadvantaged, at the core of the explanation, and the materialist explanation looks to factors that lie beyond this agency in two respects, that is, they either operate in parallel to it or lie further back in the explanatory chain and help to explain what produces and structures the subjectivities and choices of the disadvantaged. Of course a lifestyle-based explanation is not in itself a 'victim blaming' explanation. To refer to the culture, behaviour and choices of a smoker or drinker as part a causal explanation is not necessarily to ascribe moral responsibility to the smoker for the consequences of their behaviour. But in practice the focus on lifestyles can be closely linked to what people worry about under the heading of victim blaming. This is arguably the case when a body of research and practice approaches health promotion largely through the lens of what individuals can do for themselves, thereby reproducing the cultural/behavioural explanatory readings and by contrast neglecting the larger canvas. Beaglehole and Bonita, for example, argue that this individualistic orientation 'runs the risk of blaming the victim and encouraging health education strategies at the expense of social, economic and environmental changes' (Beaglehole & Bonita, 1997). The debate about the relative weight to be attached to lifestyle or structure is thus paralleled in the debate within health promotion about the relative weight to be attached to the two components of health promotion (as identified in Tones and Tilford's simplified definition) – that is, health education *or* public policy directed at broader and deeper health determinants. These two tensions between, roughly speaking, (a) education 'versus' persuasion/ compulsion and (b) individualistic 'versus' structural approaches are at the crux of the 'models debate' within health promotion (Tones & Tilford, 2001; Caplan & Holland, 1990). What I am aiming to underline here is that in many respects the ethical judgements about how to strike the proper balances between different health promotion policy approaches are made 'upstream' as we make our readings of social life. Ethical analysis needs to be applied to the related processes of knowledge construction and policy construction, and not just to the conduct of policy or practice which represents the surface feature of health promotion.

As I have signalled above, there are a range of different potentially different 'side effects' of the ways in which health promotion problems and solutions are constructed. But, for simplicity, I have divided these into two – there are the cultural effects, that is the effects on patterns of recognition and respect along with the reproduction of judgemental and moralistic discourses; and there are the direct effects on 'health outcomes' (let us say on patterns of morbidity and mortality narrowly conceived). The above critique of 'lifestylism' can serve as an example of the dangers of moralism or stigmatization. But Beaglehole and Bonita also use it to pick out the effects of this approach on the distribution of health – 'Research interventions in wealthy countries which have focused on consumption and not on production, have only added to the inequalities in health between the poor and the rich within wealthy countries, and between poor and wealthy countries' (Beaglehole and Bonita, 1997). If true, this latter claim is obviously an important one. It suggests that well meaning and perhaps, in their own terms, ethically scrupulous approaches to health promotion that focus on individual lifestyle change may serve to extend rather than reduce health inequalities. (Of course this would not necessarily make these approaches ethically unacceptable – among other things this depends upon a consideration of the ethics of relative advantage – but it does raise fundamental ethical concerns that need careful analysis.)

It would be possible to multiply this kind of example endlessly. As I have said, this issue applies whether the main purpose of the social research is descriptive, explanatory or evaluative. One dimension of the cultural effects of health promotion models is worth spelling out – it is the risk of pathologising certain properties or conditions. This can be done more or less directly or innocently. There are some choices – such as the adoption of the language of teenage pregnancy as a research focus rather than the use of a different language to point to different phenomena – such as, for example, 'high risk pregnancy', 'unwanted pregnancy' or 'disadvantaged parenting' – that immediately signal risks of moralizing and of health promoters getting caught up in highly contentious social agendas. Here teenage pregnancy can easily be treated as a disease analogue – as a physical condition which is somehow inherently 'unhealthy' and in need of social treatment or prevention. But this pathologizing can take place in other areas, though much less conspicuous processes. One example is the way in which health researchers deploy racialized categories in their work. There is a strong argument to say that the use of racialized categories (along with practices such as ethnic monitoring) may be useful for identifying potential effects of racism or institutional discrimination. But, on the contrary, some critics have raised the danger that using racialized categories (and ethnic monitoring) to explain things like educational performance, employment status or health status can contribute to racism and institutional discrimination and can obscure other factors including the role of class/socio-economic factors (Gewirtz & Cribb, 2006).

For example Davey Smith et al. (2000) have argued (a) that too much health research takes constructions of ethnicity as unproblematic, and (b) that work on health inequalities that does not open up the complex and ever changing pathways that may connect members of minority ethnic groups to experiences of ill health can lead 'to the pathologizing of minority ethnic status in itself'. As part of their discussion, for example, they critique a study of differences in stroke rates in London between what the authors (Stewart et al. 1999) refer to as 'Black' and 'White' populations arguing that the model of occupational class that the authors use to adjust for class differences simply fails to capture the full range of relevant socio-economic and other differences between the populations. Davey Smith and colleagues' worry is that this method 'produces data which apparently – but spuriously – demonstrate that health differences are due to genetic or cultural/behavioural factors' (Davey Smith et al. 2000, p. 35). They go on to say given that minority ethnic groups 'are among the most disadvantaged sections of British society' this work risks 'not only perpetuating but exacerbating disadvantage'.

I have used a few examples that relate to the ways in which the framing practices, explanatory practices and evaluative practices of social science are implicated in health promotion policy effects. And I am suggesting that the construction of health promotion knowledge through the practices of social science is one important subject matter for the study of health promotion ethics. Of course, for my purposes, it does not matter exactly how far the above examples are valid, for example, whether Beaglehole and Bonita are wrong to suggest that much health education has served to exacerbate health inequalities or whether Davey Smith and colleagues have got their analysis right and Stewart et al. wrong – all that matters is that these critiques point to potential problems. Indeed in each of these cases the empirical and ethical arguments are by no means straightforward – social scientists and health promoters who want to take them seriously will need to wrestle with dilemmas of various kinds. The central point is that we cannot neatly separate out the empirical and ethical consideration of health promotion, and ethicists cannot 'devolve' the consideration of 'the facts' to social scientists. Normative judgements are so deeply embedded in health promotion knowledge claims that ethical appraisal cannot begin by focusing on specific proposals for intervention. Besides (or as part of) seeking to critically examine the ethics of specific interventions, it must ask about the processes of knowledge construction that help frame problems and solutions in the first place. I am not taking sides here in the problem solving versus critical debate within policy analysis. I am happy to make common cause with those who stress the importance of attempting to insulate empirical readings from value assumptions and judgements but I am very conscious of how this is a permanent struggle which demands continuous epistemological and ethical reflexivity – in short I am saying that in practice one has to act as if the factual and evaluative judgements underlying health promotion policies and practices are entangled if only in order to try and disentangle them.

CONCLUSION

Having conducted a very partial review of a few facets of health promotion ethics, I will not attempt to say anything conclusive, but I can offer a small conclusion that follows from the above discussion. Ethically appraising health promotion means thinking about the specific actions that are undertaken in the name of health promotion, but it also means thinking about the 'social stage' on which these actions are undertaken. In other words, judgements about the ethical acceptability of specific health promotion interventions depend upon seeing them in the context of wider bundles of interventions and policy complexes. The best

balance between education and persuasion or compulsion, for example, depends among other things on the total 'package' of welfare goods in place and on an understanding of the full set of context-dependent reciprocal obligations between individuals, communities, institutions and the state. In this chapter I have placed emphasis upon various kinds of disadvantage or discrimination because when we are engaged in health promotion our activities are inevitably bound up with inequalities of income, wealth, status and power. In order to determine whether certain kinds and degrees of health promotion 'influence' are justified – whether and when we are right to exhort people or to attempt to enforce constraints or collective obligations upon them – we must be able to make and defend readings of the social field. In particular, I suggest, we need an empirically grounded and rich account of the kinds of pressures that different persons are under and the resources and social supports that are available to them; and we need to determine – partly through a consideration of this account – what it is feasible and fair to expect from them.

REFERENCES

Beaglehole R, Bonita R. *Public Health at the Crossroads*, Cambridge: Cambridge University Press, 1997; p. 119.

Caplan R, Holland R. Rethinking health education theory. *Health Educ J* 1990; **49**(1): 10–2.

Cribb A. *Health and the Good Society*. Oxford: Oxford University Press, 2005.

Davey Smith G, Charsley K, Lambert H, Paul S, Fenton S, Ahmad W. Ethnicity, health and the meaning of socio-economic position. In: Graham H, ed. *Understanding Health Inequalities*. Buckingham: Open University Press, 2000.

Gewirtz S, Cribb A. What to do about values in social research. *Br J Sociol Educ* 2006; **27**(2): 141–55.

Stewart J, Dundas R, Howard R, Rudd A, Woolfe C. Ethic difference in incidence of stroke: prospective study with stroke register. *Br Med J* 1999; **318**: 967–71.

Tones K, Tilford S. *Health Education: Effectiveness, Efficiency and Equity*, London: Chapman Hall, 2001.

Whitehead M. *Inequalities in Health*. Harmondsworth: Penguin, 1992.

World Health Organization. *Ottawa Charter for Health Promotion*, Geneva: WHO, 1986.

76

Preventing Disease

MARCEL VERWEIJ

It is better to prevent than to cure.

Big stories about past, present and future developments in medicine and health care almost invariably focus on new ways to diagnose and treat diseases. Indeed most expenditure in medical research goes to further the development of diagnosis and treatment options. MRI scanning, organ transplantation, reproductive technologies, new treatments for cancer, and genetic testing and diagnosis are all interesting and potentially expensive targets for research and development. In modern health care most financial resources are allocated to chronic patients for long-term care, as well as to those lacking in capacity because of illnesses such as dementia. Moreover, for decades now, bioethics has focused on questions concerning technological developments in curative medicine (e.g. separating conjoined twins and mechanical ventilation), and on dilemmas in the interaction between patients who require attention and physicians and nurses who care for them.

However, the importance of curative medicine and patient-oriented health care, and especially their impact on public health should not be overstated. When focusing on public health, on general life expectancy and morbidity, the biggest achievements have been realized – and are still to be realized – by means of preventive efforts outside the clinic. The best way to fight illness is not to diagnose disease by means of high-tech scans and to treat illness by whatever means; the best way to deal with disease is to simply prevent it. This is partly, though in a rather simplistic way, expressed in sayings 'an ounce of prevention is worth a pound of cure' or 'better to prevent than to cure'. The strong increase in life expectancy that has been realized in high-income countries during the nineteenth and twentieth centuries was not just caused by better treatment of patients (although the invention of antibiotic drugs arguably did play a large role). Improvement of living conditions, housing, the creation of sewerage systems, the provision of safe drinking water and the availability of food have had an impact that was much greater than medical technology and treatment of patients. Vaccination has led to a situation where many dangerous infectious diseases are under control in large parts of the world (e.g. measles, diphtheria, poliomyelitis) or have even eradicated completely (e.g. smallpox). In the coming decades much effect is to be expected from the growing rejection and discouragement of smoking and, especially in affluent countries, from changes in nutritional habits. Indeed, many modern public health problems like lung cancer and cardiovascular disease can only be most effectively countervailed by preventive means. Related to that, one of the most important moral concerns in public health is about health inequities: the strong correlation between ill-health, poverty and lack of education. It is unthinkable that such health inequities could be countervailed in any significant sense by means of improving the care for persons who get ill. For that matter, even apart from achievements and prospects for public health, prevention is normally preferable to cure because it helps individuals to avoid the burdens of illness as well as the burdens, risks and side-effects of diagnosis and therapy.

ETHICAL ISSUES

Notwithstanding the many reasons for praising preventive medicine, prevention also raises a number of moral concerns and other worries. First of all, the idea that prevention is always better then cure is obviously false. Politicians sometimes assume that it is cheaper to prevent diseases than to treat them. This is often not true. The reduction of mortality due to a number of infectious diseases may have led to more rather than less health care expenditures. This is

Principles of Health Care Ethics, Second Edition   Edited by R.E. Ashcroft, A. Dawson, H. Draper and J.R. McMillan
© 2007 John Wiley & Sons, Ltd

not only because preventive interventions like vaccinations often need to be targeted at the whole population and not just to the smaller group of diseased persons, but also because prevention of premature death after a short period of severe illness (as in the case of measles, smallpox and poliomyelitis) may lead to an increase in life expectance *and* concurrent chronic diseases that require a long period of staff-intensive care and support. The ultimate hope of medicine is compression of morbidity: to increase lifespan *and* reduce the average years a person is ill during his or her life (Fries, 1983). In the age of chronic diseases, however, it is not certain that the burden of disease within the average person's life will decrease. This is no reason to consider prevention unimportant or undesirable, but it does put exaggerated expectations into perspective.

There are also moral reasons for questioning the obviousness of the idea that prevention is better than cure. One has to do with issues of priority-setting. In health care, priority is often given to treating persons who are most needy; persons who, from an egalitarian perspective, may have a stronger claim on medical resources than persons who are healthy. Even if preventive interventions are considered much more efficient than interventions that satisfy actual needs, it would be controversial to decide to allocate more resources for prevention at the cost of patients who need health care now. People often intuitively accept the *rule of rescue*, that is the principle that life-saving interventions aiming to rescue assignable individuals in acute situations, demand priority above preventive efforts that only save 'statistical' lives. The 'rule of rescue' and its (alleged) justification is an ongoing topic of debate in bioethics. Arguably, in acute situations moral agents should not trade off preventive care and acute relief of needs. If there is a person in immediate need, one ought to rescue him or her if one can, and donating money to *Médicins sans Frontières* cannot be a reasonable alternative to that, even if the latter option would be more cost-effective (cf. Cullity, 2004). On a population level, however, and especially in decisions about allocating resources for public health, governments and other institutions cannot simply rely on the rule of rescue as a justification for downplaying prevention (Hope, 2001; Marseille, Hofmann & Kahn, 2002).

Preventive medicine also raises moral concerns that are especially relevant from the perspective of members of target groups. In most cases, prevention is directed at healthy persons for whom it may not be obvious that they need preventive care. Their outlook is radically different from patients who experience symptoms and who seek treatment for their ailments. Such treatment may have side-effects, but patients normally have a reasonable prospect that the benefits of therapy do outweigh such burdens. In preventive medicine, it is much more difficult for persons to assess whether or not interventions like vaccination, screening or behaviour

change are worthwhile. Indeed, burdens and risks of preventive interventions may not be justified easily, given that there is no immediate need for treatment. On a population level, the beneficial effects of a prevention programme may be beyond doubt, showing a clear reduction in morbidity; yet from the perspective of individual persons, this is less clear. The benefits of prevention are often remote, and most people only experience burdens and other side-effects of a vaccine or a screening procedure. Geoffrey Rose called this the 'prevention paradox': interventions that have a great impact on public health may have little effect on the health of an individual (Rose, 1992).

The fact that prevention is targeted at persons who do not need a medical intervention suggests that preventive programmes will need to be 'sold' to target groups in order to be successful. Prevention, therefore, necessarily takes a pro-active, outreaching approach, where persons are invited, persuaded, or even pressed to participate. One typical way is to offer prevention as a routine procedure where participation is considered more or less self-evident, and the possibility of refusing the intervention is not mentioned explicitly. Such procedures are common in programmes for childhood vaccination and neonatal screening. Obviously, these procedures raise questions as to what extent persons participate voluntarily and whether more substantive forms of informed consent, as they are common in clinical medicine, are required. Many argue that informed consent procedures are indispensable, especially because prevention is aimed at healthy persons; yet there are also good reasons to think that informed consent procedures are unfeasible and even undesirable (Nijsingh, 2007). Routine testing and vaccinations may be justified if, at least, the effectiveness and safety of these interventions are beyond doubt, because many prevention programmes aim to protect or promote the health of the public at large and not just all individual persons. It should be noted, however, that few medical interventions, including preventive treatments such as vaccination, are without any risk. In prevention, even very small risks need to be taken seriously, given that preventive interventions are often targeted at very large groups of healthy persons. For example, if several million children are vaccinated with the live oral polio vaccine (OPV), there is a reasonable chance that some individuals will develop vaccine-associated poliomyelitis (VAPP). This occurs in approximately 1 in 760000 first vaccinations with OPV (Halsey, 2003). Such risks may be justified given the large benefits on a public health scale; yet many parents might decide to forego vaccination of their child if they were informed explicitly about all small risks – which would be detrimental to all. Especially in affluent countries where diseases like polio are virtually eradicated, it may be difficult to persuade people to participate in such a prevention programme. After all, the chance that one's child will be infected with poliomyelitis will be almost (though not completely) nil. In this way, preventive programmes like vaccination may sometimes be undermined by their own success.

A further group of moral concerns about prevention focus on the fact that almost all situations and activities of human beings have some impact on health, and as a result of that, all situations and activities may be eligible for preventive concerns. If we consider illness as something undesirable and if we even can have moral duties to avoid causing illness, this might serve as a basis for virtually unlimited concern by health professionals for our lives, and potentially far reaching moral duties upon us to take care of the impact of our actions on the health of others. The first concern is often phrased in terms of *medicalization* or *healthism*: the possibilities of prevention may put all aspects of daily life in the light of concerns about health and disease, and that may be undesirable. The second concern refers to the *overdemandingness problem*: the far reaching possibilities of prevention may lead to duties to care for the health of others that are very demanding – possibly too demanding. Both issues are especially relevant for preventive medicine and have raised little concern in the field of clinical medicine.

MEDICALIZATION AND CONCERNS ABOUT THE GOOD LIFE

Preventive interventions are sometimes considered morally problematic as they contribute to *medicalization*. The term 'medicalization' was coined by Zola, denoting the trend to see social problems as medical problems, requiring medical intervention and control (Zola, 1972). In the context of prevention, considerations of medicalization or healthism are different. They are mostly put forward to criticize the fact that preventive practices invite healthy persons to medical examination, screening, preventive treatment, or to change their way of life according to medical recommendations. Authors such as Ivan Illich, Petr Skrabanek and James McCormick pointed at numerous harmful effects and other drawbacks of preventive medicine – notably screening. Illich (1977) emphasized the iatrogenic effects of medical practice and rhetorically claimed that 'the medical establishment has become a major threat to health'. Skrabanek and McCormick raised doubts about the effectiveness of mass screening programmes and pointed out that inevitably a number of participants would suffer serious harm as a result of screening (Skrabanek, 1990, 1994; McCormick, 1996).

There are however good reasons to avoid using such a vague notion of *medicalization* for such important dimensions. Obviously, vaccination and screening practices must be safe and effective, but such requirements are obscured rather than clarified if they are framed in terms of medicalization. That, however, does not imply that the concept of medicalization is useless altogether, but issues of medicalization do not warrant the critique that Illich has raised.

In the context of preventive medicine, medicalization can refer to two interrelated processes (Verweij, 1999). One is on the level of language and concepts: terms such as 'health', '(un)healthy' and 'illness' are used for other areas: a person's behaviour, and events and problems that are usually part of normal life. On a practical level 'medicalization' refers to the phenomenon that healthy persons tend to adjust their life and lifestyle according to medical information, advice and procedures. This definition is relatively free of moral assumptions. Yet, some reasons can be given for the common intuition that medicalization can be morally undesirable. These reasons are not as clear-cut as requirements of safety, non-maleficence, effectiveness, or respect for autonomy. Moreover, the phenomena of medicalization, and the moral reluctance they raise, do not normally arise in one preventive intervention carried out by one health professional. They arise as a result of the practice of preventive medicine at large. Nowadays, people are informed about numerous health risks; they are invited to participate in screening programmes; they are told to avoid unhealthy food and other risky behaviour; they are urged to get vaccinated, and so on. Moreover, these preventive opportunities are given in almost all areas in their lives: not only when they talk to their family physician, but also at school, at work, in sports clubs and through the mass media. Obviously, some level of health is extremely important for a reasonably good life, but it is not self-evident that being reminded all the time of risks and opportunities to avoid illness will contribute to well being. This process of medicalization may lead to three different moral problems. These problems cannot simply be avoided by imposing particular requirements on preventive practices – they are mainly reasons not to apply the growing possibilities of preventive medicine.

A first problem has to do with the probably inevitable effect that many forms of prevention, notably screening programmes, cause people to worry and feel uncertain about the possibility that they have or will develop a specific disease. These inconveniences will often be surmountable and can be minimized if sufficient attention is given to communication between professional and client. The worries and uncertainties caused by screening programmes will normally be taken away if a negative test result is disclosed. If the result is positive, worries will probably increase, but in that case obviously the worries are appropriate. The first moral problem of medicalization is not that such feelings are inconvenient, but that, if they are raised (and taken away) very often, this might affect a person's basic confidence in the solidity of his or her health. Nowadays, people are given information about the dangers of many activities that used to be common and normal. Numerous activities, substances and habits need to be avoided in order to reduce the risk that one will get a serious disease. Many other activities need to be performed in order to protect or promote health. The effects of preventive care programmes on people's confidence in health should not be assessed for each particular programme as such. They accumulate, so they should be evaluated as a whole. For persons who take all offers of preventive care seriously, it may come to seem that health is a fragile equilibrium and as if human beings must constantly anticipate threats against their health. Such a view of health is detrimental to feelings of confidence and security regarding one's health and well-being.

A second problem of medicalization as a result of preventive medicine concerns moral responsibility for illness. Preventive medicine gives people opportunities to reduce risk and avoid disease. If someone decides not to take the opportunity offered and later on contracts the disease in question, it will be no surprise that people will say, 'he is responsible for his illness'. To some extent, such a judgement is correct. Interventions such as health information, vaccination and screening in some sense enhance the autonomy of people as they create meaningful options for choice. Responsibility is simply the flipside of their increased autonomy. Though it often makes sense to give people a sense of responsibility so that they can make their own choices and face the consequences, in health care practice it may not always be appropriate to emphasize personal responsibility for illness. Many health care systems express values of solidarity in which the financial burdens of health care are shared by all, assuming citizens are to some extent willing to contribute to care for the unfortunate who become ill. Solidarity is most strong if it is based not only upon compassion with the worse off, but also on a common interest: the knowledge that sooner or later one might need health care as well. If we come to believe that many individuals are partly responsible for the health care they (or their children) need, this could undermine the second pillar of solidarity – a prospect that many would consider as undesirable. In short, giving people more options to prevent disease is *prima facie* a good thing, but it may have some undesirable effects as well.

A third problem of medicalization concerns the tendency that people see health as a central value in their lives. Arguably, a certain level of health is important in any account of human well-being, and prudent persons who aim to live well should not constantly neglect risks to their health. For that matter, it would be equally imprudent for individuals to endorse health as the *ultimate* value in their lives, if only because one can be certain that sooner or later one's health will decline. The manifold preventive interventions will not force people to adopt such a 'healthist' view of life,

but they may make it more and more difficult for individuals to develop a way of life in which the value of health is *not* especially prominent. Such a problem might not trouble health professions and physicians, but in a pluralistic and democratic society it is undesirable if particular reasonable ways of life cannot flourish. It is not irrational for a person 'just to live his or her life' and only bother about his or her health if he or she would feel ill or if there are apparent and clear risks. Yet the more one is confronted with the offers of screening and preventive care, the more difficult it is to develop and sustain such an attitude.

Often a person's conception of how to live is not an explicit plan of life that is ready made or deliberately chosen: it is formed, developed and adjusted in situations in which this person needs to think about his or her way of life, and consider which things he or she wants to avoid, and which things he or she wants to pursue. A person's view of life will be influenced by the kind of questions he or she is confronted with. Should I go to church or is my belief in God receding? Do I want to have children or not? Should I care for my immobile parent? Should I be faithful to my spouse? Nowadays such questions are considered to belong to the private realm and few of these questions are raised and discussed by public institutions. Choices about health and risk are notable exceptions. Through information about opportunities to reduce or avoid risks of disease, preventive health care institutions encourage people to consider how they should live. But the more a person is urged to consider his or her life in a context of opportunities for health and risks of disease (instead of contexts of religion, politics, parenthood, etc.), the more the view of life he or she is developing will get 'biased' by this theme. This bias may be positive or negative. In both cases, health-choices are a relatively important determinant for his or her view of life. Either he or she considers health as important or he or she attaches less importance to health. But even in the latter case, health is a theme that cannot simply be ignored. Obviously, in large parts of the world, people's health is threatened continuously, and ongoing concerns about these threats are inevitable and important. In affluent countries, however, it may be unreasonable for persons to focus so much on the relatively small risks they run and be concerned about their health in all aspects of their lives.

In conclusion, many preventive interventions like vaccination, screening or health promotion programmes necessarily aim to make people aware of health risks and enable them to avoid or reduce those risks. The expanding knowledge of health risks and possibilities for preventive medicine leave little room for aspects of life where concerns about health and disease are not relevant. Such developments may have negative effects on human well-being and they may turn 'health' into a value that has an unreasonably prominent place in people's conceptions of the good life. Interestingly, such considerations do not support clear obligations or limitations for public health practitioners and health care professions, though they might play an important role in reflections on good preventive practices and ideals in public health (Verweij, 2000).

THE SCOPE OF OBLIGATIONS TO AVOID CAUSING ILLNESS

Expanding knowledge about risks and how to prevent disease may not just support preventive interventions that are pervasive throughout our lives. It forces us to reconsider our obligations to other people, given that our activities may not only affect our own health, but the health of others as well. This is most apparent in cases where the behaviour of one person may directly put others at risk, as in drinking and driving, but it may equally apply to less immediate threats as in smoking. In many contexts, it is more or less accepted that one should not smoke in the company of people who do not smoke and who may not consent to passive smoking. This is just a corollary of the principle of non-maleficence. The meaning of this principle and its scope in the context of prevention is however far from clear, especially when contagious diseases like influenza, measles or hepatitis B force us to rethink to what extent we have an obligation to avoid infecting others (Harris, 1995).

It is generally accepted that hygienic measures in health care are part of standards of due care, which means that health care professionals have a professional duty to take precautions against contamination and infection. Sterilization of surgical instruments, the use of gloves and frequent hand-washing are obvious examples. Yet, it is less clear whether health professionals also have a professional and moral duty to be vaccinated against influenza and other diseases in order to avoid infecting their patients (van den Hoven & Verweij, 2003; Poland, 2005). Are such precautions also to be considered part of due care? Some health care workers might consider such requirements too demanding, especially if they have personal or religious objections to vaccination.

Questions like these do not apply only to the health care workers, but also to citizens in general. Most clearly, a person who knows he is HIV-positive should, from a moral point of view, refrain from unsafe sex practices, or disclose his HIV-status to sex partners (which does not imply that such moral obligations should be sanctioned by criminal law (cf. Chalmers, 2002; Elliot, 2002; SOAIDS, 2004). Yet, it would be inadequate to assume that such moral concerns only apply to persons who know they are HIV-positive. Many persons in HIV risk groups who have not been tested yet may be infected, and capable of infecting others. It would be unreasonable to impose all the obligating burdens of precaution upon only those who know they are seropositive and not on

others who are at risk of being HIV-positive. Moreover, HIV is not the only sexually transmitted disease that is harmful, and therefore the duty to take precautions and practise safe sex applies to a group of persons that is much broader than just members of HIV-risk groups.

Such an expanded scope of the duty to avoid infection does not have to be too demanding. First, although many persons may prefer not to use condoms, it is a relatively simple precaution that is not very burdensome. Second, protected sex is a responsibility that is shared by sex partners. In consensual sex, partners can negotiate the levels of protection they deem necessary, and this may set the limits as to what they owe to each other. For example, it is morally justified for sex partners A and B to jointly decide to have unprotected sex if they consider the risks negligible or acceptable. Or, on the contrary, they can decide to have protected sex if they prefer not to disclose their HIV-status.

Our obligations to prevent infection may have far wider implications in the case of diseases that are transmitted much more easily, such as measles, influenza, or, for that matter, the common cold. Influenza infections normally lead to relatively mild illness in young and middle-aged adults, but in elderly persons and certain chronic patients it causes serious and life-threatening disease. The viruses are spread easily, by means of aerosols of virus-laden respiratory secretions that are expelled into the air by infected persons when they cough, sneeze or talk. Vaccination offers reasonable protection to persons who are otherwise healthy, but the effectiveness in persons at high risk is relatively weak. Now, if we assume that there is a moral requirement to prevent disease and not infect others, this supports the idea that persons who feel ill should not visit nursing homes or other places where there are at-risk persons. Or, one step further, given that one may be infected but not have developed symptoms, there are moral reasons not to visit such a place altogether, during the flu season. Or, even further, the requirement supports mandatory vaccination against the flu for everyone, as this will strongly reduce the risk of transmission of influenza, and hence contribute to protection of elderly persons and immuno-compromised patients. Again, what level of precaution can be considered obligatory? What level of protection do we owe to persons for whom influenza infection involves a serious threat to their health?

It may be appealing to analyse this issue in terms of the distinction between non-maleficence, which is supposed to be obligatory, and beneficence, which can be beyond duty. Yet this will not be of help. The distinction between both principles is not particularly clear anyway, and, given that that there are clear cases of duties of beneficence (e.g. a duty to rescue), this distinction does not determine which actions or omissions are obligatory and which are not. Ethical analysis and specification of the scope of the duty to prevent infecting others requires to appeal to more general moral theories, as well as clarification of our moral intuitions about what sort of obligations are (un)reasonable. Interestingly, this issue can be considered as a practical counterpart of the recent philosophical debates about the limits of morality (Murphy 2000; Kagan, 1989; van den Hoven, 2006). Consequentialist theories are often criticized for imposing unreasonably demanding moral obligations. However, the overdemandingness problem is equally relevant for non-consequentialist theories, especially with respect to moral requirements to prevent harm (Ashford, 2003; Verweij, 2005).

CONCLUSION

Although the achievements of preventive medicine in promoting public health are beyond doubt, preventive efforts (screening, vaccination, health information and promotion) raise moral issues that need to be taken seriously. In this chapter, three groups of concerns have been discussed. First, prevention is normally offered in a proactive or routine way to healthy persons, and this raises special concerns about the weighing of harms and benefits as well as about threats to voluntary consent. Second, the possibilities for prevention can be pervasive throughout our lives, and this raises concerns about medicalization: could it be that care for health and worries about disease are acquiring a too prominent role in people's outlook? Third, to some extent people have a moral duty to avoid harming other people, for example, to prevent transmission of infectious diseases. The scope of such an obligation is not well-defined, and this is a fruitful area for theoretical and practical reflection in health care ethics.

REFERENCES

Ashford E. The demandingness of Scanlon's contractualism. *Ethics* 2003; **113**: 273–302.

Chalmers J. The criminalization of HIV transmission. *J Med Ethics* 2002; **28**: 160–3.

Cullity G. *The Moral Demands of Affluence*. Oxford: Clarendon Press, 2004.

Elliot, R. *Criminal Law, Public Health, and HIV Transmission*. Geneva: UNAIDS, 2002. http://data.unaids.org/Publications/IRC-pub02/JC733-CriminalLaw_en.pdf

Fries JF. The compression of morbidity. *Milbank Memorial Fund Q* 1983; **61**: 397–419.

Halsey NA. Vaccine safety: real and perceived issues. In: Bloom BR, Lambert P, eds. *The Vaccine Book*. San Diego: Academic Press, 2003; 371–89.

Harris J, Holm S. Is there a moral obligation not to infect others? *BMJ* 1995; **311**: 1215–7.

Hope T. Rationing and life-saving treatments: should identifiable patients have higher priority? *J Med Ethics* 2001; **27**: 179–85.

Illich I. *Limits to Medicine. Medical Nemesis: The Expropriation of Health*. Harmondsworth: Penguin Books, 1977.

Kagan S. *The Limits of Morality*. Oxford: Oxford University Press, 1989.

Marseille E, Hofmann PB, Kahn JG. HIV Prevention before HAART in Sub-Saharan Africa. *Lancet* 2002; **359**: 1851–6.

McCormick J. Medical hubris and the public health: the ethical dimension. *J Clin Epidemiol* 1996; **49**: 619–21.

Murphy LB. *Moral Demands in Nonideal Theory*. Oxford: Oxford University Press, 2000.

Nijsingh NN. Informed consent and newborn screening. In: Dawson AJ, Verweij MF, eds. *Ethics, Prevention, and Public Health*. Oxford: Oxford University Press, 2007.

Poland GA, Tosh P, Jacobson RM. Requiring influenza vaccination for health care workers: seven truths we must accept. *Vaccine* 2005; **23**: 2251–5.

Rose G. *The Strategy of Preventive Medicine*. Oxford: Oxford University Press, 1992.

Skrabanek P. Why is preventive medicine exempted from ethical constraints? *J Med Ethics* 1990; **16**: 187–90.

Skrabanek P. *The Death of Humane Medicine and the Rise of Coercive Healthism*. Suffolk: Social Affairs Unit, 1994.

SOAIDS. Executive Committee on Aids Policy and Criminal Law. *Detention or Prevention? A Report on the Impact of the use of Criminal Law on Public Health and the Position of People Living with HIV*. Amsterdam: SOAIDS, 2004; www.aidsfonds.nl/folders/strafrechtEng.pdf

van den Hoven MA, Verweij MF. Should we promote influenza vaccination of health care workers in nursing homes? Some arguments in favour of immunization. *Age Ageing* 2003; **32**: 487–9.

van den Hoven MA. *A claim for reasonable morality. Commonsense morality in the debate on the limits of morality*. Utrecht: Zeno/Utrecht University, 2006.

Verweij MF. Medicalization as a moral problem for preventive medicine. *Bioethics* 1999; **13**: 89–113.

Verweij MF. Preventive medicine between obligation and aspiration. *International Library of Ethics, Law, and the New Medicine*, vol. 4. Dordrecht: Kluwer Academic Publishers, 2000.

Verweij MF. Obligatory precautions against infection. *Bioethics* 2005; **19**: 323–35.

Zola IK. Medicine as an institution of social control. *Sociol Rev* 1972; **20**: 487–504.

Quantitative Methods for Priority-Setting in Health: Ethical Issues

DANIEL WIKLER, DAN W. BROCK, SARAH MARCHAND,
AND TESSA TAN TORRES

INTRODUCTION

Health resources are invariably scarce relative to need, especially in the developing world, where resources are few and the burden of disease is concentrated (Murray, 1996). Setting priorities among alternative uses of available resources to ensure that they are distributed efficiently and fairly is a moral responsibility for health systems (Wikler, 2003).

Setting priorities in the allocation of health resources requires the simultaneous resolution of many uncertainties and of multiple conflicting goals. Choices must be made about how to allocate resources between health and other goods, between health needs as dissimilar as infertility, autism, pancreatic cancer and cleft palate (to choose just a few examples), and between interventions that vary in cost and effectiveness. These decisions, moreover, often must be made within political, legal, regulatory and commercial constraints; and the information and expertise needed to make optimal decisions may be unavailable, uncertain or costly. As life and freedom from distress and disability hang in the balance, it is unsurprising that scholars from many disciplines have laboured to develop methods for health resource allocation that could make allocations closer to the ideal.

In what follows, we examine some of the ethical issues arising in the design and use of some quantitative methods for priority-setting, focusing primarily on cost-effectiveness analysis (CEA), a technique for comparing the health outcomes and costs of interventions. We will also contrast CEA with cost–benefit analysis (CBA), a method that (unlike CEA) explicitly permits comparison of the value of outcomes of health interventions to the value yielded by use of those resources for goods other than health. Neither CEA nor CBA are merely number-crunching exercises. Each relies upon and incorporates assumptions and choices regarding a number of difficult ethical and conceptual issues. In many instances these ethical commitments are implicit. Moreover, neither method is sufficient for priority-setting unless used in combination with appropriate regard for competing ethical concerns such as fairness. We identify a number of the moral issues raised by these methods for setting priorities. For the most part, we focus on ethical questions about CEA and CBA, with scant attention to the priority-setting dilemmas that these methods are used to resolve. Similarly, we omit discussion of several related moral dimensions of priority-setting in health, such as public deliberation and participation, and compliance with international agreements on human rights, each of which deserve extended exposition (Gruskin & Tarantola, 2001; Daniels & Sabin, 2002).

CEA AND CBA

Both CEA and CBA are used to assist in using health resources wisely. Both involve measures of the costs of interventions and of the benefit they produce. But CEA compares costs, in dollars (or other unit of resources; our exposition uses dollars for brevity's sake), to health outcomes, measured in units of health such as deaths averted, life years saved, or quality-adjusted life years (QALYs), whereas CBA compares costs, in dollars, to the *dollar value* of health (or other) outcomes. The substantial literature on these two analytic techniques and on the relationship between them is marked by controversy over their relative advantages in terms of theoretical soundness, practical usefulness and moral acceptability. After a brief discussion of similarities

Principles of Health Care Ethics, Second Edition Edited by R.E. Ashcroft, A. Dawson, H. Draper and J.R. McMillan
© 2007 John Wiley & Sons, Ltd

and differences between the two techniques, we focus on the moral issues.

The immediate goals of CBA and CEA differ. By computing the value of outcomes in dollars, CBA offers a direct assessment of whether the benefit of an intervention exceeds its costs, and, in principle, can also tell us whether using the money for purposes other than health could yield greater benefit. For example, CBA could be used to try to determine whether a given health intervention would create as much value for a population of poor children as an enhancement of their public schools would. The scope of CBA is potentially vast. An ambitious study of all spending on health in the United States from 1960 to 2000, for example, concluded that even though its costs were the world's highest, the money spent by America's health system had been worth while (Cutler, Rosen & Vijan, 2006).

CBA not only measures the value of health interventions in a way that permits comparison to the value of other uses of resources, but it can also take into account a broader range of the effects of health interventions. CEA, as used in health resource allocation, is concerned with the quantity of health benefit, such as life years or QALYs, which alternative interventions produce. But health interventions are often valued not only for the health they can provide but also for a variety of other attributes. One intervention for a stigmatized condition, for example, might be preferred to another of equal health efficacy if it would be easier to hide from public knowledge. The dollar value ascribed in CBA to these interventions to an individual is understood to reflect the totality of the (perceived) benefits to that person – that is, the degree to which the intervention satisfies all of the individual's preferences.

CBA and CEA can be – and are – used in tandem; indeed, a major stimulus to CEA in the United States was a directive from the government's Office of Management and the Budget in 2003 to supplement CB studies of the effects of regulations with several kinds of CEA (Office of Management and the Budget, 2003). Some scholars have proposed methods for translating one to the other. For example, the results of a CEA, expressed in health units (e.g. a quality-adjusted life year) can be expressed in dollar terms if we could attach a dollar value to that unit of health. CEA is often used, in actual practice, to gauge the value of a drug or intervention in relation to its cost by comparing its cost per added QALY to a benchmark dollar value for a QALY. The benchmark might be derived by averaging the maximum prices per QALY that have been deemed acceptable in the past, or by imputing a dollar value per QALY to agency decisions that have made other kinds of trade-offs between cost and health, such as in safety or environmental regulations. However, benchmark values chosen in these studies are not standardized, and those chosen in the priority-setting literature vary several fold (Polsky, 2005). Only at the extremes – 'best buys' and very cost-ineffective interventions, respectively – are

the recommendations based on CEA likely to be insensitive to this variability in the choice of benchmark values. The soundness of this method for translating CEA into CBA has also been questioned for populations whose valuations are not uniform (as they often are not) (Dolan & Edlin, 2002; Kenkel, 1997).

Nevertheless CEA, not CBA, dominates the literature on priority-setting in health economics, though the reverse is true in other fields, such as environmental regulation, that similarly require dollar-health tradeoffs. Though the use of these quantitative priority-setting methods is bound to become more common as rising health costs make these difficult choices unavoidable, their use has provoked a number of ethical concerns that could limit the acceptance of CEA and CBA by decision-makers. Although some of these may reflect misunderstandings, the usefulness of these techniques for their intended purpose requires that these concerns be explicitly addressed. We begin with some general (and perhaps ill-defined) ethical doubts and proceed to more specific concerns.

VALUE OF A LIFE

Do quantitative priority-setting methods require us to place a dollar value on a human life? Is this inherently wrong – or are there unobjectionable ways to do so?

This ethical objection applies directly only to CBA in the case of interventions that might affect mortality. CEA does not place a dollar value on anything except the costs of the intervention. CBA, on the contrary, evaluates outcomes in dollars, and if the intervention being assessed would affect the number or probability of deaths, a dollar value for the lives lost would ordinarily need to be assigned. The notion that each human life is infinitely precious, if taken literally, is in direct contradiction to this practice. But if this is an ethical offence it is not the cost–benefit analysts who are alone guilty of it. Each of us implicitly places a dollar value on life when we make spending decisions – for example, to pay extra for better brakes on a new car – that could have life-or-death consequences, be the lives our own or those of others. But the notion that lives and dollars are 'fungible', that choices among public policies should be indifferent to savings in dollars versus saving human lives, provided that the dollar value of a human life is set correctly, is for some intuitively unacceptable.

Is this intuition sound, or is it a confused sentiment? The complex web of values that govern our actions towards each other inevitably bears on our ethical response to cost–benefit analyses. Lives do not merely pop in and out of existence; if a person dies, there may have been an act by another individual that constitutes negligence or even murder, and these considerations may be decisive in our moral judgement of the change independently of the dollar value of the life of the deceased. An employer may protest against regulations that require the safest workplace that is technologically feasible (McCaffrey, 1982), if this requires very large expenditures to reduce risks only slightly, but the justification for the regulation may reflect concerns about the workers' bargaining power, or a moral judgement (sound or otherwise) that employers are responsible for avoidable deaths on the job. Public attitudes on the monetary value of risk reduction for passengers on British railways, for example, seem to vary depending on the source of those risks (Wolff, 2002).

It may be impossible to gauge the value of outcomes of public policies and health expenditures affecting risks to life unless life itself is assigned a particular value, but it should be the right value. Indirect measures such as the amount the individual is willing to pay to reduce risks (e.g. in buying safety devices for a new car) reflect the individual's wealth, tolerance of risk and perhaps age, none of which is necessarily constitutive of the value of the person's life from a moral viewpoint. It is more plausible to hold that our obligation to save lives is stronger toward those who would live many years thereafter (a consideration that CEA takes into account), than to claim that the strength of our obligation varies according to how much the individual would be willing to pay (a measure often used in CBA). The former is a more plausible measure of how much good we would do for those who are saved. These considerations are not merely academic. A cost–benefit analysis of measures to mitigate the effects of global warming for example might recommend measures that would protect a few hundred Frenchmen from heat stroke over measures that would protect many thousands of Bangladeshis from flood. If the value of saving these lives is the same irrespective of the individual's wealth, then this CBA, based on differences in ability and willingness to pay for protective measures, is a poor gauge of value (Broome, 2004).

SOURCES OF ETHICAL CONCERN ABOUT CEA

CEA would seem to be less vulnerable than CBA since it does not require the use of methods to elicit or impute dollar values for lives, but similar concerns do arise. For example, the US Public Health Service has recommended that the patient's time, counted as a cost of care, be determined by the average wage of the target population (Gold, Siegel, Russell & Weinstein, 1996; Holtgrave, 2004). CEA of interventions targeting the poor would thus count the patients' time as less valuable than if the target population had been wealthy; and the same is true, on the average, of interventions targeting women versus men or (in the United States, and on average) African–Americans versus whites. Valuing the time of people in less-advantaged groups less than that of the more advantaged may give offence, but the net effect on priority-setting might be positive for the former. The reason is that, all else being equal, this entails that interventions targeting the less-advantaged cost less for the same result (Russell, 2004).

Even when costs are computed differently for higher- and lower-income individuals, respectively, CEA typically counts the value of the outcomes of interventions, such as restoring sight, in the same manner for each person (Broome, 2002). For some authors, this is a matter of principle: equity demands that each person's health be regarded as equally important (Murray, 1996). Others contrast the ethical framework assumed by CEA and CBA, respectively, by locating CEA within a 'spheres of justice' perspective (Walzer, 1983) in which norms of equality govern health considerations even as non-egalitarian principles underlie most of the rest of social interaction (Dolan & Edlin, 2002). But it is unclear what principle is upheld by stipulating that the value of a QALY is the same for everyone, when costs are figured differently for rich and poor.

These issues raise questions regarding the interpretation of the measurement units that denominate CEA that remain unresolved: what they intend to measure, or do measure and how well they measure it. The Disability-Adjusted Life Year, a variant used by the World Health Organization (WHO), is sometimes presented and defended as a measure of health, whereas QALYs are typically understood to be a measure of the *value* of health states and health gains. It is usually taken for granted that the correct measure of the value of health states are individuals' preferences: an individual is better off in health state *a* than in health state *b* if she prefers *a* to *b*. To identify what people prefer with the goodness or badness of health states and to decide on that basis whether individuals are better or worse off in one health state than another, however, requires ethical assumptions that are controversial (Hausman, 2006).

First, it may be false that if a person prefers to be in health state *a* over health state *b*, then she is better off in health state *a* than in health state *b*. When we say that a person is better or worse off in one state than in another, a natural way to understand such statements is that the person's quality of life or well-being is improved or worsened. According to many accounts of human well-being, people can and often do prefer what is not good for them, and satisfying their preferences may make them worse off. Even when preferences are well informed, are based on a good understanding of the facts and involve no errors of reasoning, we may reject the notion that if people prefer state *a* to state *b* then people are necessarily better off in state *a*. According to some theories of well-being, people are better off if they possess certain resources, capacities and freedoms, follow certain pursuits and have certain kinds of personal relationships – whether they prefer these or not (Sen, 1999). Such 'objective' theories of well-being reject the idea that something is valuable, or makes someone better off, just because and in so far as it is desired by that person. While people may desire what is valuable or good for them, according to objective theories, they desire it because it is valuable or good for them; it is not valuable or good for them because they desire it. If such accounts are correct, then preferences can at best be evidence for, and not constitutive of, what is good or bad for people (Brink, 1989).

Second, preferences for health states, like many other kinds of preferences, reflect both the qualities of the health state and the circumstances of the chooser. As we discuss below, surveys of health state preferences usually find that people who have long had, and have adjusted to, a given disability view life with that disability as being much closer in value to healthy life than others do. Which preferences should be figured into QALY based CEA? The answer requires ethical judgements; it cannot be settled by still more data about preferences (Hausman & McPherson, 2006).

CEA, AGE AND TIME

Further ethical concerns about CEA arise in connection with the way that CEA addresses priorities for interventions as they affect people of different ages and at different times. The DALY, for example, incorporated the results of polls conducted by the WHO that showed that greater importance was attached to the years of young maturity than to those of early childhood or advancing age. A plausible explanation for these results is that respondents were concerned that those with young dependants be able to meet their needs. Although the DALY may have mirrored the preferences of much of the public in this regard, it is not clear that this practice is consistent with counting everyone's health and life as equally valuable. Apart from the implied inequality in the importance of years of life at different stages of the lifespan, this age-weighting favours some individuals because of their value to others. However benign this may seem in the case of young parents, the same principle, consistently applied, might privilege the more productive individuals in a society. WHO in many instances provided results both with and without age-weighting.

The way in which CEA assigns value to health outcomes occurring in the future raises further ethical questions. It is a standard practice in CEA to discount both health care costs and benefits at the same rate, for example 3% or 5%. There is little controversy that future monetary costs and benefits should be discounted to their present value in a CEA. The same amount of money is worth more if received today than in 10 years because it can be invested at the market rate of interest if received today, and for the same reason costs that can be deferred require fewer present dollars to meet them. The controversial issue is whether health benefits should be discounted, that is, whether the same magnitude of health benefit has progressively less social value the further into the future that it occurs.

This issue is complex and has engendered an extensive literature that cannot be reviewed here, but we can at least try to focus the issue. It is appropriate to discount for the uncertainty about whether potential beneficiaries will survive to receive a future health benefit. It is also reasonable to take into account any increased uncertainty about whether a benefit will occur because it is more distant. However, these uncertainties are reflected in the calculation of expected future benefits and do not require that future benefits be discounted. If individuals receive a health benefit, such as regaining eyesight or mobility, sooner rather than later, their total lifetime benefit may be greater, but this too is reflected in the estimation of the total benefit without discounting.

The ethical issue about discounting is whether, after taking account of such considerations, a health benefit of the same size has progressively less social value the further into the future that it occurs. To make the issue more concrete, suppose we must decide between two programmes, one of which will save 100 lives now and the other of which, say a hepatitis vaccination programme, will save 200 lives in 30 years. The vaccination programme will save twice as many lives, but if we apply even a 3% discount rate to the future lives saved then they are equivalent to only 78 lives saved now and we should prefer the first programme. This example illustrates not only the theoretical issue but also its practical import because discounting future health benefits will systematically tend to disadvantage resource allocation prevention programmes that must be undertaken now, but whose benefits only occur at some point in the future. This applies not only to many vaccination programmes but also to most programmes to change unhealthy behaviours whose benefits generally occur at some later time. When future health benefits would go to different individuals or even different generations they will raise issues of distributive justice or equity between those individuals or generations which could in some cases lead us not to prefer the larger future benefit. These issues of distributive justice are not properly addressed simply by discounting future benefits.

Arguments for discounting health benefits at the same rate as costs have ranged from consistency arguments (Weinstein & Stason, 1997), avoidance of paradoxes in allocation concerning research and deferral of spending (Keeler & Cretin 1983), individual or social rates of time preference and so forth. We cannot review these arguments here, but only insist that deciding whether to discount health benefits is squarely an ethical question about the relative moral importance of health benefits that occur now and in the future, and should be explicitly addressed as an issue of justice such as in health resource allocation.

CEA AND DISABILITY

A broad contrast between 'humanitarian' and 'economic' approaches to health economics is often found in writing that is distrustful of quantitative approaches to priority-setting in health care. Its resonances include the aversion to pricing life, discussed above, and also concern for the disabled. In this view, the disabled are at risk of being regarded as less valuable than others both because of stigma and because they are less able to defend themselves. The bottom of the slippery slope was reached by Nazi Germany, whose 'T4' programme of the so-called euthanasia had the goal of ridding the nation of the 'burden' of 'useless eaters' as it entered a period of economic strain due to the looming armed conflict (Burleigh, 1994).

Apart from this general fear of the influence of economic considerations on health care, advocates for the disabled have voiced a number of specific moral concerns about CEA. We have alluded to the fact that people who have adjusted to a disability typically view its impact on their well-being as less significant than non-disabled individuals imagine it would be if they became similarly disabled. The disabled learn how to cope with their disability, and they adjust their goals to reflect the opportunities remaining open to them. The non-disabled are less likely to be informed about what life with a given disability is actually like and may have exaggerated fears about its impact. In conducting CEA for interventions that could prevent or relieve disabilities, the results may vary considerably depending on whether the health measures used in the analysis reflect the valuations of the non-disabled or the disabled, respectively. Advocates for the disabled may insist that the latter are not only more accurate, that is, based on better knowledge, but also that priority-setting that uses the valuations by the non-disabled population of health states involving disability are prejudicial and unjust.

A careful moral analysis of the issue, however, reveals considerable complexity. Just as assigning lower value to the time of poor people in CEA may result in increasing the relative priority of interventions that target them (see above), the net effect of using the health state valuations and preferences of the disabled may be to reduce, rather than increase, the importance attached by CEA to the prevention and treatment of the disabling condition. If life with the disability is not as adversely affected as the non-disabled fear and imagine, then the ratio of cost to improvement in health outcome for interventions that prevent or relieve the disability is proportionately increased and the relative priority of these interventions is lowered (Brock, 2002).

A concern for the impact of CEA on the disabled is more sharply focused in connection with assigning relative priority to extending the lives of disabled and non-disabled people, respectively. If a disabled person and a healthy person share a meal that includes mushrooms that turn out to be poisonous, both may be in a sudden need of a liver transplant. If only one liver becomes available, and a choice must be made between the two candidates, the disabled patient may fear the results of thinking influenced by CEA. Though the need for the liver has no connection to the person's disability, it will be undeniable that the population that results from rescuing the previously healthy individual will be healthier, overall, than the population that would result from choosing the previously-disabled patient (assuming, of course, that this disability would remain after regaining his previous level of health). Concerns over this point were raised in connection with the advice that the WHO might give to member states (Arneson & Nord, 1999). To avoid this implication, some have suggested that in choosing whom to save, what is relevant is not the individual's prospective quality of life but rather whether this quality of life remains acceptable to the individual who will experience it (Harris, 1970, 1975). In its explicit statements on this issue, both then and now, WHO has urged that extending the lives of the disabled and the non-disabled be valued the same way. Careful consideration has been given by WHO to the concerns over whether its methodology for CEA embodies a contradictory implication, and if so, how this can be reconciled (Kamm, in press).

THE ROLE OF CBA AND CEA IN PRIORITY-SETTING

CBA and CEA, quantitative methods that can inform priority-setting decisions in health in distinctive ways, are not in themselves sufficient guides to responsible choices among interventions and policies. CEA, for example, seeks to identify the mix of interventions that achieves maximum health gains that can be achieved with a given amount of resources. It is not always appropriate or just to use existing resources to maximize health gains. Other goals may have greater moral importance. For example, it is not always most cost-effective to treat those who may be in greatest medical need. In a large American city, for example, the subpopulation with the greatest prevalence of life-threatening hypertension may be poor, male African-Americans living in the inner city. Because this same population is the least likely to have access to health care or to be able to afford antihypertensive drugs, the health impact of a public hypertension screening initiative targeting this group may be less favourable than one that focuses on, say, middle-class Caucasian whites. Cost-effectiveness might be disregarded by health authorities in favour of priority to the less well-off in this instance. This would be particularly appropriate if the unjust social conditions that exacerbated the inner-city men's hypertension were also a factor in their lack of access to health care and consequent inability to benefit from hypertension screening to the same extent as their more fortunate suburban counterparts.

Practitioners of CEA are often the first to emphasize the need to combine cost-effectiveness with fairness and other distributive considerations in setting priorities in health (Gold, 1996). Whether those who make priority-setting decisions and look to CEA and CBA for guidance heed this advice is less certain. A virtue of these quantitative techniques is that they summarize the implications of a confusing jumble of measurements of costs and the value of outcomes into a single number or small set of numbers. This is also a drawback. Decision-makers whose inadequate grasp of these issues leads them to heed only the numbers may miss dimensions of priority-setting that are just as essential as cost-effectiveness, even if they cannot be represented in quantitative terms. A number of significant moral uncertainties remain regarding both the foundations of these techniques and their respective uses. An ethical issue deserving first priority is whether those who use these methods understand their limitations and the indispensability of further moral judgement in achieving ethically defensible decisions.

REFERENCES

Arneson T, Nord E. The value of DALY life: problems with ethics and validity of disability adjusted life years. *BMJ* 1999; **319**: 1423–5.

Brink D. *Moral Realism and the Foundations of Ethics.* Cambridge: Cambridge University Press, 1989.

Brock D. Health resource allocation for vulnerable populations. In: Danis M, Clancy C, Churchill L, eds. *Ethical Dimensions of Health Policy.* New York: Oxford University Press, 2002.

Broome J. Measuring the burden of disease by aggregating wellbeing. In: Murray C, Salomon J, Mathers C, Lopez A, eds. *Summary Measures of Population Health: Concepts, Ethics, Measurement and Applications.* Geneva: World Health Organization, 2002; pp. 91–114.

Broome J. *Weighing Lives.* Oxford: Oxford University Press, 2004.

Burleigh M. Death and deliverance: *Euthanasia.* Cambridge: Cambridge University Press, 1994 (in Germany, c.1900–1945).

Cutler DM, Rosen A, Vijan S. The value of medical spending in the United States, 1960–2000. *NEJM* 2006; **355**: 920–7. (This study used conventional estimates of the dollar value of years of life.)

Daniels N, Sabin J. *Setting Limits Fairly: Can We Learn to Share Medical Resources?* Oxford University Press; 2002.

(a) Dolan P, Edlin R. Is it really possible to build a bridge between cost-benefit analysis and cost-effectiveness analysis? *J Health Econ* 2002; **21**: 827–843.

Gold MR, Siegel JE, Russell LB, Weinstein MC, eds. *Cost Effectiveness in Health and Medicine.* Oxford University Press, 1996.

Gruskin S, Tarantola D, Health and human Rights. In: Detels R, Beaglehole R, eds. *Oxford Textbook on Public Health.* Oxford University Press, 2001.

Harris J. The role of age and life expectancy in prioritising health care. In: Walter PJ, eds. *Coronary Bypass Surgery in the Elderly. Ethical, Economical and Quality of Life Aspects.* Dordrehtc: Kluwer Academic, 1995.

Harris J. *The Value of Life: An Introduction to Medical Ethics.* London: Routledge and Kegan Paul, 1970.

Hausman D, McPherson M. *Economic Analysis, Moral Philosophy and Public Policy,* 2nd edition. Cambridge: Cambridge University Press, 2006.

Hausman D. Valuing Health. *Philosophy and Public Affairs* 2006; **34**(3): 246–74.

Holtgrave D. HIV prevention, cost-utility analysis, and race/ethnicity: methodological considerations and recommendations. *Med Decis Making* 2004, **24**: 181–91.

Kamm FM. Disability, discrimination, and irrelevant goods. In: Wikler D, Murray C, eds. *Health, Well Being, Justice: Ethical Issues in Health Resource Allocation.* Geneva: World Health Organization; in preparation.

Keeler EB, Cretin S. Discounting of life-saving and other non-monetary effects. *Manage Sci* 1983; **29**: 300–6.

McCaffrey DP. *OSHA and the Politics of Health Regulation.* New York: Plenum Press, 1982

Murray C, Lopez A. *The Global Burden of Disease.* Cambridge: Harvard University Press, 1996.

Murray C. Rethinking DALYs. In: Murray C, Lopez A, eds. *The Global Burden of Disease.* Cambridge: Harvard University Press, 1996.

Office of Management and the Budget. *Circular A-4, Regulatory Analysis.* Washington: Government Printing Office, 2003.

On valuing morbidity, cost-effectiveness analysis, and being rude. *J Health Econ* 1997; **16**: 7490–757.

(Our exposition uses dollars for brevity's sake.)

Polsky D. Does willingness to pay per quality-adjusted life year bring us closer to a useful decision rule for cost-effectiveness analysis? *Med Decis Making* 2005; **25**(6): 605–6.

Russell L. Is cost-effectiveness analysis unfair? *Med Decis Making* 2004; **24**: 232–4.

Sen A. *Development as Freedom.* New York: Knopf, 1999.

Walzer M. *Spheres of Justice.* New York: Basic Books, 1983

Weinstein M, Stason WB. Foundations of cost-effectiveness analysis for health and medical practices. *N Engl J Med* 1997; **296**: 716–21.

Wikler D. Why prioritize when there isn't enough money? *Cost Effect Resource Alloc* 2003; **1**: 5.

Wolff J. *Railway Safety and The Ethics of the Tolerability of Risk.* London: Railway Safety Research Programme, Rail Safety and Standards Board, 2002.

Economics, Political Philosophy and Ethics: The Role of Public Preferences in Health Care Decision-Making

JEFF RICHARDSON, JOHN MCKIE

A defining characteristic of economics is that it attempts to answer the question of how best to use our limited resources to achieve social objectives. This suggests that there is an important role for public preferences to play in the evaluation of health services. Accounts of this role are provided by different theories within the disciplines of economics, political theory and ethics, and are discussed in the first three sections of this chapter. In the next two sections, a more empirical approach is outlined and defended. The last section draws together the various themes discussed and ends with some practical recommendations and theoretical conclusions.

WELFARE THEORY

The tools of orthodox Welfare Theory (WT) have been developed to a high degree of precision, and they are useful in a number of contexts. The fundamental normative assumption of WT is that the distribution of goods and services should be based upon individual preferences. At the macro- or health-system level, the theory provides the rationale for a competitive market and, at the micro-level, which is concerned with the evaluation of particular services, it provides the theoretical basis for cost–benefit analysis. The assumption enshrines the principle of 'consumer sovereignty' (Penz, 1986) at both these levels.

However, WT is based on a number of specific assumptions that make it largely irrelevant in the health context. For example, it is assumed that the preferences consumers reveal through their choices represent what is in their best interests. As Mishan (1971, p. 172) states: 'economists are generally agreed – either as a canon of faith, as a political tenet, or an act of expediency – to accept the dictum that each person knows his own interests best'. Defending consumer sovereignty (at least by implication) J.S. Mill stated: 'Most persons take a juster and more intelligent view of their own interests, and of the means of promoting it, than can either be prescribed to them by a general enactment of the legislature, or pointed out in the particular case by a public functionary' (Mill, 1994, Book V, Chapter 11, Section 9).

However, in the health context it is typically not the case that the 'consumer' is the best judge of the *means* of promoting his or her own interests. Most conspicuously, lack of knowledge is ubiquitous: consumers lack crucial information about their own health status, what treatments are available, their effectiveness, the risks involved, and so on (Rice, 2001). People may know what they want (health) but lack the knowledge to secure it (unless they are medically trained). (Further support for the tenuousness of the connection between behaviour and subjective well-being comes from psychology. Recent empirical work in psychology suggests that wanting and liking arise from two different neural systems (Berridge, 1996). Activities that arise from wanting, therefore, may not reflect what an individual likes, and may not produce subjective well-being, even assuming that subjective well-being is what people seek.)

Orthodox WT also equates rationality with the maximization of self-interest. This excludes the possibility of rational self-sacrifice or 'commitment' (Sen, 2005). It is sometimes assumed that any action aimed at achieving something – any purposeful action – *must* reflect a self-interested preference, and thus be aimed at utility maximization, or some other action would have occurred. Interpreted in this way, no conceivable action can fail to be utility maximizing, and the revealed preference criterion becomes a tautology. As Thurow comments: 'Revealed preferences ... is just a fancy way of saying that individuals do whatever individuals do, and whatever they do, economists will call it "utility maximization"' (Thurow, 1983, p. 217).

Of course, there is a wealth of everyday observation, and systematic empirical evidence, suggesting that people do not invariably seek to maximize their own self-interest, when this is not defined tautologically. For example, there is a growing body of evidence from experimental economics which suggests that people are prepared to make significant sacrifices in order to obtain other social objectives which carry no obvious personal pay-off (Krebs, 1982; Kahneman et al., 1986; Andreoni, 1995; Keser, 1996; Bolton and Ockenfels, 2000). There has also been a recent resurgence of interest in 'group selection' in evolutionary theory, which is compatible with individual self-sacrifice (Seeley, 1996; Wilson, 1997; Sober and wilson, 1998). Excluding these preferences from consideration on the ground that they are irrational is itself a normative assumption and lacks justification when applied to otherwise rational people. In the context of the provision of public health services people have strong preferences for allocating resources fairly, which should not be deemed 'irrational' and ignored.

A particularly limiting assumption of WT concerns the nature of social welfare itself: namely, the assumption that social welfare is a function exclusively of individual utilities. Sen describes the resulting doctrine as 'welfarism' and has vigorously criticized it as a normative doctrine. For example, he notes that individuals with disabilities often adjust their expectations downwards – they accommodate themselves to their condition – and, because well-being is largely determined by a person's situation relative to their expectations, they may have relatively high utility levels (Sen, 1987). But the fact that a person has learned to live with adversity should not mean that they do not have a legitimate claim for special consideration. Sen maintains there is more to social welfare than the sum of individual utilities. He recommends a focus on functionings and capabilities in economic analysis: The freedom people have to pursue valuable goals in general, including non-self interested goals. (As Cohen explains it, functionings lie mid-way between goods (or services) and utility. For example, food is not the focus of attention because this 'takes too little account of distinguishing facts about individuals' (Cohen, 1993, p. 18), nor the satisfaction that a person derives from eating food because 'this takes too much account of just such facts' (Cohen, 1993, p. 18). Rather, the focus is on how much nourishment a person gets from food. The focus is on what goods and services allow people to do or to be (being adequately nourished, having mobility, being free from avoidable disease), but not exclusively on the utility they confer.)

Efficiency in WT is defined by the Pareto criterion. A change is 'Pareto efficient' if it makes no one worse off and at least one person better off. Much of the appeal of WT stems from the fact that in the model defined by its core assumptions every competitive equilibrium results in a Pareto optimal outcome: it is not possible to make someone better off without making someone else worse off (Debreu, 1959; Arrow & Hahn, 1972). Achieving allocative efficiency in this sense has been an attractive goal in economics because it avoids the need for substantive ethical assumptions; a change that benefits at least one person without making anyone else worse off should command universal assent.

However, a major obstacle to the use of the Pareto principle in the evaluation of health services is that most decisions result in winners and losers. Introducing a health service into one area commonly means not introducing it into another, and this means that policies are seldom, if ever, Pareto efficient, and the criterion fails to apply in many contexts. Of course, this is also true in other areas of the economy. To overcome this problem, the Kaldor–Hicks potential compensation principle is usually implicitly or explicitly evoked (Hicks, 1939; Kaldor, 1939). According to this principle, one state of the world is better than another if those who are made better off could potentially compensate those who are made worse off. However, in the context of a national health scheme, the winners are the patients who receive health care and the losers are the tax payers who pay for the services. Compensation would require the taxation of patients and the return of tax revenues, which is the exact reversal of the purpose of a national health scheme. More fundamentally, the Kaldor–Kicks principle can only apply if it is *possible* to compensate those who are made worse off. For patients left with a very poor quality of life this may be impossible, and it is unequivocally impossible when a patient dies. This implies that the attempt to base policy decisions on the achievement of Pareto efficiency fails in the health sector, and with it the attempt to by-pass ethical issues in the formulation of health policy. Although the economics literature usually acknowledges the unreality of much of WT, this final conclusion is less commonly acknowledged.

LIBERTARIANISM AND EGALITARIANISM

The inapplicability of Welfare Theory in the health context creates a vacuum at the macro- or health-system level, where decisions are made with respect to the allocation of resources between services, the distribution of and access to those services, and the distribution of health care costs. Similarly, the limited applicability of Pareto efficiency and the Kaldor–Hicks potential compensation principle creates a vacuum at the micro-level, which is concerned with the evaluation of particular services or programmes, such as cancer screening programmes and transplant programmes. At both levels the exact role of public preferences (preferences for the type and content of a national health scheme) in economic analysis remains problematical although there is almost universal agreement that these preferences are of importance.

Williams clearly and persuasively identifies two major viewpoints in the literature dealing with system-level issues – namely, libertarianism and egalitarianism, and contrasts them along four dimensions (Williams, 1988). With respect to *personal responsibility*, the libertarian viewpoint holds that unearned rewards weaken the motive force that assures economic well-being and places great emphasis upon achievement. The egalitarian viewpoint places less emphasis upon personal incentives to achieve and does not equate economic failure with social worthlessness. With respect to *social concern*, libertarianism advocates private charity for those who fail despite appropriate efforts. Egalitarianism sees charity as potentially degrading and inequitable and advocates public support mechanisms to maintain self-sufficiency as a matter of entitlement. The libertarian viewpoint places great emphasis upon personal *freedom* and sees government involvement in the financing of health care as a restriction of the freedom of consumers and providers. The egalitarian viewpoint sees government involvement as necessary for real freedom, by removing economic constraints that limit opportunities for meaningful choice. With respect to *equality*, libertarians see it as less important than freedom and focus primarily on equality before the law. Egalitarians place greater emphasis upon equality of opportunity because without this the moral worth of achievement is undermined.

All public health systems incorporate elements of both viewpoints, with national health schemes differing in the subsidy they provide for different services, the relative cost of these services to government and to individual patients, the ownership of assets, the incentives and remuneration offered to service providers, and the type of regulatory controls employed. For pragmatic and ethical reasons neither unfettered freedom nor unfettered paternalism is advocated in the literature, and the extremes on the libertarianism/egalitarianism spectrum are avoided. However, this still leaves a range of feasible alternatives occupying the 'middle ground', and views differ regarding which alternative represents the right balance between these two viewpoints for a given society. This limits the amount of practical guidance that can be derived from an abstract consideration of arguments for and against libertarianism and egalitarianism. There is no simple way of trading off these theories in their more abstract form to arrive at an acceptable balance from within the theories themselves.

TRADITIONAL ETHICS

The literature applying ethical theories, and their derivative ethical principles, to the problem of fairly allocating health care resources is also characterized by disagreement. For example, utilitarianism holds that the right action, choice or policy is the one that will maximize happiness, or pleasure, or preference-satisfaction, taking everyone's interests into account. By contrast, Rawls uses social contract theory to argue that social and economic inequalities are justifiable only if they are of the greatest benefit to the least advantaged members of society (Rawls, 1971). In the health context, this may lead to a head-on collision between the distribution of resources to maximize health (e.g. minimize the cost per QALY); distributing to favour those in greatest need (e.g. those with the lowest pre-treatment QALY score); and distributing to maximize utility (as revealed by a free market supplemented to overcome market failures). (In its simplest form the QALY (Quality-Adjusted Life Year) represents a year of life that has been weighted by an index representing quality of life. By tradition, full health has a weighting of 1 and death has a weighting of 0. For example, if years on dialysis are judged to be worth only 57% as much as years of normal health (Torrance, 1986) then 20 years of dialysis would be discounted to $20 \times 0.57 = 11.4$ QALYs.) There is no clear way to resolve the impasse while debate remains at the level of philosophical analysis.

The hope has sometimes been expressed that convergence may be possible in ethics, especially with the decline of religion, but there is no evidence of this occurring (Parfit, 1984; Smith, 1994). On the contrary, new variants of the traditional ethical theories continue to appear. Of course, the desire to increase welfare and the desire to help the worst off are both important and widespread in most communities. But in practice they often pull in different directions, and it is difficult to know how to balance these various *desiderata* when they conflict. In the absence of consensus, we are again at an impasse.

THE EMPIRICAL APPROACH

Given the lack of practical guidance and uncertainty surrounding the political and ethical solutions discussed above, a good case can be made for investigating the preferences of the community as a way of arriving at the desired compromise between alternative principles.

At the microlevel there are now a large number of studies that demonstrate the existence of societal preferences that are not narrowly self-interested. For example, when informed that patients regard the health improvements from two services as being identical, people generally indicate a strong 'social' preference for giving priority to the patient with the poorer initial health state. Consequently, priority does not only reflect the utility gained from a procedure but also the distribution of health benefits. For example, in an early study, Nord examined public preferences associated with two health states A and B. These were described to survey respondents as: 'unable to work, unable to pursue family and leisure activities, strong pain, depressed' (A); and 'unable to work, moderate pain' (B). Nord found that returning one person from A to full health was regarded by respondents as being as valuable as returning 50 people to full health from B. However, the utility values for these states (assigned by the participants using a rating scale) implied that curing one person in a more severe state should be equivalent to curing two people in a less severe state (Nord, 1991, 1993, p. 33). Similarly, returning one person to full health from the first state was considered as valuable as returning 100 people to full health from a state of 'moderate pain', even though the utility associated with 'moderate pain' implied that this number should have been five. The societal value of treating the more severely ill was much higher than would be expected from only taking account of patient utilities.

The sentiment expressed in this, and other, surveys is summed up by Callahan: 'Our bias, I contend, should be to give priority to persons whose suffering and inability to function in ordinary life is most pronounced, even if the available treatment for them is comparatively less efficacious than for other conditions' (Callahan, 1994, p. 463). Support for severity can also be found in official government guidelines in several countries, and in reports of government-appointed commissions (Dutch Committee on Choice in Health Care, 1992; Campbell & Gillett, 1993; Swedish Health Care and Medical Priorities Commission, 1993). Importantly, studies of societal preferences regarding the importance of severity offer the possibility of quantifying the trade-off between minimizing the cost per QALY and giving priority to the worst off.

Several empirical studies have also observed a societal preference for giving equal consideration to patients irrespective of their potential for health improvement. For example, Nord (1993) conducted a study in which subjects were asked to choose between two 60-year-old housewives, each of whom had contracted a life-threatening disease. An operation would make Mrs Anderson 'completely healthy', whereas it would give Mrs Peterson a life 'with moderate pain and dependency on crutches for walking'. Subjects were asked whether they thought Mrs Anderson

should be operated first, or whether they should be taken in the order in which they were admitted to the hospital. The results showed that the majority of participants, 78.7%, chose the option that afforded both patients an equal chance of being treated (order of admission), whereas only 14.8% favoured the option that would maximize health (treating Mrs Anderson).

Other studies show that many citizens in Australia, the USA, England and Spain share this reluctance to discriminate against the permanently disabled, the chronically ill and others with a limited potential for health improvement (Nord et al. 1995; Abellan-Perpiñán & Prades, 1999; Dolan & Cookson, 2000; Ubel Richardson & Baron, 2002). Of course, it cannot be concluded from this that the state of health after treatment is irrelevant. When the potential for improvement is very limited subjects place considerably more weight on health outcome (Abellan-Perpiñán & Prades, 1999; Dolan & Cookson, 2000). None the less, potential for improvement does not have the importance for the general public that an exclusive focus on health maximization would suggest; the public also considers 'realizing one's potential for health improvement', whether large or small, important in social decision-making. Confirming this, in 1992 the United States Secretary for Health and Human Services rejected the Oregon plan for prioritizing the state's health services on the ground that it discriminated against the disabled when the improvement in health from a medical cure is limited by the patient's disability (Daniels, 1993). Work by Ubel et al. indicates that the public would support this rejection. Survey respondents would not prioritize (long-term) paraplegics below other patients when both groups faced a life-threatening illness even though their paraplegia meant that they would gain less health (the so-called 'double jeopardy' of those with a long-term illness) (Ubel, Richardson & Baron, 2002). Importantly, the trade-off between realizing potential and maximizing health can be precisely calculated, which is not to deny the technical problems confronting preference elicitation.

Empirical studies also suggest that many people are willing to give certain age groups priority in the competition for limited health care. For example, in one study, subjects were asked to choose between two equally costly projects that would enable patients to continue living in normal health for 10 years (Nord et al. 1996). Project A would allow the treatment of more patients, but project B would benefit younger patients. Subjects were asked to adopt the role of health administrators and say how many patients treated under project B were considered equivalent to 10 patients being treated under project A. The study found that saving the lives of 10 twenty-year-olds was considered equivalent to saving the lives of 9.5 ten-year-olds, and that saving the lives of 10 eighty-year-olds was considered equivalent to saving the life of 1 twenty-year-old.

Because all patients were stipulated to derive the same benefit (10 years in good health), this outcome is again inconsistent with health maximization. In general, Nord et al. found that 'the preference for the young is more pronounced the greater the disparity in the two age groups' (Nord et al. 1996, p. 106). Similar results were obtained for health-improving rather than life-saving treatments (see Choudhry et al. 1997; Ratcliffe, 2000; Tsuchiya, Dolan & Shaw, 2003).

Even from within this empirical literature there is evidence that indicates the need for caution in the use of survey results to guide policy. In one study, respondents were asked whether they believed that the views of the public should be adopted even when they differed from the views of the government and government departments. Results varied with the context of the question, but at least in some cases the public rejected the use of public preferences (Richardson, 2002). In contrast, evidence from other studies suggests that the public does want a role in priority-setting. However, willingness to participate varies with the level of decision-making involved (individual patient, programme or health system) and the time commitment required for participation. (Richardson, Charny & Hanmer-Lloyd, 1992; Bowling, Jacobson & Southgate, 1993; Abelson et al. 1995, Bowling, 1996; Myllykangas et al., 1996; Litva et al., 2002; Wiseman et al., 2003). In this context, it has been argued that 'where citizens would rather have professionals make decisions for them, these professionals should base their decisions on the community's values, not their own (elitist) values' (Black & Mooney, 2002). We explore the status of community preferences in the next section.

ETHICS AND SOCIAL SCIENCE

Consulting the public on priority-setting in the health sector is important in a liberal democracy and offers a way of reconciling alternative political and ethical viewpoints. In a practical sense, researchers adopting this approach typically formulate hypotheses about societal preferences, undertake both quantitative and qualitative studies to test them experimentally, and subject the results to further testing and refinement. For example, there is evidence that the public believes it is fair for the benefits of health care to be distributed widely, rather than narrowly concentrated among a few (Nord et al., 1996, Johannesson & Gerdtham, 1996). It may be, however, that the public believes it is unfair to deny the few a significant health benefit if benefits are distributed too widely, and the benefit per person becomes trivial. This hypothesis has been confirmed (Olsen, 2000; Rodríguez-Míguez & Prades, 2002).

In these cases, ethics can play an important role in clarifying population responses, drawing out the implications of policies and suggesting questions for further research. Ideally, the process should continue until relatively stable principles are derived, which can withstand (tolerably well) both ethical criticism and the test of population support. This process has been called 'Empirical Ethics' (Richardson, 2001).

As part of this process of eliciting societal preferences, techniques should be used that will encourage reflection and deliberation, and a precise statement and specification of values. These techniques might include re-interviewing and different forms of information feedback (including Delphi techniques), the triangulation of issues (eliciting responses using different techniques and comparing results), focus groups, citizens' juries and other qualitative methodologies. The hope is that the appropriate use of these methodologies will minimize 'correspondence' and 'reflection' irrationality. 'Correspondence irrationality' occurs when a person's actual choices do not correspond with his or her reasoned reflection. 'Reflection irrationality' characterizes a failure of careful reflection itself (Sen, 1985). This is particularly important for the evaluation of health services and programmes, as the opportunities people have to reflect on the worth of these, in comparison with other conventional goods and services, are limited. For example, Dolan, Cookson & Ferguson (1999) found that participants in small groups commonly changed their mind after discussion and reflection.

It is important that the results of this process are not misinterpreted. Frohlich and Oppenheimer, for example, suggest that definitive answers to ethical questions may exist, but that this requires 'moving ethical theory out of the armchair and into the laboratory' (Frohlich & Oppenheimer, 1992, Jacket). They conducted a series of experiments in Canada, Poland and the United States to identify attitudes towards fairness in the distribution of wealth and income. They conclude: 'Our results lead us to believe that cumulative progress (like that achieved in the physical sciences) may even be possible in certain branches of ethics if philosophers adopt the techniques of experimental science and move beyond speculation and debate' (Frohlich & Oppenheimer, 1992). Nord adopts the same approach when he writes: 'I define a *fair* resource allocation in health care as one that accords with societal feelings about the strength of claims of different patient groups. A resource allocation that violates such feelings is defined as *unfair*' (Nord, 1999, p. 23).

However, this interpretation of the process misrepresents the nature of ethics. If this approach was adopted it would be impossible to critique the implications of empirical research as these would define or reveal what was ethical. It would only be possible to criticize the studies on technical grounds. But one of the main functions served by the moral component of language is criticism, and the belief that there are 'scientific' solutions to moral problems threatens this role. That is, 'the autonomy of ethics' must be preserved (Pigden,

1989). Social surveys like those described above, which reveal support for the more severely ill, the disabled, the young and so on, should not be interpreted as attempts to arrive at the 'truth' concerning ethical matters, or as attempts to define away ethical problems. Rather, they are a way of reaching practical political solutions to complex social problems when there is a diversity of ethical views in the community.

CONCLUSION

'Empirical Ethics' provides one explanation of how the insights of ethics and economics can be used simultaneously to help answer policy questions. Ethics can play an important role in clarifying population responses, drawing out implications and suggesting questions for further research. Properly conducted, Empirical Ethics tells us what people *believe* is fair. However, it leaves unanswered the question of what is *really* fair, independently of the prevalence and distribution of social views. For example, community surveys may tell us that people are willing to give priority to the more severely ill, and may even allow a precise measure of the preferred trade-off between health maximization for the entire population and maximization for the worst off members of the community. But it is, and should always be, possible to ask whether or not a policy based on these results is *really* fair.

As noted above, there are numerous ethical theories and derivative ethical principles that are applicable for health policy. Thus, there will always be multiple, incompatible answers to the question of what is really fair. Utilitarians may give one answer, Kantians another, Rawlsians another and so on. Moreover, the precise nature of this question and how one understands the various answers to it will vary according to which meta-ethical theory is adopted: that is, whether moral judgements are seen as objectively true or false (Moore, 1903; Prichard, 1912; Ross, 1930), as disguised factual statements (Harman, 1977), as reports of personal opinion (Westermarck, 1932; Perry, 1954), as expressions of emotion (Ayer, 1936; Stevenson, 1945) or without foundation at all (Ruse, 1988).

For practical purposes, policy makers and their economic advisers cannot wait for such normative and meta-ethical disagreements to be resolved. As stated in the opening sentence of this chapter, a defining characteristic of economics is that it attempts to answer the question of how best to use our limited resources to achieve *social objectives*. In this chapter, we have argued that both ethics and empirical research into public preferences should have a role in this process. In this chapter, we have tried to give some insight into how this task might be conducted better.

In summing up, we offer three practical recommendations and three theoretical conclusions.

Practical Recommendations:

1. Economists involved in economic evaluations of health services and programmes should consult the public regarding their preferred services and programmes, their preferred principles and methods for distributing health care, and their preferred method of paying for these services.
2. There is a lack of data on societal preferences and the acceptable trade-offs between social goals. There is an urgent need for research into the ethical values of health care 'consumers', and a need to further develop empirical methods that elicit deliberative rather than spontaneous societal preferences.
3. Although conventional ethics does not provide unambiguous answers to ethical questions, health economists should acquaint themselves with the major ethical theories, particularly regarding distributive justice and procedural fairness, in order to interpret and critique the results of community consultations.

Theoretical Conclusions:

1. Health and health care are different from other goods and services. Orthodox welfare theory and cost-benefit analysis are based on a number of assumptions that severely limit their applicability in the health context. The 'welfarism' of welfare theory is not the only theoretical basis for health care policy.
2. Unambiguous policy recommendations cannot be derived from traditional political or ethical theories. Political and ethical disagreement will persist no matter how much discourse takes place and no matter how openly, rationally and conscientiously it is pursued.
3. Consulting the public on their ethical views does not jeopardize the autonomy of ethics. 'Empirical ethics' is a way of reaching practical solutions to complex social problems, given the diversity of ethical views in the community. It does not imply that there are 'scientific' solutions to moral problems.

REFERENCES

Abelson J, Lomas J, Eyles J, Birch S, Veenstra G. Does the community want devolved authority? Results of deliberative polling in Ontario. *Can Med Assoc J* 1995; **153**(4): 403–12.

Abellan-Perpiñán J-M, Prades J-LP. Health state after treatment: a reason for discrimination? *Health Econ* 1999; **8**(8): 701–7.

Andreoni J. Cooperation in public goods experiments: kindness or confusion? *Am Econ Rev* 1995; **85**(4): 891–904.

Arrow KJ, Hahn F. *General Competitive Analysis*. Edinburgh: Oliver and Boyd, 1972.

Ayer AJ. *Language, Truth and Logic*. London: Gollancz, 1936.

Berridge KC. Food reward–brain substrates of wanting and liking. *Neurosci Biobehav Rev* 1996; **20**(1): 1–25.

Black M, Mooney G. Equity in health care from a communitarian standpoint. *Health Care Anal* 2002; **10**(2): 193–208.

Bolton GE, Ockenfels A. ERC: a theory of equity, reciprocity, and competition. *American Economic Review* 2000; **90**(1): 166–193.

Bowling A. Health care rationing: the public's debate. *Br Med J* 1996; **312**(7032): 670–4.

Bowling A, Jacobson B, Southgate L. Explorations in consultation of the public and health professionals on priority setting in an inner london health district. *Soc Sci Med* 1993; **37**(7): 851–7.

Callahan D. Setting mental health priorities: problems and possibilities. *Milbank Q* 1994; **72**(3): 451–470.

Campbell A, Gillett G. Justice and the right to health care. *Ethical Issues in Defining Core Services*. Wellington: The National Advisory Committee on Core Health and Disability Support Services, 1993.

Choudhry N, Slaughter P, Sykora K, Naylor CD. Distributional dilemmas in health policy: Large benefits for a few or small benefits for many? *J Health Serv Res Policy* 1997; **2**(4): 212–6.

Cohen GA. Equality of What? On welfare, goods, and capabilities. In: Nussbaum M, Sen A, eds. *The Quality of Life*. Oxford: Clarendon Press, 1993; pp. 9–29.

Daniels N. Rationing fairly: programmatic considerations. *Bioethics* 1993; **7**(2/3): 224–33.

Debreu, G. *The Theory of Value: An Axiomatic Analysis of Economic Equilibrium*. New York: John Wiley & Sons, Ltd, 1959.

Dolan P, Cookson R. A qualitative study of the extent to which health gain matters when choosing between groups of patients. *Health Policy* 2000; **51**(1): 19–30.

Dolan P, Cookson R, Ferguson B. Effect of discussion and deliberation on the public's views of priority setting in health care: focus group study. *Br Med J* 1999; **318**(7188): 916–9.

Dutch Committee on Choices in Health Care. *Choices in Health Care*. Rijswijk: Ministry of Welfare, Health and Cultural Affairs, 1992.

Frohlich N, Oppenheimer JA. *Choosing Justice: An Experimental Approach to Ethical Theory*. Berkeley: University of California Press, 1992.

Harman G. *The Nature of Morality: An Introduction to Ethics*. Oxford: Oxford University Press, 1977.

Hicks JR. The foundations of welfare economics. *Econ J* 1939; **49**(196): 696–712.

Johannesson M, Gerdtham U-G. A note on the estimation of the equity-efficiency trade-off for qalys. *J Health Econ* 1996; **15**(3): 359–68.

Kahneman D, Knetsch JL, Thaler RH. Fairness as a constraint on profit seeking: entitlements in the market. *Am Econ Rev* 1986; **76**(4): 728–41.

Kaldor N. Welfare propositions of economics and interpersonal comparisons of utility. *Econ J* 1939; **49**(195): 549–52.

Keser C. Voluntary contributions to a public good when partial contribution is a dominant strategy. *Econ Lett* 1996; **50**(3): 359–66.

Krebs D. Prosocial behaviour, equity, and justice. In: Greenberg J, Cohen RL, eds. *Equity and Justice in Social Behaviour*. New York and London: Academic Press, 1982; pp. 261–308.

Litva A, Coast J, Donovan J, Eyles J, Shepherd M, Tacchi J, Abelson J, Morgan K. "The Public is Too Subjective": public involvement at different levels of health-care decision making. *Soc Sci Med* 2002; **54**(12): 1825–37.

Mill JS. In: Riley J, ed. *Principles of Political Economy*. Oxford: Oxford University Press, 1994.

Mishan EJ. Evaluation of life and limb: a theoretical approach. *J Polit Econ* 1971; **79**(4): 687–705.

Moore GE. *Principia Ethica*. Cambridge: Cambridge University Press, 1903.

Myllykangas M, Ryynänen O-P, Kinnunen J, Takala J. Comparison of doctors', nurses', politicians' and public attitudes to health care priorities. *J Health Serv Res Policy* 1996; **1**(4): 212–6.

Nord E, Richardson J, Street A, Kuhse H, Singer P. 'Maximizing Health Benefits vs Egalitarianism: An Australian Survey of Health Issues'. *Soc Sci Med* 1995; **41**(10): 1429–37.

Nord E, Street A, Richardson J, Kuhse H, Singer P. The significance of age and duration of effect in social evaluation of health care. *Health Care Anal* 1996; **4**(2): 103–11.

Nord E. *Cost-Value Analysis in Health Care*. Cambridge: Cambridge University Press, 1999.

Nord E. The relevance of health state after treatment in prioritising between different patients. *J Med Ethics* 1993; **19**(1): 37–42.

Nord E. The validity of a visual analogue scale in determining social utility weights for health states. *Int J Health Plan Manage* 1991; **6**(3): 234–42.

Olsen JA. A note on eliciting distributive preferences for health. *J Health Econ* 2000; **19**(4): 541–50.

Parfit D. *Reasons and Persons*. Oxford: Oxford University Press, 1984.

Penz GP. *Consumer Sovereignty and Human Interests*. Cambridge: Cambridge University Press, 1986.

Perry RB. *Realms of Value*. Cambridge: Harvard University Press, 1954.

Pigden C. Logic and the autonomy of ethics. *Austr J Philos* 1989; **67**(2): 127–51.

Prichard HA. Does moral philosophy rest on a mistake? *Mind* 1912; **21**(81): 21–37.

Ratcliffe J. Public preferences for the allocation of donor liver grafts for transplantation. *Health Econ* 2000; **9**(2): 137–48.

Rawls J. *A Theory of Justice*. Cambridge: Harvard University Press, 1971.

Rice T. Should consumer choice be encouraged in health care? *The Social Economics of Health Care*. London and New York, Routledge: J.B. Davis, 2001; pp. 9–39.

Richardson A, Charny M, Hanmer-Lloyd S. Public-opinion and purchasing. *Br Med J* 1992; **304**(6828): 680–2.

Richardson J. *Empirical Ethics Versus Analytical Orthodoxy: Two Contrasting Bases for The Re-Allocation of Resources*, working paper 111. Monash University, Melbourne: Centre for Health Program Evaluation, 2001.

Richardson J. Age weighting and time discounting: technical imperatives versus social choice. In: Murray CJL, Salomon JA, Mathers CD, Lopez AD, eds. *Summary Measures of Population Health: Concepts, Ethics, Measurement and Applications*. Geneva: World Health Organization, 2002; pp. 663–76.

Rodríguez-Míguez E, Prades J-LP. Measuring the social importance of concentration or dispersion of individual health benefits. *Health Econ* 2002; **11**(1): 43–53.

Ross WD. *The Right and the Good*. Oxford: Clarendon Press, 1930.

Ruse M. Evolutionary ethics: healthy prospect or last infirmity? *Can J Philos* 1988; **1988**(Suppl 14): 27–73.

Seeley TD. *The Wisdom of the Hive*. Cambridge, Massachusetts: Harvard University Press, 1996.

Sen A. *The Standard of Living*. New York: Cambridge University Press, 1987.

Sen A. Rationality and uncertainty. *Theory Decis* 1985; **18**(2): 109–27.

Sen A. Why exactly is commitment important for rationality? *Econ Philos* 2005; **21**(1): 5–14.

Smith M. Realism. In: Singer P, ed. *Ethics*. Oxford and New York: Oxford University Press, 1994; pp. 170–6.

Sober E, Wilson DS. *Unto Others: The Evolution of Altruism*. Cambridge, Massachusetts: Harvard University Press, 1998.

Stevenson CL. *Ethics and Language*. New Haven: Yale University Press, 1945.

Swedish Health Care and Medical Priorities Commission. *No Easy Choices: The Difficulties of Health Care. Sveriges offentlige utredninger, 1993*. Stockholm: The Ministry of Health and Social Affairs, 1993.

Thurow LC. *Dangerous Currents: The State of Economics*. New York: Random House, 1983.

Torrance GW. Measurement of Health State Utilities for Economic Appraisal. *J Health Econ* 1986; **5**(1): 1–30.

Tsuchiya A, Dolan P, Shaw R. Measuring people's preferences regarding ageism in health: some methodological issues and some fresh evidence. *Soc Sci Med* 2003; **57**(4): 687–96.

Ubel PA, Richardson J, Baron J. Exploring the role of order effects in person trade-off elicitations. *Health Policy* 2002; **61**(2): 189–99.

Westermarck E. *Ethical Relativity*. New York: Harcourt, Brace & Co, 1932.

Williams A. Priority setting in public and private health care: a guide through the ideological jungle. *J Health Econ* 1988; **7**(2): 173–83.

Wilson DS. Incorporating group selection into the adaptationist program: a case study involving human decision making. In: Simpson J, Kendrick D, eds. *Evolutionary Social Psychology*. Mahwah, NJ: Lawrence Erlbaum Associates, 1997; pp. 345–86.

Wiseman V, Mooney G, Berry G, Tang KC. Involving the general public in priority setting: experiences from Australia. *Soc Sci Med* 2003; **56**(5): 1001–12.

Decision Analysis: The Ethical Approach to Most Health Decision Making

JACK DOWIE

INTRODUCTION

Medical practitioners and, by implication, all those involved in health-related decisions should be able to engage in 'critical ethical thinking'. This will permit them to 'go behind', rather than 'mindlessly follow'–or try to follow – the sort of general exhortations and instructions embodied in professional codes of behaviour and ethical guidelines. This has long been the central contention of Gillon (1985).

I endorse Gillon's argument, but only in a highly qualified way: Along the lines of 'yes, provided it is part of the wider case that medical practitioners and health decision makers of all kinds should be able to engage in critical thinking *in general*, in order that they can maximize the chances of arriving at the *best* decision for those for whom they are acting as agent, or with whom they are sharing decision responsibility'. The agency or the sharing may relate to the individual patient (in the straightforward clinical context) or to a population (in the straightforward public health context) or to both individual and population (conceptualized as other individuals) in the complex case of a health service body charged with deciding which clinical interventions are to be provided or reimbursed within a resource-constrained publicly funded health service. (The National Institute for Health and Clinical Excellence in England and Wales (NICE) is leading the world in tackling this last task, but the significant advances it is making relative to the past ways of tackling it – which favour denying the problem – involve the fudging of fundamental conflicts of perspective and clashes of concept.)

I will argue that an essential ingredient of that 'general critical thinking' is competency in techniques – especially decision analysis in its various forms – which are considerably more analytical than those with which health decision makers are typically familiar. If this is accepted, it follows that they have an *ethical* obligation to understand, possess and, where appropriate, apply these techniques in their work.

A crucial aspect of such understanding will be acceptance of the paradigmatic difference between science and decision, from which it follows that research findings satisfying *scientific* standards using mainstream statistical methodologies – par excellence the randomized controlled trial – can play only a highly problematic role in the determination of the best decision for an individual or population. Members of ethics committees, whether research or practice focused, who lack this understanding, as far too many currently do, are among those likely to be culpable of unethical practice.

The goal of judgement and decision making in health care, be it clinical or public or clinical–public, is to *make the best decision*, not to be 'ethically correct' or 'scientifically correct' in some specific sense. An ability to engage in critical *ethical* thinking of the sort envisaged by Gillon is undoubtedly one of the *necessary* conditions for making the best decision, but it is not a *sufficient* condition. Any 'critical ethical thinking' must somehow be incorporated into the *general* thinking involved in the making of the decision, and failure to address the question of precisely how that ethical thinking and its results are to be integrated into the choice of action will leave it having an unknown and unknowable impact on the decision. Decision analysis – in the form of clinical decision analysis in the individual health context and (opportunity) cost-effectiveness analysis in the public health context – makes the processes of selecting and integrating both evidence and values as *coherent* and *transparent* as possible. These two attributes constitute its ethical power and the basis of its claims to be *the* ethical decision technology for the majority of decisions in which health professionals and authorities are involved.

Decision-analytic procedures, properly performed, involve drawing on ethical theory in the same way as they involve drawing on theory and knowledge of anatomy, physiology, biochemistry, statistics among others. Through the decision analysis, the quality of the ethical thinking inputs will impinge on the quality of the resulting decision in the same way as the quality of the inputs from all the other disciplines necessary for good judgement and decision-making in health.

ETHICS AND DECISIONS

The ability to engage in 'critical ethical thinking' obviously requires basic familiarity with the range of positions conventionally and loosely gathered under the 'absolutist–deontologist' and 'consequentialist–utilitarian' umbrellas. However, because thinking within these opposing categories often leads to irresolvable conflicts, Gillon, along with many others, has been led to argue that we can avoid these by identifying a set of 'guiding principles' – beneficence, non-maleficence, respect for autonomy and concern for justice are a familiar quartet – which are common to both positions (Beauchamp, 1994). It is suggested that if these four principles are 'taken into account and borne in mind' throughout a decision-making process, no relevant moral concerns will be overlooked.

It may be so. But in the absence of any coherent and transparent way of applying these principles to a specific case (clinical or public), we are left with the claim that they have been somehow *intuitively* 'taken into account and borne in mind' and 'not overlooked' in the decision. We have no audit trail of what has actually happened to them. Moreover, bilateral and multilateral conflicts among the four are logically inevitable if we try to respect all four principles simultaneously. In the absence of *any* coherent and transparent way of resolving these conflicts (i.e. establishing the trade-offs between the principles), we will have no explicit insight into either the *rating* of each of the decision options on each principle (how well each option was held to deliver each principle) or the *weighting* attached to each of the principles (what relative weight was, for example, given to 'beneficence' vis-à-vis 'non-maleficence').

The introduction of any intermediate set of 'guiding principles' can therefore do little to raise the analytical level of the decision process to that which is ethically demanded in an agency or shared decision-making context. Explicit coherence is not required and transparency remains minimal. On the other hand, coherence and transparency are ensured when decision analysis is undertaken. Taking the four guiding principles above, the technique provides the framework

within which 'respect for autonomy' can be given precise expression and within which the necessary transformation of the other three principles into the inputs needed for choice–benefits, harms and the distributions of benefits and harms among individuals–can be undertaken.

The decisions we are concerned with here are the ones that everyone agrees should be treated 'seriously'. In everyday terms, it will involve meeting the criteria implied when people say that 'we really must think this thing through'– and mean it. The underlying assumption of the chapter is that in most health decisions there is now a real option of moving to a more *analytical* mode of decision making from the customary, more *intuitive* one. The selection of the balance between analysis and intuition in relation to (1) the knowledge ('evidential') inputs into the decision, (2) the value inputs into the decision and (3) the decision-making itself, becomes the metaethical task to be answered in all health decision and policy making. With the ready availability of computer power, speed and relevant software, we should now be focusing on the ethics of *deciding how to decide*.

DECISION ANALYSIS

Any systematic analysis of a decision problem will necessarily involve the framing of the problem as a choice among alternative actions (e.g. operate or not, take the child into care or not), with each action leading to a set of possible 'small world' scenarios and outcomes. Any one scenario will reflect particular resolutions of all uncertainties along its path (e.g. the appendix was or was not the problem, the child was or was not being abused) and end in particular outcome states (e.g. good health, moderate disability or some multidimensional health state).

Decision analysis is the formal modelling of these key components of a decision, most simply in the form of a decision 'tree'. The simplest clinically relevant example is given in Figure 79.1.

This tree has been constructed on the basis of the judgement that there are two available options, here labelled 'remove' and 'leave' (e.g. a possibly diseased appendix or a possibly abused child). It further suggests that there is uncertainty about whether or not the underlying condition (appendicitis, abuse) is present. Finally, it suggests that there are four different outcomes, some of which will be regarded as more desirable than others. These four outcomes are conceptually equivalent to the consequences ('small worlds') which flow from making or not making the two sorts of error which are possible in this situation ('false positive' and 'false negative'). In other words, the four outcomes are the consequences of true and false positive judgements (a positive judgement leading, by definition, to removal) and

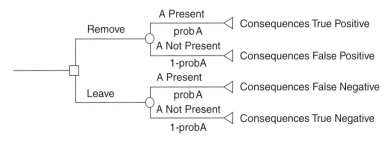

Figure 79.1. Basic decision tree.

the consequences of true and false negative judgements (a negative judgement leading, by definition, to non-removal).

This tree has also been provided (Figure 79.2) with the numerical 'fruit' necessary for establishing the optimal decision – *probabilities* on the chance branches to quantify the uncertainties and *utilities* on the outcome nodes to quantify the relative desirability/undesirability of the four outcome states. Given the numbers inserted here and given the judgement that maximizing the expected utility is the appropriate integrating principle, the optimal choice is to leave. Other numbers and other principles *could* change this (for example a probability of disease/abuse higher than 33 % is needed to make removal the optimal decision, given that with these utilities a false negative error is regarded as twice as bad as a false positive one). Decision analysis makes the selection of the ethically charged utilities and the integrating principles explicit.

This tree is easily expanded to incorporate a third 'test' branch. This will enable the decision maker to establish whether further investigation is the best decision at this point, as opposed to proceeding immediately to either remove or leave. It is crucial to see that gathering further information may or may not always be the best decision (and, it follows, the ethical one) as is sometimes assumed. Whether it is the best decision will depend on the quality characteristics of the test (sensitivity and specificity in the medical case) and the effect on the four consequences of

obtaining the extra information – including what happens during the testing or information gathering.

Fuller expositions of clinical decision analysis and cost-effectiveness analysis are to be found elsewhere (Hunink, et al., 2001). It needs to be stressed that there are few limits to the complexity of decision models. Although many real life cases are more complex than the above-mentioned illustrative one, the limitations of decision analysis lie neither in the technique nor in the computer software which is desirable for its implementation in anything but the simplest case. The quality of a decision analysis is determined by (1) the ability of human beings to think clearly about great complexity and model it and (2) the relevant data that human beings have chosen to generate. Many health professionals and authorities argue that they cannot structure a problem for modelling purposes (even with professional help) because of its 'complexity' nor provide the necessary numerical assessments of chance and desirability for such a model. It is therefore disturbing to find that they remain confident of their ability to make the decision successfully, using their *intuition* to overcome both their structuring difficulties and the data problems that they are keen to point to as a limitation of decision modelling but are actually the same for all decision technologies.

We all think we can intuitively deal with complex things. But for most of us this is a massive delusion. We *could* be much better at *systematic analysis and modelling* if we were

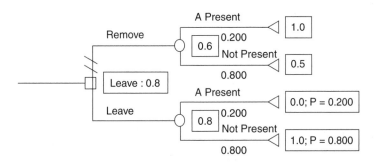

Figure 79.2. Basic decision tree populated and rolled back to identify optimal choice.

given lots of practice, lots of support and lots of reward, but at the moment we get none of these. Professional and ordinary education is devoid of any attention to systematic analysis for judgement and decision making and the career rewards in most fields go to those who show disdain for such methods, claiming to be able to make good judgements and decisions by drawing on their intuitive powers of insight, based on 'my years of experience' and on 'my *knowledge*'. Constant reinforcement of these beliefs occurs within decision contexts dominated by 'taking into account and bearing in mind' (TIABIM) processes, where social conventions prevent explicit exposure of beliefs and values other than in the most vague and general way.

Nevertheless, it is vital to recall that even though decision analysis is a significantly more analytical decision technology than TIABIM, it still requires substantial intuition-based inputs. In developing decision-analytic models it is important to distinguish the *decision structure* from the *judgements* which need to be made within the structure in order to identify the optimal choice. A decision always involves choice among two or more options. Judgements do not involve choice among options; they require assessments or valuations on some scale. Intuition will typically have a major role in generating these judgemental inputs, most obviously in relation to the utilities.

In most health decisions, and hence in decision analyses of them, judgements of four broad types are needed.

1. Judgements as to the '*availability*' of various action options – what are the possible choices? What is judged as an 'available' option for a particular patient or population may be affected by clinical, religious, ethical, legal, economic or other considerations. For example if the 'removal' concerned was of a 12-week-old foetus from the mother's womb, some people would argue that it is not an available option on the ground that abortion is simply wrong. Decision analyses are accordingly 'utilitarian' only within a specified deontological and rights framework.

    This sort of judgement will determine whether an option gets into the contest (model) and what options are being compared. The three other sorts of judgements relate to the evaluation of the contenders.
2. Judgements as to the *chances* involved wherever there is uncertainty involved in an option scenario. The uncertainty may relate to whether an event will or will not occur in the future (e.g. the abuse will continue if the child is left) or whether something is or is not the case (e.g. the appendix is or is not diseased). In the decision context, these probabilities are irredeemably subjective, though they may be subjected to intersubjectively agreed criteria (Dowie, 2006).
3. Judgements as to the *desirability* of the various possible outcome states (e.g. normal good health; confined to bed; unable to undertake self-care; dead). Providing the generic health measures necessary for most health decisions will require internal 'subjudgements', for instance, of the relative weighting of such health dimensions as mobility, mental function and pain. They will also include making judgements as to the valuation of states which will occur at different points of *time* in the future – are future effects and costs to be discounted relative to the present ones and if so at what rate? And also making judgements as to the valuation of states which will occur in different points in *space* – are effects and costs falling on different subgroups in a population to be given equal weight or differential weights? In both these cases, judgements are necessary about who has the *right* to be 'taken into the count' (future generations in the case of time, other individuals in the case of space).
4. Judgements as to the way *integration* of the foregoing judgements is to be achieved: how the uncertainty and desirability assessments pertaining to an option are to be integrated into some overall assessment for the option, so as to permit its comparison with the other available options. This will involve judgement as to whether or not 'maximizing expecting utility' – weighting utilities by their probabilities – is the appropriate rule for integration. Although the present author does not find the arguments against maximizing expected utility as a normative strategy convincing (Deber & Goel, 1990) the key point is that the explicit specification of chance and desirability judgements in decision analyses enables any alternative integration strategy *which is made explicit and transparent* to have its coherence and implications explored.

DECISION ANALYSIS AND ETHICS

It is sometimes asked 'Is decision analysis ethical?' The question is, in fact, loaded and should not be responded to in this form. One may legitimately ask about the ethicality of all decision technologies or, more usefully, about the ethicality of particular applications of all decision technologies. But this must be done in comparative terms, comparing the alternatives with each other in a specific case, not comparing one of them with a hypothetical 'nirvana standard', while leaving the others unexamined. So, one may legitimately ask whether a particular application of decision analysis is more or less ethical than a particular application of TIABIM or intuition to the same case, but not ask simply whether the decision analysis is ethical, implying that the other decision technologies need not be similarly scrutinized because they can be assumed to be superior if sufficient limitations and flaws are exposed in the analysis.

Decision analysis has particular strengths in relation to the issue of patient or population autonomy. Adopting a decision-analytic approach does not *guarantee* that claims for autonomy will be respected but it does provide the framework within which the key issue in relation to autonomy – *whose* utilities are to count and with what relative *weight* (the patient, the professional (s), the carers, the community, the nation, the globe) – is made totally explicit. In whatever way this issue is resolved for the analysis, it cannot be resolved covertly or ambiguously as it is – in many cases intentionally – when a TIABIM decision technology is employed.

The controversies are deepest when more than one party is involved in the decision (e.g. the mother and the foetus, the mentally ill patient and the family) and the question of resolving conflicting interpersonal interests arises. Alternative ways of systematically (numerically) rating and weighting the preferences of parties to a decision, as required in decision analyses, are available. Most of these procedures are instantly rejected by many practitioners on the grounds of their 'crudeness' or 'unacceptability' or 'impossibility'. For example it is customary for them to decry the analyst asking for importance weights for mother and foetus to be given in the form of two numbers that add up to 100%. To the decision analyst this reaction is a signal that such logically necessary judgements are going to be provided implicitly and covertly, using intuition or TIABIM processes.

Decision analysis accordingly imposes two heavy psychological burdens on health decision makers. First, it demands that all differences in beliefs and values which pertain to the decision, whether consequentialist or absolutist, be made explicit and resolved in the open with patient or population. Explicitness is to be taken as an ethical imperative in health decisions unless there is an *overwhelming* case against it on therapeutic or incompetence grounds. (This is apart from any legal imperatives to explicitness in clinical contexts emerging from 'informed consent' requirements, especially where the 'reasonable patient' standard applies.) Secondly, it demands that all verbal assertions of differences in magnitude be quantified. There is no prejudice or bias against expressing magnitudes on numerical scales as opposed to verbal ones. In this connection it is important to emphasize that 'number' includes 'numerical range'. There is no requirement in decision analyses for numbers to have any particular degree of precision, so that criticisms which assume that decision analysis requires one to be 'inexactly precise' are misconceived. On the contrary, decision analysis does require one to be 'precisely inexact' in the sense of quantifying one's uncertainties as probability distributions.

It is important at this point to re-emphasize that decision analysts themselves have nothing to say about what the probability or utility numbers in an actual decision should be – except that they should be coherent. Their task is to make clear that the end products of all searching of hearts, minds, emotions and literatures which should go on in relation to the case are to be such numbers. Although this requirement need not dominate every moment of the discourse in which the analysis should be embedded, it is vital that that discussion be conducted against the assumption that these numbers are what are needed at 'the moment of *decision*'–which is conceptually quite inappropriate to call the 'moment of *truth*'.

DECISION ANALYSIS AND THE ETHICS OF COHERENCE

The decision analysts, like other professionals, have ethical responsibilities. Among these, it can be argued, is the responsibility to refuse to carry out analyses in ways which are inconsistent with the ethical justification of the analysis. This is most likely to occur when they are instructed to restrict the analysis in some way for 'political' or other reasons. Being asked to exclude a 'do nothing' option from the analysis is a typically sought constraint. Refusal to accede to these demands is not a demand for decision-making power. It is a demand to design and conduct the analysis in line with the normative principles of decision analysis and the *publicly stated goals and values of the decision makers*(such as 'maximizing the health of the population'). It is important to see that the decision makers have the legal right and the political power to disregard the results of the analysis – or not to commission it in the first place – but not to say how it should be conducted.

The discipline demanded in carrying out a decision analysis and the responsibility which flows from it is, above all, a way of ensuring that *ethical incoherence* does not creep into decision making. Nowhere is incoherence more potentially inequitable than in cost-effectiveness analyses conducted to pursue the joint goals of efficiency and equity in the allocation of resources in publicly funded health services. It is worth documenting this through an illustrative example based on (but not drawn from) appraisals carried out by the NICE.

NICE is charged with establishing the clinical and cost-effectiveness of new technologies – mainly drugs, but occasionally other procedures and devices. The ethical justification for the use of a cost-effectiveness criterion is clear: the use of resources in any particular way in a resource-constrained publicly funded health service has opportunity costs in the form of the benefits foregone by other patients in the system.

NICE is mandated to appraise the cost-effectiveness of new technologies in relation to 'standard practice'. But the use in cost-effectiveness analyses of 'standard practice' comparators *which have not themselves been evaluated* undermines the ethical justification for the use of this technique in public health care systems. A fully worked numerical example can be found in Dowie (2005). In summary, assume that drug B has become the 'standard treatment' on the grounds of its *effectiveness* relative to drug A, but without passing a *cost-effectiveness* test. From retrospective cost-effectiveness analyses carried out in relation to the appraisal of new drug C, we can now see that drug B would have failed that test. The new drug C may now emerge as cost effective when compared with drug B, though it would not be cost effective if drug A had been (correctly) used as the comparator. (Of course, drug A itself may or may not have passed a cost-effectiveness test, using 'do nothing' as the comparator, if it had been properly evaluated.)

This use of unevaluated standard practice is therefore a breach of both the fundamental principles of cost-effectiveness analysis and the ethical basis for its use in a public health service. The reader is invited to speculate about the reasons for this unwillingness to stand firm on behalf of *all other patients* – the ones who experience the opportunity costs when any particular new intervention is approved – against the panoply of political, popular, professional and pharmaceutical interests ranged against ethically coherent decision making.

Even if one argues that cost-effectiveness can be outweighed by other considerations, this in no way justifies assessing cost-effectiveness incoherently. Using unevaluated standard practice as a comparator will always infringe the basic ethical principle underlying (opportunity) cost-effectiveness assessment – that the foregone benefits to other patients should be established by transparently coherent and equitable procedures. In many cases, standard practice may well, when evaluated, prove to be cost-effective relative to alternative interventions. What is ethically unacceptable, because of its incoherence, is the refusal to countenance the proper and transparent evaluation of 'standard practice'– and disinvestment in those standard practices which fail the ethical test of equitable cost-effectiveness analysis.

A parallel breach of ethical coherence relates to interventions which are cost-effective, but not (incrementally) effective. A new drug which is less effective (say 5% less effective) than an old one, but much cheaper (say 50% cheaper), is likely to emerge as the cost-effective intervention in a properly conducted analysis. It should therefore be the one which is reimbursed (at least for new patients) in an equitable service. The ethics of a public health service require that cost-effectiveness trumps effectiveness, even if the latter is

measured comprehensively using a generic health measure, as it rarely is (Dowie, 2004).

EVALUATING DECISION TECHNOLOGIES

Here are some of the statements of intention which proliferate in decision-making contexts when a TIABIM decision technology is employed:

> 'We must take into *account* all the relevant circumstances.'
> 'We must strike the right *balance* between risks and benefits.'
> 'Clearly, we need to give quality of life considerations *due weight*.'
> 'We must keep the claims of autonomy and justice in *proportion*.'
> 'We must factor all the ethical claims into the *equation*.'
> 'We must *gauge* the impact of our decision on all parties.'
> 'As chair of the committee I believe we have reached a *degree* of consensus.'

The italicized words give the impression that some form of quantification – 'weighing', 'balancing' and 'establishing proportions' – is going on – but if this is not merely metaphorical and rhetorical use of these concepts, it is certainly never intended that some underlying *intuitive* quantification is to be made overt. In contrast, decision analysis involves actual, numerical, weighing, balancing, taking into account and establishing proportions. The decision-analytic framework specifies the quantifications and the calculations – the literal equations – which are necessary for identifying the optimal choice.

We are now in a position to throw new light on an old complaint. As many who have consulted them complain, the problem with ethical advisers – and even the ethical consultants'/ethicists' increasingly found in North American hospitals – is that they do not actually tell you *how* to 'take into account' all the 'considerations' they suggest are relevant to the decision. They say that this is not their job, which is to 'raise awareness' about the various possibilities and 'factors that need to be borne in mind'. This can undoubtedly be a valuable contribution. But after the ethical consultation or counselling is finished, those involved are left trying to 'weigh up the consequences and get the right balance between doing good and doing harm' (or something along these lines) if they have been listening to any sort of utilitarian; or trying to 'do what you think is right, taking everyone's interests and obligations into account' (or something along these lines) if they have been listening to any sort of deontologist. Or most likely they are left with a confused and confusing mixture of both. A take home task clearly envisaged by the counsellor as one to be completed using an intuitive or TIABIM decision technology.

We can now see that there is an alternative.

Of course, any decision technology, including decision analysis, can be abused. But the difficulty and dangers of abuse are less the greater the openness and transparency of the procedure. The argument that an innumerate population – and profession – could be misled by numbers and equations involved in decision analyses deserves to be heeded and the appropriate remedial work begun immediately.

In the legendary TV series *The Prisoner*, the eponymous 'Number 6' sustains his morale by asserting 'I am not a number, I am a free man'. A fine sentiment, but one which, like many, is unhelpful in the real world if misinterpreted. The most prevalent misinterpretation in this case involves confusion between being treated on the basis of statistical considerations and being treated as a statistic, that is as a dehumanized object in an experiment or trial. (Every health encounter may conceptually be regarded as one or the other.) A truly free person is the one who is able to benefit from being treated on the basis of his or her set membership when the limits of current knowledge mean that attempting to go beyond this will lead to inferior treatment. As a patient I say to doctors 'I am a free man but please treat me as a statistic if it improves my odds'. And please 'accept error to make less error' (Einhorn, 1986) because although you will inevitably make *some* errors because of the irreducible uncertainty surrounding my case (Hammond, 1996), I have no logical grounds for believing that I have any less chance than any other of your patients of being one of your *unnecessary* errors'.

The ethical decision technology is the one which produces the best decisions as judged by results in a large number of similar cases. Which process does this can only be established by evaluation. In medicine the controlled trial is accepted as the ideal mode for such evaluation of competing technologies. So, as with the evaluation of drugs or imaging technologies, decision technologies too need to be evaluated by robust methods. The issue can then be clearly seen as not being whether decision analysis or any alternative mode (such as 'clinical judgement') is *perfect*, but which produces the *better* results.

What are the ethical implications of a commitment to intuitive or TIABIM decision-making processes *not* based on any systematic comparative evaluation? It involves acting on the assumption – or, more brutally, *faith* – that the results are better than those that could be produced by the alternative. It surely cannot be ethical to refuse to carry out a controlled trial of one's judgement and decision making and other alternatives simply on the ground that 'it's the way I/we as experienced practitioner/s do it' or 'it's the way things are done in this practice/hospital'. Nor can it be ethical to refuse a study on the grounds that the alternatives are obviously 'defective' and 'unacceptable' *as processes*.

There is a paradox here in that the analytical alternatives to intuitive and TIABIM decision technologies – such as decision analysis – are by definition more explicit and specific. Their potential limitations and weaknesses can be much more easily identified, even if we rule out, as we surely should in the interests of patients and populations, 'acceptability' to practitioner or decision-making authority as a key criterion.

A truly free – and truly ethical – professional decision maker or decision-making authority is one that accepts their limitations as an information processor and decides whether or not to adopt a decision technology (way of deciding) on the basis of evidence, rather than *assuming* that they must be able to outperform it because of its manifest defects when evaluated against a standard of perfection: A standard of perfection which is never applied as rigorously – or at all – to their own preferred, intuition-dominated, technology. In other words, the ethical decision maker does not maintain that 'my judgement must always take precedence' but adopts the reflective position that 'my judgement will take precedence when I have good evidence to support the view that it will outperform the judgement produced by an alternative technology, such as decision analysis'.

REFERENCES

Beauchamp TL. The 'Four Principles' approach. In: Gillon R, ed. *Principles of Health Care Ethics*. Chichester: John Wiley & Sons, Inc., 1994; pp. 3–12.

Deber RB, Goel V. Using explicit rules to manage issues of justice, risk, and ethics in decision analysis: when is it not rational to maximize expected utility? *Med Decis Making* 1990; **10**: 181–94.

Dowie J. Comparator Ethics 2005, (draft, available on request from author).

Dowie J. The Bayesian approach to decision making. In: Killoran A, Swann C, Kelly M, eds. *Public Health Evidence: Tackling Health Inequalities*. Oxford: Oxford University Press 2006; pp 309–21.

Dowie J. Why cost-effectiveness should trump (clinical) effectiveness: the ethical economics of the South West quadrant. *Health Econ* 2004; **13**: 453–9.

Einhorn HJ. Accepting error to make less error. *J Person Assess* 1986; **50**: 387–95.

Gillon R. *Philosophical Medical Ethics*. Chichester: John Wiley & Sons, Inc., 1985.

Hammond KR. *Human Judgment and Social Policy: Irreducible Uncertainty, Inevitable Error, Unavoidable Injustice*. New York: Oxford University Press, 1996.

Hunink M, Glasziou P, Siegel J, Weeks J, Pliskin J, Elstein A, *et al*. *Decision Making in Health and Medicine: Integrating Evidence and Values*. Cambridge: Cambridge University Press, 2001.

80

Health Inequities and the Social Determinants of Health

WENDY ROGERS

INTRODUCTION

The health of individuals and populations is influenced by many variables. These include genetics and biology, but perhaps more important than these are the social determinants of health. The social, political and economic circumstances in which people live their lives are critical in determining how long they live and with what burden of ill health. These differences are very marked between countries, for example a 15-year-old boy in Lesotho has about a 10% chance of living until the age of 60, compared with a 15-year-old boy in Sweden who has a 91% chance of living to 60 (Marmot, 2005). The differences are not, however, limited to those between countries; within countries, people's life expectancies vary according to where they live, their educational opportunities, what kind of work they do and how much they earn. Study of the social determinants of health has informed our understanding of patterns of health and ill health and led to discussion about the moral implications of these patterns, and possible actions to reduce disparities (Anand, Peter & Sen, 2004).

INEQUALITIES AND INEQUITIES

Health inequalities are 'differences, variations and disparities in the health achievements of individuals and groups' (Kawachi et al., 2002, p. 647). To say that a health inequality exists tells us that there is a difference in health status or health outcomes between some individuals or groups. Women have higher rates of osteoporosis than men for example, so that there is an inequality in the distribution of the incidence of osteoporosis between men and women. Men have higher rates of cardiovascular disease than women, another health inequality. Professional footballers have higher rates of some musculo-skeletal injuries than the general population. These are descriptions of states of affairs; the existence of health inequalities per se does not necessarily mean that the inequalities are unfair or unjust in a way that demands our moral attention. In general, health inequalities which are the result of social circumstances which are themselves morally wrong (for example, poverty, educational disadvantage or racial discrimination) are considered unjust. Health inequalities which are the result of bad luck (for example, biological or genetic factors over which we have little control) or the result of free and deliberate choices on the part of individuals (such as the choice to go hang gliding) may not be inequitable, although of course how we respond to them raises issues of justice. Health inequalities which are the result of unjust conditions or failures of identifiable duties are termed health inequities.

To give an example, the kinds of health differences which are inequities are those associated with social, political or economic circumstances which are in themselves morally wrong. In Australia, babies born to indigenous mothers are more likely to be of low birth weight (12.9% compared with 6.2% of babies of other mothers) and more likely to die. The perinatal mortality rate for babies born of indigenous mothers is 17.2 per 1 000 compared with 9.5 for babies of other mothers (Laws & Sullivan, 2004). These stark differences are inequities because they are the result of multiple social, economic and political wrongs including dispossession, poverty, inadequate housing, unemployment, lack of access to culturally appropriate health care and lack of educational

Principles of Health Care Ethics, Second Edition   Edited by R.E. Ashcroft, A. Dawson, H. Draper and J.R. McMillan
© 2007 John Wiley & Sons, Ltd

opportunities. All of these factors are unjust or unfair rather than the result of bad luck or free and voluntary choices, making the health disparities inequitable, rather than just unequal.

HEALTH EQUITY

The International Society for Equity in Health offers this definition of equity in health: 'the absence of potentially remediable, systematic differences in one or more aspects of health status across socially, economically, demographically or geographically defined populations or subgroups' (Macino & Starfield, 2002). Turning this around, health inequities have been defined as those health inequalities which are unfair or unjust, or stem from some kind of injustice (Kawachi et al., 2002). In her influential 1992 paper, Whitehead included the criteria that health inequities be avoidable. This has been challenged on the grounds that unfairness implies avoidability, and that it is undesirable to link equity explicitly to avoidability as this may offer reasons not to act if an inequity is deemed unavoidable (Braveman & Gruskin, 2003).

Whitehead identified seven main determinants of health differentials. Three of these, natural biological variation, freely chosen health damaging behaviour (such as dangerous sports) and early uptake of health promoting behaviour are generally accepted not to be inequities. She considers the other four to be avoidable and to be associated with health inequalities which are unjust. These are:

1. health damaging behaviour where there is severely restricted degree of choice over lifestyle;
2. exposure to unhealthy, stressful living and working conditions;
3. inadequate access to essential health and other public services; and
4. health related social mobility, reflecting the tendency for ill people to move down the social scale (Whitehead, 1992, p. 432).

There are challenges in measuring and assessing health inequalities and in translating these data into information about health inequities. One of the key issues revolves around whether to measure social group differences in health, or the distribution of health statistics across individuals in a population (Kawachi et al., 2002). Measuring individual health disparities allows comparisons between the healthier and the sicker within populations and provides flexible data for comparisons over time and space. This can be useful for international comparisons in which there are problems comparing different occupational or social groups. On the contrary, simply measuring disparities without looking at the distributions of these across social groupings does not tell us anything about equity and the effectiveness of policies to reduce inequities, and may hinder inquiries into the causes of health inequalities (Kawachi et al., 2002; Braveman & Gruskin, 2003). Although both individual and group data are complementary and useful, it is the latter which are critical in identifying health inequities and so paving the way to addressing them through policy and practice.

As well as measuring health outcomes, equity in access to health care is also important. There are two dimensions to equity of access to health care; vertical equity refers to preferential treatment for those with greater health needs, while horizontal equity refers to equal treatment for equivalent needs (Macino & Starfield, 2002). Both are necessary for comprehensive equity of access, although policy makers and service providers have found it easier to focus on horizontal equity as this does not involve the difficult process of prioritizing between competing health needs.

HEALTH EQUITY, SOCIAL JUSTICE AND RIGHTS

Health equity is a normative concept, grounded in values of fairness and justice and extending well beyond the arena of health care and health policy. Sen has argued that health equity is central to an understanding of social justice for three reasons (Sen, 2004). First, good health is a critical constituent of human capabilities, as without good health, we are limited in our opportunities for other capabilities and in achieving the things that we value. If the lack of good health is potentially avoidable and due to social, political or economic arrangements, it is an unfair limit on one's capabilities. Second, equitable processes are important in relation to access to health care services. Health equity would not be achieved, according to Sen, by discriminating against healthier groups in order to reduce their health to that of the worst off group, although this might eliminate some health inequalities. Sen's final argument is that health equity cannot be solely concerned with health capabilities or access to health care, but must also engage with the ways that resource allocation and social arrangements are linked to health. For example, health equity might require a redistributive taxation policy rather than a universally low rate of taxation if the former had a greater impact on reducing poverty, with its associated health inequities (Sen, 2004).

Braveman and Gruskin (2003) link health equity with human rights. The right to health is recognized in a number of international treaties and declarations, including the International Covenant on Economic, Social and Cultural Rights which requires recognition of 'the right of everyone to the enjoyment of the highest attainable standard of physical and mental health' (United Nations High Commisson on Human Rights, 1976). This claim has been criticized on the grounds that it does not provide a clear standard for action; however Braveman and Gruskin argue that one way of operationalizing this is to take the standard of health enjoyed by the most advantaged group in a society as the standard which should be achievable for all members of that society. Further connections between human rights and health equity can be made by grounding the notion of equal opportunities to be healthy with the right to non-discrimination, emphasizing the responsibility of governments to eliminate the discrimination which exists against social groups suffering health inequities.

On a global scale, abuses of human rights are closely associated with health inequities, ranging from the spread of HIV/AIDS among those with the least protection of their human rights, through to the adverse health effects of incarceration and torture.

THE SOCIAL DETERMINANTS OF HEALTH

The evidence for the impact of social, political and economic circumstances upon health is considerable. In all societies, there is a socioeconomic health gradient in which those who live in more comfortable circumstances have longer and healthier lives than those who are less well off (Daniels et al., 1999; Wilkinson & Marmot, 2003). Between countries, the differences are marked with life expectancies in poorer countries far lower than in richer countries. For example, in Lesotho, Swaziland and Zimbabwe, the 2003 life expectancies were less than 40 years, compared with over 80 years in Japan, Switzerland and Iceland (World Health Organization, 2004). Within countries there are also disparities which can be as large as those between countries. There is a 20 year gap in life expectancies between white men in the healthiest US states, compared with black men in the least healthy (Marmot, 2001). In Australia, the excess mortality rate for disadvantaged women is such that if the death rate could be lowered to that of the least disadvantaged, there would be a 56% decrease in the premature all-cause mortality rate for women aged 24–65; for men the reduction would be 26% (Turrell & Mathers, 2001). This social gradient effect is not limited to the poorest but operates across the spectrum, so that even among those who are employed, such as middle class office workers, lower ranking staff have higher rates of morbidity and mortality than higher ranking staff (Marmot et al., 1997; Donkin et al., 2002).

This kind of information raises interesting questions as to whether it is the socioeconomic gradient itself or poverty which causes these inequalities. Internationally, there is a clear relationship between life expectancy and per capita gross domestic product (GDPpc), but once a certain threshold level of GDPpc is reached, the relationship levels off (Daniels et al., 1999). Countries with similar GDPpcs may have quite different life expectancies. For example, both Cuba and Iraq have quite low GDPpcs, but life expectancy is over 20 years higher in Cuba than Iraq. Likewise, countries with quite large disparities in income may have similar life expectancies. The United States, for example, is far richer than Costa Rica, but the two countries had identical life expectancies in 2003 (Daniels et al., 1999; World Health Organization, 2004).

Observations of these kinds have led to debate about the definition of 'poverty' and whether this should be defined in absolute or relative terms. Absolute poverty describes the condition in which a person is unable to meet basic human needs such as food or shelter, while relative poverty relates to the standards which exist elsewhere in the society. Given the strength of the socioeconomic gradient in health across all groups, including those who are reasonably well off, the concept of relative poverty is more useful in relation to health equity (Kawachi et al., 2002).

Further work in this area has explored the links between absolute and relative incomes in relation to health inequalities. Differences in life expectancies seem to vary with the nature of income distribution within countries indicating the importance of relative income; the more equal the income distribution, the higher the life expectancy, and vice versa. This may be part of the explanation as to why Costa Rica has a life expectancy similar to that of the United States despite much lower incomes. This theory is currently under investigation through looking at the association between income distribution and individual health. To date, the results are mixed with some studies identifying an income inequality effect on either individuals or groups, while other studies have found no effects (Kawachi et al., 2002).

There is often a clustering or cascade of the health effects of socioeconomic disadvantage. Sources of exclusion from health care, particularly in poorer nations, include geographical isolation, poverty, race, language and culture. These factors go hand in hand with exclusion from other services such as safe housing, clean water and sanitation and education (World Health Organization, 2005). In more affluent nations, disadvantage also compounds, with those born into poverty more likely to have ill health and lower educational achievements, leading to lower job security, more poverty, more stress and more ill health.

The kinds of factors which are known to impact upon health include psychosocial stresses as well as material disadvantage. In practice, the two are linked as lack of material resources, such as inadequate housing or lack of income, are likely to trigger feelings of stress and distress. A range of psychosocial stresses including isolation, low self-esteem, anxiety, insecurity and lack of control over one's work are associated with poor physical and mental health (Wilkinson & Marmot, 2003).

The effects of deprivation not only reflect a person's current circumstances, but are also cumulative over the life cycle. Three possible mechanisms for this have been suggested. Latent effects refer to adult health effects associated with the early life environment, including intrauterine health, which are independent of any intervening conditions, such as the association between intrauterine growth and adult cardiac disease. Pathway effects describe the ways in which the early life environment sets individuals onto life trajectories which affect health status over time, such as exposure to high levels of pollution in childhood leading to an excess burden of respiratory disease with loss of school time, poor educational achievement and low status work in adult life. Cumulative effects relate to the intensity and duration of unfavourable exposures over time, in a dose–effect relationship, such as the cumulative effect of anxiety and stress experienced by a person with poor job security and isolation, culminating in depression.

THEORETICAL RESPONSE TO THE MORAL IMPLICATIONS OF HEALTH INEQUALITIES

As discussed above, the concept of health equity is a normative concept, raising questions about justice, fairness and the values which societies ought to promote. This has led to significant work in moral philosophy, as scholars describe and defend theories of justice in relation to health equity (Anand, Peter & Sen, 2004; Ruger, 2004). Prior to the interest in health equity, questions of resource allocation in health care were dominated by utilitarian thinking, in the form of quality-adjusted life years and cost-effectiveness analyses. These focus upon maximizing overall benefits or utility, with little regard to the degree of inequality in different distributions of benefits. Given what we now know about the nexus between disadvantage and poor health, recent accounts of justice and health care have avoided a simple maximizing approach. Two significant accounts warrant discussion here: the justice as fairness approach of Daniels and colleagues; (Daniels et al., 1999; Daniels, 2002) and the capabilities approach of Sen (1992, 2004).

Rawls' theory of justice as fairness specifies the terms of social cooperation which free and equal citizens can accept as fair. Rawls does not address questions of health and health care, but Daniels argues that justice as fairness does provide a way of addressing health inequities 'by establishing equal opportunities, a fair distribution of resources, and support for our self respect – the bases of Rawlsian justice – we would go a long way in eliminating the most important

injustices in health outcomes' (Daniels, 2002, p. 11). A society organized on Rawlsian principles would be likely to flatten the socioeconomic gradient considerably, thus eliminating a major antecedent to health inequities. In addition, the guarantee of the social bases for self-respect together with the citizens' convictions that their prospects were fair might decrease some of the psychosocial stresses of being at the lower end of any remaining socioeconomic gradient.

There are at least two areas, however, where this justice as fairness approach is problematic. The first is in connection with the Difference Principle which permits inequalities as long as the inequalities work to make those who are worst off as well-off as possible. Putting the Difference Principle into practice requires a decision about potential trade-offs between health and other primary goods, for example, risking health by taking a high paying but physically dangerous job such as underwater maintenance on an off-shore oil rig. As Daniels notes, there is no clear answer to the question as to how much health one can trade for other gains, nor how to judge any ensuing inequalities. Perhaps more importantly, it may be the wrong question in that health and other social goods are not separate and independent such that they can be traded-off in a relatively simple way. The second problem area is that of allocation, both setting fair limits to the total resources allocated to health care in relation to other goods, and prioritizing between patients. Prima facie, a commitment to fair equality of opportunity requires giving priority to the worst-off, as ill health drastically reduces one's opportunities across the board. But does this require a never-ending stream of resources to be directed to the worst off despite diminishing returns? Alternatively, we can look at who is likely to benefit most, but this takes us back to the problem of distribution – those benefiting the most may not be those with the greatest burden of ill health or disadvantage, so that the results might do nothing for health equity. Daniels notes that in the absence of an agreed set of principles of distributive justice, the question becomes one of procedural justice: under what conditions are rationing decisions legitimate? He then outlines four conditions under which limit-setting decisions might be considered fair and legitimate.

Sen takes a different path. His capabilities approach argues that health is not only central to our well-being but also that the exercise of our other freedoms and capabilities is dependent upon our health achievements. As such, health equity is central to social justice rather than being a fortunate side-effect of implementing justice as fairness (Sen, 2004). Taking the capability for health as the central goal, rather than specific health achievements or equitable distribution of primary goods, recognizes the importance of agency and the role of individual choice in influencing health outcomes. Sen notes, however, that for the most part health achievement is a good guide to the underlying capability, given almost universal preferences to be healthy.

Sen's account of capabilities engages with the complexity of health and the inter-relatedness of health with other important capabilities such as the capability to be well educated, to avoid economic vulnerability and to be self-determining. The capability for good health is obviously reliant to some extent upon the distribution of resources and primary goods, but other considerations beyond the social and economic are also important, such as personal disabilities, individual susceptibility to illness, hazards linked to geographical location, climatic variations and so on (Sen, 2004). Thus, equality in health capabilities can be distinguished from equality in the distribution of the resources necessary for health, and it is the former which is central to health equity. Ruger (2004) argues that the capability approach to health recognizes the central role of health in all of our capabilities, and the importance of addressing health needs on multiple fronts in multiple policy domains, through comprehensive strategies delivered through multiple institutions.

Other scholars have addressed the question of why health inequalities are morally important and which of these are unjust, without developing a more comprehensive theory. Brock (2002) has examined whether or not the worse off have special moral claims, and if so, how we should respond to them. In giving priority to the worse-off rather than to those with the greatest needs, it is possible or likely that there will be fewer overall gains in health care, thereby requiring some justification. Brock identifies three potential justifications for a prioritarian view. The first is that the worse off a person is, the greater the relative improvement in their condition a given benefit will provide, and so for any given health benefit, it will 'matter more' to a person who is worse off. Though this is intuitively appealing, it may be hard to find a scale which combines disadvantage and ill health in an appropriate way, or to argue that a person with diabetes, heart disease and cancer is more deserving of life saving treatment than a person with cancer alone. A second possible justification is that there are stronger moral claims generated by the ill health associated with undeserved disadvantage, just because the disadvantage and ill health are undeserved. This relies on being able to distinguish between deserved and undeserved disadvantage which is a notoriously difficult question, especially in relation to health inequities where the interconnections between social context, opportunities and choices, and health are so complex. Finally, priority to the worse off may be justified by treating the most urgent needs first on the grounds that urgency is morally relevant. Treatment of urgent needs at the expense of those with less urgent needs would need to take into account other morally relevant considerations such as the needs of the

better off and the likely diminishing returns of treating some conditions. The problem here is that, for example, a programme to treat an urgent health need such as life threatening heart attacks may have an inequitable effect in that it is the least disadvantaged who are most likely to have access to emergency services. As Brock notes, all of these arguments are complicated by the difficulty of defining who is worse off, even if we limit this to health rather than overall disadvantage (Brock, 2002).

Taking a broader approach, Beitz (2001) has looked at the reasons for thinking that global inequalities matter. In doing so, he puts aside direct reasons grounded in the view that equality is a fundamental ethical requirement and focuses upon derivative reasons. These revolve around the moral imperative to relieve the harms which are associated with inequality, including avoidable suffering, humiliation and denial of agency, curtailment of liberty and procedural unfairness. All of these are reasons which we can have for acting against inequalities which, by virtue of their moral wrongness, are also inequities. The advantage of this approach is to 'concentrate attention on the situation of those who are worse off and to emphasize the respects in which their circumstances interfere with their living what might reasonably be described as decent satisfying lives', which he takes to be a fairly uncontroversial conception of human well-being (Beitz, 2001, p. 120). Beitz also points out that many of the possible measures to alleviate the harms of global inequalities do not require some kind of levelling, but might instead focus upon alleviating specific harms through, for example, community empowerment, improved nutrition or the introduction of democratic processes.

PRACTICAL RESPONSES AND REASONS TO ACT

Alongside these philosophical investigations, practitioners and policy advisers have taken a practical approach to addressing health inequities.[1] In their discussion about the reasons to reduce health inequalities, Woodward and Kawachi (Woodward & Kawachi, 2000) emphasize the practical benefits and solutions. One of their arguments revolves around the claim that inequalities affect everyone, so that conditions which lead to significant health inequalities are detrimental to all members of society, not just the disadvantaged. This is the self-interest argument which drove many of the sanitary reforms in the nineteenth century as the affluent realized that poor living circumstances created ideal conditions for the infectious diseases which then threatened their own well-being. The threat of spread

---

[1] There is a point of terminology to be noted here. Much of the literature, especially the medical literature, uses the term 'health inequalities' 'health gap' (UK and Europe) or 'health disparities' (US) rather than health inequities, presumably to avoid the normative dimensions.

of infectious diseases from disadvantaged areas to more af-fluent ones is probably higher today, with the ease of inter-national travel and the likelihood that epidemics of diseases such as avian flu will emerge from countries with relatively poor living conditions or inadequate health services. Spill over effects are not limited to contagious diseases but ap-ply to alcohol misuse, violence and mental illness also, as high rates of these problems can affect all members of a society. Woodward and Kawachi argue that interventions to reduce social inequalities will have not only health related benefits for the whole community but also wider benefits such as reducing social exclusion which is both costly in terms of loss of potential resources and leads to increased danger from those who feel disenfranchised from the main-stream society. A second practical line of reasoning is that interventions to reduce inequalities do exist and are cost-ef-fective, although there is a current paucity of evidence, and our understanding of the underlying mechanisms linking disadvantage and ill health is incomplete. The small body of existing research evidence indicates that interventions to improve access to health care for the disadvantaged can have a potentially significant impact upon health inequalities, but as we have noted above, access to health care is only a small part of health equity. It is likely that interventions outside the health sector which improve social determinants such as income and education will have the greatest effect on health inequalities. This however requires a degree of political vision and cooperation which is not always apparent.

Whitehead and colleagues have spelled out a compre-hensive policy response to inequities in health, consisting of four elements, each with a number of strategies (White-head, Dalgren & Gilson, 2001). The four elements are:

1. establishing shared values;
2. assessing and analysing the health divide;
3. tackling root causes; and
4. building equitable health care systems.

They emphasize the importance of setting health equity objectives, not only to monitor progress and improve accountability but also for symbolic purposes, to inspire and motivate and provide political direction. This links directly with the need for accurate data. As discussed above, there has been a debate about the methods for measuring health inequalities, and, as yet, it is not standard practice to analyse health and research data by social groupings (Whitehead, Dalgren & Gilson, 2001; Rogers, 2004). Accurate data are also essential for analysing the causes and understanding the pathways between disadvantage and ill health, and so for developing effective ways to tackle the root causes of health inequities. Whitehead and colleagues draw upon a conceptual model of the main determinants of health to identify potential interventions,

ranging from healthy macropolicies through to creating supportive environments for behavioural change. Finally, building equitable health care systems requires policies which address barriers to access, the creation of an equity-oriented health system and vigilance in monitoring and protecting equity.

Internationally, there are some encouraging develop-ments with regard to health equity. The 'Target One' of the WHO European Regions Health for All strategy has helped to put equity issues onto the international stage, serving as both a symbolic and a practical goal (Whitehead, Dalgren & Gilson, 2001). More recently, the WHO Commission on Social Determinants of Health was announced in 2005 with the following goals:

1. to support policy change in countries by promoting models and practices which effectively address the social determinants of health;
2. to support countries in placing health as a shared goal to which many government departments and sectors of society contribute; and
3. to help build a sustainable global movement for action on health equity and social determinants, linking governments, international organizations, research institutions, civil society and communities (World Health Organisation, 2005).

CONCLUSION

There is a central conflict with regard to health and health care. On one hand, we have an increasingly individual and technical focus on health, with the promise of personalized treatments such as pharmacogenetic or stem cell therapies, and on the other hand, we have increasing evidence that the social determinants of health are responsible for a great burden of excess morbidity and mortality. We are continu-ously facing choices about the ways in which we address health problems. These choices will necessarily reflect our underlying ideological, political, social and economic val-ues. There are powerful moral and practical arguments as to why we should attend to the social determinants of health to improve global health and to decrease health inequities, but at present these do not seem to have captured the imagina-tions of populations and politicians around the world. The current circumstances in which global capitalism exerts a powerful influence upon the shape and functioning of our world seem to mitigate against initiatives to decrease ineq-uities. There are, however, some signs of a sea change, with increasing scholarship and practical moves to conceptual-ize, describe, analyse and act upon the social determinants of health, and increasing recognition that health equity is crucial for the health of all.

REFERENCES

Anand S, Peter F, Sen A. *Public Health, Ethics and Equity*. Oxford: Oxford University Press, 2004.

Beitz C. Does global inequality matter? In: Pogge T, ed. *Global Justice*. Oxford: Blackwell, 2001; pp. 106–122.

Braveman P, Gruskin S. Defining equity in health. *J Epidemiol Community Health* 2003; **57**: 254–8.

Brock D. Priority to the worse off in health-care resource prioritisation. In: Rhodes R, Battin M, Silvers A. *Medicine and Social Justice*. New York: Oxford University Press, 2002; pp. 362–72.

Daniels N, Kennedy B, Kawachi I. Why justice is good for our health: the social determinants of health inequalities. *Daedalus* 1999; **128**: 215–51.

Daniels N. Justice, health and health care. In: Rhodes R, Battin M, Silvers A, eds. *Medicine and Social Justice*. New York: Oxford University Press, 2002; pp. 6–23.

Donkin A, Goldblatt P, Lynch K. Inequalities in life expectancy by social class 972–1999. *Health Stat Q* 2002; **15**: 5–15.

Kawachi I, Subramanium SV, *et al*. A glossary for health inequalities. *J Epidemiol Community Health* 2002; **56**: 647–52.

Laws J, Sullivan E. *Australia's Mothers and Babies 2002*. Sydney: AIHW National Perinatal Statistics Unit, 2004.

Macino JA, Starfield B. Annotated bibliography on equity in health, 1980–2001. *Int J Equity Health* 2002; **1**(1): 1–20.

Marmot M, Bosma H, *et al*. Contribution of job control and other risk factors to social variations in coronary heart disease incidence. *Lancet* 1997; **350**: 235–9.

Marmot M. *What are the Social Determinants of Health?*, 2005; accessed on 9 Feb 2006 from: http://www.who.int/social_determinants/en/

Marmot M. Inequalities in health. *New Engl J Med* 2001; **345**(2): 134–6.

Rogers W. Evidence-based medicine and justice: a framework for looking at the impact of EBM on vulnerable or disadvantaged groups. J Med Ethics, 2004; **30**: 141–5.

Ruger J, Ethics of the social determinants of health. *Lancet* 2004; **364**: 1092–7.

Sen A. *Inequality Reexamined*. Cambridge, MA: Harvard University Press, 1992.

Sen A. Why health equity? In: Anand S, Peter F, Sen A, eds. *Public Health, Ethics and Equity*. Oxford: Oxford University Press, 2004; pp. 21–34.

Turrell G, Mathers C. Socioeconomic inequalities in all-cause and specific-cause mortality in Australia: 1985–1987 and 1995–1997. *Int J Epidemiol* 2001; **30**(2):231–9.

United Nations High Commission on Human Rights, UNHCR. *International Covenant on Economic, Social and Cultural Rights*, 1976.

Whitehead M, Dalgren G, Gilson L. Developing the policy response to inequities in health: a global perspective. In: Evans T, Whitehead M, Diderichsen F, Bhuiya A, Wirth M, eds. *Challenging Inequities in Health: From Ethics to Action*. London: Oxford University Press, 2001; 309–322.

Whitehead M. The concepts and principles of equity and health. *Int J Health Services* 1992; **22**(3): 429–45.

Wilkinson R, Marmot M. *Social Determinants of Health: the Solid Facts*, 2nd edition. Copenhagen: World Health Organization, 2003.

Woodward A, Kawachi I. Why reduce health inequalities? *J Epidemiol Community Health* 2000; **54**: 923–9.

World Health Organization. *Statistical Annex Table 1: Estimated life Expectancy at Birth and Child and Adult Mortality Risks, by Sex*. WHO Member States, 2002; World Health Report 2004, 2005.

81

Organizational Ethics in Health Care

JACOB E. KURLANDER, MARION DANIS

The complex organizational structures involved in modern health care delivery have prompted a flurry of attention to organizational ethics. The ancient discipline of clinical ethics, which has dealt mainly in the norms and values bearing on singular patient–physician relationships through the first half of the twentieth century, has proved ill-equipped, on the whole, to answer questions of another order: What responsibilities does a *health care organization* (HCO) have towards those with whom it interacts – payers, employees, suppliers, their communities, along with its dedication to, patients? These questions are hard to answer clearly and consistently, particularly in highly competitive market driven environments dominated by managed care organizations (MCOs) like those in the United States. Furthermore, HCOs are often in flux in the face of constant pressures to cut back or merge with other organizations requiring ethical analyses to be often revised.

In this chapter, we start by laying out the theoretical underpinnings of organizational ethics, still relatively young, by drawing on established work done in clinical, business and professional ethics that have contributed to it. We define organizations in order to clarify how a coordinated group of individuals can be conceived of as one moral agent that shares a health related mission and purpose. Next, we examine several spheres in which demands are made of HCOs and consider two different theoretical approaches to conceptualize their obligations – stakeholder theory and social-contract theory. Building on this theoretical base, we turn to practical aspects of designing organizational ethics programmes and provide guidance on how to initiate and run them. In the course of this discussion, we hope the reader will become aware of some of the conflicting views about organizational obligations that make this area of analysis particularly interesting.

THEORY

THE MORAL STATUS OF ORGANIZATIONS

To understand the nature and the content of the responsibilities that HCOs are subjected to, we must first provide a coherent definition of an organization. The ideas we develop in this section owe greatly to work done by Spencer, Mills, Rorty, and Werhane in their book *Organization Ethics in Health Care* (Spencer et al., 2000). As they argue, 'an organization is a subunit of the larger society, comprising individuals in various roles and authorized by the larger society to function for specific, often narrowly defined, purposes'. One approach to the analysis of organizations might be to analyse how individuals within the organization meet the demands of the roles that are set for them by their organization (role morality). This perspective, however, fails to critically evaluate what the actual purposes and demands of the organization are. Bureaucratic ethics, which asks how those many individuals interact to achieve a common goal, suffers from a similar problem in not questioning the justification of those goals. Indeed, any attempt to reduce an organization to its constituent parts threatens to overlook crucial aspects.

First, organizations, as a whole, have larger purposes that they serve in society, the foremost of which should be to provide health care to individuals and populations in the case of health care organizations (Spencer et al., 2000; Emanuel, 2000). The purpose of an organization can often be found in an organization's mission statement, which ought then to give rise to a set of guiding values (Silverman, 2000). The mission statement is not a static document. Rather, it requires constant interpretation and may even need to be amended at times. Jennings et al., following an

Principles of Health Care Ethics, Second Edition   Edited by R.E. Ashcroft, A. Dawson, H. Draper and J.R. McMillan
© 2007 John Wiley & Sons, Ltd

extensive study of not-for-profit hospital boards, write that not-for-profit trustees' primary duty is to 'use their authority and best efforts justly to promote the mission of the not-for-profit organization, and to keep that mission alive by interpreting its meaning over time in light of changing circumstances' (Jennings et al., 2002, p. 19). In addition to fidelity to mission, Jennings et al. believe that not-for-profits hospital trustees have three general principles of service in their mission: 'Service to patients by providing medical, nursing, and allied health care; service to community by, among other things, promoting health; and service to the hospital through stewardship on behalf of that uniquely valuable social institution (Jennings et al., 2002, p. 814–5)'. In for-profit organizations, the mission may be different because of a responsibility to produce profits for shareholders. We will explore this question further in our discussion of different types of institutions.

Second, organizations may have their own cultures that guide how well they adhere to their mission and values in their decision-making and behaviour (Silverman, 2000). Jacques (1951) defined organizational culture as '[t]he customary or traditional ways of thinking and doing things, which are *shared*, to a greater or lesser extent by all members of the organization and which new members of the organization must *learn* and at least partially accept in order to be accepted into the service of the firm' (from Spencer, 2000). The ethical climate is one component of organizational culture, likened to the organization's collective conscience.

The mission and culture of organizations are the focus of organizational ethics. Although other forms of ethics are deficient by failing to account for the stated values and emergent properties of organizations as a whole, the task of organization ethics is to promote and operationalize organizational integrity, the state of being whole, in which organizational behaviour lives up to professed goals (Silverman, 2000).

Organizations thus have several characteristics that liken them to individuals: they have goals, they act and are held accountable according to certain standards by various parties in society (Spencer et al., 2000, p. 26). Although organizations are not individuals, strictly speaking, and cannot be reduced to the individuals who compose them, it seems reasonable to regard them as moral agents. This position is not uncontested (Wilmot, 2000). For example, how can an organization meaningfully be said to have an intention? While granting philosophical problems with the notion of organization as moral agent in exactly the same way as an individual, organizations undeniably have collective actions and dispositions that undergo public scrutiny or praise. We take this much as a basis to cautiously apply to organizations some ethical analyses that have been applied to individuals. Following a deontological tack, we might ask whether a health care organization was well intentioned in its policy on care for the indigent. From a consequentialist

perspective, we might ask whether one hospital's merger with another nearby will be beneficial for those in a certain community. We should note that corporations are granted limited legal personhood so that they enjoy the privileges, if not always the responsibilities, of individuals under the law. This allows them to enter into contracts and own property.

At the same time, the application of ethical principles derived from individual ethics is not perfectly suited to institutions. Several authors have noted the dearth of attention in the literature to so-called 'mid-level', or institutional ethics, in favour of individual and social ethics (Khushf, 1997, 1998; Thompson, 1999). In many cases, organizations have higher standards of morality than individuals (Rie, 1991). For instance, pluralist societies do not permit organizations to discriminate against any class of people, while citizens retain that right. We demand a higher degree of tolerance from organizations.

Having considered the nature of an organization, we now turn to conceptualizing organizational decisions in situations with many interested parties. Two predominant theories derived from business ethics pertain.

STAKEHOLDER THEORY VERSUS INTEGRATIVE SOCIAL CONTRACTS THEORY

Stakeholder theory, developed in large part by R. Edward Freeman, begins with the recognition that organizations and their managers have responsibilities to many parties, and particularly in the care of for-profit organizations, parties other than exclusively their corporate shareholders (Freeman, 1991). It begins with two questions: what is the purpose of the firm, and what responsibility does management have to stakeholders (Freeman, 2004)? While shareholders provide the investments that allow corporations to operate, communities have granted corporations the permission to exist, and customers provide them with the patronage that helps them remain profitable. For these reasons, as well as the plain fact that businesses interact with and affect human beings, who have rights, stakeholder theory acknowledges the interests of a broad array of groups that come into contact with organizations. 'By calling attention to the variety of roles that can be occupied by individuals, all of whom have a moral stake in the organization, stakeholder theory can help to provide a framework for understanding and explicating the possibility of conflicts of value, of loyalty, of commitment, and of interests' (Spencer et al., 2000, p. 56).

Stakeholder theory has both descriptive and normative components. The descriptive component begins by identifying and examining the roles of stakeholders within and outside the organization. Different forms of stakeholder theory define stakeholders more or less broadly. Narrowly conceived, stakeholders are only those who are instrumental to the firm and its well-being in some way; more broadly conceived, stakeholders consist of anyone who stands to gain or suffer by corporate actions (Spencer et al., 2000, pp. 56–57). Stakeholders in HCOs likely include employees, management, owners/shareholders, customers, suppliers and the community. The normative component of stakeholder theory grants intrinsic value to the claims of all stakeholders. These components come together when the claims of the stakeholders are prioritized in terms of legitimacy and how they contribute to the organization's mission, survival, and flourishing. It is at first difficult to understand how the organization can find intrinsic value in all stakeholder claims at the same time as it elevates some and de-emphasizes others; however, the normative claim recognizes that all stakeholders have the right to make claims, not that all claims carry equal weight.

Stakeholder theory entails a reconceptualization of the role of organizations. Instead of simply enriching its owners, the purpose of an organization is understood to be the betterment of all stakeholders. Spencer writes, 'The very purpose of a firm [and thus its managers] is to serve as a vehicle for coordinating stakeholder interests. It is through the firm [and its managers] that each stakeholder group makes itself better off through voluntary exchange. The corporation serves at the pleasure of its stakeholders, and none may be used as a means to the ends of another without full rights of participation of that decision' (Spencer et al., 2000, p. 57). The moral force of the organization's responsibility comes, first, from the fact that stakeholder relationships are relationships between human beings, all of whom have certain obligations to one another – they must, for example, be treated fairly and with respect. Additionally, the organization and stakeholder are obligated to each other because the stakeholder relationship is reciprocal, that is, 'each can affect the other in terms of harms and benefits as well as rights and duties', as R. Edward Freeman, one of the originators of the theory, explains (Freeman, 1999 as found in Spencer et al., 2000, p. 57).

Stakeholder theory has the benefit of viewing ethics as an integral part of business, not simply an awkward appendage in the drive for profit (Freeman et al., 2004). The theory acknowledges that the marketplace is not value-neutral, and that acting in the name of shareholders against other parties demands justification. It sees relationships with all its stakeholders as an essential part of jointly creating the value aspired to in the organization's purpose.

Stakeholder theory has been criticized on several grounds (Donaldon & Dunfee, 1995, p. 88). It is unable to account for the important role of community standards. It is also unclear who should count as a stakeholder. Clearly, the interests of one who hopes to defraud an organization should not be counted. Donaldson and Dunfee write that the theory's most significant shortcoming is 'that it lacks a normative foundation both for assessing the ethical validity of the interests asserted by particular groups of stakeholders, as well as for identifying and prioritizing the rights and duties of

affected stakeholders'. Its crudeness, they argue, weakens it during real ethical dilemmas.

Integrative social contracts theory (ISCT) has largely been developed through the work of Thomas Donaldson and Thomas Dunfee by building on Thomas Hobbes's notion of a social contract. Hobbes's theory maintains that humans choose to form societies, which impose restrictions on their individual behaviour, on the basis of tacit agreement which allows cooperation among parties and the freedom to pursue their individual goals. Entering into this 'macrosocial contract' serves to 'preserve for individual economic communities significant moral free space in which to generate their own norms of economic conduct, through actual "micro-social contracts"' (Donaldson & Dunfee, 1995 as quoted in Spencer et al., 2000 p. 54).

Donaldson and Dunfee argue that the larger social contract generates 'hypernorms', generally agreed upon minimum standards of decent behaviour, which might include such principles as not causing gratuitous harm, honouring contracts, and treating others fairly (Donaldson & Dunfee, 1995). Although these govern relationships everywhere, there also exists a moral free space in which individual communities, including organizations, may tacitly consent to their own rules and agreements, so long as they are compatible with the previously established hypernorms. Logical rules then exist for prioritizing conflicting norms depending on their consistency with hypernorms, prevention of adverse effects, the extent of the community in which the norms hold, and how precise the norms are (Donaldson & Dunfee, 1995, p. 106). The priority rules have been praised because of the ease managers would have been applying them in the business setting (Conry, 1995).

Spencer et al. argue that ISCT is conceptually useful in organizational ethics. First, it is able to explain why society, segments of the population, and individuals have certain expectations of HCOs, for example, that they will provide adequate medical care. Society has allowed HCOs to come into existence under a tacit social contract in which the HCO commits to meeting such expectations. Although this commitment may not be written out for each patient, it flows from an HCO's mission, an agreement with society as a whole regarding the organization's responsibilities. Public frustration, when an HCO fails, makes sense because society perceives the HCO as having breached its contract.

Second, the notion of moral minimums (hypernorms) is useful in evaluating HCOs across diverse contexts. HCOs could not resort to the excuse that these minimums are only relative or that they apply only in limited contexts. Conversely, Spencer et al. argue that the analytical power of ICST may still be quite limited *within* organizations because it would allow for moral free space within.

ISCT has been praised for helping make explicit the norms that govern a certain (business) community, but a substantial criticism of ISCT questions whether clear hypernorms even exist. This question proves especially salient in the case of the health care industry, which has recently undergone rapid change and may lack clear consensus on the role of values such as egalitarianism versus libertarianism in healthcare provision.

Both theories are still in development, and work is being done to address their shortcomings. Stakeholder theory is useful in thinking through the diversity of interests involved in many healthcare decisions. We find ISCT particularly useful for its theoretical foundation which establishes norms that can serve to set priorities.

OTHER FORMS OF NORMATIVITY

Along with its reliance on business ethics, organization ethics is built on professional ethics and clinical ethics. Health care organizations are composed of professionals who are inculcated with codes of professional ethics in their training. Both in society as a whole and within HCOs, medical professionalism serves as the grounds for the moral conscience that underlies a commitment to the well-being of patients (Wynia et al., 1999). Thus organizations can expect and rely upon the ethically sound behaviour of their professional employees. It should be noted, however, that institutionalization of professions in which professionals are valued more for their technical expertise can sometime undermine this assumption (Thompson, 1999).

A place for professional ethics is preserved even in the context of an overarching theory like ISCT in which a moral free space is permitted within organizations for norms that are compatible with hypernorms. Ethical issues within organizations that are insufficiently addressed can be handled by the exercise of ethical behaviour by professionals. Some ethicists have argued that in certain circumstances when a HCO is in disarray, physicians are required to take ethically defensive actions, including exit, refusal and whistleblowing (Buchanan, 2000; Chervenak & McCullough, 2005).

Clinical ethics has been a major contributor to organizational ethics in the health care setting (Spencer et al., 2000). Indeed, while early organizational ethics was concerned mainly with economic issues, attention to clinical ethics brought with it a focus on the science and practice of medicine. For various reasons having to do in part with increasing reliance on outcomes research, cost control measures, and population-based care, the economic and clinical aspects of medicine are arguably now too finely enmeshed to make a distinction between the ethics governing the two (Khushf, 2001).

COMPLIANCE

The concepts of compliance and organizational ethics are often confused. Compliance guarantees that no infraction

of rules occurs, whereas organizational ethics is intended to provide a more positive ethical environment. Strong organizational ethics should reduce failures to comply. There is a debate in compliance literature about whether to frame compliance programmes as value-based or regulation-based. Heller argues that good compliance programmes should help employees not only to adhere to rules but also to have insight into the values of their institutions (Heller, 1999).

The relationship between ethics, compliance and the law warrants particular attention. There are several approaches an organization can take when dealing with the law ranging from a very legalistic to a more ethics oriented one. The legalistic view equates ethics with the law. It involves following the law blindly and can sometimes lead to very unfortunate organizational rules. For example, patients might be dying in the hospital parking lot, but to comply with insurance policy, a hospital may forbid its physicians to care for those patients. A better but still less than ideal approach is an efficient compliance as exemplified by investing only as much in following a rule as it calculates is efficient. Spielman (2000) argues that organizations should first consider what is the ethical approach to a problem. In doing so, an organization does not ignore the law, but it does move beyond an unreflective legalism to compliance within an ethical framework.

MARKETPLACE

The derivation of much of the underpinnings of organizational ethics for health care from business ethics becomes understandable when one considers the market-based approach to health care that has existed in the United States. In market context, HCOs struggle with the need to remain profitable while pursuing their health related missions.

HCOs should have the promotion and provision of health care as their foremost purpose, and should also be concerned with professional excellence of its staff, long-term organizational viability, and community access (Spencer et al., 2000, p. 61). In fact, studies have found that the most successful corporations, in terms of long-term survival, responsibility, *and* profitability, are those that combine profitability with other purposes (Collins & Porras, 1994).

Certain market environments may pose a greater or lesser risk of distorting organizations' attention to certain elements of mission. In the United States, persistent double-digit growth in health care costs has driven the emergence (and arguably the decline) of managed care organizations, which contain costs by using prospective payment schemes based on patient diagnosis. This has had the effect of shifting responsibility for cost containment from payers through managed care organizations, onto the provider side (Spencer et al. 2000).

HCOs have been forced to take dramatic cost containment measures, such as restriction of certain procedures, elimination of unprofitable services and, in some cases, closures or mergers. All of these decisions have ethical implications that must be carefully weighed to the extent that they affect equitable access to care for patients. Moreover, changes in the environment may force organizations to modify their organizational structure or redefine their critical task in order to relate to that environment more effectively (Wolff, 1993). Here the common phrase 'No margin, no mission', gains credence (Pearson et al., 2003). There is a danger (Shortell et al., 1996) that health care executives will lose sight of the multifocal mission and attend to fewer of their mission driven priorities (Shortell et al., 1990, as found in Wolff, 1993, p. 48).

Some of the most ethically troubling decisions that organizations face are those that arise in circumstances that may be considered non-ideal. What is the ethically right course of action in situations where others are not acting entirely ethically? Such ethical dilemmas are likely to arise in communities where access to health care is inequitable. In the health care context, a salient question might be, 'Does my hospital have to provide more care to the indigent if the hospital across town has decided not to provide any care and these individuals are turning to us?' This quandary may be best addressed by the emerging area in philosophy known as 'non-ideal theory'. Non-ideal theory asks what obligations individual actors have to comply with moral or ethical principles when others are less than fully compliant (Murphy, 2000, p. 7). Liam Murphy argues that the responsibility of individuals in a situation of partial compliance is to do as much as would be required were there perfect compliance. We would argue further that an organization could act as an advocate for those disadvantaged individuals who turn to it. In doing so, HCOs can act not only to provide services to underserved patients but also voice the need for allocation of more societal resources on their behalf.

PRACTICAL ASPECTS

Organizational ethics is a very practical endeavour involving processes and organizational structures as well as cultures and norms. Thus, having outlined its theoretical underpinnings, we turn to the pragmatic realm of organization ethics (Blake, 1999). We first consider the establishment of a comprehensive organizational ethics programme. Next, we address the process that should unfold in tackling any particular organizational ethics question.

THE STRUCTURE OF AN ORGANIZATIONAL ETHICS PROCESS

Establishing an organizational ethics programme may seem a daunting task because the ethics of an organization is

Table 81.1 Drivers of ethics initiatives

1.	Recognition of fundamental conflict between doing what is best for the group and what is best for the individual
2.	The search for additional savings, after initial, least painful, cuts in costs have been made
3.	New technology which changes practice and increases expense
4.	Mergers and acquisitions, causing conflicts in culture, values and business objectives
5.	Desire to avoid outside interference
6.	Public mistrust in Health Maintenance Organization (HMOs)

From Rovner (1998).

manifest in the behaviour and attitudes of every member of an organization. Very commonly, there is a precipitant that leads an HCO to develop an ethics programme (Table 81.1). Regardless of the stimulus that may prompt this development, there are a number of common elements that have been recommended for a comprehensive programme (Table 81.2). The programme should be equipped to influence all aspects of the operation of an HCO, including, but not limited to, policy development, business operations, and clinical care. Given the omnipresent and everyday organizational culture, however, the structural and procedural elements of an organization ethics programme are challenged not to seem intermittent and piecemeal. Those elements must represent ethics as an ongoing aspiration.

The programme should be designed to meet the challenges of everyday operation. To work effectively, it should have broad representation of key parties in the organization. The programme should be accessible to employees in the organization so that intimidation or fear of retaliation is avoided. At its best, an organization ethics committee should exercise proactive thinking and action to prevent difficulties. As

Table 81.2 Components of an ethics programme

1.	Mission statement
2.	Values
3.	Corporate code of ethics
4.	Ethics office/officer
5.	Ethics task force or committee
6.	Ethics communication strategy
7.	Ethics training
8.	Ethics help-line
9.	Measurements and rewards
10.	Comprehensive system to track data
11.	Periodic evaluation
12.	Ethics leadership

From Rovner (1998).

such, it serves as an ethics think-tank (McCullough,1998). An effective organizational ethics committee may be viewed with reservations by some members of an organization because it may challenge the status quo. In certain circumstances like a pending organizational merger, there should be mechanisms for community-wide input.

CONSULTATION AND DELIBERATION

When an organizational ethics committee is asked to consider a particular issue, it is advisable to address a consistent series of questions in the deliberative process (Table 81.3). An ethics coordinator or team should initiate the process. In complex situations, the coordinator will need to balance the need to be very inclusive because of a large number of stakeholders versus the need to be less inclusive so that the delib-

Table 81.3   Key questions for addressing an organizational ethics dilemma

1.	What is the problem?
2.	Who should participate in the deliberation? Who are the primary stakeholders?
3.	What are the facts?
4.	What is the background, and external social, political or legal climate in which this organizational issue is imbedded?
5.	What is the organization's mission and organizational culture in this case?
6.	What are the ethical issues from the perspective of various participants or stakeholders?
7.	What are the viable alternative solutions?
8.	How do you defend those alternatives?
	What core values are at stake?
	Who is harmed? Who benefits?
	What rights are at stake?
	Can you defend this action publicly?
	What kind of precedent does it set?
9.	What are the practical constraints?
10.	What is the best choice, or least harmful, all things considered?
11.	What is the implementation plan for the alternative that you have chosen?
	Which individuals need to be contacted with these recommendations?
	Who will have the responsibility communicating and carrying out recommendations?
12.	How should you follow up on the outcomes of the decision?
13.	What organizational policies, procedures, or structures would you suggest that might have prevented such a problem?

Adapted from Spencer et al. (2000).

erations do not become unwieldy. One potential approach is to hear from various stakeholders in a series of meetings.

In analysing a case, organizational ethics draws from many ethical theories, including virtue ethics, consequentialism and deontology (Spencer et al., 2000, p. 28). Here we briefly consider a number of these ethical frameworks, as suggested by Spencer et al. As in the analysis of an individual's action, each theory can be applied with some modification in an analogous fashion to organizational activities. In the course of analysing a situation, deliberation will necessarily be highly context-dependent and empirical, and the participants should have a reasonable grasp of these ethical frameworks from which to draw.

Character and Virtue Ethics: From this philosophical vantage point, one would judge organizational decisions based on the character of the decision makers, who ideally possess the civic virtues of integrity, good judgement, community spirit, honour, loyalty and, perhaps, shame (Spencer, 2000, p. 28 cites Solomon 1992). Character is then reflected in culture and climate and the daily behaviour of the organization. A virtuous organization would possess good organizational citizenship, prevent rights violations and promote the well-being of the organization's stakeholders (Spencer et al., 2000).

Consequentialism/Utilitarianism: Taking this philosophical stance, one would examine the distributed costs and benefits of an action to weigh its morality. A good decision is one which creates more benefit than harm, all things considered. Although strict utilitarianism takes a neutral stance on the distribution of the benefits and harms, in keeping with stakeholder theory, decision makers should be extremely cautious in opting for a decision that makes any one party, be it the organization, shareholders, customers or the community, worse off (Spencer et al., 2000). Some decision types, such as those with measurable effects on the parties involved, will clearly be more amenable to this sort of analysis.

Deontological/Rules based: Taking a Kantian approach, deontological forms of morality seek rules that may not be broken in any decision. Accordingly, people should never be treated merely as a means to an end, but only as ends in themselves. Respect for rights and autonomy are paramount, and organizations can institute mechanisms for guaranteeing such respect by putting in place procedures which include informed consent, procedural fairness and fair-minded contractual agreements.

Moral Minimums: Despite wide variation in social norms across societies and communities, Michael Walzer conceived of moral minimums with which almost all people would agree. Moral minimums prohibit gratuitous harm, unfair practices, processes, or outcomes; lying, breaking promises and contract; and not respecting individuals and their rights (Walzer, 1994). Applied to the organizational context, any institutional action that would controvert any of these widely held norms would be highly suspected.

Principlism: Several researchers have recently taken up the task of applying Beauchamp and Childress's *Principles of Biomedical Ethics* – autonomy, beneficence, non-maleficence and justice – to organizations. Komatsu describes how Beauchamp and Childress's four principles can be combined with two principles drawn from stakeholder theory for use by a corporate ethics team (Komatsu, 2001). Winkler and Gruen derive four principles for HCOs (provide care with compassion, treat employees with respect, act in a public spirit, and spend resources reasonably) from the roles that they are expected to play (care givers, employers, citizens and managers, respectively) (Winkler and Gruen, 2005). Their framework has the advantage that different types of HCOs, be they providers or insurers, may differentially weigh the principles based on the specific expectations of their organization. A group of leaders in health care and the humanities developed a set of ethical guidelines, known as the 'Tavistock Principles', for sorting out competing professional, clinical, quality and fiscal concerns (Sandrick, 2001). Among the principles is a right to health and health care, a balance of individual and population health, treatment of comprehensive health problems (including suffering), cooperation, quality improvement, safety and openness.

Table 81.4   Common issues in organizational ethics, by category

1.	*Patient Services:* Admitting, admitting to special units, rationing of resources within the institution, billing, maintaining confidentiality or records, and other services and activities
2.	*Business and Service Plans:* Managed care plans, plans for mergers and joint ventures, marketing and advertising strategies, plans for dealing with uncompensated care, and plans concerning the location of facilities
3.	*Business and Professional Integrity:* Resolving actual and potential conflicts of interest, employing financial incentives, setting criteria for performance review, and managing bottom-line pressures, among others
4.	*Employee Rights and Responsibilities:* Salary/ wage scales, promotion opportunity and criteria, collective bargaining, harassment, workforce diversity, privacy and downsizing
5.	*The Organization's Role in the Community:* Organization's advocacy and lobbying activities, investment practices, disposal of medical waste, participation in community projects

Adapted from Weber (1997).

Subject to the demands of the situation, these different frameworks, with a measure of commonsense, can play a useful role in organizational ethics deliberation. As Spencer et al., note, 'Each evaluative focus is based on the assumption that one can step back from a particular situation or context and make disinterested moral judgments of oneself, of one's roles and role obligations, and of organizations, their mission, culture and direction' (Spencer et al., 2000, p. 29). Some of these theories serve more as checks on decisions, while others can function as decision tools (i.e. utilitarianism). Still, at best they can only serve as rough guides in the decisions of an ethics team as it prioritizes the demands of their stakeholders in accord with the organizational mission. Many organizational ethics teams are likely to find common issues confronting them (Table 81.4). Attention to the key questions and philosophical approaches we have outlined should serve to address them.

EFFECTIVENESS OF ORGANIZATIONAL ETHICS

There are a few studies demonstrating the benefits of organizational ethics programmes. Research does indicate that physicians face substantial pressure to make decisions about how to allocate institutional resources to their patients (Hurst, 2005). Health care executives have conflict in their roles, and there is a widespread desire to address this (Jurkiewicz, 2000) and improve their organizations; but they find it difficult to do so. Given these perceived pressures on the part of clinicians and administrators in HCOs, one might expect organizational ethics programmes to fulfil an important function, but the proof still lies ahead.

REFERENCES

Blake DC. Organizational ethics: Creating structural and cultural change in healthcare organizations. *J Med Ethics* 1999; **10**: 187–93.

Buchanan A. Trust in managed care organizations. *Kennedy Instit Ethics J* 2000; **10**: 189–212.

Chervenak FA, McCullough LB. The diagnosis and management of progressive dysfunction of health care organizations. *Obstetr Gynecol* 2005; **105**: 882–7.

Collins J, Porras J. *Built to Last: Successful Habits of Visionary Companies.* New York: Harper Collins Publishers, 1994.

Conry E J. A critique of social contracts for business. *Business Ethics Q* 1995; **5**(2).

Donaldson T, Dunfee TW. Integrative social contract theory. *Econ Philos* 1995; **11**: 85–112.

Emanuel LL. Ethics and structures of healthcare. *Cambridge Q Healthcare Ethics* 2000; **9**: 151–68.

Freemn RE. *Business Ethics: State of the Art.* New York: Oxford University Press, 1991.

Freeman RE, Wicks AC, Parmar B. Stakeholder theory and the "corporate objective revisited". *Organ Sci* 2004; **15**(3).

Freeman RE. Stakeholder theory and the modern corporation. In: Donaldson T, Werhane PH, eds. *Ethical Issues in Business*, 6th edition. Upper Saddle River, NJ: Prentice Hall, 1999 (Reprinted).

Heller JC. Framing healthcare complicance in ethical terms: a taxonomy of moral choices. *HEC Forum* 1999; **11**: 345–57.

Hurst SA, Hull SC, DuVal G, Danis M. Physicians' responses to resource constraint. *Archives Intern Med* 2005; **165**: 639–44.

Jacques E. *The Changing Culture of the Factory*. New York: Dryden Press, 1951.

Jennings B, Gray BH, Sharpe VA, Weiss L, Fleischman AR. Ethics and trusteeship for health care: Hospital board service in turbulent times. *Hastings Center Report* 2002; **32**: S1–28.

Jurkiewicz CL. The trouble with ethics: results from a national survey of healthcare executives. *HEC Forum* 2000; **12**: 101–23.

Khushf G. Announcing a new section and a call for papers: Administrative and organizational ethics. *HEC Forum* 1997; **9**: 299–309.

Khushf G. Editor's introduction: The scope of organizational ethics. *HEC Forum* 1998; **10**: 127–35.

Khushf G. The value of comparative analysis in framing the problems of organizational ethics. *HEC Forum* 2001; **13**: 125–31.

Komatsu GI. A corporate ethics team: an approach to organization ethics, *HEC Forum* 2001; **13**: 171–7.

McCullough LB. Preventive ethics, managed practice, and the hospital ethics committee as a resource for physician executives. *HEC Forum* 1998; **10**: 136–51.

Murphy LB. *Moral Demands in Nonideal Theory*. Oxford: Oxford University Press, 2000.

Pearson SD, Sabin JE, Emanuel EJ. *No Margin, No Mission: Health Care Organizations and the Quest for Ethical Excellence in Competitive Markets*. New York: Oxford University Press, 2003.

Rie MA. Defining the limits of institutional moral agency in health care: A response to Kevin Wildes. *J Med Philos* 1991; **16**: 221–4.

Rovner J. Organizational ethics: It's your move. *Health Syst Leader* 1998; **5**: 4–12.

Sandrick K. Ethics: a unifying force. The Tavistock principles provide a decision-making framework for everyone. *Trustee* 2001; **54**: 24–8.

Shortell S, Morrison EH, Friedman B. *Strategic choices for American Hospitals: Managing Change in Turbulent Times*. San Francisco: Jossey-Bass, 1990.

Shortell SM, Gillies RR, Anderson DA, Erickson KM, Mitchell JB. *Remaking Health Care in America*. San Francisco: Jossey-Bass Publishers, 1996.

Silverman HJ. Organizational ethics in healthcare organizations: Proactively managing the ethical climate to ensure organizational integrity. *HEC Forum* 2000; **12**: 202–15.

Solomon R. *Ethics and Excellence*. New York: Oxford University Press, 1992.

Spencer EM, Mills AE, Rorty MV, Werhane PH. *Organization Ethics in Health Care*. New York: Oxford University Press, 2000.

Spielman B. Organizational ethics programs and the law. *Cambridge Q Healthcare Ethics* 2000; **9**: 218–29.

Thompson DF. The institutional turn in professional ethics. *Ethics Behav* 1999; **9**: 109–18.

Walzer M. *Thick and Thin*. Notre Dame, IN: Notre Dame University Press, 1994.

Weber LJ. Taking on organizational ethics. To do so ethics committees must first prepare themselves. *Health Prog* 1997; **78**: 32.

Wilmot S. Corporate moral responsibility in health care. *Med Health Care Philos* 2000; **3**: 139–46.

Winkler EC, Gruen RL. First principles: substantive ethics for healthcare organizations. *J Healthcare Manage* 2005; **50**(2): 109–19.

Wolff M. "No margin, no mission": Challenge to institutional ethics. *Business Prof Ethics J* 1993; **12**: 39–50.

Wynia MK, Latham SR, Kao AC, Berg JW, Emanuel LL. Medical professionalism in society. *N Engl J Med* 1999; **341**: 1612–6.

82

Ethical Issues in Epidemiology[1]

STEVEN S. COUGHLIN

INTRODUCTION

Epidemiology, the study of the distribution and determinants of disease in human populations, can be viewed as the basic science of public health. The results of epidemiologic research studies contribute to generalizable knowledge by elucidating the causes (aetiologies) of a specific disease or group of diseases; by combining epidemiologic data with information from other disciplines such as genetics and microbiology; by evaluating the consistency of epidemiological data with aetiological hypotheses (hypotheses having to do with causation); and by providing the basis for developing and evaluating health promotion and prevention procedures and public health practices (Lilienfeld & Lilienfeld, 1980). The primary professional roles of epidemiology are the design and conduct of scientific research and the public health application of scientific knowledge. These include the reporting of research results and the maintenance and promotion of health in communities. In carrying out these professional roles, epidemiologists often encounter a number of ethical issues and concerns that require careful consideration.

Key concepts such as ethics and professional ethics are defined in other chapters in this text. Professional ethics in epidemiology involve ethical precepts that are widely shared in the field. This chapter deals with ethical issues arising in the professional practice of epidemiology but does not deal with all ethical issues that are of interest to epidemiologists (for example, institutional rules pertaining to financial disclosures or sexual harassment are not discussed). Major developments in bioethics such as the Belmont Report (National Commission for the Protection of Human Subjects of Biomedical and Behavioral Research, 1978) and the US federal regulations governing human subjects research (Department of Health and Human Services, 1981) are mentioned in the section that follows, but this chapter does not focus specifically on the US regulatory system for the protection of research participants.

Ethical concerns in epidemiology and public health practice often relate to the obligations of health professionals to acquire and apply scientific knowledge aimed at maintaining and restoring public health although respecting individual rights. Potential societal benefits must often be balanced with risks and potential harms to individuals and communities, such as the potential for stigmatization or invasion of privacy. In this chapter, major ethical issues in epidemiology are discussed and examples provided of recent or ongoing ethical concerns in the field. A summary of developments with ethics surveys, ethics guidelines and ethics education for epidemiologists is given in the following sections.

RECENT HISTORY AND BACKGROUND

The important historical events that have occurred in bioethics and human subjects research ethics have been considered elsewhere (Levine, 1988; Coughlin & Beauchamp, 1996; Roelcke & Maio, 2004), including in other chapters in this text. Major historical developments in bioethics, as discussed elsewhere, include the Nuremberg Code and the Declaration of Helsinki (United States v. Karl Brandt, 1947; Howard-Jones, 1982; World Medical Association, 1955). Other important developments include the Belmont Report, federal regulations protecting human research participants in the United States (45 CFR 46) and training in scientific integrity required by institutions in the United States that receive funding from the National

[1]The findings and conclusions in this chapter are those of the author and do not necessarily represent the views of the Centers for Disease Control and Prevention.

Institutes of Health (National Commission for the Protection of Human Subjects of Biomedical and Behavioral Research, 1978; Department of Health and Human Services, 1981; National Institutes of Health, 2000). There have also been important bioethical developments in Great Britain, Canada and many other countries (Roelcke & Maio, 2004; Coughlin & Beauchamp, 1996).

Important events of specific interest to epidemiologists include the development of ethics guidelines and educational programmes on ethics for epidemiology graduate students and practicing epidemiologists (Coughlin, 1996a). Some of the important developments pertaining to ethics surveys, ethics guidelines, and ethics education for epidemiologists and other public health professionals are summarized below.

ETHICS SURVEYS OF EPIDEMIOLOGISTS

Ethics surveys of epidemiologists have played an important role in identifying core values in the field and helping to lay the groundwork for the development of ethics guidelines for epidemiologists. Ethics surveys have targeted epidemiologists and other public health professionals, public health students and representatives from institutions that train epidemiologists and other public health professionals. Soskolne and colleagues conducted an international ethics survey in 1994 among epidemiologists who were reached through the International Society for Environmental Epidemiology, the Italian Epidemiological Association and the Global Environmental Epidemiology Network (managed by the Office of Global and Integrated Environmental Health of the World Health Organization, Geneva) (Soskolne et al., 1996). The results of the survey helped to identify ethical issues and concerns among environmental epidemiologists and contributed to the development of ethics guidelines in the field (Soskolne & Light, 1996). Results from the survey highlighted different perspectives of environmental epidemiologists concerning their roles as dispassionate scientists and passionate advocates for the public's health. The American College of Epidemiology's Ethics and Standards of Practice Committee conducted an ethics survey among a random sample of 300 North American members of the American College of Epidemiology, the Society for Epidemiologic Research and the American Heart Association Council on Epidemiology and Prevention (Prineas et al., 1998). Results from the survey facilitated the development of ethics guidelines for epidemiologists in North America (American College of Epidemiology, 2000). Kessel (2003) conducted a survey of the nature and content of teaching of public health ethics in medical schools and public health graduate programmes in the United Kingdom. Public health ethics was taught in 75% of medical schools and 52% of institutions providing postgraduate education, although the content and nature of ethics teaching was incomplete and often minimal (Kessel, 2003). Ethics surveys have also been conducted at United States institutions

that train graduate students in epidemiology and other public health disciplines (Rossignol & Goodmonson, 1996; Coughlin et al., 1999).

DEVELOPMENT OF ETHICS GUIDELINES FOR EPIDEMIOLOGISTS

Ethical and professional norms in epidemiology have been clarified in ethics guidelines for epidemiologists (Beauchamp et al., 1991; Council for International Organizations of Medical Sciences, 1991; Soskolne & Light, 1996; American College of Epidemiology, 2000). In many respects, ethics guidelines for epidemiologists are aspirational rather than prescriptive. They generally do not provide a standard against which practising epidemiologists can be held accountable, partly because epidemiologists do not need a licence to practise. Also, epidemiologists may belong to several different disciplines or professional backgrounds including medicine, statistics, and anthropology or other social sciences. Nevertheless, guidelines such as those developed for the Industrial Epidemiology Forum, the International Society for Environmental Epidemiology and the American College of Epidemiology provide useful accounts of the obligations of epidemiologists to research participants, society, employers and professional colleagues (Beauchamp et al., 1991; Soskolne & Light, 1996; American College of Epidemiology, 2000). Ethics guidelines for environmental epidemiologists drafted by Colin Soskolne and Andrew Light, which were adopted by the International Society for Environmental Epidemiology in 1999, highlight the important obligations that epidemiologists have to communities that are affected by environmental hazards (Soskolne & Light, 1996). The ethics guidelines adopted by the American College of Epidemiology discuss core values, duties and virtues in epidemiology and the professional role of epidemiologists, minimizing risks and protecting the welfare of research participants, providing benefits, ensuring an equitable distribution of risks and benefits, protecting confidentiality and privacy, obtaining informed consent, submitting proposed studies for ethical review, maintaining public trust, avoiding conflicts of interest and partiality, communicating ethical requirements, confronting unacceptable conduct, and obligations to communities (American College of Epidemiology, 2000). International guidelines for ethical review of epidemiological studies were published by the Council of International Organizations of Medical Sciences(Council for International Organizations of Medical Sciences, 1991). The CIOMS guidelines draw a distinction between epidemiologic research and routine practice (for example, outbreak investigations and public health surveillance) and consider some of the issues associated with obtaining informed consent in epidemiologic studies.

ETHICS EDUCATION FOR EPIDEMIOLOGISTS

Courses on ethics in epidemiology and public health have been initiated at several institutions that train public health professionals. Curricula on public health ethics for epidemiology graduate students have been developed at several institutions in the United States, Canada and Great Britain. Topics dealt with in courses on ethical issues in epidemiology and public health research include a framework for ethics in health research, basic methods of moral reasoning, ethics guidelines for epidemiologists, privacy and confidentiality protection, issues surrounding informed consent, ethical issues in studies of vulnerable populations, human subjects research, communication responsibilities of epidemiologists, issues surrounding the publication of research findings, conflicts of interest and scientific misconduct (Coughlin, 1996b). Resources available for graduate courses and continuing professional education on ethical issues in epidemiology and public health-include textbooks and ethics cases for small group discussion and additional curricular materials (Coughlin et al., 1997; Association of Schools of Public Health). Model curricula in public health ethics have been developed by the Association of Schools of Public Health in the United States (Association of Schools of Public Health). Such efforts have been bolstered in the United States by educational training on ethical principles and institutional review board procedures recommended by the Office for Human Research Protections (Office for Human Research Protections).

ETHICAL ISSUES IN EPIDEMIOLOGY

In the discussion that follows, some of the major ethical issues that arise in epidemiologic research are considered and examples of recent ethical concerns that have arisen in the field are provided. The ethical issues discussed in this section are not exhaustive. Additional ethical issues arising in epidemiologic research and public health practice have been highlighted in ethics guidelines for epidemiologists and public health practitioners and in other published reviews (Soskolne & Light, 1996; American College of Epidemiology, 2000; Coughlin, 1997).

MINIMIZING RISKS AND PROVIDING BENEFITS

Epidemiologists have ethical and professional obligations to maximize the potential benefits of studies provided to research participants and to society, and to minimize potential harms and risks. In addition, these obligations are often legal or regulatory requirements, such as US federal regulations protecting human research participants (45 CFR 46). The risks of epidemiologic studies and practice activities can be minimized by rigorously protecting the confidentiality of health information, as discussed later in this chapter.

Although the risks posed by epidemiologic studies are often minor compared with those that may be associated with clinical trials and other experimental studies, participants in epidemiologic studies may be burdened by a loss of privacy, by time spent in completing interviews and examinations and by possible adverse psychological effects such as enhanced grief or anxiety (Coughlin, 1996c). Such risks and potential harms can be minimized by careful attention to study procedures and questionnaire design, for example, by limiting the length of interviews or by scheduling them on a date that is less likely to result in adverse psychological effects.

Minimizing risks and potential harms and maximizing potential benefits is particularly important in epidemiologic studies of vulnerable populations. Examples include studies of children, prisoners, some elderly persons and persons who belong to groups that are marginalized or socioeconomically deprived. Migrant farmworkers in the United States are a vulnerable population because they work in a hazardous industry, are often members of an ethnic minority, have difficulty in accessing health care and are often of lower socioeconomic status (Cooper et al., 2004). In studies of migrant farmworkers, Cooper et al. (2004) noted that epidemiologists may need to consider some modifications of procedures for conducting interviews to minimize potential harm or inconveniences.

A further obligation is the need to ensure that the burdens and potential benefits of epidemiologic studies are distributed in an equitable fashion. The potential benefits of epidemiologic research are often societal in nature such as obtaining new information about the causes of diseases. Benefits may occur through the identification of disparities in health across groups defined by race, ethnicity, socioeconomic status or other factors (Coughlin, 1996a). Research participants may receive direct benefits from participation in some studies such as when previously unrecognized disease or risk factors for disease are detected during examinations.

The balance of risks and potential benefits of epidemiologic studies are considered not only by individual researchers but also by members of human subjects committees such as institutional review boards in the United States.

HUMAN SUBJECTS REVIEW

The purpose of research ethics committees or institutional review boards is to ensure that studies involving human research participants are designed to conform with relevant ethical standards and that the rights and welfare of participants are protected (National Commission for the Protection of Human Subjects of Biomedical and Behavioral Research, 1978). Human subjects review by such committees ensures that studies have a favourable balance of potential benefits and risks, that participants are selected in an equitable fashion and that procedures for obtaining informed consent are adequate. In the United States, federal regulations for the protection of human research subjects (45 CFR 46) have resulted in a complex institutional review board system. Similar safeguards exist in many other countries.

Despite the important role played by research ethics committees and institutional review boards, researchers have sometimes expressed concern about the obstacles that human subjects review can sometimes create. For example, researchers in Great Britain and the United States have expressed concern about the time and effort required for review and approval by committees at several institutions in multi-centre studies (Warlow, 2004). Steps have been taken in some countries to streamline the process of human subjects review such as by adopting standardized forms and review processes or by centralizing review by research ethics committees (Pattison & Stacey, 2004). As previously mentioned, one of the important issues considered by research ethics committees and by individual researchers is the adequacy of provisions for obtaining the informed consent of study participants.

INFORMED CONSENT

Informed consent provisions in epidemiology studies ensures that research participants make a free choice and also provide institutions with a legal authorization to proceed with the research (Shulz, 1996). Investigators must disclose information that potential participants use to decide whether to consent to the study. This includes the purpose of the research, the scientific procedures, anticipated risks and benefits, any inconveniences or discomfort, and the individual's right to refuse participation or to withdraw from the research at any time (45 CFR 46). Informed consent requirements may be waived in exceptional circumstances when obtaining consent is impractical, the risks are minimal, and the risks and potential benefits of the research have been carefully considered by an independent review committee. For example, in some epidemiology studies involving the analysis of large databases of routinely collected information (for example, insurance claims data), it may not be feasible to recontact patients to ask them for their informed consent. Risks and potential harms in such studies may be very low, and risks may be further reduced by omitting personal identifiers from the computer databases.

Special considerations for obtaining informed consent may arise in epidemiologic studies of socioeconomically deprived persons. Persons who have limited access to health care may misunderstand an invitation to participate in a study as an opportunity to receive medical care. In addition, they may be reluctant to refuse participation when the researcher is viewed as someone in a position of authority such as a physician or university professor. Socioeconomically deprived persons may also be more motivated to participate in studies involving financial incentives for participation. Procedures for obtaining informed consent may need to be modified in such studies to protect potential research participants from

possible unintended coercion (Cooper et al., 2004). A further issue is that there is often a need to translate informed consent statements into a language other than English so that information about the study can be communicated to potential participants who do not speak English (Cooper et al., 2004). The important issues that arise in international research conducted by researchers from countries such as the United States and Great Britain in developing countries have also received considerable attention (Council for International Organizations of Medical Sciences, 1991; Macklin, 1999).

As an example of issues pertaining to informed consent in population-based research, controversy has surrounded the development of a database in Iceland to study genetic factors associated with a variety of health conditions (English et al., 2000; Greely, 2000; Palsson & Rabinow, 2001; Winickoff, 2001). In December 1998, the Icelandic parliament passed legislation to construct a database containing the health records of the entire country which could be combined with genetic data (English et al., 2000; Winickoff, 2001). Although the potential scientific and commercial benefits of the database are clear, the legislation does not require informed consent from persons in Iceland for the inclusion of their medical information in the database. An exclusive licence has been granted to one company for the creation and operation of the database. Ethical issues have been raised related to the adequacy of informed consent, privacy and confidentiality protection, and the ownership of the genomic data, in the context of rapid advances in biotechnology and genomics, public/private partnerships and commercial interests (English et al., 2000; Greely, 2000; Palsson & Rabinow, 2001; Winickoff, 2001).

PRIVACY AND CONFIDENTIALITY PROTECTION

One important way in which epidemiologists reduce potential harms and risks to the persons included in epidemiologic studies is by rigorously protecting the confidentiality of health information collected as part of research studies or included in secondary analyses. Specific measures taken by epidemiologists to protect the confidentiality of health information include keeping records under lock and key, limiting access to confidential records, discarding personal identifiers from data collection forms and computer files whenever feasible, and training staff in the importance of privacy and confidentiality protection (Coughlin, 1996b). Other measures that have been employed to safeguard health information include encryption of computer databases, limiting geographic detail, and suppression of cells in tabulated data where the number of cases in the cell is small (Wynia et al., 2001; McLaughlin, 2002).

In the United States, the Health Insurance Portability and Accountability Act (HIPAA) of 1996 privacy rules took effect early in 2004 after extensive planning and discussion (Centers for Disease Control and Prevention, 2003). The new regulations provide protection for the privacy of certain individually identifiable health data, referred to as protected health information. The privacy rules permit disclosures without individual authorization to public health authorities authorized by law to collect or receive the information for the purpose of preventing or controlling disease, injury, or disability, including public health practice activities such as surveillance (Centers for Disease Control and Prevention, 2003).

In the United States and many European countries, routine cancer surveillance is required by law and informed consent is generally not obtained from cancer patients whose medical records are abstracted for the purposes of cancer registration (McKenna et al., 2004). In the United Kingdom, the use of identifiable patient information from disease registries has generated controversy (Morrow, 2001; Illman, 2002). The United Kingdom Association of Cancer Registries has argued that it is impossible to run an effective population-based registry by relying on informed consent (Illman, 2002).

AVOIDING AND DISCLOSING CONFLICTS OF INTEREST

Other ethical issues that arise in the professional practice of epidemiology relate to how best to deal with potential conflicts of interest, in order to maintain public trust in epidemiology and sustain public support for health research. Recent media reports about previously undisclosed conflicts of interest in the United States and other countries have raised public awareness of the potential for conflicts of interest in clinical research and epidemiology, and about the need for institutions and individual researchers to address such conflicts. Conflicts of interest can affect scientific judgement and harm scientific objectivity. Studies have suggested that financial interests and the commitment that researchers have to a hypothesis can influence reported research results (Seigel, 2003). To address such concerns, steps have been taken by funding agencies and institutions at which research is carried out including the adoption of new educational training programmes for researchers about the importance of avoiding or disclosing conflicts of interest, and revised or strengthened institutional rules and guidelines. Professional societies and medical associations have also issued policy statements and recommendations about how best to address conflicts of interest in clinical research (AAMC Task Force on Financial Conflicts of Interest in Clinical Research, 2003; Morin et al., 2002). Researchers should disclose financial interests and sources of funding when publishing research results. It may also be important to disclose information about potential or actual financial conflicts of interest when obtaining informed consent from research participants.

OBLIGATIONS TO COMMUNITIES

The obligations that epidemiologists have to members of communities included in research studies have been highlighted in several reports (Soskolne & Light, 1996; American College of Epidemiology, 2000). These obligations include

communicating information about the results of epidemiologic studies at the earliest possible time, after appropriate scientific peer review, so that the widest possible audience stands to benefit from the information. Epidemiologists should strive to carry out studies in a way that is scientifically valid and interpret and report the results of their studies in a way that is scientifically accurate and appropriate.

In addition, epidemiologists should respect cultural diversity in carrying out studies and in communicating with members of affected communities. For example, following the outbreak of sudden acute respiratory distress syndrome (SARS) in cities such as Toronto, there was a need to take steps to alleviate the isolation and stigmatization of members of Asian communities who were perceived to have a higher risk of SARS (Singer et al. 2003; Gostin, 2004).

These are just some of the ways in which epidemiologists meet their obligations to members of communities who are targeted in research studies. Other obligations of epidemiologists to community members and to research participants have been highlighted in ethics guidelines for epidemiologists and other public health professionals (Soskolne & Light, 1996; American College of Epidemiology, 2000; Beauchamp et al. 1991; Public Health Leadership Society).

SUMMARY AND CONCLUSIONS

As highlighted in this chapter, a number of interesting and important ethical issues arise in epidemiologic research. These ethical issues and concerns have been examined in ethics surveys, in ethics guidelines, and in curricular materials for teaching ethics to epidemiologists and other public health professionals. Developments in ethics and epidemiology have often been related to how best to balance risks and potential harms of epidemiologic research (for example, invasions of privacy or possible enhancement of stigmatization) with potential benefits of epidemiologic research to society and to individual research participants (for example, acquiring new information about how to prevent illness or to reduce or eliminate disparities in health). As the examples provided in this chapter show, ongoing ethics training and continuing professional educational opportunities are needed to help epidemiologists deal with their obligations to research participants, society, employers and professional colleagues.

REFERENCES

AAMC Task Force on Financial Conflicts of Interest in Clinical Research. Protecting subjects, preserving trust, promoting progress. II: Principles and recommendations for oversight of an institution's financial interests in human subjects research. *Acad Med* 2003; **78**: 237–45.

American College of Epidemiology. Ethics guidelines. *Ann Epidemiol* 2000; **10**: 487–97.

Association of Schools of Public Health. *Ethics and Public Health: Model Curriculum*; http://www.asph.org/document.cfm? page=782.

Beauchamp TL, Cook RR, Fayerweather WE, *et al*. Ethical guidelines for epidemiologists. *J Clin Epidemiol* 1991; **44**(Suppl I): 151S–69S.

Centers for Disease Control and Prevention. HIPAA privacy rule and public health. Guidance from CDC and the U.S. Department of Health and Human Services. *MMWR* 2003; 52: 1–12.

Cooper SP, Heitman E, Fox EE, *et al*. Ethical issues in conducting migrant farmworker studies. *J Immigrant Health* 2004; **6**: 29–39.

Coughlin SS. Advancing professional ethics in epidemiology. *J Epidemiol Biostat* 1996(a); **1**: 71–7.

Coughlin SS. Ethically optimized study designs in epidemiology. In: Coughlin SS, Beauchamp TL, eds. *Ethics and Epidemiology*. New York: Oxford University Press, 1996(b); pp. 145–55.

Coughlin SS. Model curricula in public health ethics. *Am J Prev Med* 1996(c); **12**: 247–51.

Coughlin SS. Ethics in epidemiology and public health practice. *Ethics in Epidemiology and Public Health Practice: Collected Works*. Columbus, GA: Quill Publications, 1997; pp. 9–26.

Coughlin SS, Beauchamp TL. Historical foundations. *Ethics and Epidemiology*. New York: Oxford University Press, 1996; pp. 5–23.

Coughlin SS, Katz WH, Mattison DR. Ethics instruction at schools of public health in the United States. *Am J Public Health* 1999; **89**: 768–70.

Coughlin SS, Soskolne CL, Goodman KW. *Case Studies in Public Health Ethics*. Washington, DC: American Public Health Association, 1997.

Council for International Organizations of Medical Sciences. International guidelines for ethical review of epidemiological studies. *Law Med Health Care* 1991; **19**: 247–58.

Department of Health and Human Services. *Final Regulations Amending Basic HHS Policy for the Protection of Human Subjects*. Federal Register 46, no. 16. January 26, 1981; pp. 8366–92.

English V, Heath L, Romano-Critchley G, Sommerville A. Ethics briefings. *J Med Ethics* 2000; **26**: 215–6.

Gostin LO. Pandemic influenza: public health preparedness for the next global health emergency. *Int Comp Health Law Ethics Winter*, 2004; pp. 565–73.

Greely HT. Iceland's plan for genomics research: facts and implications. *Jurimetrics* 2000; **40**: 153–91.

Howard-Jones N. Human experimentation in historical and ethical perspectives. *Social Sci Med* 1982; **16**: 1429–48.

Illman J. Cancer registries: should informed consent be required? *J Natl Cancer Inst* 2002; **94**: 1269–70.

Kessel AS. Public health ethics: teaching survey and critical review. *Soc Sci Med* 2003; **56**: 1439–45.

Levine RJ. *Ethics and Regulation of Clinical Research*, 2nd edition. New Haven: Yale University Press, 1988.

Lilienfeld AM, Lilienfeld DE. *Foundations of Epidemiology*, 2nd edition. New York: Oxford University Press, 1980.

Macklin L. *Against Relativism: Cultural Diversity and the Search for Ethical Universals in Medicine*. New York: Oxford University Press, 1999.

McKenna MT, Wingo P, Gibson JJ. Registries and informed consent. *N Engl J Med* 2004; **350**: 1452–3.

McLaughlin CC. Confidentiality protection in publicly released central cancer registry data. *J Registry Manage* 2002; **29**: 84–8.

Morin K, Rakatansky H, Riddick FA Jr, *et al*. Managing conflicts of interest in the conduct of clinical trials. *JAMA* 2002; **287**: 78–84.

Morrow JI. Data protection and patients' consent. Informed consent should be sought before data are used by registries. *BMJ* 2001; **322**: 549–50.

National Commission for the Protection of Human Subjects of Biomedical and Behavioural Research. *The Belmont Report: Ethical Principles and Guidelines for the Protection of Human Subjects of Research*. Washington, DC: U.S. Government Printing Office, 1978.

National Institutes of Health. Required education in the protection of human research participants. *NIH Guide*, June 5, 2000; Notice: OD-00-039.

Office for Human Research Protections. U.S. Department of Health and Human Services. *Federalwide Assurance for the Protection of Human Subjects*; http://www.hhs.gov/ohrp/humansubjects/assurance/filasurt.htm.

Palsson G, Rabinow P. The Icelandic genome debate. *Trends Biotechnol* 2001; **19**: 166–71.

Pattison J, Stacey T. Research bureaucracy in the United Kingdom *BMJ* 2004; **329**: 622–4.

Prineas RJ, Goodman K, Soskolne CL, *et al*. Findings from the American College of Epidemiology ethics survey on the need for ethics guidelines for epidemiologists. *Ann Epidemiol* 1998; **8**: 482–9.

Public Health Leadership Society. *Principles of the Ethical Practice of Public Health*; http://www.phls.org.

Roelcke V, Maio G, eds. *Twentieth Century Ethics of Human Subjects Research: Historical Perspectives on Values, Practices, and Regulations*. Stuttgart, Germany: Franz Steiner Verlag, 2004.

Rossignol AM, Goodmonson S. Are ethical topics in epidemiology included in the graduate epidemiology curricula? *Am J Epidemiol* 1996; **142**: 1265–8.

Seigel D. Clinical trials, epidemiology, and public confidence. *Stat Med* 2003; **22**: 3419–25.

Shulz M. Legal and ethical considerations in securing consent to epidemiologic research in the United States. In: Coughlin SS, Beauchamp TL, eds. *Ethics and Epidemiology*. New York: Oxford University Press, 1996; pp. 97–127.

Singer PA, Benatar SR, Bernstein M, *et al*. Ethics and SARS: lessons from Toronto. *BMJ* 2003; **327**: 1342–44.

Soskolne CL, Jhangri GS, Hunter B, *et al*. Interim report on the Joint International Society for Environmental Epidemiology (ISEE)—Global Environmental Epidemiology Network (GEENET) ethics survey. *Sci Total Environ* 1996; **184**: 5–11.

Soskolne CL, Light A. Towards ethics guidelines for environmental epidemiologists. *Sci Total Environ* 1996; **184**: 137–47.

United States v. Karl Brandt. Trials of War Criminals Before the Nuremberg Military Tribunals under Control Council Law No. 10. vols. 1 and 2. *The Medical Case* (Military Tribunal I, 1947). Washington, DC: U.S. Government Printing Office, 1948–1949.

Warlow C. Clinical research under the cosh again. This time it is ethics committees (Editorial). *BMJ* 2004; **329**: 241–2.

Winickoff DE. Biosamples, genomics, and human rights: context and content of Iceland's Biobanks Act. *Biolaw Bus* 2001; **4**: 11–7.

World Medical Association. Human experimentation: declaration of Helsinki. *Ann Int Med* 1955; **65**: 367–8.

Wynia MK, Coughlin SS, Alpert S, *et al*. Shared expectations for protection of identifiable health care information. Report of a national consensus process. *J Gen Intern Med* 2001; **16**: 100–11.

83

Screening: Ethical Aspects

NIKLAS JUTH, CHRISTIAN MUNTHE

INTRODUCTION

In this chapter, we give an overview of the ethics of screening with the aim of making the chief questions clear for further investigation and discussion. Starting with a clarification of the concept of screening ('What is Screening?'), we then move to the issue of what values may be promoted (or threatened) by screening programmes ('Why Screening?'). In 'Screening – what and when?', we consider in more detail the issue of what aspects of screening are relevant for determining whether it should be undertaken or not. Assuming it is acceptable, the further question arises as to how the programme should be organized in order to remain defensible ('Screening – How?'). In 'Conclusion,' we make the some comments regarding the nature of the ethics of screening, and what this possibly implies for medical ethics.

WHAT IS SCREENING?

There is no standard definition of the term 'screening'. However, some of the following features are often mentioned: screening aims at *selecting individuals* at risk of disease(s) from a (large) *population* of individuals *not united by previously recognized risk or symptoms* of the disease(s) in question by relatively *rapid and cheap* means. Moreover, there are typical examples of screening: routine ultrasound in pregnancy care, neonatal testing for phenylketonuria (PKU), breast cancer-testing programmes through mammography, and so on.

In their classic text on screening, Wilson and Jungner (1968, p. 11), emphasized its role as a filtering device, sorting out those individuals who probably have or may have some disease(s) from a larger group for further investigation. However, due to the rapid development of genetics

the methods used for diagnosing or determining the risk of disease and those utilized in screening programmes are now often the same. Instead, emphasis is often placed on the fact that the *initiative to the investigation is not coming from the investigated individual herself*, but rather from health care professionals (The Danish Council of Ethics, 1999). This feature gives rise to many of the ethical issues concerning actual screening programmes. Furthermore, it is often presupposed that screening is directed towards a more or less large *population of people* (Shickle, 1999; Kinzler et al., 2002). It should nevertheless be observed that there is no precise limit to either how large a population has to be in order for the concept of screening to be applicable, or how unaware the members of this population have to be of the risk screened for. There are programmes where the population is not united by any recognized increase of risk at all, for instance neonatal screening (Chadwick et al., 1999). These programmes may thus be described as *pure*. However, many programmes target populations where there is some initial awareness, for example, genetic carrier screening confined to certain ethnic groups where a disease is particularly prevalent, or prenatal screening targeting pregnant women above a certain age. Even more obvious are cases where one person is tested positively and others are approached as a result of this, for example, in the management of communicable diseases, such as HIV, or so-called cascade genetic testing (when health care initiates an investigation of someone's relatives based on a positive genetic test of that individual).

Screening is traditionally thought of as a detection tool for treating disease in its early stages or, preferably, preventing it before onset. Some definitions of screening also include the condition that the test used should be rapid and/ or (relatively) cheap (Wilson and Jungner, 1968; Shickle, 1999). These features relate to the purpose of screening as

Principles of Health Care Ethics, Second Edition   Edited by R.E. Ashcroft, A. Dawson, H. Draper and J.R. McMillan
© 2007 John Wiley & Sons, Ltd

a preventive public health measure, where the cost-benefit is a relevant factor (Kinzler et al., 2002). As the benefits are often cast in terms of health, well-being or autonomy, and the costs, besides the economic ones, regard the reduction of such values, many arguments for and against screening can be analysed in a consequentialist framework (Hoedemaekers, 1999). Thus, early detection and the test being cheap and rapid should primarily be understood as a reminder of the importance of balancing various costs and benefits. However, this has more to do with ideas about what may *justify* a screening programme than what makes it *screening* in the first place.

We will, accordingly, in the rest of this chapter consider ethical issues particular to the use of medical testing methods at the initiative of health care or society for investigating the health status of individuals with the aim of selecting some of these for possible further treatment from a large population of people not united by previously recognized risks or symptoms of disease. We recognize, however, that several of these issues may also be applicable in cases where the screening is not as pure, for example, where the population is not that large or when there is some initial awareness of risk.

WHY SCREENING?

In order to determine whether a certain screening programme should be implemented or not, one has to ponder why such an effort may be worthwhile at all. In this section, the most common general basic values used to justify screening will be presented. We will also describe some of the conflicts actualized by them, as well as drawbacks or 'disvalues' in the light of these values.

The classic idea of what may make screening a good thing is that it improves *public health*, that is, the aggregated health level of a population. For public health to be promoted by a screening programme, there should be an acceptable treatment for the disease screened for. Wilson and Jungner (1968) held this criterion to be the most important one to be met in order for screening programmes to be justified.

However, it is far from clear when treatments should be judged as *acceptable* (see 'Treatments' below). Moreover, it is unclear what should be included in the concept of treatment to start with. Traditionally, the focus has been on treatment in the traditional sense of *medical* treatment, that is, treatment aimed at preventing, curing or ameliorating disease of a person identified by a screening programme. However, in the context of communicable disease management protecting public health, measures such as quarantine might be viewed as treatment, and it has been suggested that counselling in connection with genetic screening may

be seen in the same way (Shickle, 1999). This argument is based on the inclusion of other goals in medicine than the traditional ones of combating disease. This expansion is most conspicuous in areas such as reproductive medicine and genetics. These goals are almost without exception cast in terms of either some kind of *psychological well-being*, for example, the reduction of anxiety, reassurance, preparation, or in terms of enhancing *autonomy* (Juth, 2005).

Thus, somewhat roughly, there are three kinds of goals or values that can provide the rationale for introducing screening programmes:

1. Improvement of physiological health, reduction of disease or amelioration of symptoms of disease.
2. Improvement of psychological well-being or reduction of suffering.
3. Enhancement of (health-related) autonomy.

An important issue is, of course, to what extent these suggested goals really are worth promoting – not the least because the basic values underlying these goals may conflict in various ways.

WELL-BEING

Well-being can be increased (or 'ill-being' reduced) by screening in two ways: by increasing physiological health (point 1), which is the most uncontroversial rationale for screening, or by increasing psychological well-being (point 2). The most straightforward way in which an individual may be better off regarding her psychological well-being is by having her anxiety regarding her future health status removed. However, this presupposes that the individual has some initial worry or suspicion. As the initiative for the investigation is not from the individual this cannot be presupposed in the case of screening. So, reducing anxiety is primarily an argument for health care to offer medical investigations if requested, not for screening. On the contrary, screening runs the evident risk of creating more anxiety than it reduces.

Thus, regarding well-being, screening must primarily be justified with reference to physiological health. Furthermore, for *screening* to be justified, there must be reason to believe that it has some advantage beyond the standard model of letting the individual herself take the initiative to access health care. In effect, there must be some sort of *treatment*, an *advantage of early detection in terms of treatment*, and reasons to believe that *the individuals themselves have no prior suspicion of being at risk*. Because, as noted in the foregoing section, each of these factors may be present at different degrees, it may still be quite difficult to determine whether a particular screening programme is defensible or not.

In many cases of screening, promoting *public* health harmonizes well with the goal of promoting the health of individual people. There are, however, specific areas where tensions appear between these two aspects of promoting well-being. For instance, HIV testing of the known sexual contacts of an infected individual initiated by authorities may not always be followed by offers of preventive treatment, especially in less affluent countries, but may only be motivated by the need to protect society against an epidemic. This type of rationale can easily be envisaged in not too far-fetched scenarios of more pure screening programmes, for example, if there is an outbreak of a highly communicable and very aggressive and dangerous disease that is difficult to combat by ordinary medical means. Such scenarios expose clearly the potential tension between the traditional goal within health care of promoting individual well-being and the goal of public health to promote the aggregated well-being of the population.

AUTONOMY

Enhancing autonomy as a goal of health care is both of a later date and more controversial than is the goal of improving well-being. This goal has primarily been proposed in relation to prenatal screening and the goal is thus of improve reproductive autonomy by increasing the couple's reproductive options. However, testing as a means of improving autonomy need not be confined to the reproductive area.

The line of reasoning underlying this idea is that if individuals possess the knowledge that they or their offspring have an increased risk of contracting some disease, they are in a better position to plan their lives in accordance with their own plans and values. To live such a life is roughly what it means to live an autonomous life. The idea is, then, that leading an autonomous life, or at least increasing the possibility to do so, is something that screening may and should promote (Juth, 2005).

However, although the autonomy of some individuals may be promoted by receiving health information, there are special problems related to screening programmes. The fact that, in screening, the initiative for the investigation is not coming from the individual herself is problematic from the point of view of autonomy because there should be no pressure to accept or refrain from accepting medical procedures on this idea. Not only must informed consent be obtained, the individual should not be persuaded or subjected to more subtle manipulative efforts. Because health care, which occupies a position of authority on medical matters in most people's minds, is initiating screening, there always is some pressure being applied on the individual to accept rather than reject the offer (e.g. the more participation is taken for granted, the more pressure there is to participate).

In addition, screening programmes may have side effects at the societal level that are detrimental to autonomy (Hoedemaekers, 1999). Declining participation may start to be viewed as irresponsible, and screening may thus reinforce the norm that we are responsible for our own health, the health of our children or for public health. This in turn may add to the pressure to participate (see 'Prenatal screening' below).

JUSTICE

Another value that is sometimes mentioned in the context of screening is *justice* (Hoedemaekers, 1999). Even though justice is a contested concept, a basic conception common to all suggestions about justice is that *relevantly similar cases should be treated similarly*. The most common use of this notion as regards screening is to provide arguments against programmes on the basis that they imply an unjust allocation of health care resources. However, it has also been used for defending screening on the basis that if some testing procedure is offered due to its benefits for someone, all those who may gain from such benefits should receive the same procedure (Shickle, 1999).

This latter consideration of justice works only if one presupposes that the benefits befalling the initial (limited number of) people having some type of test would remain a benefit when health care professionals approach large numbers of people who would otherwise not have contacted the health care services themselves. As will be seen, there are reasons to be sceptical about this, because the downside in terms of being worried and pressured may outweigh possible advantages for some individuals. Well-being and autonomy thus remain the *primary* candidates for values that may be promoted by screening. Justice becomes relevant only as an additional argument in those cases where the other values speak in favour of screening, but it may then also provide arguments against screening.

SCREENING – WHAT AND WHEN?

Under the present heading, we will outline problems regarding what *diseases* to screen for (see 'Diseases' below), the *tests* used ('Tests' below) and available *treatments* ('Treatments' below). Having done this, we will address problems particular to various *target groups* ('Target groups' below).

DISEASES

Wilson and Jungner (1968) included in their recommendations the requirement that the disease screened for must be an 'important' health problem. The interpretation of 'important' is, however, far from obvious. Wilson and

Jungner took it to mean that the prevalence of disease must be high or that the disease is 'serious' for the individual. As they use PKU as an example of a serious disease (with low prevalence), they probably had diseases connected with much suffering or premature death in mind in the latter case. However, because suffering and premature death are matters of degrees and because what will actually occur with regard to a particular patient is hard to estimate (e.g. with Fragile X), this criterion allows for a wide range of interpretation, setting the limit for justified screening in different places on a continuum of seriousness. The same can, of course, be said with regard to prevalence, as well as the combination of these two factors.

TESTS

The properties of the testing methods applied have to be considered from an ethical point of view. One important property is the monetary cost because the practice of screening is located in a public health context, where cost-effectiveness is a crucial consideration and because costly programmes are more liable to criticism from the point of view of justice.

Another consideration is the *safety* of the testing method. In neonatal, adolescent and adult screening, this method often consists of an ordinary blood sample, or even completely noninvasive ways of collecting tissue. In contrast, prenatal testing often involves invasive methods, which bring a 0.5–1% risk of miscarriage (Connor and Ferguson-Smith, 1997). In other cases, proposed screening programmes face the problem of ignorance regarding the risks of the testing method, as is often the case when the method utilizes novel technology.

The most discussed property of tests in screening is their validity; that is their ability to identify correctly those, and only those, who have or will have a disease. A test can fail to identify individuals with disease in one of two ways: by being positive (i.e. indicating disease or high risk thereof) when there actually is or will be no disease (*false positive*) or by being negative (i.e. indicating absence of disease or low risk) when there actually is or will be a disease (*false negative*).

Screening programmes generally use tests that detect indirect indicators of the actual disease. For instance, cholesterol is an indicator for increased risk of coronary heart disease: the higher the level of cholesterol, the higher the risk. Whenever such tests are used, a threshold level has to be set in order to separate findings that should be counted as positive from those that should be counted as negative. So, the lower the level of cholesterol that is taken to indicate risk of coronary heart disease, the more test results will count as positive, and, for that reason, a larger proportion of the indicated positives will be false ones. This gives rise to a

general problem: the more the threshold is set to exclude all negative cases, the higher the risk of false negatives. Similarly, the more the threshold is set to include all positive cases, the higher the risk of false positives.

Both false positives and false negatives are associated with various downsides. False negatives have the apparent cost of delay or lack of needed treatment, in the worst case with fatal results. However, false positives have their downside too: unnecessary anxiety and stigma, as well as the burden of further investigations and/or unnecessary treatment. On a societal level, the higher the number of false positives, the higher the cost of unnecessary further investigations and/or treatment. A closer examination of various other variables seems necessary to balance these factors ethically, for example, the disease tested for, the consequences for the individuals tested as well as for society and the availability of treatments. For instance, if the diagnosis is associated with much anxiety, as is the case with many late onset disorders, such as hereditary breast cancer, few false positives are desirable. Also, if diseases are connected with societal stigma, such as sickle cell anaemia (Clarke, 1994) or HIV/AIDS, avoiding the 'disease label' when there actually is no disease becomes increasingly important. The case for the importance of few false positives is strengthened if there are no effective treatments, as in the case of Huntington's disease, or if existing treatments are very burdensome, as is the case with prophylactic mastectomy for preventing breast cancer, or abortion due to prenatal diagnosis. In contrast, it seems more reasonable to opt for minimizing false negatives if there is an effective treatment and there are severe consequences for the individual in terms of health without early diagnosis, as is the case with PKU.

Furthermore, the ability of a test to accurately, informatively and unambiguously predict the actual (future) health status of the tested individual (its *predictive value*) is crucial in order to determine whether its use for screening is warranted. The predictive value is highly important in a screening context, since the general idea is to acquire results that can guide practical decision-making (about further tests, treatments, lifestyle changes, etc.).

The problem of predictive value becomes accentuated when the results themselves are either constituted by, or based on, population-based statistical figures rather than binary results. This problem is a pressing one due to the increasing possibility of quantifying predispositions for various diseases that are the result of both complex genetic and environmental factors, for example, the so-called *multifactorial* diseases (such as Alzheimer's disease, diabetes, cardiovascular disease, various forms of cancer and schizophrenia) (Connor and Ferguson-Smith, 1997). As not one indicator determines whether or not an individual will have the disease, a single test can only deliver a probability for having (or going on to develop) the disease. This risk

determination will in most cases be estimated on the basis
of evidence that is probabilistic as well, so any figure given
is likely to be both inadequate and difficult to interpret.

TREATMENTS

The most common ethical issue in screening with regard to treatments concerns their efficacy and associated
risks. Available treatments may vary in this respect from
well-established procedures that are highly efficient with
almost no risk of side effects (such as the dietary treatment
for PKU), to complicated and rather uncertain measures
that bring a range of risks. Moreover, some treatments
merely delay certain symptoms, like treatment for HIV or
Alzheimer's disease. There is, however, no clear-cut answer
to the question as to when treatment should be deemed 'acceptable enough' to warrant screening. It seems plausible
to hold as a general view that this factor has to be balanced
against a host of other morally relevant features. For example, serious symptoms may make an otherwise burdensome
treatment acceptable, whereas risks of 'overtreatment' due
to false positives must be taken into account when the treatment brings risks of its own (as in the case of cancer).

It is crucial not to underestimate the difference between
ordinary medical testing initiated by the individual and testing done within a screening programme in relation to the
treatment aspect. In the case of screening, the possibility
of individually 'tailormade' treatments must be discounted
because the focus is not upon identifiable treatment. This
suggests a stronger responsibility to be able to offer an acceptable treatment in the screening case than in the ordinary health care situation.

TARGET GROUPS

Different target groups for screening tend to actualize
different goals and they also give rise to different ethical
problems.

Prenatal Screening

Autonomy as a goal for screening is most salient in discussions about prenatal diagnosis: if the couple can gain knowledge about the expected health status of potential children,
they are in a better position to make reproductive decisions
in accordance with their own plans (Chadwick, 1999).

However, even if one grants that reproductive autonomy
is an important goal for prenatal *diagnosis*, it is a highly
questionable argument in favour of organizing this practice in the form of *screening programmes*. The reason for
this is the same one that makes screening programmes in
general problematic from the point of view of autonomy:
because the initiative to the investigation in question is not

the individual's but the society's, there is always some pressure on the individual to undergo the investigations. Furthermore, because screening programmes single out some
of the conditions that can be tested, these conditions will
inevitably be perceived as especially problematic, which
tends to reinforce the initial pressure.

Even though reproductive autonomy is often addressed
in discussions of prenatal screening, preventing disease has
also been suggested as an important rationale (Munthe,
1996). However, as very few conditions can be treated before birth, the follow-up procedure offered in almost all
cases of a positive prenatal diagnosis is abortion. The type
of prevention is thus not that of disease but that of sick people, and this makes prenatal screening ethically controversial. The core of much current criticism is the suspicion that
the goal of prenatal screening is to 'sort out' certain types
of individuals who, due to their disabilities, are not seen
as worthy of protection to the same extent as other human
beings – possibly due to the cost to society (Munthe, 1996;
Parens and Asch, 2000).

There certainly is something to this criticism. If health
care is to implement prenatal *screening*, it has to make an
active approach and choose the conditions that are to be
the focus of testing. As this will mean significant societal
pressure to test for these things, the primary goal of such
a practice cannot be to promote autonomy. Rather, when
health care suggests a list of conditions that are especially
desirable to avoid, it is hard not to see this as an implicit
official message that the individuals that have these conditions are considered less worthy of protection (because
avoiding the conditions amounts to avoiding individuals
with the conditions). Moreover, this message will also be
likely to pressure individual pregnant women and couples, and this will be problematic from the perspective of
autonomy.

Neonatal Screening

In contrast to the prenatal case, neonatal screening has
mainly been considered for conditions that can be prevented or ameliorated. The traditional goal of promoting
health by preventing or ameliorating disease thus seems
to be paramount in this area (Gustavson, 1989; Chadwick,
1999; Wilcken et al., 2003; ACMG, 2005).

The classic example of neonatal screening is PKU. Today, most western countries have screening programmes
for this and similar diseases. These diseases all share some
common characteristics: they can be detected early and
early intervention is available and necessary for preventing
or ameliorating the disease in question. Moreover, the tests
required are reliable and safe, and the diseases themselves
are very serious. Although each disease is very rare,
because so much is at stake for the individual and because

the risk of testing is negligible, screening can be considered acceptable. In such cases, the obvious downside to neonatal screening (that those screened cannot consent themselves) will in practice be quite weak.

Nonetheless, neonatal screening is an increasing subject of controversy. An example of a recent development that has attracted much attention is tandem mass spectrometry, which facilitates rapid, cheap and simultaneous neonatal screening for a large number of metabolic disorders (Wilcken et al., 2003; Pandor et al., 2004). But to what extent this new method should be used depends on a number of factors. Take for instance the condition of there being an 'efficacious treatment' (ACMG, 2005). Even if interpreted in terms of generally accepted standards of health, such as morbidity and mortality, there is still the question of how substantial the gains must be in order for screening to be justified. This question is ethical rather than medical and cannot be settled by any number of empirical investigations. Furthermore, how 'demonstrated' must the benefits in terms of efficient treatment be in order to be judged well-founded?

So, depending on how criteria and goals are interpreted in detail, policy and practical recommendation for screening can vary widely. Accordingly, while ACMG (2005) recommends 20 metabolic disorders for screening, a report for the Health Technology Assessment Programme in the United Kingdom recommends far fewer such disorders (Pandor et al., 2004). This reflects a difference in the *evaluation of* data rather than a difference of data. To complicate things further, this evaluation is strongly connected to the legal and economic organization of health care, because it is such factors that seem to have prompted the radical expansion of neonatal screening in the Unites States (Natowicz, 2005).

Screening of Adolescents

As in the case of neonatal screening, screening children can mainly be cast in terms of traditional health care goals, although the problem of autonomous decision-making becomes more important.

However, unlike most existing neonatal programmes, in adolescent screening it is likely that some parents will be unwilling to have their children enter the programme. This raises the question of the rights of parents to deny their children potentially beneficial health care measures. On one hand, one may deny such a right with reference to the best interest of the child, or society. On the other, one may point to the fact that there are many areas where parents are allowed to make decisions on behalf of their children that may be detrimental to the interests of the child or society.

Adolescent screening is, however, further complicated by the fact that, from the point of view of autonomy, the case for letting the wishes of the child influence the decision becomes stronger in proportion to its maturity. It may be the case that a child younger than the legal cut-off point is mature enough to be an autonomous decision-maker. Because the children and their parents may not want the same thing, the stronger such reasons there are, the more probable it is that balancing conflicting choices of the children and their parents becomes a serious ethical problem.

One way in which the future autonomy of a child may be threatened by any type of medical test is that the information provided by the test affects the parents in a way that is harmful to the child. In particular, the phenomenon of so-called *stigmatization* has been suggested as one such risk: information regarding the expected future health of the child may make the parents alter radically the way they relate psychosocially to it. For example, they may perceive it as much more unhealthy and vulnerable than is in fact the case. Most seriously, this type of effect may occur even if the information only suggests a risk of future health problems – a risk that may in fact never be realized.

Screening of Adults

In addition to previously discussed issues, the case of adults sees a particular practical consideration that underlines the need for the ethics of screening to consider a wider socio-political context. This consideration has its roots in the fact that the information provided by the tests used in screening programmes may be of interest not only for health care and the individual but also for various third parties such as insurance companies and employers (Radetzki et al., 2003; Juth, 2005).

Obviously, this complicates the assessment of whether or not a screening programme is 'good enough'. Even if the goal is only to promote health, failure to realize this goal may result from the fact that a person is in the future denied work or health insurance. In view of that, autonomy seems to require that screening makes such risks apparent. On a more overarching level, this complication widens the scope of socio-political issues of relevance to screening even further. For one way to avoid the risks just pointed out is to organize society in a way that accomplishes this (such as publicly financed health insurance good enough to make private health insurance unnecessary).

SCREENING – HOW?

We will not discuss all the relevant questions, but only address the most debated ones. First, there are issues regarding how screening programmes approach and subsequently handle people. With regard to this, we will focus on the much debated and related questions of informed consent (see 'Informed consent') and counselling (see

'Counselling'). Second, we will address some 'large-scale' issues regarding funding, and if, and then how, participation should be encouraged (see 'Funding and participation').

INFORMED CONSENT

Even if a large uptake is desired, today there is a general agreement that participation in screening should be voluntary and that the patient has a right to be informed about the procedure and the possible results of acceptance or rejection (ESHG, 2003). *Informed consent* is thus considered to be an important feature of an ethically sound screening programme. Underlying informed consent is the rule of respecting autonomy. However, ensuring that autonomy is respected is a tricky question. For example, what type and amount of pressure should be seen as unacceptable infringements of autonomy? Even in the absence of overt coercion, there are more subtle forms of pressure such as social attitudes or enticement.

Moreover, the standard notion of not withholding any relevant information from the patient is the subject of much discussion. First, it should not be taken to allow that information is *forced* on to the patient without consent. The right *not* to know can also be defended with reference to considerations of autonomy (Häyry and Takala, 2000; Juth, 2005). Second, large or complicated bundles of information may *reduce* autonomy because confusion may be the result. Third, the goal of promoting health and well-being can obviously conflict with autonomy because individuals need not consent to testing and treatment beneficial to health. Thus, despite an increasing allegiance to the rule of informed consent, it might be argued that informed consent should be a secondary concern in screening programmes after all. Judging from the case of communicable diseases, acceptance of such a view might seem more tempting if the goal of screening is foremost to promote the public health.

COUNSELLING

For individuals to benefit from the medical information resulting from a screening programme, *what* information is disclosed and *how* it is disclosed is of great importance from the point of view of well-being, as well as that of autonomy. Understanding the information properly is necessary in order to undertake appropriate health care measures, to avoid unnecessary anxiety and to be able to make decisions in accordance with one's plans.

Counselling is a practice that aims at designing the situation of disclosure so that it is conducive to the well-being and autonomy of the individual. It is, in the words of Fraser's (1974) famous characterization of genetic counselling, a 'communication process which deals with the human problems associated with the occurrence or risk of occurrence of a genetic disorder'. There is some controversy as to how counselling should be performed in practice in order to achieve the goal of preserving the well-being and autonomy of the individual, as well as what values should be given most weight. However, it is unanimously agreed that it is not an easy affair to preserve and promote the autonomy and well-being of the patient in relation to the often complicated information resulting from medical tests. It takes time, effort, training and, thus, resources to facilitate the processing of the information both before and after testing. This presents a special problem for screening programmes, partly because they involve such large numbers and partly because these people are not prepared for such testing. Such counselling requirements may be so costly that screening may prove not to be cost-effective and even unjust.

FUNDING AND PARTICIPATION

This raises the further issue of how screening programmes should be funded. Public funding seems to be the default assumption, and there are good reasons for this: participation will be affected negatively if people have to pay for themselves. Moreover, it seems unjust that only those who can afford it should be able to benefit.

However, this gives rise to an issue of just allocation: to what extent should publicly funded health care spend resources on screening? Should health care primarily spend its resources on people with diseases or people who may be or become ill? How great should the benefits of screening be in comparison to the benefits of alternative health care measures? Which benefits and harms should count? Which values? How should they be weighted in cases of conflict? What role should financial savings and considerations of efficiency play?

A related question is how to ensure participation in screening programmes. Above, we touched on the issue of whether it would be acceptable to make participation in neonatal programmes obligatory. Such an aim is especially relevant when the focus is on improving *public* health.

Strategies to increase participation include public education or the design of the setting where screening is offered. For instance, the offer may be made in connection with other health care measures where uptake is already high or an explicit verbal offer is more likely to encourage participation than in handing out a written form. In addition, there is always the possibility of individual persuasion in order to increase participation. However, all of these strategies may backfire if the benefits are dubious or if people may be harmed.

However, all measures aimed at ensuring participation may be viewed as adding to the pressure applied by screening programmes in the first place. It is a difficult issue to assess when this would make a programme seriously problematic from the point of view of autonomy.

CONCLUSIONS

The subject of the ethics of screening is vast and complex, and we repeatedly argued that the ethics of screening calls for an unusually wide inquiry. Determining the ethical defensibility (or lack of such) of any screening programme involves consideration of cultural, economic, political and social, and medical considerations, basic questions of value and a host of other factual and normative factors. We would like to end this chapter by pressing this point further and challenging somewhat the picture of screening as a particular issue for *medical* ethics. Or, perhaps, our point is rather that the default view of medical ethics should be expanded; the case of screening demonstrates that, in real life, any health care professional, directly or indirectly, will have to deal with that web of complications made so salient by the case of screening.

ACKNOWLEDGEMENT

Work on this chapter was undertaken within the intersection of two projects: Presymptomatic Testing and Genetic Counselling: Goals and Ethics for Clinical Practice, Caring and Education, funded by the Swedish Ethics in Health Care Programme; and European Public Health Ethics Network (EuroPHEN), funded by the European Commission. We would also like to acknowledge the valuable assistance of Angus Dawson, Ulrika von Döbeln, Karl-Henrik Gustavson and Jan Wahlström.

REFERENCES

American College of Medical Genetics. *Newborn Screening: Toward a Uniform Screening Panel and System.* Rockville, MD: Maternal and Health Care Bureau, 2005; also available at http://mchb.hrsa.gov/screening.

Beauchamp TL, Childress JF. *Principles of Biomedical Ethics*, 5th edition. New York and Oxford: Oxford University Press, 2001.

Buchanan A, Brock DW, Daniels N, Wikler D. *From Chance to Choice – Genetics and Justice.* Cambridge: Cambridge University Press, 2000.

Bui TH, Nordeskjöld M. Prenatal diagnosis: molecular genetics and cytogenetics. *Best Pract Res Clinic Obstet Gynaecol* 2002; **16**: 629 – 643.

Chadwick R, Shickle D, Have ten H, Wiesing U, eds. *The Ethics of Genetic Screening.* Dordrecht: Kluwer Academics Publishers, 1999.

Clarke A, ed. *Genetic Counselling: Practice and Principles.* London: Routledge, 1994.

Connor M, Ferguson-Smith M. *Essential Medical Genetics.* Oxford: Blackwell Science Ltd, 1997.

Dawson A, Verweij M. The meaning of 'public' in 'public health'. In: Dawson A, Verweij M, eds. *Ethics, Prevention, and Public Health.* Oxford: Oxford University Press, 2006.

European Society of Human Genetics. Population genetic screening programmes: technical, social and ethical issues. Recommendations of the European Society of Human Genetics. *Eur J Human Genet* 2003; **11**: 5–7.

Fraser FC. Genetic counseling. *Am J Human Genet* 1974; **26**: 636–659.

Gianroli L, Magli MC, Feraretti A, Munné S. Preimplantation diagnosis for aneuploidies in patients undergoing in vitro fertilization with a poor prognosis: identification of the categories for which it should be proposed. *Fertil Steril* 1999; **72**: 837–844.

Gregg AR, Simpson JL. Genetic screening for cystic fibrosis. *Obstet Gynecol Clinic North Am* 2002; **29**: 329–340.

Gustavson K-H. The prevention and management of autosomal recessive conditions. Main example: alpha$_1$-antitrypsin deficiency. *Clinic Genet* 1989; **36**: 327–332.

Hampton ML, Anderson J, Lavizzo BS, Bergman AB. Sickle-cell 'nondisease'. *Am J Dis Child* 1974; **128**: 58–61.

Häyry M, Takala T. Genetic ignorance, moral obligations and social duties. *J Med Philos* 2000; **1**: 107–113.

Hoedemaekers R. Genetic screening and testing. A moral map. In: Chadwick R, et al., eds. *The Ethics of Genetic Screening.* Dordrecht: Kluwer Academic Publishers, 1999.

Ioannou P. Thalassaemia prevention in Cyprus. Past, present and future. In: Chadwick R, et al., eds. *The Ethics of Genetic Screening.* Dordrecht: Kluwer Academics Publishers, 1999.

Juth N. *Genetic Information – Values and Rights: The Morality of Presymptomatic Genetic Testing.* Gîteborg: Acta Universitatis Gothoburgensis, 2005.

Kinzler WL, Morrell K, Vintzileos AM. Variables that underlie cost efficacy of prenatal screening. *Obstet Gynecol Clinic North Am* 2002; **29**: 277–286.

Moran NE, Shickle D, Munthe C, Dierickx K, Petrini C, Piribauer F, Czabanowska K, Cowley H, Blancafort S, Petsetakis E. Are compulsory immunisation and incentives to immunise effective ways to achieve herd immunity in europe? In: Selgelid M, Battin M, eds. *Ethics and Infectious Disease.* London: Blackwell, 2006.

Munthe C. *The Moral Roots of Prenatal Diagnosis. Ethical Aspects of the Early Introduction and Presentation of Prenatal Diagnosis in Sweden.* Göteborg: Centre for Research Ethics, 1996.

Munthe C. *Pure Selection. The Ethics of Preimplantation Genetic Diagnosis and Choosing Children without Abortion.* Göteborg: Acta Universitatis Gothoburgensis, 1999.

Murray CJL, Salomon JA, Mathers CD, Lopez AD. *Summary Measures of Population Health: Concepts, Ethics, Measurement and Applications.* Geneva: WHO, 2002.

Natovicz M. Newborn screening – setting evidence-based policy for protection. *N Engl J Med* 2005; **9**: 867–870.

Pandor A, Eastman J, et al. Clinical effectiveness and cost-effectiveness of neonatal screening for inborn errors of metabolism using tandem mass spectrometry: a systematic review. *Health Technol Assess* 2004; **8**: 1–134.

Parens E, Asch A. *Prenatal Testing and Disability Rights.* Washington, DC: Georgetown University Press, 2000.

Radetzki M, Radetzki M, Juth N. *Genes and Insurance: Ethical, Legal and Economic Issues.* Cambridge: Cambridge University Press, 2003.

Rawls J. *A Theory of Justice.* London: Oxford University Press, 1972.

Shickle D. The Wilson and Jungner principles of screening and genetic testing. In: Chadwick R, et al., eds. *The Ethics of Genetic Screening,* Dordrecht: Kluwer Academics Publishers, 1999.

Shickle D, Harvey I. Inside-out, back-to-front: a model for clinical population genetic screening. *J Med Genet* 1996; **30**: 580–582.

The Danish Council of Ethics *Screening – A Report.* Copenhagen: The Danish Council of Ethics, 1999.

The Nuffield Council on Bioethics. *Genetic Screening and Ethical Issues.* London: The Nuffield Council on Bioethics, 1993.

Wilcken B, Wiley V, Hammond J, Carpenter K. Screening newborns for inborn errors of metabolism by tandem mass spectrometry. *N Engl J Med* 2003; **23**: 2304–2312.

Wilson JMG, Jungner G. Principles and practice of screening for disease. *Public Health Papers.* Geneva: WHO No. 34, 1968.

84

Vaccination Ethics

ANGUS DAWSON

INTRODUCTION

Strongly held, but differing, opinions are put forward about the success and acceptability of vaccination. In this chapter, I will outline a few of the key arguments about this area of public health.

I begin with some clarifications about the limits of this chapter. First, vaccination at its broadest can be taken to involve some form of artificial stimulation of the immune system as a response to actual or potential bacterial or virological infection. Vaccination might be either preventive (given prior to potential infection) or therapeutic (given in response to infection). This chapter is deliberately termed 'vaccination ethics' as I will restrict my discussion to priming of the immune system *before* contact with any disease. This means we can exclude from this chapter discussion of other forms of immunization such as the giving of immunoglobulin after possible exposure to, or after infection with, a disease. This is not because such techniques are unimportant, but because both the use of immunoglobulin and therapeutic vaccination might be thought of as clinical interventions rather than public health activities. This chapter will concentrate on preventive vaccination as this is at the core of controversy about vaccination. Second, the classic image of vaccination consists of an injection (usually into the muscle). However, in some cases the relevant material is given orally (and absorbed through the digestive tract) or in the future it might be delivered in some other way (such as by nasal spray). Lastly, most preventive vaccination is carried out in childhood. This is not only because this is the time when the immune system can be primed to the greatest advantage, but also because it is the time of greatest threat to the individual from many diseases. However, it should not be forgotten that many other vaccinations are carried out with adolescents and adults. Such vaccination might be for a number of reasons: boosters for

childhood vaccinations, because older individuals might be at threat of disease due to travel, or because they are held to be at increased risk for some other reason (e.g. medical conditions related to immune suppression or old age). I will focus on childhood preventive vaccination for the rest of this chapter unless I specify otherwise.

I outline three key arguments in the following sections: a discussion of harms and benefits; the nature of our obligation not to bring about harm to others; and the idea of best interests. I end with a short discussion of the possible grounds for compulsory vaccination.

HARMS AND BENEFITS

Arguments related to the balancing of harms and benefits are important to vaccination policies. You do not need to be committed to consequentialism to accept this, and it is important to see that this is not the only possible moral argument about vaccination. The vital and difficult issue to decide is: what are the relevant harms and benefits? In this section I will begin by suggesting some relevant considerations and then argue that in vaccination policy (as in many preventive programmes) the focus cannot just be on harms and benefits in relation to particular individuals but that any such judgement needs to take into account the consequences for populations not just individuals. This complicates the ethical discussion.

Vaccination brings potential benefit to the individual receiving the vaccination because they are less likely to develop that particular disease if they come into contact with it. However, there is also an important benefit to society if sufficient members of that population are vaccinated to create herd protection (Paul, 2004). Herd protection means that all members of the community are at reduced risk of attack by an infectious disease. This is because if such a disease enters

Principles of Health Care Ethics, Second Edition Edited by R.E. Ashcroft, A. Dawson, H. Draper and J.R. McMillan
© 2007 John Wiley & Sons, Ltd

the population, it is far less likely to become an epidemic or pandemic as any diseased individual is less likely to pass on the infection if the surrounding individuals have been vaccinated prior to contact. In addition, any unvaccinated individuals in the population are better protected, as they are less likely to come into contact with an infected individual. (At least some unvaccinated individuals are not at risk due to their own decisions. For example, neonates might not be old enough to be vaccinated; the ill and those with compromised immunity might be unvaccinated for sound medical reasons; vaccination might fail or be insufficient to give immunity; scheduled vaccinations might have been missed due to population movement, etc.). Herd protection offers all these groups their *only* vaccine-related protection against the risk of disease.

The supporters of vaccination will argue that few other medical interventions have had such a positive impact on the world's health (CDC, 2006). Smallpox could not have been eradicated without vaccination, and poliomyelitis (despite some problems) is close to eradication as a result of global efforts and a sustained vaccination programme. Much effort is going into preparation for a vaccine in response to the threat of an influenza pandemic as a direct means of preventing the spread of such a disease (should it emerge). If routine vaccination for recommended diseases were available across the world, the impact on global health would be highly significant (WHO, 2002). Despite this, some authors have expressed scepticism about the scale of the contribution of vaccination to the dramatic reduction in childhood mortality from infectious disease since the mid-nineteenth century (Keown, 1976). They suggest that improvements in nutrition, water quality and sanitation have had more impact upon the disease-related mortality figures. I would argue that these factors have certainly contributed to this fall, as a healthy child is better able to fight infection. However, Keown's thesis almost certainly underestimates the impact of vaccination in preventing, or reducing the force of, waves of disease. The (additional) impact of vaccination can be seen by looking at infection rates for such diseases as diphtheria in the United Kingdom where the number of infections (and deaths) plummeted after routine vaccination was introduced in the 1940s and 1950s (Salisbury and Begg, 1996).

Ironically, in the developed world it is the very success of vaccination in maintaining unprecedented low rates of many infectious diseases that has proved to be part of the reason why vaccination has become such a controversial issue at times. Few adults in the developed world have any experience of previously very common infectious diseases (e.g. diphtheria, measles, pertussis, etc.), and so it is easier to downplay or ignore the risks of such diseases and over-emphasize any potential risks from a vaccine. Of course, vaccinations can cause harm. Such harms range

from inflammation and pain at the site of injection to anaphylaxis and death. However, any adverse events are rare, and serious adverse events are very rare indeed for most vaccines. Occasionally, the public can lose confidence in a particular vaccine, as happened in the United Kingdom with pertussis during the 1970s and MMR since 1998. In some cases, with particular vaccines, the risks of vaccination can be higher than would be acceptable for a routine vaccination programme, and this can lead to poor uptake in target populations (e.g. recent smallpox vaccination among 'first responders' in the US was held to be disappointing. See Yih et al., 2003). Media reports, rumours and misunderstandings can feed these concerns. Vaccines are subject to the same rigorous development standards as any other medicinal products. If anything, standards are higher given the need to administer vaccines to very large asymptomatic populations. We can distinguish between the perception of risks and the statistical reality of risks, but the former matters as vaccination programmes need to be acceptable to the target population (Verweij and Dawson, 2004).

Different vaccines have different adverse event profiles depending on how they are made. Vaccines can be manufactured using live but weakened (attenuated) pathogens, dead pathogens, part-pathogens or inactivated toxins. In some cases there is a choice of vaccines for the same disease (as with polio), and they will have different modes of operation and side-effects (Paul and Dawson, 2005). In other cases, the choice of a particular strain might make a difference to the likelihood of side effect as some strains will be more virulent than others (see Kretzschmar et al., 2006 on smallpox vaccines). In addition, the vaccine will not only contain an active ingredient designed to induce immunity but also other things including adjuvants (ingredients to stimulate an immune reaction) as well as preservatives. Sometimes these elements can be the reason for concern, such as the recent discussion in the United States about the role of mercury as a preservative in vaccines (Institute of Medicine, 2004). Vaccine development involves a constant process of refinement and improvement with the aim of trying to reduce any potential risks to a minimum.

There are some other possible 'harm-related' objections to vaccination that I will leave to one side. For example, it might be claimed that there is no risk of harm involved in common childhood diseases, or that the risk of harm from vaccines is disproportionate to the threat from such diseases. Such arguments tend to be overgeneralized or involve dubious empirical claim. Much of the popular anti-vaccination material available in the public domain is based on no or poor evidence, with little attempt to consider the issues fairly (see Sorell, 2007). Objections to vaccinations *as such* will not be considered here (although I do not think they make much sense, as any harm/benefit judgement can only be focused on a consideration of an individual vaccine and disease).

As mentioned earlier, it is important that in considering harms and benefits in relation to vaccination we do not merely focus on how these issues affect individuals but also the whole population. This is vital in relation to vaccination because of the issue of herd protection. Herd protection is a good example of a benefit that exists at the population level. However, this population benefit is not an instance of a mere aggregation of individual benefits. Where herd protection exists the benefit extends much further than the sub-group of the total population that has been vaccinated. One way of conceptualizing this population benefit is in terms of seeing it as a public good. A public good is a good that cannot be created by any individual alone; it takes collective efforts. It cannot be broken down into individual goods and distributed amongst the members of a population. All benefit in a population, if it exists. None can enjoy it, unless all benefit. There are various problems associated with the creation and maintenance of public goods, but the importance for this section is that such a benefit as herd protection cannot be easily entered into any simple harm and benefits calculation in relation to individuals; the population level is relevant to such deliberations (Dawson, 2007).

It is important to see that this appeal to population benefits does not mean that individuals need to be sacrificed for the good of the population, just that the relevant benefits to the population as a whole are relevant consideration in any deliberations about harms and benefits. Although it can be argued in relation to at least some preventive public health policies that risks are run by individuals and benefits accrue to the population, this is not true of vaccination policies (Dawson, 2004). Vaccinated individuals do benefit from their participation in the programme; it is just that they will gain an *extra* benefit if herd protection exists. Where herd protection is an explicit aim of a vaccination programme and vaccination is strongly encouraged, it is very important to consider the question of compensation for any possible vaccine-related harm: even the perception of injustice, of unnecessarily sacrificing individuals for the good of the population, should be avoided if possible (Paul and Dawson, 2005).

HARM TO OTHERS

Much contemporary bioethics assumes a broadly liberal set of background commitments. How might this approach be related to vaccination? Traditional liberals (such as Mill, 1859, and Feinberg, 1973) commonly make a distinction between actions likely to cause harm only to self and those that are likely to result in harm to others. They hold that this makes a vital difference to the legitimacy of interfering in someone's freedom of action. On this approach,

third parties have fewer justifiable reasons to intervene on harm to self grounds. Although health care professionals may have a duty to warn about a risk of harm or provide relevant information, any attempt to enforce a vaccination for someone's own good will be met with the charge of paternalism.

What is paternalism? Paternalism can be defined as acting (or not acting) with the intention of reducing harm or bringing about greater good for the particular individual affected by the action (or omission). On this definition, it is left open whether a paternalistic action is morally justifiable: there are two separate judgements. Is it paternalism? If it is, is it morally justified? However, many liberals believe that we can use a distinction between hard and strong or soft and weak paternalism to settle the issue of justifiability. On this view, it is argued that strong paternalism is where an action will overrule the action or decision of a competent individual (in the liberal's view this is usually held to be unjustifiable), whereas weak paternalism is where an action is performed on behalf of an incompetent individual (e.g. a young child, an adult with serious learning difficulties; an adult with dementia, etc.). (In the liberal's view this is usually held to be justifiable.)

Routine childhood vaccinations are usually carried out on very young children; so, if we are talking about paternalism at all, we are talking about weak paternalism. The key issue under discussion will not be whether someone should make decisions on behalf of children just a few months old but who should do so. As we are talking about incompetent individuals here, we can set aside the harm to self argument and concentrate upon harm to others considerations. With young children, 'harm to self' considerations end up being, at best, only a component of a judgement of best interests (as we will see below). In the case of young children, any argument about harm to others considerations related to vaccination will focus on the potential harm (to third parties) as a result of the parents' decision not to vaccinate their child.

However, note that harm to others considerations are likely to be an important consideration in relation to decisions about the vaccination of competent adults as well as children. For example, an adult traveller might knowingly put others at risk of harm if they refuse to be vaccinated for a contagious disease. A related issue is whether certain individuals or groups have special obligations to protect others from harm. For example, in many parts of the world, health care workers are required to be vaccinated for conditions such as hepatitis B as a means not only of reducing the risk of being infected themselves but also of passing on infections to others. There has been a recent lively discussion about whether there is an obligation upon workers in care homes to be vaccinated against influenza. (See Verweij's chapter in this volume.)

As suggested above, although liberal political philosophy generally leaves it to individuals to make decisions about their own lives, there is an important exception – where actions might result in harm to others. (Such arguments are common in the public health arena, for example there are compulsory powers of detention under the Public Health Act of England and Wales when you have the potential to spread an infectious disease and you refuse treatment). We can construct a harm to others argument related to vaccinations as follows:

1. Contagious diseases that might result in (more than trivial) harm can be passed on to others through non-intentional action.
2. This could be prevented through vaccination of any potential source individual in advance (where a relevant vaccine exists).
3. We have a general moral obligation not to cause harm to others through our own actions and inactions.
4. Given 1 and 2, an individual can reduce the risk of causing (non-trivial) harm to others through vaccination for (serious) contagious disease.

Conclusion: given 3 and 4, we are morally obliged to have vaccinations for (serious) contagious diseases (where these are available).

Of course there are many issues to discuss in exploring such an argument (Dawson, 2007). However, support for this view comes from the fact that, as mentioned earlier, a decision not to vaccinate (against contagious diseases) does not just put the non-vaccinated individual's health at risk. A failure to vaccinate is not like a failure to consent to a blood transfusion. In the latter case it is only the individual himself or herself who is harmed, whereas in the vaccination case others may be harmed as a result of an individual's choice or parents' decision not to vaccinate their child. In other words, where there are serious public health issues at stake it is possible to argue that we are under a moral obligation to be vaccinated or ensure our children are vaccinated on the grounds of potential harm to third parties (Dawson, 2007).

It should be noted that harm to others arguments are not paternalistic because the reason for intervention is nothing to do with the good or potential harm relating to the particular individual we are concerned about. The justification for action is the potential harm to third parties following the parent's decision. This argument is potentially powerful in the case of vaccination, because of the highly contagious nature of many vaccine-preventable childhood diseases. However, some will object to such an argument, because they will say that the presumption in favour of parental autonomy should not be overturned on these grounds in relation to vaccination, perhaps, because the risk of harm

resulting from a particular instance of non-vaccination will be too remote. However, even if this is true, the harm to others argument will become stronger the more imminent and the greater the threat of harm resulting from the decision.

THE 'BEST INTERESTS' ARGUMENT

Liberal democracies rightly value individual liberty. As a result, competent adults are usually considered to be the appropriate persons to make decisions about their own health care treatment. This freedom is usually extended to parents in relation to decisions about their children's health. Such a position could be supported on a number of different theoretical and practical grounds. For example, parents might be considered to know better than anyone else what is in an individual child's best interests because they can reasonably be expected to know that particular child better than anyone else. They are also likely to know what will benefit their child, and be aware of the societal and cultural context within which the child will be raised. Parents might also argue that such decisional authority is part of what it is to be parents. Although this latter claim may consist of an assertion of ownership or control, it need not be so; for example, parents might, alternatively, link the idea to the responsibilities they have as parents. Ultimately, however such a view is justified, there seems a reasonable claim at its root, as it will be the parents who have to deal with any negative or positive consequences that result from any decision made. Another possible argument in support of parental authority might be based on the idea that the family is a private institution, and that it is inappropriate for the state to intervene in decision-making relevant to the family, except in exceptional circumstances. Each of these claims has different merits and problems. Luckily, we do not need to debate them here. We can just accept that liberal philosophy, however supported, will normally give parents decisional authority in relation to their children.

How does this relate to vaccinations? Parents generally make decisions about childhood vaccinations. Is it appropriate for parents to refuse vaccination on behalf of their child? The child has no say in the matter, and by the time they are competent, damage might have been caused to the child as a result of the parents' decision. Whilst most will agree that the presumption in favour of parental authority can be over turned in cases where it is a matter of potential life or death, or serious and significant harm, is there a role for the state to step in to protect the child from parental decisions and enforce vaccinations? Certainly such a power is used in other health and social contexts. Let us focus on preschool vaccinations. (If an older child is held to be competent, then we can treat them as we treat adults.) An argument can be constructed in favour of vaccinations on the grounds of best interests as follows:

1. Medical decisions about incompetent patients should be made on the basis of what is in their best interests (where prior wishes are unknown or nonexistent).
2. Preschool infants are incompetent (and have no prior wishes).
3. Therefore, decisions about the medical care of infants should be made on the basis of what is in their best interests.
4. Best interests in relation to infants should be determined by seeking to balance the potential harms and benefits of possible actions and inactions.
5. Where the parents make a decision about an infant's care which is likely to result in substantial risk of significant harm to that infant, then third parties (such as the state) have an obligation to intervene to protect the infant from the consequences of that decision.
6. Given 4, what is in the best interests of infants in relation to vaccinations is to be decided by seeking to balance the harms and benefits associated with vaccination versus non-vaccination.
7. Given 3, 5 and 6, where it is in an infant's best interests to be vaccinated (or not vaccinated) and the parents decide the other way, then the state (or other legitimate third parties) have an obligation to ensure that the infant is protected from the consequences of such a decision.

Conclusion: Parental decision-making about childhood vaccinations can be overruled legitimately in at least some cases.

This argument requires a lot of explanation and discussion over issues such as what constitutes 'best interests'. All I suggest here is that it might be possible to construct such an argument assuming that parents do not *by definition* decide what is in their child's best interests; that is, parents can *in fact* be in error about what is in their child's best interests (Dawson, 2005). On this view, best interests are decided on the basis of an overall welfare judgement, and on at least some occasions, other parties may step in to ensure that children are protected from the consequences of their parents' decision-making.

A possible objection is that a judgement about best interests is always made in relation to an individual child. In circumstances where herd protection exists in a population, it looks as though a judgement about best interests may favour non-vaccination (assuming there is *any* possibility of harm resulting from that vaccination). Some might argue that there is a potential issue of justice here and that such parental decision-making is essentially a free riding upon the actions of others (Cullity, 1995). There is a sense in which it is true, but it is not clear that objections based on free

riding are sufficient to impose an obligation to vaccinate in such circumstances (Dawson, 2007). In addition, it should not be forgotten that there will be individual benefits from vaccination as well (for example, the child might come into contact with another population where herd protection does not exist) and there will always be strong pragmatic reasons in favour of vaccination even where herd protection does exist (Dawson, 2005, 2007).

COMPULSION?

So we have seen that arguments appealing to both the idea of harm to others and best interests might provide some justification for a moral obligation to vaccinate a child (in at least some circumstances). Let us assume this is the case – does it follow that compulsion is therefore justified? It is important to see that the issue of compulsion is different from that of the existence of a moral obligation. An argument for compulsion requires a further step from our moral condemnation of a parent to inference in the family to bring about a certain end. However, in certain circumstances it might be justified: for example, where the risk of harm was great enough or perhaps where a court orders vaccinations after a parental dispute (Dawson, 2005). Of course, 'compulsion' in the everyday sense implies the use of force or of legal sanctions such as fines. However, related activities might count as 'indirect' compulsion and these can cover a range of cases from the requirement to have vaccinations before enrolment in school to a presumption in favour of vaccination with little possibility to opt out or little attempt to offer the relevant information for an informed consent. Of course, compulsion is a matter of last resort. In many cases there will be strong arguments against, and if it is not proportionate it might actually result in a decline in vaccination uptake. However, some people will be opposed to compulsion on principle, so in the rest of this section I will consider some categorical objections to compulsory childhood vaccination.

First, it might be argued that it can never be appropriate to over rule parents' decisions about vaccinations because vaccination is a preventive rather than a therapeutic measure, and in most cases the diseases are trivial and low-risk. Invoking the powers of the state to interfere in the family in such a case, it could be argued, is just inappropriate. However, it is not clear that this argument will succeed. On the one hand, any attempt to draw a morally significant difference between an action based upon the fact that it is either preventive or therapeutic is potentially problematic. It can be argued that it should be a balance between all relevant harms and benefits that matters (Dawson, 2004). On the other, any risk of disease must be balanced against the risk of vaccination. Any risks of vaccination of common diseases are low. Whilst the risk of contracting such diseases in the developed world are also usually low, if contracted, the potential impact of many of these diseases should not be underestimated. (Neither should it be forgotten that the calculations of such risks and benefits might vary widely depending upon the background societal conditions. In many parts of the developing world, childhood diseases are endemic and millions of children die each year from vaccine-preventable diseases.)

Second, it might be argued that parents can invoke a right to refuse this medical intervention. Presumably such a claim would have to involve some kind of justification for seeing this particular right as taking precedence over other rights, including the right of the child to be protected from potential harm. I do not have space to consider rights discourse in any detail here, but it is worth pointing out that the parents' refusal in this case does not govern their own care, but that of their child. This may make a significant difference to the case. Even if such a right to refuse treatment is held to be central to the debate about vaccinations, it is only likely to block any best interests argument, leaving the harm to others argument untouched.

Third, parents might use another form of appeal to rights. In this case, they may argue that the child has a right to bodily integrity, and that this will be transgressed in the case of compulsory vaccination. Once again, the important thing about rights is that there are many such rights, and that when they are invoked, it is a requirement of their defender to produce an argument not just to say why we have such a right, but to explain why that particular right is supposed to take precedence in our moral deliberations. Although such an argument can, no doubt, be produced, it can surely be contested. Once again, although such a right might, at most, have some claim in relation to arguments about best interests, it is not clear how it might deflect any harm to others argument.

Although all of these objections may be important, as the risk of harm to others from the relevant disease grows, it becomes more and more difficult to hold that any such rights take precedence. Even in relation to best interests, we might doubt whether these arguments are decisive. This is because any deliberations about best interests mean that no parent has an absolute right to do as they want with a child. Parents have a great deal of leeway about how they choose to bring up their children, but there are serious constraints on what will count as legitimately in the best interests of any child.

CONCLUSIONS

These different arguments will work in different ways depending on the nature of the particular disease, vaccine and potential recipient(s). Determining the most relevant and effective vaccination policy is not easy. However, it will certainly involve a consideration of the risks of harm and benefits from vaccination and nonvaccination, as well as more theoretical arguments about harm to others and best interests. Thinking about the ethical issues related to vaccination requires new thinking because the focus of traditional bioethics has been on the individual. This is unhelpful as it misses the fact that vaccination is not just about individuals and their choices but population health as well.

REFERENCES

CDC. Vaccine preventable deaths and the global immunization vision and strategy, 2006–2015. *MMWR* 2006; **55**(18): 511–515; http://www.cdc.gov/mmwr/preview/mmwrhtml/mm5518a4. htm (Accessed 1September 2006).

Cullity G. Moral free riding. *Philos Public Affairs* 1995; **24**(1): 3–34.

Dare T. Mass immunisations programmes: some philosophical issues. *Bioethics* 1998; **12**(2): 125–149.

Dawson A. Vaccination and the prevention problem. *Bioethics* 2004; **18**(6): 515–530.

Dawson A. Herd protection as a public good: vaccination and our obligations to others. In: Dawson A, Verweij M, eds. *Ethics, Prevention and Public Health*. Oxford: Oxford University Press, 2007.

Dawson A. The 'best interests' argument and childhood vaccinations. *Bioethics* 2005; **19**(2): 188–205.

Feinberg J. *Social Philosophy*. Engelwood Cliffs, NJ: Prentice-Hall, 1973.

Institute of Medicine. *Immunization Safety Review: Vaccines and Autism*. Washington: National Academies Press, 2004.

Kretzschmar M, Wallinga J, Teunis P, Xing S, Mikolajczyk R. Frequency of adverse events after vaccination with different Vaccinia strains. *PLoS Med* 2006; **3**(8).

McKeown T. *The Role of Medicine: Dream, Mirage, or Nemesis*. London: The Nuffield Provincial Hospitals Trust, 1976.

Mill JS. *On Liberty* (Reprinted 1974). Harmondsworth: Penguin Books, 1859.

Paul Y. Letter: herd immunity and herd protection. *Vaccine* 2004; **22**: 301–302.

Paul Y, Dawson A. Some ethical issues arising from polio eradication programmes in India. *Bioethics* 2005; **19**(4): 393–406.

Salisbury D, Begg N, eds. *Immunisation against Infectious Diseases*. London: HMSO, 1996.

Selgelid M. Battin M, Smith CB. *Ethics and Infectious Disease*. Oxford: Blackwell, 2006.

Sorell T. Parental choice and expert knowledge in the debate about MMR and autism. In: Dawson A, Verweij M, eds. *Ethics, Prevention and Public Health*. Oxford: Oxford University Press, 2007.

Verweij M, Dawson A. Ethical principles for collective immunisation programmes. *Vaccine* 2004; **22**: 3122–3126.

World Health Organization. *State of the World's Vaccines and Immunization*. Geneva: WHO, 2002.

Yih WK, Lieu TA, Rêgo V H, O'Brien MA, Shay DK, Yokoe DS, Platt R. Attitudes of healthcare workers in U.S. hospitals regarding smallpox vaccination. *BMC Public Health* 2003; **3**: 20.

85

The Patient as Victim and Vector: Bioethics and the Challenge of Infectious Diseases[1]

MARGARET P. BATTIN, LINDA S. CARR-LEE, LESLIE P. FRANCIS,
JAY A. JACOBSON, CHARLES B. SMITH

In our contemporary world, infectious diseases strike frighteningly at the forefront of public awareness, both nationally and internationally. Emerging and re-emerging diseases such as avian flu, severe acute respiratory syndrome (SARS), West Nile virus, Ebola and bovine spongiform encephalopathy, or 'mad cow disease', as well as drug-resistant strains of tuberculosis and HIV/AIDS, generate concerned discussions about national and international agendas. Infectious diseases seem to know no boundaries; environmental degradation, population growth and poverty feed transnational reservoirs of infection that elicit worries about international pandemics and raise concerns over problems of national and international law (Fidler, 1999; Farmer, 2001, 2003). Concerns about the threat of antibiotic resistance fuel fears as pathogenic micro-organisms outrun our capacity to control them. Threats of bioterrorism lead to controversial proposals for surveillance and other major new public health measures, developed, for example, in the Model Emergency Health Powers Act (Gostin, 2003).

However imperative careful attention to infectious diseases appears today, it has not always been so. In the formative years of the field of bioethics – the late 1950s through to the early 1970s – the world looked quite different. Developments in sanitation, immunization and antibiotics, successes in eliminating smallpox and nearly eliminating polio, control through immunization and treatment of diphtheria, tetanus, typhoid, yellow fever, leprosy and plague, and promising research for other diseases, combined to suggest an optimistic picture. Sometime between 1969 and 1972, the US Surgeon General purportedly said that it was time to 'close the book' on infectious diseases.[2] Recent history over the past two decades has clearly shown that the prediction that infectious diseases would be eradicated was premature. Yet, the concepts of bioethics were initially formulated during the period when concerns about decision-making at the end of life and chronic disease were foremost in mind and when ethically significant features that cluster with infectiousness were under-appreciated. This history has affected how discussions in bioethics approached decisive medical issues such as duties to treat, patient confidentiality, informed consent and what contributes to comprehensive and just patient care.

The task of developing a systematic and coherent account of the issues raised by infectious diseases is enormous. When disease is communicable, a patient cannot be seen solely as an individual. This has been the central limitation of bioethics. Infectious diseases show us that the patient must be understood as a patient in relationship to others: others who are the sources of infection, others who might become infected from the patient and others who will be affected by how the patient is treated. As human beings are vulnerable to infectious diseases, we are simultaneously both *victims* and *vectors*, both persons-in-need and persons-as-threat. This duality warrants exploration.

[1]Some of the material in this chapter also appears in *The Patient as Victim and Vector: Ethics and Infectious Disease*, by M. P. Battin, L. P. Francis, J. A. Jacobson, and C. B. Smith (Oxford University Press: in press).

[2]This phrase is quoted in many places. For an example, see the Department of Energy website, http://www.eh.doe.gov/health/news/infectious20040331.pdf (accessed 22 February, 2006). Although the quotation is typically attributed to testimony before Congress, it cannot be corroborated.

Principles of Health Care Ethics, Second Edition   Edited by R.E. Ashcroft, A. Dawson, H. Draper and J.R. McMillan

The characterization of individuals facing the possibility of infectious diseases requires us to rethink the ethical significance of many traditional concepts in bioethics. What is it to be an autonomous agent in the light of communicable disease? How do we understand harm and what do we regard as our duties and responsibilities to one another in a world where infectious diseases force us to acknowledge our shared vulnerability? We see today, all too poignantly, that the individualistic picture that has prevailed in bioethics from its beginnings is incomplete. Philosophical approaches must come to terms with the ethical implications for the concepts of autonomy and rights that infectious diseases teaches us.

INFECTIOUS DISEASES: BIOLOGICAL BASICS AND DISTINCTIVE FEATURES FOR BIOETHICS

To ask what is interestingly different about infectious diseases opens a Pandora's box. There are over 1400 pathogens that can infect human beings – viruses, bacteria, parasites, fungi and prions (von Radowitz, 2006). Some features of infectious diseases are biological; others are social responses to them; still others are combinations.

Infectious diseases are numerous and highly varied, often coming on suddenly and, if left untreated, worsening rapidly. Although some infectious diseases are non-discriminatory, attacking any human, others prey on selective groups. Some primarily affect children; others affect those of any age. Still others prey on the ill, malnourished or weak. Surprisingly, even some infectious diseases disproportionately attack the strong and healthy, such as the flu of 1918, where 18–24-year olds suffered the highest lethality rates (Berry, 2004). We never outgrow our risk of infectious diseases.

Treatment options vary widely for infectious diseases. Many are easily, safely and inexpensively treated in short duration. Most often, treatments for potentially lethal infectious diseases either result in a complete cure, restoring a person to their previous state of healthfulness, or in death. Despite the examples of polio and smallpox, permanent disability is uncommon. Many infectious diseases are easily preventable or limited to a one-time occurrence. However, the unappealing opposite is true for some types of infectious diseases: they can be extraordinarily difficult to manage or can remain entirely untreatable. For example, cold sores caused by the herpes virus can recur over a lifetime and chickenpox can appear in one form only to reappear six to seven decades later in another excruciating form, shingles. Many types of infectious diseases occur in epidemics, produce high mortality rates and often provoke intense fear and emotional and irrational responses.

What distinguishes infectious diseases from other diseases is human interaction with another living organism. Sometimes, complex interactions take the form of communicable or transmissible diseases. One factor that affects whether exposure to an infectious agent results in disease is whether or not antibodies – specific proteins that target and/or neutralize an infectious agent – have formed. Vaccines can stimulate an asymptomatic person to develop antibodies that make them immune to the infectious agent. Vaccines now have been developed for diseases that include measles, mumps, rubella, polio, influenza, diphtheria, tetanus and bacterial meningitis and pneumonia.

We turn to some of the characteristic themes that make up the core of the challenge of infectious diseases for bioethics. These can be broadly classified into discussions about issues of high morbidity and mortality, invasiveness, acuity, communicability, preventability and treatability, host and community susceptibility, and high socio-economic impact.

HIGH MORBIDITY AND MORTALITY

Despite remarkable advances in the eradication, control and treatment of infectious diseases such as smallpox, polio and bacterial infections, infectious diseases continue in the twenty-first century to be among the leading worldwide causes of death and disability (World Health Organization, 2001). Other diseases such as cancer and heart disease have high morbidity and mortality rates, to be sure, but infectious diseases display this quality to both a greater degree and with greater rapidity than most other types of disease. This characteristic sparks ethical debate when government organizations, health professionals or individuals react fearfully to outbreaks – real or potential – altering their own behaviour, or requiring others to alter their behaviour in ethically questionable ways.

When fear of disease becomes a principal decision-making force in clinical and public health decision-making, concerns over just distribution of resources and human rights arise. For example, social programmes that support education, nutrition or economic development (Garrett, 1994) may be shortchanged when funds are redirected to control and treat infections and infectious threats. This occurred in the 2003 outbreak of frequently fatal SARS and in outbreak cases of the highly fatal and contagious Ebola virus, essentially holding commerce and social spending hostage when resources were diverted to intensive hospital care, quarantine and travel and immigration restrictions.

Perceived needs of the community to utilize quarantine and forced therapy to control potentially fatal infectious diseases such as HIV/AIDS and tuberculosis may conflict with rights of autonomy and privacy. In the early 1990s, for example, when New York City public health officials saw that many avoidable deaths were occurring from normally treatable tuberculosis, they instituted mandatory directly observed therapy, significantly restraining people to treat their cases of drug-resistant tuberculosis (Gasner et al., 1999).

Complex dilemmas arise about the proper ethical responsibilities of clinical health care workers. Do health care workers have a duty to treat even though they themselves might become infected or infectious? Do physicians, nurses and hospital employees have a duty to be vaccinated against smallpox – or other infectious diseases – in order to protect themselves, their patients and the public, particularly when there are well-defined potential risks associated with live-virus vaccination? Some of these risks include serious, even fatal illness in those vaccinated, as well as the potential spread of these risks to family, friends or immune-deficient patients.

High morbidity and mortality rates for infectious disease are at least in part attributable to the ability of micro-organisms to mutate rapidly to become resistant to antimicrobials and vaccines (Lappe, 1995). Resistant pathogens have been attributed to increasing and inappropriate usage of antimicrobials in patient care and by the agricultural industry. Both individual patient desire for maximum antibiotic therapy, and the meat and poultry industries' practice of speeding animal weight gain by using antibiotics in animal feed, conflict with community health interests in reducing inappropriate antimicrobial use that contributes to development of resistant microbial pathogens.

INVASIVENESS

Infectious diseases are caused by invasion or attack on humans by foreign micro-organisms. 'Killer viruses', 'flesh-eating strep', 'black death' and other war metaphors capture the notion of enemy attack that pose ethical questions similar to those faced in actual warfare. Consider these questions: what rights do individuals and communities have in defending themselves against such attacks? To what extent are different defensive measures justified? May individuals refuse to defend themselves if this refusal endangers others? Is a paternalistic response ever justified to force people to defend themselves? How are the rights of the individual and of the community to protection from attack at stake in many examples? The experience in 2001 with the 'anthrax letters' and the possibility of bio-terrorism in the United States raised policy and ethical concerns about who should be screened for infection, who should receive limited supplies of prophylactic antibiotics, who should receive a vaccine of uncertain effectiveness and safety profile and what services, such as the mail, should be shut down to protect the public (Rosenbaum and Stolberg, 2001). Ethical discussion abounds on whether increasing funds for public health laboratories and programmes will reduce fearfulness (Fraser and Brown, 2000) or possibly undermine confidence in the effectiveness of the military, FBI and other government officials if fear of the risks of bioterrorism result in exaggerations and lies (Sidel et al., 2002).

In the case of diseases such as HIV/AIDS, public opinion may sometimes see the infected individual who transmits as the attacker, a victim not of some foreign aggressor but of their own behaviour, and the person to whom it is transmitted as the true victim – though often also a victim of their own behaviour. The notion of patient as victim *and* vector exposes this point of view as simplistic and reveals a more complex picture. The characteristic of invasiveness – the idea of enemy attack – suggests an obligation to the victim of infectious diseases despite the fact that this victim is also the 'attacker' or vector.

ACUITY

Infectious diseases such as meningitis, pneumonia, bacterial septicaemia and haemorrhagic viral infections can develop and progress to fatal outcomes in less than 24 h. This acuity leads to fear and rapid decision-making, often before a definitive diagnosis is available. Hasty decisions may make poor public health policy: schools may be closed, communities evacuated or people may flee, making it difficult for public health officials to conduct needed prophylaxis and immunization programmes. Infected individuals may be deprived of their rights as rapid progression of the disease prohibits the time necessary for reasoned, informed consent.

The rights of autonomous agents to choose maximum therapy may also conflict with community rights to discourage antibiotic prescriptions in an effort to curtail development of resistant pathogens. In cases of acute infectious diseases of unclear aetiology, for example, therapeutic efficacy may initially require that a patient be treated with multiple antibiotics (Jacobs, 1999).

COMMUNICABILITY

Different patterns of communicability may raise different ethical issues when the patient is a risk to the community in general, when the patient is a risk to health care providers, and when health care providers pose a risk to their patients. In each type of situation, who poses the risk, who can best avoid the risk, who should take preventive measures and who should bear the costs of prevention, need to be addressed.

Whenever infectious diseases strike, interactive behaviours must be altered at some point. Difficult questions of individual choice and public health and safety must be weighed to determine which behaviours can justifiably be required to be altered and what degree of force can be used to achieve the altered behaviour. The case of a hospital that refuses to accept smallpox patients should an outbreak occur shows that institutions as well as individuals may react fearfully to communicable diseases. Questions about who should bear the costs of requirements cannot be ignored.

Sometimes behavioural associations with infectious diseases have led to effective but controversial public health practices that conflict with particular community religious and moral values. Examples include condom use to reduce the spread of venereal diseases such as syphilis, gonorrhoea and HIV, and needle exchange programmes that provide clean syringes to drug addicts to decrease the spread of HIV and hepatitis.

Sometimes the public's fear of communicable infections far exceeds the actual risk. Exiled leper communities are an historical example. Debate among medical ethicists and political leaders over quarantine proposals for drug-resistant tuberculosis or avian flu home in on this concern (Campio, 1999). We must keep in mind that fear-induced, overly restrictive practices may make victims of those they affect. When HIV-infected children such as Ryan White were excluded from school, or when some physicians and other health care workers refuse to care for HIV/AIDS patients, we ought to keep in mind that these patients are victims as much as they are potential vectors of the disease they carry, and are deserving of our respect.

The complexity of the concept of patient seen as victim and vector is brought into particularly stark relief when a physician, nurse or other caregiver becomes the patient with a potentially lethal infectious disease (Ippolito et al., 1999). When caregivers refuse to treat infected patients because of the risks of communicability and yet when infected with these viruses continue to practise their profession in ways that increase risk of transmission to their patients, the ethics of professionalism are challenged (DeVille, 1994).

PREVENTABILITY AND TREATABILITY

Most infectious diseases are preventable and treatable. Heated ethical discussions centre on the dilemma that if we have effective therapies and preventive measures, why are infectious diseases still major causes of mortality? Sometimes preferences of the communities themselves are cited to explain this dilemma: religious convictions to refuse immunization, personal fears about side effects or concerns about the actual effectiveness of immunizations. In explanations of this sort, the ethical debate turns to questions about the extent to which comparatively disease-free nations, or nations in which a particular disease has not spread, should impose preventative measures on disease-afflicted countries that prefer to opt out? On the contrary, many patients in underdeveloped nations are unable to receive appropriate therapy for their infections due to the high cost of antimicrobials. The desire of drug manufacturers to protect their patents and related profits, citing intellectual property rights for antibiotics, conflicts with the therapy needs of ill patients in poor countries. The recent heated dialogue over availability of much less expensive generic anti-HIV medications in developing countries, such as Brazil, India, Kenya and South Africa, arises from these ethical tensions.

An additional concern centres on the concept of 'herd immunity'. Vaccines for infectious diseases such as polio,

measles, chickenpox and smallpox have been effective not only for individual recipients, but also in reducing the incidence of these infections in whole communities. Due to herd immunity, the minority who for allergic, immune-compromised or sensitivity issues cannot be vaccinated, receive protection. Ethical issues arise when individuals, families or religious groups assert the right to refuse vaccination for non-health-related reasons, essentially refusing to accept the rare but unavoidable risks vaccinated people take, receiving a 'free ride' and increasing the overall risks to the remaining population to infection (Ross and Aspinwell, 1997). Should vaccination be required?

HOST AND COMMUNITY SUSCEPTIBILITY

The general health of the host determines the susceptibility and resulting morbidity and mortality rates of many infectious diseases such as tuberculosis, enteric pathogens and acute respiratory tract diseases. High mortality rates for common infant diarrhoeas and childhood respiratory tract infections seen in malnourished children in poor African nations (Rosenstein et al., 2001) and in wartime refugee camps exemplify this. This realization leads to debates over the just distribution of community resources where it has been argued that limited resources should be spent on adequate nutrition before more expensive, possibly less effective medical services.

Ethical discussions about treatment of infectious diseases in end-of-life cases also recognize that patients dying of cancer or other debilitating diseases are often more susceptible to infectious diseases such as pneumonia. Treatment of the infection may simply prolong a deteriorating status quo, which has prompted some patients to refuse antibiotics in episodes of pneumonia much as they might refuse respirators, chemotherapy and other life-prolonging therapy.

The general health of the community environment – sanitation, hygiene, availability of clean air, water and food, adequate nutrition and control of mosquitoes and other vectors of infectious diseases – determines susceptibility to many infectious diseases, raising issues of justice and human rights (Whitman, 2000). WHO estimates that at least two-thirds of the world's population lacks safe sanitation and one quarter lacks access to safe water (Whitman, 2000). Poverty-related lack of hygiene and increased susceptibility to infectious diseases are problematic in developed countries such as France and the United States where outbreaks of tuberculosis, diphtheria and louse-borne trench fever have occurred among the homeless (Brouqui et al., 1999). So, too, are war-associated refugee camps with high attack rates and mortality from measles, cholera, infantile diarrhoeas, acute respiratory tract diseases and malaria (Whitman, 2000). In most wars, morbidity and mortality from infectious diseases have exceeded those of military actions.

HIGH SOCIO-ECONOMIC IMPACT

Infectious diseases can wreak havoc on economies and communities. Recent 'mad cow' outbreaks in British and Canadian cattle of the fatal neurological disease, bovine spongiform encephalopathy, associated with over 130 cases of variant Creutzfeldt-Jakob disease, a similar fatal neurological disease in humans (Probable Variant Creutzfeldt-Jakob disease in a US resident-Florida, 2002), demonstrated the economic impact of infectious diseases when hundreds of thousands of cattle were slaughtered and imports of beef from infected herds and countries were embargoed. The deterioration of community socioeconomic status is seen most strikingly in those countries where as many as 25% of the working age population are taken out of the workforce due to HIV/AIDS. The 2002 Macroeconomics and Health Report to the WHO recognized that economic growth is not possible without a healthy population (Banta, 2002). This testifies to the need for a more just distribution of resources between rich and poor nations. In the 2002 meeting of the World Health Assembly, the Commission on Macroeconomics and Health reported that the world now has the capability of ending poverty and poverty-associated diseases for the first time in history: the cost to the rich, developed countries would only be one cent out of every $10 of gross national product (Banta, 2002). By 2005, the United Nations had increased the suggested level of support to five cents (0.5%) out of every $10 of GNP, and five countries (Norway, Denmark, Luxembourg, Sweden and the Netherlands) had each achieved a higher level by giving 0.7% of GNP (Dugger, 2005). Countries of the EU had agreed to meet the 0.7% funding level by 2015 (World Summit Examines Progress, 2005).

NEW PARADIGMS FOR BIOETHICS: EMBEDDED AUTONOMY

In the light of what infectious diseases teach us, our paradigms for bioethics are in urgent need of expansion. To better understand how critical lessons of infectious diseases failed to be incorporated into the traditional paradigms bioethics uses today, it behooves us to travel back to the late 1950s through to the early 1970s when bioethics was developing conceptually. Civil rights, environmental protection and aspirations of ending human poverty were the focus of activism and legislation. *Brown* v *Board of Education* (1954), the Civil Rights Act of 1964, the National Environmental Policy Act of 1964, the 1965 institution of Medicare, the Age Discrimination in Employment Act of 1967, the Clean Air Act of 1970 and the Clean Water Act of 1972 are representative examples of these concerns. Public health was increasingly addressing environmental hazards and problematic health behaviours such as asbestos exposure, smoking and obesity. Infectious diseases were almost nowhere to be found.

Bioethics, firmly grounded in the hallmark doctor–patient relationship and the individualism of clinical medicine, originated as a contrast to the aggregative, population-based approaches of public health. Bioethics studied dilemmas physicians faced at the bedside – whether to tell dying patients the truth, whether to reveal confidential information, or whether to limit patients' liberties for their own good. Issues explored arose in situations like coma and terminal illness, organ transplantation and dialysis, and reproductive failure, including abnormal pregnancy and neonatal deficit and human experimentation. Conditions at issue were congenital anomalies, brain injuries, cancers, renal failure and heart disease. Challenges included life-extending technologies in compromised persons, problems of social justice such as access to health care, and discrimination based on race, disability or age.

Infectious diseases caught the attention of bioethics when the cause of HIV/AIDS was identified as a virus in the early 1980s, but instead of spearheading an exploration into the theoretical challenges that infectious diseases that are communicable from person to person poses more broadly for bioethics, HIV/AIDS was treated as 'exceptional'. Perhaps because HIV/AIDS did not press other challenging characteristics of infectious diseases, such as rapid lethality or widespread transmission among strangers, or perhaps because both the areas of inquiry for bioethics and a core set of normative principles defined as the prevailing philosophical approach were already established by the time HIV/AIDS came on the scene, concern with the characteristic features of infectious diseases continued to play virtually no role in the development of bioethics.

To be sure, the Tuskegee studies of deliberately untreated syphilis in black men, the Willowbrook studies of institutionalized children intentionally infected with hepatitis, and end-of-life controversies about letting terminally ill patients succumb to pneumonia ('the old man's friend') were addressed in bioethics during this time. But the consuming focus of bioethics in each of these matters of concern was *not* the characteristics of infectiousness, but rather the vulnerability of the study populations, coercion in institutional settings, civil rights and racial discrimination and exploitation. That the diseases involved were transmissible from one to another was largely overlooked. Gregory Pence (1990) observed, virtually alone, that 'an especially troubling fact to critics was that no effort was made to survey syphilis in wives and children of subjects, and that the researchers took a chance on the possibility that wives of subjects might be infected or re-infected or children might be born with congenital syphilis'. Another illustrative example of this pattern of ignoring infectiousness during this period is a case discussion, 'The Homosexual Husband and Physician Confidentiality', in *The Hastings Center Report* (Kuschner, 1982). In analysing what is appropriate for physicians to discuss with patients, the issue is framed as one about homosexuality and confidentiality, not one about infectiousness and confidentiality. In a discussion of whether a physician should reveal a fiancé's sexual orientation to his prospective spouse, that the fiancé presents with sexually transmitted diseases is completely ignored.

These illustrations are not unique. Our review of 19 of the most widely used texts in bioethics, dating from the 1950s to 1984 (before the advent of HIV/AIDS), and confirmed by a survey of the traditional dilemma cases and histories of the field of bioethics, found that systematic discussion of ethical problems raised by communicable infectious diseases was manifestly absent in early texts, mentioned infrequently, if at all. Jonsen et al. (1982) is the one exception that presents acute infectious diseases as a model of clinical care and addresses the ethical concerns of the model (MacKensie and Stoljar, 2000). But their discussion neither presents the kind of sustained treatment other types of examples receive, such as the withdrawal of life-sustaining treatment in a patient in a persistent vegetative state, nor recognizes the full range of characteristics of infectious diseases.

By the mid-1980s texts began to discuss HIV/AIDS, but AIDS 'exceptionalism' discouraged investigations into infectious diseases more generally. HIV/AIDS provoked attention to some issues raised by communicable infectious diseases – attention to confidentiality, duty to warn, risks to providers and the just distribution of resources when people pose risks of harm to each other – but these were treated inadequately due to AIDS' particular mode of transmission and activism about civil liberties. Theoretical developments in bioethics remained untested by some features typical of many infectious diseases, high acuity, for example, often associated with airborne or waterborne diseases. Were bioethics to have been so tested, the issues raised by communicable infectious diseases would have forced us to recognize that individuals are socially and physically situated in a distinctive way – not just as individuals who are located in a social nexus, but as transmitters and receivers of each other's pathogens, foci of victimhood and vectorhood in relation to others.

The complexities of infectious diseases challenge bioethics to develop more complicated accounts of at least four aspects of traditional liberal concepts: the individual agent, autonomy, the harm principle and responsibility. Bioethics must reassess the conventional notion of the individual agent to capture the complexity and vulnerability our biology demands. We cannot think of ourselves as independent, individual agents whose liberties are to be restricted. We are not independent, but all live together in a web of potential and actual disease, all the time, even when we are

not aware of the possibility of transmission. We must think of ourselves as agents who are constantly 'embedded' in potential circumstances of microbial exchange, whether this exchange is reciprocal, linked sequentially in a series of transmissions or exponentially widespread. The picture of human reality informed by infectious diseases cannot dichotomize the individual against the community as communitarian accounts do, for in an important sense, we *are* our microbial environment. Essentially, this account of individual agency takes the feminist emphasis on relationality (MacKensie and Stoljar, 2000) from a local to a universal level: the individual, in addition to standing in an interconnected nexus of social and biological relationships that include family, ancestry, reproduction and societal and cultural ties, is shown by the characteristics of infectious diseases also to include physical, biological relationships that are accidental and among strangers (May, 2005). We are all constantly and simultaneously victims and vectors, interconnected as individuals, community members and as inhabitants of a global world.

Individual agency seen in this light acknowledges our universally shared, inescapable vulnerability based on the complexity of our interconnections with constellations of other vulnerable organisms – other people like ourselves. As long as unpreventable, uncontained infectious diseases exist, we cannot fully insulate ourselves and may pose urgent threats to one another. We all share in the burdens and benefits of these biological facts. The expanded awareness of this new picture invites needed attention to issues such as confidentiality and privacy, for example, in disease-containment strategies like mandated reporting, contact tracing, mandatory immunization and global surveillance.

Traditional accounts of autonomy posit the ideal of a thoughtful, rational chooser who decides on a course of action according to personal preferences and interests. This picture is undercut by the concept of the embedded agent, for it fails to adequately account for the possibilities of unknown and interlocking risks that transmissible infectious diseases pose. So are our accounts of harm and responsibility. For example, the acuity of some infectious diseases militates against reflective decision-making; the capacity for permanent prevention may reshape assessments of risk and benefit; and the complex infective mechanisms of communicable disease may work against some philosophical accounts of autonomy as informed by plans. Our interests are not always clearly distinct from those of society or of the world at large. We are non-electively related in our vulnerability. We need to think through how to deal with potentially harmful situations so that we all are protected from infectious diseases and so that the burdens of protection are fairly shared. We must enhance our understanding of autonomy, harm, responsibility and their implications

always to consider the general point that we are always potential victims and potential vectors in relationship to each
other and to the natural world.

It is time for bioethics to carefully reassess the full social
and physical character of our relationships with each other
in the context of communicable infectious diseases. Protecting our individuality and autonomy, the traditional hallmark
goal of bioethics, expands to protecting our interrelatedness
once we recognize the risks that we pose to one another
as victims and vectors. Our embeddedness among others
who, like us, are way-stations of disease, cuts against binary
judgments that we are either responsible or not responsible,
blameworthy or not blameworthy. Judgments about what
people ought to do, when we can restrict their liberties and
what we owe them in return must be seen not only as individual but also as shared distributive problems. Judgments
of individual responsibility appropriate in the cases of deliberate transmission or known risks must be supplemented
by judgments about how we together are responsible for
reservoirs of infectiousness. We must respond fairly to
these burdens, recognizing both parts of our human reality, victimhood and vectorhood. As members of the public,
we must understand and keep in mind our individuality as
victims as well as vectors, and that as autonomous agents,
we must understand and keep in mind our interconnectedness as *vectors* as well as victims.

RESPECT, COMPENSATION AND RECIPROC-
ITY: DEVELOPING A POSITIVE THEORY OF THE
OBLIGATIONS OF PEOPLE TO EACH OTHER IN
A WORLD OF TRANSMISSIBLE INFECTIOUS
DISEASES

In public policy issues, extensive debate centres on the
justice of quarantine, isolation, involuntary immunization
and other highly restrictive measures to contain infectious
threats. There has been endless discussions of whether constraints may be used and if so, in what contexts. What has
not been significantly discussed in the literature is what we
owe to those who are being or have been constrained (Harris
and Holm, 1995). Responses to constraint appropriately include adequate and rapid diagnosis, effective treatment and
compensation for identifiable losses, including, but not limited to, losses of income, destroyed property and business or
financial interests. But this does not exhaust what we owe
each other in cases of willing or unwilling constraint. There
is much work to be done in exploring these issues and in
developing a positive theory. As infectious diseases teach
us that we are all both victims of and vectors to one another, we come to recognize that simple compensation for
constraint, where it is even possible, may not be adequate
and that something more is called for when individuals voluntarily participate, or are required to participate, or are

physically or legally forced to participate in measures to
reduce the transmission of infectious diseases.

At a minimum, we owe each other mutual respect, not
just as victims but because we are at the same time cast in
the role of largely unwilling potential vectors, a role we do
not normally choose but which carries with it substantial
ethical implications. It is spelling out the tangible manifestations of respect for each other as both victims *and* also
vectors that requires further reflection. As we see ourselves
in these dual and unavoidable roles, notions of reciprocity
capture some of the sense that we must act in mutually cooperative ways – even in submitting to constraints – if we
are to reduce the burdens of disease that threaten us all and
with which we threaten each other. Obligations of reciprocity also ground the claim that we must also act coopera-
tively in the face of disease if we are to protect our mutual
liberties. Yet duties of reciprocity may not fully address the
issue of what we owe those who have been or are being constrained, and the theoretical question remains as follows:
what more we ought to do for the victims and vectors of infectious diseases – not only others, of course, but ourselves
as well. This is uncharted territory for bioethics, territory
that, in our contemporary world – as we face emerging and
re-emerging diseases as well as familiar plagues, as we see
the risks of antibiotic resistance and the threat of weapons
utilizing infectious diseases – it is newly imperative to
explore.

REFERENCES

Banta D. Economic development: key to healthier world. *J Am Med
Assoc* 2002; 287: 3195–3197.

Berry JM. *The Great Influenza*. New York: Penguin Books, 2004.

Brouqui P, Lascola B, Roux V, Raoult D, Chronic bartonella quintana
bacteremia in homeless patients. *NEJM* 1999; **340**: 184–189.

Brown v. Board of Education of Topeka. 347 U.S. 483, 1954.

Campio EW. Liberty and the control of tuberculosis. *N Engl J Med*
1999; **1340**: 385–386.

DeVille KS. Nothing to fear but fear itself: HIV-infected physicians and the law of informed consent. *J Law Med Ethics* 1994;
22: 163–175.

Dugger CW. U.N. Panel urges doubling of aid to cut poverty. *New
York Times*, International section, January 18, 2005; p. A1;
A18.

Farmer P. *Infections and Inequalities: The Modern Plagues*.
Berkeley, CA: University of California Press, 2001.

Farmer P. *Pathologies of Power: Health, Human Rights, and the
New War on the Poor*. Berkeley, CA: University of California
Press, 2003.

Fidler DP. *International Law and Infectious Diseases*. Oxford:
Clarendon Press, 1999.

Fraser MR, Brown DL. Bioterrorism preparedness and local public
health agencies: building response capacity. *Public Health Rep*
2000; **115**: 326–330.

Garrett L. *The Coming Plague: Newly Emerging Diseases in a World Out of Balance*. New York: Penguin Books, 1994; pp. 192–221.

Gasner MR, Maw KL, Feldman GE, *et al*. The use of legal action in New York City to ensure treatment of tuberculosis. *N Engl J Med* 1999; **340**: 359–366.

Gostin LO. The model state emergency health powers act: public health and civil liberties in a time of terrorism. *Health Matrix* 2003; **13**: 3–32.

Harris J, Holm S. Is there a moral obligation not to infect others? *BMJ* 1995; **311**: 1215–1217.

Ippolito G, Puro V, Heptonstal J, et al. Occupational human immunodeficiency virus infection in health care workers: worldwide cases through September 1997. *Clin Inf Dis* 1999; **28**: 365–383.

Jacobs MR. Emergence of antibiotic resistance in upper and lower respiratory tract infections. *Am J Manage Care* 1999; **5**: S651–661.

Jonsen AR, Siegler M, Winslade WJ. *Clinical Ethics*. New York: Macmillan, 1982.

Kuschner H. The homosexual husband and physician confidentiality. In: Levine C, Veatch RM, eds. *Cases in Bioethics from The Hastings Center Report*. New York: The Hastings Center, 1982; p. 20.

Lappe M. *Breakout: The Evolving Threat of Drug-Resistant Disease*. San Francisco, CA: Sierra Club Books, 1995; pp. 69–92.

MacKensie C, Stoljar N. *Relational Autonomy: Feminist Perspectives on Autonomy, Agency, and the Social Self*. New York: Oxford University Press, 2000.

May T. The concept of autonomy in bioethics: an unwarranted fall from grace. In: Taylor JS, ed. *Personal Autonomy: New Essays on Personal Autonomy and its Role in Contemporary Moral Philosophy*. Cambridge: Cambridge University Press, 2005, pp. 299–309.

Pence G, *Classic Cases in Medical Ethics*. Boston, MA: McGraw-Hill, editions 1990, 1995, 2000, 2004.

Probable Variant Creutzfeldt-Jakob disease in a US resident-Florida, 2002. *Mortal Morbid Weekly Rep* 2002; **51**: 927–929.

Rosenbaum DE, Stolberg SG. A Nation Challenged: The Vaccine. *New York Times*, section B, column 5, 20 December, 2001; p.1.

Rosenstein NE, Perkins BA, Stephens DS, et al. Meningococcal disease. *NEJM* 2001; **344**: 1378–1388.

Ross LF, Aspinwell T. Religious exemptions to the immunization statutes: balancing public health and religious freedom. *J Law Med Ethics* 1997; **25**: 202–293.

Sidel VW, Gould RM, Cohen HW. Bioterrorism Preparedness: Cooptation of Public Health. *Med Global Survival* 2002; **7**: 82–89.

von Radowitz J. Animals *Spreading Many More Diseases to Humans*. Press Association Newsfile, 20 February 2006 (quoting Mark Woolhouse speaking at meetings of the AAAS).

Whitman J, ed. Refugee infections. *The Politics of Emerging and Resurgent Infectious Diseases*. NY: St. Martin's Press, 2000; Chapter 6.

Whitman J, ed. *The Politics of Emerging and Resurgent Infectious Diseases*. New York: Palgrave Macmillan, 2000.

World Health Organization. *The World Health Report*. Geneva, Switzerland: The World Health Organization, 2001; pp. 144–155.

World Summit Examines Progress in Meeting Development Financing Commitments Made Five Years Ago in Monterrey. U.S. Fed. News, 14 September, 2005.

86

Bioterrorism, Society and Health Care Ethics

MICHAEL J. SELGELID

INTRODUCTION

This chapter reviews the history of biological weapons, explains why the threat of bioterrorism is taken so seriously at the beginning of the twenty-first century and examines ethical issues associated with bioterrorism most relevant to those working in health care. Health care ethical issues related to bioterrorism fall into two main categories: those related to patient treatment and those related to biomedical research. Ethical issues in treatment include questions about education, triage and health care workers' duties to expose themselves to danger in order to care for patients. Ethical issues in research include questions about the extent to which dual-use research – that which could be used for both beneficent and malevolent purposes – should be controlled.

HISTORICAL BACKGROUND

Though concerns about biological weapons and bioterrorism have grown dramatically since 11 September 2001 and the anthrax attacks that followed, the use of biological agents as weapons is not a new phenomenon. Biological weapons have a long, dark history. Partly due to recent advances in biomedical science, however, there is reason to fear that the danger of biological weapons is greater than ever before.

The earliest examples of biological weapons' use go back to ancient times. Hannibal, for example, 'ordered the launch of viper-filled vessels upon enemy ships of Pergamus in 190 B.C.' (Sutton, 2005); and ancient Greeks and Romans poisoned the wells of enemies with carrion (Block, 2001). Alexander

the Great is believed to have 'catapulted the bodies of dead men over the walls of besieged cities, possibly as a means of spreading disease and inciting terror' (National Research Council, 2004, p. 34); and on the Crimean Peninsula in the mid-fourteenth century, the Tartars catapulted dead bodies of plague victims over the walls of Caffa to Genoese adversaries. The latter's subsequent return home on plague-infested ships is the standard explanation of how the Black Death reached Europe in 1346, sparking an epidemic that killed one third of the European population in just four years.

Other salient historical episodes involve the use of smallpox as a weapon in the New World. During the French and Indian Wars, for example, Sir Jeffrey Amherst famously made the request:

> 'Could it not be contrived to Send the *Small Pox* among those Disaffected Tribes of Indians? . . . We must, on this occasion, Use Every Stratagem in our power to Reduce them.' In response to Amherst's recommendation, [Colonel] Bouquet replied . . . 'I will try to inoculate . . . by means of some blankets that may fall in their Hands, taking care however not to get the disease myself' (Tucker, 2001, p. 20).

The British Army was also accused of using smallpox against the colonial army during the Revolutionary War, and US government agents allegedly gave smallpox-infected blankets to Plains Indians during the 1800s (National Research Council, 2004).

Major twentieth-century examples include Germany's use of anthrax and glanders against enemy livestock during the First World War; the Japanese poisoning of over 1000 wells in Chinese villages with typhus and cholera, and the Japanese aerial bombing of Chinese cities with jars

Principles of Health Care Ethics, Second Edition   Edited by R.E. Ashcroft, A. Dawson, H. Draper and J.R. McMillan
© 2007 John Wiley & Sons, Ltd

containing plague-infested fleas, during the Second World War (Frischknecht, 2003).

BAN ON BIOLOGICAL WEAPONS

Though the United States and other major industrialized countries had signed the Geneva Protocol of 1925 which ruled out the *use* of biological weapons, the United States was actively engaged in offensive biological weapons research, on anthrax and its dispersal among numerous other things, from 1942 until 1969 when President Nixon called for a ban on offensive biological weapons research. The reasons for getting out of the business of biological weapons included the fact that biological weapons are so unpredictable and hard to control and the fact that they are relatively cheap and easy to make in comparison with nuclear weapons. The latter point was that this was not a good area to become involved in an arms race insofar as biological weapons have the potential to serve as poor countries' weapons of mass destruction (Miller et al., 2001). Such thinking soon led to the Convention on the Prevention of the Development, Production and Stockpiling of Bacteriological (Biological) and Toxin Weapons and on Their Destruction, which was signed in 1972 and came into effect in 1975. Known as the BTWC, this treaty requires in Article I that

> Each State Party to this Convention undertakes never in any circumstances to develop, produce, stockpile, or otherwise acquire or retain:
>
> Microbial or other biological agents, or toxins whatever their origin or method of production, of types and in quantities that have no justification for prophylactic, protective or other peaceful purposes;
>
> Weapons, equipment or means of delivery designed to use such agents or toxins for hostile purposes or in armed conflict (BTWC, 1972).

Though the BTWC also required that any already existing biological weapons be destroyed or diverted to peaceful purposes, it did (and does) allow for possession of and research on biological agents for defensive purposes (Nixendorff and Bender, 2002). A well-known, and currently controversial, weakness of the BTWC, in the meanwhile, is its lack of teeth insofar as it fails to call for verification mechanisms.

SOVIET SCIENCE

Perhaps, (partly) as a result of this weakness, the BTWC unfortunately failed to bring an end to biological weapons development. Though a signatory to the BTWC, the former Soviet Union secretly ran an enormous biological weapons

programme called 'Biopreparat' until its fall in the early 1990s. Developing and producing a long list of biological weapons agents, at peak levels they had the capacity to produce 1500 (metric) tonnes of tularemia, 4500 tonnes of anthrax, 150 tonnes of Venezuelan equine encephalitis virus, 1500 tonnes of *Yersinia pestis* (bubonic plague), 100 tonnes of smallpox, 2000 tonnes of glanders and 250 tonnes of Marburg virus (similar to Ebola) yearly (Miller et al., 2001). Their research and development efforts included a project aimed at engineering a 'chimera' of smallpox and ebola – with the hope of producing a virus as contagious as the former and as deadly as the latter.

The Soviets reportedly succeeded in engineering a vaccine-resistant strain of anthrax and multidrug–resistant strains of anthrax, glanders and plague (Alibek and Handelman, 1999). These and other horrors were revealed by former Deputy Director of Biopreparat Ken Alibek who defected to the United States and revealed all to the CIA – and then to the public in a book titled *Biohazard: The Chilling True Story of the Largest Covert Weapons Program in the World – Told from the Inside by the Man who Ran it*.

A central reason why the threat of bioterrorism is taken so seriously at present relates to the fact that, given the small size of microbes, proliferation is so much easier in the context of biological weapons in comparison with nuclear weapons. Destruction of Soviet biological weapons, including intercontinental missiles loaded with smallpox, has never been verified. The whereabouts of most of the 60 000 Biopreparat scientists – who would obviously make attractive recruits for, or potential suppliers of, 'rogue nations' or terrorist organizations – are presently unknown.

SMALLPOX

The possibility of smallpox proliferation is especially troubling. Smallpox usually tops lists of feared biological weapons agents. This disease, for which there is no known treatment, is highly contagious and kills a third of its victims. Smallpox is believed to have killed more people than any other infectious disease in history and 300–500 million people during the twentieth century alone – that is, three times more people than were killed in all the wars of that period (Oldstone, 1998). As routine vaccination ended worldwide when eradication was declared in 1980, and earlier in many industrialized nations, the world population now lacks smallpox immunity. Most of the world's population has never been vaccinated against smallpox, and the immunity of those who have been vaccinated has probably worn off with time. Experts believe that if smallpox is in fact used as a weapon, this could spark a global epidemic causing the devastation expected from (perhaps a series of) nuclear attack(s).

That the United States takes such threats seriously is revealed by its post -11 September stockpiling of smallpox vaccine, its mandatory vaccination of hundreds of thousands of military personnel against smallpox and its failed attempt (starting in 2003) to have 10 million 'first-responders' (i.e. health and emergency workers) vaccinated on a voluntary basis. The latter programme failed because very few health and emergency workers volunteered to be vaccinated because of fears about dangerous vaccine side effects, uncertainty about the extent to which compensation would be provided if such complications were suffered and because specific details regarding smallpox proliferation – and thus the likelihood of a smallpox attack – remained largely unknown.

RECENT INCIDENTS

Current concern about bioterrorism can also be partly explained by a number of more recent incidents involving biological weapons use. In 1984, for example, the Rajneeshee cult poisoned salad bars with *Salmonella* in The Dalles, Oregon, with the hope of winning an election by making those who would vote for political opponents sick. Another cult organization called Aum Shinrikyo – perhaps most famous for the sarin gas attack on the Tokyo subway in 1995, killing 13 people and injuring 5000 – 'staged as many as a dozen unsuccessful germ attacks [with anthrax and other agents] in Japan from 1990 to 1995' (Miller et al., 2001, p. 154). Last but not the least, of course, were the anthrax attacks in the United States in 2001. In this case, anthrax powder sent through the mail to government and media offices led to 22 infections, five deaths and significant social disruption. Though none of these incidents caused large-scale casualties, they reveal terrorists' willingness to use biological weapons to cause death and disorder.

MODERN SCIENCE

The final reason why the threat of bioterrorism is taken so seriously is the fact that recent advances in the life sciences may enable production of more dangerous biological weapons than previously would have been possible. Scientific developments which enable better understanding and control of human health can also facilitate biological weapons development. Genetic engineering techniques might lead to the development of preventative or life-saving 'genetic therapies', for example, but they could also be used to develop more dangerous strains of disease. The growing understanding of the mechanisms of disease can likewise be used for both beneficial and sinister purposes. In an unclassified document titled 'The Darker Bioweapons Future', the CIA (2003) claims that:

A panel of life sciences experts convened for the Strategic Assessments Group by the National Academy of Sciences concluded that advances in biotechnology . . . have the potential to create a much more dangerous biological warfare (BW) threat. The panel noted [that] the effects of some of these engineered biological agents could be worse than any disease known to man . . . The same science that may cure some of our worst diseases could be used to create the world's most frightening weapons.

It is, among other things, possible that increased understanding of human genetics will enable development of a 'new generation' of biological agents that target specific individuals or ethnic groups. (Targeting of the latter, however, is generally considered less scientifically feasible.)

BIOTERRORISM AND HEALTH CARE ETHICS

PATIENT CARE

Education

The increased threat of bioterrorism poses significant ethical challenges and duties for those working in health care. Physicians need to look out for unusual symptoms in patients and report suspect cases to authorities (in accordance with local guidelines), for example, because reduction of impact in the event of a biological attack will depend on early recognition of disease outbreak. In order to recognize diseases most likely to result from biological attack, those working in health care need to familiarize themselves with the nature and symptoms of (perhaps rare or exotic) diseases they would otherwise not likely have experience with. The first duty of health workers related to the bioterrorist threat is thus educational. Primary care physicians must increase their own awareness of the bioterrorist threat, the kinds of diseases likely to be used as biological weapons, and the ways in which such diseases would present in clinical cases.

Triage

In the event of a massive disease outbreak that could potentially result from a successful biological attack, it is possible that hospitals and the health care system will lack the capacity to provide care for everyone who needs it. If there are not enough medical personnel, drugs or other resources such as beds to provide for everyone in need, then a different – and more severe – kind of triage than that usually employed in hospital emergency rooms will be required. While standard emergency room triage involves making decisions about *the order* in which patients will be treated based on the urgency of patients' needs; in a catastrophic situation that could result from a bioterrorist attack, triage may require making decisions that some patients will not receive treatment at all. In extreme situations, '[p]ractitioners must prioritize intervention to those who will benefit most from the fewest resources' (Pesik et al., 2001, p. 644). If there are not enough resources for everyone, then some must be turned away or simply, but sadly, left to die. Though familiar to military medical personnel on battlefields, ordinary domestic health workers will not have faced this kind of situation on such a scale before. In contrast to the ethical basis of other aspects of health care – where there is an emphasis on things like the primacy of each patient and patient autonomy – the ethics of triage is widely considered to be inherently utilitarian. '[S]ystems of triage', according to Childress, 'were designed to produce the greatest good for the greatest number by meeting human needs most effectively and efficiently under conditions of scarcity' (Childress, 2003). (Alternative forms of rationing – on a first-come first-served basis, or by lottery, for example – are imaginable. And even a utility-maximizing triage might be justified on non-utilitarian grounds, e.g. via social contract.)

Insofar as the importance of each person's health is given equal weight in utilitarian triage calculus, an egalitarian element is central to the ethics of triage. A difficult question, however, is the extent to which *social utility* should be taken into account when making decisions about who will receive limited medical resources. Should special priority be given to health care workers themselves, for example, when allocating limited drug and/or vaccine supplies? Because the health of such personnel is a precondition of others receiving treatment, this kind of priority would often be called for. Insofar as possible, however, relevant policy should be debated and formulated ahead of time via public, transparent processes in order to increase public trust in both the capacity and fairness of the health care system (Pesik et al., 2001; Childress, 2003).

Duty to Treat

A major ethical issue relevant to infectious diseases in general, and thus bioterrorism in particular, is the question of the extent to which health care workers should be expected to expose themselves to danger when caring for patients. In the event of a biological attack or other infectious disease outbreak, treating patients may involve risks of exposure to contagious deadly diseases. When the disease suffered by patients is (perhaps novel and) not well understood, with regard to the degree and mechanisms of contagion, the extent of risk to health workers will be uncertain. This situation was common both in the early days of HIV/AIDS and also more recently during the SARS crisis of 2003. Should health care workers be expected to – and do they have ethical duties to – treat patients when doing so could endanger their own lives and also the lives of their family members who may subsequently become infected?

Facing some danger is undoubtedly part of a health worker's job; and the fact that risks are involved with this kind of work is something that any health care worker should have already been aware of when she chose to enter the profession. Though there may be differences of degree, the situation of health workers in this respect is not altogether different from that of fire-fighters or military personnel. Although health care professionals have implicitly or explicitly agreed to face (some) danger in their work, however, the harder question asks: what are the limits to the dangers they have agreed to face or the dangers they should actually face?

If it was known that treating a particular patient would *very likely* cost a physician her life, then should we expect her to do it? Imagine, for example, a contagious patient infected with smallpox. Should a physician who has not been vaccinated against smallpox care for such a patient if no vaccine (which can be used as a prophylactic) is available in the context in question? To deny that a supposed duty to treat covers cases like this is reasonable. Even if a health care worker has duties to promote human health, it is unreasonable to expect her to do so at all costs to herself. In the case in question, furthermore, the general duty to promote human health would itself be frustrated if the physician is killed, for she would then be unable to care for any additional patients. The duty to treat any given patient should be balanced against the right to protect oneself and duties to treat *other* patients.

The situation where a patient presents with an unknown condition with an unknown aetiology is, however, a different matter that is not easily settled. That physicians have a duty to treat even when there is (some) danger to their own lives was held by the 1847 American Medical Association *Code of Ethics*:

> When pestilence prevails, it is [physicians'] duty to face the danger, and to continue their labours for the alleviation of suffering, even at the jeopardy of their own lives (Huber and Wynia, 2004, p. W6).

Although versions of this statement remained in the AMA code for 130 years, it was dropped in 1977, at a time when the threat of infectious diseases had subsided (in developed nations at least) and when the health care profession was struggling to defend its autonomy (Huber and Wynia, 2004).

While significant ethics debate surrounded the question of the duty to treat early in the HIV/AIDS epidemic, much attention then focused on the issue of discrimination in particular. Norman Daniels, for example, argued that the duty to treat contagious patients ultimately rests on physicians' own consent to face such risks. Because the overall risk (of death) associated with treating patients infected with HIV were (prior to the availability of hepatitis B vaccine, anyway) no greater than the risk of treating patients infected with hepatitis B (which is much more contagious, though less deadly), the fact that physicians routinely treated the latter without qualms revealed consent to face the level of risk involved with the former. Refusal to treat patients infected with HIV/AIDS, therefore, according to Daniels, involved either ignorance about the level of risk involved or ethically unacceptable discrimination against a particular patient population (Daniels, 1991).

Lynette Reid has more recently argued that the SARS epidemic revealed additional complexity involved with the question of health workers' duty to treat (Reid, 2005). It is not just a matter of a health worker's duty to treat patients potentially conflicting with a right she has to autonomy and the protection of her own safety that is relevant here; there is a complex web of duties to be taken into consideration when considering the duty to treat. A health worker's duty to treat patients may come into conflict with other duties she has to care for family members who depend on her. Moreover, she has duties to society, her employer (the hospital) and co-workers who will be called in to do her job if she refuses. The large influx of patients during the SARS epidemic had the potential to overwhelm health care institutions – and the functioning of hospitals depended on each person fulfilling her role. If one refused to treat SARS patients to protect her own safety – or to protect her family members – then someone else (who might also have a family) would have to face the danger; and if too many refused, then the hospital would no longer function. The important thing revealed by SARS, according to Reid, is the importance of solidarity – a mutually dependent health care team working together for a common cause. The fact that so few health care workers actually refused to care for SARS-infected patients, according to Reid, is best explained by social cohesion rather than heroism in the face of danger.

Society as a whole, of course, depends on health care workers to provide medical treatment when necessary, and perhaps the best argument that can be given in support of health workers' duty to treat appeals to a social contract. Society provides numerous exclusive benefits and privileges to health care workers, and the social expectation is that health care workers will provide health care in return (Huber and Wynia, 2004; Clark, 2005). When a health care worker refuses to treat, she then reneges on her side of the bargain. Although this does not settle questions about the level of risk that health care workers should face (which are beyond the scope of this chapter), it does support a strong duty to treat in times of emergency.

The idea of a social contract also reveals something else of importance. If society as a whole depends on health care workers to provide health care, then it should support their efforts as far as possible. It is not unreasonable, that is, for health care workers to demand that their working conditions are made as safe as is feasible. Special facilities, protective clothing and equipment, and access to drugs and vaccines, for example, make treatment of contagious patients less dangerous. If society expects health care workers to 'do their job', then it should make it possible for them to work under reasonable conditions of safety. Individual health care workers should not be expected to bear exceptional burdens that can be avoided. It would likewise be reasonable for health workers, or their families, to expect and receive compensation from society when harms result from fulfilment of dangerous duties (University of Toronto Joint Centre for Bioethics, 2005).

RESEARCH

As noted above, one reason that the bioterrorist threat is taken to be so serious at present relates to the fact that recent advances in science may facilitate production of more dangerous biological weapons than previously would have been possible. The ethical phenomenon in question is often referred to as 'the dual-use dilemma'. Given that the very same knowledge or technological developments that might be used for beneficial purposes can also be used for malevolent purposes, how should research that could potentially result in potentially dangerous discoveries be controlled? And what, if any, regulation should be placed on the dissemination of information in such cases? These questions have been central to ethical debate related to bioterrorism.

Much of this debate has focused on the publication of two studies in particular. In the first case, Australian scientists used standard genetic engineering techniques to insert the IL-4 gene into the mousepox virus. Though their hope was that infection with the resultant virus would cause infertility in mice – and thus provide a means of pest control – they accidentally discovered that they had produced a super-strain of mousepox. The genetically engineered virus killed both mice that were naturally resistant to mousepox and mice that had been vaccinated against mousepox. They went on to publish their findings, along with description of materials and methods, in the *Journal of Virology* in 2001 (Jackson et al., 2001).

In a second study, American scientists constructed a DNA template of the polio genome by stringing together strands of DNA purchased over the internet in accordance with the RNA polio genome which is published on the internet. The addition of protein resulted in synthesis of a 'live' polio virus that paralysed mice. Upon publication of their findings, again including description of materials and methods, in *Science* in 2002 (Cello et al., 2002), they said their purpose was 'to send a warning that terrorists might be able to make biological weapons without obtaining a natural virus' (Pollack, 2002).

Critics complain that neither of these studies should have been published. In addition to providing would-be bioterrorists with ideas about new ways of making biological weapons, the worry is that these publications provide explicit instructions for doing so. At the very least, it is objected, the materials and methods sections should have been omitted from the published articles. The danger of the mousepox publication is that it might be possible to make vaccine-resistant smallpox using the very same techniques as those employed by the Australian scientists. A danger of the polio study is that it might be possible to produce smallpox (the genome of which is admittedly much larger than polio's) – or other dangerous microbes, such as Ebola – using similar methods to those employed by the Americans. Related techniques have already enabled scientists to 'resurrect' the 1918 flu virus, which killed 40–100 million people (Kaiser, 2005).

Scientists and editors involved with these two publications, on the contrary, hold that it was important to publish in order to alert the scientific community of the need to develop defences against what were shown to be new kinds of threats. Defenders of publication also appeal to the importance of scientific openness more generally, holding that the free sharing of information is crucial to the progress of science and that omission of materials and methods, for example, would conflict with the need for replication and verification in science.

The debate which has surrounded these studies and others like them highlights dangers related to the fact that there has been a long history of complete openness in the sharing of information in the life sciences – especially in comparison to nuclear science, where discoveries with weapons implications are 'born classified'. The fact that biological weapons are so much easier to make in comparison with nuclear weapons makes the public availability of relevant information in the former context all the more worrisome. The methods used in the mousepox study, for example, are described in standard microbiology textbooks, and nothing in the way of extraordinary equipment was required.

Part of the aftermath of this debate, following meetings between the security and scientific communities, has been the publication of a 'Statement on Scientific Publication and Security' by the 'Journal Editors and Authors Group' in *Science, Nature,* the *Proceedings of the National Academy of Sciences* and the American Society for Microbiology journals. Among other things, the statement says that these journals will screen submissions for cases where the potential harm of publication would outweigh benefits and that they will prevent publication – that is, censor – when necessary (Journal Editors and Authors Group, 2003).

The US National Research Council has since advocated increased oversight of potentially dangerous research through expansion of Institutional Biosafety Committee (IBC) monitoring. The review of research proposals will thus target research with potential weapons implications in addition to other (environmental) dangers these committees traditionally aimed to screen for.

Another development is the American Medical Association's adoption of 'Guidelines to Prevent Malevolent Use of Biomedical Research', which hold that

' . . . before participating in research, physician-researchers should assess foreseeable ramifications of their research in an effort to balance the promise of biomedical innovation against potential harms from corrupt applications of the findings' (Green et al., 2006).

While it is often thought by scientists that the generation of knowledge is good in and of itself – and that it is the way that knowledge is applied that might be good or bad – the AMA holds that scientists have a responsibility to avoid generating knowledge that would forseeably do more harm than good. In addition to the education imperative addressed above, it thus is important that medical researchers increase their own awareness of the ways in which their work has potential for abuse by would-be bioterrorists.

FOR FURTHER STUDY

This chapter has examined the history of biological weapons, reasons why the bioterrorist threat is taken so seriously at present and major ethical issues associated with bioterrorism most relevant to health care workers. There are, of course, additional ethical issues associated with bioterrorism to those covered above. In the event of a major disease outbreak that could result from a terrorist attack, for example, it is possible that isolation, quarantine, travel restrictions, mandatory treatment and/or vaccination, privacy-intruding surveillance and so on will be called for by public health authorities. The ethical issue here is that the public health policy measures that might be needed to protect the greater good of society in the way of public health could conflict with basic rights and liberties, such as freedom of movement. Rather than giving absolute priority to either the promotion of public health or individual liberty, it is ethically important that a balance be struck between these two legitimate goals. (Because these are primarily questions of public health ethics – as opposed to health care ethics – such issues have been set aside for the purpose of this chapter.)

Other ethical issues relevant to bioterrorism, 'the war against terrorism' and war more generally relate to physician involvement in harsh interrogations – that is, torture – of prisoners. The concern here is that physicians working for the military might be confronted with 'dual loyalties' if they are asked by superior officers, for example, to monitor the 'fitness for questioning' of those being tortured. In cases like this, following orders (and potentially promoting national interests, in ticking bomb scenarios) may come into conflict with international law and the basic obligation of health workers to do no harm (Gross, 2006).

Additional ethical issues involving research, finally, relate to human subject protection and biological weapons research. In the former case, a worry is that less protection will be afforded to human subjects involved in (possibly classified) research considered vital to national interests during times of national emergency (Moreno, 2002). The latter issue relates to the fact that, as indicated above, offensive biological research is banned by the BTWC; and although purely defensive research is legal, it is often hard to draw a clear line separating the former from the latter. As the BTWC is still in effect, it is important that scientists become familiar with it lest they unwittingly engage in illegal research contrary to its requirements. Because purely defensive (legal) research may often look like offensive research to potential adversaries, furthermore, the fact that it has the potential to promote a biological arms race makes even this kind of research ethically problematic (though perhaps not always wrong all things considered).

REFERENCES

Alibek K, Handelman S. *Biohazard: The Chilling True Story of the Largest Covert Weapons Program in the World – Told from the Inside by the Man who Ran it.* New York: Delta, 1999.

Block SM. The growing threat of biological weapons. *Am Sci* 2001; **89**: 28–37.

Cello J, Paul AV, Wimmer E. Chemical synthesis of poliovirus cDNA: generation of infectious virus in the absence of natural template. *Science* 2002; **297**: 1016–1018.

Central Intelligence Agency. *The Darker Bioweapons Future*, 2003; available at http://www.fas.org/irp/cia/product/bw1103.pdf.

Childress JF. Triage in response to a bioterrorist attack. In: Moreno JD, ed. *In the Wake of Terror.* Cambridge, MA: The MIT Press, 2003; pp. 77–93.

Clark CC. In harm's way: AMA physicians and the duty to treat. *J Med Philos* 2005; **30**, 65–87.

Convention on the Prohibition of the Development, Production and Stockpiling of Bacteriological (Biological) and Toxin Weapons and on Their Destruction (BTWC), 1972; available at: http://www.opbw.org/convention/documents/btwctext.pdf.

Daniels N. Duty to treat or right to refuse. *Hastings Center Rep* 1991; **21**(2): 36–46.

Frischknecht F. The history of biological warfare. *EMBO Rep* 2003; **4**: S47–S52.

Green SK, Taub S, Morin K, Higginson D, for the Council on Ethical and Judicial Affairs of the American Medical Association. Guidelines to prevent malevolent use of biomedical research. Camb Q Health Ethics 2006, **15**: 432–447.

Gross M. Bioethics and Armed Conflict. Cambridge, MA: MIT Press, 2006.

Huber SJ, Wynia MK. When pestilence prevails … physician responsibilities in epidemics. *Am J Bioethics* 2004; **4**(1): W5–11; available at: www.bioethics.net.

Jackson RJ, Ramsey AJ, Christensen CD, Beaton S, Hall DF, Ramshaw IA. Expression of mouse interleukin-4 by a recombinant ectromelia virus suppresses cytolytic lymphocyte responses and overcomes genetic resistance to mousepox. *J Virol* 2001; **75**(3): 1205–1210.

Journal Editors and Authors Group. Uncensored exchange of scientific results. *Proc Natl Acad Sci* 2003; **100**(4): 1464, available at: www.pnas.org/cgi/doi/10.1073/pnas.0630491100.

Kaiser J. Resurrected influenza virus yields secrets of deadly 1918 pandemic. *Science* 2005; **310**: 28–29.

Miller M, Engelberg S, Broad W. *Germs: The Ultimate Weapon.* London: Simon and Schuster, 2001.

Moreno JD. Bioethics after the terror. *Am J Bioethics* 2002; **2**(1): 60–64.

National Research Council. *Biotechnology Research in An Age of Terrorism.* Washington, D.C.: National Academies Press, 2004.

Nixendorff K, Bender W. Ethics of university research, biotechnology and potential military spin-off. *Minerva* 2002; **40**: 15–35.

Oldstone MB. *Viruses, Plagues, and History.* New York: Oxford University Press, 1998.

Pesik N, Keim ME, Iserson KV. Terrorism and the ethics of emergency medical care. *Annals Emerg Med* 2001; **37**: 642–646.

Pollack A. Scientists create a live polio virus. *The New York Times on the Web*, 2002; available at http://www.nytimes.com/2002/07/12/science/10POLI.html?ex=102750869&ei=1&en=9c90f7f35631fbcd.

Reid L. Diminishing returns? Risk and the duty to care in the SARS epidemic. *Bioethics* 2005; **19**(4): 348–361.

Sutton V. A multidisciplinary approach to an ethic of biodefence and bioterrorism. *J Law Med Ethics* 2005; **33**: 310–322.

Tucker. *Scourge: The Once and Future Threat of Smallpox.* New York: Grove Press, 2001.

University of Toronto Joint Centre for Bioethics. *Stand on Guard for Thee: Ethical Considerations in Preparedness Planning for Pandemic Influenza* (a report of the University of Toronto Joint Centre for Bioethics Pandemic Influenza Working Group), 2005; available at: http://www.utoronto.ca/jcb/home/documents/pandemic.pdf.

Drug Addiction, Society and Ethics

WAYNE HALL, ADRIAN CARTER

Addiction or drug dependence is characterized by a pattern of drug use in which individuals use drugs in large amounts–typically daily or near daily–and for substantial periods of time, require increasing doses of the drug to achieve the desired effects, experience withdrawal symptoms if they stop drug use abruptly and continue to use the drug in the face of problems caused by its use, such as health and psychological problems, adverse effects of drug use on partners and children or workmates, and legal problems, for example, drink or drug driving, fights and assaults, and being arrested for drug and property offences.

These patterns of behaviour raise important ethical questions: are people who use drugs in these ways morally responsible for their behaviour? How should we respond to people who use drugs in ways that harm themselves? Is it ethically justified to prohibit the use of some drugs (e.g. cannabis, cocaine and heroin) in order to prevent addiction and reduce the social and economic burdens that addiction to alcohol, tobacco and other drugs imposes upon society? Is it morally justifiable to legally coerce addicts into treatment? Should we use genetic information to identify young people who are at increased risk of addiction and vaccinate them against the effects of drugs like cocaine and nicotine? Under what circumstances is it justified to screen individuals for drug use? The answers that we give to these questions depend critically on how we understand drug use and addictive behaviour.

SCEPTICAL VIEWS OF ADDICTION

A 'common-sense' view is that 'addicts' are simply drug users who use 'addiction' as an excuse for continuing to use drugs; they could stop using drugs if they 'really' wanted to. A sceptical view is also expressed by some social scientists who argue that 'addiction' is an attribution that enables drug users to avoid responsibility for the social consequences of their drug use (Szasz, 1997; Davies, 1997).

Sceptical views make sense of a number of features of 'addictive behaviour' (as described above). Drug use typically begins as a voluntary act, with addictive patterns of drug use emerging gradually over time in a minority of users and in ways that make it difficult to draw a bright, sharp line between drug use that is voluntary and that which is addictive. Among the minority of drug users who do become addicted, most stop using drugs by themselves (Peele, 2004).

Sceptical views of addiction are less successful in explaining a number of dependable empirical relationships between drug use and addictive behaviour.

First, the minority of drug users who become addicted to a drug can be substantial. Addiction affects a third of tobacco smokers, one quarter of heroin users and a sixth of alcohol users, for example (Anthony, 1994).

Second, these differences in addiction risk are, in part, a consequence of the mode of action and the different ways in which these drugs are used. Short-acting drugs that are smoked (nicotine or crack cocaine) or are injected (amphetamine, heroin or cocaine) are much more likely to produce addictive behaviour than longer-acting drugs that are swallowed (alcohol) or smoked (cannabis) (Anthony, 1994).

Third, there is an identifiable subset of individuals who we can predict with reasonable accuracy and who are more likely to show addictive behaviour if they use drugs. This includes people who have more opportunities to use drugs, who take these opportunities at an earlier age, who are from socially disadvantaged backgrounds; who perform poorly in school, who have peers who use drugs, who have a family history of addictive behaviour, who have other mental disorders, and so on (Hawkins et al., 1992).

Principles of Health Care Ethics, Second Edition   Edited by R.E. Ashcroft, A. Dawson, H. Draper and J.R. McMillan
© 2007 John Wiley & Sons, Ltd

Fourth, although many addicts stop their drug use without assistance, others do not. Only a minority of addicts seek help, but most of those who receive treatment return to drug use in the year after cessation. Over time, repeated attempts to stop do result in a substantial proportion of addicts successfully quitting, but most addicts who seek treatment still find it difficult to stop (Teesson et al., 2002).

Fifth, 'common-sense' sceptical views of addiction have not been successful in reducing drug use. Those who regard addiction as an excuse for bad behaviour tend to favour the imprisonment of those who use prohibited drugs and those who engage in crimes to finance their drug use. These policies have led to imprisonment of substantial numbers of drug users, who typically return to drug use and reoffend on release from imprisonment (Gerstein and Harwood, 1990; National Research Council, 2001).

NEUROBIOLOGICAL THEORIES OF ADDICTION

Neurobiological theories of addiction attempt to identify the molecular and cellular mechanisms of how drugs act on the brain in ways that may impair control over drug use. Such a theory of addiction now in ascendance in the United States is the 'chronic, relapsing brain disease model', as described by the National Institutes on Drug Abuse (NIDA). According to NIDA, addiction is caused by chronic self-administration of drugs that produce enduring changes in brain neurotransmitter systems that leave addicts vulnerable to relapse after abstinence has been achieved (Leshner, 1997; Volkow and Li, 2005).

Over the past several decades, neuroscience research has shown that the major drugs of dependence act on key neurotransmitter systems in the brain (Koob, 2001). Repeated drug use produces changes in the brain receptor systems that may explain the phenomena of drug tolerance, whereas adaptive responses by the brain to chronic drug administration explain the withdrawal symptoms that addicts experience when they abruptly cease their use (Hyman and Malenka, 2001; Koob and Le moal, 2001). The actions of the different receptors on which various psychoactive drugs act also converge on a common neural pathway centred on the nucleus accumbens in the forebrain where many of the rewarding effects of these drugs appear to be mediated (Hyman and Malenka, 2001; Koob and Le moal, 2001).

There is also evidence from twin and adoption studies that there is a substantial genetic contribution to addiction vulnerability (Goldman et al., 2005). This vulnerability may be mediated by genes that regulate the metabolism of psychoactive drugs and the brain neurotransmitter systems on which they act (Goldman et al., 2005). Neuroimaging studies in human addicts have also found changes in brain pathways which, it is claimed, explain the loss of control and compulsive behaviour of addicts (Volkow et al., 2004).

Proponents of neurobiological theories of addiction see their research as providing more effective ways of helping addicts to withdraw from their drugs of dependence and better pharmacological methods to help them remain abstinent (Volkow et al., 2004). Genotyping of people seeking help to deal with addiction may also enable patients to be matched to the pharmacological treatments that have the best chance of assisting them to become and remain abstinent, for example, nicotine replacement or bupropion for smoking cessation (Munafo et al., 2001).

Addiction neuroscientists also hope that their work will reduce community scepticism about the 'reality' of addiction (Leshner, 1997). They hope that the neurobiological model of addiction as a 'chronic, relapsing brain disease' (Leshner, 1997, p. 33) will supplant the 'common-sense' moral view of addiction and that the punitive policies it encourages will be replaced by more humane policies, such as reducing stigmatization and providing better access to more effective forms of treatment.

More sceptical social scientists point to a number of potentially less welcome social uses of the 'brain disease' model of addiction. The 'chronic brain disease' view may be seen as warranting heroic interventions in the brain's function, such as ultra-rapid opiate detoxification for heroin dependence (Hall, 2000), or the neurosurgical treatment of addiction (Hall, 2005). Moreover, if addicts are seen as suffering from a 'brain disease', they may need to be coerced into treatment because they will be viewed as incapable of acting in their own best interests.

If taken literally, the 'brain disease' model of addiction may also undermine the capacity of neuroscientists to undertake research on addiction (Hall, 2002). Some bioethicists in the United States have argued, for example, that addicts lack the capacity to give free and informed consent to participate in (1) experimental neurobiological studies of addiction, for example, scanning the brains of addicts who are given drugs of dependence (Cohen, 2002); and (2) clinical trials of injectable heroin as a treatment for opioid dependence (Charland, 2002). There are good reasons to question the validity of these arguments (Hall et al., 2003), but if they are accepted by ethics review committees, they will severely constrain the type of neurobiological research that it is permissible to conduct.

The findings of behaviour genetics may also be used to support misguided social policies towards drug use that we may expect to be enthusiastically embraced by suppliers of legal drugs. If, for example, 'alcoholism' comes to be seen as a 'brain disease' that affects a genetically predisposed minority of drinkers, then the alcohol industry may advocate that we should identify this genetically vulnerable minority so that the rest of the population can drink alcohol with impunity (Hall, 1996). Such a policy would ignore the serious adverse public health effects of alcohol intoxication in binge drinkers, most of whom are not alcohol-dependent (Room, 2007).

Addiction neurobiologists have an ethical obligation to ensure that the public, and their political representatives, understand what does and does not follow from their research (Hall and Carter, 2004). They need to make it clear that addiction is not a simple Mendelian disorder, that is, it is not the case that if you have 'the gene' then you will become addicted and that you would not if you do not. Addiction is more likely to be a polygenic disorder, that is, it is the result of complex interactions between social environment and the actions of a large number of genes, each with a small effect, that affect drug metabolism, brain neurotransmitters levels, risk-taking, school performance, susceptibility to peer influence, and so on. It will be a major challenge to explain this more complex model of addiction genetics to a community that has largely been exposed to media stories about such simple Mendelian models of the genetics of human disease.

Another major challenge will be avoiding genetic understandings of addiction (Ball et al., 2007) which could undermine social policies that reduce drug use and addiction risk. Behaviour genetic, epidemiological and sociological research all show that drug use and addiction are affected by social and environmental factors. These include the cost (Cave and Godfrey, 2007) and availability of drugs, the degree of social approval or disapproval of different types of drug use, peer drug use, social disadvantage and many other factors (McKeganey et al., 2007). These social influences provide important policy opportunities – the use of taxation and restrictions on drug availability and use – to prevent addiction and moderate the harmful effects of drug use and intoxication (McKeganey et al., 2007). Such policies are likely to be more cost-effective than pharmacological interventions given the minority of drug users who become addicted and seek treatment (Hall and Teesson, 1999).

ADDICTION AND PATERNALISM

Most developed societies prohibit adults from using cannabis, cocaine and heroin on penalty of imprisonment. In prohibiting the use of these drugs by adults, these laws are paternalistic, that is, they override the free choices of adults in order to prevent them from harming themselves (Childress, 1982). Paternalism is rejected by libertarians who argue that the sole purpose for restricting the free choices of autonomous adults is to prevent harm to others (Mill, 1998 [1862]; Szasz, 1997).

If one accepts that paternalism is sometimes ethically acceptable (e.g. if one supports compulsory seat belt laws

or the regulation of pharmaceutical drugs), a major ethical problem remains in explaining why adults are permitted to use alcohol and nicotine, although the use of cannabis, cocaine and heroin is prohibited (Husak, 2004). There is no obvious neurobiological justification for the fact that alcohol and tobacco are legal whereas heroin, cocaine and cannabis are not (Ashcroft et al., 2007). Nor does the legal status of these drugs correspond to the relative harms caused by their current use because alcohol and tobacco clearly cause much greater societal harm than cannabis, heroin or cocaine (Room, 2007). Even when we take account of the fact that many fewer people use illegal than legal drugs (in part because of their illegality), alcohol and tobacco cause much more harm to users than does cannabis (Room, 2007).

Some neuroscientists (e.g. Blakemore, 2002; Iversen, 2002; Iverson et al., 2007) are hopeful that their research will allow the development of policies towards drugs that reflects their prevalence of use and their capacity to harm users and others. They may be overly optimistic to do so. International drug control agreements and opposition in most developed societies to any liberalization of policies towards illicit drugs have prevented even minor changes to penalties for cannabis, the illicit drug where the case for a more liberal policy seems the strongest (MacCoun and Reuter, 2001). Indeed, one can more easily imagine addiction neuroscience being selectively used to justify more coercive policies towards illicit drug use in the name of preventing adolescents from acquiring a 'chronic brain disease'.

ETHICAL ASPECTS OF CONTROVERSIAL ADDICTION POLICY OPTIONS

COERCED ADDICTION TREATMENT

Legally coerced addiction treatment is entered into by addicts who have been charged with or convicted of an offence to which their addiction has contributed. It is most often provided as an alternative to imprisonment, with the threat of imprisonment being used to encourage compliance with addiction treatment (Hall, 1997; Spooner et al., 2001). Coerced treatment is often justified as an effective way to reduce the chances of an addicted offender returning to drug use and reoffending (Gerstein and Harwood, 1990). It has been most often used to treat offenders who are addicted to heroin (Leukefeld and Tims, 1988) and cocaine (National Research Council, 2001).

Coerced treatment raises ethical and human rights issues because it involves the state using the threat of imprisonment to force addicts to receive treatment for their addiction (Mann, 1999). Some authors reject any form of coerced addiction treatment. Szasz, for example, denies that addiction exists, arguing that as drug use is voluntary, any drug user who commits a criminal offence should be punished (Szasz, 1997). Others, such as Newman, accept that addiction exists, but oppose coerced treatment because they claim it does not work (Newman, 1974). If treatment under coercion is ineffective (as Newman claims), then there would be no ethical justification for providing it.

A consensus view prepared for the World Health Organization (Porter et al., 1986) concluded that drug treatment under coercion was legally and ethically justified if and only if (1) the rights of the individuals were protected by 'due process' (in accordance with human rights principles), and (2) effective and humane treatment was provided. In the absence of due process, coerced treatment could become *de facto* imprisonment without judicial oversight. In the absence of humane and effective treatment, coerced drug treatment could become a cost-cutting exercise to reduce prison overcrowding.

DRUG SCREENING AND TESTING

Drug testing involves biochemical testing of blood, urine or hair for metabolites of drugs. It can be used to tell if an individual has used a drug within a particular time period and, in some cases, whether they were intoxicated. Drug testing arguably does not raise any major ethical issues if a person's drug use puts others at risk, for example, when they are driving a motor vehicle, flying a plane or operating machinery. In these cases, drug testing is ethically justified if there is evidence that (1) drug use impairs performance in ways that endanger others, (2) the drug testing provides valid assessment of impairment and (3) drug testing deters people from using drugs in ways that put others at risk. These conditions are satisfied when blood alcohol concentration is used to test for impairment in automobile, train and truck drivers, or pilots.

Testing in the workplace and other settings for drug use rather than intoxication raises additional ethical issues (Allsop, 1997). The aim of this type of drug testing is to reduce employer costs (health and sick leave) and increase productivity, as opposed to ensuring the safety of employees or the public; but there is very little evidence that this kind of drug testing produces these effects (Allsop, 1997). Moreover, in the American workplace, drug testing is often confined to testing for metabolites of illegal drugs (particularly cannabis, which is easiest to detect) (DeCew, 1994) rather than alcohol which is much more commonly used and much more likely to impair work performance. In this type of testing, impairment has not been demonstrated (Allsop, 1997), and concerns are raised about the right to privacy and confidentiality, workers' freedom to consent to testing, and discrimination and stigmatization of workers who screen positive for drug use rather than impairment (Allsop, 1997).

PREDICTIVE TESTING OF GENETIC RISK OF ADDICTION

If susceptibility genes are identified for addiction risk, then children and adolescents could be genetically tested and those at higher risk could be given preventive behavioural and pharmacological interventions to reduce their likelihood of using drugs (Collins, 1999). There is an obvious objection to this proposal in the case of cigarette smoking: it is not good public health policy to encourage people to smoke tobacco, regardless of their genetic risk of dependence (Hall, 2002). An alternative rationale is that such screening would allow individuals who were at highest genetic risk of addiction to make informed decisions about whether to avoid drug use. Even if we place a high value on individual autonomy, there are a number of good reasons why on current information genetic screening for addiction is unlikely to be a good policy (Holtzman, 2000).

First, when multiple genes predispose to a common disease, individual susceptibility alleles only predict a very modestly *increased risk* of dependence (Hall and Carter, 2004). Testing multiple genetic variants that were individually weak predictors would improve prediction if the results of multiple genetic tests were combined (Khoury et al., 2004). However, the larger the number of genes that are involved in disease susceptibility, the less useful *most* individuals will find the information about their genotype (Hall and Carter, 2004; Khoury et al., 2004). It also means that a very large number of individuals need to be screened to identify the few at highest risk (Vineis et al., 2001).

Second, predictive genetic testing may have unintended adverse effects. This would be the case, for example, if testing adolescents for susceptibility to addiction *increased* their preparedness to try drugs, as could happen, for example, if they were prompted to test the accuracy of the genetic predictions (Hall, 2002).

Third, screening is only ethically justifiable if there is an effective intervention to prevent the disorder in those who are identified as being at increased risk (Khoury et al., 2003). No such interventions currently exist, but the prospect of preventive vaccination against cocaine and nicotine may raise this possibility in the future (Hall and Carter, 2004).

THE PREVENTIVE USE OF A NICOTINE VACCINE

A 'nicotine vaccine' induces the immune system to produce antibodies that bind to nicotine and prevent it from crossing the blood-brain barrier to act on receptors in the brain (Vocci and Chiang, 2001). Animal studies have shown that antibodies can be raised that have a high affinity for nicotine and that attenuate nicotine's effects, abolish self-administration of nicotine and suppress dopamine release in the *nucleus accumbens* (Hall, 2002).

Active vaccination against nicotine could reduce relapse into smoking in abstinent smokers during the first few months after quitting when most smokers relapse (Vocci and Chiang, 2001). A nicotine vaccine could be circumvented by increasing the dose of nicotine, however, attenuating the rewarding effects of nicotine may be enough to reduce rates of return to daily smoking (Vocci and Chiang, 2001; Hall, 2002).

The term 'vaccine' inevitably prompts discussion about its possible preventive use. Misconceptions that a vaccine will produce lifelong immunity against nicotine may prompt parents to vaccinate their children (Cohen, 1997). As minors, children would not be legally able to consent to vaccination, but as parents already make choices for their children about other vaccines and other interventions that affect their lives (e.g. their diet and education), some have argued that vaccination against nicotine and other drugs is simply another decision that parents should be able to make on behalf of their children (Cohen, 1997). This argument is likely to be contested by civil libertarians and others who place a high value on personal autonomy (Hasman and Holm, 2004), as well as adolescents who disagree with their parents' wishes.

Even if we set aside the ethical issues, there are major practical obstacles to the preventive use of a nicotine vaccine in children. First, the limited period of protection provided by existing vaccines would require booster injections, perhaps every two or three months throughout adolescence (Kosten et al., 2002). Second, the fact that the vaccine could be circumvented by using higher doses of nicotine means that vaccination could be counterproductive if adolescents were prompted to test its efficacy. Third, it would be costly to universally vaccinate children against nicotine with a vaccine of modest preventive efficacy (Hall, 2002).

Vaccination of 'high-risk' adolescents seems a more plausible and less expensive option. However, the feasibility of even this approach is doubtful, given the low predictive validity of genetic screening for smoking risk (outlined above), the doubtful preventive efficacy of a nicotine vaccine and the possible adverse effects of vaccination, such as, stigmatization of those who screened positive, and discrimination against them by third parties, such as life or health insurance companies.

The 'off label' use of a nicotine vaccine by a physician acting at the request of a parent is the most likely way in which a vaccine will be used preventively. It is difficult to see how this could be prevented if a nicotine vaccine is approved for therapeutic use, other than by education of physicians and parents about the limitations of this approach (Hall, 2002).

THE TASKS AHEAD FOR ETHICISTS

A major challenge for addiction policy and ethics will be finding ways to acknowledge the neurobiological contribution to drug use and addiction although recognizing that both are nonetheless affected by individual and social choices. Individual choices about drug use are not always wisely made given that they are often made by young people with temporal myopia, a sense of personal invulnerability, scepticism about their elders' advice about drug use, and an exquisite sensitivity to adult hypocrisy about different drugs. Older adults must recognize their complicity in some of these choices by their willingness to allow drugs like alcohol and tobacco to be readily available, heavily promoted and provided at a low cost to young people.

In the best of all possible worlds, addiction neurobiology may allow us to reconsider our social responses to the minority of drug users who become addicted by reducing their stigmatization and increasing their access to more effective psychological and biological treatments. But an improved understanding of the neurobiology of addiction will not relieve us of the obligation to do what we can to prevent problem drug use by youth by reducing the number of troubled young and otherwise vulnerable people who are susceptible to the appeal of all forms of drug use and reducing the social conditions that contribute to their vulnerability (Spooner and Hall, 2002).

REFERENCES

Allsop S. Drug testing in the workplace: an unfortunate marriage. In: Midford R, Heale P, eds. *Under the Influence? Issues and Practicalities of Alcohol and Other Drug Testing in the Workplace: Proceedings of a Forum*, 8 October 1996, Perth, Western Australia. Perth: National Drug Research Institute, 1997; pp. 1–20.

Anthony JC, Warner L, Kessler R. Comparative epidemiology of dependence on tobacco, alcohol, controlled substances and inhalants: basic findings from the National Comorbidity Survey. *Exp Clin Psychopharmacol* 1994; **2**: 244–268.

Ashcroft R, Campbell A, Capps B. Ethical aspects of developments in neuroscience and drug addiction. In: Nutt D, Robbins T, Stimson G, Ince M, Jackson A, eds. *Drugs and the future: Brain science, addiction and society*. London: Academic Press, 2007; pp. 439–466.

Ball D, Pembrey M, Stevens D. Genomics. In: Nutt D, Robbins T, Stimson G, Ince M, Jackson A, eds. *Drugs and the future: Brain science, addiction and society*. London: Academic Press, 2007; pp. 89–132.

Blakemore C. From the public understanding of science to scientists' understanding of the public. In: Marcus SJ, ed. *Neuroethics: Mapping the Field*. New York: The Dana Press, 2002; pp. 211–221.

Cave J, Godfrey C. Economics of addiction and drugs. In: Nutt D, Robbins T, Stimson G, Ince M, Jackson A, eds. *Drugs and the future: Brain science, addiction and society.* London: Academic Press, 2007; pp. 389–438.

Charland LC. Cynthia's dilemma: consenting to heroin prescription. *Am J Bioethics* 2002; **2**: 37–47.

Childress JF. *Who Should Decide? Paternalism in Health Care.* New York: Oxford University Press, 1982.

Cohen PJ. Immunization for prevention and treatment of cocaine abuse: legal and ethical implications. *Drug Alcohol Depend* 1997; **48**: 167–174.

Cohen PJ. Untreated addiction imposes an ethical bar to recruiting addicts for non-therapeutic studies of addictive drugs. *J Law Med Ethics* 2002; **30**: 73–81.

Collins FS. Medical and societal consequences of the Human Genome Project. *N Engl J Med* 1999; **341**: 28–37.

Davies JB. *The Myth of Addiction.* Amsterdam: Harwood Academic, 1997.

DeCew JW. Drug testing – balancing privacy and public safety. *Hastings Center Rep* 1994; **24**: 17.

Gerstein DR, Harwood HJ. *Treating Drug Problems Volume 1: A Study of Effectiveness and Financing of Public and Private Drug Treatment Systems.* Washington, DC: Institute of Medicine, National Academy Press, 1990.

Goldman D, Oroszi G, Ducci F. The genetics of addictions: uncovering the genes. *Nat Rev Genet* 2005; **6**: 521–532.

Hall WD. The role of legal coercion in the treatment of offenders with alcohol and heroin problems. *Austr N Z J Criminol* 1997; **30**: 103–120.

Hall W. UROD: an antipodean therapeutic enthusiasm. *Addiction* 2000; **95**: 1765–6.

Hall WD. The prospects for immunotherapy in smoking cessation. *Lancet* 2002; **360**: 1089–1091.

Hall WD. Minimising the chances of another great and desperate cure: neurosurgical treatment of heroin addiction. *Addiction*, in press.

Hall WD, Carter L. Ethical issues in using a cocaine vaccine to treat and prevent cocaine abuse and dependence. *J Med Ethics* 2004; **30**: 337–340.

Hall W, Carter L, Morley K. Heroin addiction and the capacity for consent: a reply to Charland. *Addiction* 2003; **98**: 1775–1776.

Hall WD, Carter L, Morley KI. *Ethical Implications of Advances in Neuroscience Research on the Addictions.* Sydney: National Drug and Alcohol Research Centre, 2002b.

Hall WD, Carter L, Morley KI. Neuroscience research on the addictions: a prospectus for future ethical and policy analysis. *Addict Behav* 2004a; **29**: 1481–1495.

Hall W, Madden P, Lynskey M. The genetics of tobacco use: methods, findings and policy implications. *Tobacco Contr* 2002a; **11**: 119–124.

Hall WD, Morley KI, Lucke JC. The prediction of disease risk in genomic medicine. *EMBO Rep* 2004b; **5**(Suppl 1): S22–26.

Hall WD, Sannibale C. Are there two types of alcoholism? *Lancet* 1996; **348**: 1258.

Hall WD, Teesson M. Alcohol use disorders: Who should be treated and how? In: Andrews G, Henderson AS, eds. *Unmet Need in Psychiatry: Problems, Resources, Responses.* Cambridge: Cambridge University Press, 1999; pp. 290–301.

Hasman A, Holm S. Nicotine conjugate vaccine: is there a right to a smoking future? *J Med Ethics* 2004; **30**: 344–345.

Hawkins JD, Catalano RF, Miller JY. Risk and protective factors for alcohol and other drug problems in adolescence and early adulthood: implications for substance abuse prevention. *Psychol Bull* 1992; **112**: 64–105.

Holtzman NA, Marteau TM. Will genetics revolutionize medicine? *N Engl J Med* 2000; **343**: 141–144.

Husak DN. The moral relevance of addiction. *Subst Use Misuse* 2004; **39**: 399–436.

Hyman SE, Malenka RC. Addiction and the brain: the neurobiology of compulsion and its persistence. *Nat Rev Neurosci* 2001; **2**: 695–703.

Iversen L. *The Science of Marijuana.* Oxford: Oxford University Press, 2002.

Iverson L, Morris K, Nutt D. Pharmacology and treatments. In: Nutt D, Robbins T, Stimson G, Ince M, Jackson A, eds. *Drugs and the future: Brain science, addiction and society.* London: Academic Press, 2007; pp. 169–208.

Khoury MJ, McCabe LL, McCabe ER. Population screening in the age of genomic medicine. *N Engl J Med* 2003; **348**: 50–58.

Khoury MJ, Yang Q, Gwinn M, Little J, Flanders WD. An epidemiological assessment of genomic profiling for measuring susceptibility to common diseases and targeting interventions. *Genet Med* 2004; **6**: 38–47.

Koob GF, Le Moal M. Drug addiction, dysregulation of reward, and allostasis. *Neuropsychopharmacology* 2001; **24**: 97–129.

Kosten TR, Rosen M, Bond J, Settles M, Roberts JS, Shields J, Jack L, Fox B. Human therapeutic cocaine vaccine: safety and immunogenicity. *Vaccine* 2002; **20**: 1196–1204.

Leshner AI. Addiction is a brain disease, and it matters. *Science* 1997; **278**: 45–47.

Leukefeld CG, Tims FM. Compulsory treatment: a review of the findings. In: Leukefeld CG, Tims FM, eds. *Compulsory Treatment of Drug Abuse.* Rockville, MD: National Institute of Drug Abuse, 1988; pp. 236–251.

MacCoun R, Reuter P. *Drugwar Heresies: Learning from Other Vices, Times and Places.* Cambridge: Cambridge University Press, 2001.

Mann JM. Medicine and public health, ethics and human rights. In: Mann JM, Gruskin S, Grodin MA, Annas GJ, eds. *Health and Human Rights: A Reader.* London: Routledge, 1999; pp. 439–452.

McKeganey N, Neale J, Lloyd C, Hay G. Sociology and substance use. In: Nutt D, Robbins T, Stimson G, Ince M, Jackson A, eds. *Drugs and the future: Brain science, addiction and society.* London: Academic Press, 2007; pp. 359–388.

Mill JS. *On Liberty and Other Essays: Edited with an Introduction and Notes by John Gray.* Oxford: Oxford University Press, 1998 [1862].

Munafo M, Johnstone E, Murphy M, Walton R. New directions in the genetic mechanisms underlying nicotine addiction. *Addict Biol* 2001; **6**: 109–117.

National Research Council. *Informing America's Policy on Illegal Drugs: What We Don't Know Keeps Hurting Us.* Washington, DC: National Academy Press, 2001.

Newman RG. Involuntary treatment of drug addiction. In: Bourne PG, ed. *Addiction.* New York: Academic Press, 1974; pp. 113–126.

Peele S. The surprising truth about addiction. *Psychol Today* 2004; 43–46.

Porter L, Arif A, Curran WJ. *The Law and the Treatment of Drug and Alcohol Dependent Persons: A Comparative Study of Existing Legislation.* Geneva: World Health Organization, 1986.

Room R. Social policy and psychoactive substances. In: Nutt D, Robbins T, Stimson G, Ince M, Jackson A, eds. *Drugs and the future: Brain science, addiction and society.* London: Academic Press, 2007; pp. 337–358.

Spooner C, Hall WD. Preventing drug misuse by young people: we need to do more than 'just say no'. *Addiction* 2002; **97**: 478–481.

Spooner C, Hall WD, Mattick RP. An overview of diversion strategies for Australian drug-related offenders. *Drug Alcohol Rev* 2001; **20**: 281–294.

Szasz T. *Ceremonial Chemistry: The Ritual Persecution of Drugs, Addicts and Pushers.* Holmes Beach, FL: Learning Publications, 1997.

Teesson M, Degenhardt L, Hall WD. *Addictions.* New York: Taylor and Francis, 2002.

Vineis P, Schulte P, McMichael AJ. Misconceptions about the use of genetic tests in populations. *Lancet* 2001; **357**: 709–712.

Vocci FJ, Chiang CN. Vaccines against nicotine: how effective are they likely to be in preventing smoking? *CNS Drugs* 2001; **15**: 505–514.

Volkow ND, Fowler JS, Wang GJ. The addicted human brain viewed in the light of imaging studies: brain circuits and treatment strategies. *Neuropharmacol* 2004; **47**(Suppl 1): 3–13.

Volkow ND, Li TK. Drugs and alcohol: Treating and preventing abuse, addiction and their medical consequences. *Pharmacol Ther* 2005 [Epub ahead of print].

88

Smoking: Is Acceptance
of the Risks Fully Voluntary?[1]

ROBERT E. GOODIN

Obviously, people cannot voluntarily accept the health risks of smoking if they do not know what they are. Despite tobacco companies' best efforts, though, the great majority of people – smokers included – know, in broad outline, what health risks smoking entails. In a 1978 Gallup poll, only 24% of even heavy smokers claimed that they were unaware of, or did not believe, the evidence that smoking is hazardous to health (U.S. FTC, 1981; Anonymous, 1986). That figure might somewhat overstate the extent of their acceptance of the statistics. There are various other false beliefs smokers sometimes employ to qualify their acceptance of those statistics and, hence, to rationalize their continued smoking (e.g., that the lethal dose is far in excess of what they smoke, however many that may be) (Marsh, 1985). Still, we can reasonably suppose that, in some sense or another, well over half of smokers know that what they are doing is unhealthy.

It is worth pausing at this point to consider just how we should handle that recalcitrant residual of smokers who deny the evidence. Having smoked thousands of packets containing increasingly stern warnings, and having been exposed to hundreds of column inches of newspaper reporting and several hours of broadcasting about smoking's hazards, they are presumably incorrigible in their false beliefs in this regard. Providing them with still more information is likely to prove pointless (cf. Feinberg, 1971/1983). People will say, 'if they are so bad for you as all that the government would ban cigarettes altogether'. Or they will say, 'the government

says that nearly everything is bad for you'. Or they will find still some other way of rationalizing the practice.

Ordinarily, it is not the business of public policy to prevent people from relying on false inferences from full information which would harm only themselves. Sometimes, however, it is. One such case comes when the false beliefs would lead to decisions that are 'far-reaching, potentially dangerous, and irreversible' – as, for example, with people who believe that when they jump out of a tenth-storey window they will float upward (see Feinberg, 1971/1983; Dworkin, 1972/1983).

We are particularly inclined towards intervention when false beliefs with such disastrous results are traceable to familiar, well-understood forms of cognitive defect (Sunstein, 1986). There is something deeply offensive – morally, and perhaps legally as well – about the 'intentional exploitation of a man's known weaknesses' in these ways (White, 1972).

One such familiar form of cognitive defect is 'wishful thinking': smokers believing the practice is safe because they smoke, rather than smoking because they believe it to be safe (Pears, 1984). There is substantial evidence that smokers believe, groundlessly, that they are less vulnerable to smoking-related diseases (Leventhal et al., 1987). More surprising, and more directly to the 'wishful thinking' point, is the evidence that smokers came to acquire those beliefs in their own invulnerability and to 'forget' what they previously knew about the dangers of smoking, *after* they took up the habit.[2]

[1]Reprinted from Robert E. Goodin, *No Smoking: The Ethical Issues* (Chicago: University of Chicago Press, 1989), pp. 20–30, with permission of University of Chicago Press, copyright holders.

[2]In a crucial study Alexander et al. (1983) administered a 28-item questionnaire about the health risks of smoking to 6000 school children aged 10–12. Then they exposed them to a health education programme informing them, among other things, about the health consequences of smoking. When administering the same 28-item questionnaire to the same children a year later, the researchers came upon this startling discovery: those children who had taken up smoking over the course of the year showed a decrease in knowledge on that test compared to their previous year's score, whereas other children who had not begun to smoke showed significant increases.

Principles of Health Care Ethics, Second Edition   Edited by R.E. Ashcroft, A. Dawson, H. Draper and J.R. McMillan
© 2007 John Wiley & Sons, Ltd

Another cognitive defect is the so-called anchoring fallacy (Kahneman et al., 1982). People smoke many times without any (immediately perceptible) bad effects. Naturally, people extrapolate from their own experience. They therefore conclude – quite reasonably, but quite wrongly – that smoking is safe, at least for them.

Yet another phenomenon, sometimes regarded as a cognitive defect, is 'time discounting'. Sometimes the ill-effects of smoking would be felt almost immediately. Tonight's cigarette will make me short of breath when jogging tomorrow morning, for example. To ignore such effects, just on the grounds that they are in the future, is obviously absurd when the 'future' in question is so close; it would imply a discount rate of 100% per hour, 'compounding to an annual rate too large for my calculator', as Schelling (1980, p. 99) sneers. But most of the really serious consequences of smoking are some decades away for most of us. And as young smokers will not suffer the full effects of smoking-related diseases for some years to come, they may puff away happily now with little regard for the consequences, just so long as they attach relatively little importance to future pains relative to present pleasures in their utility functions (Fuchs, 1982). Economists, of course, are inclined to regard a 'pure time preference' as a preference like any other, neither rational nor irrational. But reasons can be given for thinking that a lack of due regard for one's own future truly is a form of cognitive defect.[3]

All of these cognitive defects point to relatively weak forms of irrationality, to be sure.[4] In and of themselves, they might not be enough to justify interference with people's liberty, perhaps. When they lead people to take decisions that are far-reaching, potentially life-threatening, and irreversible, though, perhaps intervention would indeed be justifiable.

Interfering with people's choices in such cases is paternalistic, admittedly. But there are many different layers of paternalism (Sartorius, 1983; Feinberg, 1986). What is involved here is a relatively weak form of paternalism, one that works within the individual's own theory of the good and merely imposes upon him a better means of achieving what after all are only his own ends.[5] It is one thing to stop people who want to commit suicide from doing so, but quite another to stop people who want to live from acting in a way that they falsely believe to be safe (Feinberg, 1971/1983; Dworkin, 1972/1983). Smokers who deny the health risks fall into that latter, easier category.

The larger and harder question is how to deal with the great majority of smokers who, knowing the risks, continue smoking anyway. Of course, it might be said that they do not *really* know the risks. Although most acknowledge that smoking is 'unhealthy', in some vague sense, few know exactly what chances they run of exactly what diseases. In one poll, 49% of smokers did not know that smoking causes most cases of lung cancer, 63% that it causes most cases of bronchitis, and 85% that it causes most cases of emphysema (U.S. FTC, 1981; see similarly Marsh, 1985).

Overestimating badly the risks of dying in other more dramatic ways (such as car crashes, etc.), people badly underestimate the relative risks of dying in the more mundane ways associated with smoking. This allows them to rationalize further their smoking behaviour as being 'not all that dangerous', compared to other things that they are also doing.

Of course, logically it would be perfectly possible for people both to underestimate the extent of a risk and simultaneously to overreact to it. People might suppose that the chances of a snakebite are slight but live in mortal fear of it nonetheless. Psychologically, however, the reverse seems to happen. People's subjective probability estimates of an event's likelihood increase the more they dread it, and the more 'psychologically available' the event therefore is to

---

[3]Daniels(1985, p. 99) tries to show its irrationality by inviting us to construct a notion of a 'hypothetical agent … abstract[ing] from certain features of individuals' as we know them. He then argues that it would be prudent for (i.e. rationally incumbent upon) such agents to take a strong interest in their futures. That amounts to a quasi-Rawlsian appeal against the injustice of time-discounting, though. It does not, strictly speaking, demonstrate its imprudence or irrationality. My preferred argument is this: suppose, plausibly enough, that your later self will prefer that your earlier self had taken its later interests more seriously. Then want-regarding moralities (utilitarianism, certainly) would put this later claim fully on a par with that of the earlier self (Goodin, 1982). So long as earlier and later selves are instantiations of one and the same person, we can say that the earlier one is therefore 'irrational' not to take properly into account his later interests. (If they are not the 'same person', it is indeed appropriate to appeal to norms of justice: It is unjust for one person to take advantage of another in this way, whether or not they share the same body at different moments.)

[4]The addiction evidence surveyed below is evidence of genuine, full-blown irrationality; and it might explain why people are so prone to these more modest cognitive errors when it comes to smoking as well.

[5]One of a person's ends – continued life – at least. Perhaps the person has other ends ('relaxation', or whatever) that are well served by smoking; and insofar as 'people taking risks actually value the direct consequences associated with them…it is more difficult to intrude paternalistically' (Daniels, 1985, pp. 158, 163). But assuming that smoking is not the only means to the other ends – not the only way to relax, etc. – the intrusion is only minimally difficult to justify.

them (Kahneman et al., 1982). Smoking-related diseases, in contrast, tend to be 'quiet killers' of which people have little direct or indirect experience, which tend to be under-reported in newspapers (typically not even being mentioned in obituary notices) and which act on people one at a time rather than catastrophically killing many people at once (Lichtenstein et al., 1978). Smoking-related diseases being psychologically less available to people in these ways, they underestimate their frequency dramatically – by a factor of 8, in the case of lung cancer, according to one study (Slovic et al., 1982).[6]

Besides all that, there is the distinction between 'knowing intellectually' some statistic and 'feeling in your guts' its full implications. Consent counts – morally, as well as merely legally – only if it is truly informed consent, that is to say, only if people really know what it is to which they are consenting. That, in turn, requires not only that we can state the probabilities, but also that we 'appreciate them in an emotionally genuine manner' (Dworkin 1972/1983). There is a reason to believe that smokers do not (U.S. FTC, 1981).

It may still be argued that, as long as people had the facts, they can and should be held responsible if they chose not to act upon them when they could have done so. It may be a folly for utilitarian policymakers to rely upon people's imperfect responses to facts for purposes of constructing social welfare functions and framing public policies around them. But there is the separate matter of who ought to be blamed when some self-inflicted harm befalls people. Arguably, the responsibility ought to be on people's own shoulders (Knowles, 1977; Wikler, 1987). Arguably, we ought to stick to that judgement, even if people were 'pressured' into smoking by the bullying of aggressive advertising or peer group pressure (cf. Gewirth, 1980; Daniels, 1985).

What crucially transforms the 'voluntary acceptance' argument is evidence of the addictive nature of cigarette smoking. Of course, saying that smoking is addictive is not to say that all smokers are hooked and none can ever give it up. Clearly, many have done so. By the same token, though, 'most narcotics users...never progress beyond occasional use, and of those who do, approximately 30% spontaneously remit' (U.S. DHHS, 1988, p. v). Surprisingly enough, studies show that more than 70% of American servicemen addicted to heroin in Vietnam gave it up when returning to the United States (Robins, 1973; Fingarette, 1975; Pollin, 1984). We nonetheless continue to regard heroin as an addictive drug. The test of addictiveness is not the impossibility but rather the difficulty of withdrawal.

There is a tendency, in discussing *volenti* or informed consent arguments, to draw too sharp a distinction between 'voluntary' and 'involuntary acts' and to put the dividing line at the wrong place, at that (Feinberg, 1986). The tendency is often to assume that any act that is in the least voluntary – that is, in any respect at all, to any extent at all, within the control of the agents themselves – is to be considered fully voluntary for the purposes. If we want to claim that some sort of act was involuntary, we are standardly advised to look for evidence of 'somnambulism' or 'automatism' or such like (Prevezer, 1958; Fox, 1963). Thus, US Supreme Court justices wanting to argue for more humane treatment of addicts felt obliged to assert that 'once [the defendant] had become an addict he was utterly powerless' to refrain from continuing to service his addiction (Fortas, 1968, p. 567). That is an implausibly strong claim, given the above evidence.

There is no need to make such a strong claim, though, to vitiate arguments that the conduct was 'voluntary' and the harm self-incurred. For purposes of excusing criminal conduct, we are prepared to count forms of 'duress' that stop well short of rendering all alternative actions literally impossible. It is perfectly possible for bank tellers to let a robber break their arms instead of handing over the money, but no one expects them to do so. A credible threat of serious pain, or perhaps even very gross discomfort, is ordinarily regarded as more than sufficient to constitute duress of the sort that excuses responsibility for otherwise impermissible behaviour.

So, too, I would argue should be the case with addiction-induced behaviour. The issue is not whether it is literally impossible, but merely whether it is unreasonably costly, for addicts to resist their compulsive desires. If that desire is so strong that even someone with ' "normal and reasonable" self-control' (Watson, 1977, p. 331) would succumb to it, we have little compunction in saying that the addict's free will was sufficiently impaired that his apparent consent counts for naught.[7]

---

[6]Thus, health education campaigns have begun focusing on the risks of contracting Buerger's disease from smoking, the amputation of limbs being, like snakebites, psychologically more accessible to people (especially teenagers, before they start to smoke) than rotting lungs.

[7]Some would question whether drug withdrawal symptoms in general are really so severe as to justify claims of involuntariness by reason of 'pharmacological coercion'. Fingarette(1975, p. 437)(see also Fingarette, 1970) may well be right that the effects of withdrawal are largely in the addict's own mind and that they loom much larger in prospect among addicts contemplating withdrawal than they turn out to have been in retrospect after withdrawal has been successfully accomplished. Still, it is the agent's beliefs that are always the keys to coercion: If the bank tellers believed the robber's gun was loaded, they handed over the money under duress and are excused for that reason, even if it turns out that the gun's chambers were empty.

This is arguably the case with nicotine addiction. To establish a substance as addictive, we require two sorts of evidence. The first is some sort of evidence of 'physical need' for the substance among its users. That evidence is widely thought necessary to prove smoking is an addiction, rather than just a 'habit' (U.S. DHEW, 1964), a psychological dependence, or a matter of mere sociological pressure (Daniels, 1985) – none of which would undercut, in a way that addictiveness does, claims that the risks of smoking are voluntarily incurred. That physical link has now been established, though. Particular receptors for the active ingredients of tobacco smoke have been discovered in the brain; the physiological sites and mechanisms by which nicotine acts on the brain have now been well mapped, and its tendency to generate compulsive, repetitive behaviour in consequence has been well established. Such evidence (summarized in the Surgeon General's report (U.S. DHHS, 1988; see also Leventhal and Cleary, 1980; Winsten, 1986)) has been one important factor in leading the World Health Organization (1978) and the American Psychiatric Association (1987) to classify nicotine as a dependence-inducing drug. (Strictly speaking, the term 'addiction' is out of favour in these circles, with 'dependence' taking its place; in what follows, I shall continue using the more colloquial term in preference to the more technical one, though.)

None of that evidence proves that it would be literally impossible for smokers to resist the impulse to smoke. Through extraordinary acts of will, they might. Nor does any of that evidence prove that it is literally impossible for them to break their dependence altogether. Many have. Recall, however, that the issue is not one of impossibility but rather of how hard people should have to try before their will is said to be sufficiently impaired that their agreement does not count as a genuine consent.

The evidence suggests that nicotine addicts have to try very hard indeed. This is the second crucial fact to establish in proving a substance addictive.[8] Central among the WHO/APA criteria for diagnosing nicotine dependence is the requirement of evidence of 'continuous use of tobacco for at least one month with...unsuccessful attempts to stop or significantly reduce the amount of tobacco use on a permanent basis' (APA, 1987, sec. 305.1).

The vast majority of smokers do indeed find themselves in this position. The Surgeon General reports the results of

various studies showing that 90% of regular smokers have tried to quit (see U.S. DHHS, 1979, quoted in Pollin, 1984). Another 1975 survey found that 84% of smokers had attempted to stop, but that only 36% of them had succeeded in maintaining their changed behaviour for a whole year (Benfari et al., 1982; see also Leventhal and Cleary, 1980). Interestingly, graphs mapping the 'relapse rate' – the percentage of ex-addicts that are back on the drug after a given period of time – is almost identical for nicotine and for heroin (Winsten, 1986; U.S. DHHS, 1988).[9]

On the basis of all these evidences, the Surgeon General has been led to three 'major conclusions' contained in his 1988 report:

1. Cigarettes and other forms of tobacco are addicting.
2. Nicotine is the drug in tobacco that causes addiction.
3. The pharmacologic and behavioral processes that determine tobacco addiction are similar to those that determine addiction to drugs such as heroin and cocaine (U.S. DHHS, 1988, p. 9).

Evidence of smokers trying to stop and failing to do so is rightly regarded as central to the issue of addiction, philosophically as well as diagnostically. Some describe free will in terms of 'second-order volitions' – desires about desires – controlling 'first-order' ones (Frankfurt, 1971). Others talk of free will in terms of a person's 'evaluational structure' controlling his 'motivational structure' – a person striving to obtain something if and only if he thinks it to be of value (Watson, 1975, 1977). Addiction – the absence of free will – is thus a matter of first-order volitions winning out over second-order ones and surface desires prevailing over the agent's own deeper values. In the case of smoking, trying to stop can be seen as a manifestation of one's second-order volitions, or one's deeper values, and failing to stop as evidence of the triumph of first-order surface desires over them. The same criteria that the WHO and APA use to diagnose nicotine dependence also establish the impairment of the smoker's free will, philosophically.

For certain purposes, at least, even the courts now treat nicotine as addictive. Social security benefits are not payable to those claimants whose disabilities were voluntarily self-inflicted. But the courts have held that

[8]There are other physical needs that we would have trouble renouncing – such as our need for food – that we would be loath actually to call 'addictions'. Be that terminological issue as it may, we would also be loath, for precisely those reasons of physical need and the difficulty of renouncing it, to say that we eat 'of our own free will'. (We would have no hesitation that someone who makes a credible threat of preventing us from eating has thereby 'coerced' us.) As involuntariness and impairment of free will are what is really at issue here, those thus do seem to be the aspects of addictiveness that ground the conclusion that we do not voluntarily consent to the risks associated with addictive substances.

[9]It might be wrong to make too much of that fact, however. Perhaps heroin addicts find both that it is harder to give up and that they have more reason to do so. Then relapse rates would appear the same, even though heroin is more addictive, in the sense of being harder to give up.

'smoking can be an involuntary act for some persons', and that those benefits may not therefore be routinely withheld from victims of smoking-related diseases on the grounds that they are suffering from voluntarily self-inflicted injuries.[10]

Various other policy implications also follow from evidence of addictiveness, though. One might be that the over-the-counter sales of cigarettes should be banned. If the product is truly addictive, then we have no more reason to respect a person's voluntary choice (however well-informed) to abandon his future volition to an addiction than we have for respecting a person's voluntary choice (however well-informed) to sell himself into slavery (Mill, 1859/1975). I am unsure how far to press this argument, because after all we do permit people to bind their future selves (e.g. through contracts). But if it is the size of the stakes or the difficulty of breaking out of the bonds that makes the crucial difference, then acquiring a lethal and hard-to-break addiction is much more like a slavery contract than it is like an ordinary commercial commitment (cf. Feinberg, 1986).

In any case, addictiveness thus defined makes it far easier to justify interventions that on the surface appear paternalistic. In some sense, they would then not be paternalistic at all. Where people 'wish to stop smoking, but do not have the requisite willpower…we are not imposing a good on someone who rejects it. We are simply using coercion to enable people to carry out their own goals' (Dworkin, 1972/1983, p. 32).[11]

There is, of course, a genuine difficulty in deciding which is the 'authentic' self. With whom should we side, when the person who asks us to help him to 'enforce rules on himself' repudiates the rules at the moment they come to need to be enforced (Schelling, 1980, 1983, 1984a, 1984b, 1985).[12] But at least we have more of a warrant for interference, in such cases, than if we were never asked for assistance by the agent at all.

Much of the assistance that we have to render in such situations will necessarily be of a very personal nature, and it will be outside the scope of public policy for that reason. There is nonetheless a substantial role for public policy in these realms. Banning or restricting smoking in public places (especially the workplace) can contribute crucially to an individual's own efforts at smoking cessation, for

example (Etzioni, 1978; Leventhal and Cleary, 1980; U.S. DHHS, 1986).

The real force of the addiction findings, in the context of *volenti* or informed consent arguments, though, is to undercut the claim that there is any *continuing* consent to the risks involved in smoking. There might have been consent in the very first instance – in smoking your first cigarette. But once you were hooked, you lost the capacity to consent in any meaningful sense on a continuing basis (White, 1972). As Hume (1760) says, to consent implies the possibility of doing otherwise; and addiction substantially deprives you of the capacity to do other than continue smoking. So once you have become addicted to nicotine, your subsequent smoking cannot be taken as indicating your consent to the risks.

The most that we can now say with confidence, therefore, is that 'cigarette smoking, at least initially, is a voluntary activity', in the words of a leading court case in this area (Brown, 1987). If there is to be a consent at all in this area, it can only be a consent in the very first instance, that is, when you first began to smoke. That, in turn, seriously undercuts the extent to which cigarette manufacturers can rely upon *volenti* or informed consent defences in product liability litigation and its moral analogues.

It does so in two ways. The first arises from the fact that many of those now dying from tobacco-induced diseases started smoking well before warnings began appearing on packets in 1966 and were hooked by the time those warnings reached them. Their consent to the risks of smoking could only have been based on 'common knowledge' and 'folk wisdom'. That is a short-term problem, though, because that cohort of smokers will eventually die off.

The second and more serious problem is a continuing problem in a way the first is not. The vast majority of smokers began smoking in their early to middle teens. Evidence suggests that 'of those teenagers who smoke more than a single cigarette only 15% avoid becoming regular dependent smokers' (Russell, 1974). Studies show that, 'of current smokers, about 60% began by the very young age of 13 or 14' (Blasi and Monaghan, 1986), and the great majority – perhaps up to 95% – of regular adult smokers are thought to have been addicted before coming of age

---

[10]*Gordon v Schweiker*, 725 F.2d 231, 236 (4th Cir. 1984).

[11]That is one way of explaining an apparent paradox surrounding 'sin' taxes in general: 'items such as alcohol [and cigarettes] are so commonly consumed, and so little complaint is made about large excise taxes' on them, that microeconomists are led to conclude that it simply must be in the individual's own perceived interest, somehow, to be so taxed Crain et al. (1977).

[12]It begs this question to say that the one reflects an 'evaluational' and the other merely a 'motivational' judgement (Watson, 1975, 1977) or that the one reflects a 'second-order preference' and the other merely a 'first-order' one (Frankfurt, 1971). In the intrapersonal bargaining game that Schelling envisages, each side typically claims the superior status for its own preference ranking. From the wanton self's point of view, wanton preferences enjoy evaluational rather than merely motivational status.

(Califano, 1981; Lewit et al., 1981, Pollin, 1984; Leventhal et al., 1987; Davis, 1987; U.S. DHHS, 1988).

The crux of the matter, then, is just this: being below the age of consent when they first began smoking, smokers were incapable of meaningfully consenting to the risks in the first instance.[13] Being addicted by the time they reached the age of consent, they were incapable of consenting later, either.

REFERENCES

Alexander HM, Calcott R, Dobson AJ. Cigarette smoking and drug use in schoolchildren. IV. Factors associated with changes in smoking behaviors. *Int J Epidemiol* 1983; **12**: 59–65.

American Psychiatric Association (APA). *Diagnostic and Statistical Manual of Mental Disorders*, 3rd edition. Washington, D.C.: APA, 1987.

Anonymous. Note: Plaintiff's conduct as a defense to claims against cigarette manufacturers. *Harvard Law Rev* 1986; **99**: 809–827.

Benfari RC, Ockene JK, McIntyre KM. Control of cigarette-smoking from a psychological perspective. *Annu Rev Public Health* 1982; **3**: 101–128.

Blasi V, Monaghan HP. The first amendment and cigarette advertising. *J Am Med Assoc* 1986; **256**: 502–509.

Brown JR. Opinion of the U.S. Court of Appeals. *Palmer v. Liggett Group, Inc.* 825, F.2d 620 (1st Cir. 1987), 1987.

Califano JA Jr. *Governing America.* New York: Simon & Schuster, 1981.

Crain WM, Deaton T, Holcombe R, Tollison R. Rational choice and the taxation of sin. *J Public Econ* 1977; **8**: 239–245.

Daniels N. *Just Health Care.* Cambridge: Cambridge University Press, 1985.

Davis RM. Current trends in cigarette advertising and marketing. *N Engl J Med* 1987; **316**: 725–732.

Dworkin G. Paternalism. *Monist* 1972; **56**(1): 64–84 (Reprinted in Sartorius, ed. 1983, pp. 19–34).

Etzioni A. Individual will and social conditions: toward an effective health maintenance policy. *Annals Am Acad Polit Soc Sci* 1978; **437**: 62–73.

Feinberg J. Legal paternalism. *Can J Philos* 1971; **1**:106–124 (Reprinted in Sartorius, ed. 1983, pp. 3–18).

Feinberg J. *Harm to Self.* New York: Oxford University Press, 1986.

Fingarette H. The Perils of *Powell:* In search of a factual foundation for the 'disease' concept of alcoholism. *Harvard Law Rev* 1970; **83**: 793–812.

Fingarette H. Addiction and criminal responsibility. *Yale Law J* 1975; **84**: 413–444.

Fortas A. Dissenting Opinion. *Powell v. Texas.* 392 US 514, 1968; pp. 554–570.

Fox SJ. Physical disorder, consciousness and criminal liability. *Columb Law Rev* 1963; **63**: 645–668.

Frankfurt HG. Freedom of the will and the concept of a person. *J Philos* 1971; **68**: 5–20.

Fuchs VR. Time preference and health: an exploratory study. In: Fuchs VR, ed. *Economic Aspects of Health.* Chicago: University of Chicago Press, 1982; pp. 93–120.

Gewirth A. Health rights and the prevention of cancer. *Am Philos Q* 1980; **17**: 117–125.

Goodin RE. *Political Theory and Public Policy.* Chicago: University of Chicago Press, 1982.

Hume D. Of the original contract. *Essays, Literary, Moral and Political.* London: A. Millar, 1760.

Kahneman D, Slovic P, Tversky A, eds. *Judgment under Uncertainty.* Cambridge: Cambridge University Press, 1982.

Knowles JH. The responsibility of the individual. *Daedalus* 1977; **106**(1): 57–80.

Leventhal H, Cleary PD. The smoking problem: a review of the research and theory in behavioral risk modification. *Psychol Bull* 1980; **88**: 370–405.

Leventhal H, Glynn K, Fleming R. Is the smoking decision an 'informed choice'? *J Am Med Assoc* 1987; **257**: 3373–3376.

Lewit EM, Coate D, Grossman M. The effects of government regulation on teenage smoking. *J Law Econ* 1981; **24**: 545–569.

Lichtenstein S. Slovic P, Fischhoff B, Layman M, Combs B. Judged frequency of lethal events. *J Exp Psychol (Human Learning and Memory)* 1978; **4**: 551–578.

Marsh A. Smoking and illness: what smokers really believe. *Health Trends* 1985; **17**: 7–12.

Mill JS. On liberty. In: Wollheim R, ed. *Three Essays.* Oxford: Oxford University Press, 1859/1975, pp. 1–141.

Pears D. *Motivated Irrationality.* Oxford: Clarendon, 1984.

Pollin W. The role of the addictive process as a key step in causation of all tobacco-related diseases. *J Am Med Assoc* 1984; **252**: 2874.

Prevezer S. Automatism and involuntary conduct. *Criminal Law Rev* 1958; pp. 361–367, 440–452.

Robins L. *A Follow-up of Vietnam Drug Users.* Interim Final Report, Special Actions Office for Drug Abuse Prevention. Washington, D.C.: Executive Office of the President, 1973.

Russell MAH. Realistic goals for smoking and heath. *Lancet* 1974; **7851**: 254–258.

Sartorius R, ed. *Paternalism.* Minneapolis: University of Minnesota Press, 1983.

Schelling TC. The intimate contest for self-command. *Public Interest* 1980; **69**: 94–118 (Reprinted in Schelling 1984a, pp. 57–82).

Schelling TC. *Choice and Consequence.* Cambridge, MA: Harvard University Press, 1984a.

Schelling TC. Ethics, law and the exercise of self-command. *Tanner Lectures on Human Values* 1983; **4**: 44–79 (Reprinted in Schelling 1984a, pp. 83–113).

---

[13]Strictly speaking, ability to consent is not predicated – legally or morally – upon attaining some arbitrary age but, rather, upon having attained the capacity to make reasoned choices in the matter at hand (Anonymous, 1986). The level of understanding manifested by teenagers about smoking clearly suggests that their decision to start smoking cannot be deemed an informed choice, however (Leventhal et al., 1987).

Schelling TC. Self-command in practice, in policy, and in a theory of rational choice. *Am Econ Rev* (Papers and Proceedings) 1984b; **74**: 1–11.

Schelling TC. Enforcing rules on oneself. *J Law Econ Organ* 1985; **1**: 357–374.

Slovic P, Fischhoff B, Lichtenstein S. In: Tversky KS, eds. *Fact vs. Fears: Understanding Perceived Risks*, 1982, pp. 463–89.

Sunstein CR. Legal Interference with the Private Preferences. *Univ Chicago Law Rev* 1986; **53**: 1129–1174.

U.S. Department of Health, Education and Welfare (U.S. DHEW). *Smoking and Health*. Report of the Advisory Committee to the Surgeon General of the Public Health Service. Washington, D.C.: Government Printing Office, 1964.

U.S. DHHS. Surgeon General. *Smoking and Health*. Washington, D.C.: Govenret Printing Office, 1979.

U.S. DHHS. Surgeon General. *The Health Consequences of Involuntary Smoking*. Washington, D.C.: Government Printing Office, 1986.

U.S. DHHS. Surgeon General. *The Health Consequences of Smoking: Nicotine Addiction*. Washington, D.C.: Government Printing Office, 1988.

U.S. Federal Trade Commission (U.S. FTC). In: Meyers ML, chairman. *Staff Report on the Cigarette Advertising Investigation* (Public version). Washington, D.C.: FTC, 1981.

Watson G. Free agency. *J Philos* 1975; **72**: 205–220.

Watson G. Skepticism about Weakness of Will. *Philos Rev* 1977; **86**: 316–339.

White AA. The intentional exploitation of man's known weaknesses. *Houston Law Rev* 1972; **9**: 889–927.

WHO. *International Classification of Diseases*, 9th edition. Geneva: WHO, 1978.

Wikler D. Personal responsibility for illness. In: van de Veer D, Regan T, eds. *Health Care Ethics*. Philadelphia: Temple University Press, 1987; pp. 326–358.

Winsten JA. *Nicotine Dependency and Compulsive Tobacco Use*. A Research Status Report, Center for Health Communication. Harvard School of Public Health, 1986 (Reprinted in *Tobacco Prod Liab Rep* **1**(7)).

89

Doctors and Human Rights[1]

DORIS SCHROEDER

When hearing 'Doctors and Human Rights', one is inclined to think of doctors rushing to disaster zones to provide emergency medical aid, running out of hospitals to help bomb victims or tackling contagious diseases at a risk to their own lives. An air of heroism emanates from the words 'doctors' and 'human rights', when used in the same phrase. But doctors' engagement with human rights is often much more mundane. Besides, it is rather striking that none of the people listed at the German Resistance Memorial Center (2005) are doctors (the overwhelming majority are jurists, politicians, aristocrats or military officers). Likewise, the e-book summarizing the proceedings of the South African Truth Commission does not show any hits for 'doctor', although it does for other professions (Christie, 2000). So, let us ignore the heroic overtones of this topic and concentrate on the straightforward links between doctors and human rights.

It will be taken for granted that doctors respect human rights implemented through national or international legislation in their countries. For an overview of selected principles for doctors, see Table 89.1.

What we are interested in goes beyond legal requirements into more fundamental questions, such as 'Can doctors play a role in justifying human rights?' or 'Is the human rights framework sufficient for the morally aware and conscientious doctor?' This chapter is divided into six sections. A brief outline of human rights classifications (1) precedes questions about the justification (2), the types (3) and the enforcement (4) of human rights. The last section looks at the limits of the human rights framework (5) to be followed by a conclusion (6).

Table 89.1. Ethical codes and principles for doctors

400 BC / 1964	The Hippocratic Oath at: http://classics.mit.edu/Hippocrates/hippooath.html, accessed: 12 August 2005; The Modern Hippocratic Oath at: http://www.pbs.org/wgbh/nova/doctors/oath_modern.html, accessed: 12 August 2005.
1947	Nuremberg Code, 1947.
1964 / 2002	World Medical Association Declaration of Helsinki at: http://www.wma.net/e/policy/b3.htm, accessed: 12 August 2005.
1993 / 2002	Council for International Organizations of Medical Sciences, International Ethical Guidelines for Biomedical Research Involving Human Subjects at: http://www.cioms.ch/frame_guidelines_nov_2002.htm, accessed: 12 August 2005.
1997	Council of Europe Convention on Human Rights and Biomedicine, at: http://conventions.coe.int/treaty/en/treaties/html/164.htm, accessed: 12 August 2005.

HUMAN RIGHTS

'Human rights' is a global topic. As soon as one agrees that a right is a *human* right, one cannot restrict it to certain groups. People have human rights by virtue of their humanity, not by virtue of their nationality, their status, their gender, their ethnicity, etc. But what are these rights and how can they be defined? According to the *New Oxford Dictionary of English*, 'rights' are 'moral or legal entitlements to have or obtain something or to act in a certain way'. If we add the domain to which this definition applies – humans – we receive the following minimal definition:

---

[1] This chapter deals with 'Doctors and Human Rights'. Although many of its passages could be applied to other health care professionals, this will not be indicated in the text.

Principles of Health Care Ethics, Second Edition   Edited by R.E. Ashcroft, A. Dawson, H. Draper and J.R. McMillan
© 2007 John Wiley & Sons, Ltd

Human rights are moral or legal entitlements held by human beings by virtue of their humanity to have or obtain something or to act in a certain way.

Questions that immediately pose themselves are as follows: Why should human beings have certain entitlements? And if they do, what are these entitlements and how can they be enforced? The topic of 'human rights' is not only one of the most exciting but also one of the most contentious topics in the twenty-first century. Agreement and divergence can be found in three areas covering concept, content and enforcement (see Figure 89.1).

On the conceptual level, one needs to ask whether there is a foundation for human rights: a justification for their supposed existence. Affirmative answers range from a confident 'yes' based on human dignity or rationality (e.g. Kant, 1965; Gewirth, 1984) to 'This is the way it is with rights. You want' em, so you say you got' em, and if nobody says you don't then you do' (Danto, 1984). Non-affirmative answers focus mostly on the claim that human rights are a western invention, which cannot be universalized across the rest of the world (Muzzafar, 1999; Sakamoto, 1999).

Should one agree that human rights exist, the next question is which *particular* rights do human beings have by virtue of being human: political and civil rights (often called 'first-generation rights'), economic, social and cultural rights ('second-generation'), rights to international solidarity ('third-generation') or right to peace ('fourth-generation'). And the questions continue within these categories. For instance, if we agreed on freedom of the press as a political right, where would we draw the line with another right we might want to include, namely the right to privacy?

The last category of questions on human rights concerns enforcement. Without effective laws and enforcement agencies, human rights discourse can easily decline into fantasizing about rights without careful consideration of equivalent obligations and implementation (O'Neill, 2001). For instance, in November 2002, the United Nations Committee on Economic, Cultural and Social Rights took the unusual step of agreeing that water is a human right (Hartl, 2002).

Water is fundamental for life and health. The human right to water is indispensable for leading a healthy life in human dignity. It is a pre-requisite to the realization of all other human rights.

Without wanting to criticize this UN Committee, one has to consider the following points. The 145 countries which signed the UN International Covenant on Economic, Social and Cultural Rights will henceforth have to ensure access to safe drinking water to their citizens without discrimination. What if governments cannot afford to provide safe water to all? What if they decide they have other, equally pressing, priorities? The United Nations has very few enforcement mechanisms, which means that rights declared by UN committees do not easily translate into reality. Also, the United Nations currently has 191 members, which means that 46 did not sign the covenant. Do citizens of these countries have a human right to water or not? They are human after all.

DOCTORS AND THE JUSTIFICATION OF HUMAN RIGHTS

Doctors are not philosophers. Their main tasks are as follows:

- to promote and safeguard the health of the people (Declaration of Helsinki A1);
- to promote respect for all human beings (ibid., A8);
- to protect the life, health, and dignity of the human subject in research (ibid., B10); and
- to promote advances in medical achievement.

It is not their task to ponder the justification or foundation of human rights. However, in recent decades, philosophical debates and scientific medical research have become increasingly entangled in two areas, namely the beginning and end of life decisions. And given the immediate relevance of such topics to doctors in practice, their interest is unsurprising.

Human rights

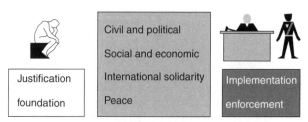

Figure 89.1.   Human rights topics

Table 89.2   Prominent human rights declarations

1948	Universal Declaration of Human Rights at: http://www.un.org/Overview/rights.html, accessed: 4 August 2005.
1950	European Convention on Human Rights at: http://www.hri.org/docs/ECHR50.html, accessed: 4 August 2005.
1981	The Universal Islamic Declaration of Human Rights at: http://www.alhewar.com/ISLAM-DECL.html, accessed: 4 August 2005.
1981	African Charter on Human and Peoples' Rights at: http://www.hrcr.org/docs/Banjul/afrhr.html, accessed: 4 August 2005.
1998	Asian Human Rights Charter at: http://www.ahrchk.net/charter/mainfile.php/eng_charter/, accessed: 4 August 2005.

Imagine you were asked to pick one human right above all others, which would you choose? It would probably be the right to life, which is the first substantial right in all modern human rights proclamations (Table 89.2).

If human beings have a right to life as one of their most fundamental rights, abortion and euthanasia become immediately problematic. And increasingly, doctors involved in medical research have been drawn into the debate. So, instead of getting involved in questions such as 'Why should human beings have special rights?' they get drawn into almost equally metaphysical questions such as 'Who is a human being?', 'Is a blastocyst a human being, is an embryo a human being and is somebody with brain stem death in a vegetative state, a human being?' Of course, doctors are in no better position to give *easy* answers to such questions as other professionals. However, depending on the exact phrasing of the ethical question involved, they can supply medical information to advance the debate as the following imaginary dialogue between Aristotle and a modern doctor mediated by Prof. Schroeder shows:

Schroeder   Is taking the morning-after pill murder, that is, the unlawful, premeditated killing of a human being?

Aristotle   In order to answer this question, we need to look at the essence of human beings first.

Schroeder   What do you mean by 'essence'?

Aristotle   'Essence' is what makes an object or a being fundamentally what it is, its spirit, its core, its most important feature.

Doctor   So what is the essence of human beings?

Aristotle   The essence of human beings is rationality (Aristotle, 1985: p. 1178a).

Schroeder   How does this help us find an answer to the question raised?

Doctor   Perhaps I can help. If Aristotle is right and we define human beings via their rationality, brain function is required to make an entity a human being. It is only in week three of a pregnancy that the brain begins to develop. In contradiction to its name, the morning-after pill is usually effective taken up to 72h after, well …. let's call it the 'incident' in the presence of our esteemed philosophy colleague. This means that taking the morning-after pill cannot ever be regarded as murder, because the destroyed entity is not a human being.

Schroeder   Thank you very much. This was a helpful clarification.

With the increase of modern medical technologies (e.g. embryonic stem cell research, cloning and xenotransplantation), fruitful cooperations between doctors and philosophers are on the rise. In fact, a good number of medical ethicists are doctors or nurses with a background or training in philosophy, and vice versa. Doctors rely on such cooperations (as do policy makers) to define and understand the legal and moral limits of their practice. Philosophers, in turn, can benefit from the cooperation because answers to seemingly mundane questions about the morning-after pill can lead to insights into eternal topics.

A serious note of caution: if one involves modern medical research in debates about fundamental questions of human rights, as in the above example, one clearly endorses a particular framework of thought based on strict individualism, secular humanism and the belief that technology equals progress. One needs only to question Aristotle's belief in the essence of human beings and replace it with, for instance, a spiritual belief that the essence of human beings is an unintelligible soul, which enters the world on conception, and most medical research becomes redundant within the argument.

DOCTORS AND THE TYPE OF HUMAN RIGHTS

Human rights are usually categorized according to generations, as outlined in the section on 'Human Rights'. Political and civil rights; economic, social and cultural rights; rights to international solidarity and a right to peace. At first sight, it might seem as though only a small number of these rights were relevant to the work of doctors. However, this is not so.

First-generation rights: A violation of civil liberty rights (e.g. torture) translates directly into increased morbidity or mortality. At the same time, public health measures (e.g. compulsory vaccinations) can infringe civil liberties.

Second-generation rights: With the exception of the United States, all affluent industrialized nations offer universal access to health care to their citizens (Benatar and Fox 2005). When this is not the case, as in the United States or developing countries, doctors cannot easily discharge their duty of promoting and safeguarding the health of people; they either restrict their help to the affluent, or they turn into a Good Samaritan offering their services free during their leisure time.

Third-generation rights: Rights to international solidarity are relevant to doctors in two aspects: by providing health care services beyond national welfare states (e.g. health-related development aid) and by cooperating towards the preservation of a healthy environment (e.g. tackling global climate change).

Fourth-generation rights: Finally, violations of the right to peace lead invariably to increased morbidity and mortality as experienced in war as a result of both fighting and shortages of goods.

In an ideal world, every human being would have access to adequate health care, provided through national or international solidarity in a setting of peace. This is not the case. For those who believe in the above rights, rights violations occur more often and in more unexpected places than one would assume. The following examples give an overview of common rights violations relevant to the first three generations of rights,[2] which can put doctors into very difficult positions:

First-generation rights: Article 5 of the Universal Declaration of Human Rights demands that 'no one shall be subjected to torture or to cruel, inhuman or degrading treatment or punishment'. But how exactly does one define 'torture' and which punishment is degrading or inhuman? In some Islamic countries, amputation is a type of punishment ordered by sharia law for theft. Many readers will categorize this as inhuman punishment, others might not. But what clearly emerges from this example are the serious problems of conscience for physicians. Why? Those who regard amputation as inhuman punishment will have the duty to care for the sick. Maimed patients clearly belong to this category. By distancing themselves from amputation in a strict manner, doctors would make suffering much worse. As a result, the International Red Cross forbids its staff

to perform amputations, but encourages the treatment of maimed patients who require care (Gross, 2004). A similar problem arises for physicians in Israel, which has set standards for the so-called 'moderate physical pressure' as opposed to torture during interrogation. This includes 'beating and slapping, forcefully shaking the upper torso causing the neck and head to "dangle and vacillate rapidly" and excessive tightening of handcuffs' (Gross, 2004). Doctors play an important role in such interrogations by, for instance, certifying a suspect's fitness for various types of questioning. In this context, the so-called 'necessity defence' is invoked, which means that the prevention of imminent and grievous harm to others (e.g. bomb victims) justifies interrogations, which exert moderate physical pressure on suspects. Again, the conflict for physicians is clear. Their duty to care might be compromised by acquiescence to inhuman punishment or torture, but it still exists (Gross, 2004).

Second-generation rights: Health is expensive in the United States: 16.6% of GDP was spent in 2002 to provide health care services across the country. This compares to 10.9% for Germany, 9.7% for France, 7.9% for Japan and 7.7% for the United Kingdom (WHO, 2002). At the same time, an estimated 15.2% of the population, or 43.6 million people, were without health insurance coverage (DeNavas-Walt et al., 2003). This combination of high costs and low accessibility which – in the Western hemisphere – is unique to the United States has been called 'a national scandal' (Schwartz, 1996, p. 226). Within such a setting, doctors are faced with cases that are normally restricted to developing countries. 'A man in his early 20s with a worsening dental infection who was unable to afford a dentist ... finally saw a physician who prescribed an antibiotic, but the patient was unable to pay for the prescription. He presented to our clinic [a charity-funded clinic for those without health insurance] with sepsis and spread of the infection to his mediastinum. He died soon after admission' (Ferrer, 2001).

Third-generation rights: According to the World Health Organization (WHO, 1999) most of the 13 million deaths a year from infectious diseases could be prevented with low-cost health interventions. For instance, childhood vaccinations against the six major killer diseases (diphtheria, whooping cough, tetanus, polio, measles and tuberculosis) could prevent 1.6 million deaths a year among children under five, costing $15 per child (Unicef, 1998). One Viagra pill costs between $8 and $12 (predictable comparison, I know). As a doctor if one subscribes to the human right to life combined with a right to international solidarity, such comparisons will have to be made (also see the last section).

The above examples show that doctors can be placed in Catch-22 positions, which require an extraordinarily high

---

[2]If one makes THE right to peace a human right, one has to ensure world peace. The right to world peace is such a utopian right at the outset of the twenty-first century that one might as well argue for a right to happiness. Hence, this right will not be discussed in detail.

degree of good judgement. In fact, some doctors will not be able to arrive at morally satisfactory decisions, as in the amputation or torture cases. And some doctors, for instance in an Alpine town hospital, could be blissfully unaware or even complacent about the difficult choices their colleagues in other countries might face.

DOCTORS AND THE IMPLEMENTATION/ ENFORCEMENT OF HUMAN RIGHTS

Article 25 of the Universal Declaration of Human Rights demands that 'everyone has the right to a standard of living adequate for the health and well-being of himself and of his family, including food, clothing, housing and **medical care** and necessary social services, and the right to security in the event of unemployment, sickness, disability, widowhood, old age or other lack of livelihood in circumstances beyond his control' (my emphasis).

But is the Universal Declaration of Human Rights not just an optimistically written piece of paper signed by many but adhered to by few? Do human rights really exist? The easy answer to this question is 'Yes they exist, if they are implemented through national legislation as legal rights'. For instance, the first core principle of the British National Health Service is to 'provide a universal service for all based on clinical need not ability to pay' (NHS, 2005). In this regard, the right to medical care as envisaged by Article 25 has been implemented in Britain. If a doctor refuses to treat a patient without appropriate justification, the right to medical care can be enforced through the courts. However, it does not make sense to restrict human rights to legal rights. During the apartheid era Black South Africans were disenfranchised through legal regulations forbidding them to vote. Taking part in the government of one's country, either directly or indirectly through freely chosen representatives, is a human right (Art. 21). If only legal rights were accepted as human rights, it would have been impossible to argue that the rights of Black South African citizens were violated by unjust legislation. Human rights have to exist outside individual legal systems to have any power in situations of injustice. Ideally, though, they would be realized through implementation in national or international legal codes.

Some doctors engage in human rights activism of this type. For instance, Physicians for a National Health Program (PNHP) is a US advocate organization, which lobbies for the introduction of a national health system (www.pnhp. org). PNHP – a nonprofit organization – coordinates the activities of physicians, medical students and other health care professionals pressing the US government for the introduction of a single-payer system. This system would involve government-financed health care for all, although the delivery would remain mostly under private control.

Organizations such as Médecins Sans Frontières (MSF) or Médecins du Monde help to progressively realize a right to medical care – at the moment mostly a right to emergency medical assistance. MSF is an international humanitarian aid organization which provides emergency medical assistance to populations in danger in more than 70 countries (www.msf.org). More political in its approach, Médecins du Monde is an international humanitarian aid organization which provides health care to vulnerable populations around the world, at the same time as bearing witness to human rights abuses. In doing so, they hope to give a voice to vulnerable people whose stories may not otherwise be heard (http://www.medecinsdumonde.org).

Most closely linked to the topic of this chapter is Doctors for Human Rights, an organization which aims to investigate health and human rights violations worldwide, promote international health and human rights standards, advocate on behalf of victims of human rights violations, and advise international bodies on measures to attain high standards of health (http://www.doctorsforhumanrights.org/).

However, one should note that lobbying for the legal implementation of human rights is a highly time-consuming and complex task, which lies outside the immediate realm of a physician's power.

DOCTORS AND THE LIMITS OF HUMAN RIGHTS

So far, we have looked at the potential involvement of doctors in human rights debates and action. But is it enough for doctors to follow blindly human rights principles and codes laid down by others? No. Human rights principles have not been revealed to us by an omniscient, benevolent, wise entity whom we can entirely trust to give us perfect professional codes. They are human-made with two potential corollaries. First, it makes sense to monitor and potentially improve human rights principles (note: the Declaration of Helsinki has been revised seven times since 1964). Second, the human rights framework itself might have to be critically examined and defended against opponents. Ideally, doctors need to be aware of such efforts.

On the one hand, human rights are heralded as a promising concept that can transcend religions, borders and cultures with the potential to flourish around the globe (Benatar et al., 2003). On the other hand, Hyakudai Sakamoto (1999), the President of the Japanese Association of Bioethics, as well as the Asian Bioethics Association, argues that the human rights discourse is a specifically western approach to problems in health care ethics, which should not be imposed on other parts of the world.

This divide is not easily bridged. One could say that western health care ethics relies almost exclusively on the concepts of individualism and human rights, and can often be described as anthropocentric (i.e. focused on human life rather than plant or animal life). In contrast, the African world-view has been described as 'eco-bio-communitarian' (Tangwa, 1999), implying a preference of community values over individualistic values as well as a recognition of the interdependence of all forms of life on earth. Similarly, the essence of the Asian world-view in bioethics has been described as 'a holistic harmony' (Sakamoto, 1999) with a higher esteem for social values over individual values and no strict dichotomy between humans and nature.

What are the strengths and the limits of a world-view framed around individualism and human rights as relevant to doctors? It is important that some elements of human life are framed with individuals in mind. For instance, 'life' is – above all – an individual asset. A mother who starves so that her children can live might make an invaluable community contribution, but she loses the one life she has. Similarly, 'bodily integrity and health' are individual assets. The pains of violent attacks, torture, rape, hunger, cold and disease are individual pains of separate human beings. Whatever the merits of altruism, modesty, humility and willingness for self-sacrifice, there is a need to set limits to what one human can inflict on another (through action, e.g. violence, or non-action, e.g. refusal of solidarity and beneficence). In this regard, it is important that doctors respect and protect the life, bodily integrity and health of individuals.

Problems arise when (1) the rights of individuals collide with other important goods and (2) a strict focus on individual human rights veils more general, systemic questions of, for instance, social justice. Particularly in the first instance, doctors need to make carefully considered, measured judgements instead of blindly following codes, as though one was ticking off items on a shopping list.

HUMAN RIGHTS AND PUBLIC HEALTH

The following example illustrates possible tensions between the rights of individuals and the broader social good (Fox and Goemaere, 2006). As part of a mission to explore the feasibility of treating HIV/AIDS in economically disadvantaged settings, Médecins Sans Frontières launched a project providing antiretroviral drugs to inhabitants of Khayelitsha, a township near Cape Town, South Africa. One of the many ethical dilemmas encountered within the project was the potential development of multi-drug-resistant infections due to patient's non-adherence

to the treatment regime. In the context of HIV/AIDS, antiretroviral drugs need to be taken on a life-long basis and according to a specified regime. Non-compliance can lead to the emergence of resistance, with high public health costs and implications for other individuals (Benatar, 2006). The problem can be illustrated with a case from the Khayelitsha project (Fox and Goemaere, 2006).

> L., a 32-year-old, male patient, was among the first to be enrolled in the Khayelitsha ARV programme. Although the selection committee was aware that he was violent towards his girlfriend, and that he abused alcohol, they believed that he would be able to turn his life around and stabilize it. Their confidence in his capacity was based on their admiration for his dedicated involvement in the Treatment Action Campaign (TAC). L. had organized a TAC branch close to his home, and worked hard to promote access to treatment for HIV/AIDS. However, he was never able to find regular paid employment.
> Shortly after starting ARV treatment, L. ceased to adhere to the mandatory drug regimen. Subsequently, clinic staff learned that this was due to the fact that he had been hospitalized for a broken arm caused by a gunshot wound. Therapy was rapidly resumed, and he improved significantly; but after 6 months of therapy, his non-adherence to the treatment became manifest. His CD4 count was barely improving, and his viral load remained detectable at 3- and 6-month routine checkups. Shortly after 9 months on ARV medications, his clinical status worsened, and he developed pulmonary tuberculosis. He was urged by the staff to attend intensive counselling sessions, which he did. He improved once more for a short while, but 'defaulted' again in the taking of his medications, and vanished from sight. When he reappeared, his clinical status had deteriorated still further. At this point, the Khayelitsha team painfully decided to withdraw ARV treatment, not only because the clinical signs indicated that it was not benefiting him any more, but also because they hoped that this would produce a 'reality shock' that would forcefully remind him about the importance of 'regularity' and 'adherence'. Their strategy did not work. L. died from disseminated tuberculosis, 18 months after he had received his first dose of antiretroviral drugs.

The promotion and safeguarding of the health of their patients is usually considered the prime duty of physicians. But what if trying to safeguard the health of one patient (L) risks the health of others, who could be exposed to drug-resistant strains of the HIV/AIDS virus as a result? In this instance, both the rights of other individuals to have their health safeguarded as well as the overall social good of society are at risk. According to the human rights framework, which is non-utilitarian in spirit, individual rights trump the social good, in this context public health. What is called 'clinical fidelity' (Bloche, 1999), the allegiance to the patient in one's care, conflicts with the social purposes of medicine, particularly public health goals. There are no straightforward answers to such dilemmas. Doctors need to be aware of the benefits and limits of the human rights approach as based on strict individualism and, in particular, the possible tension between clinical fidelity and public health goals.

VEILING THE GLOBAL PERSPECTIVE

The human rights framework with its focus on individuals has the potential to distract from some of the most pressing ethical questions of our time, namely those that concern whole populations. For instance, US bioethicists have, by and large, concentrated their efforts on ethical questions related to cloning, genetics and new reproductive technologies (Benatar and Fox, 2005). Instead of concentrating on the billions who *do not* have access to health care, the sophisticated problems of the millions who do have access dominate ethical debates. In this regard, the concern of ethicists mirrors the famous 90/10 gap, referring to the fact that 10% of funding is targeted at diseases accounting for 90% of the global disease burden (Global Forum for Health Research, 2005). The 'obscene disparities' between those with 'too much care' and those with 'no care at all' (Farmer, 2003) are being veiled by an overly strong focus on individual human rights, where the definition of rights only starts when the doctor meets the patient (e.g. informed consent). Those who cannot benefit from meeting a doctor in the first place are potentially excluded.

CONCLUSION

To be a doctor is a task heavy with responsibility, requiring a good understanding of human rights as well as good judgement when rights come into conflict with other important goods. The emergence of new medical technologies has increased the need to find not only moral and legal limits to the medical practice but also the involvement of physicians in unusual questions ('what is a human being?'). Likewise, the conscientious doctor will take a stance when civil, social or beneficence rights are violated, without forgetting that the human rights framework needs to be critically monitored and improved where appropriate.

The possible tensions between individual human rights and public health goals and the potential neglect of obscene disparities in health care access should not distract from the achievements of human rights activism over the last 100 years. Imagine being stranded in a foreign country with a false accusation of armed robbery and a diabetic attack. Where would you want to be? In a country that adheres in a pedantic manner to individual human rights or one with a communal focus on societal well-being? You choose. As for the role of doctors to provide leadership in human rights promotion, in supporting public health measures *and* in looking beyond their own patients to global problems, one might say: 'This is too much; doctors are only human'. However, as Solomon Benatar and Renée Fox have rightly noted, in many western countries, physicians are the 'conscience of society', an observation which thrusts them into a privileged position to achieve change. So, perhaps a little heroism is required after all.

REFERENCES

Aristotle. *Nikomachische Ethik*. Hamburg: Felix Meiner Verlag, 1985.

Benatar S. Facing ethical challenges in rolling out antiretroviral treatment in resource poor countries. *Cambridge Quarterly of Healthcare Ethics* (2006); **15**(3): 302–312

Benatar S, Daar A, Singer P. Global health ethics: the rationale for mutual caring. *International Affairs* 2003; **79**: 107–138.

Benatar S, Fox R. Meeting threats to global health. *Perspect Bio Med*; **48**(3): 344–361.

Bloche MG. Clinical loyalties and the social purposes of medicine. *JAMA* 1999; **281**(2): 268–274.

Christie K. *The South African Truth Commission*. , Basingstoke: Palgrave Macmillan, 2000.

Danto AC. Constructing an epistemology of human rights: a pseudo problem? In: Paul EF, Paul J, Miller Jr FD, eds. *Human Rights*. Oxford: Blackwell, 1984, pp. 25–34.

DeNavas-Walt C, Proctor BD, Mills RJ. *Income, Poverty, and Health Insurance Coverage in the United State*. Washington: US Census Bureau, 2003. At http://www.census.gov/prod/2004pubs/p60-226.pdf, accessed 14 August 2005, p. 14.

Farmer P. *Pathologies of Power: Health, Human Rights and the New War on the Poor*. Berkeley, CA: University of California Press, 2003.

Ferrer R. Within the system of no-system. *JAMA* 2001; **286**(20): 2513–2514.

Fox R, Goemaere E. They call it 'patient selection' in Khayelitsha. *Cambridge Quarterly of Healthcare Ethics* (2006 forthcoming); **15**(3): 322–330.

German Resistance Memorial Center. *Biographies*, 2005. At http://www.gdw-berlin.de/index-e.php, accessed 28 July 2005.

Gewirth A. The epistemology of human rights. In: Paul EF, Paul J, Miller Jr FD, eds. *Human Rights*. Oxford: Blackwell, 1984, pp. 1–24.

Global Forum for Health Research. *The 10/90 Gap*, 2005. At http://www.globalforumhealth.org/site/000 Home.php, accessed 12 August 2005.

Gross M. Doctors in the decent society: torture, ill-treatment and civic duty. *Bioethics* 2004; **18**(2): 181–203.

Hartl G. Water for health enshrined as human right. World Health Organization, 2002. At: http://www.who.int/mediacentre/news/releases/pr91/en/, accessed 28 July 2005.

Kant I. *Grundlegung zur Metaphysik der Sitten*. Hamburg: Felix Meiner Verlag, 1965.

Muzzafar C. From human rights to human dignity. In: van Ness P, ed. *Debating Human Rights*, London: Routledge, 1999, pp. 25–31.

NHS. *NHS Core Principles*, 2005. At http://www.nhs.uk/England/AboutTheNhs/CorePrinciples.cmsx, accessed 15 August 2005.

Nuremberg Code. In: Mitscherlich A, Mielke F, eds. *Doctors of Infamy: The Story of the Nazi Medical Crimes*. New York: Schuman, 1947, pp. xxiii–v.

O'Neill O. Agents of justice. In: Pogge T, ed. *Global Justice*. Oxford: Blackwell, 2001, pp. 188–203.

Sakamoto H. Towards a new 'global bioethics'. *Bioethics* 1999; **13**: 191–197.

Schwartz RL. Life style, health status, and distributive justice. In: Grubb A and Mehlman MJ, eds. *Justice and Health Care*. Chichester: John Wiley & Sons, Ltd, 1996, pp. 225– 249.

Tangwa G. Globalisation or westernisation? Ethical concerns in the whole bio-business. *Bioethics* 1999; **13**: 218–226.

Unicef. *Health Commentary – Immunization, Going the Extra Mile*, 1998. At http://www.unicef.org/pon98/14-21.pdf, accessed 14 August 2005.

WHO. *Removing Obstacles to Healthy Development*, 1999. At http://www.who.int/infectious-disease-report/pages/ch4text.html#Anchor1, accessed 14 August 2005.

WHO. *Countries*, 2002. At http://www.who.int/countries/en/, accessed 14 August 2005.

Duties to Refugees and Asylum Seekers in Host Countries' Medical Systems

PASCALE ALLOTEY, HILARY PICKLES, VANESSA JOHNSTON

INTRODUCTION

Health care professionals undertake their practice within the boundaries of the ethical standards of their professional organizations. However, like all individuals, they are also influenced by their own cultural and personal backgrounds and the social and political context of the societies in which they live. It is inevitable therefore that interaction with their patients will be influenced to some degree by these externalities. The assessment and care of refugees present a major challenge to health care professionals and health services, more generally, for two major reasons. First, as a subpopulation, their experiences prior to arrival in countries of resettlement (host countries) create a set of unique vulnerabilities. Second, discourses on refugees and migration in host countries, such as Australia and the United Kingdom, have become increasingly emotive and politically controversial, influencing policies relating to refugees and asylum seekers. These have significant implications for health. This chapter raises and discusses some of the broad ethical challenges in meeting the health needs of asylum seekers and refugees, drawing on examples largely from the United Kingdom and Australia.

BACKGROUND

The 1951 Convention Relating to the Status of Refugees (Refugee Convention), the foundation document of international refugee law, was drafted in the spirit of humanitarianism in the wake of the Second World War. The internationally recognized definition of a refugee provided in the Convention is a person who

owing to well-founded fear of being persecuted for reasons of race, religion, nationality, membership of a particular social group or political opinion, is outside the country of his nationality and is unable or, owing to such fear, is unwilling to avail himself of the protection of that country; or who, not having a nationality and being outside the country of his former habitual residence as a result of such events, is unable or, owing to such fear, is unwilling to return to it (UNHCR, 1951).

Countries that ratified the Refugee Convention accepted in good faith the obligation and responsibility to provide refuge, and the entitlements and supports that they afford their own citizens. In addition a country is obliged not to return refugees or asylum seekers to the country from which they fear persecution, a principle known as *non-refoulement* (Allotey, 2003, 2004). Once outside their country of origin, people who meet the conditions specified under the Convention may lodge an application for asylum through the United Nations High Commissioner for Refugees (UNHCR) or a potential host country's government for refugee status. The term 'asylum seeker' applies to a person who has applied for recognition as a refugee in another country and is awaiting the outcome on his/her application. (*see* UNHCR 'Definition and Obligations' http://www.unhcr.org.au/basicdef.shtml).

Although this strictly legal definition of a refugee continues to be used to assess an applicant's eligibility for refugee protection (see the protocol relating to the Status of Refugees 1967) the current political context in which people are compelled to flee their countries of habitual residence or nationality has changed considerably from the circumstances of the mid-twentieth century. Forced migration in the new millennium encompasses several legal, social and political categories, and in contrast to the Cold War

Principles of Health Care Ethics, Second Edition   Edited by R.E. Ashcroft, A. Dawson, H. Draper and J.R. McMillan
© 2007 John Wiley & Sons, Ltd

era, most forced migrants today flee for reasons that are not formally defined by the international protection regime. This includes displacement resulting from environmental devastation, natural disasters and large-scale development projects, as well as the mass exodus of populations resulting from protracted civil conflict (Castles, 2003). In addition, globalization and ease of travel have had a significant effect on global movements of people, in general, and the ability of people to pursue a more secure future for themselves and for their families (Allotey and Zwi, In Press). With the resultant increase in the number of people seeking asylum, the legitimacy of claims, other than those specified under the Convention, is often contested (Johnston and Murray, 2003). Many governments in both high- and low-income countries are concerned about the frequent misuse of the asylum claims process, the need to restrict immigration, border security and 'dilution of national identity' by culturally diverse immigrants (Allotey, 2003, 2004). There has therefore been a tightening of both refugee and migration policies in several countries. The move over recent years towards the harmonization of immigration and refugee policies, within the European Union for instance, has had the clear aim of restricting the number of asylum seekers gaining entry (Overbeek, 1995; White, 2000). The resultant public debate has raised concerns about xenophobia, rights to citizenship and the humanitarian obligations of states towards those in need of protection versus the desire to protect national sovereignty. In addition, images of refugees and asylum seekers portrayed in the mass media are mixed and not necessarily positive. They range from the portrayal of powerless vulnerable people, living in deplorable conditions, harbouring diseases long eradicated, to those taking perilous journeys to cross borders without legal documentation (Allotey, 2004). These representations are powerful and important in developing public opinion (Kleinman and Kleinman, 1997) and towards the type of reception refugees and asylum seekers receive in host countries. It is not uncommon, for instance, for the terms refugees and asylum seekers, and even in some cases, illegal immigrants, to be used interchangeably in the media and political discourse (Steiner, 2000; de Bousingen, 2002). Illegal or undocumented immigrants are those who do not have the legal documentation to remain in the country of current residence.

Contemporary policy discourse on refugees and asylum seekers is therefore more centred on tightly defined administrative categories than addressing legitimate human rights and humanitarian concerns. Refugees, whose claims for asylum have been legally accepted and who resettle in host countries, are entitled, for the most part, to the rights and protections offered to citizens and permanent residents of the host country. This is often not the case for asylum seekers. The distinctions between the categories are therefore important because they form the basis for policy decisions about the levels of government-subsidized access to health and other social support and welfare services, and the rights to seek employment. In this chapter, we trace the ethical issues of care for asylum seekers and refugees from the period of assessment of claim for asylum to ongoing health care needs of refugees in the host country. In the first section on asylum seekers, we focus more on the ethical dilemmas faced by health professionals. In the following section on resettling refugees, we concentrate on the ethical issues in the broader context of health service provision and allocation of resources for their care. We do not cover the specific issues of illegal immigrants, although it is worth noting that the ethical dilemmas may be at their most extreme for those to whom they present for health care. Although specific policies and procedures may differ from one country to another, the broad ethical issues remain largely similar.

ASSESSMENT OF CLAIMS FOR ASYLUM

The starting point for a potential refugee is the granting of appropriate status, either through the UNHCR or at a national port of entry. The standard processing procedure includes a medical assessment (the 'Istanbul protocol' provides helpful advice on the assessment). Health professionals play a critical role in this process in providing support and care for applicants who may have undergone physical and psychological torture and trauma. Depending on the nature and duration of the circumstances preceding flight or displacement, some may have experienced conditions that have resulted in malnutrition and poor health. Women have often been at particular risk of exploitation and sexual assault if they have been without the protection of male family members (Callamard, 1999). Communicable diseases such as tuberculosis and malaria are also a concern if the refugee applicants are from or have fled through disease-endemic countries (Toole, 2003).

The medical assessment may be undertaken or is repeated in many host countries (Silove et al., 2000). The purpose is primarily to screen and provide early or ongoing treatment for diagnosed conditions, notably infectious diseases. However, this health assessment has also been used to authenticate the signs and symptoms of prior physical and psychological torture and trauma in claims for asylum (Summerfield, 1999; Summerfield; 2001, Herlihy et al., 2002). One of the tests for deceit is based on the inconsistencies in the accounts of the experiences of persecution despite evidence that suggests that patients suffering from high levels of post–traumatic stress disorder have particular difficulties in recall. Recall is particularly affected if the application process is prolonged (Herlihy et al., 2002).

That notwithstanding, there are undoubtedly abuses of the asylum and international protection systems. Aspiring immigrants may gain an advantage by being untruthful about their country of origin, health status, pregnancy, family relationships and age, as well as history of torture or other maltreatment. Therefore, the opinion of the health practitioner about the truth of the claim can provide the definitive evidence of whether the asylum seekers are granted leave to remain in the host country or have their claim rejected, leading to deportation. Reports of coercion of health professionals to provide evidence to support the rejection of a claim are not uncommon (Harding-Pink, 2004). Although in the United Kingdom, 'the medical examination must not be used to determine the veracity of statements that may have been made' to other officials (Department of Health, 1992), more junior colleagues still face the tension between support for the asylum seeker/patient and the demands of their employer and the law. Like all health professions, responsibilities go wider than just the presenting patient and include the population at large and third parties, for example child protection, where claimed relationships may be untrue (Laming, 2003).

Those involved in the assessment of asylum seekers may need to reconcile competing tensions: Professional ethics would support assisting the asylum seeker challenge the system and make the best case possible, but would not support active collusion in an untruth or any breach of confidentiality. If in doubt in the face of a difficult judgement, advice should be available through defence unions and professional bodies, with ethical committees available in some institutions(RCP, 2005).

IMMIGRATION DETENTION

The application-processing period has other implications for the health and care of asylum seekers. Over recent years, several countries have introduced immigration policies of mandatory detention of asylum seekers, pending the outcome of their applications. The duration of detention can range from a few days to indefinite periods, and detention may take the form of restricted movements within the community to incarceration in purpose-built detention centres (Koopowitz and Abhary, 2004, Steel et al., 2004b, Fazel and Silove, 2006). Delays in the process can result from difficulties in obtaining supporting documentation to verify claims or from inefficient administrative processes. Furthermore, if the application for asylum is rejected, the applicant may be required to remain in detention until deportation. This can again be a long drawn-out process, complicated by the principle of *non-refoulement*, and in some instances lack of knowledge of the country to which a person should be returned.

The reasons given for the need for detention vary from the defence of national security and public health protection to administrative convenience and expediency of the application process (Crock, 1993; Mackinolty, 2001). Regardless of intention, immigration detention carries inherent health risks, that exacerbate the mental health status of people who may have had prior traumatic experiences (Silove et al., 2000; 2001a; 2003; Steel et al., 2006). The poor conditions in detention centres have been extensively documented by human rights activists, health researchers and health practitioners involved in the care of asylum-seeking detainees (Steele and Silove, 2001; Bhagwati, 2002; Loff et al., 2002; Silove, 2002). Reports of poor quality of health care and degrading treatment by staff at the detertion centres are not uncommon (HREOC, 1998, 2004; Loff et al., 2002). Harding-Pink (2004) reports cases of doctors tendering their resignations because their position as ethical practitioners had been compromised: they had witnessed the violation of the rights of detainees and had been refused access to detainees who required medical care; confidentiality of patients (detainees) was not guaranteed and they felt at the limits of international humanitarian law and human rights with no recourse or ability to protect their patients. When the cost of medical care has to be found from the same budget as the cost of running the detention facility, there are perverse incentives to neither diagnose nor treat the conditions, especially those that might prevent deportation because of either the risks during transit (infectious TB) or inadequacies of treatment at the destination (HIV). Furthermore, incidents are reported of treatments being discontinued once it is know that the asylum seeker's claims have been rejected (Hall, 2004; Arnold et al., 2006). The regulation of health care to those held in immigration detention centres in England is under the Inspectorate of Prisons and outside the standards set by the Healthcare Commission. The sanctions for ignoring their recommendations appear insufficient (HM Chief Inspector of Prisons, 2006).

Depression and self-harm are commonly reported amongst children and adult asylum detainees (Keller et al., 2003, Mares and Jureidini, 2004; Steel et al., 2004a;). For example, public self-mutilation is consistently reported in Australian immigration detention centres (Steele and Silove, 2001; Loff et al., 2002; Silove, 2002). Images of detainees with their lips stitched to demonstrate their resolve in abstaining from food have been shown in the media. Self-harm and practices such as hunger strikes are invariably emotive, ethically complex and politically charged with suggestions that these behaviours are manipulative and akin to blackmail rather than acts of desperation (Topsfield, 2005). Debates on the ethics of health care for people on hunger strike, recently raised by incidents among the Gulf War detainees in Guantanamo, are rife (Okie, 2005). The management of self-harm presents major legal and ethical challenges for health professionals working with asylum seekers in detention.

Hunger strikes in asylum-seeking detainees often occur either to protest their detention or as a suicide attempt expressing a preference for death over deportation to the country of origin (Brockman, 1999). Hunger strikes are, therefore, by definition, a political statement, made by a person who is mentally competent despite some evidence of high levels of clinical depression (Kalk et al., 1993; Silove and Mollica, 2001b; Sultan and O' Sullivan; 2001). There are a number of international declarations that outline guidelines for the treatment of hunger strikers. Notably, the World Medical Association's Declaration of Tokyo (1975) unequivocally states that when a hunger striker is assessed as medically competent, he/she should not be artificially fed (see Declaration of Malta (1991, revised in 1992)). Presented with a hunger striker, the medical professional has two choices: (1) assess him/her as mentally impaired and therefore requiring treatment for depression and medically enforced feeding; or (2) if mentally competent, refrain from force-feeding in accordance with respect for the autonomy of the individual who chooses to assert his/her agency by seizing control of his/her life through this choice of protest (Kenny et al., 2004b). British law affirms the right of the detainee to refuse enforced feeding under the principle of self-determination and autonomy. A number of concerned organizations such as the Medical Justice Network have produced guidance notes to support practitioners who work in these settings.[1]

In Australia, authorities in relevant government departments are legally empowered to authorize non-consensual medical treatment for immigration detainees if there is a risk of physical harm. (Migration Regulations 1994 (commonwealth), Regulation 5.35). This is enforced by contracted health workers. Although practitioners cannot be compelled under this law to enforce treatment if it is contrary to their ethical, moral and religious standards, it does highlight the ethical obligations to a patient in this context and the pressures of policies that are predicated on maintaining order and security inside detention (Kenny and Steel, 2004a). This is an example of 'dual loyalty' whereby there is a 'clinical role conflict between professional duties to a patient and obligations, express or implied, real or perceived, to the interests of a third party such as...the state' (PHR, 2003; Zion, 2004).

A number of other forms of self-harm have been recorded in immigration detention. Cases in the United Kingdom have been reported of detainees increasing their risk of infection to communicable diseases such as tuberculosis to extend their residence for the duration of a further appeal process.

A further concern has been the short- and long-term effects of mandatory detention on the health and well-being of children (Zwi et al., 2003, Mares and Jureidini, 2004,

Fazel and Silove, 2006, Steel et al., 2006b). The conditions in detention centres have been described as violating several human rights treaties and thus endangering children (Bhagwati, 2002; Zwi et al., 2003). A child detainee diagnosed with chronic post-traumatic stress disorder has little chance of recovery if he remains within the confines of the detention centre (Zwi et al., 2003). Other studies have documented the effects on children of watching their parents withdraw and become increasingly depressed, self-harm in adults around them and the use of solitary confinement as punishment (Pittaway and Bartolomei, 2003). Health professionals have met with resistance in attempting to act in the best interests of the child. This has prompted some professional bodies to make public statements about the compromised ethics of health providers within detention (MHA, 2005).

The reaction to the detention of children in Australia was an intensive lobby process through professional, political and human rights organizations, culminating in the release of children and their families into protected community facilities (Fazel and Silove, 2006). However, with less stringent guidelines for children, there are ongoing problems of having to establish the age of some asylum seekers who may be on the cusp of adulthood (Human Rights and Equal Opportunity Commission, 2004). Health practitioners are again at the forefront of these decisions as they undertake and review the necessary investigations in age determination. The objective evidence on age determination remains controversial (Mali, 2004; Physicians for Human Rights, 1999). The use of X-rays is also not without risk from radiation, albeit small, and is justified only if there is a personal benefit, and like any other medical procedures, it requires informed consent. The European Council on Refugees and Exiles (ECRE) provides clear guidance on working with refugee children, particularly those who are unaccompanied. (http:// www. ecre.org/positions/children.shtml).

ASYLUM SEEKERS IN THE COMMUNITY

Although the detention of asylum seekers receives the most political and media coverage, the large majority of asylum seekers live in the community while their claims are being processed. The support they receive is largely dependent on the policy of national governments towards asylum seekers. Most countries have some restrictions in what is available to non-citizens (Tiburcio, 2001), and under a system of universal health coverage or of government safety nets, governments can decide who has access to health care by stipulating citizenship. However, in the attempt to overcome the potential fraud and abuse of the asylum system, it can be argued that the restriction of citizenship rights and limited access to social goods and services establishes a hierar-

---

[1]http://www.medicaljustice.org.uk/gfx/Fluidandfoodrefuserspaper.pdf

chy of vulnerability and institutionalizes marginalization. Indeed, the economics of restricting primary care may result in higher emergency and hospital admission costs (Hull and Boomla, 2006).

In Australia, depending on when an individual lodges a claim or what stage they are in an appeal process, asylum seekers may be denied access to government-funded primary health care and the right to earn an income to pay for health services. In countries like the United Kingdom that offer universal health care coverage, there have been ongoing public debates about the extent to which access should be granted to asylum seekers. Since 2004, 'failed asylum seekers' have been made ineligible for free-nonurgent in-patient NHS hospital care. The government is currently considering a proposal to further restrict access to Accident and Emergency departments in order to limit the burgeoning health care budget (Vernon and Feldman, 2006). Similar debates are running throughout Europe (Hogan and Matthews, 1999; Dobson, 2005). In Australia and the United Kingdom health professionals have attempted to address the need for care by forming networks outside the national health care systems to provide mostly *pro bono* medical health care to the disadvantaged asylum seekers who have no other support. The Refugee and Asylum Seeker Health Network in Melbourne, Australia, and the Médicins du Monde in France and more recently in the United Kingdom have growing support from practitioners and civil society who have concerns about withholding care from those who may be the most in need (Johnston, 2003; Hull and Boomla, 2006). Although such groups are critical, the ethical dilemma arises when the development of alternative services for refugees and asylum seekers results in governments abrogating their responsibility to provide basic care. Additionally, although individual health workers can waive their fees on a discretionary basis, they may not be able to secure the free cost of other resources, such as medicines or pathology services, which may also not be subsidized for asylum seekers in this situation. This begs the question: how far do the ethical obligations of a health worker to their patient extend in such a scenario? More generally, to what extent is a health worker responsible for ensuring access to the care of marginalized population? (Mann, 1997).

RESETTLING REFUGEES

Refugees are a widely diverse population originating from countries across the world and displaced by varying crises. Their demographic profiles are as diverse as the profiles found in host populations across socioeconomic status, gender, age, education and religion. Ultimately, individual refugees would therefore present with their unique set of circumstances. Lack of familiarity with mainstream health services, lack of proficiency in the language of the

host community, cultural differences, poverty and marginalization, combined with previous experiences of physical or psychological trauma all contribute to social and health disadvantage and vulnerabilities of refugees (Toole, 2003; Zwi and Alvarez-Castillo, 2003). The reported prevalence of previous torture and trauma in resettling refugee communities ranges from 30% to 70% (Allotey, 1998; Jaranson et al., 2004). Added to these are the 'normal' migration stresses of settling in a new country (often not of choice) and finding acceptable food, shelter, education and employment. Rediscovering safety and developing social networks and a sense of stability and trust in people and their environment are critical in the early years, and the importance of policies in host countries to facilitate this process cannot be overemphasized (Allotey, 1998; Beiser, 1999).

The health of resettling refugees is an ongoing concern. There is a tendency towards resettlement in areas that perpetuate the cycle of poverty and disadvantage, where health services are non-existent or overstretched (Hull and Boomla, 2006) and therefore the quality of care required to identify and address the needs cannot be provided. These marginalizing factors are also the main barriers to accessing health services. For instance, although psychiatric assessments are often part of the on-arrival screening process to identify those at risk of post-traumatic stress disorder, the evidence suggests that mental health disorders occur in the post-settlement period (after two years), after the more immediate settlement needs are met (Allotey, 1998, Carlsson et al., 2006, Schweitzer et al., 2006). Problems with resettlement, such as continuing social isolation, perceived discrimination and unemployment, further add to psychiatric disorders (Gerritsen et al., 2006). There are important gender differences, although the findings are not always consistent across countries and refugee groups. In broad terms, female refugees report more mental and other chronic health symptoms (Akhavan et al., 2004, Blight et al., 2006, Gerritsen et al., 2006, Schweitzer et al., 2006,). However, studies in some resettling refugee communities suggest that, particularly when unemployed, mental health outcomes may be worse for refugee men than women (Blight et al., 2006). This is manifest, for instance, in the dynamics of gender-based violence in refugee communities (Kaplan and Webster, 2003). Qualitative studies have also highlighted gender-based strategies for coping and resilience in refugee women (McMichael, 2003). There is a clear need for similar work to be carried out with refugee men.

Research on the experiences of refugees within the health services highlights the complex interaction of their previous and current experiences with other social determinants of health and disease. Torture and trauma experiences can leave permanent physical and mental scars that influence their ability to trust those around them and to interpret what to others are unremarkable social interactions. Problems have been identified, for instance, in promoting the uptake of regular cervical screening in refugee women who have had previous experiences of brutal sexual assault (Allotey, 1998; Kaplan and Webster, 2003). Patients undergoing dental treatment have displayed behaviours characterized as a 'severe over-reaction' when the reaction had resulted from a triggered memory of torture experiences involving their teeth being pulled out. Similar reactions have been reported from refugees undergoing EEG and ECG investigations who have previously been tortured by electrocution (Allotey, 1992). In addition, patients often present with symptoms that mask underlying psychological distress. Careful consideration therefore needs to be given to the meaning of symptoms with which patients present. However, it is also important to avoid the assumption that an unusual presentation is necessarily psychological. Despite guidelines written for refugee and cross-cultural groups, ultimately, patients are their best cultural experts and they may need the time to develop a sense of trust with their health care professionals.

ETHICAL IMPLICATIONS FOR PRACTICE

Any discussion of the ethical issues faced by heath services and health workers regarding refugee care cannot be divorced from the wider social and political context, especially given the framing of forced migrants in 'security', rather than humanitarian terms in contemporary global discourse. There is a need for universal ethical standards or guidelines that specifically consider the evolving political agenda in dealing with refugees and asylum seekers. These would be particularly critical to health care in detention, assessment of effects of torture, which will determine migration outcome, expulsion to countries with no health facilities and psychological disturbances in unaccompanied children or in children whose families face uncertainty (Harding-Pink, 2004).

Some have argued that given the above, there needs to be a paradigm shift from traditional notions of bioethics to incorporate more normative principles of human rights (Mann, 1997; Farmer and Gastineau, 2002). This has been contested on the grounds that there are difficult challenges ahead in the interpretation, implementation and credibility of such frameworks (Faunce, 2005). Nonetheless, there are some interesting advances in this area. For example, Physicians for Human Rights in the United States released a report in 2003 on 'Dual Loyalty and Human Rights' which contains guidelines for prevention of complicity by health workers in human rights

violations (PHR, 2003). Additionally, the British Medical Association edited a book entitled *The Medical Profession and Human Rights* which was published in 2001 (BMA, 2001) and contains a section dedicated to 'Doctors and asylum seekers'. Most recently, the United Nations Education, Cultural and Scientific Organization (UNESCO) adopted at its General Conference in October 2005 the 'Universal Declaration on Bioethics and Human Rights'. According to Article 1(1) 'this declaration addresses ethical issues related to medicine, life sciences and associated technologies as applied to human beings, taking into account their social, legal and environmental dimensions' (UNESCO, 2005). This document does bring sharply into focus the intersection between bioethics and human rights (Faunce, 2005). The European Convention on Human Rights and its reflection in UK law, the Human Rights Act 1998, create further tensions for those officials expected to match the requirements of the state with their obligations to asylum seekers.

The health care of this population also highlights the stronger need for political engagement and advocacy from health systems and health care providers who have traditionally perceived themselves solely as either clinicians or service providers (Mann, 1997; McNeil, 2003). This might be characterized as what Callahan and Jennings term 'advocacy ethics' which emphasizes a strong orientation towards equality and social justice (Callahan and Jennings, 2002).

Finally, in broad terms, the policy environment dictates the allocation of resources that enable health services to respond to the client group. Within health service provision for refugees, health service delivery models have ranged from specialized ethno-or refugee-specific services to mainstream services. Refugee-specific services provide targeted service to the client groups, ensuring that the providers are either from the same ethnic backgrounds or specialized in the needs of refugee communities. They include dedicated clinics that recognize the special health needs of these groups who may present with conditions not endemic within the host population. It has been argued, however, that although these services may meet a need, they are not an efficient use of health care resources and they further marginalize refugees from the host communities (Kelaher and Manderson, 2000). On the other hand, providing refugee care within the mainstream services risks the failure to identify and respond to special needs due to the cultural chasm between service providers and refugees (Allotey, 2004). These issues need to be explored comprehensively to determine the most appropriate models. As the years pass, many initially disadvantaged and dependent asylum seekers emerge as creative and productive citizens, repaying in kind and taxes the state which provided refuge at the time of need. This argues for a broad vision and long time-frame for judging the reallocation of resources away from the indigenous population to refugee groups.

REFERENCES

Akhavan S, Bildt C, Franzön E, Wamala S. Health in relation to unemployment and sick leave among immigrants in Sweden from a gender perspective. *J Immigrant Health* 2004; **6**: 103–118.

Allotey P. Perceived health status, health needs and utilization of health services among Latin American Refugees in Perth. *Community Health Research and Training Unit, Department of Medicine*. Perth: University of Western Australia, 1992.

Allotey P. Travelling with 'excess baggage': Health problems of refugee women in Western Australia. *Women Health* 1998; **28**: 63-81.

Allotey P, ed. *The Health of Refugees: Public Health Perspectives from Crisis to Settlement*. Melbourne: Oxford University Press, 2003.

Allotey P. Refugee health. In: Ember CR, Ember M., eds. *Encyclopaedia of Medial Anthropology. Health and Illness in the World's Cultures*. New York: Kluwer Academic/Plenum Publishers, 2004.

Arnold F, Beeks M, Fluxman J, Katona C. *Unmet Medical Needs in Detention*. London: BMJ. (Rapid response to Fazel M & Silove D, 2006.)

Beiser M. *Strangers at the Gate: The Boat People's First Ten Years in Canada*, Toronto: University of Toronto Press, 1999.

Bhagwati P. Report of the regional advisor for Asia and the Pacific of the UNCHR: Human rights and immigration detention in Australia. *Mission to Australia 24 May–2 June*. Geneva: United Nations High Commissioner for Human Rights, 2002.

Blight KJ, Ekblad S, Persson J-O, Ekberg J. Mental health, employment and gender. Cross-sectional evidence in a sample of refugees from Bosnia-Herzegovina living in two Swedish regions. *Soc Sci Med* 2006; **62**: 1697–1709.

BMA. *The Medical Profession and Human Rights: Handbook for a Changing Agenda*, London: Zed Books in association with the British Medical Association; New York: Palgrave, 2001.

Brockman B. Food refusal in prisoners: a communication or a method of self killing? The role of the psychiatrist and resulting ethical challenges. *J Med Ethics* 1999; **25**: 451–456.

Callahan D, Jennings B. Ethics and public health: forging a strong relationship. *Am J Public Health* 2002; **92**: 169–176.

Callamard A. Refugee women: A gendered and political analysis of the refugee experience. In: Ager A, ed. *Refugees: Perspectives on the Experience of Forced Migration*. London: Continuum, 1999.

Carlsson J, Mortensen E, Kastrup M. Predictors of mental health and quality of life in male tortured refugees. *Nord J Psychiat* 2006; **60**: 51–57.

Castles S. Towards a sociology of forced migration and social transformation. *Sociology – J Brit Sociol Assoc* 2003; **37**: 13–34.

Crock M. *Protection or Punishment? The Detention of Asylum-Seekers in Australia*. Sydney: The Federation Press, 1993.

de Bousingen DD. Health issues and the rise of Le Pen in France. *The Lancet* 2002; **359**: 1673.

Department of Health. Instructions to Medical Inspectors. Medical Examination under the Immigration Act 1971. London: HMSO, 1992.

Dobson R. Ten out of 25 EU countries restrict health care for asylum seekers to emergencies only. *BMJ* 2005; **331**: 986b.

Farmer P, Gastineau N. Rethinking health and human rights: time for a paradigm shift. *J Law Med Eth* 2002; **30**: 655–666.

Faunce TA. Will international human rights subsume medical ethics? Intersections in the UNESCO Universal Bioethics Declaration. *J Med Eth* 2005; **31**: 173–178.

Fazel M, Silove D. Detention of refugees. *BMJ* 2006; **332**: 251–252.

Gerritsen A, Bramsen I, Devilla© W, Van Willigen L, Hovens J, Van der Ploeg H. Physical and mental health of Afghan, Iranian and Somali asylum seekers and refugees living in The Netherlands. *Soc Psych Psych Epid* 2006; **41**: 18–26.

Hall M. Frontline nursing in detention. *Aust Nurs J* 2004; **11**: 32–33.

Harding-Pink D. Humanitarian medicine: Up the garden path and down the slippery slope. *BMJ* 2004; **329**: 398–399.

Herlihy J, Scragg P, Turner S. Discrepancies in autobiographical memories – Implications for the assessment of asylum seekers: Repeated interviews study. *BMJ* 2002; **324**: 324–327.

HM Chief Inspector of Prisons. Report of an unannounced inspection of Harmondsworth Immigration Removal Centre. HM Inspectorate of Prisons: London 2006.

Hogan H, Matthews P. Meeting health needs of asylum seekers. *BMJ* 1999; **318**: 671.

HREOC. *Those Who've Come Across the Seas: Detention of Unauthorised Arrivals*. Sydney: Human Rights and Equal Opportunity Commission, 1998.

HREOC. *A Last Resort? National Inquiry into Children in Detention*. Sydney: Human Rights and Equal Opportunity Commission, 2004.

Hull SA, Boomla K. Primary care for refugees and asylum seekers. *BMJ* 2006; **332**: 62–63.

Jaranson JM, Butcher J, Halcon L, Johnson DR, Robertson C, Savik K, Spring M, Westermeyer J. Somali and Oromo refugees: Correlates of torture and trauma history. *Am J Public Health* 2004; **94**: 591–598.

Johnston V. Mobilizing the chattering classes for advocacy in Australia. *Development* 2003; **46**: 75–80.

Johnston V, Murray S. Musings and mutterings on migration, citizenship, identity and rights. *Development* 2003; **46**: 124–129.

Kalk W, Felix M, Snoey E, Veriawa Y. Voluntary total fasting in political prisoners: clinical and biochemical observations. *S Afr Med J* 1993; **83**: 391–394.

Kaplan I, Webster K. Refugee women and settlement: Gender and mental health. In: Allotey P, ed. *The Health of Refugees: Public Health Perspectives From Crisis to Settlement*. Melbourne: Oxford University Press, 2003.

Kelaher M, Manderson L. Migration and mainstreaming: Matching health services to immigrants'; needs in Australia. *Health Policy* 2000; **54**: 1–11.

Keller AS, Rosenfeld C, Meserve C, Sachs E, Leviss JA, Singer E, Smith H, Wilkinson J, Kim G, Allden K, Ford D. Mental health of detained asylum seekers. *The Lancet* 2003; **362**: 1721–1723.

Kenny MA, Silove DM, Steel Z. Legal and ethical implications of medically enforced feeding of detained asylum seekers on hunger strike. *Med J Aust* 2004b; **180**: 237–240.

Kleinman A, Kleinman J. The appeal of experience: The dismay of images: cultural appropriations of suffering in our times. In: Kleinman A, Das V, Lock M, eds. *Social Suffering.* Berkeley: University of California Press, 1997.

Koopowitz LF, Abhary S. Psychiatric aspects of detention: Illustrative case studies. *Aust Nz J Psychiat* 2004; **38**: 495–500.

Laming L. *The Victoria Climbié Inquiry.* London: HMSO, 2003.

Loff B. Detention of asylum seekers in Australia. *The Lancet* 2002; **359**: 792.

Loff B, Snell B, Creati M, Mohan M. 'Inside' Australia's Woomera detention centre. *The Lancet* 2002; **359**: 683.

Mackinolty C. Detention curbs disease risk, says Ruddock. *The Age.* Melbourne, 2001.

Mali W. Skeletal maturation in assessing underage asylum seekers. *Ned Tijdschr Geneeskd* 2004; **148**: 2259–2261.

Mann J. Medicine and public health, ethics and human rights. *The Hastings Centre Report* 1997; **27**: 6–13.

Mares S, Jureidini J. Psychiatric assessment of children and families in immigration detention – Clinical, administrative and ethical issues. *Aust Nz J Public Health*, 2004; **28**: 520–526.

McMichael C. Narratives of forced displacement. In: Allotey P, ed. *The Health of Refugees. Public Health Perspectives From Crisis to Settlement.* Melbourne: Oxford University Press, 2003.

McNeil PM. Public health ethics: Asylum seekers and the case for political action. *Bioethics* 2003; 17, 487–502.

Medical Justice Network MHA. *Immigration Minister Still Failing on Mental Health*, 2005.

Okie S. Glimpses of Guantanamo – Medical ethics and the war on terror. *N Engl J Med* 2005; **353**: 2529–2534.

Overbeek H. Towards a new international migration regime: Globalization, migration and the internationalization of the state. In: Miles R, Thranhardt D, eds. *Migration and European Integration: The Dynamics of Inclusion and Exclusion.* London: Pinter, 1995.

PHR. *Dual Loyalty and Human Rights in Health Professional Practice*, 2003, www.phrusa.org

Pittaway E, Bartolomei L. Double jeopardy: Children seeking asylum. In: Allotey P, ed. *The Health of Refugees: Public Health Perspectives from Crisis to Settlement.* Melbourne: Oxford University Press, 2003.

RCP. Ethics in Practice. Royal College of Physicians in London: London, 2005.

Schweitzer R, Melville F, Steel Z, Lacherez P. Trauma, post-migration living difficulties, and social support as predictors of psychological adjustment in resettled Sudanese refugees. *Aust Nz J Psychiat* 2006; **40**: 179–188.

Silove D. The asylum debacle in Australia: A challenge for psychiatry. *Aust Nz J Psychiat* 2002; **36**: 290–296.

Silove D, Steel Z, Mollica R. Detention of asylum seekers: Assault on health, human rights, and social development. *The Lancet* 2002a; **357**: 1436–1437.

Silove D, Steel Z, Watters C. Policies of deterrence and the mental health of asylum seekers. *JAMA* 2000; **284**: 604–611.

Silove DZS, Mollica RF. Detention of asylum seekers: assault on health, human rights, and social development. *The Lancet* 2001b; **357**: 1436–1437.

Steel Z, Momartin S, Bateman C, Hafshejani A, Silove D. Psychiatric status of asylum seeker families held for a protracted period in a remote detention centre in Australia. *Aust Nz J Public Health* 2004a; **28**: 527–535.

Steele Z, Silove D. The mental health implications of detaining asylum seekers. *Med J Aust* 2001; **175**: 596–599.

Steel Z, Silove D, Brooks R, Momartin S, Alzuhairi B, Susljik I. Impact of immigration detention and temporary protection on the mental health of refugees. *Brit J Psychiat* 2006; **188**: 58–64.

Steiner N. *Arguing About Asylum: The Complexity of Refugee Debates in Europe.* New York: St Martin's Press, 2000.

Sultan A, O'Sullivan K. Psychological disturbances in asylum seekers held in long term detention: a participant observer account. *Med J Aust* 2001; **175**: 593–596.

Summerfield D. Sociocultural dimensions of war, conflict and displacement. In: Ager A, ed. *Refugees: Perspectives on the Experience of Forced Migration.* London: Pinter, 1999.

Summerfield D. The invention of post-traumatic stress disorder and the social usefulness of a psychiatric disorder. *Brit Med J* 2001; **322**: 95–98.

The World Medical Association Declaration of Tokyo. *Guidelines for Physicians Concerning Torture and other Cruel, Inhuman or Degrading Treatment or Punishment in Relation to Detention and Imprisonment.* World Medical Association, 1975.

Tiburcio C. *The Human Rights of Aliens under International and Comparative Law.* The Hague: Martinus Nijhoff, 2001.

Toole M. The health of refugees: An international public health problem. In: Allotey P, ed. *The Health of Refugees. Public Health Perspectives From Crisis to Settlement.* Melbourne: Oxford University Press, 2003.

Topsfield J. Vanstone plays down self-harm. *The Age.* Canberra, 2005.

UNESCO. *Universal Declaration on Bioethics and Human Rights*, 2005.

UNHCR. *Convention Relating to the Status of Refugees.* Geneva: United Nations High Commissioner for Refugees, 1951.

Vernon G, Feldman R. Government proposes to end free health care for failed asylum seekers. *Brit J Gen Pract* January 2006; **2006**: 59.

White PJ. The global refugee crisis. *Migration Action* 2000; **22**: 4–11.

Zion D. Caring for detained asylum seekers, human rights and bioethics. *Aust Nz J Public Health* 2004; **28**: 6–8.

Zwi A, Alvarez-Castillo F. Forced migration, globalization and public health: getting the big picture into focus. In: Allotey P, ed. *The Health of Refugee. Public Health Perspectives from Crisis to Settlement.* Melbourne, Oxford University Press, 2003.

Zwi KJ, Herzberg B, Dossetor D, Field J. A child in detention: Dilemmas faced by health professionals. *Med J Aust* 2003; **179**: 319–322.

Medical Aid in Disaster Relief

SØREN HOLM

INTRODUCTION

Disasters occur for many different reasons: some have an initial cause in a physical phenomenon – tsunami, earthquake, draught – and some are more directly caused by human agency – war, civil war, genocide, some types of famines. (In the present chapter, I will not discuss the special issues raised by war, but I will touch on the issues raised by civil war, especially concerning the neutrality of helpers. I will also bracket issues raised by disasters caused by infectious diseases, whether or not these are natural or caused by bioterrorism.) But what turns the initial event into a disaster is always a complex net of prior and subsequent decisions made by human agents. If people did not choose to live close to volcanoes or in earthquake-prone areas, the primary consequences of volcanic eruptions and earthquakes would be much less catastrophic, and if other people chose to be more active in disaster relief, the secondary consequences could be very different. It is the element of choice that makes disaster relief an ethical question. Without the ability to help or the knowledge that the disaster has happened, there could not be an ethical question concerning whether we should engage in disaster relief (we will look at the question of wilful ignorance below).

In this chapter, I will generally use the term 'victims' to describe those who have been afflicted by the disaster and 'helpers' for those who are in a position to help. In the more technical literature on the methodology of disaster relief, there are a number of different ways to define a disaster and estimate its magnitude, and here I will follow the approach in Redmond (2005), which assesses the scale of a disaster by mortality rates and only rates situations with mortality rates above 2 a day per 10 000 adults as 'out of control' and only those with mortality rates above 4 as major catastrophes (for comparison, the mortality in the United Kingdom is less than 1 a day per 10 000 population even in the age group of 85 years and above). This means that true disasters very rarely occur in rich countries outside of wartime, except on the first day of the event. Rich countries are shielded from catastrophes, not necessarily because fewer natural disasters occur, but because their infrastructure is better (fewer people, for instance, die or are injured by an earthquake of similar magnitude) and their indigenous abilities to provide fast relief is much more developed.

Health-affecting disasters thus primarily afflict poor countries and when, in the remainder of this chapter, I use the word 'disaster' it will only be to denote disasters of this kind.

ETHICAL THEORY AND DISASTER RELIEF

Almost all ethical theories generate some obligation to help the victims of disasters, the only exception being strict libertarianism which will see helping victims of disasters as a good thing to do, but not as an obligation and especially not an enforceable obligation. This position is succinctly summarized by the prominent libertarian Jan Narveson:

> 'Finally, a word may be said on the subject of disasters, tragedies at the hands of nature or one's fellow man.
>
> . . .
>
> With regard to such things, we should all be ready to help if we can – and most of us do, I should note. Natural disasters can happen to anyone, regardless of politics, culture, religion, and the like. At such times, the need for help from others can be desperate, and sometimes the help needed can be supplied more readily, or perhaps only, by the comparatively well off. It is, of course, a virtue to be disposed to help in such cases, if useful help is possible and affordable.
>
> . . .
>
> But there is a temptation to turn this kind of help, which is charity in the strictest and literal sense of the term, into something else – to

Principles of Health Care Ethics, Second Edition Edited by R.E. Ashcroft, A. Dawson, H. Draper and J.R. McMillan
© 2007 John Wiley & Sons, Ltd

bureaucratize it, to turn to the compulsions of taxation rather than the market freedom of independent aid agencies. This temptation is very strong – but it should be resisted. When disaster strikes, it is between ourselves and our hearts and consciences how much, if at all, we will respond' (Narveson, 2005, p. 343).

In the subsequent discussion I will ignore the libertarian arguments because I think that the denial of an obligation to help the really needy very nearly amounts to a *reduction* of the libertarian position as a *bona fide* ethical stance. Consequentialism can easily generate an obligation to help, simply because attempting to help will, in almost all circumstances, maximize the expected utility, and most non-consequentialist ethical theories contain strong obligations to act beneficently and to uphold justice, including distributive justice.

Given the role of prior choice in who is affected by disasters and to what extent, the question immediately arises whether the element of 'option luck' as opposed to 'brute luck', to use Ronald Dworkin's distinction (Dworkin, 2000), entails that victims of disasters do not have a legitimate claim in justice for some redistribution of resources. If I climb Vesuvius to see the magma crater and am injured by an eruption, it may be claimed that this is my own fault and simply bad option luck which should not be compensated. There are many other ways in which I could have spent my holiday, most of them much less risky. But if I choose to live close to the beach, because that is where the tourists are and therefore the best possibilities for making a living, it is difficult to claim that my house being hit by a tsunami is primarily bad option luck, because there is a very significant element of bad brute luck in my having to live there.

It is therefore unlikely that a justice-based claim will be vitiated by option luck considerations in the case of most disaster victims in poor countries.

THE REQUIREMENTS OF JUSTICE AND BENEFICENCE

What does justice and beneficence require of us in the context of disaster relief? The first, fairly obvious and strict requirement is that even if we decide not to help ourselves,

we should not prevent others from helping, or hinder them in their relief efforts. We should not put in place structural obstacles to disaster relief in advance, and we should not interfere negatively in the actual relief effort. (This obligation holds even within a libertarian framework.)

If country A has a dispute with country B, and a disaster happens in country B the least country A is morally obliged to do is not to prevent country C from helping in any way (I leave it to the reader to fill in country names for the placeholders). No country should, for instance, prohibit aircraft carrying aid from using its airspace. But this obligation to remove obstacles also holds in cases where a country has actually decided to help. There are often structural obstacles, for instance preventing the release of suitably trained health care professionals from their jobs that impede the relief effort. There is a strong moral obligation to identify and remove such obstacles in advance (partly because the occurrence of disasters is fully predictable, see below). How much should we help? How much does justice require? This initially looks like a very complicated question. How much should the United Kingdom for instance, have allocated to help Indonesia cope with the 2004 tsunami, or how much should I as an individual give to Oxfam to feed the victims of the current African draught crisis?

However, one of the reasons why these questions are truly very complicated is that they are pitched at the wrong level(s). They are asking about the response to a specific disaster as if disasters are unpredictable and each new one requires a new response or new complex moral reflection. But the occurrence of disasters and their costs are no more unpredictable than any other events that we insure ourselves against. It is unpredictable whether my house will burn down during the next year, but the estimate of the total costs of rebuilding those houses that will burn during a year and that are insured by the insurance company I am insured with can be calculated with great precision. If that was not the case the insurance company would quickly go out of business. It is therefore not beyond the wit of man or of any half-decent actuary to calculate the average annual cost of disasters that are so large that they require outside relief.[1]

[1] The United Nations Statistics Division has, for some years, collected statistics on an indicator entitled 'Economic and human loss due to natural disasters' defined as 'The number of persons deceased, missing, and/or injured as a direct result of a natural disaster; amount of economic and infrastructure losses occurred as a direct result of the natural disaster. Natural disaster is the consequence of the impact of natural hazard on a socioeconomic system with the given degree of vulnerability, which overwhelms local capacity to respond to the emergency and has disruptive consequences on human, social and economic parameters' (http://unstats.un.org/unsd/indicatorfoc/indsearchpage.asp?cid=195). Although this indicator is not perfect, it is a good beginning. The global reinsurance firm (i.e. a firm which insures insurance companies) Munich Re publishes an annual review of natural catastrophes, which estimates both the total economic losses and the insured losses of natural disasters. For 2005, it estimates the total economic losses from natural disasters as $31 million in Africa and $21 717 million in Asia. Apart from the numbers these reports also contain interesting insights into the reality of disasters in poor countries; in an analysis of the Kashmiri earthquake in October 2005 in which 88 000 people lost their lives we read: 'One of the biggest natural catastrophes in recent decades was practically a non-event for the insurance industry. In Pakistan, most of the risks covered by earthquake insurance are large industrial plants. Because the region affected is very rural, the insured loss was low' (Munich, 2006, p. 32).
For a more technical discussion concerning whether disaster costs are insurable and for other methods for hedging against disaster risk see Linnerooth-Bayer and Amendola (2005).

What looks like a complicated ethical problem is to a large extent a coordination problem.

The only ethical consideration that comes into the calculation is to what level disaster relief should be provided, that is, what is the end state where helpers can justifiably say that they have helped enough. In ordinary insurance this will often be a return to the state before the insured event, for example the rebuilding of my burnt–out house, but that is a contractual matter and not a question of (natural) justice; I could for instance have insured for a fixed sum. What end state does justice require in disaster relief? The minimum requirement of justice must be that the community affected by the disaster should receive a sufficient amount of help to become economically and socially self-sustaining.[2] For some communities this will mean that they are not brought back to the *status quo ante*, whereas other more deprived communities that were not self-sustaining previously may actually be improved. The justification for claiming that this is the minimum requirement is, first, that if a helper is in a position to provide complete and definitive help, but chooses not to do it, there is a problem of justification, unless the differences in costs between the two options is large. Analogously, if a doctor can cure a patient, but chooses only to palliate, we would require a very good explanation. Sustainability as a community is the first point at which it can be claimed that complete help has been provided.

Second, there is also good pragmatic justification. If the community is left in a state where it cannot sustain itself, someone will have to provide ongoing aid or someone will have to bear the costs when the community eventually fails or disintegrates. Analysing the problem of disaster relief in this way also shows that it is distinct from the more general question of the extent of any obligations to provide help to the poor and/or needy in third world countries. Peter Singer and others have argued convincingly that there are such obligations of significant scope (Singer, 1972; Unger, 1996), but even a rejection of their mainly consequentialist arguments does not necessarily affect the justification of personal or state obligations to provide disaster relief.

Let us now assume that we have calculated the average amount needed for disaster relief per year; what share of this amount ought every (rich) country and every (rich) individual to contribute? This is a slightly more tractable question than the one we started with.

By saying that the question is more tractable I do not want to imply that it has an easy answer, but there are at least some possibilities to make headway.

Let us first try a simple suggestion. Let us posit that every country above a certain level of income per inhabitant has an ethical obligation to pay in to an independent disaster relief fund (or one of a number of independent funds)[3] and that the payment is assessed as a percentage of gross domestic product. What would be wrong with such a system? In one sense it is arbitrary and is vulnerable to all the objections raised against any form of taxation system. Let me just list some of the possible questions in no particular order: Should the system be progressive? Should it have a ceiling? Should the amount of internal inequality in the rich countries be factored into their payment? Should countries that did not have any colonies or had relatively few colonies pay less? How should private philanthropy count and so forth. The right-wing American think-tank The Hudson Institute, for instance, urges us to include both philanthropy and private remittances when calculating the total US contribution to aid (Hudson Institute, 2006). These questions are all relevant, but also intractable. There is no non-contentious way of designing a tax system and no non-contentious way of establishing the exact payment required from a given country to a comprehensive global disaster relief fund.

What we can say without any doubt is that the current allocation of resources to disaster relief is insufficient, simply because many people who could have been saved, die from lack of aid every single year and many communities are left destitute. It is also unlikely that there is any country in the world that pays the amount it should pay under an equitable system, whatever the specific features of that system is. The countries that pay most in development aid pay around 1% of their GDP, but that is for all development aid, and less than 5% of development aid goes to disaster relief (OECD, 2005). Furthermore, this includes disaster relief provided in situations where the disaster is caused by military conflict.

Every rich country and most rich individuals therefore need to do better. Because a large part of the general problem of disaster relief is a series of coordination problems, there may be an argument for collecting contributions through national tax systems.

For an individual who does not contribute regularly to a disaster relief organization there may be considerable transaction costs involved in giving a one-off donation. There will be the time costs involved in making the decision and making the actual donation (although charities have found clever ways to reduce the last cost, including donation by SMS), and the organization will also have larger costs in handling such donations. This means that a one-off donation is less efficient than a regular donation and that there may

[2]In the parable the Good Samaritan provided both first aid and what was necessary to assure sustainability (Luke 10: 33–35).

[3]Because these funds would have to invest the surplus in years with less-than-average costs of disasters, we might for instance have to have Islamic and non-Islamic funds, the first only investing according to the sharia law.

be situations where a small one-off donation is not actually helping anyone.

The same argument does not apply to governments, except if they are extremely stingy and give very small donations. It may thus, for efficiency reasons, be better to raise disaster relief from national taxation.

There is another coordination problem that affects government relief efforts, and that is that they are often less then perfectly integrated with the relief efforts of other governments, and there is clearly an obligation on governments to try to achieve maximum coordination and its attendant efficiency gains.

WILFUL IGNORANCE

Does the duty – those who are (relatively) resource of rich to act as helpers to disaster victims imply a duty to actively seek knowledge about disasters? There are after all pragmatic reasons to remain in ignorance. The more ignorant I am, the less effort and resources do I have to expend on fulfilling my obligations. (This is one of the problems which would be solved if we had a proactive international disaster relief fund as outlined above, because no government would then be able to claim ignorance.)

There are probably no strong obligations on individuals to actively seek information about disasters elsewhere, partly because it is unclear whether the time spent seeking information could not be used better in other ways and partly because there will be many situations where, for instance, doing something in the local community will discharge (other) important obligations and create (almost) the same amount of good (see the argument concerning transaction costs above). That line of argument is, however, not nearly as convincing in the case of governments. Governments already monitor the situation in other countries, for instance to issue up-to-date travel advice, and there will be little (if any) extra effort involved in collecting the additional information necessary to determine the scale of an (impending) disaster.

THE KLEPTOCRATIC EXCUSE

A possible excuse for not helping is that the help will be inefficient because all, or large amounts of, the resources will never reach the victims but will be diverted by the kleptocratic regimes in the country where the disaster has happened, and will only fill the coffers of those who have already enriched themselves illegitimately (Narveson, 2005). It is undoubtedly true that this is a problem and that if we knew that no help

would reach the victims, we would have perfect legitimation for not helping. But what about the situation where some help will get through, but most will be diverted? Let us consider the situation where the agent getting fat on the aid to the victim is not a human but a rodent. If rodents ate most of the aid before it reached its final destination, and some rodents are almost completely omnivorous and will at least nibble at the tents as well, we would not see that as a strong reason not to send aid, but as a reason to do something about the rodents. I am not suggesting that we should apply the same extermination methods to kleptocratic elites, but maybe we should consider other methods to keep them under control or make them disappear. As noted above, the occurrence of disasters in poor countries is not unpredictable, although the exact timing and place may be so; we are already in a situation now where we have good reason to target kleptocratic elites for extinction, for instance by removing their resource privileges (for a more in-depth discussion of causes and remedies for kleptocracy, see Pogge, 2002).

If we have not succeeded in removing kleptocracies prior to the disaster, we have an obligation to think creatively about ways in which kleptocrats can be persuaded not to lay their hands on the aid deliveries. This could, for instance, be done by defining interference with aid in major disasters as a 'crime against humanity' and penalize those indicted in the same way as other persons indicted such crimes (restrict their travel and that of their close family, freeze their international assets etc.).[4] In failed states where even the kleptocracy is disorganized we may simply have to buy it off. This may be an unpalatable approach but would further the immediate goal of helping the victims, and would not bar us from indicting the people in question later.

USING RELIEF FOR POLITICAL ENDS AND THE NEUTRALITY OF HELPERS

Is it legitimate to use disaster relief for political ends, for instance by requiring economic restructuring or the introduction of democracy? If the political ends are extraneous to the relief situation and no convincing argument can be found that they are actually good ends to pursue in themselves, seen from a neutral perspective, it is highly problematic to attach them as conditions to disaster relief. If a rich country requires a poor country to open its market to the rich country's goods as a condition for receiving disaster relief, there is a problem. The rich country is essentially saying: we will help you, but only as a *quid pro quo*. But if this is a situation where there is an obligation to help, it is immoral to add such conditions.

---

[4]This would even be compatible with libertarian thinking because the enrichment activities (read 'theft') pursued by kleptocracies are clearly illegitimate transfers.

The question is more complicated if the political end being sought is good in itself, like changing from dictatorship to democracy or introducing freedom of the press. Another related issue concerns the neutrality of helpers in situations where a disaster involves several groups who are in conflict. The International Red Cross has traditionally maintained absolute neutrality and many other aid organizations have also followed this approach. The justification is first that taking sides will almost always complicate or hinder aid efforts and second that it is often difficult to decide which side in a conflict is right. Even though someone has a just cause, they may, for instance, use ethically problematic means to pursue that cause. But how far should neutrality be pursued? We may agree that everyone in need should be treated equally and without preference to one group, but does neutrality, for instance, entail that a helper should not publicize human rights abuses perpetrated by one group against another?

The neutrality paradigm is currently under criticism and many now argue that whereas there should be neutrality in aid distribution, helpers have a moral obligation to act as public advocates for groups that are oppressed or subject to human rights abuses and who may not be able to advocate for themselves (see, for instance, Pasic and Weiss, 1997). The critics argue *inter alia* that in conflict situations strict neutrality will almost always be of net benefit to one of the parties in the conflict, usually the strongest party.

OBLIGATIONS TO DONORS

In respect of nongovernmental aid organizations like Oxfam we have to ask what obligations they have towards their donors, apart from the obvious one of using the resources they have received effectively. Should donors' views concerning who should be helped, for instance, matter in the allocation of disaster relief? In the Principles of Conduct for the International Red Cross and Red Crescent Movement and NGOs in Disaster Response Programmes, to which many NGOs have signed up, principle 3 states that (IFRC, 1994):

> **Aid will not be used to further a particular political or religious standpoint**
> Humanitarian aid will be given according to the need of individuals, families and communities . . .

On an expansive interpretation of this principle, an NGO has an obligation to use the resources received from donors to help the most needy, wherever they might be. But this expansive definition is clearly not the one used by most NGOs; they collect money for the needy in specific regions, countries or parts of countries and do not redirect the money, even if there might be more needy people in other parts of the world.

But how far can the principle be restricted? Is an organization absolutely bound by the purposes that the donors have specified (if we assume that these purposes are not overtly discriminatory) or for which it has collected the money?

This depends on a number of factors including (1) how specific the targeting of the donation was, (2) whether the original intended recipients are still needy, but no longer the most needy, (3) whether it is generally known that the organization may redirect targeted donation, and (4) whether the redirection happens in a transparent way with a publicly stated justification.

If the needs of the initial intended recipient community have been met, we have the simplest case where it is probably morally obligatory to redirect in a transparent manner. If these needs have not been met, a much stronger justification for redirection is necessary.

TRIAGE IN DISASTERS

Disasters are among the situations where the issue of the appropriateness of triage may arise. Triage is a procedure originally developed in military medicine to prioritize treatment when not all can be treated, or not all can be treated immediately. There are now many different triage systems, but they all aim at dividing wounded persons into four groups:

1. Those that are so severely injured that they will die even if treated with the available medical resources.
2. Those that require immediate medical attention to prevent deterioration.
3. Those that require medical attention, but not immediately.
4. Those that are so lightly injured that they are able to manage for themselves or can be dealt with immediately with little use of resources.

Persons in group 1 receive no treatment and persons in group 4 only very little, whereas those in group 2 are prioritized. The aims of triage are to maximize the medical benefit from the available resources and to get lightly wounded soldiers back to the battlefield. In certain triage systems developed for civilian disaster in industrialized countries, the first group is omitted, so that everyone who is injured and still alive will be treated, even if it is very likely that treatment will be ineffective. (This is, for instance, the case in the SMART Incident Command System, a commercial system used by many emergency services in the United States and the United Kingdom and provided by TSG Associates (http://www.tsgassociates.co.uk/English/Civilian/about_us.htm). But in the type of disaster under discussion in this chapter, it is likely that harsher triage systems will be used with a fairly broad definition of those excluded from treatment. But is the use of a triage system, which has the effect that some of the people who could have benefited from health care will not receive it and will die as a result, justified in a disaster situation? It could clearly be justified on purely consequentialist grounds if it maximizes either the number of survivors or the aggregate health gain, and because this is a situation where true and often extreme scarcity exists, it may be one of the situations where even the deontologically inclined will accept consequentialist reasoning.

THE SPECIFIC OBLIGATIONS OF HEALTH CARE PROFESSIONALS

What are the specific responsibilities of health care professionals in the context of disaster relief?

I will not reiterate the general issues concerning the extent and basis of professional responsibility, but just state that I think that although health care professionals have specific obligations, these do not flow from a particular codified professional ethic or oath but primarily from their specific skills and secondarily from whatever implicit promises they have made to obtain social recognition as a high-status profession. It is because health care professionals can avert and alleviate certain health consequences of disasters that they have specific obligations (Harris and Holm, 1993, 1995). A few may, of course, have made specific and recent promises to their patients, such as 'I will stay with you throughout the eruption', and are bound by these promises to the same extent as others who make promises, but most will not have made such promises, and discussing the strength of such promises is outside the scope of this chapter.

What are the obligations of health care professionals close to the disaster? The simple answer is that they have an obligation to use their own skills and other health care resources at their disposal in the most effective way, at least in the acute phase of a disaster. A nurse working in a private cosmetic surgery clinic cannot, for instance, claim that her obligations to her current patients outweigh her obligations to more needy disaster victims in the locality.

What about health care professionals far from the disaster? It is important to note first that most health care professionals are not trained to act effectively in disaster situations. Because of this lack of training they may actually hinder the relief effort if they try or succeed to get to the place where the disaster has taken place. Such health care professionals have a strong obligation to stay at home and not waste valuable resources. They can contribute positively in their normal role as citizens and, more specifically, by making it easy for those who are appropriately trained to leave their normal work and go to the disaster area.

Health care professionals who are trained in disaster relief have an obligation to make themselves available to participate in the relief effort, but as with many other of those positive obligations that require specific, personal performance, it is difficult to provide any rule concerning how strong the obligation is in each individual case. It has often been highlighted in recent years that many rich countries are net importers of health care staff from poorer countries, without contributing to the education of those health care professionals (Harris and Holm, 1995). Making it easy for such staff to return temporarily to their region of origin to participate in disaster relief would partially remedy the injustice in poaching them in the first place.

What level of risk should health care professionals engaged in disaster relief be willing to take? There is no reason why health care professionals should take greater risks than other helpers, but there are general reasons why helpers should be willing to take somewhat greater risks than they would otherwise do in 'normal life'. The first is the simple consequentialist reason that the expected utility of risk-taking is often, but not always, higher in disaster situations. The second is that although risks in the normal day-to-day work of health care professionals can be shared out, disasters are locally specific and often disrupt the possibility to move both patients and health care professionals.

But the obligations of health care professionals outlined here may, in some cases, raise the general issue of the possible excessive demands of our moral obligations. What if the sacrifices required are great or the risks very large? Is there no limit to what morality can require of the individual agent? A complete answer to that question is far beyond the scope of this chapter, but it may be useful to distinguish between the acute and the chronic phase of a disaster. In the acute phase it is often true that there is no one else who can perform the actions in question and that this is nobody's fault, but in the chronic phase it can only be the case that there is no one else if many other moral agents have not fulfilled their moral obligations to help. Although this may not reduce the magnitude of the moral obligation, it may reduce the blameworthiness of anyone who is unable to discharge it.

REFERENCES

Ahmad OB. 2005. Managing medical migration from poor countries. BMJ 2005 **331**: 43–45.

Dworkin R. *Sovereign Virtue: The Theory and Practice of Equality.* Cambridge, MA.: Harvard University Press, 2000.

Harris J, Holm S. If only AIDS was different! *Hastings Center Report* 1993; **23**(6): 6–11.

Harris J, Holm S. Is there a moral obligation not to infect others? *BMJ* 1995; **311**: 1215–1217.

Hudson Institute. *Index of Global Philanthropy.* Washington, DC: Hudson Institute, 2006.

International Federation of Red Cross and Red Crescent Societies. *Principles of Conduct for the International Red Cross and Red Crescent Movement and NGOs in Disaster Response Programmes.* Geneva: IFRC, 1994.

Linnerooth-Bayer J, Amendola A. Global change, natural disasters and loss-sharing: Issues of efficiency and equity. *The Geneva Papers on Risk and Insurance* 2000; **25**(2): 203–219.

Munich Re. *Topic Geo – Annual Review: Natural Catastrophes 2005.* München: Munich Re Group, 2006.

Narveson J. Welfare and wealth, poverty and justice in today's world. *J Eth* 2005; **8**: 305–348.

OECD. *Development Cooperation Report,* Paris: OECD, 2005, p. 161.

Pasic A, Weiss TG. The politics of rescue: Yugoslavia's wars and the humanitarian impulse. *Eth Int Affairs* 1997; **11**: 111–131.

Pogge T. *World Poverty and Human Rights.* New York: Polity Press, 2002.

Singer P. Famine, affluence and morality. *Philos Public Aff* 1972; **1**(Spring): 229–243.

Unger P. *Living High and Letting Die.* Oxford: Oxford University Press, 1996.

PART IV

RESEARCH ETHICS AND ETHICS OF NEW TECHNOLOGIES

Research ethics is in some ways the cutting edge of medical ethics. Not only are most innovations in medicine introduced through scientific research and technological development, many of the issues now considered to be at the core of medical ethics proper were first debated in detail in the context of the ethics of medical research. For instance, it is arguable that the centrality of informed consent within post-Second World War medicine comes about because of its importance in the Nuremberg Nazi Doctors Trial of 1946–1947.

This part introduces the principal ethical debates around research ethics and around some of the main new medical technologies of the next 10–20 years. We can distinguish between the ethics of research and the ethics inherent in a technology (Ashcroft, 2000). While all technologies have ethical features through the decision choices embodied in them or through the selection of problems they are designed to address or through the context in which they are taken up, the evaluation of these features can usually be distinguished from the ethical issues involved in testing these new technologies with human research 'subjects'. Nonetheless, society has sophisticated methods for evaluating the ethical burdens of medical experimentation and other research methods, but it has not developed methods for evaluating technologies as such except in a few rare cases. Hence, asking questions about the ethical status of a technology is often handled by questioning the experimental methods for testing the effectiveness of the technology.

In the opening chapter of this part, Ashcroft introduces research ethics and research governance as an attempt to solve the double problem of ensuring that innovation proceeds in the interests of the common good while protecting individuals from the risks and burdens of research. The next chapters examine different aspects of the medical research process. De Grazia presents an overview of the debates about the ethics of using animals in medical research. This is normally considered an essential precursor to studies in humans, but is controversial in many countries because of differing views of the moral status of sentient animals. Another essential precursor to research with human subjects is to ensure that the research question is well posed, that we do not already know the answer to it, and that we have a well-founded risk assessment of the procedures in the planned research. These issues are discussed by Clarke, arguing for the importance of systematic review of the scientific literature as a necessary precursor to new research. Flory, Wendler and Emanuel examine the ethical requirements for valid informed consent in research, and Miller and Weijer analyse the evaluation of risk–benefit trade-offs in research. Consent and fair risk–benefit ratios have been considered essential components in the ethics of research in humans since the Nuremberg Code of 1947 and the Declaration of Helsinki (1964, subsequently revised several times). While much of the debate in research ethics has been essentially about protecting research participants' rights, interests and welfare, some recent work has argued that we need also to consider patients' duties in research. Woods considers this argument, and puts it into the context of a wider debate about the duties of patients in public health care systems.

Some of the most heated recent debates in research ethics concern not consent or risk but the fairness of research. The next three chapters consider this debate in international context. Lie discusses the fairness of the choice of control treatment and control group in randomized controlled trials in the developing world, where standards of care may be dramatically worse than those available in the West. Benatar puts this debate into the context of a wider debate about research priorities for global health: are we researching the right medical problems and the right kinds of ways of addressing them, given global inequalities in health and wealth? Schüklenk and Gallagher consider how far the pharmaceutical industry which sponsors much medical research has a collective or firm-level obligation to research participants or to poor world populations in general.

One of the main outcomes of research is publication, and this is a major context of possible unethical behaviour – from suppression of adverse results, to fraud, to plagiarism or denial of authorial contribution. Yet more seriously, patient care and welfare can be seriously biased by the failure to publish or by misleading publication. These issues are considered by Smith and Chalmers.

Moving to the evaluation of new medical technologies themselves, the remaining chapters consider ethical debates about some key future technologies. One of the most controversial is embryonic stem cell research. Jones and Galvin consider the debates about reproductive cloning, and Draper looks at the ethics of obtaining ova from women for research. Embryo research is an interesting area where the ethics of the research and the ethics of the proposed new technology overlap and are considered together. Similarly, the field of xenotransplantation research brings together the safety of the treatment for patients, the public health risks of zoonosis, the ethics of using animals for human benefit, and the evaluation of clinical trial protocols. These issues are discussed by Hughes.

Genetic medicine is a major focus of both biomedical research and bioethical reflection. In her chapter Chadwick considers the ethical aspects of research and treatment using genetic 'personalized medicine' (pharmacogenetics and pharmacogenomics). Juengst and Grankvist discuss the ethical and social issues involved in contemporary gene therapy. In the future gene therapy and pharmacogenomics may be used not only for treating disease but for extending life, improving human performance, or modifying other valued human traits. Cutas and Harris look at the debates concerning techniques for extending the human life span, while ter Meulen, Nielsen and Landeweerd examine the wider debates on the distinction between treatment and enhancement.

Another major area of research is neuroscience. Gillett discusses the ethical and philosophical issues concerned in psychological modification through modifying brain structure by surgery or device implantation in the brain. Hasman considers the ethics of behaviour modification through using vaccines, for example to lower people's susceptibility to developing addictive behaviours.

These chapters only cover a selection of the many ethical issues in new technologies and medical research. By our next edition some of these technologies will have become well established and moved to other sections in the book, reflecting their status as standard practice. Others will have become seen as false trails or empty dreams. But the general issues will remain with us.

REFERENCES

Ashcroft RE Health technology assessment. In Chadwick R (ed.) *Concise Encyclopedia of Ethics of New Technologies*. San Diego, CA: Academic Press, 2000; pp. 235–244

Richard E. Ashcroft

92

The Ethics and Governance of Medical Research

RICHARD E. ASHCROFT

Research Ethics Committees (RECs) serve an important social function: they protect the interests of research participants and, more generally, regulate research in the public interest. In recent years they have become a much debated phenomenon. To understand why, consider research as a topic of social concern.

RESEARCH AS A TOPIC OF SOCIAL CONCERN

Medical research is advocated using two basic styles of argument. First, research is argued to be a continuous search for improvements which leave the basic structures of medical care (such as the doctor–patient relationship) untouched in principle, but better in practice. In this vision of medical research, research techniques are 'the same as usual, but better monitored and formalized'. Hence, the techniques require no special discussion or consideration, and the involvement of non-researcher stakeholders is minimal, requiring input only through consumption and periodically reaffirmed legitimation. A good example of this is the representation of the use of patient data by epidemiologists as continuous with the use of routine data in audit and clinical care and management of patients.

The other language of research is the language of novelty and innovation – research offers new, unexpected solutions; hence the existing regulatory or methodological standards are held to apply only weakly, if at all, to these techniques (Brown, Rappert and Webster, 2000). This is the language of breakthroughs and change (which needs to be managed). Much bioethics concentrates on this kind of research, but (in my opinion) in some fairly unreflective ways. What may be overlooked is the way any research constructs worlds, reorders societies, reinforces or disrupts systems of power and influence, and does all this in ways which can be hard to foresee or predict. This is obvious in some contexts – hence the furore over cloning bundles together responses to risk, religion, potential for reinforcing old forms of human domination over other humans and inventing new forms, suspicion of the role of scientists in adjudicating moral, technical and human change, and suspicion of the political economy of biotechnology. Yet all of these factors are, or could be, present in response to any research proposal. Some research proposals appear more stable and black boxed than others, yet even these are negotiable. Consider, for instance, pathological research on organs and tissues taken from patients who have died or who have had them removed as part of surgery, or the inspection of medical records for epidemiological purposes. Both of these forms of research, entirely traditional for many years, have in the past two years become matters of loud, and sometimes bitter, public debate.

It is this greyness or unsealability of the supposedly black-boxed techniques which has caused such surprise and dismay to the affected sectors of the scientific community. Techniques they thought uncontroversial and widely accepted have become open to social challenge.

A HISTORICAL CONTEXT FOR STRUGGLES OVER MEDICAL RESEARCH IN SOCIAL CONTEXT

This echoes debates more than 30-years-old. As is well known, in the aftermath of the Second World War, a number

Adapted from Ethics and Governance of Medical Research, Reproduced by permission of Taylor and Francis Group Ltd. http://www.tandf.co.uk/journals

of prominent German scientists and doctors were tried at one of the Nuremberg Trials for crimes against humanity, in particular for a series of experiments on humans in the concentration and extermination camps. Part of the trial proceedings was the promulgation of the Nuremberg Code, which is reputed to be the first full statement of the human rights of subjects of human experimentation. Ironically enough, it was not actually the first, as laws and state decrees had been promulgated in Prussia and Germany in the late 1890s and again in the early 1930s. And although being a statement of human rights implied that it was universal, recent scholarship has shown that the Code was not universally applied even by the Allied powers, either in war crimes and crimes against humanity trials of the defeated Axis powers (the Japanese biological warfare experiments in Manchuria being now a notorious example), or indeed 'at home' (Moreno, 1999; Harris, 2002). It became clear in the 1960s that human experiments in the United States and the United Kingdom were being carried out, which were not compliant with the Code. The publication of a number of exposés of this non-compliance brought a furious (and embarrassed) response from the medical professions of both countries. The essence of the response was that the exposés were mere muckraking and that there was a difference between the acts of well-intentioned doctors, acting in the public interest, often with state authorization, trying to promote medical care in a democracy, and acts of ill-intentioned doctors acting in the service of a discredited biological ideology working for a criminal state (Rothman, 1992). The techniques used were widely accepted within the scientific community. The proposal that they were being misused or were even intrinsically problematic was profoundly disconcerting to a scientific community which regarded them as taken-for-granted elements of professionally warranted practice.

Nevertheless, various professional and official responses began to emerge. The principle of 'informed consent' began to be more widely applied; at this time it was generally agreed that there was an important difference between research procedures and routine treatment, and the rapid growth in the number of randomized controlled trials appeared to imply that this distinction was now wider than before (administration of an experimental drug to a patient for whom nothing else worked was not seen as 'experimenting' on them, whereas randomized assignment to treatment or control was, as it did not – apparently – place the best interests first) (Doyal and Tobias, 2000).

The 1960s was also the period in which the regulation of the testing and manufacture of pharmaceuticals was being modernized and formalized. This had two consequences: the growth of randomized trials for regulatory purposes, and the development of quality standards and cross-industry standards for the management and reporting of trials, par-

ticularly for safety of data and proof of efficacy. This in turn had the consequence of there being more research funding for academic centres, and the extension of the regulatory standards to academic-based work, and the increased internationalization of pharmaceutical research and development work. The rapid growth in this period of the numbers of Investigational New Drugs (this being the golden age of discovery of effective antibiotics and steroids) meant that in this period the sheer quantity of research and development work was growing rapidly, as were the numbers of doctors and patients involved in research.

The research, professional, public and official communities began seriously to debate a range of research risks: direct harm from research procedures; adverse reactions to experimental drugs, trade-offs between incidence and severity of side effects or adverse reactions and the severity of the disease treated, access to experimental drugs within and outwith research protocols, when to terminate trials on favourable or unfavourable interim data, the possibility of research involving incompetent or incapacitated subjects, the integrity of researchers and sponsors in recording data, recruiting subjects and publishing papers based on the research (Abraham, 1996; Le Fanu, 1999). What responses were made to these risks?

I suggest, following Kutcher (2001) and Stevens (2000), that the development of social controls over research had as much to do with concerns internal to the research and industrial communities about exposure to legal risk as to do with the rise of civil rights movements, as was suggested by Rothman (1992) and Jonsen (1998). Our social emphasis on a discourse risk makes more explicit the uneasy balance that has been struck between regarding doctors and researchers as morally culpable for their mistakes and their consequences, and regarding them as unwitting agents of systemic risks already inherent in the medical and research enterprise, and which can be managed and reduced but not altogether removed. One consequence of this risk-oriented approach has been to emphasize safety and governance over the means used in medical research over moral evaluation of the ends of such research, as has been argued by Evans (2002).

PROFESSIONAL-ORIENTED RESPONSES

One approach to the management of the risks posed to subjects by research is to concentrate on the researcher (Jamrozik, 2000). This involves elaborating and developing the professional ethics of the researcher and, through education, professional debate and the dissemination of guidelines, to ensure that these standards become universally known across the profession. This approach fits with what I call the 'moral' discourse of medical ethics: it concentrates on individual agency, the personal responsibility of doctors for the relationship between them and the patient's well-being, and the importance to the individual of the good name of the profession and his or her standing within it.

Within this form of response, guidelines have a special place; they are presented as an elaboration of the essential core ethics of medicine, whose tradition has evolved over time. The period between 1960 and the present has been an age of guidelines (Hurwitz, 1998). However, in the present context, it is important to realize that until the mid-1990s, the guidelines produced are different from those we are beginning to see now. The older type of guideline was a statement of general principles, occasionally declaring that a certain act or attitude was wrong or prohibited, but generally leaving wide scope for interpretation under particular circumstances and after due consideration and discussion. Hence guidelines were normally an aid to moral judgement, rather than a constraint on action. There was rarely, if ever, any attempt to enforce guideline standards. Thus, although clinical guidelines have been occasionally thought to prescribe clinical conduct or used to define what 'a responsible body of medical men skilled in that art' would recommend for the situation in hand, this has only begun to look like a serious possibility in recent years. There is no case law in the United Kingdom on clinical research and its impact on patients (in part because of the difficulty of proving negligent harm). There are few instances of research activity involving a doctor in General Medical Council (GMC) misconduct hearings, and whatever there are tend to relate to fraud (often forgery of consent forms to create records for nonexistent patients) (Lock, Wells and Farthing, 2001).

The other feature of the agent-oriented moral approach is that it leaves room for considerable discretion on what is taken to be a moral issue, and what is not. Thus, it is for the doctor to judge when accepting certain kinds of grant or per capita payment for recruitment would place him or her in a conflict of interest, which should be declared (Rodwin, 1993; Davis and Stark, 2001). The personal risk is that others might not see it that way; the magnitude of the risk is controlled by whether those 'others' in the profession would concur with the doctor's own judgement that acceptance would be morally and professionally viable. Hence the social functioning of the agent-oriented moral approach depends largely on trust between doctors, patients and peers, and on a common professional culture. This culture underwrites the way judgements are made and supports the professional's own reliance on the likelihood that others would judge in the same way or would accept that honest difference with him or her is possible and tolerable. The apprentice model of medical training and the hierarchical nature of a profession which has tended to be internally deferential to authority and professional tradition would tend to make this culture stable and transmissible.

PROCESS-ORIENTED APPROACHES

However, the response to research risk can be understood from the regulatory viewpoint too. The regulatory approach I take to be broadly process-oriented, rather than person-oriented. There are three principal process-oriented approaches to which I would like to draw attention. The first is peer review of research at the grant application stage, which subjects a proposal to scientific and professional review – is the question well posed, important and feasible with this method, staff and resources? Is it medically a good practice? This process tends not to concentrate on the 'ethical' issues, although it can do. However, many of the judgements of clinical relevance and safety are ethical inasmuch as they relate to the welfare of the subjects and to the welfare of future patients. This kind of review and the subsequent review of the data generated by the project's Data and Safety Monitoring Board, and by the regulatory agencies where relevant, might be seen as 'classic' regulation, aimed at securing public safety and protecting the public goods of health care innovation and a functioning economy.

The second process-oriented approach is the informed consent of the subject. This might seem rather an odd way of looking at informed consent. Nonetheless, the informed consent of the subject is a process which functions as a gate through which the research must pass; the request for consent is a routinized process, with information leaflet and form, to ensure that all subjects are aware of the project and agree to assume such risks as are foreseeable and reasonable. The regulatory role of consent as a sort of ritual and as an auditable moment with its own paperwork and accessibility to judicial scrutiny, has received little attention (Mason and Megone, 2001).

Of course, informed consent is also morally important, and much ink has been spilt on why this is so. In medical teaching, I spend a lot of time impressing on students the importance of patients' autonomy and the legal foundations of consent as a protection against physical and psychological harm. Yet this moral and legal view has a history and an impact on social relations between doctor and patient. Two views of what informed consent has done in clinical (as well as specifically research) practice are that it has amoralized medicine, rendering it a consumer transaction and making the doctor a sort of salesperson, or alternatively that it has remoralized medicine, focusing attention on medical care as a relationship between the vulnerable but competent patient and the skilled but finite and human doctor (Rothman, 1992; Katz, 1997; Hogg, 1999; Evans, 2002).

The third process-oriented approach is the REC. This will be the focus of the rest of my chapter. I will concentrate on the British model, as there is much international variation, and many countries lack this process (Brody, 1997; Smith,

1999; Department of Health, 2001). The idea of a REC is that a group of professionals, scientists and lay members of the public sit and review the protocol, and evaluate the question, design, management and information to patients, to determine whether the research is ethically sound (rather than giving a scientific review) (McNeill, 1992). The typical committee is constituted of 8–12 people, of whom two are lay, at least one is a nurse, and at least one a general practitioner, with a chair and a vice-chair (one of whom is usually lay). Usually committees have at least a part-time administrator, who runs the committee, deals with the applications and takes the minutes.

The moral function of the committee is to ensure that the protocol is given an objective and disinterested review, appropriately informed by knowledge of medical science and practice. The principal issues that a committee is concerned with are (1) is the patient appropriately informed? (2) is the balance of risks and benefits posed by the research fair and reasonable? (3) are the patients likely to be worse-off for participating in the research, and if so, does their consent represent a sufficient protection of their interest (i.e. are they being exploited)? and (4) is the research likely to be useful and informative?

A BRIEF HISTORY OF RESEARCH ETHICS COMMITTEES IN THE UNITED KINGDOM

RECs were initially established in the United States in the early 1960s as institutional review boards – that is, they were committees of the institution hosting the research. The first RECs were established in the United Kingdom shortly afterwards, apparently because UK university hospitals seeking US industry-sponsored research funds were asked to ensure that their research projects were reviewed by a committee in order to satisfy the US Food and Drug Administration's requirements for licensing trials. The UK committees made representation to the Royal College of Physicians for some guidelines on appropriate committee structure, which were produced, and the Medical Research Council soon followed up by producing guidelines on research in human subjects, initially applicable only to Medical Research Council grant applicants but widely taken as authoritative. The Ministry of Health took no official notice for some time, but did eventually give its blessing, without taking any formal role in the process of establishment of or guidance to committees. Committees grew up, initially in teaching hospitals, but eventually in other sites, and although notice was taken by the Ministry and (later) the Department of Health (DoH), it was not until 1991 that official guidelines for NHS RECs were issued and made binding on all research projects taking place in NHS institutions (including general practices) or using NHS staff or patient records

and certain other categories of subjects or materials. Until the late 1990s any project taking place in more than five centres had to be reviewed in every single centre; in 1997 the so-called 'multicentre' committees were established, to review projects taking place in five or more centres. These projects still had to be given a review in all local sites, but only relating to a limited list of 'local' questions. This process and the guidelines for all RECs were formalized under the Clinical Trial Regulations (2004), which implemented the European Clinical Trials Directive (2001) in UK law. As part of a seemingly continuous process of review of research ethics review, in 2005 the DoH published a report recommending further revisions to the REC system. At the time of writing, it is not clear how the system will be further modified in response to this report. One proposal is to involve prescreening of proposals by expert 'ethics officers', who will determine whether or not a proposal involves substantial ethical issues, with referral to a committee only taking place if the proposal does involve such issues (or if referral is a statutory requirement).

RESEARCH ETHICS COMMITTEES AND THE REGULATION OF RESEARCH

I have presented RECs as a process-oriented approach to the promotion of ethical standards and practice in research, and implied that this fits best into what I called the regulatory discourse of medicine.

In the first place, note that RECs have many functions and stakeholders similar to classic regulatory agencies in the pharmaceutical and medical sectors. They are intended to be universal in coverage. They are meant to be independent of the sponsor/researcher interest and to give an independent evaluation of the research against declared standards. Those standards represent a balance of the interests of all parties (in particular, the DoH requires committees both 'to protect the dignity, rights, safety and well-being of all actual or potential research participants' (2.2) and to 'take into account the interests, needs and safety of researchers who are trying to undertake research of good quality' (2.3)), which involves them in a judgement of risk, and on whom risk falls, on how that risk can be minimized, and what the opportunity costs for present and future patients will be (Department of Health, 2001). They are not meant to judge some issues as being outside their competence, such as scientific merit, the impact on host institution resources, or the likely effect on the sponsors' income streams or the researcher's career. Nonetheless, they have an obligation to ensure that the host institution (as part of the NHS) has reviewed the proposal to ensure that non-participants will not be adversely affected and that the research budget is adequate; moreover, the slogan that 'bad science is bad ethics' and the likelihood that ethics-driven changes to the protocol will change the science somewhat do imply that an evaluation of the science is involved. They are meant to review confidentially and with due diligence and fair process. Here fairness relates to the treatment of the researcher. Although technically they have no corporate existence and are advisory rather than holding any decision-making capacity, they are subject to administrative law and members are indemnified against the consequences of their decisions. Their ability to monitor research post-approval is minimal, but they do have (and occasionally use) the power to require researchers to desist from further recruitment and to retrospectively withdraw approval.

Besides these formal similarities, they are perceived as regulatory agencies by their users (researchers and sponsors). Periodically there is a blitz of articles and letters complaining about the behaviour of committees. There is a small literature of articles giving quantitative measures of time to review, time to approval, variation between committees or within committees, consistency of judgements with published guidelines. There are proposals for audit of committee process (I have been involved with one such audit). Researchers routinely complain about committees, and the view of them as 'hurdles' is entirely standard. On the contrary, researchers seek out some sites as being more 'pro-research'. Standard techniques of regulatory management such as sharing information on how to manage contacts with the chair and administrator of the committee and how to use sponsorship and participation in educational meetings are well known. Researchers are often members of the RECs, although conflict of interest guidelines require them not to discuss work in which they have a personal involvement or financial stake.

The culmination of the regulatory model of the nature and role of a REC is the inclusion of the REC system in the NHS research governance framework (Department of Health, 2000). This achieves a number of things: it brings all existing NHS RECs formally under the control of the DoH, rendering them formally answerable to the DoH (or one of its NHS delegates) for compliance with the published official guidelines (until 1998 the DoH did not know even how many RECs there were or where they were). It inserts RECs formally into the new NHS clinical quality management (governance) structure and ensures that the hitherto sporadic reporting on REC activity will now be actively sought and that the performance of committees will be audited. It also ensures that there are systems in place for ensuring that all research under the NHS umbrella is reviewed by a REC.

Note that placing 'all research' under the NHS umbrella involves an important set of social processes. REC review now covers a much wider range of types of research than it did originally. Many projects which would once have been regarded as audits are now regarded as research; much that

remains audit is now reviewed by an audit committee which has a kind of ethical gate-keeping function in that it has to decide which studies are 'research' and which are not, and so which audit-like studies are referred to a REC. Innovations in surgery and experimental uses of drugs 'off-label' are now potentially within the REC's remit. This has a number of impacts – on patients, who now become 'research subjects', on professionals, who now become 'researchers', and on hospital management and clinical treatment processes, which now intersect with a different governance system (REC review). More broadly, the REC process reconstitutes certain kinds of work as acceptable or unacceptable, reconfigures certain kinds of work in order that they can fit with REC requirements and redefines certain kinds of person, patient or procedure. For instance, certain patients are defined as 'vulnerable subjects', which is both a putative metaphysical state and a bureaucratic category. This is done in various ways, through citation of relevant law or guidelines and through the now widely shared requirement that all researchers submit applications to the committee using a standardized and highly structured application form, which can have implications for the selection of research methods (in order to 'get through' a REC review or avoid the need for it) and for how researchers conceive their work.

Placing RECs in the governance framework effects the completion of a conceptual transformation of RECs from peer-led 'ethical committees' close in spirit to if distant in form from the professional-oriented model, to management- and institution-oriented quality management systems. (Note that quality in the NHS includes patient safety). On the face of it, this means that RECs are part of a risk management framework, albeit the risks are research risks, which overlap with clinical risks but are not a simple subset of them. And this means that they should be open to analysis and redesign using the tools of risk analysis.

EVALUATING AND MEASURING RECS

It might be possible to evaluate RECs by estimating the cost of REC work (and they are already being encouraged to charge for their work), and considering their economic impact and the implicit utility weights they place on the risks they evaluate, and the trade-offs they make between risks. The pharmaceutical industry has for many years done comparative cost analysis on different regulatory regimes, including evaluations of the nominal loss they make every month and what they lose on the patent clock due to decision-making delay. It would be easy to do the same for RECs (if only we had the cost data). It is already possible to audit committees against criteria such as time to review compared with mean time to review in the committee population, and compliance with the published guideline standards.

One exciting possibility would be to consider RECs as public health interventions; in essence they act as risk assessment and control mechanisms to reduce, control or allocate the exposure of the population to the relative risks of research participation (and, by the same token, the exposure to the relative benefits). On this model, it should be possible to assess the REC model (and particular instances of it) for such characteristics as risk-aversity or proneness, uneven allocation of risks among or within groups defined by disease/condition, age group, sex/gender and socioeconomic group.

RECs are already invited to evaluate the suitability of the local site as a location for proposed research, the exposure of the proposed study population to previous or ongoing research and the suitability of the local researcher to carry out the research. They may lose the operational responsibility for these tasks, but under the draft new guidelines, they will retain the administrative responsibility for ensuring that the host institution has carried out this assessment.

Hence, in research governance, the REC is open actively to be assessed for its efficiency, effectiveness and relative cost-effectiveness. It will have a certain management responsibility. And it will be 'managed'.

THE MORAL AND THE REGULATORY DISCOURSES OF RESEARCH ETHICS COMMITTEES

I have sketched why the regulatory version of RECs is both a widely held perception of the committees by their users and has been operationalized within the NHS.

Many people are profoundly unhappy at this move. Part of the rationale for the revision of the existing guidelines and the construction of research governance in its present form has to do with a conflict between the existing RECs and the DoH (and many in the world of medical research and the pharmaceutical industry) over variations between RECs in the evaluation of research. This is often considered a serious inconsistency in moral judgement. Although some of this variation can be attributed to ignorance on the part of committees of the relevant guidance and a lack of training in ethical principles and method of analysis, there may be deeper reasons for it.

The 'moral discourse' reading might help: circumstances might differ between localities, moral disagreement is possible and interpretation of broad guidelines is inevitably variable (Edwards, Ashcroft and Kirchin, 2004). This clue leads to the view that the governance model of REC review is misleading because it substitutes administrative norms of efficiency, effectiveness and cost-effectiveness for moral norms of judgement, reflection and integrity. Closing a committee because it is too slow

is a terrible solecism; the committee might be morally reflective and penetrating in a way that its more rapid, and literal-minded, committee peers were not. One cannot, it is said, trade ethical thinking against cost in this way.

Notwithstanding this objection, regulatory thinkers about RECs are right about a number of things. Some of these stand up as moral arguments, others challenge the moral arguments to justify their credentials.

Recently, it was reported that *Le Monde* alleged that it was impossible to have a serious intergovernmental discussion about the ethics of biotechnology with the British because all they would talk about was the cost. I sympathize. However, against *Le Monde*, cost is a consideration. It matters how you count it, what discounting you use and so on. And if we are in the business of protecting the public, defining and assessing the public interest is a consideration, and cost is one way to do that. More aggressively, one might say that the assessment of opportunity costs is always relevant in ethics, but rarely is done, and assertions of principle are sometimes self-defeating because if we considered all the options we would realize that the best options from the principled point of view was one we ruled out too hastily. (Utilitarian arguments are visibly vulnerable here.) More strongly still, appeal to moral principle will often win arguments when the principle itself is unjustified, incoherent or irrelevant. Many researchers feel that their work has been blocked on just such ill-considered grounds.

Another approach to the moral and practical significance of REC variation is to say that from a regulatory point of view, due process and fair consideration take very high priority. Hence, one of the key challenges is to ensure that the process of review is carried out appropriately with reference to the norms of procedural justice. Amongst other things, this includes a right of appeal, reference to public and accessible standards, reasons given for decisions and decision within a reasonable time. Of course, justice also requires that the participants be treated fairly. But it might require that non-participants and future patients be not unfairly excluded or delayed from accessing the benefits of research, a burden of responsibility which might arguably fall on a REC as much as on the researcher or sponsor. Fair process should be evaluable (and is evaluable in law), even if proper outcome is not (because ethics is not a science). However, manifest refusal or inability to justify decisions or an irrational degree of flexibility in interpretation of widely accepted guidelines, laws and standards might fall outside the domain of legitimate moral disagreement. (Cf. debates on abortion and embryo research where, *pace* the Human Fertilisation and Embryology Authority, they are hardly likely to appoint someone with pronounced 'pro-life' views to chair the Authority.)

Related to this is a more complex argument about disagreement under liberalism. In principle, a committee could block a proposal on moral grounds – indeed, if an ethics committee cannot, who can? Yet there are difficult questions on how far their power to veto extends – in many cases, where there is disagreement, civil peace and a right to private life (in the US sense) should dictate freedom to research without hindrance from arbitrary or prejudiced authorities (Ashcroft, 2002). This is analogous to the classical debates about how far the state is legitimate in drawing limits to the freedom of contract doctrine. Another way to look at the issue is to see it as a debate about the proper limits of liberal paternalism in protecting patients from research risk (Edwards, Kirchin and Huxtable, 2004; Garrard and Dawson, 2005).

CONCLUSION

The moral discourse and the regulatory discourse converge, in an attempt to define appropriate goals, fair trade-offs, the competing private interests and the indefinite public interest. I have argued how RECs can be seen as combining moral and regulatory features, and how the REC process constitutes and shapes what is research, how it is organized and how the relationship to patients is structured. The REC is not a simple gatekeeper, applying a simple pass/fail test of ethical correctness, which might be implicit in seeing it as a pure regulatory mechanism. Yet its ability to do ethics, in the sense of fuzzy, vague, tentative, reflection on processes leading to a future state of knowledge and action only partly defined and only dimly foreseeable, is also challenged by its place in a regulatory mechanism which has a significant role in the health services and in industry's product cycle. Sociologically and normatively it has many features of both models.

REFERENCES

Abraham J. *Science, Politics and the Pharmaceutical Industry: Controversy and Bias in Drug Regulation*. London: UCL Press, 1996.

Ashcroft RE. Ethical considerations in outsourced clinical trials. In: Drucker R, Hughes G, eds. *Outsourcing in Clinical Drug Development*. Denver, CO: Interpharm Press, 2002, pp. 73–86.

Brody B. *The Ethics of Biomedical Research: An International Perspective*. Oxford: Oxford University Press, 1997.

Brown N, Rappert B, Webster S, eds. *Contested Futures: A Sociology of Prospective Techno-Science*. Aldershot: Ashgate, 2000.

Davis M, Stark A, eds. *Conflict of Interest in the Professions*. New York: Oxford University Press, 2001.

Department of Health. *Research Governance Framework*. London: Department of Health, 2000.

Department of Health. *Governance Arrangements for Research Ethics Committees*. London: Department of Health, 2001.

Doyal L, Tobias JS. *Informed Consent in Medical Research*. London: BMJ Books, 2000.

Edwards SJL, Ashcroft RE, Kirchin S. Research Ethics Committees: Differences and moral judgement. *Bioethics* 2004; **18**: 408–427.

Edwards SJL, Kirchin S, Huxtable R. Research ethics committees and paternalism. *J Med Ethics* 2004; **30**: 88–91.

European Parliament and Council (2001) Directive 2001/20/EC of the European Parliament and of the Council of 4 April 2001 on the approximation of laws, regulations administrative provisions of the Member States relating to the implementation of good clinical practice in the conduct of clinical trials on medicinal products for human use. *Official Journal of the European Communities* L121, 01/05/2001, 0034-0044.

Evans JH. *Playing God? Human Genetic Engineering and the Rationalization of Public Bioethical Debate, 1959–1995*. Chicago: University of Chicago Press, 2002.

Garrard E, Dawson AJ. What is the role of the Research Ethics Committee? Paternalism, inducements and harm in research ethics. *Journal of Medical Ethics* 2005; **31**: 419–423.

Harris SH. *Factories of Death: Japanese Biological Warfare, 1932–1945, and the American Cover-up*, 2nd edition. London: Routledge, 2002.

Hogg C. *Patients, Power and Politics: From Patients to Citizens*. London: Sage, 1999.

Hurwitz BS. *Clinical Guidelines and the Law: Negligence, Discretion and Judgement*. Oxford: Radcliffe Medical Press, 1998.

Jamrozik K. The case for a new system for oversight of research on human subjects. *J Med Ethics* 2000; **26**: 334–339.

Jonsen AR. *The Birth of Bioethics*. New York: Oxford University Press, 1998.

Katz JS. *The Silent World of Doctor and Patient*, 2nd edition. Baltimore, MD: Johns Hopkins University Press, 1997.

Kutcher GJ. Clinical Ethics and Research Imperatives in Human Experiments: A Case of Contested Knowledge. Cambridge: University of Cambridge, unpublished doctoral dissertation, 2001.

Le Fanu J. *The Rise and Fall of Modern Medicine*. London: Abacus, 1999.

Lock S, Wells F, Farthing M, eds. *Fraud and Misconduct in Biomedical Research*. London: BMJ Books, 2001.

Mason SA, Megone C, eds. *Informed Consent in Neonatal Research in Europe*. Aldershot: Ashgate, 2001.

McNeill PM. *The Ethics and Politics of Human Experimentation*. Cambridge: Cambridge University Press, 1992.

Medicines for Human Use (Clinical Trials) Regulations 2004. Statutory Instrument 2004 No. 1031 http://www.opsi.gov.uk/si/si2004/20041031.htm

Moreno J. *Undue Risk: Secret State Experiments on Humans from the Second World War to Iraq and Beyond*. New York: W.H. Freeman, 1999.

Rodwin MA. *Medicine, Money and Morals: Physicians' Conflicts of Interest*. New York: Oxford University Press, 1993.

Rothman DJ. *Strangers at the Bedside: How Law and Bioethics Transformed Medical Decision Making*. New York: Basic Books, 1992.

Smith T. *Ethics in Medical Research: A Handbook of Good Practice*. Cambridge: Cambridge University Press, 1999.

Stevens MLT. *Bioethics in America: Origins and Cultural Politics*. Baltimore: Johns Hopkins University Press, 2000.

On The Ethics of Animal Research

DAVID DEGRAZIA

INTRODUCTION

Few moral issues are as polarizing as the use of nonhuman animals in biomedical research. Contrary to some at the poles, this issue is also enormously complex. Moreover, the stakes are high. From 50 to 100 million animals are involved in such experiments annually (Orlans, 1998, p. 400). And, according to many proponents of animal research, biomedical progress requires the continuation of experiments upon live animals. The purpose of this chapter is to convey some of the complexity of this important issue, sketch and evaluate leading positions, and offer several ethical and policy recommendations.

Reflection on the ethics of animal research inclines most people towards neither absolute abolitionism nor a pure *laissez-faire* approach, but to something (perhaps not well defined) in between. From such a moderate standpoint, it may seem obvious that some animal research is justified. Imagine an experiment that would cause mild pain or distress to 100 rats before they are painlessly killed, and is very likely to succeed, thereby validating a cure for a disease that currently kills tens of thousands of children every year; no scientifically promising alternative to this experiment is known. Although it may seem perfectly obvious that this experiment passes moral muster, this judgement is not self-justifying. After all, most of us would condemn an experiment that caused pain or distress – not to mention death – to human subjects *who neither consented to participate nor stood to benefit from their participation*. Yet, the rats in the imagined study neither consent nor stand to benefit. They are sacrificed for the benefit of others. The judgement that the experiment is justified while similar coercive use of humans would not be justified implies that the *moral status* of rats is, in some sense, less than that of humans.

More generally, any justification of animal research requires assumptions about moral status. Naturally, the same is true of principled opposition to animal research, because such opposition assumes that animals' moral status is too substantial to permit their sacrifice for others' (humans' or animals') benefit. My first thesis, then, is that consideration of animals' moral status is inescapable in any responsible investigation of the ethics of animal research.

In its admirable, well-researched report, the Nuffield Council on Bioethics (NCB) disagrees:

> 'The debate is not best characterized in terms of the relative moral status of humans and animals but in terms of what features of humans and animals are of moral concern . . . Once those features are identified, the question [is] how they should be taken into account in moral reasoning. Are they factors to be weighed against others, or do they function as absolute prohibitions?' (NCB, 2005, p. 57; cf. Rachels 2004).

The NCB identifies *sentience, higher cognitive capacities, the capacity to flourish, sociability, and possession of a life* as morally relevant features (NCB, 2005, p. 41).

However, this proposal is deeply problematic. First, deciding which features are morally relevant can be as controversial as debates about moral status. For example, contrary to the NCB's list, I do not believe that an amoeba's being alive is morally relevant – just as I doubt that life *per se* confers moral status. Second, even if we confidently endorsed a list of morally relevant features, as the NCB notes, we must decide how to take these features into account. If sentience is morally relevant, we must ask whether, say, rats' sentience justifies (1) an absolute prohibition against causing rats pain, (2) a presumption against causing them pain *equal* to the presumption against causing humans (unconsented) pain, or (3) a presumption against causing pain that is *weaker* than that against causing humans pain. The NCB notes that we must decide between absolute constraints and balancing considerations. But on what basis? Note that any endorsement of balancing will be unhelpful without a specification of *how* to balance different factors. Should a rat's pain count as much as a human's pain, or less? And, if less, how much less? Answers to the questions raised in this paragraph, I suggest, are intelligible only on the basis of assumptions about animals' moral status.

Before we take up the issue of moral status, some background should be helpful.

BACKGROUND

In this chapter, 'animal research' will refer to two broad endeavours. First is animal usage in the *pursuit of original scientific knowledge*. This category divides into *basic research*, which pursues new knowledge of biological processes and functions, and *applied research*, which seeks new biological, medical or veterinary knowledge in order to promote human, animal or environmental health. Second, *testing* on animals evaluates chemicals and other products for safety.

Animal research dates back to classical Greece and Rome and, further east, to early Arabic medicine after the fall of Rome (NCB, 2005, pp. 15–29). Although little animal research was conducted in medieval Europe, animal experiments led to several important discoveries – for example, about blood circulation and the function of lungs – in the seventeenth and eighteenth centuries. The volume of animal research greatly increased in the nineteenth century. Partly in response to the pioneering experiments of François Magendie and Claude Bernard in that century, a notable antivivisection movement emerged in Britain. The 1876 (British) Cruelty to Animals Act, the world's first legislation regulating animal research, established a system requiring licences for experimentation on animals.

Despite continuing protests, animal research grew steadily for most of the twentieth century. Responding to both society's interest in animal research and its ethical concerns, British scientists William Russell and Rex Burch published in 1959 a landmark work that established the 'three Rs' – *Refinement* of techniques to reduce suffering, *Reduction* of numbers of animal subjects and *Replacement* of live animals wherever possible – as central concerns for conscientious members of the profession (Russell and Burch, 1959). Public pressure for increased regulation in Great Britain led to the 1986 Animals (Scientific Procedures) Act, which regulates the research use of all vertebrates and, by a subsequent modification, octopi. Prominent in this legislation is a requirement of harm/benefit assessments of proposed experiments.

In the United States, the (Laboratory) Animal Welfare Act became law in 1966, following widespread outrage that pet dogs were being stolen and sold to research laboratories. At first, it was primarily a pet protection bill. Subsequent amendments significantly increased the requirements for the care and use of research animals. Although this legislation has never covered farm animals, or even rats and mice – the animals most commonly used in research – Public Health Service (PHS) policy covers all vertebrate animals in PHS-funded research. But PHS policy leaves rats and mice unprotected in privately funded research – a major gap in American regulation.

Today, member states of the European Union are legally bound by the 1986 EU Directive EEC 86/609. Among its provisions are a requirement for special authorization to conduct experiments likely to cause severe, prolonged pain in animals; requirements for breeders and suppliers; and the prohibition of animal use where a valid alternative exists. A more recent ban on the use of animals in cosmetics testing has passed and is due to take effect in 2009.

Is the policy status quo morally defencible? That depends, in significant measure, on how we should understand animals' moral status.

MORAL STATUS

A being has *moral status* if he or she is morally important in his or her own right, and not merely because how he or she is treated may affect others' interests. All *moral agents* – that is, all beings who have moral responsibilities – have moral status. Rocks do not. They have no conscious or sentient life (even potentially), so nothing we do to them can possibly matter to them. We cannot harm or benefit rocks. Similarly with cars (although what one does to a car can matter to its owner), because our treatment of a car does not matter to it and therefore does not harm or benefit it in any morally significant sense. Common sense suggests that only beings who have interests – or a welfare – have moral status. So having interests is necessary for moral status. If having interests is also sufficient for moral status, then many animals have moral status. Do they?

One historically prominent view answers negatively. According to this *no-status view*, animals' interests have no moral importance except where our treatment of animals affects human interests. That kicking a dog may upset some people, or damage an owner's property, is morally important on this view; that it hurts the dog does not directly matter. The no-status view is enormously implausible in the case of sentient animals, who have interests, and its historical prominence seems to have more to do with humans' self-interested bias and power over animals than with moral insight. Here, I quickly suggest two reasons to reject the no-status view. First, it does not adequately account for our considered judgement that cruelty to animals is wrong; an adequate account must acknowledge the moral status of cruelty's victims. Second, it has trouble explaining why it is wrong to mistreat those human beings who are sentient yet, due to injury or genetic anomaly, lack (even potentially) advanced capacities such as moral agency and linguistic competence – capacities commonly believed to confer special moral status on human persons (DeGrazia, 1996, pp. 40–3, 54–6). Hereafter in this chapter, I will assume that (sentient) animals have at least some moral status, that how we treat them has non-derivative moral importance and that they are beings to whom moral agents can have obligations.

Among the theories ascribing moral status to animals, significant differences appear. Let us first distinguish *equal-consideration views* and *unequal-(less-than-equal-) consideration views.*

The language of 'consideration' focuses on how important, morally, animals' interests are in comparison with prudentially comparable human interests. Take for example, one's interest in not suffering (to some degree, however measured), an interest humans and animals share. How important is animal suffering (in its own right)? Equal-consideration (EC) views maintain that comparable interests have equal moral weight, regardless of the interest bearer's species. This implies that sentient beings have *equal moral status at the level of basic consideration*, but perhaps not with respect to certain interests that do not seem prudentially comparable across species. For example most commentators agree that death typically harms a person more than it harms, say, a mouse, so that their interests in staying alive are not prudentially comparable (not presumptively equal) – in which case equal consideration is consistent with the judgement that killing persons is generally worse than killing mice. (For a fuller discussion of noncomparable interests, see DeGrazia, 1996, ch. 8). Unequal-consideration (UC) views hold that animals' interests have some (non-derivative) moral importance but less than what persons' comparable interests have – implying that animals have moral status, but less than persons.

The major representatives of EC views are *utilitarianism* and *animal rights theories*. Utilitarianism grants sentient beings equal consideration by counting everyone's comparable interests equally in its directive to maximize utility or net welfare (Singer, 1990 although here he stresses equal consideration more than utilitarianism). Animal rights theories afford stronger protection for the vital interests of humans and certain animals (those claimed to have rights), generally resisting appeals to utility as a justification for sacrificing those interests. In this chapter I use the term *animal rights views* somewhat narrowly to refer to views in which rights generally trump appeals to utility (Regan, 1983; Pluhar, 1995). Some use the term more broadly to refer to all equal-consideration views or even all views granting moral status to animals.

UC theories have received less attention in the literature than EC views and the no-status view. One UC theory is the *two-tier theory*, according to which persons or humans deserve full, equal consideration whereas other sentient beings deserve some nontrivial, but less-than-equal, consideration (Warren, 1997; McMahan, ch. 3). Another UC theory is a *sliding-scale model* of moral status, according to which sentient beings deserve consideration in proportion to their level of cognitive, emotional and social complexity. (I describe this model, without endorsing it, in DeGrazia 1996, ch. 3) This model is likely to stipulate that beyond some threshold of complexity such as personhood, one deserves full consideration – consistent with two-tier theories and the considered judgement that all persons deserve equal consideration.

Each theory of moral status just sketched is, unlike the no-status view, a serious contender. Each is supported by substantial arguments and each faces important challenges. In this chapter, I assume that both EC and UC theories are fairly reasonable and will not attempt to adjudicate between them. Before exploring the implications of these theories, let us examine the possible benefits and harms associated with animal research.

THE ISSUE OF BENEFITS

Proponents of animal research stress its benefits, which accrue mostly to humans but also to animals. The claim of benefits extends to the use of animals in basic research, in modelling diseases and developing therapeutic interventions, in pharmaceutical research and development, and in toxicity testing. Now, in the case of many advances in biomedicine and veterinary science, animal research has certainly been part of the pathway to progress. But it does not logically follow that animal research was necessary for such progress. There may be multiple paths to a particular goal. In justifying animal research, we tend to focus on the path actually taken; relatively little attention (and even less funding) has been given to other possible paths. This raises the issue of alternatives to animal research.

Some critics of animal research hold that it impedes biomedical progress. They doubt that nonhuman animals are reliable models for human beings. Obviously, mice, rats and dogs are not the same as humans. And surely the methodological difficulties of extrapolating data from nonhuman subjects to the human situation are substantial. It is probably fair to assert that animal models can be misleading, with serious consequences. Some critics argue, for example, that reliance on animal models delayed the development of an effective polio vaccine for many years (LaFollette and Shanks, 1996, ch. 8). And critics often cite the disaster involving thalidomide, which was licensed following animal research for use by pregnant women (a group on which the drug was not tested) as a treatment for morning sickness, leading to the birth of thousands of children with major limb deformities.

Nevertheless, it seems reasonable to assume that, due to many continuities and similarities across species, well-chosen animal models often furnish valuable data on the road to biomedical advances. But what if there are other, non-animal roads to progress? It would greatly vitiate the moral case for animal research if the latter were unnecessary. So how extensive are the benefits that *only* animal research can provide?

Confronting this complex issue requires comparing (1) progress that results, or has resulted, from use of animal subjects with (2) progress that could result, or could have resulted, from optimal non-animal methods. But progress of type (2) is hypothetical because investments in the study of alternatives pale in comparison with investments in animal research. So, we must speculate to estimate the value of (2). Yet, unless proponents of animal research can compare the values of (1) and (2) rather persuasively – as seems doubtful – then, although they can assert that animal research has yielded benefits, they are in no position to say that it was *necessary* for those benefits.

We must also remember that particular benefits from animal studies are only *possible and hoped for*, whereas the harms to animals are typically immediate and certain. (Countless animal studies harm animals without producing benefits.) Any honest cost/benefit analysis must multiply the value of hoped-for benefits *by the (<1) probability of achieving them*, before considering the predictable costs and harms. This often overlooked fact is critical not only to utilitarianism but also to all positions that regard costs and benefits as relevant to the justification of animal research. In light of both (1) the need to factor in likelihood of success in any honest cost/benefit analysis and (2) the issue of non-animal alternatives, the value of animal research would seem to be less than what proponents typically claim.

Yet its value may sometimes be sufficient to justify the associated costs and harms. Perhaps an animal experiment is the only possible way to achieve some important benefit – such as knowledge about a new veterinary technique's viability. Or perhaps non-animal means to some human benefit would be so costly or harmful to humans as to be unacceptable. (In principle, we *could* always use human subjects to learn about human biology, effective therapies and toxicity, but doing so might require coercion of human subjects or unacceptable risks to them.) Suppose we assume that animals can be useful models in pursuit of some substantial benefit *and* that no non-animal alternative is both scientifically viable and morally acceptable. Does this justify animal research? Not necessarily, for we must also consider harms and costs.

HARMS AND COSTS

In addressing harms and costs associated with animal research, we are likely to think first of harms caused in experimental procedures. These harms range from none (e.g. in simply observing animals) to severe (e.g. in prolonged deprivation of food, water or sleep; force-feeding a substance until subjects die; induction of cancer tumours; brain damage). Intermediate cases include the taking of frequent blood samples, holding an animal in restraints in an inhalation chamber and performing a caesarean section on a pregnant animal.

Additional sources of harm for animal subjects include the following:

- *Acquisition* – usually through breeding but sometimes through the capture of wild animals;
- *Transportation to the research facility*;
- *Housing conditions*, which typically confine animals to small spaces, often without enrichment or access to conspecifics;
- *Handling* of animal subjects, sometimes including the use of restraints; and
- *Death* – if continued life for the animal subject would be worth living.

In cost/benefit assessments, harms count as 'costs'. Of course, so do costs in the ordinary sense. Government-funded research uses taxpayers' money. Research funded by for-profit companies – say, in product testing – uses stockholders' money.

Where non-animal research methods are employed, harms to animal subjects are avoided whereas financial costs are not. Wherever animal methods are not replaced, the other two Rs, reduction and refinement, loom large. Harms and costs are minimized by using the smallest possible number of animals consistent with scientific objectives. Refinements, meanwhile, involve fine-tuning experimental conditions and procedures in light of a sensitive appreciation of animal subjects' needs. Providing an instructive illustration of the latter, the NCB offers this list of rats' and mice's husbandry needs: housing in stable, compatible groups; enough space for exercise and normal social behaviour; a solid floor with a wood-shaving substrate; sufficient height for rearing; nesting material; material to gnaw; and refuges (NCB, 2005, p. 211).

With the benefits, harms and costs associated with animal research in view, let us return to theories of moral status and explore their ethical implications.

SOME DIFFERING IMPLICATIONS

The animal rights approach has almost no interest in cost/benefit considerations because it opposes harming some individuals (without their valid consent) for others' benefit. Although this approach might seem to preclude animal research, it does not. For it can consistently permit (1) research that does not harm its subjects at all and (2) research that promotes animal subjects' best interests – therapeutic veterinary research. Moreover, insofar as current policy permits *minimal-risk* research on human children, who cannot consent in the relevant sense, an animal rights theory might permit this third category as well. But it would preclude the vast majority of animal experiments currently conducted. It would also reject the hypothetical experiment described earlier in this chapter despite its extraordinarily favourable benefit/cost ratio.

The other EC view, utilitarianism, would embrace the hypothetical experiment because its expected utility is higher than that of any known alternative. Utilitarianism would also justify some animal research conducted today. Even more-than-minimal-risk, non-therapeutic research is acceptable on this view so long as the expected benefits – factoring in the likelihood of achieving them and giving animals' interests equal weight to humans' comparable interests – outweigh the total costs, and no alternative offers a better benefit/cost ratio. Then again, utilitarianism's commitment to equal consideration entails that rather little animal research is justified. Meanwhile, utilitarians must grapple with the fact that their theory seems open, in principle, to the coercive use of human subjects in some circumstances.

Compared with utilitarianism, UC theories will be considerably more welcoming of animal research because they grant animals' interests (e.g. avoiding suffering) less weight than comparable human interests. The main difference between the two-tier theory and the sliding-scale model, both UC views, is this: the former would give all sentient nonhuman animals' interests the same weight, whereas the latter would give their interests more weight if the animals in question are more complex. But, more importantly, no UC theory will be *laissez-faire* about animal research. Recognizing that animals have moral status and that they are not mere tools for research, UC views would likely reject a great deal of current research. Examples include frivolous experiments lacking real benefits (e.g. the infamous cat sex experiments (Wade, 1976)), research offering non-essential benefits (e.g. testing new cosmetics), research causing excessive harm (e.g. Harry Harlow's maternal deprivation studies on monkeys (Harlow and Zimmerman, 1959)) and experiments that are clearly replaceable (cosmetics testing in general). UC views would also seek to minimize the harms associated with acquisition, transport, handling, housing and experimental procedures. The challenges of accommodating the needs of animal subjects' might lead such views to ban or severely limit the use of certain 'higher' mammals, such as primates, whose social and psychological needs are especially hard to meet.

These implications of EC and UC theories motivate another thesis: no reasonable view of animals' moral status can justify the full extent of animal research conducted today. Moreover, all reasonable views would permit some animal research, though animal rights theories would permit precious little. But our discussion of the theories' implications has tacitly assumed that there are no viable alternatives to animal research. Is that so?

WHAT ABOUT ALTERNATIVES?

Although the term 'alternatives' is often used to refer to the *replacement* of live animal use with non-animal techniques, the term is sometimes used more broadly to refer to the other Rs as well: *reduction* in the number of animals used to that needed for scientific validity and *refinement* of techniques to minimize suffering. It is difficult to imagine morally serious opposition to reduction and refinement, so let's focus on replacement.

Replacement alternatives can be either 'complete' or 'incomplete'. Complete replacements use no animal-derived materials. Examples include mathematical and computer modelling studies of biological processes, predictions based on chemical properties of molecules, analyses of epidemiological data, research on human cell or tissue cultures, and studies directly involving human volunteers. Incomplete replacements use some biological materials derived from living or humanely killed animals – for example, cell or tissue cultures from a small number of sacrificed animals – or use animals thought to be insentient such as horseshoe crabs or insects.

The alternatives movement has made considerable progress in recent years (Stephens, Goldberg and Rowan, 2001). With respect to replacements, the most progress has been made in the area of testing. Since the late 1990s several alternatives have achieved regulatory acceptance and widespread adoption. Examples include an *in vitro* test for phototoxicity and Corrositex, a kind of synthetic skin, to test skin corrosivity. Providing an indication of progress, the Netherlands and Great Britain have stopped using animals for testing cosmetics – and the European Union has banned cosmetics testing with effect from 2009 (NCB, 2005, p. 235).

Although alternatives, including replacements, have made significant inroads in testing, one might doubt the feasibility of replacing animals in original biological research. Nevertheless, there have been advances in this area as well. For example, an *in vitro* method has proven to be a viable substitute for mouse-based methods of producing monoclonal antibodies. Sometimes computer modelling is effective in simulating biological systems. Meanwhile, some progress has involved and will continue to involve the use of human beings. Volunteers sometimes participate in physiological studies or in testing diagnostic techniques. Epidemiological studies can help identify factors contributing to particular diseases. Human tissue and cell cultures (e.g. tumour cell lines, neuronal cell culture lines) represent an important growth area. Though often overlooked, the use of new imaging technology – such as PET scans and magnetic resonance imaging – permits study of the live human brain without invasive procedures on people or animals. Finally, the use of stem cells derived from embryos or, less controversially, from adults has enormous research promise.

Inasmuch as regulatory and financial support for alternatives to animal research is in its infancy, it is very difficult to predict how far, scientifically, alternatives can lead. What is clear is that heavy investment in and development of alternatives should be a very high priority on any reasonable view of animals' moral status.

SOME SUGGESTIONS

The ethics of animal research is enormously complex. Even if we settled the hard factual issues (e.g. the validity of animal models, the prospects for alternatives, the sentience or insentience of particular animals) and conceptual issues (e.g. how to evaluate the harm of death in the case of animals), the issue of moral status would remain. I have discussed representatives of both EC and UC views not out of politeness to representatives of different views; I honestly find all of these views reasonable. Even if one theory is the most reasonable, several others are within reason and none is an obvious winner.

Although this plurality of reasonable views impedes the quest for a detailed ethics of animal research, it does not prevent us from identifying points of overlapping consensus or palatable compromises where consensus is unavailable. In this spirit, I close with several policy suggestions:

1. *There should be a massive public investment in alternatives research.* Inasmuch as animals have moral status, they cannot be regarded – merely or even primarily – as tools for human use. On any reasonable view, there must be a presumption against animal research. And, at this time, we know relatively little about the full promise of alternatives. (Apparently, the NCB shares the spirit of my suggestion: 'The Working Party therefore agrees that there is a moral imperative to develop as a priority scientifically rigorous and validated alternative methods for those areas in which Replacements do not currently exist' (NCB, 2005, p. XIX).)
2. *Animal experiments should not be permitted where viable replacement alternatives are known to exist.*
3. *Where animal research is permitted, housing conditions must meet the basic needs – physical, psychological and social – of animal subjects.* Barren housing is a source

of major harm to research animals. Although meeting the basic needs of animal subjects is costly, nothing less is appropriate for beings with moral status. Presumably, this requirement will be considerably easier to satisfy in the case of rodents, the animals most commonly used in research, than in the case of 'higher' mammals, especially primates.

4. *Wild animals should never be captured for laboratory research.* Breeding avoids the harms associated with forcing an animal to transition from one form of life to a radically different sort of existence.
5. *Great apes should not be used in research unless their participation is voluntary and/or compatible with the best interests of individual research subjects.* Some great apes currently live in captivity. If all their basic needs are met – which is far from easy to ensure – they may be appropriately used in two circumstances: (1) where they freely choose to participate (e.g. by accepting an 'invitation' to take part in language-learning exercises and not resisting continued participation) and (2) where there is no other known means to help them (therapeutic veterinary research). As I have argued elsewhere, the cognitive, emotional and social complexity of great apes suggests that they are 'borderline persons' who deserve protections comparable with those afforded to humans of uncertain personhood (DeGrazia, 2005). (The same is true for dolphins. But as it appears impossible to meet their basic needs while they are held captive, I reject any research on dolphins that maintains them in captivity longer than necessary to benefit the dolphin subjects themselves.)
6. *Toxicity testing on live animals should be banned.* We have made much progress in developing alternatives to animal testing. With a massive public investment in alternatives, progress should accelerate. Although some representatives of business may chafe at this suggested ban, their priority – maximizing profits – is less important than minimizing harm to beings with moral status.
7. *Public funding for animal research that aims at original scientific knowledge, both basic and applied, should be reduced to some relatively small fraction – say, 10% – of current levels.* That seems a reasonable compromise between EC views, which would justify little animal research, and UC views, which would preserve considerably more of the status quo. This requirement would strongly encourage consideration of alternatives and greatly reduce harm to animal subjects while protecting the very best, most important animal research. The money saved here could more than pay for the massive increase in public funding for alternatives research recommended above.

REFERENCES

DeGrazia D. *Taking Animals Seriously: Mental Life and Moral Status*. Cambridge: Cambridge University Press, 1996.

DeGrazia D. On the question of personhood beyond *Homo sapiens*. In: Singer P, ed. *In Defense of Animals*, 2nd edition. Oxford: Blackwell, 2005; pp. 40–53.

Harlow H, Zimmerman R. Affectional responses in the infant monkey. *Science* 1959; **130**: 421–432.

LaFollette H, Shanks N. *Brute Science*. London: Routledge, 1996.

McMahan J. *The Ethics of Killing*. Oxford: Oxford University Press, 2002.

NCB. *The Ethics of Research Involving Animals*, London: 2005.

Orlans B. History and ethical regulation of animal experimentation: an international perspective. In: Kuhse H, Singer P, eds. *A Companion to Bioethics*. Oxford: Blackwell, 1998; pp. 399–410.

Pluhar E. *Beyond Prejudice*. Durham, NC: Duke University Press, 1995.

Rachels J. Drawing lines. In: Sunstein C, Nussbaum M, eds. *Animal Rights*. Oxford: Oxford University Press, 2004; pp. 162–74.

Regan T. *The Case for Animal Rights*. Berkeley CA: University of California Press, 1983.

Russel W, Burch R. *The Principles of Humane Experimental Technique*. London: Methuen, 1959.

Singer P. *Animal Liberation*, 2nd edition. New York: New York Review, 1990.

Stephens M, Goldberg A, Rowan A. The first forty years of the alternatives approach. In: Salem D, Rowan A, eds. *The State of the Animals 2001*. Washington, DC: Humane Society Press, 2001; pp. 121–135.

Wade N. Animal rights: NIH cat sex study brings grief to New York museum. *Science* 1976; **194**: 162–167.

Warren MA. *Moral Status*. Oxford: Oxford University Press, 1997.

The Ethical Requirement for Systematic Reviews for Randomized Trials

MIKE CLARKE

Systematic reviews of the effects of health care interventions are now common, but many more are needed, especially in the context of new randomized trials. There are more than 3000 full Cochrane reviews in *The Cochrane Library*, alongside published protocols for 1600 more. Thousands of systematic reviews have also been published in other journals. However, randomized trials are much more common than this. Hundreds of thousands have been conducted over the last few decades, having recruited many millions of participants. Unfortunately, it is likely that most of these trials will not have been designed in the light of a systematic review of the existing evidence and most will not have been reported in the context of the totality of the relevant, related evidence; ideally in the form of an updated systematic review incorporating the new trial. In this chapter, I will argue that not only is this situation unfortunate, it is unethical and bad science. Systematic reviews should be regarded as primary research, done before a trial, to help design and justify it; and as primary findings, done after the new trial, to provide an updated, overall summary of the best available evidence. This applies not only to randomized trials but also to other types of research. Studies of all designs can be systematically reviewed.

INTRODUCTION

When making choices between health care interventions, we should all want to be able to turn to high quality research for reliable estimates of their relative effects on outcomes of relevance to us. How we use these findings in making our decision will depend on many factors that may not have been considered in the research, but an important starting point must be whether one intervention is more beneficial or less harmful, or both are similar. Researchers have a scientific and ethical responsibility to ensure that, as far as possible, the findings from their research are reliable enough to help people in making these decisions. In order to do so, they need to minimize the effects of systematic biases and chance.

In an individual randomized trial, biases are tackled through the appropriate choice of the comparison groups in the trial, by applying a robust and secure method of treatment allocation to ensure that the only differences between participants in the intervention groups arise from the interventions under study, or chance, and by ensuring high quality in other relevant aspects of the conduct of the trial. Chance is minimized through recruiting a sufficiently large number of participants. However, chance is still likely to affect every trial in such a way that it over- or under estimates the true differences between the interventions. In such circumstances, there is a danger that bias will be introduced after the trial, through undue emphasis on the single trial because of its results. Systematic reviews help to overcome these problems by bringing together as much of the relevant evidence as possible, appraising and summarizing it. This chapter discusses the practice and science of systematic reviews to show how these are relevant to randomized trials, and describes why systematic reviews should be regarded as an ethical necessity for the design, reporting and interpretation of these trials.

THE SCIENCE AND PRACTICE OF SYSTEMATIC REVIEWS

Systematic reviews and the statistical averaging – or meta-analysis – of the results of trials are not a new feature in

---

Principles of Health Care Ethics, Second Edition   Edited by R.E. Ashcroft, A. Dawson, H. Draper and J.R. McMillan
© 2007 John Wiley & Sons, Ltd

health research. Examples exist from the beginning of the twentieth century (Chalmers, Hedges and Cooper, 2002). Before then, Lord Rayleigh, at the meeting of the British Association for the Advancement of Science in Montreal in 1884, had described a process of systematic reviewing for scientific research in general:

'If, as is sometimes supposed, science consisted in nothing but the laborious accumulation of facts, it would soon come to a standstill, crushed, as it were, under its own weight.

The suggestion of a new idea, or the detection of a law, supersedes much that has previously been a burden on the memory, and by introducing order and coherence facilitates the retention of the remainder in an available form. Two processes are thus at work side by side, the reception of new material and the digestion and assimilation of the old. One remark, however, should be made. The work which deserves, but I am afraid does not always receive, the most credit is that in which discovery and explanation go hand in hand, in which not only are new facts presented, but their relation to old ones is pointed out' (Lord Rayleigh, 1885).

However, it is only in the last couple of decades that systematic reviews have become a common form of research in health care. Several factors have been responsible for this, and many are interconnected: the desire for evidence-based health care in which the results of research are combined with other knowledge, including values and preferences, to inform decision-making; the overwhelming amount of health information available; and the growth in organizations preparing systematic reviews. These include individual Health Technology Assessment agencies in many countries and, since the early 1990s, The Cochrane Collaboration, which is the world's largest organization dedicated to preparing, maintaining and promoting the accessibility of systematic reviews of the effects of health care interventions (http://www.cochrane.org/).

The Cochrane Collaboration was established in 1993 and includes more than 14 000 active members in nearly 100 countries. These people come from a wide range of health care disciplines but are not restricted to health care professionals or academic researchers. Patients, carers and policymakers are all involved as well. Cochrane systematic reviews are published in full in the *Cochrane Database of Systematic Reviews* (*CDSR*), as part of *The Cochrane Library*. This is available on the internet (www.thecochranelibrary.com) and CD-ROM. In 1995, *CDSR* contained 36 full Cochrane reviews, rising through 500 in 1999, to 1000 in 2001, and 2000 in April 2004. As of mid-2007, more than 3000 full Cochrane reviews have been published. Published protocols are also available for 1600 Cochrane reviews that have not yet brought together the information from eligible studies. Hundreds of newly completed reviews and protocols appear each year, and a

couple of hundred existing reviews are updated so substantively that they can be considered to be the equivalent of new reviews. Hundreds more are brought up-to-date annually, with the addition of new information. Thousands of other systematic reviews have also been published elsewhere during the last 20 years and structured abstracts for many of these available in the Database of Abstracts of Reviews of Effects (www.york.ac.uk/inst/crd/darefaq.htm). Several of these reviews are likely to cover the same topics, and the accumulated evidence in some will be out-of-date.

However, despite this considerable number of systematic reviews, the majority of randomized trials of health care interventions conducted over the last half century and more are not yet the subject of any systematic review. This probably represents millions of participants and billions of dollars of research funding. For example, the *Cochrane Central Register of Controlled Trials* (*CENTRAL*), the most comprehensive source of reports of randomized trials, contains more than 450 000 records (http://www.thecochranelibrary.com/) (Dickersin et al., 2002) and only a minority of these have been included in systematic reviews. At the start of 2001, when there were approximately 300 000 records in *CENTRAL* and 1 000 Cochrane reviews, it was estimated that at least 10 000 separate systematic reviews would be needed to cover all of the existing research which might be relevant to people making decisions about health care (Mallett and Clarke, 2003)

As with all scientific research, a key step in preparing a systematic review is deciding on its objective and scope. This process of question formulation also needs to be followed when a new trial is designed. The similarity of this process and the potential benefits of using a systematic review to help refine the question for a new trial are the arguments made in this chapter for the conduct of systematic reviews before all new trials. When the question for a review has been determined, the reviewer then decides on the most appropriate types of study to tackle this and tries to identify, appraise and include as much of the relevant research as possible. Whatever topic is chosen for the review, the researchers are likely to be faced with a vast amount of information, not just in journals, books and conference proceedings but increasingly on the internet. Although tackling this may seem daunting, the same task would be faced by any person wishing to make a health care decision in the light of the totality of the relevant evidence, if a systematic review is not available to her.

When the researchers have identified studies for possible inclusion in their systematic review, they appraise these studies. They need to satisfy themselves that the studies are of the correct design and included the relevant interventions, participants and outcome measures, so that they are eligible for the review. The reviewers might also wish to determine that the studies were good enough to be included in their attempt to provide a reliable answer to the question they have posed. On the contrary, if the objective for the systematic review is to describe all existing research on a particular topic (so as, for example, to learn from successes and failures of the past when designing a new study), the reviewers might actively seek studies across a broad spectrum of quality.

Having chosen the studies to be included, the reviewers might wish to decide if these trials are similar enough for their results to be combined in a meta-analysis in order to produce an average estimate of the relative effects of the treatments. As with any numerical average, if the items being combined to generate it are too different, this average will be meaningless, and it needs careful consideration by the people doing the review. This may be especially important when researchers are deciding whether to combine the results of their new trial with other trials in an updated meta-analysis. However, an advantage of basing this decision within a transparent systematic review process is that readers who disagree with the researchers' decision about doing, or not doing, a meta-analysis, should have sufficient information available to them to investigate the alternative approach, should they so wish.

ETHICS, RANDOMIZED TRIALS AND SYSTEMATIC REVIEWS

A fundamental ethical and scientific responsibility for all researchers is to do the best possible research. Systematic reviews can help to meet this responsibility through all steps in the conduct of a randomized trial; from conception and design, through recruitment and follow-up, to reporting and interpretation. As such, a systematic review should be regarded as an ethical requirement for new research. It should underpin the rationale for the trial and provide the justification for the randomized comparison of the interventions to be assessed. This justification relates to ensuring both that the question posed in the trial is appropriate (and has not already been answered) and that the trial is built upon the experiences of previous researchers.

The ethical and scientific responsibility for doing the best possible research does not end with the analysis of the trial. The researchers need to ensure that their results are placed in appropriate context. People making decisions about health care on behalf of others also have a responsibility to ensure that these decisions are informed by the best available evidence. Systematic reviews are necessary when considering the totality of the relevant research on a particular topic. If included in the report of a randomized trial, they make this information readily available to the reader of the report.

SYSTEMATIC REVIEWS IN THE DESIGN OF RANDOMIZED TRIALS

Embarking on a new study, without first systematically reviewing what has been done before, not only runs the risk of doing research for which the answer is already known, but it also means that the researchers have denied themselves the opportunity to learn from the successes and failures of others when designing their own study. Researchers have a responsibility to the participants in their research that it will be of the most appropriate design possible. To help make sure that this is the case, they should have ensured that they were adequately informed about what research had been done previously when they design their new study (Clarke, 2004).

A systematic review of the existing research might reveal that the question to be posed in the new trial has already been answered satisfactorily and that the new trial would be unnecessary and unethical because of this. At least two examples of where systematic reviews of the existing evidence might have prevented unnecessary research or, at least, led to properly informed decisions about its legitimacy have been published. The first of these looked at trials comparing prophylactic antibiotics to placebo or no such treatment in colon surgery, up to 1980. It showed that the benefits of antibiotics would have been clear before several of the trials began, if systematic reviews had been done as part of their design (Baum et al., 1981). A similar point was made a quarter of a century later in regard to aprotinin in cardiac surgery (Fergusson et al., 2005).

Even if a systematic review of the existing evidence does not reveal that the question to be posed in the new trial has already been answered, it may reveal that modifications of the trial design might lead to a better, and hence more ethical, piece of research. A systematic review might help to refine the eligibility criteria for participants in the trials, to modify the interventions to be compared, or to recalculate the sample size that will be needed for the trial to succeed. As an example, the Early Breast Cancer Trialists' Collaborative Group overview, which has produced meta-analyses of individual patient data from randomized trials of treatments for breast cancer on five-year cycles since the mid-1980s, has greatly influenced not only routine practice in cancer but also the design of new research. This influence has arisen from the robustness of these systematic reviews and the engagement of breast cancer researchers in the overview process, and has led to modifications in ongoing trials and the design of many new ones (Clarke, 2003).

A systematic review of existing evidence which does not produce definitive answers on the effects of interventions being considered for a new trial would still make a valuable contribution to its design. The systematic review might confirm the need for the new trial by proving that the necessary evidence is lacking (Alderson and Roberts, 2000). It might also reveal ways in which earlier research was done which should be copied or avoided in the new trial. This might relate to strategies for recruiting participants (Mapstone, Elbourne and Roberts, 2002), or greater clarity on the outcome measures to collect, in particular if standardization of these measures would improve the applicability of the trial's findings (Woodworth et al., 2002).

Thus, researchers who wish to meet their ethical duty to do the best possible research need to conduct a systematic review before embarking upon it. They need to do this to ensure that their trial is relevant and appropriate. They also need to do it to ensure that the people they will try to recruit to their trial are given adequate, up-to-date information about the interventions to be investigated and are protected from participation in research that might be unnecessary or potentially harmful (Evans, Thornton and Chalmers, 2006).

SYSTEMATIC REVIEWS IN THE REPORTING OF RANDOMIZED TRIALS

If the researchers did a systematic review before their trial, the task of placing its findings in context at its conclusion would be made much easier. They would need to update their original review to take account of other research that had taken place at the same time as their trial and add the findings of their own trial. In this way, they would minimize the dangers for readers who might otherwise find themselves reliant on the out-of-context results of a single study in a high-profile journal. If this is all that readers have access to, they are likely to find only those trials whose findings are the most striking or atypical and miss similar research that was less fortunate with its results. It must be remembered that however good the conduct of a piece of research, chance effects will mean that some studies will produce an overestimate and some an underestimate of the true effects, but the easy to find literature is likely to be dominated by the former (Counsell et al., 1994). Furthermore, using a sample, rather than the whole body of relevant research will have less statistical and evidential power to answer the question of interest to the user. Even if the reader is able to access much more of the health care literature than the highest profile journals, the sheer size of this task is likely to overwhelm her. There are tens of thousands of health care journals, publishing millions of articles each year; and over the last few decades, hundreds of thousands of randomized trials have been reported, mostly in isolation.

If researchers discussed their findings in the light of previous, relevant research, many of the problems of information overload would be eased. One would only need to find the most recent report of a relevant study and its discussion section would place that study within the context of an updated systematic review. This was suggested by the original CONSORT statement on the reporting of randomized trials (Begg et al., 1996). However, studies of five well-known general medical journals – *Annals of Internal Medicine, BMJ, Lancet, JAMA* and the *New England Journal of Medicine* in 1997 and 2001 revealed that this was not the case, at least for these journals. Only two of the more than 50 reports of randomized trials reported in these journals in May, in these two years, included an updated systematic review in their Discussion section (Clarke, Alderson and Chalmers, 2002).

CONCLUSION

Systematic reviews should be regarded as an ethical requirement for the design of new trials and the foundation for the scientific rationale for ensuring that the trial is of the highest possible quality. In this context, systematic reviews are the true 'primary research'. They need to be done, first, before the trial. They should also be regarded as 'primary research' in the context of reporting the findings of a new trial because it is only by placing the results of the trial in the context of an updated overall summary of the best available evidence that readers are provided with the evidence they need to make well-informed decisions. This applies not only to randomized trials but also to other types of research because the systematic review process is suitable for studies of all designs.

It is now much easier for researchers to prepare or access a systematic review of the effects of health care interventions than it was even 10 years ago. They are able to benefit from the greater ease of finding reports of randomized trials, for example within the *Cochrane Central Register of Controlled Trials* (Dickersin et al., 2002), and might even be able to draw on a systematic review done by someone else, given the tremendous increase in the number of these.

This chapter has argued that by not doing a systematic review before embarking on their trial and by failing to report their new results in the context of an updated systematic review, researchers are failing both ethically and scientifically to conduct the best possible research. They are also likely to fail to achieve the ultimate aim for their trial, which should be to do good research to generate reliable evidence that will support better health care and lead to improved health.

REFERENCES

Alderson P, Roberts I. Should journals publish systematic reviews that find no evidence to guide practice? Examples from injury research. *BMJ* 2000; **320**: 376–377.

Baum ML, Anish DS, Chalmers TC, Sacks HS, Smith H Jr, Fagerstrom RM. A survey of clinical trials of antibiotic prophylaxis in colon surgery: evidence against further use of no-treatment controls. *N Engl J Med* 1981; **305**: 795–799.

Begg C, Cho M, Eastwood S, Horton R, Moher D, Olkin I, et al. Improving the quality of reporting of randomized controlled trials. The CONSORT statement. *JAMA* 1996; **276**: 637–639.

Chalmers I, Hedges LV, Cooper H. A brief history of research synthesis. *Eval Health Prof* 2002; **25**: 12–37.

Clarke M. The Early Breast Cancer Trialists' Collaborative Group: systematic reviews of treatments for women with breast cancer. In: Perry MC, ed. *American Society of Clinical Oncology Educational Book*. 39th Annual Meeting of the American Society of Clinical Oncology; 31 May–3 June, 2003; Chicago (IL). Alexandria (VA): American Society of Clinical Oncology, 2003; pp. 751–758.

Clarke M. Doing new research? Don't forget the old: nobody should do a trial without reviewing what is known. PLoS Med 2004; **1**: 100–102.

Clarke M, Alderson P, Chalmers I. Discussion sections in reports of controlled trials published in general medical journals. *JAMA* 2002; **287**: 2799–2801.

Counsell CE, Clarke MJ, Slattery J, Sandercock PAG. The miracle of DICE therapy for acute stroke: fact or fictional product of subgroup analysis? *BMJ* 1994; **309**: 1677–1681.

Dickersin K, Manheimer E, Wieland S, Robinson KA, Lefebvre C, McDonald S. Development of the Cochrane Collaboration's CENTRAL Register of controlled clinical trials. *Eval Health Prof* 2002; **25**: 38–64.

Evans I, Thornton H, Chalmers I. *Testing Treatments: Better Research For Better Healthcare*. London: British Library, 2006.

Fergusson D, Glass KC, Hutton B, Shapiro S. Randomized controlled trials of aprotinin in cardiac surgery: could clinical equipoise have stopped the bleeding? *Clin. Trials* 2005; **2**: 218–229.

Mallett S, Clarke M. How many Cochrane reviews are needed to cover existing evidence on the effects of healthcare interventions? *Evid Based Med* 2003; **8**: 100–101.

Mapstone J, Elbourne D, Roberts I. Strategies to improve recruitment to research studies. *The Cochrane Database of Methodology Reviews* 2002, **Issue 3**.

Lord Rayleigh. Address by the Rt. Hon. Lord Rayleigh. In: *Report of the 54th Meeting of the British Association for the Advancement of Science*, August–September 1884, Montreal, Canada. London: John Murray, 1885; pp. 3–23.

Woodworth TG, Furst DE, Strand V, Kempeni J, Fenner H, Lau CS, Miller F, Day R, Lipani J, Brooks P. Standardizing assessment of adverse effects in rheumatology clinical trials. Status of OMERACT Toxicity Working Group March 2000: towards a common understanding of comparative toxicity/safety profiles for antirheumatic therapies. *J Rheumatol* 2001; **28**: 1163–1169.

Informed Consent for Research

JAMES FLORY, DAVID WENDLER AND EZEKIEL EMANUEL

INTRODUCTION

In theory and practice, informed consent is considered a requirement of ethical clinical research. Since the late nineteenth century it has been a recognized ethical goal that people not only decide freely whether to participate in clinical research, but decide with an understanding of the relevant facts. This requirement helps to protect the autonomy of research participants and avert serious research abuses.

This simple doctrine – that consent should be not just voluntary but informed – has proved difficult to realize in practice. The data show that research participants can have significant misconceptions about the nature of research even when researchers diligently follow consent procedures required by regulation. Truly informing research participants is very hard, and therefore the goal of truly informed consent poses serious challenges in policy and ethics. To help to address these challenges, we consider three relevant empirical questions: How well do participants understand their research participation? Is there any way to predict who will have the most trouble in understanding? And which interventions might improve participants' understanding? We will start with the first of these questions.

UNDERSTANDING THE PURPOSE OF RESEARCH

Empirical data on research participants' understanding of the study purpose is typical of the data on participants' understanding in general. These data suggest that participants' understanding varies considerably from study to study but in general is relatively poor. At the encouraging end, a study of parents enrolling their children in a trial of malaria drugs in Uganda found that 80% of the parents knew that the study purpose was 'determining which malaria drugs are most effective for children' (Pace et al., 2005). In a rather different setting, a survey of people enrolled in oncology research in Boston found that 75% of participants agreed with the statement that 'the main reason cancer clinical trials are done is to improve the treatment of future cancer patients' (Joffe et al., 2001). But much of the data reflects poorer understanding. A study that focused on phase I oncology research participants in Chicago found that only 27% could correctly describe the purpose of the research as dose finding/toxicity determination (Daugherty et al., 2000). In rural Bangladesh, half of the women in a study of iron supplements thought that participation in research was part of routine health care (Lynoe et al., 2001).

These numbers, and similar data from other studies, provide a glimpse at the state of understanding in research studies across the world. Generalizing from data like this must be done cautiously, but we can at least note that the percentage of participants who seem to understand the purpose of the studies in which they participate varies a great deal from study to study. It is rare for all participants to understand a study's purpose, and common for fewer than 75% to understand it. In addition, there is no consistent evidence that people from poor nations understand less than those from affluent countries (Pace et al., 2005).

But the data are more difficult to interpret than they appear at first. In most of the examples given above, there is a more complicated story to tell. In the Uganda study, most parents knew that the study was meant to answer a scientific question about which malaria drugs are most effective for children (Pace et al., 2005). But in contrast to the high rate of correct responses to the purpose question, only 19% of these parents realized that different children in the study were being assigned to different treatments. Did these parents understand that the design of the study meant doctors would be unable to make treatment decisions based on what was deemed best for the child?

Principles of Health Care Ethics, Second Edition   Edited by R.E. Ashcroft, A. Dawson, H. Draper and J.R. McMillan
© 2007 John Wiley & Sons, Ltd

The Boston oncology study addressed this point more directly, asking whether participants agreed that the study was designed primarily to benefit future patients (Joffe et al., 2001). The statement that a study is designed primarily to benefit future patients is a truism of research ethics, and one's first reaction is concern about the 25% of participants who did not agree with it. Yet that 25% were in good company: only a minority of health care providers (46%) agreed with this statement when they were given the same survey. Were providers more poorly informed than the participants they recruited? A more likely explanation is that in much of oncology research, the care participants receive on-protocol is arguably better than they would receive off-protocol, and it is reasonable to think of the protocol as partly or even primarily intended to benefit its own participants. How is one to be sure that the remaining 25% of participants were really ill informed about the study's purpose?

In the study of phase I oncology research participants, researchers asked a more specific question about the scientific question addressed by the study (Daugherty et al., 2000). Only a third of participants correctly identified dose finding and toxicity as the purpose of this protocol; 61% of participants believed that the purpose of the study was to evaluate the efficacy of the cancer drug. How far wrong were these participants, and did their confusion make their consent invalid? In the same study, nearly 90% of participants realized that they were in research. Is this good news, or should we focus on the bad news that most of them failed to make a further distinction between screening for safety and screening for efficacy?

The point of these examples is that the purpose of a research study is a surprisingly complex article of information. One can understand it at different levels, from the simple appreciation that a study is meant to create scientific knowledge to more detailed knowledge of the type of knowledge in question and the specific scientific issues involved.

In fact, to discuss study purpose clearly, one has to step back to consider the ambiguous relationship between investigators and research participants. One influential idea in bioethics is that research participants often suffer from the 'therapeutic misconception', defined as conflation of the goals and principles of clinical research with those of clinical care (Appelbaum, 2004). It is generally assumed that this conflation is bad because it leads research participants to think that research studies are meant to benefit them in the same way that clinical care does. Although this is an entirely reasonable concern, it can also lead us to lose sight of the fact that many studies have a dual effect, both generating scientific information and providing superior care for participants. This is especially true in settings where individuals have access to little or no standard medical care.

Many questions about study purpose assume that participants should recognize that the researchers' purpose is to create generalizable knowledge and that anyone who fails to answer in this way fails to understand. But the fact that researchers' purpose is to create generalizable knowledge does not exclude the possibility that they also intend to benefit those who enrol in the research. Investigators at some sites may participate in the research with the primary purpose of helping their own patients. And, of course, many individuals enrol in research with the explicit purpose of receiving treatment. Therefore, questions about intentions and purpose can have more than one right answer.

Moreover, it is not always clear that understanding of the purpose of the research is necessary for a valid informed consent – at least, not for every study. Imagine participants who enrol in a phase II treatment study of a new medication for a disease without any currently effective treatment. How important is it for participants to recognize that the purpose of the study is not to treat them *per se*, but to create generalizable knowledge on the efficacy of treating groups of patients (Sreenivasan, 2003)?

UNDERSTANDING VOLUNTARINESS

Where study purpose is a complex topic, relating to deep questions about the differences between patients and research subjects, voluntariness stands out at first as simple. The topic has its complexities, but there is no fundamental ambiguity: participants should be free to refuse research participation and to withdraw from research without pressure or coercion. This right to withdraw should be understood by 100% of participants. Against such simplicity, it is striking how many people do not fully appreciate that their participation in research is voluntary. In general, studies have shown that most but by no means all participants were aware that they did not have to join a study and that they had the right to withdraw from it. In some cases, however, the percentage of participants aware of these rights was below 50% (Lynoe, 2001).

Studies which delved deeper into the right to withdraw revealed that in many cases, participants' understanding is worse than it appears at first. In one case, 65% of parents knew they had the right to withdraw their children from research, but only 17% knew they could exercise that right at any time. Essentially, they thought that they had the right to withdraw as long as investigators said that they could (Pace et al., 2005). In another case, 91% of parents knew that they had the right to withdraw their children from research, but 25% of them still felt obliged to continue their participation (Van Stuijvenberg et al., 1998). In a third case, while 93% of participants thought they were free to quit a perinatal HIV transmission study, only 2% believed that the hospital would allow them to quit. In addition, 32% felt their care would be compromised if they did not participate

(Abdool Karim et al., 1998). In each of these cases, the initial impression that participants understood their rights is complicated by aspects of the responses which suggest that participants' participation may be less free than when they first appeared.

It is difficult to know for certain what these participants were thinking, but several possibilities present themselves. A relatively benign possibility is that participants were quite aware of the right to withdraw, yet felt they had to continue to participate because of external factors, as opposed to pressure from researchers. For example, they might feel that the study was the best or the only way for them to get needed medical care (Pace et al., 2005). This possibility does not imply poor informed consent, coercion or inappropriate pressure from researchers.

A second possibility is that participants thought the right-to-withdraw language was an empty promise. This is illustrated by those who thought they were free to quit at any time as long as investigators gave permission. A variation is shown by those who thought they were free to quit but that there would be adverse consequences to their medical care. This reveals confusion about the nature of the right to withdraw that has a parallel in everyday life. I have the right to say unflattering things about my boss; even so, there will be some unpleasant consequences if I exercise this right. Without specific information to the contrary, research participants may assume that the right to withdraw does not protect them from negative consequences if they exercise this right.

Thus, it turns out that voluntariness is in its own way a complicated concept. There are different degrees of freedom. Research participants should have the highest degree of freedom, namely, the ability to refuse or quit a study whenever they want, with the knowledge that doing so will not compromise their routine medical care. Accordingly, investigators need to offer this freedom and should take care to communicate it fully. Investigators and regulators should also be careful not to mistake participants who feel obliged to participate by external circumstances, like the severity of their illness or limited options, for participants who feel that they are being coerced or inappropriately pressured by researchers. The fact that individuals feel compelled to enrol in research due to the severity of their illness, and the absence of alternative treatments, does not necessarily undermine the validity of their informed consent, any more than patients' experiencing respiratory distress undermines the validity of their consent to intubation (Wertheimer, 1987; Hawkins and Emanuel, 2005). The data do not always clearly distinguish pressure from one's illness from more ethically worrisome pressure, especially pressure from the research investigators.

UNDERSTANDING PROTOCOL DESIGN AND RANDOMIZATION

Research on how well participants understand protocol design almost invariably focuses on randomization and placebo control. Although there are exceptions, the majority of studies show that fewer than half of participants understand these issues. There is far less evidence on how well participants understand prosaic but important details like whether a study drug is oral or injected, or the length and frequency of clinic visits they need to make as part of their participation. The limited available data suggest that investigators may do a good job communicating this information, yet fail to get the concept of randomization across to participants.

The malaria study in Uganda offers a detailed example of this point (Pace et al., 2005). Of those participating, 78% knew that they would have to make seven visits to the clinic in the course of the study, 79% knew their children would be taking drugs orally, and 98% knew that the study involved blood samples. Only 19% knew that children were being assigned to different treatments, and only 7% went further to understand that assignment would be random.

What is one to make of such a striking shift, from the majority of patients understanding practical details of the protocol to a tiny minority understanding randomization? There are several possible explanations. First, randomization may simply be a hard concept to understand. Few studies assess whether most people fail to grasp randomization due to the therapeutic misconception, as opposed to simple confusion about a complicated concept. Another possibility might be that participants must understand practical details in order to comply with the protocol, so investigators and participants find it easier to focus on them. Finally, investigators might gloss over the subject of randomization. Against this possibility, one study in which consent procedures were videotaped and compared against participants' later understanding found that understanding of randomization continued to be poor even when investigators devoted significant time to explaining it (Kodish et al., 2004).

UNDERSTANDING OF RISKS AND BENEFITS

The literature approaches understanding of risks and benefits in two ways. The broad approach asks research participants how much they expect to benefit from or be harmed by their study participation. Here, the literature suggests that research participants tend to be quite optimistic, possibly unreasonably so, about their potential to benefit from research participation. The narrow approach assesses how well participants remember specific details about the risks and benefits of their trial. The data here show that participants have difficulty absorbing and retaining lists of potential adverse events, but occasionally they have good retention of particular facts (Penman et al., 1984; Miller et al., 1994).

There are several examples of what seems to be excessive optimism. In one survey, 43% of patients stated that they had no doubts at all about benefits from a treatment, even though most of their consent forms stated that no benefit could be assured (Penman et al., 1984). A study specifically designed to identify the prevalence of unreasonable optimism reported that 51% of the participants expressed an unreasonable belief in the likelihood of benefit (Appelbaum, 2004). It seems reasonable to expect that many research participants will tend to overestimate the likelihood that they will benefit. In spite of these results, it is hard to determine whether this is a widespread problem or not. At least in oncology, it is clear that some participants can be realistic. In one example, only 22% of participants thought they would receive benefit in a phase I trial (Daugherty et al., 1995). The rest of the participants appeared to have faced up to a difficult reality. It is hard to be sure whether understanding was a problem among the 22% who thought they would benefit. A key issue in the communication of risk and benefit is the difficulty of distinguishing a patient who is mistaken about the prospect of benefit from one who is simply hopeful, and prefers to make positive statements about the future (Horng and Grady, 2003). Confusion implies inadequate informed consent; hope does not.

Given this ambiguity about the meaning of broad expressions of optimism or pessimism, the narrow approach of seeing how many facts about risks and benefits participants are able to absorb has obvious appeal. Studies taking this approach make it clear that retaining long lists of possible adverse events is difficult for participants (Bergler et al., 1980; Penman et al., 1984; Miller et al., 1994; Daugherty et al., 1995). In one oncology study, only a minority of participants were able to remember three side effects within 1–3 weeks of receiving that information. Although most participants were aware of the risk of vomiting or nausea, only 20–30% were aware of more abstract risks, like lowered white cell counts (Penman et al., 1984). In another study looking at retention of information for up to 60 days after informed consent, only about half of participants could recall even one of the 12 side effects. In a study looking at recall of two side effects from heart failure drugs, only 28% of participants could name both side effects shortly after the study was explained to them, although an additional 44% could name one (Bergler et al., 1980).

These data raise a question as to whether it is reasonable to expect research participants to benefit from long lists of potential adverse events, when it is clearly difficult to remember more than a few side effects. A telling example from the literature is a study of hospital employees who were asked to consider joining a sham protocol in which they would take an experimental drug. Employees were randomized to one of the three consent forms for this trial. Each consent form described the side effect profile of the sham experimental drug in a different level of detail, and in each case the profile was an accurate description of the potential side effects of aspirin. Employees who were given the most detailed description grossly overestimated the risk of taking the drug; those given the brief description formed a much more accurate conception of the drug's risk even though they had less raw information to work with (Epstein and Lasagna, 1969).

These data suggest investigators should be careful about encouraging too much optimism in research participants. They also indicate that expecting participants to recall a laundry list of risks is unrealistic, and they cast doubt on the utility of loading consent forms with long lists of side effects.

THE EFFECT OF DEMOGRAPHICS ON UNDERSTANDING

Several demographic factors have been shown to be associated with better understanding in informed consent. The literature offers strong evidence that better education is associated with better understanding. A more limited evidence base indicates that advancing age (over 50) and mental illness are risk factors for low understanding. Other basic demographic characteristics, including sex, minority status and income have not been consistently linked with poor understanding. Importantly, there is no evidence that participants from poor countries understand less well than participants from industrialized nations.

At least 14 studies have shown that higher education and reading levels are significantly associated with increased overall understanding scores. Frequently these differences are striking. In a study of parents who were considering paediatric leukaemia trials for their children, 7% of parents with less than a high school education understood randomization, whereas 78% of parents who were college graduates understood it ($p < .001$) (Kodish et al., 2004). Another study of advanced cancer patients enrolling in phase I trials found that 69% of college graduates correctly stated the purpose of phase I trials as a determination of dose toxicity, while only 26% of non-college graduates were right about this ($p = .002$) (Daugherty et al., 1995). The relationship between education and understanding is robust across many settings and studies, and it is strong enough to be of major practical significance.

Increased age was associated with significantly lower understanding in five studies that enrolled participants with mean age older than 50 years (all $p < .05$) (Taub, 1980; Taub et al., 1986; 1987; Aaronson et al., 1996; Coyne et al., 2003). However, two other studies have reported no association between understanding and age (Kucia and Horowitz,

2000; Dunn et al., 2002). In addition, mental illness, particularly schizophrenia, has been associated with lower understanding in four studies that compared mentally ill research participants with healthy or medically ill volunteers (all $p < .05$) (Benson et al., 1988; Carpenter et al., 2000; Stiles et al., 2001; Dunn et al., 2002).

A review article comparing informed consent in research in poor countries to that in affluent democracies found no evidence that participants from the poor countries understood less (Pace, unpublished). In the light of generally lower levels of education in poorer countries, this is a surprising finding. One possibility is that international studies might have more heavily monitored and effective consent processes than is the norm in industrialized countries. It is worth noting that saying understanding in poor countries is as good as it is in developed countries is not the same as saying it is good on an absolute scale.

INTERVENTIONS TO IMPROVE UNDERSTANDING

Helping research participants understand better is a challenge. An extensive and growing literature has tested diverse approaches. At least 42 trials have compared the understanding of research participants who had undergone a standard informed consent process with the understanding of those who had received an intervention to improve their understanding. Unfortunately, no clearly effective solutions have emerged. Here, we briefly outline the available evidence and its implications. For a more detailed argument and justification, we refer to the reader to a review article discussing the same data (Flory and Emanuel, 2004).

Interventions that have been tested can be categorized into five groups: (1) multimedia, including computer-based informed consent; (2) enhanced consent form; (3) extended discussion; (4) test/feedback; and, (5) miscellaneous. Overall, 12 trials tested multimedia interventions, using computer or video technology in place of (Llewellyn-Thomas et al., 1995; Dunn et al., 2002; Agre et al., 2003) or in addition to (Benson et al., 1988; Weston et al., 1997) the usual written informed consent form. A further 15 trials evaluated consent forms with modified content, writing style, format or length (Epstein and Lasagna, 1969; Taub, 1980; Taub et al., 1986; Taub et al., 1987; Young et al., 1990; Davis et al., 1998; Ragers et al., 1998; Bjorn et al., 1999; Murphy et al., 1999; Dresden and Levitt, 2001; Stiles et al., 2001; Coyne et al., 2003; Agre and Rapkin 2003; Agre et al., 2003). Five trials of extended discussion evaluated interventions in which a member of the study team or a neutral educator scheduled additional time to discuss the disclosed information with research participants (Benson et al., 1988; Tindall et al., 1994; Aaronson et al., 1996; Kucia and Horowitz, 2000; Fitzgerald et al., 2002). These interventions ranged from a 30-min telephone conversation with a nurse (Aaronson et al., 1996) to multiple counselling sessions lasting up to 2 h (Fitzgerald et al., 2002). Another five trials evaluated test/feedback interventions, in which research participants were quizzed about the information disclosed to them and were given a review of questions that they answered incorrectly (Taub et al., 1981; Taub and Baker, 1983; Wirshing et al., 1998; Stiles et al., 2001; Coletti et al., 2003). Five trials of miscellaneous interventions were not readily comparable with any of the other interventions that were tested (Rikkert et al., 1997; Carpenter et al., 2000; Stiles et al., 2001; Agre et al., 2003; Coletti et al. 2003). For example, one trial put research participants through a week-long tryout for the procedures in the protocol before asking for consent (Rikkert et al., 1997).

THE EFFECTIVENESS OF INTERVENTIONS

Overall, 12 trials of multimedia interventions revealed that such interventions often failed to improve research participants' understanding (Benson et al., 1988; Llewelly-Thomas et al., 1995; Fureman et al., 1997; Weston et al., 1997; Dunn et al., 2002; Agre & Rapkin, 2003; Agre et al., 2003). One published trial showed a statistically significant improvement in understanding using a computerized presentation of information. The population for this trial was primarily patients with mental illness, with a few healthy volunteers. In addition, two unpublished trials reportedly produced increases in understanding, one from a video presentation and the other from a computerized presentation; but the significance of these results is difficult to assess prior to complete analysis, peer review and publication of the data. None of the other nine trials reported a significant improvement in understanding, although two trials of video interventions that showed no increase in understanding immediately after disclosure did show improved retention of information weeks later.

Of the 15 trials with enhanced consent forms, six studies showed significant gains in understanding while nine did not. Of the six studies that showed significant gains, five evaluated simulated consent processes with no discussion of the information in the consent form; the consent form was the only means used to disclose information to participants. Because in most real consent processes research participants receive some information through discussion, the effect of improvements to the consent form is likely to be larger in such a hypothetical scenario than in a real research context.

Extended discussion between study staff and research participants resulted in statistically significant increases in understanding in three of the five trials. Both the negative trials showed trends towards improved understanding ($p = .054$ and $p = .08$, respectively). Three of the trials in this category have questionable validity due to their small sample sizes and non-randomized designs.

The test/feedback approach, in which participants were evaluated for understanding and then given additional explanation if their understanding was inadequate, had significant impact (all $p < .05$) in all the five trials that evaluated this approach. But each study in this category measured the outcome using the same questionnaire that was used in the test/feedback intervention itself. This is a serious methodological flaw because any improvement in the test score could reflect rote memorization of the answers to questions rather than increases in real understanding.

Among the five miscellaneous interventions, two were combinations of more common approaches. One trial compared a standard consent process with a process enhanced by a combination of extended discussion time, additional written information and simple teaching aids. A second trial used extended discussion time and teaching aids that included computerized presentation. Both the trials simulated a consent process and resulted in significant gains to understanding. A one-week tryout period in which research participants underwent some protocol procedures before deciding whether to give consent was also associated with a significant improvement in understanding. Two other trials did not show a significant increase in understanding.

This review suggests several conclusions and recommendations for policy and future research. First, although multimedia interventions may have the potential to improve understanding, this potential has not been realized in practice. Of the 12 trials, only one published and two unpublished trials of such interventions have documented an improvement in understanding among research participants.

The lack of consistent improvement in understanding due to video and computer technology may seem surprising, partly because previous studies have suggested that multimedia interventions increase patients' understanding in routine medical care. This disparity may result from the fact that in research, the informed consent process is already formalized through federal regulations that require a written consent form. Video-based and computer-based interventions may not add much to this relatively thorough disclosure process. Indeed, in previous studies, when a decision aid was compared with standard medical care, increases in understanding were quite large; but when a more elaborate decision aid was compared with a simple one, increases were small. In the same way, multimedia interventions could be much better than nothing, but not necessarily better than the disclosure processes already common in clinical research.

Second, the data indicate that enhanced consent forms do not typically yield significant increases in understanding. Although enhanced consent forms seemed to have a significant effect in several trials, most of these trials simulated the consent process unrealistically; they included no discussion, only a reading of the form. In such a setting, the form becomes the participant's only source of information and this exaggerates the impact of changes in the form. The one realistic trial that showed an effect suggests that shortening forms by removing unnecessary standardized content appears to improve understanding.

Third, limited evidence suggests that more person-to-person contact, rather than videos or paper forms, may be the best way to improve understanding. Extended one-on-one interaction with another person may offer more opportunity for active engagement and responsiveness to the individual needs of the research participant. This hypothesis would support the idea that informed consent is more than just the action of reading a form and signing it. It is better thought of as a process, ideally a dialogue, that takes place over time and largely depends on interactions between humans.

Fourth, lower educational attainment, mental illness and, perhaps, advanced age are associated with lower understanding. Indeed, the differences in understanding between well-educated and less well-educated individuals outweigh any improvement in understanding from the various interventions. These results may reflect poorer test-taking skills among less educated research participants, causing them to score lower on tests of understanding even when their understanding is actually adequate. It may also indicate that these interventions are still not effective for individuals with less education and that disclosure processes need to be more appropriate for individuals with lower cognitive skills.

CONCLUSION

This chapter synthesizes the empirical literature on informed consent to answer the following questions: How much do research participants understand? Do some participants understand more than others? How can understanding be improved?

The reason for asking these relatively simple questions is to help answer more complicated ethical and policy questions. Were this not primarily an empirical review, we might dwell further on questions like 'Are research participants well enough informed that their participation is ethical?' and 'What should investigators do to improve understanding?' Hopefully the evidence accumulated here will be useful to anyone who wants to explore these questions in greater depth.

These are important questions for anyone involved in research, partly because researchers are as tightly bound by regulations as they are by financial and technical concerns. Research must have a satisfactory consent process for a conscientious Institutional Review Board (IRB) to approve it. But nobody knows for certain what is and is not a satisfactory consent process. There is no evidence on what steps are necessary to achieve a given level of understanding in a given population. There is no way to show whether an IRB's demands are reasonable; there is no way to show whether an investigator's efforts to inform potential participants are adequate. IRBs lack consistent standards to apply, investigators have no reliable tools to achieve informed consent, and it is not clear whether the participants are adequately protected by a system of informed consent that is flying blind.

This situation is dangerous. It retards valuable research and consumes the time of IRB members and investigators in unproductive debates lacking valid answers. Particularly in international research, where everyone struggles with the challenge of communicating information to people from a different culture, this process can be a major logistical barrier. Meanwhile, inadequately informed research participants are less able to protect themselves either from exploitation or from the inherent risks of research.

We propose that participants will be safer and regulatory processes will run more smoothly if informed consent can become an evidence-based discipline. At this point, it is essentially never evidence-based. The information summarized here is still insufficient to design a consent process to achieve any given goal. But we now have testable hypotheses, and we can identify the further research needed to develop a reliable set of ways to help research participants understand. If this research is conducted, we can hope that the demands of IRBs and the capabilities of investigators will become closely matched, and that the volunteers who make research possible will more often be well enough informed to be true partners, rather than passive subjects.

DISCLAIMER

The opinions expressed are the authors' own. They do not reflect any position or policy of the National Institutes of Health, Public Health Service, or Department of Health and Human Services.

REFERENCES

Aaronson NK, Visser-Pol E, Leenhouts GH, et al. Telephone-based nursing intervention improves the effectiveness of the informed consent process in cancer clinical trials. *J Clin Oncol* 1996; **14**: 984–996.

Abdool Karim Q, Abdool Karim S, Coovadia H, Susser M. Informed consent for HIV testing in a South African hospital: Is it truly informed and truly voluntary? *Am J Public Health* 1998; **388**: 637–640.

Agre P, Campbell FA, Goldman BD, *et al.* Improving informed consent: the medium is not the message. *IRB: Ethics Human Res* 2003; **25**(Suppl 5): S11–19.

Agre P, Kurtz RC, Krauss BJ. A randomized trial using videotape to present consent information for colonoscopy. *Gastrointest Endosc* 1994; **40**: 271–276.

Agre P, Rapkin B. Improving informed consent: A comparison of four consent tools. *IRB: Ethics Human Res* 2003; **25**(6): 1–7.

Appelbaum PS, Lidz CW, Grisso T. Therapeutic misconception in clinical research: Frequency and risk factors. *IRB: Ethics Human Res* **2004**; 26(2): 1–8.

Benson PR, Roth LH, Appelbaum PS, Lidz CW, Winslade WJ. Information disclosure, subject understanding, and informed consent in psychiatric research. *Law Human Behav* 1988; **12**: 455–475.

Bergler JH, Pennington AC, Metcalfe M, Freis ED. Informed consent: How much does the patient understand? *Clin Pharmacol Therap* 1980; **27**: 435–440.

Bjorn E, Rossel P, Holm S. Can the written information to research subjects be improved: An empirical study. *J Med Ethics* 1999; **25**: 263–267.

Carpenter WT Jr, Gold JM, Lahti AC, et al. Decisional capacity for informed consent in schizophrenia research. *Arch General Psychiatry* 2000; **57**: 533–538.

Coletti AS, Heagerty P, Sheon AR, et al. Randomized, controlled evaluation of a prototype informed consent process for HIV vaccine efficacy trials. *J Acquir Immune Defic Syndr* 2003; **32**: 161–169.

Coyne CA, Xu R, Raich P, et al. Randomized, controlled trial of an easy-to-read informed consent statement for clinical trial participation: a study of the Eastern Cooperative Oncology Group. *J Clin Oncol* 2003; **21**: 836–842.

Daugherty C, Ratain MJ, Grochowski E, et al. Perceptions of cancer patients and their physicians involved in phase I trials. *J Clin Oncol* 1995; **13**: 1062–72. [Erratum in: *J Clin Oncol* 1995; **13**: 2476.]

Daugherty CK, et al. Quantitative analysis of ethical issues in phase I trials: A survey interview study of 144 advanced cancer patients. *IRB: Ethics Human Res* 2000; **22**(3): 6–14.

Davis TC, Holcombe RF, Berkel HJ, Pramanik S, Divers SG. Informed consent for clinical trials: a comparative study of standard versus simplified forms. *J Natl Cancer Inst* 1998; **90**: 668–674.

Dresden GM, Levitt MA. Modifying a standard industry clinical trial consent form improves patient information retention as part of the informed consent process. *Acad Emerg Med* 2001; **8**: 246–252.

Dunn LB, Lindamer LA, Palmer BW, et al. Improving understanding of research consent in middle-aged and elderly patients with psychotic disorders. *Am J Geriat Psychiatry* 2002; **10**: 142–150.

Epstein LC, Lasagna L. Obtaining informed consent: Form or substance. *Arch Inter Med* 1969; **123**: 682–688.

Fitzgerald DW, Marotte C, Verdier RI, *et al*. Comprehension during informed consent in a less-developed country. *Lancet* 2002; **360**: 1301–1302.

Flory J, Emanuel E. Interventions to improve research participants' understanding in informed consent for research: a systematic review. *JAMA* 2004; **292**(13): 1593–1601.

Fureman I, Meyers K, McLellan AT, Metzger D, Woody G. Evaluation of a video-supplement to informed consent: injection drug users and preventive HIV vaccine efficacy trials. *AIDS Educ Prevent* 1997; **9**: 330–341.

Hawkins JS, Emanuel EJ. Clarifying confusions about coercion. *Hast Center Rep* 2005; **35**(5): 16–19.

Horng S, Grady C. Misunderstanding in clinical research: Distinguishing therapeutic misconception, therapeutic misestimation, and therapeutic optimism. *IRB: Ethics Human Res* 2003; **25**(1): 11–16.

Joffe S, et al. Quality of informed consent in cancer clinical trials: A cross-sectional survey. *Lancet* 2001; **348**: 1772–1777.

Kodish E, Eder M, Noll RB, *et al*. Communication of randomization in childhood leukemia trials. *JAMA* 2004; **291**: 470–475.

Kucia AM, Horowitz JD. Is informed consent to clinical trials an 'upside selective' process in acute coronary syndromes? *Am Heart J* 2000; **140**: 94–97.

Llewellyn-Thomas HA, Thiel EC, Sem FW, Woermke DE. Presenting clinical trial information: A comparison of methods. *Patient Educ Counsel* 1995; **25**: 97–107.

Lynoe N, et al. Obtaining informed consent in Bangladesh. *N Engl J Med* 2001; **344**: 460–461.

Mason V, McEwan A, Walker D, Barrett S, James D. The use of video information in obtaining consent for female sterilization: A randomized study. *BJOG* 2003; **110**: 1062–1071.

Miller C, Searight HR, Grable D, et al. Comprehension and recall of the informational content of the informed consent document: An evaluation of 168 patients in a controlled clinical trial. *J Clin Res Drug Dev* 1994; **8**: 237–248.

Murphy DA, O'Keefe ZH, Kaufman AH. Improving comprehension and recall of information for an HIV vaccine trial among women at risk for HIV: reading level simplification and inclusion of pictures to illustrate key concepts. *AIDS Educ Prev* 1999; **11**: 389–399.

O'Connor AM, Stacey D, Entwistle V, et al. Decision aids for people facing health treatment or screening decisions [Cochrane Review]. In: Cochrane Library, Issue 1. Chichester: John Wiley & Sons, 2004.

Pace C, et al. Unpublished manuscript.

Pace C, et al. Quality of parental consent in a Ugandan malaria study. *Am J Public Health* 2005; **95**: 1184–1189.

Pace C, Emanuel EJ, Chuenyam T, et al. The quality of informed consent in a clinical research study in Thailand. *IRB: Ethics Human Res* 2005; **27**(1): 9–17.

Penman DT, Holland JC, Bahna GF, et al. Informed consent for investigational chemotherapy: Patients' and physicians' perceptions. *J Clin Oncol* 1984; **2**: 849–855.

Rikkert MG, van den Bercken JH, ten Have HA, Hoefnagels WH. Experienced consent in geriatrics research: a new method to optimize the capacity to consent in frail elderly subjects. *J Med Ethics* 1997; **23**: 271–276.

Rogers CG, Tyson JE, Kennedy KA, Broyles RS, Hickman JF. Conventional consent with opting in versus simplified consent with opting out: an exploratory trial for studies that do not increase patient risk. *J Pediatr* 1998; **132**: 606–611.

Sreenivasan G. Does informed consent to research require comprehension? *Lancet* 2003; **362**: 2016–2018.

Stiles PG, Poythress NG, Hall A, Falkenbach D, Williams R. Improving understanding of research consent disclosures among persons with mental illness. *Psychiatr Serv* 2001; **52**: 780–785.

Taub HA. Informed consent, memory and age. *Gerontologist* 1980; **20**: 686–690.

Taub HA, Baker MT. The effect of repeated testing upon comprehension of informed consent materials by elderly volunteers. *Exp Aging Res* 1983; **9**: 135–138.

Taub HA, Baker MT, Kline GE, Sturr JF. Comprehension of informed consent information by young-old through old-old volunteers. *Exp Aging Res* 1987; **13**: 173–178.

Taub HA, Baker MT, Sturr JF. Informed consent for research: Effects of readability, patient age, and education. *J Am Geriat Soc* 1986; **34**: 601–606.

Taub HA, Kline GE, Baker MT. The elderly and informed consent: effects of vocabulary level and corrected feedback. *Exp Aging Res* 1981; **7**: 137–146.

Tindall B, Forde S, Ross MW, et al. Effects of two formats of informed consent on knowledge amongst persons with advanced HIV disease in a clinical trial of didanosine. *Patient Educ Couns* 1994; **24**: 261–266.

van Stuijvenberg M, Suur MH, de Vos S, et al. Informed consent, parental awareness, and reasons for participating in a randomized controlled study. *Arch Dis Child* 1998; **79**: 120–125.

Wertheimer A. *Coercion*. Princeton, NJ: Princeton University Press, 1987.

Weston J, Hannah M, Downes J. Evaluating the benefits of a patient information video during the informed consent process. *Patient Educ Counsel* 1997; **30**: 239–245.

Wirshing DA, Wirshing WC, Marder SR, et al. Informed consent: assessment of comprehension. *Am J Psychiatry* 1998; **155**: 1508–1511.

Young DR, Hooker DT, Freeberg FE. Informed consent documents: increasing comprehension by reducing reading level. *IRB: Rev Human Subjects Res* 1990; **12**(3): 1–5.

Evaluating Benefits and Harms in Clinical Research

PAUL B. MILLER AND CHARLES WEIJER

INTRODUCTION

Authoritative statements of principle are commonplace
in research ethics. *The Belmont Report* has unquestionably been most influential. Issued in 1978 by the National
Commission for the Protection of Human Subjects of Biomedical and Behavioural Research (hereafter: National
Commission), it provides that the interests of research
subjects should be protected in accord with principles
of beneficence, justice and respect for persons (National
Commission, 1978a).

Predictably, over time, problems generally attending authoritative statements of principle have come to afflict *The
Belmont Report*. Ritual invocation of *Belmont* principles
now has all the appearance of a mantra. Of the three *Belmont* principles, the principle of beneficence has suffered
most. It is least likely to be invoked in contemporary debate.
Further, there is no shared understanding of the foundation
of the principle. Finally, there is little concern evident over
specification of the principle.

Most go no further than the abstract formulation in
The Belmont Report, according to which the principle of
beneficence combines maxims to refrain from harming
others and to act for their benefit. At this level, the principle
is bedevilled by ambiguity. It fails to specify the scope of
those subject to obligation. Nor does it specify the scope of
the beneficiaries of obligation. Further, the principle fails to
resolve questions resolution of which is requisite to provision
of clear direction. Allowing that the principle may apply to
an individual beneficiary (e.g. a particular research subject),
it is unclear whether and when the promise of benefit to
that beneficiary justifies exposing them to risk of harm.
Allowing that the principle may apply to a single group or
class of beneficiaries (e.g. groups of research subjects, or

communities), it is unclear whether and when the promise of benefit to that class justifies exposing the group or
class to risk of harm. More vexing still, to the extent that
the principle may allow of multiple beneficiaries, it is unclear whether and when benefit to one may justify risk of
harm to another. Further and finally, the principle does not
specify what kind of harms or benefits are embraced by it,
nor whether differences in kind are salient to the implementation of the principle.

The ambiguity of the principle of beneficence detracts
from its normative force. For the principle to play a stronger
role, two hurdles need first to be cleared. First, its foundation must be clarified. Second, it must be specified by a
set of norms that adequately guide practical reasoning. We
aim presently only to partially meet these hurdles, focusing
on the implications of the principle for the regulatory oversight of clinical research. Our focus enjoys interpretive justification. The principle of beneficence, like other *Belmont*
principles, was articulated for purposes of informing the
development of *policy* for the *protection of research subjects*. The state is first and foremost obliged by the principle
because it alone enjoys the authority to specify to whom
the principle of beneficence applies and what it requires.
The research subject is the principal beneficiary because
protection of research subjects was and is the avowed aim
of regulatory oversight of clinical research.

THE INFLUENCE OF THE NATIONAL COMMISSION ON CURRENT SPECIFICATION OF THE PRINCIPLE OF BENEFICENCE

The Belmont Report failed to specify the principle of
beneficence. That said, it did emphasize that the regulatory

Principles of Health Care Ethics, Second Edition   Edited by R.E. Ashcroft, A. Dawson, H. Draper and J.R. McMillan
© 2007 John Wiley & Sons, Ltd

evaluation of research benefits and harms called for by the principle ought to be done in a systematic and rigorous manner:

> the idea of systematic, nonarbitrary analysis of risks and benefits should be emulated insofar as possible. This ideal requires those making decisions about the justifiability of research to be thorough in the accumulation and assessment of information about all aspects of the research, and to consider alternatives systematically. This procedure renders the assessment of research more rigorous and precise, while making communication between review board members and investigators less subject to misinterpretation, misinformation and conflicting judgments.

Although the principle of beneficence was left unspecified in *The Belmont Report*, work on systematic regulatory specification of the principle has a long, if little known, history. A leading role was played by the National Commission itself and by its members, especially Robert J. Levine (Weijer, 2000).

The National Commission sat from 1975 to 1978 and issued a total of ten reports on differing aspects of research involving human subjects. Its work represents the first sustained, in-depth exploration of the evaluation of benefits and harms in research. Little recognized is the fact that the National Commission's views on the evaluation of benefits and harms evolved over its four-year term (Weijer, 2000). Three distinct views can be found in its opus: analysis of entire protocols; analysis of protocols with particular components; and analysis of components. In turn, each underlies aspects of the current US federal regulation governing institutional evaluation of the benefits and harms of research.

The earlier works of the National Commission focused on the evaluation of benefits and harms of research involving particular vulnerable populations (National Commission, 1975; 1976; 1977; 1978b). In them, the National Commission articulated different models for the evaluation of benefits and harms. These models represented variations on the three views mentioned above, and they eventually came to be reflected in the various subparts of the Department of Health and Human Services regulations devoted to distinct vulnerable populations (Title 45, *Code of Federal Regulations*, Part 46: Subparts B, C, D).

The later works of the National Commission are typified by a move towards a model calling for analysis of the benefits and harms of components of studies. In *Institutional Review Boards*, the National Commission for the first time articulated norms to govern the evaluation of benefits and harms for all human subjects research (National Commission, 1978c). The report acknowledges explicitly that a protocol may contain therapeutic procedures, nontherapeutic procedures or both:

> A research project is described in a protocol that sets forth explicit objectives and formal procedures designed to reach those objectives. The protocol may include therapeutic and other activities intended to benefit the subjects, as well as procedures to evaluate such activities. (National Committee, 1978c, p. xx)

Risks must be evaluated systematically and should involve a procedure-by-procedure review of risks, benefits and alternatives. In the words of the National Commission, '[t]his evaluation should include an arrray of alternatives to the procedures under review and the possible harms and benefits associated with each alternative' (National Committee, 1978c, p. 23). The risks associated with particular procedures are acceptable only if:

> risks to subjects are minimized by using the safest procedures consistent with sound research design and, wherever appropriate, by using procedures being performed for diagnostic or treatment purposes; [and] risks to subjects are reasonable in relation to anticipated benefits to subjects and importance of knowledge to be gained ... (National Committee 1978c, pp. 19,20).

Levine renders the thinking of the National Commission clearer in two papers in the Appendix to *The Belmont Report*. In 'The boundaries between biomedical or behavioural research and the accepted and routine practice of medicine', the existence of 'complex activities' in research is recognized (National Committee, 1978c, p. 23). Such activities involve a mixture of procedures, some appropriately classified 'therapeutic', others 'nontherapeutic'.

The view is further elucidated by Levine in *Ethics and Regulation of Clinical Research*. He states:

> the Commission calls for an analysis of the various components of the research protocol. Procedures that are designed solely to benefit society or the class of children of which the particular child-subject is representative are to be considered as the research component. Judgements about the justification of the risks imposed by such procedures are to be made in accord with other recommendations. For example, if the risk is minimal, the research may be conducted as described in Recommendations 3 and 7 [of Research Involving Children], no matter what the risks are of the therapeutic components. The components of the protocol that hold out the prospect of direct benefit for the individual subjects are to be considered precisely as they are in the practice of medicine (Levine, 1988, 250–251).

It is this last model of benefit/harm evaluation, 'component analysis', that serves as the conceptual framework for the standards governing risk evaluation in the *Common Rule* (45 *C.F.R.* 46). Risks associated with non-therapeutic procedures must be minimized and must be 'reasonable in relation to...the importance of the knowledge that may reasonably be expected to result' (45 *C.F.R.* 46.111(a)). Risks associated with therapeutic procedures must be 'reasonable in relation to anticipated benefits ... to subjects' (45 *C.F.R.* 46.111 (a)).

While the work of the National Commission helpfully reveals an array of models for regulatory specification of the principle of beneficence, it did not ultimately secure its wish that REC/IRB evaluation of research benefits and harms be made 'systematic and rigorous'. For that to happen, REC/IRB review must be guided by a single model providing clear standards for the evaluation of benefits and harms. Current US regulations are incoherent by the virtue of incorporation of inconsistent models of harm/benefit evaluation advanced by the National Commission in its various reports. Further, standards for the evaluation of benefits and harms have been left overly vague. As noted above, the central part of the *Common Rule* requires that research be approved only where 'risks to subjects are minimized' and 'risks to subjects are reasonable in relation to anticipated benefits, if any, to subjects, and the importance of the knowledge that may be reasonably expected to result'. However, these standards raise more questions than they answer (Weijer and Miller, 2004). Which risks, to which subjects, must be minimized? To what extent must they be minimized? Which risks and which potential benefits are to be considered under the reasonableness determinations? By what measure is the IRB to determine that risks are reasonable in relation to benefits to subjects? By what measure is it to determine that risks are reasonable in relation to the knowledge that may reasonably be expected to result?

We are not alone in recognizing these problems. In its report *Ethical and Policy Issues in Research Involving Human Participants*, the US National Bioethics Advisory Commission (NBAC, 2001) raised similar concerns. NBAC recognized that regulatory norms governing evaluation of benefits and harms are inconsistently formulated and inadequately specified. It commented that:

> [an] IRB's assessment of the risks and potential benefits of research is central to determining whether a research study is ethically acceptable. Yet, this assessment can be a difficult one to make, as there are no clear criteria for IRBs to use in judging whether the risks of research are reasonable in terms of what might be gained by the individual or society (2001, p. 13).

NBAC also recognized that '[t]he lack of a single coherent, fully developed conceptual framework hinders the efforts of IRBs to assess and evaluate risks and potential benefits of research studies' (2001, p. 76). Lacking adequate direction, IRBs generally fail to devote due attention to evaluating research harms and benefits and, so, to protecting the welfare of research subjects. As NBAC concluded, 'IRBs often tend to focus more on matters where clearer regulatory direction is available—for example, reviewing the language used for consent forms' (2001, p. 70).

Frustrated by inconsistent and unclear regulatory guidance, IRBs are essentially left with two choices. They can either neglect their obligation to ensure due protection of the welfare of research subjects or simply make an intuitive judgement about the acceptability of research risks. In either event, research subjects fail to receive the protection to which they are entitled. This is clearly not satisfactory. As we explain in below, through public declarations of principle such as *The Belmont Report*, the state establishes an important bond of trust with research subjects. To satisfy the obligation it has undertaken in respect of the principle of beneficence, it must establish a coherent and comprehensive framework of substantive regulatory norms promising effective protection of the welfare of research subjects. Component analysis, reviewed below, was developed to fill this void.

POLITICAL TRUST AS THE FOUNDATION OF *BELMONT* PRINCIPLES AS APPLIED TO THE STATE

The ethics of trust relationships is a neglected topic (Baier, 1986). Nevertheless, at least four categories of trust relationship may be distinguished. In the first, one entrusts another with specific power over specific personal interests (Baier, 1986). Trust may be reposed on grounds of personal familiarity or social roles. In the second, people entrust each other with specific power over specific common interests. Trust in this sense is essential to cooperation, which in turn underlies the realization of genuine community and joint projects (Luhmann, 1979; Blackburn, 1998). In the third category, people entrust each other with unspecified and wide-ranging power over equally unspecified and wide-ranging personal interests (Baier, 1986). Trust in this sense is essential to long-term relationships of the most personal kind. The fourth and final category alone is pertinent presently. It is distinct from the others in encompassing political rather than private and public trust relationships. It covers relationships established where citizens in democratic states entrust power over public interests to political representatives and other public officials (Pettit, 1998). This category includes relationships between individual citizens and the state (e.g. wards and the state), discreet communities and the state (e.g. aboriginal peoples and the state), and citizens in aggregate (i.e. the public) and the state.

There are important differences between these categories. However, for present purposes, it is important only to recognize a structural feature that they share, namely the dependence generated by entrusting another with power over important shared or personal interests. This feature founds an obligation common to all trust relationships – namely, that requiring the entrusted party to exercise the power in question to protect or advance the interests over which it was entrusted.

In our view, *The Belmont Report* and comparable state-endorsed declarations of principle may be interpreted as establishing a relationship of trust between research subjects and the state in which the latter assumes an obligation to protect the interests of research subjects. We think several reasons of principle support our conclusion, but we first need to show it is possible for the state to undertake an obligation of this sort.

If we understand democratic states as exercising power on trust in the public interest on behalf of citizens in aggregate, we understand government officials as acting under a trust-based duty to exercise their powers in the public interest. But if so, there is potential for conflict between this duty and duties the state may undertake in the other subcategories of political trust relationship. That is, if the state can owe trust-based duties to individuals or communities, it is conceivable – indeed, likely – that these duties may conflict with its duty to act in the public interest. What are the implications of this? One response is to say that because the state's duty to act in the public interest is paramount, it is barred from undertaking trust-based duties to act in the interests of individuals or communities. Another is to allow that the state may undertake these duties, but only on the condition that where they conflict with the duty to the public, the latter is paramount. Yet another approach is to allow that the state may undertake trust-based duties to act in the interests of individuals and communities without conditions where government officials judge this to be *bona fide* in the public interest (i.e. consistent with, or demanded by, the state's duty to act in the public interest).

We think the latter approach best. The first is problematic, for it fails to square with the moral intuition, reflected in law, that the state ought in certain circumstances to be permitted to subject itself to trust-based duties to act in the interests of individuals or communities (e.g. to wards of the state or aboriginal communities). The second approach is better, but fails to square analytically with the core normative implication of trust relationships; that is, the obligation to act in the interests of another (rather than merely to balance competing interests). The third approach is best as it enables the state to enter into perfectly binding relationships of trust with individuals and communities on the basis of its duty to act in the interests of the public.

As indicated above, we believe that the state has undertaken a relationship of trust with research subjects. This undertaking is best seen as one made for furtherance of its duty to act in the public interest. The public has a clear interest in the scientifically rigorous conduct of clinical trials. Such trials may result in knowledge of great theoretical interest and obvious practical importance. Further, trials that are carefully designed and conducted provide the

evidentiary basis for evaluating the safety and efficacy of therapeutic products, from drugs to medical devices, used daily by countless people. Properly conducted, clinical trials help to ensure that medicine rests on a sound scientific foundation. The public interest in improved health through advancements in medical knowledge and technology is clearly served by the clinical trials enterprise.

It is equally clear that, conscription aside, the public interest in clinical trials could not be served without the voluntarism of research subjects. The public would be unreasonable to expect potential subjects to consider participating in clinical trials without grounds for the belief that their own interests will receive due consideration and protection. The commitment undertaken by the state to protect subjects' interests through regulatory oversight structures and standards serves as such grounds. In choosing to regulate clinical trials in the name of protecting subjects, the state effectively invites prospective research subjects to trust protection of their interests to its regulatory apparatus. To the extent that realization of the public benefits of clinical trials is contingent upon subjects' continuing trust in the ability and inclination of the state to protect their interests, the public has an interest in ensuring that this trust is well-founded and not disappointed. This trust will be met where the state clearly articulates and rigorously enforces regulatory norms protecting the rights and welfare of research subjects.

In most western democratic countries, state governments have made express representation of their intent to protect the public interest in clinical trials by developing regulatory apparatus to protect the rights and welfare of research subjects. The United States demonstrated clear leadership. It established the National Commission and other advisory bodies whose reports have, in turn, profoundly influenced the development of regulatory protections for research subjects. The US government has publicly declared its intention that the interests of research subjects be protected in accord with the *Belmont* principles. It has also acted upon *Belmont* principles in developing its regulatory apparatus (Office for Human Research Protections, 2004). In doing so, it invited and accepted the trust of research subjects, undertaking accordingly a moral obligation to ensure that their interests receive due regulatory protection in accord with declared principles.

COMPONENT ANALYSIS AS SPECIFICATION OF THE PRINCIPLE OF BENEFICENCE

The US government has not met this obligation to date. That is because, as recognized by NBAC, it has yet to develop and implement a coherent and comprehensive framework of substantive regulatory norms promising effective protection of the

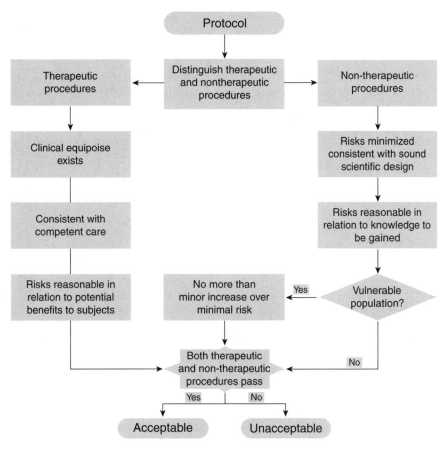

Figure 96.1. The ethical analysis of benefits and harms in research by the REC. Reproduced with permission from Miller and Weijer (2004).

welfare of research subjects. Just such a framework has, however, recently been articulated by the authors (Weijer, 2000; Weijer and Miller, 2004). Called component analysis, the framework (see Figure 96.1) answers the above-noted questions stemming from the *Common Rule* and does so by building directly on the work of the National Commission. To our knowledge, component analysis is the only systematic framework for the evaluation of research benefits and harms based on the *Belmont* principle of beneficence and consistent with US regulation. It was endorsed by NBAC in *Ethical and Policy Issues in Research Involving Human Participants*, and it has also been endorsed by a variety of commentators in the research ethics literature (Emanuel, Wendler and Grady, 2000; Karlawish, 2003; Truog, 2005; Liddell et al., 2006).

In component analysis, definitions of risk, benefit and harm track those adopted by the National Commission. Benefit is defined as a favourable outcome, harm as an adverse outcome and risk as the probability and magnitude of

an adverse outcome. Importantly, benefits and harms are not taken merely to refer to physical outcomes. Rather, benefits and harms are understood as concepts broad in scope, encompassing physical, psychological, social and economic outcomes (Levine, 1988).

Following Levine and the National Commission, component analysis is built on recognition of a basic distinction between the kinds of procedures administered to subjects in clinical trials (Weijer, 2000). It defines the distinction in terms of therapeutic warrant (Weijer, 2000, fig. 1). Some interventions, such as drug, surgical or behavioural interventions, may be administered with therapeutic warrant – that is, on the basis of evidence making it reasonable to believe administration of the procedure will yield therapeutic benefit to the research subject (Weijer and Miller, 2004). These interventions are classified as therapeutic procedures. Other interventions, such as venepuncture for pharmacokinetic drug levels, imaging procedures or questionnaires not used in clinical practice, in the absence of therapeutic warrant, are administered solely to answer a scientific question (Weijer and Miller, 2004). These interventions are accordingly classified as non-therapeutic procedures.

The distinction between different kinds of procedures is reflected in the provision of separate standards for the evaluation of the harms and benefits of therapeutic and nontherapeutic procedures in component analysis. Therapeutic warrant is understood as founding a morally salient distinction between kinds of procedures because research subjects who are patients enjoy a right to competent care. This entitlement is to be distinguished from that which all research subjects enjoy, namely to protection from exposure to undue harm solely in the interest of others.

In light of this, note that classification of the placebo control is a special case. Most would agree that placebo ought not to be classified as a therapeutic procedure on the basis of therapeutic warrant, notwithstanding evidence of possible therapeutic benefit associated with its administration (i.e. the placebo effect). The placebo control is, nevertheless, classified as a therapeutic procedure under component analysis. It is so classified by reason of its special normative and epistemological role in determining the standard of care to which those subject to the duty of care are held. In medicine, the standard of care requires provision of competent care. Care is assessed competent in the light of expert custom, in turn assessed in light of available evidence. The administration of treatment for which there is sound evidence of acceptable levels of safety and efficacy is consistent with competent care. However, where proven treatments do not exist or the evidentiary foundation for existing treatments is now doubted, new or now questioned treatments must be compared to non-treatment (i.e. placebo). The placebo control is classified a therapeutic procedure precisely because of its indispensable role in establishing and arbitrating standard of care.

As we have noted, component analysis establishes distinct standards for the evaluation of therapeutic and non-therapeutic procedures. Therapeutic procedures are evaluated according to the clinical equipoise requirement (Freedman, 1987a; Miller and Weijer, 2003). Clinical equipoise is a research-friendly response to the question: When is a physician morally permitted to offer enrolment in a clinical trial to a patient? Clinical equipoise provides that she may do so when the administration of the various therapeutic procedures in a clinical trial is consistent with competent care. It formalizes this condition by requiring the REC to certify that at the outset of a trial there exists a state of honest, professional disagreement in the community of expert practitioners as to the preferred treatment. Procedurally, in making this determination, the REC does not survey practitioners. Rather, it scrutinizes the study justification, reviews relevant literature and, where appropriate, consults with independent clinical experts. Clinical equipoise is

satisfied if the REC concludes that the evidence supporting the various therapeutic procedures is sufficient that, were it widely known, expert clinicians would disagree as to the preferred treatment for the condition.

Non-therapeutic procedures are, by definition, not reasonably judged to offer the prospect of therapeutic benefit to study participants. When assessing risks associated with non-therapeutic procedures under component analysis, the REC must ensure that two standards are met: (1) non-therapeutic risks must be minimized consistent with sound scientific design; and (2) such risks must be reasonable in relation to the knowledge that may be gained from the study. The REC implements the first standard by ensuring the elimination of unnecessary nontherapeutic procedures and by requiring, where feasible, the substitution of 'procedures already being performed on the subjects for diagnostic and treatment purposes' (45 C.F.R. 46.111(a)(1)(ii)). The implementation of the second standard requires the REC to judge the study's scientific value sufficient to justify the risks nontherapeutic procedures pose to subjects. As this judgement involves an appraisal of scientific priorities in social context, IRB membership must include community representatives (Freedman, 1987b).

When research involves a vulnerable population such as children, an important additional norm is applied to non-therapeutic procedures under component analysis. In such cases, risks associated with non-therapeutic procedures are limited to a 'minor increase over minimal risk'. This standard requires that RECs ensure that non-therapeutic risks posed to children in research are no more than a minor increase over the risks 'ordinarily encountered in daily life' (45 C.F.R. 46.406(a), 102(i)). To determine whether this standard is met, the IRB reasons by analogy (Freedman et al., 1993). It must determine that the non-therapeutic risks posed are in fact the same as those encountered in daily life – for instance, 'during the performance of routine physical or psychological examinations or tests' – or that they are sufficiently similar to such risks (45 C.F.R. 102(i)). The minimal risk threshold aims to protect the welfare of children and other vulnerable populations through shielding them from exposure to atypical levels of risk while allowing important research to proceed. It remains controversial whether the referent for minimal risk ought to be the daily lives of healthy or sick research subjects (Kopelman 1981; Miller and Weijer 2000).

CONCLUDING REFLECTIONS

Like other *Belmont* principles, the principle of beneficence is in need of sustained attention to questions concerning its foundation and specification. The implications of the principle for clinical research are currently little appreciated. Some suggest that it requires nothing more than that

RECs exercise intuitive judgement on the acceptability of research risks. We disagree. Considered reflection yields greater specificity. In our view, component analysis provides needed improvement upon existing regulatory specification of the principle of beneficence. If adopted and enforced, it would enable the state to fulfil the obligation it has undertaken to protect the interests of research subjects in accord with the *Belmont* principles.

That being said, further work remains to be done on component analysis. That work will explore outstanding questions concerning the proper referent for the minimal risk threshold. It will also consider whether adoption of a similar threshold is appropriate for research involving competent adults. Finally, it will determine whether there ought to be further specification of the requirement that risks of nontherapeutic procedures be deemed reasonable in relation to the value of the knowledge expected to result from the research.

ACKNOWLEDGEMENTS

Paul Miller gratefully acknowledges the support of a doctoral fellowship from the Social Sciences and Humanities Research Council of Canada. Charles Weijer acknowledges with appreciation the support of a Tier I Canada Research Chair and a Canadian Institutes of Health Research Operating Grant.

REFERENCES

Baier AC. Trust and anti-trust. *Ethics* 1986; **96**: 231–260.

Blackburn S. Trust, cooperation, and human psychology. In: Braithwaite V, Levi M, eds. *Trust and Governance*, New York: Russell Sage Foundation, 1998; pp. 28–45.

Emanuel EJ, Wendler D, Grady C. What makes clinical research ethical? *JAMA* 2000; **283**: 2701–2711.

Freedman B. Equipoise and the ethics of clinical research, *New England Journal of Medicine* 1987a; **317**: 141–145.

Freedman B. Scientific value and validity as ethical requirements for research, *IRB: Rev Hum Subj Res* 1987b; **9**: 7–10.

Freedman B, Fuks A and Weijer C. *In loco parentis:* minimal risk as an ethical threshold for research upon children, *Hastings Cent Rep* 1993; **23**: 13–19.

Karlawish JH. Research involving cognitively impaired adults. *N Engl J Med* 2003; **348**: 1389–1392.

Kopelman L. Estimating risk in human research, *Clin Res* 1981; **29**: 1–8.

Levine RJ. The boundaries between biomedical or behavioral research and the accepted and routine practice of medicine. In: National Commission for the Protection of Human Subjects of Biomedical and Behavioral Research, *The Belmont Report: Ethical Principles and Guidelines for the Protection of Human Subjects of Research, Appendix 1*, Washington: Department of Health, Education and Welfare, 1978.

Levine RJ. *Ethics and the Regulation of Clinical Research*, 2nd edn., New Haven, CT: Yale University Press, 1988.

Liddell K, Douglas Chamberlain, David K. Menon, Erwin J. O. Kompanje *et al*. The European clinical trials directive revisited: the VISEAR recommendations. *Resuscitation* 2006; **69**: 9–14.

Luhmann N. *Trust and Power*, Toronto: John Wiley & Sons Canada Ltd, 1979.

Miller PB and Weijer C. Moral solutions in assessing research risk, *IRB: Rev Hum Subj Res* 2000; **22**: 6–10.

Miller PB and Weijer C. Rehabilitating equipoise, *Kennedy Inst Ethics J* 2003; **13**: 93–118.

National Bioethics Advisory Commission. *Ethical and Policy Issues in Research Involving Human Participants*, Bethesda: National Bioethics Advisory Commission, 2001.

National Commission for the Protection of Human Subjects of Biomedical and Behavioural Research. *Research on the Foetus: Report and Recommendations*, Washington: Department of Health, Education and Welfare, 1975.

National Commission for the Protection of Human Subjects of Biomedical and Behavioural Research *Research Involving Prisoners: Report and Recommendations*, Washington: Department of Health, Education and Welfare, 1976.

National Commission for the Protection of Human Subjects of Biomedical and Behavioural Research. *Research Involving Children: Report and Recommendations*, Washington: Department of Health, Education and Welfare, 1977.

National Commission for the Protection of Human Subjects of Biomedical and Behavioural Research. *The Belmont Report: Ethical Principles and Guidelines for the Protection of Human Subjects of Research*, Washington: Department of Health, Education and Welfare, 1978a.

National Commission for the Protection of Human Subjects of Biomedical and Behavioural Research. *Research Involving Those Institutionalized as Mentally Infirm: Report and Recommendations*, Washington: Department of Health, Education and Welfare, 1978b.

National Commission for the Protection of Human Subjects of Biomedical and Behavioural Research *Institutional Review Boards: Report and Recommendations*, Washington: Department of Health, Education and Welfare, 1978c.

Office for Human Research Protections, United States Department of Health and Human Services. *Oral History of the Belmont Report and the National Commission for the Protection of Human Subjects of Biomedical and Behavioural Research – Interview with Tom Lamar Beauchamp*, Washington: Department of Health and Human Services, 2004. Also available on the World Wide Web: http://www.hhs.gov/ohrp/docs/InterviewBeauchamp.doc.

Pettit P. Republican theory and political trust. In: Braithwaite V, Levi M, eds. *Trust and Governance*, New York: Russell Sage Foundation, 1998; pp. 295–314.

Truog RD. Will ethical requirements bring critical care research to a halt? *Intensive Care Med* 2005; **31**: 338–344.

Weijer C. The ethical analysis of risk. *J Law Med Ethics* 2000; **28**: 344–361.

Weijer C, Miller PB. When are research risks reasonable in relation to anticipated benefits? *Nat Med* 2004; **10**: 570–573.

97

Patients' Obligations?

SIMON WOODS

In medical ethics, it is usual to emphasize the rights and interests of patients and the duties and responsibilities of health professionals. However, there has been a long history in which the obligations of patients have been discussed and described. Albury and Weisz (2001) describe how Erasmus and Galen each believed that patients had an obligation to cooperate with their doctor and to show appropriate gratitude for their care and treatment. In 1847, the American Medical Association's first code of ethics included a section on patients' obligations, reiterating the requirement for cooperation and gratitude, and grounding patient–doctor relations in a form of social contract in a fitting reflection of the time and context of its writing (Benjamin, 1985). More recently, medical ethics has been concerned almost exclusively with the rights and responsibilities of doctors and other health professionals, and as Draper and Sorell (2002) point out, one reason for this is that medical ethics literature is directed mainly at a professional audience. A second reason why the focus is almost exclusively upon the rights and interests of patients is because the dominant discourse in medical ethics, post-Second World War, has focused upon the concept of patient autonomy. Draper and Sorell comment that

> Traditionally, medical ethics has asserted that, as autonomous agents, competent patients must be allowed to decide for themselves the course of their medical treatment, and even whether to be treated at all. It is for the doctor to communicate effectively all the relevant information, assess the patient's competence, persuade without coercing, and abide by whatever decision the patient makes. Little or nothing is said about what kinds of decisions patients *ought* to make. Nor is much said about their responsibilities for making good rather than bad decisions. (Draper and Sorell, 2002, pp. 337–338)

If this is a tradition then I believe that it is a recent one, and it is therefore worth exploring how the norms of contemporary medical ethics have evolved to a point at which

this account of doctor–patient relations has become the dominant one. The account given by Draper and Sorell gives a particular view of patient autonomy in the context of consent, one that combines ethical and legal conceptions of consent. Although consent has a long history in doctor–patient relationship, the 'informed' portion is something which has evolved in purpose over time. Informing the patient was very often a pragmatic consideration when performing surgery, the patient needed to know what was about to happen to them. However as Katz notes, this was more to do with the patient's preparation than the recognition of a 'right for patients to decide, after having been informed, whether an intervention was agreeable to them in light of its risks and benefits as well as available alternatives' (1984, p. 28). If this information was selective or euphemistic, then this, in keeping with medical paternalism, was left to the discretion of the doctor to determine what in his (as it usually was) opinion was in the patient's best interests, an approach described by Beauchamp and Faden (1986) as a 'beneficence model'. However, the beneficence model was exposed as problematic and open to challenge when patients who were unhappy with the results of their treatment turned to due process. In law, there was a tangible tension between the patient's right to self-determination and the acceptance of a doctor's therapeutic discretion of disclosure to patients. The patient's right to self-determination had been confirmed in the now famous and influential decision by Justice Benjamin Cardozo in which he noted: 'Every human being of adult years and sound mind has a right to determine what shall be done with his own body; and a surgeon who performs an operation without his patient's consent commits an assault, for which he is liable in damages' (*Schloendorff v Society of New York Hospital* 21 NY 125 (1914)). Yet this position stands in palpable tension with other legal opinions. The right to self-determination can be seen as running up against the decision in *Bolam v*

Principles of Health Care Ethics, Second Edition   Edited by R.E. Ashcroft, A. Dawson, H. Draper and J.R. McMillan
© 2007 John Wiley & Sons, Ltd

Friern Hospital Management Committee (1957) and confirmed in later cases such as *Sidaway v Governors of Royal Bethlem Hospital* [1985] AC871 that what was deemed appropriate for patients to know was a matter of medical opinion and not the patients'. In his outright critique of informed consent, Robert Veatch (1995) argued that the very concept of informed consent is premised upon an assumption of the traditional authoritarian medical model rather than the principle of autonomy. Veatch points out, when informed consent is required, that what the doctor chooses to impart to the patient is based on the information the *doctor* regards as pertinent for the patient to know. The aim of informing is to get the patient to agree to what the doctor considers to be in the patient's best interests. This challenging claim is at odds with, for example, Gillon's conception of informed consent. Gillon contends that 'the doctor should be trying to meet his patient's wishes rather than his own' and to achieve that, 'it is understanding what it is like for that other person to be in his or her own shoes that is morally important' (1994, p. 115). Gillon's faith in empathic understanding is a kind of position which Veatch treats sceptically, arguing that 'doing what is best for the patient' has become an unquestioned platitude of medical ethics (Veatch, 1995, p. 7). Veatch's criticism seems to ring true with the many examples where authoritative medical opinion has been imposed on patients in the name of their best interests. Moreover, there is a long line of criticism of the wrongs of medical paternalism; Illich's critique of medicalization, Goffman's (1961) analysis of institutionalization and stigma, and Szasz (1964) and Laing's antipsychiatry (Boyer, 1972) position have all attacked in one way or another the power of doctors over patients and identified the particular vulnerability of the patient. The potential of a grossly unequal power relationship between doctor and patient, therefore, goes some way to explaining the emphasis, perhaps over-emphasis, upon patient autonomy.

However, vulnerability notwithstanding, it is also the case that patients too have obligations and responsibilities, and in this chapter I shall outline a plausible case remaining mindful of the transgressions of the past and the fact of patient's potential vulnerability.

The claim that patients have obligations is, on reflection, less startling than obvious because we are all potential patients and we all have obligations. This is of course a modest point but becomes a more interesting and more complex matter if one begins to distinguish between different kinds of obligation. Obligations can, quite reasonably, be divided into three kinds: obligations that are *hypothetical imperatives*, general moral obligations and substantive moral obligations. Although the second and third kinds of obligations have considerable overlap, I shall draw a distinction between them because I wish to make a particular case with respect to the third kind: substantive moral obligations.

First, I shall explain what I mean by obligations as *hypothetical imperatives*. A hypothetical imperative is a prescription of a very practical kind and could be described as taking the form that '*if you desire x then do y*'. The reason why I believe this characterizes a certain type of patient obligation is because it arises out of self-interest and most people seek medical attention out of self-interest, a desire to be cured or palliated or cared for. The implications for the patient are therefore several-fold; patients ought to cooperate with their doctor, act truthfully and adhere to the prescribed treatment. So Erasmus, Galen and the American Medical Association share a similar conviction that patients have obligations if they wish to be beneficiaries of medical attention, a point also made by Parsons (1964) in his account of the sick role. One may wish to characterize the hypothetical imperative, as I have described it as a species of obligation to self although this seems an overly moralistic way of describing what is in effect self-interested behaviour. Of course, it may be argued that out of self-interest a patient may lie and behave deceitfully, for example, by exaggerating symptoms to accelerate their treatment. This is true, but where lying and deceit are involved, the next category of obligations is engaged.

The second category of obligation can also be dealt with briefly. As there are moral obligations of a very general kind that require us all to respect others and refrain from harming others, these apply equally to people as patients. As Draper and Sorell (2002) argue, these range from matters of etiquette and general politeness to strict prescriptions on behaviour and expectations of individual responsibility. Indeed, many hospitals within the National Health Service (NHS) have, quite rightly, developed policies on the expected etiquette and conduct of patients and hospital visitors. Patients and visitors who swear and assault staff, who abuse property and fail to consider others can expect to be held to account. This is of course reasonable and what ought to be expected, but are there obligations that go beyond these general expectations? I believe there are and I shall spend the remainder of this chapter making this case with regard to patients' obligations as users of health care and with the particular special case of obligations to participate in research.

The claim that patients should not merely be concerned with their own interests and welfare, but with their moral obligations also, is a particular species of a more general issue in political and moral philosophy. So first, I will describe this problem before going on to explore how and in what way the problem may be applied to patients.

Political and moral philosophers have often considered the question of which moral obligations hold for everyone by focusing upon the context of 'strangers'. What right do I have to expect from a stranger, and what right does the stranger have to expect from me, and in general what society ought to expect from individuals in terms of their obligations to others?

There are several archetypes of 'stranger ethics', one of which is exemplified in the Biblical story of the Good Samaritan, a story in which a man rescues a stranger who has been robbed and badly beaten (Beauchamp and Childress, 2001). The story is usually cited as an example of, amongst other things, the virtue of charity, when an individual takes it upon him or herself to act benevolently towards another to whom they are not obligated. Most people would regard the Good Samaritan as acting out of common decency; albeit an intuitive and perhaps unreflective conception of 'doing the right thing' a traditional ethical analysis is that one is not *required* to be a Good Samaritan, and therefore this might be taken to imply that *patients* are not required to act for the benefit of others. Moral philosophers have argued that to set the level of expectation at the standard of the Good Samaritan is not only setting the standard too high but also setting a standard that is intrusive of individual liberty, and hence wrong in this particular respect. From this perspective, the Good Samaritan standard is a standard which should only be a matter for individual conscience and is therefore an *imperfect* obligation. The more reasonable level, it is argued, is that of a universal ethic of non-interference, on this view I have a *perfect* obligation not to do harm to another person and not to interfere in their life unless this is justified by the threat they pose to others. In the health context, I may therefore be justified in imposing quarantine upon a person with an infectious disease but may not justified in treating them against their will. The philosopher John Stuart Mill puts the matter this way:

> The only purpose for which power can be rightfully exercised over any member of a civilised community, against his will, is to prevent harm to others. His own good, either physical or moral, is not a sufficient warrant (Mill, 1985, p. 135).

Liberals who follow this Millian principle do so because they believe that the right to choose and live by values of their own choice is an extremely important social good. Therefore, the right each person has not to be interfered with is regarded as the base level for ethics. Non-interference does have a strong appeal because we all have an interest in living our lives as successfully as possible: we all, therefore, expect of others that they will respect our endeavours by not preventing us in this pursuit. The only constraining factor is when my freedom to live my life encroaches upon another person's right to live theirs. The freedom of the individual is, therefore, premised upon a principle of mutual respect, so that mutual respect and freedom from interference become the cornerstones of ethical behaviour between strangers. Of course, many will see this position as unsatisfactory in all sorts of ways. For example, do we not have a duty of care towards others at least to take some minimal steps to prevent harm befalling them? In one analysis, the talk of duty or obligation in this context is misplaced because the

motive to act for the good or benefit of another, it is argued, cannot be translated into an obligation but remains entirely optional, a voluntary undertaking. For one thing, we may agree that the right not to be interfered with translates into an obligation not to interfere but there is no parallel right to be benefited with the attendant *obligation* to benefit. One of the concerns about denying this claim is that it has implications on how society is structured and governed; although it seems right and justified to legislate to protect the freedom from interference with penalties against those who would interfere, it is an entirely different matter to enforce benevolence; some jurisdictions have in fact been legislated for the so-called 'Good Samaritan' laws in the context of a duty to rescue. Most European jurisdictions regard the failure to attempt to rescue a person in peril as criminally liable whilst in English law, in the absence of a specific duty to act, this remains a matter for individual judgement.

The idea that we are morally culpable when we fail to do good is often regarded as making too great a personal demand. By way of illustration of this point, the argument proffered by Peter Singer regarding the moral obligations to distant strangers is much criticized (Singer, 1995). Singer argues that citizens of affluent countries who fail to remedy the poverty of those who suffer from absolute poverty commit a profound wrong because 'allowing someone to die is not intrinsically different from killing someone, it would seem that we are all murderers' (Singer, 1995, p. 222). Although Singer makes his case in this most dramatic way, he does, however, have a less dramatic formulation that 'if it is in our power to prevent something very bad from happening, without thereby sacrificing anything of comparable moral significance, we ought to do it' (Singer, 1995, p. 229).

Singer makes his point in the strongest possible terms, and I do not intend spending time criticizing or defending his position. I will, however, argue that patients nevertheless have positive obligations, some of which can be regarded as substantive moral obligations arising in the particular context of the collective pursuit of a common good. I shall now explore this claim using three specific examples: taking responsibility for one's own health, using health resources prudently and participating in medical research where the personal risks are low. But first what do I mean by 'the common good'?

THE COMMON GOOD PROPOSAL

Space does not allow me to develop this argument as fully as it undoubtedly needs to be. So I shall present it in the form of a naïve yet entirely plausible 'common good' argument. The idea that there is a common good, the realization of which entails a common responsibility, flies in the face of the Anglo-American liberalism that dominates political and ethical thought. Individualism emphasizes the importance of

individual goods, and individualism is the *sine qua non* of
the liberal position which, as I have argued, forms one source
of the opposition to the idea of obligations of beneficence
in favour of non-interference. Consistent with this approach
is the liberal view of the good life which is also construed
in negative terms. Liberals are sceptical that there can be
an adequate positive account of the good life for human
beings, believing that any account of the good life will be
undermined by competing individual accounts of the good
life; hence, the liberals emphasis upon individual autonomy
and the freedom from interference. But the emphasis upon
the individual nature of the good life can go too far, after
all human beings are a homogeneous species with remarkably similar needs and requiring certain conditions to be
satisfied before they can begin to flourish and pursue their
wider interests. Dworkin (1993) has drawn a distinction between what he calls *experiential* and *critical* interests as a
way of capturing, if not the substance, then the framework
upon which individual accounts of the good life cohere. For
Dworkin, experiential and critical interests differ in kind and
importance. Experiential interests are the interests we have
in experiencing pleasurable things and although we may
be driven to experience more and better, a life devoted exclusively to this pursuit would be shallow and unfulfilling.
Critical interests are, for Dworkin, what matter in making
a life meaningful; they represent values that shape and underpin our aspirations and life-plans, and hence autonomy
is instrumentally vital in realizing one's critical interests. It
also follows that respect for a person's autonomous interests
is necessary to enable individuals to realize their good life
strategy. Whatever the strengths of Dworkin's account are,
there is a significant omission that it fails to acknowledge
that there are, in addition to autonomy, other common interests, the shared enabling factors which must be in place as a
condition of pursuing any kind of life at all. These conditions
must therefore be acknowledged as 'goods' and not merely as
modus vivendi to be tolerated as a condition of coexistence.
This matter *is* addressed in the political liberalism of John
Rawls (1996) where he argues that all citizens must be provided with the 'primary goods' as the prerequisites of any
life whatsoever. There is, therefore, a common interest in ensuring the widest and most equal distribution of such goods.
These 'primary goods' are what I shall refer to as common
goods and if anything can claim the status of a common good
then it is health, and therefore we all share a common interest
in protecting, preserving and restoring health. The problem
for this claim is that health is not a candidate resource for
redistribution because there is an element of brute luck in
whether we are healthy or not. However, the mechanism for
preserving health, preventing ill health and treating illness is
such a resource. A publicly funded health care system such
as the NHS aims to provide equal access to every UK citizen:
each according to his or her need.

However, the right of individuals to access health care
must be premised upon a degree of personal responsibility.
The backlash against autonomy-as-freedom has emphasized
the role of autonomy as coupled with personal responsibility
(Morreim 1991; Draper and Sorell, 2002). Although it may
be true that individuals have some responsibility for their
own health, given our vulnerability to trauma, disease and
infirmity, the enterprise of protecting and restoring health
must be a social one. Good health is a feature of a good life,
but providing for this is a feature of a good society. The
achievement of a good society is something which demands
the participation of all members of society. But what do I
mean by 'demand' and 'participation'?

By 'demand' I mean an ethical demand, and rather than
talk of this as a perfect obligation, I prefer to talk in terms
of a reasonable moral expectation that a society may have
of each of its members. This sets the default moral position
in 'positive mode' so that in the context of health, there is
an expectation that each person will participate by making
a contribution to the improvement of health care and make
fair use of a common resource.

Of course in writing this, I have in mind the sort of general provision of health care that is exemplified in the UK's
National Health Service (NHS) where, for all its faults, the
NHS succeeds in providing a high standard of health care,
free at the point of delivery, and from cradle to grave. The
raison d'être of the NHS is to meet the expectations of the
UK citizens to receive the best medical treatment and care.
Whilst it is in everyone's interests that health care delivery
is of the highest possible standard, it should also be recognized that these high standards could only be achieved with
the cooperation of the beneficiaries. As I write this chapter, the UK Prime Minister, Tony Blair, has been speaking to the media in advance of delivering a speech 'Our
Nation's Future' in which he will argue that although health
is a personal responsibility, the government will help the
public to take responsibility. The speech will emphasize the
problems of obesity, smoking and lack of exercise on the
nation's health and the likely pressure this will bring upon
NHS resources. A Downing Street spokesperson stated:

> Government is not best placed to communicate with people
> about a lot of the issues that really matter to them, in lifestyle
> issues . . . but, on the other hand, government has a responsibility
> to be engaging in these conversations . . . It is really important
> you should take more exercise, it is really important you should
> worry about children's obesity, but we are not the ones who
> should make you do it (ITV News 2006).

Although this seems to be a reasonable position in line with
my general argument that individuals have and therefore
ought to take responsibility for their own health, the detailed
implications need to be more cautiously drawn. The idea
that patient autonomy and choice in the context of health

care should be balanced against individual responsibility is not something which can be easily converted into an overall policy which enforces this responsibility in practice. Therefore, although insisting on patient's responsibility may be justified, enforcing consequences must be carefully balanced. For example, the demographics of obesity in the United Kingdom are associated with known factors of deprivation (Department of Health, 2002). An individual is more likely to be obese, to smoke and to have certain health problems according to where they live, and such inequalities in health are well established. Therefore, to deny such individuals access to health care or to challenge individuals as failing in their responsibility would be to take the concept of individual responsibility too far and fail to make an appropriate political response to a social problem. This is not to say that a patient's individual responsibility has no place in tackling such problems.

The idea of individual responsibility is not only important, but also challenging in other health contexts, and I shall explore a number of examples.

Case 1

Jack is a 67-year-old retired council worker who smokes and drinks alcohol and has done so since early adulthood. Since retiring, Jack has become an alcoholic and now, in addition to his alcohol dependency and smoking, he has a degree of liver failure, leaving him prone to bleeding disorders including severe nosebleeds (epistaxis). He also has arterial disease and is showing the first stages of gangrene in his right foot. Jack is a frequent visitor to his general practitioner as he needs dressings to his foot, injections of vitamins to help with his liver failure and regular monitoring and adjustments to his medications. Jack has at times been abusive to the staff at the surgery and has disturbed other patients by turning up inebriated for appointments. As a consequence, Jack has been barred from attending the surgery. Jack now has a severe epistaxis and a neighbour, who is familiar with Jack's history, now wonders whether to telephone the GP, call an ambulance or leave Jack to his own devices.

Case 2

Sylvia is a 39-year-old university lecturer who developed breast cancer. Although the cancer was at a very early stage, she required surgery. Sylvia had conducted her own research into treatment options and strongly preferred to have a local excision rather than a mastectomy. Sylvia discussed this with her surgeon who informed her that although there was unlikely to be any difference in survival there might be differences in psychological adjustment: lumpectomy potentially having a worse adjustment. Although Sylvia recovered well from her surgery and returned to work, she has since developed a deep depression, has been hospitalized on one occasion, and is now unable to work and is being

treated by a psychiatrist. Is it honouring her autonomy to hold her to the consequences of her earlier decision?

Case 3

James is 18 and was diagnosed as a diabetic when he was a child. James has recently been inattentive to his dietary restrictions and has been going out with friends to drink alcohol. His blood sugar levels have been fluctuating, and he has on one occasion been admitted to hospital by ambulance following a late night drinking party. James is very knowledgeable about his condition and treatment and is fully aware of the implications of mismanaging his diabetes. What responsibility ought to go with James's autonomy to live his own life?

In each of these cases, it is possible to argue that there is a degree of responsibility that goes along with the autonomy of the patient and their right to treatment and care. In case 1, it would be easy to argue that Jack's condition is to a large extent self-inflicted and his antisocial and disrespectful behaviour justifies the degree of intolerance resulting in his ban from the surgery. Yet, his health needs are quite severe, and his alcoholism is the sort of condition which clearly influences the capacity needed to be regarded as autonomous enough to take full responsibility for his actions; and therein lays one of the problems. Morreim attacks autonomy without responsibility as itself a profound moral insult to the patient, treating him as less than a competent adult and presupposes 'that he is not entitled to the full measure of dignity and respect reserved only for those who are moral agents' (1991, p. 137).

When patients are themselves unwilling to participate in decision-making by refusing to be informed of relevant details regarding their condition, or refusing to take responsibility to do what is required to improve their health, this becomes a self-fulfilling prophecy of infantile behaviour. Morreim goes on to argue that one of the wider consequences of this approach is that any behaviour that may be reclassified as 'disease' rather than 'offence' permits the health professional to offer help without condemnation. She cites examples of the drug abuser and the excessive gambler, where the consequences of declaring this behaviour a product of a disease 'rather than free choice, is to presuppose that that person is less than a full moral agent' (1991, p. 137). This may be a valid observation in some cases, but it is one that involves sufficient ambiguity about cause, choice and autonomy that there is a need for more caution. There does seem to be good grounds for distinguishing the incautious gambler from the person who has an uncontrollable compulsion to gamble, and similarly the recreational drug user from the addict or alcoholic. One way of drawing this distinction is based on autonomy itself because some gamblers or addicts have a clear second-order preference to stop their behaviour but are unable to do so because of the compulsive nature of their condition.

So how ought we respond to Jack? If Jack's epistaxis is so severe that it warrants emergency treatment then it seems reasonable, given this vulnerability, to call an ambulance and provide the emergency care. However, his further management may well warrant the drawing up of a specific contract in which conditions of behaviour, compliance with treatment, and the consequences of breaching such a contract are agreed with Jack at a point in time where his capacity is unimpaired by alcohol or a health crisis makes this a reasonably autonomous choice.

In case 2, there is complexity of a different kind. It has, for example, been argued that a health system which shields patients from the economic cost of their treatment choices is one which is inherently undermining of patient autonomy (Menzel, 1990; Morreim, 1991). This, it is argued, is a necessary feature of any third party payment scheme including publicly funded health systems such as the NHS, where patients are rarely confronted with the actual cost of their treatment choice. Both Menzel and Morreim argue that it is a condition of respecting patient autonomy that we make them aware and hold them to the cost implications of their treatment choices. This is of a course a difficult claim to apply to the context of the NHS; but with respect to Sylvia's choice, would it be reasonable to inform her also of the potential cost differences between the treatment options open to her? My own response is to say both 'yes' and 'no'. Yes, in the sense that users of health care may be usefully informed of the actual cost of their choices when it is a failure to attend a clinic or to insist upon a form of treatment that is not routinely available within the NHS, and 'no', if informing patients of the cost implications of their treatment becomes a substitution for the prudent management of health resources by the government and its administration. So although there is a higher cost attached to allowing Sylvia's preference for one treatment over another, this is nevertheless within the range of what ought to be available to individuals who require the treatment of a serious condition.

In case 3, James is a well-informed adult who is aware of the likely consequences of his actions; should we therefore respect his autonomy-with-responsibility and abandon him to his fate? To react in this way is, I believe, to act prematurely and would be to apply a concept of autonomy that is too blunt an instrument. James has a chronic disease which will have a severe impact on his life if it is not properly managed. Because his condition is incurable, it is imperative that he maintains a good relationship with health professionals and that he develops a stable approach to managing his disease over a lifetime. It is, therefore, essential that if this is a period of adolescent rebellion, a common occurrence in a young person's adjustment to a chronic illness, then it is essential that he is not alienated from health professionals. Maintaining contact and offering safety advice and guidance on how to 'rebel within limits' may

be the most effective way of enabling James to accept and manage his disease effectively in the future. This approach is, I believe, most consistent with the duty of care health workers have to patients without treating them in an overly paternalistic manner. The time for emphasizing responsibility will be when James comes to the realization that he has a lifetime challenge to deal with his condition.

Having discussed a number of clinical cases, I shall now turn to consider other aspects of health care where there are substantive moral obligations.

The best treatment and care for individuals cannot be achieved without proper research and audit, and whilst I have discussed both topics elsewhere (Harris & Woods 2000; Hagger, Woods & Barrow, 2004; Hagger & Woods, 2005) it is with respect to research that I shall explore the implications of the common good thesis.

To claim that there is a legitimate expectation that patients should participate in research may seem a retrograde step in the post-Nuremberg era in which the major drive of medical ethics has been to advance patient autonomy and protect the interests of vulnerable patients. The Declaration of Helsinki (World Medical Association, 2004) states that 'the well-being of the human subject should take precedence over the interests of science and society'. Of course talk of a 'moral demand' sounds anachronistic, at odds with contemporary notions of human rights and their instantiation in laws and codes of practice that have evolved to prevent abuses in the area of medical research. As I have discussed, autonomy-centric ethics has, quite rightly, challenged the assumption that paternalistic interventions in medical care are justified. However, I also agree that this has been taken too far at the expense of acknowledging the responsibility that goes with autonomy.

For clinical research to be of most benefit, it requires the cooperation of a significant number to render the research both valid and generalizable. Willingness to participate is an expectation that can reasonably be had of everyone because everyone can do something usually of low risk and moderate inconvenience that will make an important contribution to clinical knowledge (Harris, 2005).

So what is the upshot of my proposal and what will its impact be? Perhaps it is easiest to begin with what I am *not* proposing. I am not proposing that we adopt the notion that everyone has a perfect obligation to act beneficently in the health context, but I do want to move away from the idea that beneficence is an optional virtue and change rather the starting premise that individuals are bound to refrain from harming to the expectation that everyone ought to contribute to a common good. Are we ready to accommodate such a change in the context of research? I think not. For one thing the change will require a programme of work to ensure that the expectation is set against a background of safeguards – a point to which I shall return. Nor am

I proposing that the expectation that patients should participate in research entails the abandonment of the requirement for consent, although in some instances of research, I believe that consent could be abandoned with no net detriment to ethical rigour of the research. Consent is too often relied upon to do the bulk of the ethical work in circumstances when consent functions as a mere nod to ethics. It may, of course, be right to insist upon what we now regard as voluntary. There are many instances in which we recognize the legitimacy of placing even severe restrictions upon personal autonomy, where the interests of the community require this (Harris & Woods, 2000; Harris, 2005). Of course, the fact that we may be *morally* justified in insisting upon an obligation does not mean that we ought to convert this into coercive public policies or a legal requirement. There are contravening reasons as to why coercion should always be a last resort. However, pointing out that the common good is sufficiently important to sometimes justify compulsory measures may demonstrate the justification of less severe measures to achieve equally important ends.

Does my proposal go further than Martyn Evans' 'modest proposal' of requiring patients to participate in research where this coincides with a treatment that their doctor would have prescribed for them anyway? (Evans, 2004). Although I share most of the concerns that Evans expresses, I believe that his proposals are too modest and would make no, or very little, impact on furthering the common good. The idea that patients should only be required to participate in research from which they stand to benefit may mean that areas of research where there is most need of a breakthrough is further frustrated. We already expect people with terminal illness to participate in clinical trials of toxic drugs with no probability of personal benefit and many conditions which affect only children might be successfully treated if we permitted non-therapeutic research, albeit in restricted circumstances, on children.

Indeed my claim that it is right to have an expectation that every person will contribute to a common good also extends to children. Children like adult patients do not have an elevated moral status in virtue of being a child or a patient. Children and patients, like all individuals, deserve the highest care and concern for their welfare, but this does not diminish any expectation we may have of them to contribute to a common good. Having such an expectation, even of children, should be construed as part of the initiation into good citizenship (Hagger & Woods, 2005). Children should grow up socialized into a world in which the society in which they thrive has legitimate expectations in return. Of course, this is not to say that a person may not grow up to criticize and ultimately reject the values of their own culture. However, if health has the status of a common good in the way in which I have suggested, this is not a value which can be rejected.

This is, of course, an unpopular and admittedly difficult argument to make in the light of Bristol and Alder Hey scandals and the subsequent collapse in the trust of health professionals that has ensued (The Report of the Royal Liverpool Children's Inquiry). A society can only begin to insist upon such expectations where it has gained and is proved worthy of the trust of its citizens (O'Neill, 2002). To pick up on my earlier point, to advance the view that society can legitimately expect its members to contribute positively to advancing a common good does not diminish the responsibility of that society. If anything, having such an expectation of individuals raises the expectations that individuals have of society to actively safeguard their interests. I do not believe that we should routinely insist upon the legitimate expectation that people ought to participate in research, but this prospect is reasonable *if* there are measures in place to ensure that researchers are scrupulous in applying agreed protocols, that all research is rigorously assessed by competent ethics committees and that the agreed research protocols are also policed and evaluated. This of course is no small undertaking.

The alternative to my moral expectation approach is the view that the only legitimate grounds upon which people should be permitted to consent to research are those of self-interest and altruism. But this approach would be a less effective means of achieving the good that the research seeks to promote. This approach is not equal to the task, and what is worse, it also raises serious ethical issues. Self-interested volunteers, that is, those whose interest concerns their own benefit, would only participate in research in which they stood the best chance of benefiting, thus ruling out early phase clinical trials and probably blind placebo studies also. This would mean that we could only rely upon the truly altruistic volunteer, if indeed such persons exist, to participate in some of the most challenging research and to carry an unfair burden of responsibility and risk.

It could be observed that my claim about expectation is still too demanding given that people who turn to the health care services do so out of need and are inherently vulnerable as patients. It should be emphasized that my claim does not diminish the moral importance of each individual patient, including the right to have his or her personal interests taken into account. Nor does it give licence to health professionals to pursue their research interests without due consideration of their moral and legal responsibilities; if anything, such responsibilities are emphasized.

There are, of course, areas of research where a great deal more work is needed to be done to ensure that adequate safeguards are in place and that there is robust ethical governance and transparency with regard to the purpose and potential exploitation of research. One such area is that of genetic research.

In the post-Human Genome Project era, the promise of genetics as a contributor to advancing human good has never been greater. The so-called 'genetics revolution' has the potential for making serious inroads not only in relation to the relatively rare single-gene disorders but also in curing major diseases that shorten life and diminish quality of life for many. Diseases such as cancer, coronary heart disease and diabetes are diseases that have a complex genetic and environmental aetiology, and an important key to their prevention and cure is likely to be found in genetic epidemiology studies. Such studies require national-scale projects with wide participation over several years, yet with little prospect that individuals will realize any direct benefit. UK Biobank is a long-term national project to build the world's largest information resource for medical researchers. It will follow the health of 500 000 volunteers aged 45–69 in the United Kingdom for up to 30 years. However, Khoury (2004) has pointed out that national studies are unlikely to be adequate to the task, and therefore research into complex genetics also requires the pooling and synthesis of international cohort studies. This observation not only may usefully emphasize the need for common human endeavour but also points to the challenges of conducting such research in a global context where there are very big differences between the various national standards with regard to the protection of the rights of research participants.

Some would argue that the need for caution cannot be overemphasized because donating one's DNA has become the contemporary equivalent of selling one's soul (Nelkin, 1995). However, the fact that we may be selling our souls is rather less important than taking the precaution not to sell it to the devil particularly, as there is no international consensus on the sponsorship of genetic research, for example by tobacco companies, or for the protection of genetic information, for example, from routine forensic use. So, although genetic research is one possible route to advancing a common good, there is a need for serious advances in the regulation and governance of the field before talk of an expectation to participate is appropriate. Nothing I say, therefore, shows any weakening resolve to protect the research participant, but nor does it diminish from the expectation; but without such safeguards, it is difficult to convert the expectation into action.

In this chapter, I have only really begun to sketch out what we might understand by the notion of patients' obligations. Of course, it should by now be clear that we should move from talk specifically of 'patients' to include everyone who enjoys the benefits of a common good. I have dwelt upon a number of examples as a way of exploring the possible implications of my approach to patient obligation.

The claim that we each have an obligation to contribute towards common goods, for example reliable and better health care, stems from a very basic account of what it is to act morally and not simply from an argument about self-interest, although self-interest, as I have argued, can be construed as the origin of one kind of patient obligation. I may quite reasonably gamble that a sufficient number of people will participate in research to the extent that I can benefit in all the ways necessary for my health without the need to participate in research myself. Whereas, to act morally is to act in such a way that not only do we recognize the constraints on our actions but also recognize what positive acts are required. Hence, we are not only required to refrain merely from harming others, but, other things being equal, to do good also. The positive force of moral obligation also stems from a consideration of fairness. It seems only fair that with respect to a common good from which we are all beneficiaries, there stems an obligation to contribute to the common good and not slipstream behind the efforts of others.

REFERENCES

Albury WR, Weisz GM. The medical ethics of Erasmus and the physician-patient relationship. *J Med Eth: Med Humanities* 2001; **27**: 35–41.

Beauchamp T, Faden R, King N. *A History and Theory of Informed Consent*. New York: Oxford University Press, 1986.

Beauchamp TL, Childress JF. *Principles of Biomedical Ethics*, 5th edition. Oxford: Oxford University Press, 2001.

Benjamin M. Lay obligations in professional relations. *J Med Philos* 1985; **10**: 85–103.

Boyers R, ed. *Laing and Anti-Psychiatry*. London: Penguin, 1972.

Department of Health. *Health Survey for England: Health & Lifestyle Indicators for Strategic Health Authorities 1994–2002*. London: Dott, 2002.

Draper H, Sorrell T. Patients' responsibilities in medical ethics. *Bioethics* 2002; **16**: 335–352.

Dworkin R. *Life's Dominion: An Argument About Abortion, Euthanasia and Individual Freedom*. New York: Alfred A. Knopf, 1993.

Evans HM. Should patients be allowed to veto their participation in clinical research? *J Med Ethics* 2004; **30**: 189–203.

Gillon R, ed. *Principles of Health Care Ethics*. London: John Wiley & Sons, Ltd, 1994.

Goffman E. *Asylums: Essays on the Social Situations of Mental Patients and Other Inmates*. New York: Anchor Books, 1961.

Hagger L, Woods S. Children and research: a case of double jeopardy. *Int J Child Rights* 2005; **13**(1–2): 51–72.

Hagger L, Woods S, Barrow P. Laws of confidentiality. *Int Med Law Rev* 2003; **6**: 105–116.

Harris J. Scientific research is a moral duty. *J Med Ethics* 2005; **31**: 242–248.

Harris J, Woods S. What are the responsibilities of the individual when participating in medical research? In: Doyal L, Tobias J, eds. *Informed Consent in Medical Research*. London: Blackwell BMJ Books, 2000; pp. 286–92.

ITV News http://www.itv.com/news/britain_b18816287aaa460cc9c519d8c0ef85e3.html.

Katz J. *The Silent World of the Doctor and Patient*. New York: Free Press, 1984.

Khoury MJ. The case for global human genome epidemiology. *Nat Genet*. 2004; **36**(10): 1027–1028.

Menzel PT. *Strong Medicine: The Ethical Rationing of Health Care*. New York: Oxford University Press, 1990.

Mill JS. On liberty. In: Warnock M, ed. *Utilitarianism*. Glasgow: Fontana, 1977.

Morreim EH. *Balancing Act. The New Medical Ethics of Medicine's New Economics*, Dordrecht: Kluwer Academic Publishers, 1991.

Nelkin L. *The DNA Mystique: The Gene as Cultural Icon*. New York: Freeman, 1995.

O'Neill O. *Autonomy and Trust in Bioethics*. Cambridge: Cambridge University Press, 2002.

Parsons T. *The Social System*. New York: Free Press, 1964.

Rawls J. *Political Liberalism*. New York: Columbia University Press, 1996.

Singer P. *Practical Ethics*, 2nd edition. Cambridge: Cambridge University Press, 1995.

Szasz T. *The Myth of Mental Illness*. London: Paladin, 1964.

The Report of the Public Inquiry into Children's Heart Surgery at the Bristol Royal Infirmary 1984–1995 (Cm 5207(1)).

The Report of the Royal Liverpool Children's Inquiry, January 2001 (http://www.rlcquiry.org.uk).

Veatch RM. Abandoning informed consent. *Hastings Center Rep* 1995; **25**(2): 5–12.

World Medical Association. *The Declaration of Helsinki*. Tokyo: WMA, 2004.

Standard of Care Owed to Participants in Clinical Trials: Different Standards in Different Countries?

REIDAR K. LIE

THE CONTROVERSY OVER THE PERINATAL HIV TRANSMISSION STUDIES

Perhaps the most contentious issue in research ethics during the past few years has been the question of what standard of care is owed to participants in clinical trials. At issue is whether there is an ethical obligation to provide participants in trials, irrespective of differences in economic circumstances, interventions that are at least as good as those that would be provided to participants in resource-rich countries. This debate started with the controversy over trials to test treatment regimens to prevent perinatal HIV transmission, and it is therefore useful to take this controversy as a point of departure.

In 1994, the so-called 076 trial established that treating the mother with AZT during the last trimester of pregnancy, intravenously during delivery, and treating the newborn child for six weeks after birth dramatically reduced perinatal HIV transmission, but at a cost of about 800 dollars per pregnancy (Conner et al., 1994). This made the 076 regimen unaffordable in all of sub-Saharan Africa, in countries with the highest number of perinatal transmissions. The regimen was also logistically difficult to implement in routine prenatal care in high prevalence countries. There was therefore an urgent need to develop affordable and feasible alternatives for these countries, and a number of trials with shorter versions of the regimen were initiated. All of these, except one trial in Thailand, used placebo in the control group. In June 1997, before the controversy had erupted in major medical journals, the design was defended by the major sponsors of the trials:

The CDC is not using the ACTG-076 regimen in the current studies because although those results have changed the standard of care in the United States and other industrialized countries, the standard of care for treating HIV infected pregnancies remains "no intervention. The intent in the current studies is to answer the question which is most relevant for public health decision makers in developing countries: 'Does AZT, when given at this specific dose for four weeks, result in a lower perinatal HIV transmission rate compared to untreated women.' There is consensus at WHO, UNAIDS, and in countries where these trials are being conducted that the full regimen of ACTG-076 could not currently be implemented as standard of care. Another reason that placebo trials have been recommended is because it is necessary to change multiple parameters from the ACTG-076 regimen. . . A placebo trial is the most scientifically valid way to determine the effect of these changes. Moreover, a placebo design . . . allows for a 'streamlined study' which can provide an answer within one to two years after the start of the study . . .. A study design that compares a short AZT regimen with the long ACTG-076 AZT regiment would not meet the study objectives, in other words, it would not answer the question, 'Does short course AZT work to prevent perinatal transmission?' This would not indicate whether the short AZT regimen was better than the currently available intervention – nothing at all . . . One of the most important ethical considerations in conducting clinical trial research is that participants in the research should not receive less care than would be available to them if they were not involved in the research. Since AZT is not currently available for perinatal HIV prevention in Thailand and Ivory Coast, the placebo-controlled trial design is consistent with that principle (CDC, 1997).

Not everyone agreed with this position, however. Already in 1995, the investigators responsible for one non-placebo-controlled trial in Thailand wrote in a letter to *Science*:

We firmly believe that it would be unethical to incorporate a placebo arm in our study in Thailand . . .. Adding a placebo arm to our study design could provide added reassurance that the 076 regimen is as effective in the Thai population as in the original study and a more definite estimate of the degree of efficacy of the shortened regimen over no treatment. However, we believe that this scientific justification does not outweigh the ethical imperative to provide all subjects with a treatment that is consistent with current scientific knowledge about the efficacy of AZT in preventing transmission and with the emerging standard of care in the country in which the study is undertaken (Lallemant et al., 1995).

Although the criticism of the placebo studies was voiced in the literature from 1995 (see, for example, Cohen, 1995), not much happened until the Public Citizens Health Research Group criticized the trials in a congressional hearing on bioethics (Cohen, 1997). There were a number of news reports of these hearings, but they went largely unnoticed by the general media until Marcia Angell criticized the trials in an editorial in the *New England Journal of Medicine*, (Angell, 1997b). The editorial was accompanied by a Sounding Board article by Lurie and Wolfe from the Public Citizens Health Research Group (Lurie and Wolf, 1997). They argued that the placebo-controlled trials were unethical as they denied the control group a proven beneficial treatment. According to the then current version of the Declaration of Helsinki, all the participants 'should be assured of the best proven diagnostic and therapeutic method'. They also claimed that a placebo trial might not require fewer subjects nor would it take longer to get the necessary results. In their article, Lurie and Wolf countered the arguments that, as no treatment is the standard of care in developing countries, research subjects in the placebo group would not be denied the available treatments in that country, by pointing out that the reason for this standard of care is economic. However, it would not be difficult for economic reasons to provide the participants in the study with AZT in the required amount: this would not add much to the cost of the study. They recognized that it might not be justifiable to provide more expensive forms of care, such as treatment in coronary care units.

In a subsequent Op-Ed letter, Joseph Saba of UNAIDS and Arthur Amman of the American Foundation for AIDS research defended the trials (Saba and Amman, 1997). They argued that the trials conformed to international guidelines, had been approved by ethics committees in the countries concerned and were necessary in order to find an effective intervention for great health problems. Critics would be guilty of 'imposing their standards of care on developing countries. Local health experts, bioethicists and affected groups are best qualified to judge the risks and benefits of any medical research', and the trials 'adhere to one of the basic ethical principles of any

study, regardless of locale: that the planned intervention can be applied in the country in which it is tested'. In a reply, Marcia Angell pointed out that the trials did not conform to the requirement of the Declaration of Helsinki that 'in any medical study, every patient – including those of a control group, if any – should assured of the best proven diagnostic and therapeutic method'; it was therefore not a matter of imposing US standards on others, but breaking an international agreement. She also maintained that 'researchers knowingly consign many newborns to HIV' (Angell, 1997a). A member of the *New England Journal of Medicine* editorial board, David Ho, criticized Angell, and he subsequently resigned from the editorial board in protest against the editorial (Ho, 1997). The editorial was defended in a subsequent editorial authored by both the editor-in-chief and Angell (Kassirer and Angell, 1997).

Varmus and Satcher reiterated the position of the CDC and NIH in a subsequent article (Varmus and Satcher, 1997). In this article, they argued that

'the most compelling reason to use a placebo-controlled study is that it provides definite answers to questions about safety and value of an intervention in the setting in which the study is performed, and these answers are the point of research . . . comparing an intervention of unknown benefit – especially one that is affordable in a developing country – with the only intervention with a known benefit (the 076 regimen) may provide information that is not useful to patients. If the affordable intervention is less effective than the 076 regimen – not an unlikely outcome – this information will be of little use in a country where the more effective regimen is unavailable. Equally important, it will still be unclear whether the affordable intervention is better than nothing and worth the investment of scarce resources' (1997, pp. 1004–1005).

THE CENTRAL ELEMENTS OF THE CONTROVERSY

The main argument of those who defended the placebo-controlled trials and the need to adapt standards of treatment in trials to local circumstances was that under certain specific conditions a placebo-controlled trial is scientifically necessary in order to obtain knowledge that is relevant for the country in which the trial takes place. Those who criticized the trials essentially had two arguments. First, they maintained that valid results could be obtained by using equivalence trials. Second, they objected to the trials because researchers withheld known, effective interventions from the trial participants, interventions they could easily provide in the context of the trial.

The first argument is central in the sense that although scientific need in and of itself would not justify the trials, without any scientific need to do the trials with a lesser standard of care, there seems to be no good reason why the control group should not be offered state-of-the-art intervention, even though it is not routinely available outside the clinical trial context, if it can easily be provided without adding much to the cost of the trial. Some might worry about undue inducement to participate in the trial because the trial participants would receive interventions that would not be available to them outside the trial. However, given the clear advantages of entering such a trial, it cannot be construed as a case of being pressured to participate against one's better judgement.

Those who argued that it was necessary to include a placebo group in the perinatal HIV transmission trials pointed out that there was no reliable knowledge from African countries about the transmission rate in an untreated population, and it was known that the transmission rate varied over time, even in the same location. In such circumstances an equivalence trial, comparing the long 076 treatment with the short course treatment, would not be able to provide the crucial data of interest to developing countries: how much better is the short course treatment compared with placebo? In general, for a placebo-controlled trial to be scientifically necessary, then, two conditions need to be fulfilled. First, there has to be a variable response rate in the untreated group, or the group receiving whatever is the local standard of care. Second, it is impossible to know beforehand what the response rate is for any given population (Ellenberg and Temple, 2000; Temple and Ellenberg, 2000). If both of these conditions are fulfilled, a trial comparing the universal standard of care with a proposed cheaper alternative will not answer the question whether the proposed cheaper alternative to the universal standard of care is not significantly better than the local standard of care. If that is the question one wants to be answered, the trial has the wrong design.

Consider the following hypothetical trial. The trial has three arms: a local standard of care, a proposed more effective cheaper standard of care, and the expensive universal standard of care. Table 98.1 shows two possible outcomes of the trial in two different populations with different death rates utilizing the local standard of care. Let us first assume that we carry out a trial with only two arms, the cheaper standard of care and the universal standard of care, giving us the results provided in Table 98.1. From this trial we would conclude that the cheaper standard of care is significantly worse than the universal standard of care. We could, however, not conclude anything about how it compared with the local standard of care, if we know that the death rate in response to local standard of care can vary between 20% and 30%, and if we have no way of knowing what the death rate is in the population being studied (the two conditions above). If the death rate happens to be 20%, the

cheaper standard is no better than the local standard of care. If, however, the death rate is 30%, the cheaper standard is indeed better than the local standard of care. If we are interested in answering the question whether the proposed cheaper standard of care is better than the local standard of care, a trial with only two arms, universal standard of care and the cheaper standard of care, will not be able to answer *that* question.

The crucial question is therefore whether there is no reliable knowledge about the effect of the local standard of care, in this case perinatal transmission rates without any interventions. Given the evidence from both before the trials started and the results of the various trials that were conducted, a strong case can be made that this was indeed the case (Karim, 1998; Wendler, Emanuel and Lie, 2004). This does not, of course, in and of itself justify the placebo-controlled trials. It only establishes that in certain circumstances, if one wants a specific question answered, one has to do a trial in a certain way. Those who defended the placebo-controlled trials could point out that doing the trials with placebo controls, or a local standard of care, would leave nobody worse off than they were already, and had the potential of producing knowledge of great benefit to the countries in which the trials took place. It remains the case, however, that if the premise is that one could easily provide the intervention to the participants of the trial, one does not provide a proven beneficial intervention to people who need it, in this case, for the sake of the common good, and some people do find that objectionable.

This brings us to the second argument against the trials. Even if one could establish a scientific need for the studies, there may be something inherently wrong with not providing people in trials with interventions that are established to be effective, if they are available to people with greater access to resources, and if they could easily be provided in the context of the trial. This possible counter-argument is considerably weakened, however, because it would also be an argument against an equivalence trial: in such a trial, the control group would receive a treatment that was known to be inferior to the established standard of care. The equivalence trial therefore would violate the same ethical standards as the placebo trial. One might, of course, want to argue that the equivalence trial is superior

Table 98.1 Two possible outcomes of the trial in two different populations with different death rates utilizing the local standard of care

Population	Local standard	Cheaper standard	Universal standard
1	20%	15%	8%
2	30%	15%	8%

because everyone is at least getting *something*. This may very well be the case, but it remains a fact that one also in this case does sacrifice the interests of some of the people in the trial for the sake of the common good; so if one accepts the equivalence trial, one has at least in principle accepted that this is justified in some cases. Irrespective of the argument about scientific necessity of the placebo-controlled trials in the case of the perinatal HIV transmission studies, the central issues in the debate are therefore (1) is it ever justified to offer participants in trials interventions that are known to be inferior to what is considered a state of the art intervention? and (2) if so, under what conditions would it be justified?

EXAMPLES OF TRIALS PROVIDING LESS THAN THE UNIVERSAL STANDARD OF CARE

In order to answer these questions, it might be helpful to consider in what types of trials one may want to provide a lesser standard of care. The perinatal HIV transmission study was, of course, one such trial, but the evaluation of that trial is complicated by the fact that it was placebo-controlled and has been subject to an already highly emotional debate. It may be morally relevant that one provides nothing rather than something to the control group, although the standard of care debate is only peripherally related to the debate of the use of placebos. The central issue in the standard of care debate is whether it is ever justified to provide an intervention known to be inferior to that which is provided to participants in trials in resource-rich settings.

Consider trials to study effects of interventions to prevent transmission from mother to child during breast feeding. Even if one is able to prevent transmission from mother to child during pregnancy and delivery, there still is a substantial risk of transmission during the breast feeding period. In rich countries, this transmission is prevented by insisting that mothers should formula-feed their babies. In poor countries, because of inadequate access to clean water, breast feeding could still be recommended for HIV-positive mothers. Even with the risk of HIV infection, the risk of other life-threatening infections from contaminated water is greater. There is therefore a need to identify interventions that might prevent transmission in mothers who breast feed their babies. Several trials are underway to compare various combinations of drugs. If one takes the position that participants in trials should not be denied known effective interventions that could easily be provided to the participants in the trial, it would seem that these trials are all unethical. There is a known, effective intervention available that could easily be provided to the mothers without much cost in the context of a trial. This intervention is close to

100% effective in preventing transmission during the normal breastfeeding period.

Those who defend this trial would point out that it is essential to identify interventions that can be implemented given the realities of the lack of clean water supply in resource poor settings. Realistically, even though one might wish otherwise, clean water is not going to be readily available in the foreseeable future. There is thus an urgent need to identify interventions that can prevent HIV transmission given that context. Insisting on providing all participants in trials state of the art interventions would make trials that could identify such interventions impossible.

Consider another example provided by Killen et al. (2002). The gold standard for monitoring the effect of treatment is measurement of viral load. This is expensive and difficult to carry out in resource-poor settings. There is therefore an urgent need to develop treatment monitoring that can be more easily implemented, in particular now that the drugs themselves are affordable and are being made available even in the most resource poor settings. One might therefore wish to propose at trial to compare viral load measurements with an alternative such as measurements of total lymphocyte count. Again, having such an arm in the trial accepts that it is legitimate to provide some of the participants with a standard that is less than that which would be routinely provided in resource rich settings, as nobody expects the alternative monitoring scheme to be as good as viral load measurements. The point of doing the trial, however, is to decide if it is good enough to be used as an alternative where the gold standard cannot be implemented for economic or logistical reasons.

REVISIONS OF GUIDELINES

The debate that erupted in 1997 led to a revision process of established guidelines, such as the Declaration of Helsinki and the CIOMS guidelines. The World Medical Association adopted a revised Declaration in 2000, essentially affirming the universal standard of the 1996 version. Article 29 now says that

> The benefits, risks, burdens and effectiveness of a new method should be tested against those of the best current prophylactic, diagnostic, and therapeutic methods. This does not exclude the use of placebo, or no treatment, in studies where no proven prophylactic, diagnostic or therapeutic method exists.

Other guidelines have, however, not followed the recommendation of the World Medical Association. This is the case for the UNAIDS Guidance Document for HIV preventive vaccine research, the 2002 CIOMS guidelines, the report issued by the National Bioethics Advisory Committee (NBAC) in the United States, the report published by the Nuffield Council on Bioethics and the recommendation by the European Group on Ethics of the European Commission (Council for International Organizations of Medical Sciences, 2002; European Group on Ethics in Science and New Technologies, 2003; National Bioethics Advisory Commission, 2001; Nuffield Council on Bioethics, 2002; UNAIDS, 2000). Common to all of these guidelines is the presumption that researchers have an obligation to provide participants with a universal standard of care in the control group, but under certain circumstances exceptions might be allowed.

For our purposes here, the 2002 version of the CIOMS guidelines is the most interesting, because it provides specific conditions for the exception to be justified. Although guideline 11, which deals with the choice of control in clinical trial itself, does not mention the possibility of the type of exception considered here, the commentary is quite clear that ethics committees can, after careful considerations and under certain conditions, approve studies with less than universal standards of care. The placement of the exception in the commentary rather than in the guideline itself is perhaps a reflection of the difficulty of this issue. According to CIOMS, if the ethics committee is satisfied that the trial is responsive to the health needs of the population and that there is assurance that the intervention will be made reasonably available if it proves to be safe and effective, and if the trial design is scientifically necessary, then

> an ethical committee can approve a clinical trial in which the comparator is other than an established effective intervention, such as placebo or no treatment or a local remedy

According to CIOMS, then, in the special circumstances when a trial design is scientifically necessary, the trial is likely to yield knowledge relevant to the host country, *and* there is reasonable assurance that the results will indeed be used for the benefit of the country in terms of availability of interventions, one can allow for an exception to the general rule.

We have argued that the guidance provided by the CIOMS guidelines now should be regarded as the international consensus opinion (Lie et al., 2004). It seems to be endorsed by all major guidelines and recommendations, except the Declaration of Helsinki. Not all have agreed with this position, although little documentary evidence has been provided to support the view that there is no such emerging consensus (Schüklenk, 2004). A further indication of the emerging consensus is the report of the consultation in 2004 by the Nuffield Council, again with representatives from a wide range of countries. According to the report, 'the use of a regional or local standard of care as a comparator is now seen to be acceptable in some situations, as set out in the guidance of [the 2002 CIOMS guidelines]' (p. 33) and 'During discussion, delegates reported that local ethics committees

appear to be increasingly sympathetic to the use of regional and local standards as a comparator, rather than a universal standard, for clinical trials' (Nuffield Council on Bioethics, 2005, p. 27).

CONCLUDING REMARKS

What can one conclude from this brief overview? All the international guidelines examined, except the Helsinki Declaration, allow for exceptions to a universal standard of care. All of the guidelines also affirm strongly that the ideal should be to provide the universal standard of care, and that any exceptions require careful justification. There is some variation in the types of reasons accepted, and some variation in the minimum standard of care that can be provided during the trial. However, all guidelines accept that the main justification for making an exception would be that a design using a local standard of care is necessary in order to obtain results that are useful in the setting in which the trial takes place.

Finally, one should note that the main concern of those who are critical of allowing different standards of care in different countries is that this will lead to an exploitation of poor countries. If one allows exceptions to a universal standard of care, then studies which are not allowed in rich countries, because they are too risky or involve denying participants established interventions, can be carried out in countries with less stringent oversight procedures. Not only might research with potential benefits for the host country be approved, but the fear is that research where the primary beneficiaries are in rich countries will also be approved. This is not just a theoretical possibility; the critics can point to trials where this has actually happened. As is evident from the guidelines referred to above, however, all of the guidelines that allow exceptions do so with the presumptions that the approved trial design is necessary in order to obtain useful knowledge for the community in which the trial takes place. The crucial issue is therefore whether one can be certain that the system of research ethics approval will approve only this type of trials, and reject the others. The related question is whether it is possible to propose specific enough criteria that will be useful for research ethics review committees in terms of what constitutes sufficient guarantee that the proposed intervention will become available if it is found to be safe and effective. That is perhaps the greatest challenge, and a satisfactory account of how one should think about the benefits of research would probably do much to diminish the differences between those who are sceptical of different standards and those who think they are necessary to develop useful interventions for health problems that the majority of the people in the world face.

One might speculate that the placement of the exception in the CIOMS commentary reflects a certain degree of unease with the conclusion and the choices one is forced to make. In an *ideal* world, of course, everyone would have access to the best possible care, independent of local circumstances, and independent of the availability of funds. *Our* world, however, is an unjust world characterized by huge disparities in access to health care. Responsible people everywhere should see it as their responsibility to reduce these disparities. Some of us may conclude that the best way to do this at this moment is to identify interventions that right now are affordable in resource poor settings, even if the means to do so involves using different standards of care in research in different settings. Others may conclude that the risks in terms of abuse of this strategy are too great, and that one should instead work directly towards the long-term goal of reducing health disparities. Ultimately, it seems that the disagreement about whether we allow exceptions or not depends on these perhaps more fundamental disagreements about what the most appropriate global health policy should be. If this is correct, it also means that neither side should accuse the other of taking a morally unacceptable position, but should recognize that reasonable people can and will disagree about these issues.

DISCLAIMER AND ACKNOWLEDGEMENT

The opinions expressed in this chapter are the author's own. They do not reflect any position or policy of the National Institutes of Health, US Public Health Service, or Department of Health and Human Services.

This research was supported by the Intramural Research Program of the NIH Clinical Center.

REFERENCES

Angell M. AIDS studies violate Helsinki rights accord. *New York Times*, 24 September 1997; A26.

Angell M. The ethics of clinical research in the third world. *N Engl J Med* 1997; **337**: 847–849.

CDC. CDC studies of AZT to prevent mother-to-child HIV transmission in developing countries. *The Body* (http://www.the-body.com/hivatis/devlques.html), June 1997.

Cohen J. Bringing AZT to poor countries. *Science* 1995; **269**: 624–626.

Cohen J. Ethics of AZT studies in poorer countries attacked. *Science* 1997; **276**: 1022.

Conner EM, Sperling RJ, Gelber R, et al. Reduction of maternal–infant transmission of human immunodeficiency virus type 1 with zidovudine treatment. *N Engl J Med* 1994; **331**: 1173–1180.

Council for International Organizations of Medical Sciences. *International Ethical Guidelines for Biomedical Research Involving Human Subjects*. Geneva: CIOMS, 2002.

Ellenberg SS, Temple R. Placebo-controlled trials and active control trials in the evaluation of new treatments. Part 2. Practical issues and specific cases. *Ann Intern Med* 2000; **133**: 464–470.

European Group on Ethics in Science and New Technologies. *Ethical Aspects of Clinical Research in Developing Countries*. Brussels: European Commission, 2003.

Ho DD. It's AIDS, not Tuskegee. Inflammatory comparisons won't save lives in Africa. *Newsweek*, 29 September 1997.

Karim SSA. Placebo controlled trials in HIV perinatal transmission trials: a South African's viewpoint. *Am J Public Health* 1998; **88**: 564–566.

Kassirer JP, Angell M. Controversial journal editorials. *N Engl J Med* 1997; **337**: 1460–1461.

Killen J, Grady C, Folkers GK, Fauci AC. Ethics of clinical research in the developing world' *Nat Rev Immunul* 2002; **2**: 210–215.

Lallemant M, Le Coeur S, McIntosh K, Brennan T, Gelber R, Lee T-H, et al. AZT trial in Thailand. *Science* 1995; **270**: 899–900.

Lie RK, Emanuel EJ, Grady C, Wendler D. The standard of care debate: the international consensus opinion versus the Declaration of Helsinki. *J Med Ethics* 2004; 30: 190–193.

Lurie P, Wolf SM. Unethical trials of interventions to reduce perinatal transmission of the human immunodeficiency virus in developing countries. *N Engl J Med* 1997; **337**.

National Bioethics Advisory Commission. *Ethical and Policy Issues in International Research: Clinical Trials in Developing Countries*, Vol. I. Bethesda, MD: National Bioethics Advisory Commission, 2001.

Nuffield Council on Bioethics. *The Ethics Of Research Related to Research in Developing Countries*. London: Nuffield Council on Bioethics. London: Nuffield Council, 2002.

Nuffield Council on Bioethics. *The Ethics of Research Related to Healthcare in Developing Countries. A Follow-Up Discussion Paper*. London: Nuffield Council, 2005.

Saba J, Amman A. A cultural divide on AIDS research. *New York Times*, 20 September 1997.

Schüklenk U. The standard of care debate: against the myth of an 'international consensus opinion'. *J Med Ethics* 2004; **30**: 194–197.

Temple R, Ellenberg SS. Placebo-controlled trials and active-control trials in the evaluation of new treatments. Part 1. Ethical and scientific issues. *Ann Intern Med* 2000; **133**: 455–463.

UNAIDS. *Ethical Considerations in HIV Preventive Vaccine Research. UNAIDS Guidance Document*. Geneva: UNAIDS, 2000.

Varmus H, Satcher D. Ethical complexities of conducting research in developing countries. *N Engl J Med* 1997; **337**: 1003–1005.

Wendler D, Emanuel EJ, Lie RK. The standard of care debate: can research in developing countries be both ethical and responsive to those countries' health needs? *Am J Public Health* 2004; **94**: 923–928.

99

Justice and Priority Setting in International Health Care Research

SOLOMON R. BENATAR

INTRODUCTION

The current state of wide disparities in health across the world represents the backdrop against which the challenge of resource allocation for international health research must be viewed. However, in order to work towards constructive changes in resource allocation for medical research, it is first necessary to understand the role of powerful global forces in shaping health care systems and the medical research agenda. It is also necessary to consider what is meant by progress and development if new ideas are to be successfully applied to the medical research agenda and to improving health.

THE GLOBAL SETTING FOR RESEARCH

DISPARITIES IN WEALTH AND HEALTH

Despite unprecedented economic growth (seven-fold in the latter half of the twentieth century) and impressive progress in science, technology, wealth creation and in social governance, the world at the beginning of the twenty-first century is characterized by seemingly endless widening disparities in wealth and health and the recrudescence of infectious diseases that profoundly threaten life everywhere.

At the beginning of the twentieth century, the wealthiest 20% of the world's population were nine times richer than the poorest 20%. This ratio has grown progressively to 30 times by 1960, 60 times by 1990 and to over 86 times by 2000. Such economic disparities are associated with similar wide disparities in health and longevity (Benatar, 1998) that have been described as a form of global apartheid (Alexander, 1996).

Life expectancy at birth ranges from well over 70 years in highly industrialized countries to below 50 years in many poor countries, and in some countries in Africa it is 40 years and dropping – largely due to the HIV/AIDS pandemic (United Nations Development Report, 2000). Disparities in health and life expectancy are also observed between rich and poor in rich countries (Wilkinson, 1996).

The World Health Organization (WHO) estimated that in 1998, 10 million children and adults of working age died of six infectious diseases that could have been prevented at the cost of $20 per life saved. Among the poorest quintile of people in the world, 55% of the deaths are from communicable diseases, as compared with 5% of the deaths among the richest quintile (WHO, 1995).

Demographically developing countries bear over 80% of the global burden of disease in disability-adjusted life years, and these include about 4.5 billion of the world's people. This burden is likely to increase as the epidemiological transition progresses, with added disability and suffering resulting from non-communicable causes such as vascular disease, malignant neoplasms (especially of the lung associated with smoking), neuropsychiatric diseases, accidents and trauma.

In the late 1990s, global expenditure on health care amounted to about US$2.2 trillion. Of this, 87% was spent on about 16% of the world's population and on those bearing 7% of the global burden of diseases expressed in DALYs (Iglehart, 1999). Per capita expenditure on health ranges from over $3000 annually in advanced modern societies down to less than $15 in countries containing half the world's population.

About 1 billion people have access to most of what modern medicine can offer, while the remaining 5 billion people

Principles of Health Care Ethics, Second Edition   Edited by R.E. Ashcroft, A. Dawson, H. Draper and J.R. McMillan
© 2007 John Wiley & Sons, Ltd

make do with much less. The poorest 1 billion people in the world benefit so little from modern medicine that, from their perspective, most of the progress made in the last 100 years is almost irrelevant.

A DISTORTED AGENDA FOR MEDICAL RESEARCH

Examination of expenditure on medical research reveals a similar pattern with 90% of annual global expenditure on medical research (over US $75 billion in the early 2000s) being spent on those diseases that account for 10% of the global burden of disease (Commission on Health Research for Development, 1990). These imbalances in expenditure of resources on research (and on medical care) are augmented by the degree to which they have been driven increasingly by commercial interests in the United States and other so-called developed countries (Relman and Angell, 2002).

Of 1393 new chemical entities marketed between 1975 and 1999, only 16 were for tropical diseases and tuberculosis, despite the fact that these latter diseases account for enormous mortality and morbidity (Troullier et al., 2002). The pharmaceutical industry (through provision of almost 50% of global medical research expenditure) has an inappropriately large role in shaping the agendas for research and medical care around the world (Angell, 2000; Angell and Relman, 2002).[1] This research agenda is strongly influenced by the pharmaceutical market (which was worth about $406 billion globally in 2002), with 60% of the profits being made in the United States (5% of the world's population). The search for blockbuster drugs that could be used by many, even the well, for example to prevent baldness, osteoporosis and ageing or to improve sexual function, is more appealing economically than research on new drugs for tuberculosis or other diseases that predominantly affect the poor.

Industry expenditure on clinical trials has increased from US$3.2 billion in 1994 to $10 billion in 2004, with the proportion of this expenditure allocated to academic medical centres falling during this period from 63% to 26% in 2004. Given the competitiveness of the marketplace, it is also not surprising that industry attempts to control research data and

its publication. Standards set by academic medical centres to limit restrictions imposed by sponsors vary greatly across institutions in the United States (Mello, 2004). Attempts by the American medical colleges to develop standardized contracts to limit gag clauses and protect academic freedom have not yet been successful (Steinbrook, 2005). A recent report outlining the conflict of interest between physicians' commitment to patient care and pressure from pharmaceutical companies to sell their products (Brennan and Rothman, 2006) has achieved a high media profile (Harris, 2006). It thus seems that market forces are a dominant shaper of the research agenda and a powerful influence on researchers (Lemmens, 2004).

Another force shaping research activities is scientific curiosity. Advances in science and technology have allowed exploration of very large structures (the universe) and very small structures (for example, viruses, genetic structures, and nano-particles). Growth of knowledge in these fields has been stimulated by military and space research, and by human and plant genetic biotechnology. Because advances in these areas contribute to national power and dominance, they are given high priority and attract vast sums of money (Burrows, 2002).[2]

The research agenda is also influenced by consideration of whose lives are important and valued. In general terms favoured lives are those of the wealthy and powerful, as illustrated by the patterns of expenditure on medical care and research. Despite the much acclaimed Universal Declaration of Human Rights and the ongoing hand-wringing by wealthy nations about reducing poverty and improving health in developing countries, the paucity of resources devoted to such activities and the inadequacy of methods used belie any serious major commitment to human wellbeing at a population level (The Global Fund, 2002/2003; Changing Course, 2005). We should face the fact that the way the global economy works is a vivid indication that some lives are valued much more than others. It seems that the pursuit of ever-increasing wealth, luxuries and the esoteric interests of a small segment of the world's population outweighs the value placed on achieving access to even the basic needs for human existence for a large majority (Benatar, 2005).

[1]The pharmaceutical industry enjoys an almost unique place as a business. Its marketing and administrative costs amount to 30% of revenue, whereas research and development costs amount to only 12% of revenue. Profits, at 19% of revenue, exceed profits of commercial banks (15.8%) and those of other industries (0.5–12.1%). Moreover, the tax rate for the pharmaceutical industry (16.2% for 1993–1996) is much lower than for major American industries (27.3%). As 60% of global pharmaceutical industry profits are made in the USA, and Federal Drug and Administration links to industry are growing (with funding and staffing conflicts of interest implications, and with neither the FDA nor the US patent office taking action against abuses of the patent system), it is not surprising that American interests in market-based individual health care dominate globally, and that public health is neglected.

[2]The attractiveness of military and space research to governments is illustrated by the fact that in the 1980s, 64% of $487 billion research and development expenditure in the United States was devoted to military research, 7% to space research and only 22% to various forms of civilian research. In the same decade the then European Council spent 26% of $320 billion research and development expenditure on the military and 5% on space, with 59% on civilian research. Since the events of 9/11, there have been massive increases in expenditure on bio-terrorism research.

All of the above considerations illustrate that the pursuit of knowledge is not value-free. In general terms it is true to say that the questions that are asked and researched by scientists are those that attract resources.

THE UNDERLYING CHALLENGE

The challenge of achieving improved health for a greater proportion of the world's population is one of the most pressing moral problems of our time and is starkly illustrated by the threat of infectious diseases. A few decades ago, there was hope that the major infectious diseases plaguing humankind could be eliminated. The World Health Organization's unprecedented success with smallpox was a remarkable model. However, the recrudescence of tuberculosis and malaria in multiresistant forms, the appearance of HIV infection and other new infectious diseases such as SARS have dashed such hopes and have illustrated the limitations of a narrowly focused scientific approach to public health. Communicable diseases continue to be a leading cause of loss of human life and potential, as illustrated by the threat of the next pandemic of avian flu (Osterholm, 2005; Fauci, 2006).

The adverse historical, political and economic factors that sustain poverty and contribute to the ecological niches conducive to the rise and spread of these diseases cannot be ignored. The control of infectious diseases is not merely a problem for individual nations but for the whole world (Kassalow, 2001). Infections have no respect for geographic boundaries, particularly in an era of extensive and rapid transportation.

Chronic diseases are also becoming more prevalent in both developed and developing countries, producing a double burden of disease. So health is also being impaired by consumption of mass-produced, highly processed western foods that contribute to obesity and diabetes, and by the relentless marketing of tobacco that has such adverse effects on the heart, blood vessels, lungs, and indeed many other organs. Violence associated with the trade in small arms, illicit drugs and commercial sex are additional factors adversely affecting health (Friman, 1999).

THREATS TO THE SOCIAL REPRODUCTION OF CARING INSTITUTIONS

Political scientists Isabella Bakker and Stephen Gill postulate that a global political economy hospitable to a neoliberal economic ideology, favoured by transnational corporations and large investors, has led to progressive disintegration of previous structures of community (Bakker and Gill, 2003). As a consequence, there is an emerging contradiction between the global accumulation of capital and the provision of stable conditions for social reproduction of caring insti-

tutions – for example, those that provide equitable access to education and heath care.

They argue that changes in social relations are intensifying exploitation of labour by expansion of a primitive labour market characterized by (i) disposable (part-time) labour, (ii) the feminization of survival (women are required to work to ensure adequate family income) and (iii) racialized /gendered patterns of exploitative migration (attracting cheap labour, usually people of colour, from other countries). Thus accumulation of resources and the social reproduction of the caring institutions required for societies to flourish have become different and contradictory forces in the same system. This contradiction is being locked in by neoliberal constitutional governance mechanisms, with damaging effects on the ability to reproduce social support systems for the majority of world's population.

Transformations associated with these contradictions in the field of health care include the reprivatization of social reproduction of medical research, health education and health care and intensification of exploitation of patients, health professionals and researchers. These transformations result in increasing use of migrant health workers, exploitation of labour, conversion of medicine into a marketable commodity accessible predominantly to those with resources, feminization of labour (a growing proportion of women in medicine), privatization of risk through rising premiums and reduced cover and deflection of medical research towards profitable markets.

At the broader social level, there is erosion of socially supported health care, removal of the automatic social stabilizers of the Keynesian era, and enclosure and appropriation of the commons. An example of the enclosure of the commons is the patenting of knowledge about the human genome instead of preserving such knowledge in the public realm for wider benefit.

The consequent impact on health of these trends is manifest in widening disparities in health and life expectancy, within and between countries. Gill and Bakker conclude that 'There is an urgent need to develop new, critical approaches to human development, human security and human rights as a credible alternative to dominant market-based forms of governance'.

THE PROBLEM OF DEVELOPMENT

It is now more clearly evident than ever that efforts to address serious global problems are both dominated and thwarted by a conception of development that is predominantly focused on economic growth. It is also increasingly acknowledged that rather than there being a significant trickle-down effect, economic growth is predominantly funnelled upwards towards the wealthy. Against a backdrop of ideologically driven discourses on growth, free trade and security on a global scale, with increasing health disparities between rich and poor *between* and *within* countries, and evidence of flaws in the economic conception of development, new ideas and forces for development are urgently required.

A new model for development has been proposed that transcends the North–South dichotomy and that goes beyond a narrow conception of development as an economic process. This requires a paradigm shift towards a new metaphor that *develops* sustainability, rather than sustains development (Bensimon and Benatar, 2006).

This new paradigm of development abandons four flawed assumptions lying behind previous approaches: (i) that developing countries' problems are entirely internal; (ii) that developed countries are an example to be globally emulated; (iii) that the role of developed countries in promoting development is defined by altruism; and (iv) that the poor lack the potential to improve their own lives significantly.

Among the features of this new paradigm is explicit inclusion of the ethical challenge of effectively addressing wide disparities in global health. It would be hard to deny that the vast numbers of global poor and their lower life expectancy represent a clear and significant injustice. One way to analyse this injustice is through the lens of global distributive justice – for example, in terms of an obligation to redistribute resources from rich countries to poor countries. If we can agree, against the background of the above scenario, that this is an ethical solution, then the challenge becomes to determine how to pursue this goal.

JUSTICE IN THE ALLOCATION OF RESOURCES

As not much has been written about justice in allocating resources for medical research, I begin here by discussing resource allocation for health care as a potential model for thinking about resource allocation for medical research.

Because resources are inadequate to provide all that medicine can offer to all in need and because of growing concern about equity, priority setting in the use of public resources for medical care within countries has become essential in many countries. It has also been argued that priority-setting is a requirement of democracy as it encourages academics, professionals, scientists, politicians and administrators to reflect on allocation decisions, to attain deeper insights into their implications and to take public responsibility for decisions. Moreover, explicit priority-setting facilitates moral development of citizens by encouraging them not to believe that they are entitled to everything that is technically possible in health care, especially when benefits are only marginal (Doyal, 1997).

Explicit rationing requires the use of such techniques as cost-effectiveness analysis, systematic reviews of outcomes, scoring systems such as QUALYs (quality adjusted life years), as well as clarity about objectives, information about costs and outcomes and the ability to measure performance. These techniques place emphasis on such values as effectiveness and efficiency – both important social values but not the only ones.

Central to priority-setting is the question of distributive justice. However, ideas of what distributive justice means substantively and how it can be achieved vary greatly. Some believe in individual freedom as the most important political value to promote in the pursuit of fairness. Others are more concerned about equity, solidarity and contractual theories of justice that could contribute to achieving the ideal of a harmonious public life. Perspectives on justice also differ across disciplines. For example, philosophers are mainly interested in developing comprehensive and justifiable theories of distributive justice, while lawyers concentrate on promoting the right to health care, non-discrimination, and the obligations of health care practitioners. Political scientists reflect on the fairness of decision-making processes. Health professionals tend to be caught up with the evidence base for medical practice as well as with considerations of best clinical judgement, while economists stress efficiency.

In the absence of a satisfactory theory of justice that can be applied in everyday life, American scholars Norman Daniels and James Sabin have proposed a process for priority-setting that they have called 'accountability for reasonableness' (Daniels and Sabin, 1997). This framework requires that four conditions be met. First, the data used and the values incorporated in the rationale for decisions must be publicly accessible. Second, decisions made about which health care needs are relevant to local needs must be made by fair-minded people. Third, allowance must be made for appeals so that previous decisions can be reconsidered in the light of new evidence or arguments. Fourth, there must be a process of enforcement that facilitates the implementation of the last three conditions.

Priority-setting needs to be addressed at several levels, and there will be different implications and even different approaches at each level. At national levels the budget for public health services is determined largely by the fiscal policy of governments – hopefully influenced in democratic countries by the 'will of the people' and the priority they give to health care. Within regional geographical areas, allocation decisions are potentially influenced by policies of both national and regional governments. For particular diseases (for example, tuberculosis or malaria) or forms of treatment (for example, chronic dialysis), resource allocation decisions are shaped by central, regional and local health authorities. It has been proposed that equity can be preserved to some extent against considerations of effectiveness and efficiency by introducing the principle of non-abandonment at the macro level of resource allocation. This requires that a relevant proportion of the overall health budget be allocated to each speciality in medical practice to ensure that all patients, even those requiring expensive treatments, have at least some opportunity to be treated (Landman and Henley, 1999).

The framework proposed by Daniels and Sabin is of potential value at each level. Although this framework was developed in the context of the United States' privately funded health care system, Martin and colleagues have shown that it is workable and acceptable within the Canadian publicly funded system (Martin, Giacomini and Singer, 2002). The centrality of fairness in priority-setting became clear in their empirical study of priority-setting processes for new technologies in cancer and cardiac care in Ontario. They identified the importance of seeking multiple perspectives on the problem under review, ensuring transparency and honesty in the decision-making process, identifying potential conflicts of interest and achieving consensus. The recent detailed qualitative study by Martin and colleagues of how the framework of 'accountability for reasonableness' can be applied to access to ICUs for neurosurgery patients provides evidence that such a process improves the fairness of priority-setting (Martin, Singer and Bernstein, 2003).

Little is known about how resource allocation decisions are made in many countries, but some countries, for example, The Netherlands, Sweden, New Zealand, the United Kingdom and the state of Oregon in the United States, have moved to explicit rationing processes. Although the specific approaches in each of these countries differ, the common themes include the value of using well-publicized individual cases to bring priority-setting to public attention and the need to consult and involve the public to ensure that their views and values contribute to making judgements (Ham, 1997).

It is doubtful whether more than a few people know how resources are allocated at national, regional or institutional levels. Even at the level of major hospitals, such decisions seem to be made covertly and within a vacuum. Although many are acutely aware of the challenges at the micro level of the doctor–patient interaction, there is not yet an established medical institutional culture of trying to make such decisions in a rational and accountable manner.

It needs to be acknowledged that priority-setting is a complex process for which there is no simple or technical solution. The process is an exercise in policy learning, a struggle for power with varying implications at each of the levels described above, and is undertaken in different ways in different countries (Martin et al., 2000). Although significant progress is being made towards improving fairness

in the use and distribution of health services, much remains to be done.

In a world in which we all face common threats and in which democracy and social justice are being promoted, the argument for explicit priority-setting procedures, and accountability for these could also be applied to the global medical research agenda. However, as the procedures described above are best applied at the horizontal level of comparing different treatments for the same disease and it is more difficult to apply them vertically across different diseases, a balance needs to be shaped between favouring the good of individuals and the common good. A balance would also need to be established regarding the needs of different populations.

Giving due consideration to the burden of diseases within countries and across the world in allocating resources for medical research could facilitate achievement of such a balance. Embarking on procedures resembling those described by Daniels and Sabin could contribute to sensitizing leaders in global health to the need for moral development in decision-making at a level that has profound consequences for health.

NARROWING INJUSTICE – IS IT POSSIBLE?

Although the theoretical basis for, and extent of, any obligation to narrow injustice at the global level is controversial, such controversies should not eclipse the moral urgency of the practical problem that must be faced. Given the state of world health and widening disparities that threaten us all, it is entirely appropriate to seek practical means of reducing injustice (Changing Course, 2005; Pogge, 2005).

We have previously suggested that the principle of distributive justice in the research context requires that the burdens and benefits of research be fairly distributed among all involved. So, for example, we claimed that research initiatives themselves should not introduce new inequalities or further exacerbate existing inequalities in health in the community where research is being conducted, and that in the absence of an adequate theory of international distributive justice, it could be feasible to reduce gross injustices through reasonable and practical means (Shapiro and Benatar, 2005).

We also agree with the cogent arguments advanced by Pogge that richer sponsoring countries (governments, aid agencies, academic institutions and the pharmaceutical industry) have an ethical obligation to transfer resources to poorer nations on the grounds that they have long been and remain intimately involved with sustaining such poverty (Pogge, 2002, 2005). Contrary to the views of some that distributive justice and beneficence require continued transfer of resources so long as disparities exist, we also expressed the view that reasonable lines can be drawn.

We recommended that a minimum of 1% of the cost of a research project be allocated towards improving the standard of care in association with a project in developing countries. Although we did not unrealistically propose that research be shackled by excessive demands for associated medical care, we claimed that conducting research as though in a vacuum, oblivious to the basic health needs of research participants in developing countries, does not meet the ethical requirements of justice and beneficence (Pogge, 2002, 2005).

Taking considerations of social justice to a higher level, Gopal Sreenivasan has suggested the need to seek minimum interim measures, on which reasonable agreement should be possible, to enable urgent practical action to be undertaken. He has described this idea as an exercise in non-ideal theory and has proposed an obligation on the major seven countries in the Organisation for Economic Cooperation and Development to transfer 1% of their GDP to developing countries as an example of a minimal interim measure. Suitably targeted on basic health care and on the fundamental social determinants of health, this sum of money would make possible a significant improvement in life expectancy among the global poor (Sreenivasan, 2002).

In pursuit of social justice at the global level, Alan Buchanan has written a magisterial text outlining a systematic vision of an international legal system based on the commitment to justice for all persons (Buchanan, 2004). Others, writing in a recent special issue of *The Journal of Ethics* about the pursuit of cosmopolitan justice, have examined how such a project could be advanced (*Current debates in global justice,* 2005).

These endeavours represent early stages in the process of seeking imaginative moral and practical solutions to pervasive global injustice. We should not imagine that progress will take place easily or rapidly. However, honest recognition of the problem, scholarly approaches to defining how these important issues could be addressed and the development of practical solutions that could be implemented without undue delay would represent major steps forward. It is not too much to hope that in the next 50 years injustice could be somewhat diminished through redistribution of resources both for health care and for medical research.

CONCLUSIONS

Injustices in the allocation of resources for health and medical research are signs of systematic injustice at global and national levels that arise from the way in which the global economy operates. Powerful social and economic forces over many centuries, with escalating impact in the past 50 years, lie at the heart of the problem. While the successes

of economic growth and scientific advances should not be denied, suggestions that there may now be some evidence of entropy in the global economic and social system should not be ignored. Associated erosion of professionalism in medical practice (and in other professions) has serious adverse effects for society (Freidson, 2001; Global Forum for Health Research, 2002).

Striving for and achieving improvements in population health will require introspection about current values and seeking of imaginative new agendas. One of the most pressing moral challenges for the twenty-first century is to reduce gross inequities in health. Encouraging a universal ethical approach to medical care by placing equal value on the lives of all people through greater justice in health research and health care is one way of working towards such an ambitious goal.

REFERENCES

Alexander T. *Unravelling Global Apartheid: An Overview of World Politics.* Cambridge: Polity Press, 1996.

Angell M. The pharmaceutical industry – to whom is it accountable? *N Engl J Med* 2000; **342**: 1902–1904.

Bakker I, Gill S, eds. *Power, Production and Social Reproduction. Human in/Security in the Global Political Economy.* New York: Palgrave Macmillan, 2003.

Benatar SR. *Moral Imagination: The Missing Factor in Global Health. Public Library of Science Medicine* 2005; **2**(12): 1207–1210 (e200). Also available: http://medicine.plosjournals.org/perlserv/?request=get-document&doi=10%2E1371%2Fjournal%2E0020400

Benatar SR. Global disparities in health and human rights: a critical commentary. *Am J Public Health* 1998; **88**: 295–300.

Bensimon CM, Benatar SR. Developing sustainability: A new metaphor for progress. *Theor Med Bioeth* 2006; **27**(1): 59–79.

Brennan RA, Rothman DJ, Blank L, et al. Health industry practices that create conflicts of interest. *JAMA* 2006; **295**: 429–433.

Buchanan. A. *Justice, Legitimacy and Self-Determination.* Oxford: Oxford University Press, 2004.

Burrows G. *The No-Nonsense Guide to the Arms Trade.* Oxford: New Internationalist Publications Ltd, 2002.

Changing Course: Alternative Approaches to Achieve the Millennium Development Goals. Washington DC: Actionaid International USA, 2005, http://www.actionaidusa.org.

Commission on Health Research for Development *Health Research: Essential Link to Equity in Development.* Oxford: Oxford University Press, 1990.

Current debates in global justice The Journal of Ethics. a special issue 2005; **9**(1–2): 1–300.

Daniels N, Sabin J. Limits to health care: fair procedures, democratic deliberation and the legitimacy problem for insurers. *Philos Publ Aff* 1997; **26**(4): 303–350.

Doctors in Society: Medical Professionalism in a Changing World. Royal College of Physicians of London Supplement No. 1 Vol. 5 (6) S1-S40, 2005.

Doyal L. Rationing within the NHS should be explicit: the case for. *Br Med J* 1997; **314**: 1114–1118.

Fauci AS. *Emerging and Reemerging Infectious Diseases: The Perpetual Challenge.* New York: 2005 Robert H Ebert Memorial Lecture Milbank Memorial Fund, 2006.

Freidson E. *Professionalism: The Third Logic: On the Practice of Knowledge.* Chicago: University of Chicago Press, 2001.

Friman HR, Andreas P, eds. *Illicit Global Economy and State Power.* New York: Rowman and Littlefield, 1999.

Ham C. Priority setting in health care: learning from international experience. *Health Policy* 1997; **42**: 49–66.

Harris G. Doctors back ban on gifts from drug makers. *New York Times,* 25 January 2006 p. A14.

Iglehart J. American health services: expenditures. *New England Journal of Medicine* 1999; **340**: 70–76.

Kassalow JS. *Why Health is Important to U.S. Foreign Policy.* New York: Council on Foreign Relations and Milbank Memorial Fund, 2001.

Landman WA, Henley LD. Equitable rationing of highly specialised services for children: a perspective from South Africa. *J Med Ethics* 1999; **25**: 224–229.

Lemmens T. Leopards in the temple: restoring scientific integrity to the commercialised research scene. *J Law Med Ethics* 2004; **32**(4): 641–657.

Martin DK, Giacomini M, Singer PA. Fairness, accountability for reasonableness, and the views of priority setting decision-makers. *Health Policy* 2002; **61**: 279–290.

Martin DK, Singer PA, Bernstein M. Access to ICU beds for neurosurgery patients: a qualitative case study. *J Neurol Neurosurg Psychiatry* 2003; **74**: 1299–1303.

Martin DK, Singer PA, Giacomini M, and Purdy L. Priority setting for new technology. *Br Med J* 2000; **321**: 1316–1318.

Mello MM, Claridge BR, Studdert DM. Academic medical centres' standards for clinical-trial agreements with industry. *N Engl J Med* 2004; **352**: 2202–2210.

Osterholm MT. Preparing for the next pandemic. *N Engl J Med* 2005; **352**: 1839–1842.

Pogge T. *World Poverty and Human Rights.* Cambridge: Polity Press, 2002.

Pogge T. Real world justice. *J Ethics* 2005; **9**(1–2): 29–53.

Relman AR, Angell M. How the drug industry distorts medicine and politics: America's other drug problem. *The New Republic*; 16 December 2002; 27–41.

Shapiro K, Benatar SR. HIV prevention research and global inequality: towards improved standards of care. *J Med Ethics* 2005; **31**: 39–47.

Sreenivasan G. International justice and health: a proposal. *Ethics Int Aff* 2002; **16**: 81–90.

Steinbrook R. Gag clauses in clinical-trial agreements. *N Engl J Med* 2005; **352**: 2160–2162.

The Global Fund. Annual Report 2002/2003. Geneva, http://www.theglobalfund.org

Troullier P, Oliaro P, Torreele E, Orbinski J, Laing R, Ford N. Drug development for neglected diseases: a deficient market and a public health failure. *Lancet* 2002; **359**: 2188–2194.

United Nations Development Report (UNDP). Human Development Report 2000: Human Rights and Human Development. New York: Oxford University Press, 2000.

Wilkinson RG. *Unhealthy Societies: The Afflictions of Inequality.* London: Routledge, 1996.

World Health Organization. *Poverty and Health in Developing Countries. No. 16 WHO series Macroeconomics, Health and Development.* Geneva: World Health Organisation, 1995.

100

Obligations of the Pharmaceutical Industry

UDO SCHUKLENK AND JIM GALLAGHER

INTRODUCTION

Pharmaceutical companies have been on the receiving end of much criticism from patient activist groups, as well as government regulators, the media and academics (Cohen, 2006; Olesen, 2006). They have been criticized for alleged unethical marketing practices (Peppin, 2006), profiteering at the cost of people living in developing countries (Schuklenk, 2002) and market – as opposed to health – needs-driven research agendas (Cohen, 2003). Fairly recently, innovative pharmaceutical companies' behaviours as sponsors of clinical research in developing countries have also received serious public attention (De Zulueta, 2001). This contribution will focus on these issues in the order of their relative importance, starting with the 10/90 gap in international health research, investigating the industry's responsibility to provide affordable drugs to the world's poor and concluding with an analysis of the industry's ethical obligations towards participants of the trials it sponsors in developing countries.

COMPANIES' CORPORATE SOCIAL RESPONSIBILITIES

Simply put, pharmaceutical companies are profit-driven private organizations. Their primary reason for existing is to maximize shareholder value. In that sense there is not much difference between companies manufacturing pharmaceuticals, cars, cigarettes or coffee machines. Their products might be different, and the means by which they reach the stated objective might be different, but their primary objective is pretty much the same. These companies are very large and highly successful businesses operating in a heavily consolidated sector dominated by a small number of transnational corporations, which generate large profits from sales in the rich world. What are their ethical obligations to the poor and the diseases that affect them? This analysis begins with obligations, rather than what might be desirable or praiseworthy, in a supererogatory sense, for these companies to do.

Answering this question must start from the understanding that these businesses are joint stock companies with large numbers of stockholders, typically representing the savings or pensions of very large numbers of individuals. One does not have to agree wholly with Friedman (1962; 1970) that 'the social responsibility of business is to make profits' to accept that ethical obligations are owed to stockholders. Their funds are accepted on the promise that the management will run the business to maximize returns. This is often described as a fiduciary relationship. And management's success in meeting this promise is assessed hourly by the markets. There is a practical argument for these profits, too. As Adam Smith noted, it is this incentive that makes the market system work, creating successful enterprises that provide useful employment, pay taxes and deliver products, in this case, valuable drugs (Smith, 1776).

The pharmaceutical industry delivers on its obligations to owners over a generation (Sterckx, 2004). The US pharmaceutical sector, for instance, has been more profitable than comparable industries. A US study (US Congress 1993) concluded that the returns to the sector were between 2% and 3% annually, better than the returns to comparable industries. Similarly, returns to this sector in the United Kingdom and Germany have exceeded the returns in the market generally, as shown in Figure 100.1.

Principles of Health Care Ethics, Second Edition   Edited by R.E. Ashcroft, A. Dawson, H. Draper and J.R. McMillan

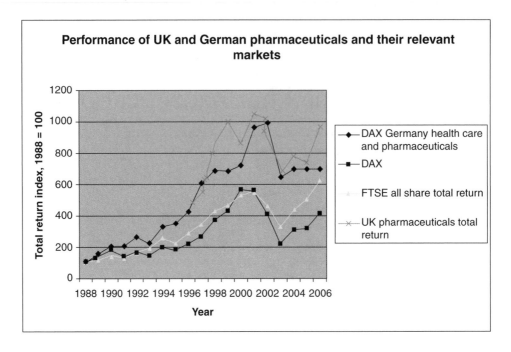

Figure 100.1. Performance of UK and German pharmaceuticals and their relevant markets (source: Abbey National Asset Managers, own calculations).

The commercial and innovative success of pharmaceutical companies is not the exclusive result of an unfettered market. Pharmaceutical companies work in a highly regulated sector in many respects. What stops competition from driving prices down to marginal cost levels, as classic economics would predict, is the operation of intellectual property law. This too has ethical and practical justifications, but profits are heavily dependent on its precise form and geographical application, both of which are contestable: the length of a patent is a matter of judgement and such judgements can reasonably vary over time and in different places.

The pursuit of profit is possible only within certain limitations: even Friedman recognized that corporations have to obey legal rules and ethical norms. These have been described as obligations to stakeholders, including employees, customers and the communities in which they operate or which might be adversely affected by their activities. The reach of these obligations extends beyond current generations (Evan and Freeman, 1998). Some of these obligations will be legally defined and well understood, such as health and safety; others are more contested and matters of judgement, such as when do highly profitable sales become an abuse of a monopoly position?

It is not self-evident, however, that enterprises have any ethical *obligations* to people who are not stakeholders. The obligations of companies have been described as negative (in pursuit of their primary aim, there are things they must not do) rather than positive, or passive responsibilities (there are acts for which they will be held accountable) rather than active ones (there are virtues they must pursue) (Bovens, 1998). Does, say, a successful software company have any obligations to starving people who cannot buy its products? Helping them would be philanthropy, but in effect with someone else's, namely its stockholders', money. Philanthropy is praiseworthy, but may be supererogatory. Carnegie (1889) argued in *The Gospel of Wealth* that business should pursue profit, but that the wealth created should be used philanthropically by individual owners for the benefit of the community.

A strong argument can be made that the rich (mostly in the western world) are obliged to provide aid in the situations of extreme need that obtain today (Unger, 1996). But it is not self-evident that there is such a duty on joint stock companies. Leisinger, for instance, argues that 'private enterprises have neither the societal mandate nor the organizational capabilities to feed the poor or provide health care to the sick in their home countries or in the developing world' (Leisinger, 2005).

Serious reputational damage to the pharmaceutical industry was self-inflicted when, among other incidents, its umbrella organization sued the South African government over its intention to set aside patents in order to permit the local production and importation of cheaper generic drugs to deal with an overwhelming AIDS epidemic in the country (Schuklenk, 2002). Today seemingly altruistic behaviour by pharmaceutical companies can be observed in many countries (Raymond, 2004). Most major pharmaceutical companies operating in the developing world as research organizations and/or manufacturers of drugs have begun myriad schemes designed to demonstrate that they are responsible corporate citizens. Among the schemes developed are access initiatives including drug donation schemes and health education programmes, as well as some investment in research and development targeting neglected diseases (Bristol-Myers Squibb, 2006; Hoffman-LaRoche, 2006; Astra Zeneca, 2006). Pharmaceutical companies have accepted the need to respond in an ethically responsive manner to the challenges people in developing countries face.

Major pharmaceutical industry players, such as GSK, Pfizer or Akzo Nobel, explicitly ground their acknowledgement of such social responsibilities in contractarian terms. Akzo Nobel, for instance, states that it considers unprofitable activities in developing countries as 'sustainable business models, a contribution to society and access to new markets in developing and emerging countries are two sides of the same coin' (Akzo Nobel, 2006). In defence of such policies one could also argue that shareholder interests are not violated even if there is a suboptimal outcome in financial terms. One could argue that investors in pharmaceutical companies are aware of the fact that these companies invest in non-profitable activities when they decide to purchase shares. Indeed, there are strong indications that shareholders support potentially unprofitable company policies on ethical grounds (Buhl, 2006).

In return for patent protection and high returns on investment in drug research and development, companies agreed to provide communities with efficient drugs at affordable prices (Dukes, 2002). Communities continue to provide support for commercial research agendas of pharmaceutical companies because much of the basic research underlying development breakthroughs has actually been financed by taxpayers (Cragg, 1996). It has been shown that

'taxpayers, not shareholders, have borne most of the [research and development] cost. Publicly funded research organizations have contributed hundreds of millions of taxpayers' dollars to AIDS drug research. Indeed, the Pharmaceutical Research and Manufacturers of America, an industry lobby group, estimates that private industry finances only about 43% of drug development. Five commonly used drugs against AIDS – didanosine, lamivudine, nevirapine, stavudine and zidovudine – were developed largely as a result of public funds' (Schull, 2000).

Arguments are sometimes made about the special circumstances of pharmaceutical companies. First, they should provide funds to make available life-saving drugs to those who cannot afford to pay for them, notably in relation to HIV/AIDS. Or second, they should invest in research into the diseases that are predominant in the developing tropical countries (Global Forum, 2004). These are clearly glaring injustices; the pharmaceutical industry has the capacity to help deal with them and, as the argument runs, is under an ethical obligation to do so. Perhaps this is best conceptualized via an example of the duty to aid. In Singer's famous example: if you see a young child drowning in a pond on your way to work, you are ethically obliged to help provided the costs to you are not unreasonably high (Singer, 1993). Such arguments are never wholly straightforward as it is not as clear, even is in the abstract, on whom the obligation falls when we try to apply this argument to long-term, systemic and global issues such as those that we are concerned about.

Does the duty to aid apply here? Arguably pharmaceutical companies meet the test of proximity: they are in a position to help in some respects, and they might well be the only moral actors who could help. Indeed, the majority of pharmaceutical multinationals are engaged in ventures they describe as non-profit in developing countries. These companies have voluntarily acknowledged that they have moral obligations towards the poor of the developing world (within the confines of the products they develop) (Schuklenk, 2002). Doing what is morally required does not necessarily maximize shareholder value. The companies argue in defence of their actions that in the long term their strategies will deliver a maximization of shareholder value. Whatever one might make of the industry's voluntary acknowledgement of moral obligations in this context, the question inevitably arises: If an obligation to aid does apply to them, what is it?

NEGLECTED DISEASE RESEARCH

One of the areas where the pharmaceutical industry's competence and resources could be put to good use is that of neglected disease research. According to the Global Forum for Health Research, 'every year more than US$70 billion is spent on health research and development by the public and private sectors. An estimated 10% of this is used for research into 90% of the world's health problems. This has been what is called the 10/90 gap' (Global Forum, 2004). A review by a team of researchers from Médecins sans Frontières concluded that 'despite an ever-increasing need for safe, effective, and affordable medicines for the treatment of these [tropical] diseases, drug development has virtually stopped' (Trouiller, 2002). An ethical allocation of research resources that takes into account global health needs should arguably help to bridge this gap, and reduce the consequences of the current misallocation. This would be of benefit not only to the researchers involved but also to their countries and the global community in general. The question is what role pharmaceutical companies have to play in this context and what their moral obligations are to confront this problem.

Neglected disease research is not obviously a duty of innovative pharmaceutical companies. After all, although they are in a position to help, they are not the only ones. States could equally step in and fill the research lacunae. Nor can the pharmaceutical companies do so without breaching to some degree their fiduciary obligations to stockholders: research would be expensive and unprofitable. However, arguing that there is no compelling ethical duty on pharmaceutical companies does not imply that they face no need to act. Companies do need to consider their own long-term and enlightened self-interest. They may expect pressure from an increasing number of their owners and from their wider existing stakeholder community, which undoubtedly includes governments as major customers – and to whose defence of wide intellectual property rights they owe their capacity to make profits. A wise industry would reflect on the long-term possibilities here and would move individually on differential pricing and collectively on neglected disease research before finding itself forced to do so in an unmanaged way.

Ultimately, however we think that solutions to these global injustices are properly located primarily in the realm of government not companies. In Lindblom's (1977) terms these are issues of politics not markets. Politics should express the ethical stances of populations. So far as drug supply and research are concerned, two potential governmental actions stand out. The first is an internationally binding and enforceable agreement to support differential pricing by restricting leakage to developed countries, and so agreeing in effect to support industry research (as the United States already arguably does). The second would be to incentivize neglected disease research, for instance via the tax system, in a concerted way and in consultation with the industry.

On an international level, new trade frameworks for health care research and development have been proposed, for instance by the US-based Consumer Project Technology (CPTech, 2006). Love argues that 'trade agreements should be reframed to focus on standards for sharing the costs of R&D' and that we 'need business models for financing R&D that do not depend on marketing monopolies for approved products' (Love, 2003).

There seems to be a consensus among industry, governments and NGOs that industry has an important role to play in research on neglected diseases. Industry has clearly accepted that it has non-supererogatory moral obligations towards the world's poor. How far these obligations reach is a matter of ongoing discussion. There can be little doubt that if states, as the institutions properly thought to be primarily responsible for health care delivery, would take their responsibilities in terms of drug research and development seriously, the discussion about industry obligations would all but disappear.

AFFORDABLE ACCESS TO LIFE-SUSTAINING DRUGS

An important ethical challenge to pharmaceutical companies is that the medication available is, more often than not, too expensive to permit affordable access to those most in need. This has been the case in many African countries such as South Africa and Uganda, where the majority of people suffering from HIV/AIDS have no access to treatment drugs because of their extreme poverty. In Uganda, for example, where more than 2 million people are infected with the virus, it is estimated by UNAIDS that not more than 2000 people have access to drugs (Cochrane, 2000). As Tina Piper argues, 'there is a growing recognition in the international and domestic context that the patent system may not function well for the equitable and affordable delivery of health care goods, and its strict operation may have to be altered by enacting accompanying regulation or changing patent laws themselves' (Piper, 2004).

At issue is the fact that pharmaceutical multinationals charge prices for patented drugs that prevent the overwhelming majority of people in developing countries from access to their products.

Various approaches to justifying patents have been discussed (Stercky, 2004). No doubt, the primary reason for the protection of intellectual property rights and patents is a public-interest-based argument. In a nutshell it states that in order for such companies to be able to achieve a desirable public objective, that is to research and produce new drugs, they must be able to reap or anticipate a profit from their products sufficiently high to support a significant research effort (Schull, 2000). Precisely this reason, however, provides a possible justification for overriding some patents in some countries. If patents are protected to ensure that the public has continuing access to privately developed drugs, something is going wrong when the public cannot actually afford access to those drugs. This is not to say that private companies which spend enormous amounts funding research should not recoup their investment from patented drugs. However, if the owners of those patents price their drugs out of the reach of the majority of those in need, so goes the argument, there is very little point in protecting those patents any longer (Schuklenk, 2002). Of course, the issues are more complicated than this. For a start, in developed countries, many people in need of expensive, patented, life-extending drugs are able to access those drugs. The same, however, cannot be said for developing countries.

Here the argument in favour of setting aside patents seems to succeed. After all, where there is no market for a patented product, little point is served by protecting patent and preventing access. Indeed, the World Trade Organization's TRIPS agreement expressly permits developing countries to override the patents for drugs that could be utilized in public health emergencies such as AIDS, TB and malaria. The problem with TRIPS-related policies is – so the pharmaceutical companies argue – that without such internationally recognized patent rights, there would be no funds and incentives for further research and development.

Currently, patent owners already battle for market share for their existing products. The argument from financial incentives to engage in R&D investment may not necessarily jeopardize drug research, as they do not tamper with the patent rights in place in the developed world. Furthermore, it is worth noting that the profits at which the industry is aiming have never been generated in the developing world.

The issue of drug supply differs in important respects from neglected disease research. The case for a duty to aid can be made on the basis that it is possible for companies to do this with existing patented products by differential pricing. Using AIDS as a paradigmatic case, it has been pointed out that even AIDS drugs sold at marginal costs in the developing world would yield profits for pharmaceutical companies simply because the industry's research investments have long been recouped from sales in the developed world (Biehl, 2006). They can cover marginal costs and do so without tying up large amounts of capital (maybe by licensing manufacture to third party suppliers in the countries concerned) and so without failing to meet their stockholder obligations. Companies routinely operate differential or Ramsey (1927) pricing in different market segments, as this is a highly regulated market and they cannot simply charge a market-clearing price. This already happens in at least one significant case.

COMPANIES' POST-TRIAL OBLIGATIONS TO PARTICIPANTS IN DEVELOPING COUNTRIES

Part of the ethical rationale for subjecting competent and informed volunteers in developed countries to certain risks in clinical trials is that possibly they, or certainly the communities in which they live, would benefit from a new drug discovery. Current and future patients in developed countries would benefit because most of them would be able to access these medications through public health care or because most of them would be covered by private health insurance schemes. There might be a few exceptions to this, but by and large this still holds true for developed countries. The same rationale cannot be straightforwardly applied to developing countries. Pharmaceutical companies may well sponsor clinical research there, yet usually trial participants are not guaranteed post-trial access. There are two reasons for this. The first and most obvious reason is that few, if any, developing countries can provide public sector health delivery services that are free at the point of delivery and sufficiently well financed to provide access to the latest state-of-the-art treatments. The second reason is that the two-tier health care systems that most developing countries rely on prevent the vast majority of these countries' citizens from having affordable access to newly patented and marketed drugs. The public sector cannot afford except such drugs, and the private sector is inaccessible to most the very well off (Wilson, 2006). In effect, a crucial component of the ethical justification for clinical trials is falling away. One might still argue that *some* patients *somewhere* would benefit, but it is obviously inequitable to conduct trials in developing countries that would mostly benefit patients in the developed world. Hence, the question arises as to what type of post-trial obligations trial sponsors have to the developing world-based trial participants, and possibly their communities. The World Medical Association's Declaration of Helsinki, the internationally most influential ethical guideline on biomedical research, states 'that it is necessary during the study planning process to identify post-trial access by study participants to prophylactic, diagnostic and therapeutic procedures identified as beneficial in the study or access to other appropriate care' (World Medical Association, 2004). The organization exhorts ethical review committees to ensure that such arrangements are considered when a trial protocol is reviewed. Others have argued that although it is ethically required that some benefits are accrued by trial participants or their wider communities, it is far from clear that such benefits should necessarily be of a clinical nature. If the issue is about ensuring that no exploitation takes places, it is conceivable that non-drug-related benefits are locally more appropriate (Wendler, 2004). In this context there has been concern that offering continuing free access to otherwise unaffordable drugs, or other benefits of similar magnitude, could constitute a perverse or undue incentive. An undue incentive is offered whenever participants are incentivized to engage against their better judgement in an activity they would not engage in except for the incentive offered. There is an important flaw in this argument: if competent adults, who are fully comprehending of the risks involved in a particular trial, choose to participate because of money offered, because they want to assist future generations or for any other reasons that are authentically their own, they are not doing so against their better judgement. Even poor, possibly poorly educated persons participating in a high-risk trial because of incentives offered, if doing so voluntarily and if they are fully informed, are not necessarily the victims of a perverse incentive.

People can reasonably hold different views on the matter of what types of benefits ought to be provided to trial participants in developing countries, but the rationale for some kind of benefit is convincing. In the absence of the developed world ethics rationale for subjecting trial participants to trial-related risks, some other kind of benefits should accrue to trial participants in the developing world. Pharmaceutical companies, if they sponsor such trials, are responsible for ensuring that such benefits are made available and that they are adequate.

CONCLUSIONS

Pharmaceutical companies, although not without any obligations to assist the poor, should not be considered to be obliged to step in altruistically when the market fails. Although they are moral actors that have some limited obligations to assist the poor where they can without risk to their own capacity to develop profitable drugs, it seems reasonable to suggest that the primary obligation to help falls onto states as opposed to private actors.

ACKNOWLEDGEMENT

We thank Darragh Hare for assisting in sourcing relevant information for this contribution as well as for editorial assistance.

REFERENCES

Akzo Nobel. Personal communication from Andre Veneman, Director of Corporate Social Responsibility, 18 April 2006.

Astra Zeneca. www.astrazeneca.com. Accessed 5 May 2006.

Beauchamp TL, Bowie NE. *Ethical Theory and Business*. Englewood Cliffs, NJ: Prentice Hall, 1998.

Biehl J. Pharmaceutical governance. In: Petryna A, Lakoff A, Kleinman A, eds. *Global Pharmaceuticals*. Cambridge MA: MIT Press, 2006, pp. 206–239.

Bovens M. *The Quest for Responsibility*. Cambridge: Cambridge University Press, 1998.

Bristol-Myers S. www.bms.com. Accessed 5 May 2006.

Buhl L. Ford shareholders uphold LGBT rights, 16 May 2006. http://news.yahoo.com/s/po/20060517/co_po/fordshareholdersupholdlgbtrighs. Accessed 26 May 2006.

Carnegie A. *The Gospel of Wealth*, 1889, quoted in Carroll AB, Buchholtz AK. *Business and Society, Ethics and Stakeholder Management. Mason.* Ohio: Thomson South Western, 2003; p. 34.

Cochrane J. Narrowing the gap: Access to HIV treatments in developing countries. A pharmaceutical company's perspective. *J Med Eth* 2000; **26**: 47–50.

Cohen J, Illingworth P. The dilemma of intellectual property rights for pharmaceuticals: the tension between ensuring access of the poor to medicines and committing to international agreements. *Developing World Bioethics* 2003; **3**: 27–48.

Cohen J, Illingworth P, Schuklenk U, eds. *The Power of Pills*. London: Pluto, 2006.

Consumer Project Technology, 2006. http://www.cptech.org

Cragg GM, Simon JE, Jato JG, Snader KM. Drug discovery and development at the NCI. In: Janick J, ed. *Progress in New Crops*. Arlington: ASHS Press, 1996, pp. 554–560.

De Zulueta P. Randomised placebo-controlled trials and HIV-infected pregnant women in developing countries. Ethical imperialism or unethical exploitation? *Bioethics* 2001; **15**: 289–311.

Dienhart JW. *Business, Institutions and Ethics*. New York: Oxford University Press, 2000,

Dukes MNG. Accountability of the pharmaceutical industry. *The Lancet* 2002; **360**: 1682–1684.

Evan WM, Freeman RE. A stakeholder theory of the modern corporation Kantian capitalism. In: Beauchamp TL, Bowie NE. *Ethical Theory and Business*. Englewood cliffs, NJ, Prentice Hall, 1998.

Friedman M. *Capitalism and Freedom*. Chicago: University of Chicago Press, 1962.

Friedman M. The social responsibility of business is to make profits, *New York Times Magazine*, 13 September 1970 (reprinted Dienhart JW. *Business, Institutions and Ethics* NewYork: Oxford University Press, 2000.

Global Forum for Health Research. http://www. globalforumhealth. org/FilesUpld/36.pdf. Accessed 28 April 2004.

Hofman-LaRoche. www.roche.com. Accessed 5 May 2006.

Leisinger KM. The corporate social responsibility of the pharmaceutical industry: Idealism without illusion and realism without resignation. *Business Ethics Quarterly* 2005; **15**: 577–594.

Lindblom C. *Politics and Markets*. New York: Basic Books, 1977.

Love J. A new framework for healthcare R&D, 2003. http://www. earthinstitute.columbia.edu/cgsd/documents/love_000.pdf (accessed 30 April 2004).

Médecins sans Frontières. *Fatal Imbalance: The Crisis in Research and Development for Drugs in Neglected Diseases*. MSF: Geneva, 2001.

Olesen T. In the court of public opinion. *Int Sociol* 2006; **21**: 5–30.

Peppin P. Directing consumption. Bennett B, Tomossy GF, eds. In: *Globalization and Health*, Dordrecht: Springer, 2006, pp. 109–28.

Piper T. Commentary. *Journal of Medical Ethics* 2004; **30**: 475–477.

Ramsey F. A contribution to the theory of taxation. *Economic J* 1927; **37**(March): 47–61.

Raymond SU. *The Future of Philanthropy: Economics, Ethics, and Management*. Hoboken, N J: John Wiley & Sons, Inc., 2004.

Schuklenk U, Ashcroft RE. Affordable access to essential medication in developing countries: Conflicts between ethical and economic imperatives. *J Med Philos* 2002; **27**: 179–195.

Schull M. Effect of drug patents in developing countries. *BMJ* 2000; **321**: 833.

Singer P. (1993) *Practical Ethics*. Oakley: Cambridge University Press, 1993.

101

Ethics and Medical Publishing

RICHARD SMITH AND IAIN CHALMERS

INTRODUCTION

In 1997, a group of editors of British medical journals founded the Committee on Publication Ethics. They did so because they found that they were encountering many ethical problems and wanted a source of advice. COPE was thus a sort of self-help group for editors, but its work provides insights into the ethical problems that arise with the publication of research. COPE has now dealt with some 250 cases, but an analysis of the first 137 cases showed that the commonest problem was publishing or submitting similar material more than once (43 cases), followed by problems with authorship (24 cases), falsification (17 cases), failure to get informed consent from patients (14 cases), 'unethical research' (for example, doing research that did not need to be done or doing it so badly that no conclusion would be possible) (14 cases), failure to get ethics committee approval (13 cases), fabrication (nine cases) and plagiarism (six cases). The committee also saw cases of editorial and reviewer misconduct, undeclared conflicts of interest, breaches of confidentiality, clinical misconduct, attacks on whistleblowers, deception and failure to publish.

We cannot in the space available deal with all these issues, but we have chosen to concentrate on the biased under-reporting of research results, peer review, authorship, conflict of interest and research misconduct. Those who would like to read more should consult books on ethical issues in biomedical publication (Hudson Jones and McLellan, 2000), peer review (Godlee and Jefferson, 2003), fraud in medical research (Lock et al., 2001) and medical journals (Smith, 2006).

BIASED UNDER-REPORTING OF CLINICAL RESEARCH

Why do patients and other volunteers accept invitations to take part in research? There are a number of reasons, which are not mutually exclusive. Sometimes the motivation is money: each of the young men who volunteered to receive a monoclonal antibody that had never previously been used in humans apparently received £2000 for their participation in a study which proved life-threatening (Goodyear, 2006). Sometimes people participate to support research in the institution in which they work: Ellen Roche, a 24-year old technician at the Johns Hopkins Allergy and Asthma Center, died after volunteering to participate in a physiological experiment designed to elucidate the development of airways sensitivity (Clark et al., 2001). Other people participate in research because they hope to benefit from novel treatments for serious health problems: for example, Jesse Gelsinger, who suffered from a very rare genetic disorder, died after gene therapy was used in an attempt to improve his prognosis (Smith and Byers, 2002). It seems probable, however, that the vast majority of people who accept invitations to participate in research do so partly or mainly because they want to play their part in contributing to a growth in knowledge that might help others or themselves in future.

This more or less altruistic motivation for participating in research has ethical implications. It implies that those who have invited people to participate in research have a responsibility to ensure that the findings of the research are made publicly available, and that this is done honestly. Unless the results of research are reported honestly, the evidence contributed by volunteers cannot contribute to a growth in knowledge, and this, therefore, breaks the contract with them implied by their agreement to participate in the research.

One of the reasons for mentioning some examples of serious adverse consequences of participating in research is to invite consideration of whether failure to publish those results of research could ever be regarded as ethical. Had these tragic consequences of participation in research not been reported, other researchers might have proceeded

Principles of Health Care Ethics, Second Edition   Edited by R.E. Ashcroft, A. Dawson, H. Draper and J.R. McMillan

in ignorance of the possibility that they were planning to expose volunteers to known dangers of which they were unaware.

In contrast to the experiences of Ellen Roche and Jesse Gelsinger, however, most adverse effects detected in research are more subtle. They are no less important, however, because they may have implications for tens of thousands of people. This is because biased under-reporting of research tends to lead to conclusions that medical treatments are more useful than they are in fact, and they can, therefore, result in unnecessary suffering and death and in wasted resources spent on ineffective or dangerous treatments (Chalmers, 2004).

For example, it has been estimated that, at the peak of their use in the late 1980s, prophylactic use of anti-arrhythmic drugs in myocardial infarction were causing tens of thousands of deaths every year in the United States – comparable annual numbers of deaths to the total number of Americans who died in the Vietnam War (Moore, 1995). The hazards associated with these drugs could have been recognized at least a decade earlier had not some studies remained unpublished because their results were disappointing to their sponsors. To their great credit, researchers in Nottingham revealed in the 1990s one example of this phenomenon related to a trial done 13 years earlier. In their paper, they reported as follows:

> Nine patients died in the lorcainide group and one in the placebo group.... When we carried out our study in 1980 we thought that the increased death rate that occurred in the lorcainide group was an effect of chance.... The development of lorcainide was abandoned for commercial reasons, and this study was therefore never published; it is now a good example of publication bias. The results described here...might have provided an early warning of trouble ahead (Cowley et al., 1993).

Biased under-reporting of research is scientific misconduct and unethical (Chalmers, 1990). It has been recognized for centuries (Dickersin, 2004), and there is now a large body of evidence confirming that it is a substantial problem (Chalmers, 2006). Biased under-reporting of research results principally from researchers not writing up or submitting reports of research for publication, not because of biased rejection of submitted reports by journal editors (Dickersin, 1997). Recent research has also revealed that, if estimates of treatment effects on some of the outcomes studied do not support the conclusions of researchers, data on those outcomes is under-reported as well (Chan et al., 2004).

Research ethics committees, medical ethicists and research funders have so far done little to acknowledge biased under-reporting of research, let alone protect patients and the public from its adverse effects (Savulescu et al., 1996;

Chalmers, 2002). Indeed, it was only after the attorney general of New York State drew attention to the way that one of the world's largest pharmaceutical companies had withheld evidence relevant to the safety of one of its products that medical journal editors began to take concerted steps to require prospective, public registration of clinical trials – one of the most basic measures needed to get to grips with the problem. The understandable and reasonable expectations of those who agree to participate in research will remain unfulfilled just as long as this form of research misconduct is tolerated by governments, research ethicists and others who should be protecting the interests of the public.

PEER REVIEW

Peer review is central to science. It is the process that is used to decide which research grant applications will be funded and which studies published. Researchers must publish to progress. Yet, despite its centrality, peer review was until recently little studied. This seems paradoxical in that science is based on experimentation and collection and analysis of data. Even stranger is that the studies that have been done demonstrate deep flaws with peer review and struggle to show its effectiveness (Lock, 1985; Jefferson et al., 2002; Demicheli and Di Pietrantonj, 2003; Jefferson and Godlee, 2003; Jefferson et al., 2006). 'If it was a drug', says Drummond Rennie, deputy editor of JAMA, 'it would never get onto the market'. Yet faith in peer review is as strong as ever. Faith not evidence supports this process that is central to science.

The essence of peer review is that the peers of a scientist will critique his or her grant application or manuscript, but the process comes in many forms. The reviewer might be asked to make an overall judgement on whether the grant application should be funded or the manuscript published, or might simply advise a research committee or an editor. Sometimes 'peer review' might be used to describe simply the contribution of the peer, but more often it denotes the whole process of deciding which applications to fund and which papers to publish. Thus in the case of journals, editors will screen out some manuscripts, select one or more reviewers and then make the final decision on publication in the light of the reviewers' comments. We would also include the scrutiny that follows publication to be part of peer review: many studies that are deemed scientifically sound enough to publish collapse when exposed to thousands of readers.

The aim of peer review might be to decide which grant applications to fund or manuscripts to publish, or it might be to improve the quality of the grant application or published paper. Often it is a combination of the two.

A systematic review of all the available evidence on peer review concluded that 'the practice of peer review is based on faith in its effects, rather than on facts' (Jefferson et al., 2002). Reviewers often do not agree much more often than would be expected by chance on whether a paper should be published (Lock, 1985), and evidence that peer review improves published papers is sparse. Studies that have inserted deliberate errors into papers show that reviewers usually do not spot most of the errors (Godlee et al., 1998). And peer review is a poor defence against fraud because it works on trust. If an author writes that there were 200 patients in a study then the reviewer assumes that to be the case: he or she does not ask to see patient records or signatures. The weakness of peer review explains why medical journals are filled with studies that are scientifically poor and statistically unsound (Altman 1991; Haynes, 1993).

Sadly, there is much stronger evidence on the defects of peer review. It is slow, usually taking months, expensive and profligate with academic time. It is prone to bias – against, for example, those from less prestigious institutions (Peters, Ceci, 1982) and women (Wennerås and Wold, 1997) and easily abused (Rennie, 1999). Reviewers may steal ideas from manuscripts sent to them or be deliberately slow or harsh in their criticisms in order to steal a competitive advantage.

Despite the lack of evidence of effectiveness and the deficiencies of peer review, it is almost unthinkable that a scientific body would abandon peer review in processing grants or a journal stop using it to help make decisions on papers. Peer review is often compared with democracy in being the least bad system available.

Attempts have been made to improve peer review. For historical reasons, rather than because of evidence, reviewers usually know the identity of authors, but authors do not know the identity of reviewers. A randomized trial suggested that blinding the reviewers to the identity of authors meant that reviewers produced higher quality reviews (McNutt et al., 1990), but two larger studies found no such improvements (Justice et al., 1998; van Rooyen et al., 1998). Studies were then done letting authors (but not readers) know the identity of reviewers (van Rooyen et al., 1999; Walsh, 2000). This improved the quality of reviews very slightly. Some journals moved to 'open peer review' (letting authors know the names of reviewers) on the grounds that it would increase the accountability of reviewers and that it was right that such an important judgement should be made openly; a hidden judge is a terrible thing. Few biomedical journals have followed.

The next logical step might be to open up peer review entirely. The whole process could be conducted openly on the World Wide Web. Peer review could become a scientific discourse rather than a somewhat arbitrary judgement. Many doctors are nervous of such a process because 'half-baked' and possibly dangerous ideas might endanger the public. But these doctors are ignoring the ineffectiveness of peer review, given the fact that papers presented at conferences usually receive little or no peer review and yet may be widely reported, and that increasing numbers of researchers are willing to present their results first to the mass media. Furthermore, science would in a sense be returning to its roots when scientific papers were presented at meetings and critically discussed rather than peer reviewed and then published.

AUTHORSHIP AND CONTRIBUTORSHIP

Disputes over authorship of research papers is one of the commonest problems dealt with by the office for academic affairs at Harvard University (Wilcox, 1998). It is probably the same in all universities (Eysenbach, 2001). Publishing is crucially important for academics. They must publish to develop their careers and reputations. They thus tend to think of authorship mostly in terms of credit: the more papers on which you can have your name the better. Editors, in contrast, think of authorship primarily in terms of accountability. Putting your name on a research paper is, says Richard Horton, editor of the *Lancet*, like signing a cheque (Horton, 1997). If there turn out to be serious problems with a paper, then all the authors must accept responsibility.

Problems arise with authorship because few scientific or medical studies are undertaken by one person. There are usually many people involved, and often those people may have contributed something very different to the study. One person may have thought of the idea, another designed the study, another collected and analysed the data, and yet another written the paper. Increasingly, research teams are multidisciplinary, including basic scientists, physicians, statisticians and even economists. Who then should be an author?

The International Committee of Medical Journal Editors (a self-appointed group known as the Vancouver Group after the city where it first met) has attempted to define who should be an author (International Committee of Medical Journal Editors, 2006). The definition has evolved, but the following definition is where it started:

Authorship should be based only on a substantial contribution to
  i conception and design or analysis and interpretation of data,
  ii drafting the article or revising it critically for important intellectual content and
  iii final approval of the version to be published.

Authors should, in other words, be able to take full intellectual responsibility for a study. If one author was on his or her way to a meeting and was suddenly taken ill, then any other author should be able to attend the meeting, present the paper and answer any questions. People who had simply collected data or who headed the unit in which the study was undertaken should not be authors.

The Vancouver Group developed this definition without consultation, and several studies showed that substantial proportions of authors on papers did not meet the definition (Shapiro et al., 1994; Goodman, 1994; Flanagin et al., 1998; Lock, 2001). Authors who had done little or nothing were included. This has been called 'gift authorship'. Often these 'authors' were heads of units or departments, and there was a time when it was normal to include such people as authors. They gave a 'stamp of approval' to the paper. Many research groups also included people who had done a lot of work collecting the data as authors. Often these people had spent more time working on the study than anybody else. It seemed right to include them.

The problem of authorship became particularly acute when studies proved to be fraudulent and yet included eminent authors (Lock, 2001). The eminent authors would not accept responsibility for the fraud. Editors thought it quite wrong that these authors should enjoy the benefits of authorship and yet refuse to accept responsibilities.

Editors have also been much concerned with the opposite problem of 'ghost authorship'. The person who wrote the paper is not named. Often these 'ghost authors' are employees of pharmaceutical companies. In extreme cases, the ghostwriter may write a review article to be submitted to a journal and then ask prominent doctors to sign the article – usually for a substantial fee.

We know less about how often people who should be included as authors are not included, but a study of authors showed that many thought that they should have been included as authors but had not been (Bhopal et al., 1997). That same study showed that most researchers did not know about the Vancouver Group's definition of authorship and when they were told about it they did not support it.

There are thus considerable problems around authorship, and various attempts have been made to solve the problem. Academic institutions have drawn up rules on authorship. Editors have asked authors to sign to certify that all authors meet the Vancouver Group criteria and that there are no other individuals who meet the criteria who are not included.

These 'solutions' have not worked, however, because the definition of authorship is inevitably subjective. Furthermore, many researchers do not accept the Vancouver Group definition. They think it reasonable to include authors who have done a great deal of work but cannot take full intellectual responsibility for a study. This is particularly true when research may include people from widely differing disciplines: if a study includes molecular biologists, cardiologists and economists, then nobody can accept full intellectual responsibility.

Reflecting on these problems, Drummond Rennie, deputy editor of *JAMA*, and others came up with a radical proposal. Instead of trying to sort people into authors and non-authors everybody should be named as a contributor – with a clear account of what each person did (Rennie et al., 1997). It should be straightforward to describe each person's contribution, no matter whether it was major or minor. This proposal thus avoids the deception of suggesting that somebody can take full intellectual responsibility for a paper when he or she made only a minor contribution or a contribution within one specialty.

Rennie and others also solved the problem of accountability by arguing that somebody should act as guarantor to the paper. They imagined that this person would inspect all the data. Others, however, accept that a guarantor can be rather like a government minister and be accountable for confidence in the team rather than inspection of all data. This latter proposal avoids the difficulty of molecular biologists having to take full intellectual accountability for the work of economists, or vice versa.

The proposal of replacing authorship with contributorship seemed radical when first suggested, but it has been adopted by many journals – and the Vancouver Group has modified its statement. It now reads:

> An 'author' is generally considered to be someone who has made substantive intellectual contributions to a published study, and biomedical authorship continues to have important academic, social, and financial implications. In the past, readers were rarely provided with information about contributions to studies from those listed as authors and in acknowledgments. Some journals now request and publish information about the contributions of each person named as having participated in a submitted study, at least for original research. Editors are strongly encouraged to develop and implement a contributorship policy, as well as a policy on identifying who is responsible for the integrity of the work as a whole.

Nevertheless, the group continues with its criteria for attributing authorship. It looks as if for some time to come we will continue to live in a world of authors and contributors.

CONFLICTS OF INTEREST

Conflict of interest has been defined as 'a set of conditions in which professional judgement concerning a primary interest (such as patients' welfare or the validity of research) tends to be unduly influenced by a secondary interest (such as financial gain)' (Thompson, 1993). It is important to understand that it is a *condition* not a *behaviour*. It often operates unconsciously, and there is substantial and growing evidence of its influence on how doctors prescribe and treat patients, what research is undertaken and how research is interpreted (Smith, 2006).

Conflicts may arise from many causes – academic, political or religious, for example – but the best-studied conflicts are financial. Probably the commonest source of financial conflict of interest in biomedical research is interaction with the pharmaceutical industry. About a quarter to a third of authors of original studies in medical journals have financial ties with the pharmaceutical industry (Krimsky et al., 1996, Bekelman et al., 2003).

A systematic review of the effect of financial sponsorship found 11 studies that compared the outcome of studies sponsored by industry and those that were not sponsored (Bekeleman et al., 2003). In every one of the included studies those that were sponsored were more likely to have findings favourable to industry. When the results were pooled, the sponsored studies were almost four times more likely to find results favourable to industry. One study included in the review looked at 69 randomized trials of non-steroidal anti-inflammatory drugs, which are prescribed on a huge scale for arthritis (Rochon et al., 1994). All of these trials were sponsored by industry, and the sponsor's drug was deemed to be as good as the comparative treatment in three-quarters of the studies and better in a quarter. In not a single case was the drug being investigated worse than the comparative treatment.

The main determinant of whether reviews find passive smoking to be harmful or safe is whether the authors have ties with the tobacco industry (Barnes and Bero, 1998). In the intense debate over whether third-generation contraceptive pills increased women's chance of developing thromboembolic disease, all industry-sponsored studies concluded that the pills were safe, whereas all publicly funded studies found that they increased thromboembolic disease (Vandenbroucke, 2000).

Despite the evidence that financial conflicts of interest have a powerful effect on the results and interpretation of studies, authors did not until recently declare conflicts of interest. The International Committee of Medical Journal Editors stated that authors should do so as long ago as 1993 (ICMJE, 1993), but a study in 2001 looked at 3642 articles in the five leading general medical journals (*Annals of Internal Medicine*, *BMJ*, *Lancet*, *JAMA* and the *New England Journal of Medicine*) and found that only 52 (1.4%) declared authors' conflicts of interest (Hussain and Smith, 2001). Yet most authors have a conflict of interest. A study in the *New England Journal of Medicine* looked at the financial conflicts of interest of authors of 75 pieces in prominent medical journals on calcium channel antagonists (Stelfox et al., 1998). The investigators asked the 89 authors of the articles whether pharmaceutical companies had provided them with reimbursement for attending a symposium, fees for speaking, fees for organising education, funds for research, funds for a member of staff or fees for consulting. They also asked about the ownership of stocks and shares in companies. Sixty-nine (80%) of the authors responded, and 45 (63%) revealed that they had financial conflicts of

interest. Yet in only two of the 75 articles had conflicts of interest been exposed.

Journals have become steadily stricter in requiring authors to declare conflicts of interest, but newspaper stories appear regularly showing that authors have undeclared conflicts of interest (Monmaney, 1999). Such stories damage the credibility of journals, and there is increasing anxiety – particularly in the United States – that, in the words of an editor of the *New England Journal of Medicine*, academic medicine is 'for sale' (Angell, 2000).

The main response to conflict of interest has been disclosure, but is that always adequate? There must come a point where the conflict is so substantial that more is required. No journal, for example, would have an editorial on a new drug written by an employee of the company that manufactured the drug. Most journals deem disclosure adequate for original studies but are stricter with review articles. Few journals, however, are transparent on what the cut-off point is for excluding authors. Nor do journals tend to disclose the scale of conflicts of interest. Yet a financial conflict worth tens of thousands of pounds may have a much greater impact than having lunch bought by a pharmaceutical company.

Conflict of interest is best studied among authors, but it also arises with reviewers, editors and owners of journals. Conflict of interest among reviewers is poorly studied, but it is likely to be common as most reviewers are also authors. Disclosure cannot work here, because reviewers are rarely revealed to readers. Many journals ask reviewers about conflicts of interest, but how they use the information is usually unclear.

A study of 30 journals found that only nine had explicit policies on editors' conflicts of interest, and only one publicly declared editors' conflicts (Haivas et al., 2004). Yet editors can have substantial conflicts of interest. For example, many editors are responsible for the budgets of their journals, and if they accept a study funded by the pharmaceutical industry the journal may make hundreds of thousands of pounds from sales of reprints. We do not know of any study of conflicts of interest of the managers and owners who publish medical journals.

It is largely accepted now that conflicts of interest can have a substantial influence on studies in many journals. Authors' conflicts of interest were not usually disclosed until recently, but journals have made considerable progress with disclosing those conflicts. Journals are not clear, however, on when disclosure is not an adequate response, and they have made little progress with managing the conflicts of interest of reviewers, editors, managers and owners.

RESEARCH MISCONDUCT

'Research misconduct' is defined by the Federal government in the United States 'as fabrication, falsification, or plagiarism in proposing, performing, or reviewing research, or in reporting research results (Office of Science and Technology Policy, 2000). Fabrication is making up data or results and recording or reporting them. Falsification is manipulating research materials, equipment or processes, or changing or omitting data or results such that the research is not accurately represented in the research record. Plagiarism is the appropriation of another person's ideas, processes, results or words without giving appropriate credit. For the Americans 'research misconduct does not include honest error or differences of opinion'.

A finding of research misconduct depends on three requirements: (1) there must be 'a significant departure from accepted practices of the relevant research community'; (2) the misconduct must be 'committed intentionally or knowingly, or recklessly'; and (3) the allegations must be proved 'by a preponderance of evidence'.

American scientists have thought it important to try to define research misconduct as exactly as possible, so that researchers can be very clear about when they may be overstepping the mark. The Europeans, in contrast, have opted for broad definitions. The Norwegian Committee on Scientific Dishonesty defines research misconduct as 'all serious deviation from accepted ethical research practice in proposing, performing, and reporting research' (Nylenna et al., 1999). A consensus conference of all the British bodies that might be concerned with misconduct in biomedical research went for something still broader: 'Behaviour by a researcher, intentional or not, that falls short of good ethical and scientific standards' (Joint Consensus Conference on Misconduct in Biomedical Research, 1999). This definition does not include anything about falling 'seriously' or 'significantly' short of good standards and does not depend on 'intention'. Traditionally in law 'ignorance is no defence', and this definition places an onus on researchers to know what are 'good ethical and scientific standards'.

The incidence of research misconduct clearly depends crucially on how it is defined. If redundant publication, misdemeanours around authorship and failure to disclose conflicts of interest are defined as research misconduct, then it is extremely common. If, however, it is restricted to the classic triad of 'fabrication, falsification, or plagiarism', then it is much less common, particularly as the degree of falsification or plagiarism must be substantial to count as research misconduct.

A survey conducted in 2002 among American researchers achieved a 40% response rate, and 2% of the 3247 respondents admitted to falsifying data, plagiarism or ignoring major aspects of rules for conducting studies with humans (Martinson et al., 2005). Nearly 8% said, however, that they had circumvented what they judged to be minor aspects of such requirements. Some 13% had overlooked

'others' use of flawed data or questionable interpretation of data' and nearly 16% reported they had changed the design, methods or results of a study 'in response to pressure from a funding source'.

The response to research misconduct has been driven not by such surveys but by high-profile cases of misconduct. In 2006, for example, Seoul National University concluded that Hwang Woo-suk, a pioneer in stem cell research and a national hero in Korea, had fabricated much of his research. His claim in 2005 to have produced stem cells from adult cells had reverberated around the world because it opened up new ways to treat Parkinson's disease and other degenerative diseases. His disgrace was equally high-profile.

The United States has experienced the most high-profile cases of research misconduct in modern times – probably not because it has more misconduct than other countries but rather because it has more research than other countries and has been energetic in exposing cases (Lock, 2001). For example, William Summerlin from the Sloan-Kettering Institute in New York, one of the world's leading biomedical research centres, claimed in the 1970s to have transplanted human corneas into rabbits. He also faked transplantation experiments in white mice by blackening patches of their skin with a pen, an extraordinarily crude form of forgery. Eventually Summerlin's misconduct could no longer be ignored, but his behaviour was attributed to a mental health problem. This is a response that is seen repeatedly. It is a form of 'scientific denial'. The United States experienced many serious cases in the 1970s and 1980s, and pressure from Congress eventually led to the creation of the Office of Research Integrity.

The Nordic countries also established national bodies to lead the response to research misconduct (Nylenna et al., 1999), but most countries, including Britain, have failed to respond to the problem nationally. Six years ago, the editors of the *Lancet* and the *BMJ* said that the United Kingdom urgently needed a body capable of investigating allegations fairly, efficiently and fast (Farthing et al., 2000). Yet allegations of misconduct still hang over the heads of 34 doctors who sought parental consent for randomized trial of neonatal care more than 12 years ago. It is high time that the public received an authoritative statement about whether the allegations are true or false (Hey and Chalmers, 2006).

Scientists have been very slow to accept the problem of research misconduct and the need to establish mechanisms to prevent and investigate it. They often argue that it is rare, happens only among those who have some sort of mental health problem, and does not matter too much – because science is 'self-correcting'. These arguments have become steadily less convincing as more high-profile cases have emerged and because of surveys suggesting high levels of misconduct – albeit that much of it is 'minor'.

Indeed, it is arguably the high level of minor misconduct that is more damaging to science than the smaller number of very serious cases.

In many countries the management of research misconduct is left to local institutions – universities or hospitals – and yet they lack experience in knowing how to respond and are often inclined to bury the cases for fear of bad publicity. That is why a national body is needed to lead. The body should not only investigate cases of misconduct but also promote good practice and deepen understanding of research misconduct through research and education.

REFERENCES

Altman DG. Statistics in medical journals: developments in the 1980s. *Stat Med* 1991; **10**: 1897–1913.

Angell M. Is academic medicine for sale? *N Engl J Med* 2000; **324**: 1516–1518.

Barnes DE, Bero LA. Why review articles on the health effects of passive smoking reach different conclusions. *JAMA* 1998; **279**: 1566–1570.

Bekelman JE, Li Y, Gross CP. Scope and impact of financial conflicts of interest in biomedical research: a systematic review. *JAMA* 2003; **289**: 454–465.

Bhopal R, Rankin J, McColl E, Thomas L, Kaner E, Stacy R, Pearson P, Vernon B, Rodgers H. The vexed question of authorship: views of researchers in a British medical faculty. *Br Med J* 1997; **314**: 1009.

Chalmers I. Under-reporting research is scientific misconduct. *JAMA* 1990; **263**: 1405–1408.

Chalmers I. Lessons for research ethics committees. *Lancet* 2002; **359**: 174.

Chalmers I. In the dark: drug companies should be forced to publish all the results of clinical trials. *N Sci* 2004; **181**: 19.

Chalmers I. From optimism to disillusion about commitment to transparency in the medico-industrial complex. *J Royal Soc Med* 2006; **99**: 337–340.

Chan A-W, Hròbjartsson A, Haahr M, Gøtzsche PC, Altman DG. Empirical evidence for selective reporting of outcomes in randomized trials: comparison of protocols to publications. *JAMA* 2004; **291**: 2457–2465.

Clark O, Clark L, Djulbegovic B. Is clinical research still too haphazard? *Lancet* 2001; **358**: 1648.

Committee on Publication Ethics. www.publicationethics.org.uk

Cowley AJ, Skene A, Stainer K, Hampton JR The effect of lorcainide on arrhythmias and survival in patients with acute myocardial infarction. *Int J Cardiol* 1993; **40**: 161–166.

Demicheli V, Di Pietrantonj C. Peer review for improving the quality of grant applications. The Cochrane Database of Methodology Reviews 2003, Issue 1. Art. No.: MR000003. DOI: 10.1002/14651858.MR000003.

Dickersin K. How important is publication bias? A synthesis of available data. *AIDS Educ Prev* 1997; **9** (1 Suppl): 15–21.

Dickersin K. Publication bias: recognising the problem, understanding its origins and scope, and preventing harm.

In: Rothstein H, Sutton A, Borenstein M, eds. *Handbook of Publication Bias*. New York: John Wiley & Sons, Inc., 2004.

Eysenbach G. Medical students and scientific misconduct: survey among 229 students bmj.com/cgi/eletters/322/7281/274#12443, 3 February 2001.

Farthing M, Horton R, Smith R. Research misconduct: Britain's failure to act. *Br Med J* 2000; **321**: 1485–1486.

Flanagin A, Carey LA, Fontanarosa PB, Phillips SG, Pace BP, Lundberg GD, Rennie D. Prevalence of articles with honorary authors and ghost authors in peer-reviewed medical journals. *JAMA* 1998; **280**: 222–224.

Godlee F, Gale CR, Martyn CN. Effect on the quality of peer review of blinding reviewers and asking them to sign their reports: a randomized controlled trial. *JAMA* 1998; **280**: 237–240.

Godlee F, Jefferson T. Peer review in health sciences. 2nd edition. London: BMJ Books, 2003.

Goodman N. Survey of fulfilment of criteria of authorship in published medical research. *Br Med J* 1994; **309**: 1482.

Goodyear M. Learning from the TGN1412 trial. *Br Med J* 2006; **332**: 677–8.

Haivas I, Schroter S, Waechter F, Smith R. Editors' declaration of their own conflicts of interest. *CMAJ* 2004; **171**(5). doi:10.1503/cmaj.1031982.

Haynes RB. Where's the meat in clinical journals? *ACP J Club* 1993; **119**: A23–24.

Hey E, Chalmers I. Are any of the criticisms of the CNEP trial true? *Lancet* 2006; **367**: 1032–1033.

Horton R. The signature of responsibility. *Lancet* 1997; **350**: 5–6.

Hudson Jones A, McLellan F. Ethical issues in biomedical publication. Baltimore, MD: Johns Hopkins University Press, 2000.

Hussain A, Smith R. Declaring financial competing interests: survey of five general medical journals. *Br Med J* 2001; **323**: 263–264.

International Committee of Medical Journal Editors. Conflict of interest. *Lancet* 1993; **341**: 742–743.

International Committee of Medical Journal Editors. Uniform requirements for manuscripts submitted to biomedical journals: writing and editing for biomedical publication. http://www.icmje.org/ (accessed 15 April 2006).

Jefferson T, Alderson P, Wager E, Davidoff F. Effects of editorial peer review: a systematic review. *JAMA* 2002; **287**: 2784–2786.

Jefferson T, Rudin M, Brodney Folse S, Davidoff F. Editorial peer review for improving the quality of reports of biomedical studies. The Cochrane Database of Methodology Reviews 2006, Issue 1. Art. No.: MR000016. DOI: 10.1002/14651858. MR000016.pub2.

Joint Consensus Conference on Misconduct in Biomedical Research. Consensus statement. 28 and 29 October 1999. http://www.rcpe.ac.uk/esd/consensus/misconduct_99.html (accessed 10 July 2003).

Justice AC, Cho MK, Winker MA, Berlin JA, Rennie D. The PEER investigators. Does masking author identity improve peer review quality? A randomised controlled trial. *JAMA* 1998; **280**: 240–242.

Krimsky S, Rothenberg LS, Stott P, Kyle G. Scientific journals and their authors' financial interests: a pilot study. *Sci Eng Ethics* 1996; **2**: 395–410.

Lock S. Research misconduct 1974–1990: an imperfect history. In: Lock S, Wells F, Farthing M, eds. *Fraud and Misconduct in Biomedical Research*. 3rd edition. London: BMJ Books, 2001.

Lock S, Wells F, Farthing M. eds. Fraud and misconduct in biomedical research. 3rd edition. London: BMJ Books, 2001.

Lock S. *A Difficult Balance: Editorial Peer Review in Medicine*. London: Nuffield Provincials Hospital Trust, 1985.

Martinson BC, Anderson MS, de Vries R. Scientists behaving badly. *Nature* 2005; **435**: 737–738.

McNutt RA, Evans AT, Fletcher RH, Fletcher SW. The effects of blinding on the quality of peer review. A randomized trial. *JAMA* 1990; **263**: 1371–1376.

Monmaney T. Medical journals may have flouted own ethics 8 times. *Los Angeles Times*, October 21, 1999.

Moore T. *Deadly Medicine*. New York: Simon & Schuster, 1995.

Nylenna M, Andersen D, Dahlquist G et al. On behalf of the National Committees on Scientific Dishonesty in the Nordic Countries. Handling of scientific dishonesty in the Nordic countries. *Lancet* 1999; **354**: 57–61.

Office of Science and Technology Policy, Executive office of the President. Federal policy on research misconduct. Federal register 6 December 2000, pp 76260-4. http:// frwebgate.access.gpo. gov/cgi-bin/getdoc.cgi?dbname=2000_register&docid=00-30852-filed (accessed 10 July 2003).

Peters D, Ceci S. Peer-review practices of psychological journals: the fate of submitted articles, submitted again. *Behav Brain Sci* 1982; **5**: 187–255.

Rennie D. Misconduct and journal peer review. In: Godlee F, Jefferson T, eds. *Peer Review in Health Sciences*. London: BMJ Books, 1999.

Rennie D, Yank V, Emanuel L. When authorship fails: a proposal to make contributors accountable. *JAMA* 1997; **278**: 579–585.

Rochon PA, Gurwitz JH, Simms RW, Fortin PR, Felson DT, Minaker KL et al. A study of manufacturer supported trials of non-steroidal anti-inflammatory drugs in the treatment of arthritis. *Arch Int Med* 1994; **154**: 157–163.

Savulescu J, Chalmers I, Blunt J. Are research ethics committees behaving unethically? Some suggestions for improving performance and accountability. *Br Med J* 1996; **313**: 1390–1393.

Shapiro DW, Wenger WS, Shapiro MF. The contributions of authors to multiauthored biomedical research papers. *JAMA* 1994; **271**: 438–442 (abstract).

Smith L, Byers JF. Gene therapy in the post-Gelsinger era. *JONAS Healthcare Law Ethics Reg* 2002; **4**: 104–110.

Smith R. *The Trouble with Medical Journals*. London: RSM Press, 2006.

Stelfox HT, Chua G, O'Rourke K, Detsky AS. Conflict of interest in the debate over calcium channel antagonists. *N Engl J Med* 1998; **338**: 101–105.

Thompson DF. Understanding financial conflicts of interest. *N Engl J Med* 1993; **329**: 573–576.

van Rooyen S, Godlee F, Evans S, Black N, Smith R. Effect of open peer review on quality of reviews and on reviewers' recommendations: a randomised trial. *Br Med J* 1999; **318**: 23–27.

van Rooyen S, Godlee F, Evans S, Smith R, Black N. Effect of blinding and unmasking on the quality of peer review: a randomised trial. *JAMA* 1998; **280**: 234–237.

Vandenbroucke JP. Competing interests and controversy about third generation oral contraceptives. *Br Med J* 2000; **320**: 381.

Walsh E, Rooney M, Appleby L, Wilkinson G. Open peer review: a randomised controlled trial. *Br J Psychiatry* 2000; **176**: 47–51.

Wennerås C, Wold A. Nepotism and sexism in peer-review. *Nature* 1997; **387**: 341–343.

Wilcox LJ. Authorship. The coin of the realm. The source of complaints. *JAMA* 1998; **280**: 216–217.

102

Human Reproductive Cloning

D. GARETH JONES AND KERRY A. GALVIN

CLONING: A BRIEF HISTORY

The cloning of human beings is the one subject capable of eliciting almost universal condemnation. For many, human cloning is a step no civilized society would ever take, and any move by scientists or legislators in this direction would bring the whole of the scientific enterprise into disrepute. Such negative views on human cloning are widespread, coming from parliaments, governments, scientific bodies, countless interest groups as well as the lay public. Diverse as these groups are, the bond that unites them is the belief that human cloning would imperil the dignity not only of the clones themselves but also in some indefinable way the human race as a whole.

The object of this repugnance is 'human reproductive cloning', the asexual reproduction of an individual by somatic cell nuclear transfer. Integral to this form of cloning is the placement of the cloned embryo in a woman's uterus for development to term. Reproductive cloning should not be confused with therapeutic or research cloning, where the cloned embryo is not allowed to develop further, instead being used for research or therapeutic purposes (including serving as a source of stem cells).

For most people the current debate on human cloning commenced in February 1997 with the intense publicity that surrounded the publication of the now famous paper reporting the birth of Dolly the sheep (Wilmut et al., 1997). Dolly showed that an adult mammalian cell can be reprogrammed to form an entirely new individual, overturning the fundamental scientific dogma that it is impossible to clone mammals.

Cloning, however, was not solely a phenomenon of the 1990s. Scientific interest in cloning existed well before 1997, commencing in the late nineteenth century and continuing unabated throughout the twentieth century.

Ethical and social debate on human cloning has also been ongoing for at least 40 years. Initial debate can be traced to the 1960s when JBS Haldane and Joshua Lederberg (Lederberg, 1966) were speculating on uses of cloning in social engineering and evolutionary terms. Although these speculations were more akin to science fiction than scientific reality, they elicited serious responses from theologians at the time (Fletcher, 1970; Ramsey, 1970).

The 1970s and early 1980s were characterized by more relevant contributions to the cloning debate. Willard Gaylin of the Hastings Center thought the Frankenstein myth would become a reality through cloning. However, he was perceptive enough to realize that a Mother Theresa clone could evolve into a tyrant, whereas a Hitler clone could turn into a saint. Richard McCormick, a Roman Catholic theologian and bioethicist, viewed cloning entirely in eugenic terms, with its potential for maximizing traits like intelligence, creativity and artistic ability (McCormick, 1981). These views were shared by many others involved in the cloning debate at that time. In the early 1990s, there was renewed interest in human cloning with the demonstration that early human embryos could be duplicated in a manner akin to the natural production of identical twins (Hall et al., 1993). This mediocre scientific achievement elicited a surprising amount of ethical debate.

While this academic debate was going on, considerable scientific progress was quietly being made in a few agricultural research laboratories, including the Roslin Institute outside Edinburgh. This institute produced Dolly and other cloned sheep. Dolly's cloning from an *adult* cell raised the spectre of human cloning and was instantly transformed into something shocking and abhorrent. This was despite the fact that the Roslin research was directed towards understanding fundamental developmental processes, not the cloning of humans.

Principles of Health Care Ethics, Second Edition   Edited by R.E. Ashcroft, A. Dawson, H. Draper and J.R. McMillan
© 2007 John Wiley & Sons, Ltd

THE INTERNATIONAL RESPONSE TO CLONING

The birth of Dolly evoked an immediate and profoundly negative response towards the cloning of human individuals from the international community. Within weeks the European Parliament had called for a ban on human cloning (European Parliament, 1997), which it saw as a serious violation of fundamental human rights and as offence against human dignity. Similarly, the General Assembly of the World Health Organization (WHO) adopted a resolution affirming that human cloning is contrary to human integrity and morality. The 186 member states of UNESCO (1997) unanimously passed a declaration towards the end of 1997 calling for a cloning ban. Similar sentiments were expressed by the Council of Europe, the Royal Society, the National Bioethics Advisory Commission in the United States and the Academy of Science in Australia.

These early resolutions against the cloning of humans have been repeated countless number of times in the intervening years. Although the initial opposition was principally to reproductive cloning, the ethical and legal waters have become muddied by those countries and groups who oppose therapeutic (research) cloning as vigorously as they oppose reproductive cloning. Hence, the current situation is that it is only the banning of reproductive cloning for which the international community displays any form of single-mindedness.

The United Nations has debated how best to regulate human cloning for several years without reaching a consensus, despite unanimous support from member states for a global ban on human reproductive cloning. The lack of consensus reflects divided opinion over the way forward for therapeutic (research) cloning. The United States has experienced similar problems in attempting to legislate against *all* forms of human cloning and as a result has no national legislation on the issue (see Pattinson and Caulfield, 2004). Other countries with no such legislation include Thailand, Portugal and China.

Other countries have drawn up laws to regulate human cloning. For example, the United Kingdom's Human Fertilisation and Embryology Act (1990) permits therapeutic cloning under licence of the Reproductive Cloning Act (2001), but it prohibits any research with reproductive cloning as its aim. Other countries with legislation prohibiting reproductive cloning include Australia, New Zealand, Germany, Austria, Spain, Norway, Japan and Switzerland.

A MISTRUST OF SCIENTISTS?

To some extent, opposition to cloning may be tied up with opposition to scientific, especially biomedical, advances at the beginning of human life. Cloning is viewed as perhaps the quintessential way in which scientists are attempting to radically transform human nature and tamper with what makes us unique as human beings. Initial responses to the advent of IVF technology voiced many of these same fears, although the far more extensive ethical debates that are now encouraged magnify the concerns many times over.

Scientists are seen to be misleading the general public and to be transgressing boundaries that should never be breached. As a result cloning has become a metaphor for unbridled science, for the unforgivable scientific sin and for the temptation of scientists to play God. The fears such scenarios instil in ordinary people appear to be justified when so-called fertility experts like Drs Panayiotis Zavos and Severino Antinori publicize their ongoing plans to clone a human being (Zavos, 2003). Mistrust in scientists was further cemented in 2004 following false claims by South Korean scientists that they had successfully cloned human embryos. Unfortunately, charades like this hurt the public perception of science and scientists, and they cast a dark shadow over cloning as a legitimate scientific pursuit.

Journalists and the media also play a role in the promulgation of this picture, and this was overtly so following the announcement of the birth of Dolly. *Time* magazine referred to Ian Wilmut as 'the first man to create fully formed life from adult body parts since Mary Shelley's mad scientist'. It could not help but compare him to Dr Frankenstein (*Time*, 1997). Another theme that shone through repeatedly was the desire of scientists to usurp God's control by becoming creators in their own right. The *Time* article compared Dolly's birth to the biblical account of creation: 'Not since God took Adam's rib and fashioned a helpmate for him has anything so fantastic occurred'.

Cloning appears to frighten and appal most people who are suspicious of scientists and science because of the 'worst-case scenarios' of cloning published in the media. Cloning with its apparent ability to produce humans to order is seen as something that threatens our identity. Hence, the front page photographs of identical babies, Hitlers, Einsteins or Mozarts being spewed out of grotesque-looking laboratory machines. This is the myth of reproductive cloning, with its powerful message that humans are able to produce *exact* replicas of living and no-longer-living human beings. But this is science fiction, and it is aeons removed from Dolly the sheep or Snuppy the dog (the one cloning success of the now discredited Korean scientists). Nevertheless, we need to ask one question: are there any serious grounds put forward for the cloning of human beings?

WHY CLONE A HUMAN BEING?

In the current debate, a majority of reasons given for cloning tend to be of a reproductive nature, and include:

- infertile, gay or lesbian couples wishing to have genetically related children;
- parents wishing to replace an aborted foetus, a dead baby or a child killed in an accident;
- parents looking for a sibling to be a compatible tissue or organ donor for a child dying from leukaemia or kidney failure;
- a couple with a recessive lethal gene, who wish to have a genetically related child and, therefore, want to avoid the use of donor genes or selective abortion;
- a wife whose husband is dying and who wishes to have biological offspring of the dying husband.

In some of these cases, children would be born to satisfy the desires or wishes of adults. Where this is the case, and even if we are sympathetic to the reasoning behind it, it prompts us to ask whether these children are being loved primarily for their usefulness, rather than for what they have to offer as unique individuals. There is no doubt that this potential does exist, but it is not inevitable. Indeed, it may be no more likely to occur than when a child is conceived for a given purpose by natural means.

More deceptive is the assumption sometimes encountered that the clone will be an exact replacement for a child who has died. This is gravely misleading because the parents would not be 'getting back' the original child. The cloned child would probably differ in countless ways and would be at least as unique and distinctive as are identical twins. There is no such thing as a replacement child; they are not interchangeable commodities, either biologically or culturally.

A particularly spurious reason for the use of cloning is as a means of cheating death. It is foolhardy to believe that cloning provides a route to some form of immortality; the clone is a different person from his or her progenitor and will die as inevitably as the rest of us die. In no sense would mortality be bypassed by reproductive cloning, even in the unlikely event of its being perfected biologically. The individual will live on in his or her clone only to the extent that we currently live on in our naturally conceived children. Death cannot be cheated, cloning or no cloning.

THE CASE AGAINST CLONING

As we have seen, there appears to be an all-pervasive feeling that cloning is inherently tainted. However, it is necessary to probe further and examine the reasons underpinning such a feeling. How convincing are these? Much of the controversy surrounding cloning stems from a focus on extreme scenarios. A popular fear is that of mass cloning in a totalitarian society, where clones will be used as slaves. Another is the production of clones as mere playthings, in order to satisfy the ego or whims of their progenitors

(Jones, 2001). As already mentioned, this is yet another frequently encountered scenario in the replication of someone who has already lived (a tyrant, a genius, a famous musician, a loved one). Confronted by such nefarious reasons for cloning, with the assumption that clones will inevitably be downtrodden and demeaned, it is hardly surprising that the very possibility of reproductive cloning releases a welter of moral antibodies. Such motives are foolhardy and reprehensible, and would almost certainly undermine human dignity.

Extreme scenarios of this order should be taken seriously, but it is distinctly unhelpful to confine all discussions of reproductive cloning (let alone therapeutic or research cloning) to these possibilities. Scenarios such as these do nothing to further contemporary scientific debate, which is far removed from cloning on a mass scale or from ego cloning. This is merely science fiction. Despite this, cloning is regarded as a despicable act. What are the major reasons given?

CLONING IMPERILS HUMAN DIGNITY

The terms 'human cloning' and 'human dignity' have been linked by a number of groups (the United Nations, the European Parliament and the WHO) when speaking out against the procedure. Examples include: human cloning is 'incompatible with human dignity', it is 'a serious violation of fundamental human rights and ... offends against human dignity' and it is 'contrary to human dignity and morality'. Indeed, an enduring association between these terms was ensured by the President's Council on Bioethics with its 2002 report entitled *Human Cloning and Human Dignity*. Why is it that so many feel that cloning is a fundamental threat to human dignity?

One concern is that cloning will lead to an instrumentalization of human beings, who will be treated as objects to be bought and sold in the marketplace. These are valid concerns, as the temptation to control the future direction of children's lives is very high. However, this may be no more inevitable for a cloned child than for a child conceived naturally. In both instances, children should be accepted and loved for who they are. Existence should be in the best interests of the children by allowing them the freedom to develop as unique individuals.

A second and compelling concern is that a clone will be forced to walk in the footsteps of another. The genetic similarity between a clone and its older progenitor raises the possibility that the clone will be pressured to live up to a set of preconceived expectations: to be exactly like 'daddy' or 'mummy'. Were this to be the case, it can be argued that the clone's own sense of uniqueness and autonomy would be undermined by adults who feel they have ordered a predetermined product. These are legitimate concerns, but they would probably only eventuate to any degree when cloning had been undertaken for egotistical reasons. However, in order to achieve this end-result, enormous behavioural pressures would have to be exerted on the child, what we might call 'behavioural cloning'. Biological cloning by itself would prove ineffective. In other words, this is not a phenomenon that has to await the advent of reproductive cloning. It exists today when behavioural pressures are exerted on children conceived by natural means; it is in no way limited to the domain of the cloned child.

A related concern is that individuals would be denied an open future because a clone would know in advance the nature of his or her future life. The concern is that a clone could do nothing but repeat a life already lived by the 'original' individual. In this manner, Kass and Callahan (2001, p. 10) describe cloning as 'an unethical experimentation on the child-to-be . . . threatening individuality, by deliberately saddling the clone with a genotype that has already lived and to whose previous life its life will always be compared'. Assertions such as these assume that clone and progenitor would be identical. This is simply not the case (see below). It would indeed be tyrannical of any third party (whether parent or 'progenitor') to impose a predetermined fate on any child, cloned or not. But this form of control would be unlikely in a healthy and nurturing family environment.

A further fundamental concern is that clones would lack genetic uniqueness because they are identical to someone already in existence (Kahn, 1997). This is worrisome if we accept that our uniqueness as individuals stems entirely from our genetic uniqueness. This cannot be true, however, because identical twins who are genetically indistinguishable demonstrate an unequivocal human uniqueness. Similarly, clones with identical genetic make-up would have different brains. This is because the organization of the brain is as much dependent upon soft wiring (influenced by the environment) as upon hard wiring (built in genetically). Environmental influences are essential for the final form of any brain (Eisenberg, 1999), and no two people will ever be exposed to exactly the same combination of events, environments or experiences. Thus, they would have different phenotypes (just like identical twins), a different sense of self, different thought processes and ultimately different personalities. Their biological uniqueness would be plain for all to see.

By itself, a lack of genetic uniqueness cannot be a threat to our freedom or human dignity. A threat would eventuate only if behavioural pressures were applied simultaneously, forcing an individual to perform in a preordained manner. But this would not be a threat unique to cloned individuals.

Controversially, it has been suggested that the lack of genetic uniqueness argument against cloning could be circumvented by combining cloning with genetic modification (Strong, 2005). This would mean that the clone would have unique genetic material. Further still, the genetic modification could be tailored so that the child would share genetic characteristics of both parents. Some may argue that this is a futuristic scenario not worthy of debate, or that it is an approach more redolent of designer babies than human cloning. However, human cloning and the slippery slope to genetic enhancement are often seen as intertwined (Bowring, 2004), and so it may be an argument worthy of attention.

An alternative perspective on the issue of human cloning and human dignity is presented by John Harris. This bioethicist argues that human dignity will be harmed more dramatically by dismissing cloning on spurious grounds than by its realization. He writes: 'if there is an issue of human dignity engaged by cloning in any of its forms, it is the huge indignity of permitting the legislative and regulatory agenda to be set by a combination of panic and prejudice' (2004, p. 143). He also contends that an added indignity is done by the promulgation of arguments by those in positions of influence, no matter how tenuous, poor or implausible, to bolster the opposition to cloning.

What has become apparent is that human dignity is more likely to be undermined by society and individuals within society than by the process of cloning itself. It is our attitudes, responses and motives that are crucial. Human dignity is unlikely to be threatened if we treat others (including cloned individuals) as equals and as beings of dignity. For all intents and purposes cloned individuals would be the same as us, and indeed indistinguishable from the uncloned majority. Any downgrading of human clones that may occur would be imposed throughout their lives, by other human beings, rather than through their inception by cloning. True as this may be, it does force a re-examination of reasons for cloning in the first place.

CLONING REPRESENTS A TECHNOLOGICAL MANIPULATION OF REPRODUCTION

A very real fear for many is that through cloning the reproductive process is being manipulated by technological means and transformed into an impersonal form of manufacture. In this scenario, clones would be seen as products made to order, rather than unpredictable or 'surprise' gifts emerging from the union of man and woman. These concerns are encapsulated by Leon Kass, American bioethicist and inaugural head of the President's Council on Bioethics. For him, any human intrusion into reproduction is a violation because it blurs the distinction between the natural and artificial. He claims that any such intervention will jeopardize the dignity and status of human beings (Kass, 1972; 2001).

Cloning is not alone in attracting this sort of criticism. Indeed, many new technological developments, particularly those in the reproductive realm such as IVF and donor insemination, initially elicited similar responses, but they have later been accepted. However, the presence of an artificial element in reproduction has not imperilled the dignity or the status of children conceived in this manner. They are ordinary individuals, who develop normally and are indistinguishable from the rest of us (Golombok et al., 1996).

Condemnation of cloning on the basis that it is an artificial intrusion into reproduction has neither basis nor consistency, unless all artificial intrusions into reproduction (any form of fertility treatment, for example) are condemned on the same grounds. Why stop with reproduction? In order to be completely consistent, all technological elements in our modern lives should be similarly criticized.

CLONING WILL LEAD TO THE FACTORY PRODUCTION OF BABIES

A related concern to that of the intrusion of an artificial element into reproduction is the picture of cloning leading to the factory production of babies. This common depiction of cloning is as misleading as it is disconcerting. Such impersonal biological manufacture is a misnomer because an environmental component is implicit in the production and subsequent development of all human beings, whether cloned or not. It is this that separates human reproduction from the type of factory manufacture that produces a particular model of car, washing machine or microwave. There is no room for individuality on the production line and no development subsequent to initial manufacture. This is in direct contrast to the human situation where a genetic blueprint undergoes constant environmental modification. Any given human being, clone or no clone, will be an individual shaped by a myriad of influences and never a reproducible 'product'.

But what if scientists and parents adopt a technocratic attitude towards cloned children, treating them as artefacts? The respect, love and recognition expressed by parents towards their children might be undermined by the *expectations* they have of them, who are treated as predetermined products or 'artefacts' (Bowring, 2004). This is a possibility, but once again, not one unique to cloning. Indeed, parents impose their will on children in a variety of ways by selecting particular foods, schools, hobbies and even professions for them. Despite admonitions that children should never be simply projects of our will, it happens every day. Current reproductive technologies do not of necessity increase the likelihood of this, and neither will cloning.

CLONING WOULD DAMAGE FAMILY RELATIONSHIPS

Human cloning could damage family relationships by introducing uncertainty and confusion into the family unit. A more specific fear is that cloning is a transgression of the natural boundaries between generations, leading to a

weakening of the social ties between them. The traditional designations of mother, father, sister and brother would be turned upside down. For example, fathers could become 'twin brothers' to their sons, mothers could give birth to their genetic twins and grandparents could be the 'genetic parents' of their grandchildren (President's Council on Bioethics, 2002).

There is no doubt that a wedge would be driven between traditional biological and family relationships. This concern has to be taken seriously, although whether it sets cloning as dramatically apart from the gamut of other parenting possibilities currently in existence is a matter for debate. For example, it has been shown that IVF children or adopted children can live happy and fulfilled lives. However, in their 2002 report, the President's Council on Bioethics argues that these family scenarios all have one thing in common, that is, they attempt to emulate the model of the 'natural' or 'traditional' family. They state that family relations involving cloned children run contrary to this model because they represent a 'unique, one-sided and replicative biological connection to only one progenitor' (p. 110).

Counter-arguments could claim that just because a family relationship is unique or untried, is not a reason to automatically condemn it. Families with cloned children should be able to deal with this in the same way that families deal with adopted children or step-children (who share a biological connection to only one parent). It is likely that it will be the social relationship, with bonds cemented through rearing and shared life experiences, that will be central, not the genetic relationship. Nevertheless, this consideration should lead to caution, as the presence of clones within a family would add to the complexity of family relationships.

CLONING INVOLVES EXPERIMENTATION ON HUMAN EMBRYOS

Within some circles (predominantly some Christian ones), opposition to cloning stems from the total moral rejection of using human embryos for research purposes. The driving principle here is that cloning is undermining the welfare and dignity of human embryos, which as the weakest and most vulnerable of human beings should never be experimented upon. For many, this is a non-negotiable position, which seeks to outlaw any form of cloning (therapeutic as well as reproductive). Others reject cloning-associated research because they fear embryos are being treated as commodities.

The theological and ethical issues raised by this position are identical to those encountered in any situation where human embryos are used in research. Whatever principles are accepted in other areas will apply equally in regard to cloning. This argument against cloning is usually directed more against therapeutic than reproductive cloning. This is because embryo destruction is intrinsic to therapeutic cloning, whereas the sole intention of reproductive cloning is to produce a new human life. A surprising consequence of this argument is that the destruction of embryos has emerged as just as significant ethically as the production of cloned individuals. It is for this reason that the tenor of the cloning debate has changed since the initial flurry of opposition to reproductive cloning alone.

CLONING IS NOT SAFE

Aside from all these arguments, it is imperative to consider the current risks associated with human reproductive cloning. With the myriad of unknowns surrounding this procedure, any attempt to clone humans at this time would be exceedingly dangerous and ethically irresponsible. Studies with mammals have shown that the overall success rate is of the order of 2% of cloned embryos producing live births (Solter, 2000). Of those born alive, many suffer from a wide range of debilitating conditions and others die prematurely. Indeed, Dolly died at the young age of six and suffered from premature arthritis at the time, although it has to be admitted that one should not base a whole safety argument on one initial case like this. In scientific terms, it remains unknown what distinguishes 'cloning lottery winners' from clones that develop abnormally, and human clones could be expected to experience similar problems (Rhind et al., 2003). These possibilities provide more than enough justification for condemning human reproductive cloning at present and in the foreseeable future.

However, this is a pragmatic argument, and the same applies to any other scientific or clinical development. There is no difference between cloning and, say, a surgical operation; if the disadvantages or risks outweigh the potential benefits then it is unethical to proceed. It could be suggested that an objection to cloning on the grounds that it is unsafe is merely a temporary argument that will disappear once techniques are improved. Others feel that this is an enduring argument against cloning because the risks imposed on children born in the course of testing the method's safety would be unacceptable, and there would be a breach of research ethics.

The President's Council on Bioethics (2002) has stated that 'there is no ethical way to try to discover whether cloning-to-produce-children can become safe, now or in the future' (p. 94). Compelling as this sounds, it was also used as an argument against the introduction of IVF. Although it should be taken seriously, it is the sort of argument that carries little weight in scientific circles, as it appears to stand in opposition to the exploratory thrust of science. When reproductive cloning is the development in question, it highlights the fragility of the interface between science and ethics. For most commentators, rejection of human cloning on the grounds of safety is the definitive argument against the procedure at present. Whether this is an argument against cloning for time immemorial remains to be determined.

CONCLUDING REMARKS

We have adopted a sceptical stance in assessing the arguments against human cloning, not in an attempt to promulgate cloning as a desirable reproductive alternative, but because accepting seriously insubstantial reasons against it may have detrimental effects on the standing of science in the eyes of the public and policy makers. Therapeutic cloning and stem cell technologies have already been hindered, even though the ultimate aim of these procedures is the alleviation of disease and suffering (Jones, 2001).

Human reproductive cloning should not be attempted at present because it is neither technically nor clinically safe. Even if it was to become feasible at some future time, one has to question whether it should be encouraged because the temptation to make other people in one's own image is very great. It may also coax us into thinking increasingly of children as products. These possibilities are far from inevitable, but cloning could heighten the risk. Allied with this is the distinct probability that cloning would be closely linked with commercial drives, akin to the market for surrogacy, embryos and gametes.

Running throughout this discussion has been an underlying question. Is cloning as distinct from the other artificial reproductive technologies as frequently suggested? There is little doubt that it is found towards one extreme end of the reproductive technology continuum, but many of the arguments against human cloning are also arguments against other reproductive manipulations such as IVF and its more recent offshoots. However, this is not often the case in practice. It follows that opposition to cloning has to be far more nuanced when there is general acceptance of the artificial reproductive technologies, whereas acceptance of the latter under certain conditions does not entail automatic acceptance of cloning. Each is to be assessed on its merits and on the individual circumstances and perspectives of those contemplating their use.

The debate over cloning (in the general sense) has been almost totally skewed by the spectre of the cloning of humans. The impression is given that the dignity of all humans will be imperilled by the existence of a small number of cloned individuals and equally by research on cloned human embryos. Although such possible threats should not be summarily dismissed, they should also be seen in the light of the myriad ways in which the dignity of naturally fertilized humans is imperilled repeatedly today by the inequitable distribution of medical resources in countless societies.

REFERENCES

Bowring F. Therapeutic and reproductive cloning: a critique. *Soc Sci Med* 2004; **58**: 401–409.

Eisenberg L. Experience, brain and behaviour: the importance of a head start. *Pediatrics* 1999; **103**: 1031–1035.

European Parliament. Cloning animals and human beings. *Bull Med Ethics* 1997; **128**: 10–11.

Fletcher J. Response to Lederberg. In: Vaux K, ed. *Who Shall Live? Medicine, Technology, Ethics*. Philadelphia: Fortress Press, 1970; pp. 60–103.

Golombok S, Brewaeys A, Cook R, Giaruzzi MT, Guerra D, Mantovani A, van Hall E, Crosignani PG, Dexeus S. The European study of assisted reproduction families: family functioning and child development. *Hum Reprod* 1996; **11**: 2324–2331.

Hall JL, Engel D, Gindoff PR. Mottla GL, Stillman RJ. Experimental cloning of human polyploid embryos using an artificial zona pelucida. *Fertil Steril* 1993, **60** (Supp 1): 1 (Abstract).

Harris J (2004) *On Cloning*. London: Routledge.

Jones DG. *Clones: The Clowns of Technology?* Carlisle: Paternoster, 2001.

Kahn A. Clone mammals ... clone man? *Nature* 1997; **386**: 119.

Kass L. Making babies. In: Kass L, ed. *Toward a More Natural Science*: *Biology and Human Affairs*. New York: The Free Press, 1972; pp. 43–79.

Kass LR. Why we should ban human cloning now: preventing a brave new world. *New Republ* 2001; **224**: 30.

Kass LR, Callahan D. Ban stand redux. *New Republ* 2001; 224: 10–2

Lederberg J. Experimental genetics and human evolution. *Am Nat* 1966; **100**: 519–531.

McCormick RA. *How Brave a New World? Dilemmas in Bioethics*. London: SCM Press, 1981.

Pattinson SD, Caulfield T. Variations and voids: the regulation of human cloning around the world. *BMC Med Ethics* 2004; **5**: E9.

President's Council on Bioethics. *Human Cloning and Human Dignity: An Ethical Enquiry*. Washington, DC: President's Council on Bioethics, 2002.

Ramsey P. *Fabricated Man: The Ethics of Genetic Control*. New Haven, CT: Yale University Press, 1970.

Rhind SM, Taylor JE, De Sousa PA, King TJ, McGarry M, Wilmut I. Human cloning: can it be made safe? *Nat Rev Genet* 2003; **4**: 855–864.

Solter D. Mammalian cloning: advances and limitations. *Nat Rev Genet* 2000; **1**: 199–207.

Strong C. Reproductive cloning combined with genetic modification. *J Med Ethics* 2005; **31**: 654–658.

Time. A special report on cloning. 10 March, 1997, pp. 40–53.

UNESCO. Universal Declaration on the Human Genome and Human Rights. Article 11, November 1997.

Wilmut I, Schneike AE, McWhir J, Kind AJ, Campbell KHS. Viable offspring derived from fetal and adult mammalian cells. *Nature* 1997; **385**: 810–813.

Zavos PM. Human reproductive cloning: the time is near. *Reprod Biomed Online* 2003; **6**: 397–398.

103

Obtaining Human Eggs for Stem Cell Research: Ethical Issues

HEATHER DRAPER

Traditionally, eggs for stem cell research in the United Kingdom have been surplus eggs from IVF donated for the purposes of research. The advantage of using surplus eggs is that the donors are already, and for their own purposes, undergoing the procedures necessary for eggs to be harvested. Harvesting eggs does carry some risks of harm, but in the context of IVF, these risks are thought to be outweighed by the potential benefit of having a child. The advantage for stem cell research of donated eggs over donated embryos is that it enables good quality embryos to be created and selected for the purposes of research rather than the researcher relying on poorer quality embryos that have been rejected for IVF purposes. But many eggs are needed to create even a single cell line, particularly when the so-called therapeutic cloning[1] is part of the research project.

An alternative, arguably more plentiful, source is to pay healthy female volunteers for their eggs, but paying for eggs is regarded as unethical. It is argued that trade in any kind of human tissue is inherently undignified. There are concerns, as there are in all kinds of trade in human tissue, that the poor will be prime targets and that the relationship with the person paying for the eggs will be an exploitative one. That the poor in this case will be women only heightens concerns about exploitation, given that in some countries, sub-communities and cultures, women already exercise very limited control over their bodies, particularly their reproductive capacities. A related argument concerns the extent to which financial reward can induce or coerce a person to agree to parting with tissue that they would otherwise not part with. Then there are arguments about what moral model of the human body, tissue or even genetic material is most appropriate, and whether, even if these can be viewed as property, they are property of the kind that can be freely traded. (Commodification and exploitation are discussed at length by Wilkinson and Wertheimer in Chapters 38 & 32 in this volume). Such arguments are fairly evenly met by their critics, but for good or ill, an international consensus seems to have developed in the stem cell research community that buying eggs renders stem cell research unethical, and this view was reinforced in commentaries on the Dr Woo Suk Hwang scandal. Even though trade in eggs was not illegal in Korea at the time the women were paid for them, it was still frowned upon, and the fact that members of Hwang's own research team had donated eggs was taken to make things worse, a situation which was compounded by Hwang's false denials. The scandal underlined the fact that how researchers obtain human eggs for stem cell research is still regarded as an important part of the ethics of stem cell research.

It is widely recognized, however, that the supply of eggs will be too small if the only available source is those that are surplus to IVF requirement. In the United Kingdom, two measures that might solve this problem are being debated. The first possibility is to extend egg sharing arrangements – which are increasingly common in the United Kingdom – to include the possibility of sharing eggs (and IVF treatment costs) with researchers rather than infertile couples. The second option is to encourage women who are not undergoing IVF to donate eggs altruistically and solely for the purpose of supporting stem cell research. This chapter concentrates on the ethical issues raised by these two possibilities.

---

[1] It has been pointed out that this is something of a misnomer as therapies are not yet available. See Magnus (2005).

Principles of Health Care Ethics, Second Edition   Edited by R.E. Ashcroft, A. Dawson, H. Draper and J.R. McMillan
© 2007 John Wiley & Sons, Ltd

EGG SHARING ARRANGEMENTS

Egg sharing arrangements (sometimes referred to as compensated egg sharing[2]) allow a woman to share her eggs with one, or at most two, other women in exchange for a reduction in the cost of her own infertility treatment. Egg sharing has been used in UK clinics since the 1990s. This system has increased the number of eggs available for donation and seems to have been affected rather less than sperm donation by the change in the law in the United Kingdom lifting donor anonymity. This may well be because of the cost of infertility treatment in the United Kingdom and the limited and uneven access to state funded treatment.[3] For some patients, egg sharing is the only affordable avenue available. The costs to recipients are no greater than they would be if they provided their own known donor or used donated eggs from some other source because recipients are expected to cover the cost of egg donation.

Egg sharing is to be distinguished from egg *giving*. In egg giving, eggs are exchanged for reduced treatment costs, but the provider undergoes one harvesting cycle from which all the eggs are given to recipients and then undergoes a second cycle from which she keeps all the eggs for use in her own treatment. Egg giving is considered to be less ethical than egg sharing because it requires the woman to go through two harvesting cycles, the first solely for the benefit of the recipient, and she runs the risk of having no eggs for her own use if the second cycle is unsuccessful. In egg sharing arrangements, where there are too few eggs for sharing, the provider keeps all of the eggs, and where eggs are more plentiful, the provider gets, as it were, first pick of the eggs.

The Human Fertilization and Embryology Authority (HFEA), the UK regulatory body, does not consider egg giving a 'suitable practice',[4] and egg sharing is only tolerated. The ambivalent attitude towards egg sharing is perhaps based on a tension between, on the one hand, accepting that in principle donors ought not to be expected to contribute towards the cost of donation (and reducing the total cost of IVF by the cost of the donation for egg share is consistent with this position), and on the other hand, a sense that as there is some financial gain involved, the arrangements appear, at least on the surface, to be a form of trade. Other issues are that the financial element might act as inducement, that sharing might decrease the sharers' chances of success and that there might be psychological damage or regret if the sharer's attempt is unsuccessful. Recent research suggests that egg sharers are just as likely to achieve a successful pregnancy as their recipient sisters (Thum et al., 2003), which dispenses with concerns about increased risks.[5] The HFEA sought to limit psychological harms by insisting that no more than two recipients should be involved. The HFEA point out that regret following autonomously made decisions is no reason to question the autonomy of those decisions at the time they were made: regret may signal a change of values held, rather than being indicative of incapacity. With respect to inducement, the HFEA is keeping a watching brief following the introduction of guidelines that aim to minimize the possibility of its occurring (HFEA, 2006).

EGG SHARING FOR THE PURPOSES OF STEM CELL RESEARCH

If egg sharing with infertile couples is permissible, why not egg sharing with researchers, again in return for reduced IVF costs?[6] Such arrangements are no more likely to act as an inducement to donation (and could be covered by the same protections, namely counselling and consent), and the arguments about compensation would also apply: sharers should be no more liable for the cost of donation than any other donors are. Indeed, sharing eggs with a researcher may be less harmful than sharing with an infertile couple. Eggs shared with a researcher are not intended to make babies, so women who share eggs but are not themselves able to

---

[2] To distinguish it from non-compensated egg sharing when women altruistically donate eggs surplus to their own needs during IVF treatment.

[3] Although the NHS is supposed to fund infertility treatment according to NICE guidelines, many PCTs have yet to implement these guidelines and some are unable to show that they have plans to implement them such that provision in the United Kingdom remains something of a postcode lottery (http://www.bionews.org.uk/new.lasso?storyid=3166).

[4] See HFEA Practice Guidance Note Egg Share. Online available at http://www.hfea.gov.uk/AboutHFEA/HFEAPolicy/SEEDGuidance-andDirections/HFEA%20Practice%20Guidance%20Note%20-%20Egg%20sharing.pdf (accessed 5 May 2006).

[5] Although it obviously remains the case that sharers part with eggs that could be used to generate additional embryos, which in turn could be frozen and used in subsequent IVF attempts if the initial attempts fail.

[6] This kind of egg sharing has been suggested for several years; see, for instance, Heng (2005), and the first licence to stem cell researchers proposing egg sharing arrangements was granted by the HFEA in July 2006 - something of a surprise given the Authority's ambivalence to egg sharing in general.

achieve a successful pregnancy will not be exposed to the potential psychological harms suggested by the HFEA.

Given the association in the minds of many people – particularly those undergoing infertility treatment – between genetic relatedness and parenthood, egg sharing has long struck me as a recipe for problems in the future. Egg sharers are undergoing infertility treatment precisely because they want a genetically related child, yet to do so they give away genetic material for others to have babies with. Those who donate gametes, or who engage in straight (as opposed to host) surrogacy, tend to be less concerned about genetic relatedness as a marker of parental rights and responsibilities. They instead tend to focus on the social, moral or nurturing relationships as decisive markers (see for instance van den Akker (2003), van den Akker (2005) and Golombok (2000)). Whilst my own view is that genetic relatedness is neither necessary nor sufficient in any definition of 'mother' or 'father' (see Draper (2007) and Draper (2005)), this is not a view supported by public policy, which still, for instance, relies on paternity testing to determine fiscal responsibility for children. It does not seem likely, then, that the psychological problems that concern the HFEA would be limited only to those eggs sharers who are unsuccessful in their attempts to have a genetically related child. Those who are successful might also experience difficulties in adjusting to the potential existence, *in another family*, of a genetically related child. For this reason, those who see egg sharing as a means to access what would otherwise be a financially inaccessible service might welcome an egg sharing arrangement with researchers for it comes without the cost of participating in the creation of a genetically related child for someone else to rear.

Not everyone accepts that because donors are not expected to cover the cost of donation, egg sharers ought to receive benefits-in-kind for their donations. It could be argued that egg sharing is a form of trade because the eggs are only given on the understanding that there will be a reduction in the cost of treatment; indeed, cost saving is arguably the prime motivation for compensated sharing.

Different people have different views about what constitutes trade. Lawyers may argue that if I remove a £10 note from your wallet and replace it with a £10 pound note from mine, this is arguably a form of trade. Accordingly,

paired donation[7] in the case of kidney transplantation may be regarded as a form of trade even though no finances are involved and the actions are essentially altruistic.[8,9] To the less pedantic, paired donation is only a form of trade in the sense that my exchanging the £10 notes is; it is more of a swap than a trade. The notion of trade in tissue is generally considered suspect when goods or money change hands, and clearly in the case of egg sharing money does change hands, albeit through a third party (the clinic). However, in the case of conventional egg sharing, we find the very kind of mutual aid that is found in the case of paired donation.[10] Both provider and recipient want children, and neither is readily able to achieve their goal without the help of the other. Mutual aid, if it is to be considered a form of trade, is a special kind of trade that relies on specific shared goals and aims – it is based on mutuality of interests. Babysitting circles are another example of this kind of reciprocity. All the members would like a night away from their children, none can afford to pay for a babysitter, so each agrees to do babysitting on the understanding that someone in the circle will babysit for them, in return.

Reciprocal altruism unlike pure altruism is motivated by the strong expectation that others will behave in a similar fashion. But it is not like trade either. Let us explore this further, taking the example used in 1998 by the HFEA (1998): would we be happy for someone to sell a kidney in order to fund their infertility treatment? Of course, some of us would be – those of us who do not object to trade in human tissue and consider it to be the individual's right to do with his body as he sees fit, including selling parts of it if he so chooses. But let us leave aside these more general arguments for a moment. If A sells B a kidney in order to fund infertility treatment the goals of A and B, except in the general sense that they both want something that they are currently unable to achieve, are quite different. They are dependent to some degree on each other to achieve these goals, but they need not have shared goals or even goals about which they are in mutual agreement. For instance, what if A is selling her kidney to raise funds for the Quakers but B wants a kidney primarily so that he can play a more active role in a terrorist movement? A is not typically entitled to know this – in trade all she needs to concern herself with is what she will get in return – even though

---

[7]Paired donation is when two people, one of whom needs a kidney and the other of whom is willing to donate one, are tissue incompatible. This pair is tissue matched with a pair in the same position so that the donor from both pairs gives a kidney to the recipient in both pairs.

[8]The altruism is not directed at the stranger with whom she is compatible, this is true, but it is directed towards the partner with whom the donor is incompatible

[9]In some countries, cross-donation, as it has been termed, exists for egg donation too, with couple exchanging the eggs for their respective donors to keep a genetic distance between themselves and a known donor. See Pennings (2005).

[10]Though not to the extent as would be found if Penning's suggestions were acted on.

she is unlikely to approve of the aim if she were to find out about it, and she may very well object to the uses to which the recipient puts his newfound freedom from the constraints of dialysis. But, in some sense this really is none of her business – once she has parted with the kidney, is does not belong to her and what the recipient does with his life post-transplantation is his business. Now there would be a certain reciprocity if C, a supporter of terrorism, gives B who wants to play a more active role in the same terrorism, a kidney not as an expression of altruism to B, but in place of money she does not have but would have given to his organization if she did. Here we also see mutuality because both B and C are trying to achieve the same ends, albeit by a different route. Likewise, if D gave E a kidney so that E could achieve a successful pregnancy, and in exchange for this E funded D's infertility treatment or shared eggs with her, we would again see the same mutuality. When, however, Z gives eggs to a stem cell researcher in exchange for financial help with infertility treatment, this kind of mutuality is absent and it is much more like selling a kidney to fund infertility treatment. This difference makes it less like mutual aid and more like conventional trade.

Why does this difference matter? It would make a difference to an egg sharer who did not approve of the goals of the stem cell researcher. But this is not a decisive objection. Leaving aside the coherence of accepting IVF but rejecting stem cell technology on the grounds that it destroys embryos, someone who did not approve would presumably not knowingly enter into such an agreement, but would instead prefer to egg sharing with an infertile woman. In the United Kingdom, it is not possible to donate gametes without explicitly consenting to the use to which these gametes will be put. It would therefore be unlawful for a clinic to offer an egg sharing arrangement without making explicit whether the gametes concerned were destined for procreation or research. Laws requiring similar disclosures could be introduced in other countries before extended egg sharing schemes are recognized internationally as an ethical source of eggs for stem cell research. This is not a significant objection.

A stronger argument can be based on the differing moral worth of reciprocity and trade. Reciprocity is a form of mutual aid, whereas trade is based in contract, which gives individuals rights and liabilities purely because of the contract, and not because of any recognition of mutuality. This is, of course, linked to the previous argument about goals. Reciprocity is more amenable to notions of shared human worth than trade and is more

likely to foster non-exploitative relationships of a Kantian kind, where people do not view each other purely as means to an end. At the satisfactory completion of a contract, both parties depart with what they bargained for (whether or not it was a fair deal). Mutual gratitude and/or respect are not a necessary part of trade. Mutuality of this kind is built on shared human need rather than financial or personal gratification. It is for these reasons, perhaps, that conventional egg sharing arrangements are not viewed as trade, but where the fine boundary between reciprocity and trade is crossed in the proposed egg share with stem cell researchers.

Another kind of argument is based on the value of sacrificial giving. Altruistic giving is often, but not always, considered to be the best form of giving, but another morally admirable form of giving occurs when some personal sacrifice is involved. Because of the predominant views about genetic relatedness, conventional egg sharing is sometimes viewed as a form of sacrificial giving: the sacrifice is related to the surrendering of a possible, wanted and genetically related child.[11] So, although the provider does benefit, she also sacrifices something people normally value, and this sacrifice can be thought to counteract, morally speaking, the financial gain. Extending egg sharing arrangements to stem cell researchers means that there is no such sacrifice. This does not mean that such arrangements are wrong, but it does distinguish them morally from conventional egg sharing arrangements.

If, however, genetic relatedness is misconceived or misplaced in significance in parenting, as I have argued elsewhere, then the whole notion that conventional egg sharing is sacrificial giving is also misplaced, as is the idea of mutual aid based on shared needs – as opposed to preferences. However, this might not reflect how it currently *feels* to those taking part, even if – as I would argue – these feelings are misplaced.

There is a further argument, not related to the trade/mutuality distinction, which could be used against extending egg sharing arrangements. This is that conventional arrangements are more beneficial because they result in the creation of a child, and all the good that flows from this for the parents and the child through her lifetime. Stem cell research, on the contrary, may ultimately save life, but substantial therapeutic progress is many years away. Thus, if extending egg sharing arrangements leads to a decrease in the number of eggs available for IVF, this would result in a net loss of overall good, at least in the short term. We can only speculate about the future success of stem cell research,

---

[11] I am not, of course, arguing that egg sharers give up a child. Rather they give up gametes. But if a child results from the use of their gametes by another, they will have no rights to parent this child or play any part in its childhood.

but it is not impossible that it will eventually save many lives and decrease suffering in other ways. However, even if this were not the case, it is difficult to argue that recipients have a greater right of access to eggs than researchers do. First, it would be hard to mount an argument that recipients have any *right* as such to eggs at all. Second, the preferences of those providing the eggs have to be taken into account. Given that the recipients have no formal right to be provided with eggs, there is no reason why the providers should not provide eggs for researchers if this is what they prefer – perhaps because of their views about genetic relatedness – to do.

In summary, whilst the harms to the providers of eggs are likely to be lessened if egg sharing is extended to stem cell researchers, the quality of the relationships involved is altered and a transaction results which is much closer to a trade than to mutual aid. If there is nothing wrong with trade in human tissue, particularly gametes, then this is not a problem. But the reaction to the Hwang scandal suggests that trade is still not an acceptable option to the international community. Given, then, that extending egg sharing to stem cell researchers makes it a form of trade, we ought to oppose such an extension, whilst continuing to tolerate conventional egg share arrangements. Extending egg sharing arrangements, however, does have the significant advantage of not exposing the providers to harms that they would not, in any case, have been exposed to. Egg sharers, unlike altruistic egg donors – the subjects of the next section – have to undergo all the procedures for harvesting to meet their own needs for infertility treatment. In this respect, whilst *compensated* extended egg sharing might not be an ethical option, *non-compensated* (altruistic) egg sharing with researchers might be thought better than altruistic donation for research purposes, effectively supporting the status quo. Moreover, we have to consider that traditionally donors are not expected to cover the costs of their donation, and this position is reflected in both conventional and extended egg sharing arrangements.

ENCOURAGING ALTRUISTIC EGG DONATION FOR STEM CELL RESEARCH

That women participating in non-compensated egg sharing are not exposed to additional risks in order to donate eggs for research is in not a decisive argument against altruistic donation. Take the case of live kidney donation. People who donate a kidney to a family member, friend or even altruistically to the general transplant pool in order to help a stranger are all exposed to risks – for no direct benefit to themselves – that are not present when cadaver kidneys are used. But the fact that this form of donation has greater risks and harms is not considered to be a decisive argument against live donation – though it might give us pause for

thought about whether we should do more to ensure that fewer cadaver kidneys are wasted rather than donated, thus negating the need for as many live donations.

Whilst there are other sources of eggs for stem cell research, this is also not a decisive objection to altruistic donation *per se*. Using eggs surplus to IVF is unlikely to produce enough eggs for the so-called therapeutic cloning. If, however, the alternative sources are unethical, we must reconcile ourselves to progress at a reduced pace. On the contrary, if it is permissible for women to act as altruistic volunteers of eggs, then the fact that there is an alternative source is not a necessarily an argument against altruistic donation. However, assuming sufficient eggs, which we cannot, using artistic donors is unnecessary, and the risks donors run in donating are taken unnecessarily. What makes using altruistic donors unethical under such circumstances is not, then, the level of risk *per se*, but the fact that this risk is not considered necessary. But assuming that there is *not* an adequate alternative source, we then have to decide if altruistic donation poses too great a risk to donors for them to be permitted to donate.

One way of looking at risk is in terms of the risk/benefit ratio. Risk-taking is justified if and only if the benefits outweigh the risks. But whose view about the risk/benefit ratio should be taken as authoritative? Suppose that it is unlikely that my grandmother will benefit from a kidney and, for this reason, she is not placed on the transplant register. I, however, would like her to have the chance of benefit, however small, so I offer my kidney, despite the known harms and risks of harms associated. I think on balance, the possibility of benefit *is* worth the risk, and surely this is a judgement only I can make. Thus, we could argue that it is up to women to decide for themselves, based on the available evidence, whether the potential benefit to others of a piece of research is worth the potential risks and actual harms to themselves of donating eggs. Such a calculation would have to take into account that the particular piece of research their eggs will be used for might fail, for there is never a guarantee of success, but the process of stem cell research in general might succeed. It is likely, indeed, that in discovering more about stem cells and the uses for which they can be put, experiments will take place that are unsuccessful: this is generally true of all research and scientific progress. So far so good, but to continue with the analogy; my grandmother may, of course, decline my offer, on the grounds that she does not consider the potential benefits to her – even if they are actualized – to outweigh the harms and risks of harms to me, as she judges things. Certainly, I cannot insist that she takes the kidney. In the same way, then, a researcher can refuse to take eggs from altruistic donors if they judge that the benefits are too unlikely in a specific experiment to outweigh the actual and potential harms to donors, or alternatively that the harms for a specific donor are too great to outweigh the possible benefits. Given their assessments of the risk and harms and likely benefits, they may prefer when conducting a specific piece of research only to use surplus eggs that have been donated following harvesting for IVF treatment.

But what if my grandmother is willing to take the kidney, but my surgeon disagrees with my assessment and refuses to remove it because in his own assessment of the risk/benefit ratio the risk is too great? Is it reasonable for him to refuse? Here we come up against a common difficulty in biomedical ethics; something that it might be permissible for someone acting alone to do might be unacceptable to someone whose help they request, and if their aid is crucial the individual's desires can be frustrated unless they have the right to insist upon the aid. In general, we do not think that patients can insist that doctors act against their consciences. The disapproving clinician referring the patient to someone who is more sympathetic often resolves the problem. The question of whether the other clinician *ought* to be sympathetic is often addressed with reference to other risks that individuals are permitted to take for themselves, and it is difficult to argue that it is not paternalistic to decide for others what a risk/benefit ratio ought to be to make a risk worth it.

Thus, even if the likely benefits are small, providing the altruistic donor, the researcher and the clinician harvesting the eggs consider that the risk is worth it, there seems nothing wrong with altruistic donation. Of course, all the usual caveats have to be added in relation to informed agreement on all sides.

If it is reasonable for a woman to decide that altruistic egg donation is worth the risks, should some women be denied the opportunity to act as donors for other reasons? What about women on a stem cell research team – should they be denied the opportunity to donate if they choose? My answer to this question as an issue of policy is that they should *not* be denied the opportunity to donate eggs. As scientists involved in stem cell research, they are extremely well placed to make a decision about potential benefits, and these benefits might not simply include the potential benefits to human kind. There could be other benefits, like keeping going a promising project that is becoming non-viable because sufficient eggs from alternative sources cannot be found. The researcher's career and livelihood might also be bound to the completion of such a project.

There are also several issues of equity that need to be mentioned in this context. First, why should these women scientists not be willing to expose themselves to the same risks and harms that their research requests of altruistic volunteers? Surely if they are willing to use donated eggs, then all things being equal they should be prepared to give them too. One concern is that there might be institutional or even contractual pressure to donate – for instance, researchers might be told at interview or even as part of their job description that annual donation is an expectation of all members of the research team; another is that pressure can be brought to bear on junior members of research teams by senior members because of the influence they have, or are perceived to have, over the careers of juniors. These kinds of concerns often surface in discussions about the circumstances required for an action to count as truly voluntary or even autonomous (see Stoljar in Chapter 3 of this volume). The important issue here, though, is whether the possibility of undue pressure or inducement is best addressed by dictating a policy that forbids women stem cell researchers (or at least junior stem cell researchers) from donating, or whether it is best addressed by looking at the ways in which more powerful members of a research team generally use this power to exert unreasonable pressure on less powerful ones. Second, it is questionable whether it is the fact that women researchers are the potential donors here that makes such a paternalistic policy seem acceptable. Would or should such a policy be considered necessary if the potential donors were likely to be only men? This leads to one final issue under equity. It could be argued that this is a gender issue because only women stem cell scientists are able to donate eggs for stem cell research. It is true that only women produce eggs, but both men and women produce gametes. If the principal concern about the use of members of the research teams is that the burden falls only on women, this is easily addressed. In the United Kingdom, the lifting of donor anonymity has severely affected supplies of sperm for infertility treatment. According to a BBC survey in September 2006 (http://news.bbc.co.uk/1/hi/health/5341982.stm.) around 70% of clinics in the United Kingdom either had no supplies of sperm or almost no supplies of sperm.Perhaps we should consider an alternative form of egg sharing arrangement, one where eggs are donated to stem cell researchers in exchange for sperm rather than reduced treatment costs. Such a scheme would ensure that both male and female stem cell researchers were afforded the same opportunity to donate gametes for stem cell research albeit with different potential harms (assuming that some men might feel harmed by the prospect of a genetically related child being brought up by another family).[12]

---

[12] However, such a scheme – even though devoid of financial implications – would be open to some of the objections to extended egg sharing arrangements, namely that there would be a move away from mutual aid as described in the previous section.

It has frequently been noted that many women in Korea volunteered to be donors as a matter of national pride when the Hwang scandal broke. We might ask whether this pride was misplaced, or whether the Korean team was really likely to be the first to crack the secrets of human cloning at all given the fraudulent practices exposed. Such observations, however, do not amount to evidence that the women concerned were incompetent to make a decision to donate for themselves. Nor do such observations help to ensure that mechanisms are in place to guarantee that it was their *own* national pride that motivated them and not the national pride of their fathers, sons, husbands or brothers. These concerns based on the processes of ensuring autonomous and informed participation apply equally well to the female relatives of those who suffer from degenerative conditions, whom it is also, and not infrequently, supposed (Magnus and Cho, 2005) will want to volunteer as egg donors in projects aimed at treating these same degenerative conditions. Again, the question should be how well they are informed about the risks and possible benefits, not whether by virtue of being a family member – with more to gain if the research pays off – they should be encouraged to donate or excluded altogether.

CONCLUSIONS

Non-compensated egg sharing is undoubtedly the most ethical method of obtaining eggs for stem cell research. The donors will in any event be exposed to the risks and altruism is generally, though not always, ethically superior to giving for gain. But this does not mean that other methods are unethical. Extending compensated egg sharing arrangements to stem cell researchers similarly only exposes sharers to risks that they would in any event be taking. Extended egg sharing arrangements, however, are more like trade than mutual aid. This is not a problem for those who think that trade in human tissue or gametes permissible; however, trade does not seem to be acceptable to the international community. Using altruistic donors has the disadvantage of exposing women to harms and risk of harms that they would not otherwise be exposed to. Altruistic donation is still defensible, particularly as alternative methods fail to meet legitimate demand. Of course, those who decide they would like to donate cannot act alone;

they can only act in cooperation with the researchers – who must be clear and realistic about what the potential benefits might be – and doctors – who must be clear about the potential and actual harms. It is unreasonable to have a blanket ban on female members of stem cell research teams donating eggs for stem cell research. However, it is important to make certain that mechanisms are in place to ensure that neither they – nor any other woman – is coerced into donating eggs.

REFERENCES

Draper H. Why there is no right to know one's genetic origins. In: Athanssoulis N, ed. *Philosophical Reflections on Medical Ethics.* Basingstoke: Palgrave/Macmilian, 2005; pp. 70–87.

Draper H. Payments to gamete donors. In: Horsey K, Biggs H, eds. *Human Fertilisation and Embryology: Reproducing Regulation.* London: UCL Press, 2007; pp. 69–82.

Golombok S. *Parenting: What Really Counts?* London: Routledge, 2000.

Heng BC. Egg-sharing in return for subsidized fertility treatment – an ethically justifiable and practical solution to overcome the shortage of donor oocytes for therapeutic cloning. *Med Hypotheses* 2005; **65**(5): 999–1000.

HFEA. *Consultation on the Implementation of the Withdrawal of Payment to Donors.* 1998 (http://www.hfea.gov.uk/cps/rde/xbcr/SID-3F57D79B-DFC7C800/hfea/Consultation_on_the_Implentation_of_Withdrawal_of_Payment_to_Donors.pdf).

HFEA. *Sperm, Egg and Embryo Donation (SEED) Review.* 2006 (http://www.hfea.gov.uk/cps/rde/xbcr/SID-3F57D79B-DFC7C800/hfea/SEEDReport05.pdf).

Magnus D, Cho MK. Issues in oocyte donation for stem cell research. *Science* 2005; **308**: 1747–1748.

Pennings G. Gamete donation in a system of need-adjusted reciprocity. *Hum Reprod.* Accessed ed online doi:10.1093/humrep/dei2005.

Thum MY, Gafar A, Wren M, Faris R, Ogunyemi B, Korea L, et al. Does egg-sharing compromise the chance of donors or recipients achieving a live birth? *Hum Reprod* 2003; **18**: 2363–2367.

van den Akker OBA. Genetic and gestational surrogate mothers' experience of surrogacy. *J Reprod Infant Psychol* 2003; **21**(2): 145–61.

van den Akker OBA. A longitudinal pre-pregnancy to post-delivery comparison of genetic and gestational surrogate and intended mothers: confidence and gynaecology. *J Psychosom Obstet Gynaecol* 2005; **26**(4): 277–84.

104

The Ethics of Xenotransplantation

JONATHAN HUGHES

INTRODUCTION

Xenotransplantation can be defined as the transplantation of live cells, tissues or organs between members of different animal species. This chapter is concerned with the ethics of animal-to-human xenotransplantation, a technology that not only offers potentially huge benefits but also raises serious ethical problems.

The most widely discussed application of the technology involves the transplantation of whole organs from animals into humans. The scarcity of organs from human donors, according to UK Transplant (2005), is such that approximately 8000 people in the United Kingdom are in need of organ transplants while only 2800 transplants take place each year. As a result, in the United Kingdom alone approximately 400 people die each year while waiting for a kidney, lung, heart or liver to become available, and many more die before even getting onto the transplant list. In addition, prolonged waiting times can have a severe impact on quality of life. The potential benefits of making animal organs available for transplant into humans are therefore very significant.

Whole organ transplantation is, however, the least immediately promising application of xenotransplantation. Although experimental animal-to-human organ transplants date back to the seventeenth century, no recipient has survived more than a few months, and in most cases much less. Most have died either because of the rejection and destruction of the transplanted organ by the recipient's immune system, or from infections resulting from the suppression of the immune system that is carried out in order to reduce the likelihood of rejection.

Although progress has been made in the development of better immunosuppressive drugs and in the use of genetic modification to make the donor animal's cells appear less alien to the human immune system, it is generally believed that successful whole-organ transplants are some years away.

It does not follow, however, that ethical consideration of xenotransplantation should be delayed until whole-organ transplants become medically viable. First, it would be a huge waste of scientific expertise, financial resources and animal research subjects to continue investigating a technology whose use could already be seen to be ethically unacceptable, and second, there are other applications of xenotransplantation that have already been used experimentally with some success.

In particular, there are a number of promising avenues of research involving the transplantation of cells rather than whole organs (for example, pancreatic islet cells for the treatment of diabetes and neural cells for the treatment of Parkinson's disease) and the use of animal cells for *ex-vivo* perfusion (for example, treatment of liver failure by perfusion of the patient's blood through an external device containing porcine liver cells).[1] These further kinds of xenotransplantation add to the potential benefits of the technology, increasing not only the range of conditions potentially treatable by it but also the urgency of ethical appraisal.

This chapter will consider four basic objections to xenotransplantation: (1) that it is an unethical violation of the natural order; (2) that it poses unacceptable risks for the xenograft recipient; (3) that it involves an unacceptable use of animals; and (4) that it poses unacceptable risks to the wider population.

---

[1]The latter intervention does not fall strictly within the definition of xenotransplantation given above, but does fall within regulatory definitions in force in the UK and US.

Principles of Health Care Ethics, Second Edition   Edited by R.E. Ashcroft, A. Dawson, H. Draper and J.R. McMillan
© 2007 John Wiley & Sons, Ltd

VIOLATION OF THE NATURAL ORDER

The idea that the 'unnaturalness' of certain procedures renders them morally wrong is common in public discourse on new biotechnologies, but is regarded with suspicion by many bioethicists. In its pure form this objection does not rest on the claim that anyone's interests are adversely affected by the procedure in question but on the thought that certain kinds of interference with the natural order are intrinsically wrong. As Veatch (2000, p. 261) puts it, '[t]he first problem that is unique to xenografts is whether the intermixing of biological material from different species somehow violates fundamental morality in and of itself'. Alternatively, the objection may rest on empirical assumptions about the beneficence or stability of nature, such that actions which radically change the natural state of things are believed more likely to have harmful consequences than those which leave things relatively unchanged.

One objection to such arguments is that people's views about what is natural often change as they become accustomed to new technologies. Thus allotransplantation (the transplantation of organs from human to human) once seemed unnatural, as did other technologies such as IVF that are now considered normal. In this respect accusations of unnaturalness are no more than expressions of an instinctive cautiousness about the unfamiliar, and our present intuitions about what is natural represent an arbitrary point in our continuing acclimatization to new technologies. It is therefore incumbent on proponents of the unnaturalness objection to provide a less arbitrary account of the natural/unnatural distinction.

John Stuart Mill famously argued that the terms 'natural' and 'unnatural' are ambiguous. In one sense, 'nature' is used to refer to everything that exists (barring the supernatural). In this sense, as nature includes humans and their powers, it is impossible to act other than in conformity with nature. In another sense, the natural is opposed to the artificial, and 'nature' refers to 'that which takes place without human intervention'. In this sense, to act at all, or at least 'with forethought and purpose', is to violate the natural order (Mill, 1904, pp. 13–14) Mill contends that the injunction to act in accordance with nature is therefore either meaningless (because we cannot do otherwise) or irrational and immoral (because it forbids any attempt to curb the violence and destructiveness of nature) (Mill, 1904, p. 32).

It might be argued that Mill presents a false dichotomy and that there can be other accounts of the natural, falling between these extremes. For example, in contemporary bioethical debates charges of unnaturalness are frequently levelled against procedures that are seen as undermining the integrity of species and the boundaries between them – xenotransplantation is one example, but a more prominent one is genetic engineering, which involves moving genes between different species and especially between plants, animals and bacteria. However, aside from the objection that this appeals to an obsolete pre-Darwinian idea of species as unchanging entities and ignores the ways in which species boundaries are constantly breached without human intervention (in horizontal gene transfer, for example), Mill's argument challenges the proponent of the unnaturalness objection to explain why the unnatural should be equated with the unethical, because, as Mill points out, much of what is widely considered to be human progress has consisted in interfering with nature in order to protect ourselves from such natural phenomena as infectious diseases, droughts and hurricanes.

Even if there are no rational grounds for equating the unnatural with the unethical, it is sometimes suggested that the *perception* of xenotransplantation as unnatural is sufficient to render it ethically problematic (Nuffield Council on Bioethics, 1996, Section 9.12). For example, if it is believed by a patient or others that receiving a xenograft will somehow make the patient less human, this could have a real impact upon her welfare, even if there is no rational basis for that view. Note, however, that this is no longer a claim about the intrinsic wrongness of tampering with nature, but about patient welfare. As such it has the same role in ethical decision-making about xenotransplantation as the other patient welfare issues that will be considered in the next section; and indeed as an element of patient welfare this is likely to be outweighed by other elements such as significant health benefits, especially as the technology becomes more familiar and accepted.

RISKS TO THE XENOGRAFT RECIPIENT

All surgery involves risks to the patient, but, despite doctors' fondness for quoting the Hippocratic slogan 'first do no harm', this is not considered to be a fundamental ethical obstacle to the practice of surgery. The imposition of what may be quite serious risks is justified by a combination of the doctor's judgement that on balance it is in the patient's interests to undergo the surgery and the patient's consent to the procedure based on an understanding of the risks and benefits. The relation between these two elements is interesting and controversial, but for present purposes let us take the conservative view that both are necessary in the case of competent patients and that where the patient is not competent to consent, the undertaking of a risky procedure is justified either by a judgement of best interests alone or by such a judgement combined with some form of proxy consent.

In addition to the general risks associated with surgery, xenograft recipients will be subjected to additional risks specific to xenotransplantation. One such risk – that of psychological harm associated with a changed self-image or social harm resulting from others' perceptions of the procedure – has just been mentioned. Other risks, however, are likely to be more significant. These include: the risk of rejection of the transplanted tissue or organ by the body's immune system (a risk that is present but less severe in the case of human-to-human transplants); the increased risk of infections and cancers resulting from the use of powerful immunosuppressive drugs; and the risk that infections (known as zoonoses) may be passed from the donor animal to the xenograft recipient.

As noted above, advances have been reported in the development of techniques to tackle the risk of rejection. In addition, better understanding of the infection agents present in donor animals and the creation of 'specified pathogen-free' herds have reduced the risk of infections being transmitted from animal to human. Nevertheless, as with many new medical technologies, it is likely that the risks for early recipients will remain significant, especially for early recipients of whole-organ transplants. The question, however, is whether these risks render xenotransplantation different in ethically significant ways from other forms of surgery.

Clearly the balance of risks and benefits will vary from one kind of intervention to another, and the high level of risk associated with experimental (and perhaps even of established) xenograft procedures will mean that the potential benefits have to be large in order to satisfy the best interests criterion. This, however, is no reason to judge the technology in general to be unethical, but merely reinforces the need for case-by-case assessment.

Another possibility is that the severity of the risks is such that the patient's capacity to consent is thrown into question. It might be suggested, for example, that a patient's willingness to consent to such a risky procedure would be evidence of a desperation that is incompatible with rational decision-making. But, although acceptance of high risks may sometimes indicate an impaired capacity for rational choice, this is not always the case. For example, it can be perfectly rational to accept high risks if the alternative is even worse (certain death, for example), or for altruistic reasons (because one wishes to contribute to the development of medical science). At most, then, the acceptance of a high-risk treatment would indicate the need to assess the rationality of the deliberative processes by which the patient arrived at that decision. Moreover, although the stakes are high for a patient faced with such a decision, there need not be anything particularly complex about the judgement to be made, and therefore, no reason to set the threshold of competence higher than usual.

THE ANIMAL RIGHTS OBJECTION

Transplantation necessarily involves a donor as well as a recipient, and whereas the risks and harms that accrue to

the xenograft recipient may be justified by their consent and the fact that the procedure is in their overall best interests, the first of these, at least, does not apply to the donor, since non-human animals lack the capacity to give valid consent.

General questions about the ethics of using animals for human ends are addressed elsewhere in this volume. However, the permissibility of xenotransplantation may also turn on empirical facts about the welfare of the donor animals. On the one hand it has been argued that the need for organs that are healthy and free of infections will ensure that donor animals are raised in conditions that are conducive to their welfare. On the other hand, it may be that in order to prevent infection or injury the animals are raised in conditions that restrict their ability to behave according to their instincts, and that the genetic modification used to control rejection will cause them to suffer.

One widely used argument in favour of xenotransplantation depends on a comparison between xenotransplantation and other uses of animals. Veatch, for example, holds that 'if there is ever a case for using an animal for the benefit of humans, it would be when the sacrifice of one animal will offer the possibility of saving an identifiable human life' (2000, p. 262). This contrasts with medical research, in which many animals may be harmed in pursuit of benefits for humans that are far from certain (although it should be noted that if a new drug is successfully developed the number of human beneficiaries is likely to far exceed the number of animals used in the research and could easily be greater than the number benefited by xenotransplantation), and with meat-eating, for which animals are killed to serve a human interest far less important than the medical needs served by xenotransplantation. A problem with this style of argument is that even if it shows xenotransplantation to be morally preferable to animal experimentation or meat-eating it will only show it to be morally permissible if these other uses are morally permissible, and this is disputed by many opponents of xenotransplantation.

Another kind of argument depends on comparisons of the mental capacities of humans and animals. It is widely held that primates, because of their presumed capacity for a level of self-awareness similar to that of humans, should not be used as xenograft donors, whereas animals with less developed mental capacities, such as pigs, may be so used (Nuffield Council on Bioethics, 1996, Section 4.42; Advisory Group on the Ethics of xenotransplantation, 1997, Sections 4.28–4.30). This, however, overlooks a well-known counterargument, which forms the basis for many 'pro-animal' perspectives (e.g. Regan, 1988; Singer, 1993). The 'argument from marginal cases' starts from the observation that mental capacities vary within as well as between species, so that although the capacities of a normal adult human exceed those of a pig, the same is not true of humans suffering from severe mental impairments. Thus, an argument that justified using pigs as a source of organs and tissues on the basis of their limited mental capacities would also justify taking organs and tissues from severely impaired humans. Conversely, if we are unwilling to abandon the intuition that using impaired humans as sources of organs and tissues is ethically unacceptable then we should similarly reject the use of pigs and other animals with similar capacities.

The argument from marginal cases is most often used in the second of these ways, to argue against the sacrifice of animals for human benefit. Frey (1996), however, argues that the range of experiences that normal humans are capable of is so far in excess of those available to non-human animals as to justify the sacrifice of the latter for the former, even though that means that we must also accept the sacrifice of severely impaired humans. Although this may seem intuitively unacceptable, two things should be noted: first, Frey's conclusion would apply only to humans with *extremely* severe mental impairment (those with mental capacities similar to or less than those of pigs or whatever other animals are proposed as xenograft donors), and second, we cannot rely on intuitions about marginal cases any more than intuitions about meat-eating or pharmaceutical research to provide uncontentious premises for arguing for or against xenotransplantation.

RISK TO PUBLIC HEALTH

The ethical issue that has been most widely debated in relation to xenotransplantation is the risk of zoonosis: that is, the transmission of infections from donor animals to human xenograft recipients. As argued above, the risk that this imposes on the xenograft recipient may be justified by the fact that taking the risk may be in the recipient's overall best interests together with the fact that they will have consented to it. However, what has generated particular controversy, and led some to conclude that xenotransplantation will be or should be abandoned, is the possibility that zoonotic infections will prove to be transmissible between humans and will spread into the general population. This is a much more difficult ethical problem for proponents of xenotransplantation, because it involves a risk to people who have not consented to any involvement in xenotransplantation, and greatly increases the potential scale of the problem, leading, as several commentators have noted, to the possibility of 'another HIV epidemic or worse' (Veatch, 2000, p. 269).

One of the difficulties in determining the proper ethical response to this scenario is that its likelihood is a matter of controversy. In the view of (Nuffield Council on Bioethics, 1996, Section 6.14),

[i]t will be very difficult to identify organisms that do not cause any symptoms in the animal from which they come. Previous experience indicates that infectious organisms are normally identified only after the emergence of the disease they cause . . . Put bluntly, it may be possible to identify any infectious organism transmitted by xenografting only if it causes disease in human beings, and after it has started to do so.

Although more recent reports have suggested that the risk of zoonosis may lower than previously feared (e.g. Günzberg and Salmons, 2000; Yang et al., 2004), it seems clear that the risk cannot be altogether eliminated and that its magnitude will remain quite uncertain for the foreseeable future. Questions therefore arise concerning the circumstances in which it is permissible to impose risks on non-consenting parties. What ethical framework should we use to assess the acceptability of a particular level of risk, and how should we proceed in the absence of a clear consensus about the probability of a zoonotic epidemic?

One approach to these questions that is widely invoked in other contexts of technological risk, and is recommended as an approach to xenotransplantation by the Nuffield Council amongst others, is the 'precautionary principle'. This is formulated in various ways, but the Nuffield Council (1996, Section 6.21) defines the principle in a manner typical of those who invoke it, as the view 'that action should be taken to avoid risks in advance of certainty about their nature' and that 'the burden of proof should lie with those developing the technology to demonstrate that it will not cause serious harm'. Like many accounts, however, this lacks precision and, depending on how it is interpreted, is either too strong in its opposition to new technologies to be plausible, or else too vague, without supplementation by other principles, to provide an answer to practical questions about the permissibility of particular technologies.

The injunction to take precautionary action in advance of scientific certainty is in itself unobjectionable. As various authors (e.g. Shrader-Frechette, 1991) have pointed out, 'scientific certainty' is often taken to mean that a hypothesis is supported by the evidence at a 95% confidence level. This is a high threshold, which may be appropriate in pure science, where the aim is to ensure that erroneous results are not accepted into the body of accepted scientific fact, but in a regulatory context it would seem culpably incautious to ignore risks of serious harm until established with this degree of confidence. (Imagine what the roads would be like if drivers refrained from using their brakes until 95% certain that an accident would otherwise result.) Without further specification, however, the injunction to act in advance of scientific certainty gives us no guidance as to the level of evidence that *would* be sufficient to justify precautionary action.

A possible answer is suggested by the second part of the principle, as formulated above. This states that in considering whether a new technology should be permitted the burden of proof should lie with its advocates to show that it will not cause serious harm. One interpretation of this is that *safety* should be demonstrated with 95% confidence before the technology is approved. But although this level of precaution may be appropriate for some risks (and the possibility of a new HIV-like epidemic may be one of them) it will be too strong for others, given that the decision *not* to employ a new technology will have opportunity costs which may themselves be very serious. In the case of xenotransplantation, these would include deaths and suffering among patients whose conditions might be cured or alleviated by xenotransplantation.

An indiscriminately strong precautionary principle is therefore unjustified, while a weaker version may provide us with a general orientation (ruling out a gung-ho approach which would ignore all risks until resolved into near-certainty) but needs other principles to help us determine what counts as an acceptable degree of risk in specific cases. Once we have such principles, however, it is questionable whether the precautionary principle serves any useful function.

A rights-based or deontological approach to risk is likely to suffer from similar problems to the precautionary principle (McCarthy, 1997). A theory that asserted an absolute right not to have risks imposed on us without our consent (or an absolute duty not to impose such risks on others) would be excessively restrictive, rendering impermissible many activities essential to the functioning and well-being of society, while a weaker version that allowed such rights or duties to be weighed against the benefits of risk-taking activity would need to refer to some factor other than rights in order to determine when such overriding is permissible.

A consequentialist approach would avoid this dilemma, being more permissive than a strong version of either the precautionary principle or a rights-based approach and, in theory at least, offering a precise answer to the question of when it is permissible to impose risk on others without their consent. Consequentialism would permit xenotransplantation provided that the expected benefit (the sum of possible benefits multiplied their probabilities) exceeded the expected harm (similarly calculated). Such an approach is the basis for the cost-benefit analysis that informs many policy decisions, but faces both ethical and practical problems in contexts like xenotransplantation.

The practical problem arises because expected utility is calculated on the basis of the probabilities of benefits and harms, which in many risk situations, including that of xenotransplantation, are not known with any precision, if at all. In the case of xenotransplantation the problem is exacerbated by the large magnitudes of the potential benefits and harms, so that the overall utility could range from a high positive to a high negative value (Veatch, 2000, pp. 268–9).

The ethical objection usually raised against consequentialism in contexts such as this is that it does not attribute any intrinsic significance to the way in which harms and benefits are distributed, and as a result is too permissive, allowing the interests of some people to be sacrificed to secure the interests of others, even when doing so produces only a marginal gain in aggregate expected utility. It can also be argued, however, that consequentialism is *insufficiently* permissive and that imposed risks that do not maximize utility may be justified where the beneficiaries have a claim to priority consideration under a principle of justice.

There are of course numerous competing principles of justice that could in principle underpin such an argument, but I will focus on Veatch's argument, which is best understood as based on a version of Rawls' difference principle applied to overall welfare rather than just socioeconomic primary goods.[2] Rawls states that 'social and economic inequalities are to be arranged so that they are . . . to the greatest benefit of the least advantaged' (Rawls, 1971, p. 83), while Veatch formulates his principle as follows:

> the principle of justice supports arranging social practices to benefit [the] worst-off people or to give them opportunities to be as well-off as others insofar as that is possible. It would support such practices even if the effect were a net decrease in the amount of good in the society – provided that was necessary to improve the lot of the worst off (Veatch, 2000, p. 269).

Veatch argues that the circumstances that make someone a candidate for xenotransplantation also put them into the category of people whose welfare is to be prioritized under his Rawlsian principle of justice:

> People so ill that they are candidates for transplant are surely not well-off. Those on waiting lists who are so ill that they are willing to volunteer to be pioneers in an experiment to transplant organs from pigs or other nonhuman animals are probably particularly poorly off. They would be members of the kind of group that would have a special claim grounded in the principle of justice, a claim for society to adopt social practices that are designed to benefit them, even if the interests of others in the society are to the contrary (Veatch, 2000, p. 269).

The problem is that although this shows that xenograft recipients are likely to be badly off, it does not show that they are necessarily *worse* off than the others against whose

---

[2]Veatch's formulation is in fact ambiguous between this Rawlsian interpretation and a more strict egalitarianism. However, I have argued elsewhere (Hughes, 2007) that the former is the most plausible interpretation.

interests theirs need to be balanced. One consideration is that members of the general public who contract an infection transmitted from an animal via a xenograft recipient might thereby be made worse off than the xenograft recipient. As Veatch acknowledges, anyone in such a position 'would have a legitimate claim to block the xenograft experiment'. Veatch responds that – though possible – this scenario is unlikely:

> First, the xenograft recipient would be in double jeopardy. He or she would be very poorly off from organ failure – a failure so severe that the individual is willing to risk experimental xenograft. Second, if it should turn out that some virus was indeed a danger to humans, that recipient would also be a victim of the virus. If we are trying to identify who is the worst off, the person with severe organ failure combined with the serious viral infection is surely worse off than the one contending only with the virus (Veatch, 2000, p. 270).

This, however, fails to rescue Veatch's argument for a permissive approach to xenotransplantation.

First, it is easy to construct scenarios in which the infected third party ends up worse off than the xenograft recipient. The xenograft recipient may pass on an infection without succumbing to it, or the infected third party may be suffering from worse health than the xenograft recipient even before becoming infected. Given that the Rawlsian principle instructs us to focus on the worst-case scenario, irrespective of its probability, this would be sufficient to render xenotransplantation impermissible. There is, however, a more fundamental objection to this part of Veatch's argument, which would apply even if zoonosis would inevitably leave all xenograft recipients worse off than infected third parties.

The harm incurred by xenograft recipients would be the result of a risk voluntarily undertaken in the hope of obtaining a benefit. This is what is referred to in the literature as 'option luck' (Dworkin, 1981, p. 293). Controversy exists about whether bad option luck should ever be compensated by society, or whether people should be held responsible for their own choices and bear the resulting costs themselves (Wolff, 1998; Anderson 1999); in the case of xenotransplantation, however, it seems clear that the possibility of suffering bad option luck should not be accepted as justification for choices that put third parties at risk.

The claim that those who stand to benefit from xenotransplantation should be allowed to undergo the procedure notwithstanding the risks to others because in the event of zoonosis occurring they are likely to be as seriously harmed as anyone else is analogous to the claim that dangerously fast driving should be permitted because in the event of a crash the fast drivers are likely to end up at least as badly as anyone else affected. What makes the xenograft candidate's claim look more plausible is the desperate situation that she faces if she does not take the risky action. That is, it is the xenograft candidate's bad *brute* luck that gives her a reason to accept the risk of a xenograft. But what this shows is that any claim the xenograft candidate has to special consideration depends on her situation *prior* to the procedure rather than that resulting from it. Veatch's double jeopardy claim is therefore irrelevant. The question for someone who subscribes to Veatch's Rawlsian principle of justice is whether third parties infected by zoonosis could be worse off than potential xenograft recipients will be if they are not permitted to receive a xenograft. Veatch asserts that this is unlikely but gives us no reason to think that it cannot happen. As a Rawlsian he should therefore conclude that xenotransplantation should not be permitted.

The fact that a Rawlsian principle of justice does not lead to the conclusion that Veatch hopes for does not, of course, show that the principle is flawed. However, reflection on the way that the principle works in the case of xenotransplantation may lead us to conclude that, like strong versions of the precautionary principle, it has implausibly conservative implications. Its conservatism arises from the fact that it instructs us to give priority to mitigating the worst possible outcome for any individual, irrespective of how rare or unlikely that outcome may be, whereas intuitively it seems that if the worst possible outcome is sufficiently unlikely and preventing or mitigating it would cause serious detriment to a sufficiently large number of people who are only slightly better off, then it must be right to focus on the better-off group. This might lead us back towards consequentialism, or, if we hold that the distribution of welfare matters, but not in the way that the Rawlsian principle implies, to a different principle of distributive justice. One possibility would be a form of prioritarianism which gives more weight to the welfare of the worse off without giving it absolute priority over the welfare of the less badly off, but I have argued elsewhere that the approaches put forward by Dworkin and Scanlon are also worthy of investigation in this context (Hughes, 2007).

CONCLUSION

It has been suggested in this chapter that objections to xenotransplantation on grounds of unnaturalness should be rejected and that those based on risk to the xenograft recipient are best considered on a case-by-case basis, taking into account the patient's consent and overall best interests in the same way as for other surgical procedures. Objections based on the harm suffered by donor animals may depend on arguments about the moral status of animals which are beyond the scope of this chapter; however, it was suggested, following Frey, that the marginal cases argument, at least, is not conclusive against the permissibility of xenotransplantation.

The most controversial objection to xenotransplantation, however, arises from the risk of transmitting infections from donor animals to the general (non-consenting) population, and here no clear conclusion was reached. None of the approaches considered was found entirely satisfactory. Precautionary or rights-based approaches were found to be either implausibly restrictive given the risks that we routinely impose on others in everyday life or, in weaker interpretations, incapable of providing useful guidance about particular cases. Veatch's Rawlsian approach was similarly found to be implausibly restrictive, whereas a consequentialist approach is problematic to apply where the probabilities of different outcomes are unknown, and ignores the distribution of risks and benefits in a way that could be either too permissive in allowing some to be sacrificed for the benefit of others, or not permissive enough in restricting developments that would be of particular benefit to the badly off. It seems likely, therefore, that the most plausible approach to the problem of zoonosis and to the broader problem of when it is permissible to impose risk on nonconsenting bystanders, will turn out to be a justice-based one, which takes account of how risks and benefits are distributed, in a way which allows the interests of badly off to carry extra weight but does not give absolute priority to the worst off in the manner of Rawls' difference principle.

REFERENCES

Advisory Group on the Ethics of Xenotransplantation. *Animal Tissue into Humans: A Report by the Advisory Group on the Ethics of Xenotransplantation*, London: Stationery Office 1997.

Anderson E. What is the point of equality? *Ethics* 1999, **99**: 287–337.

Dworkin R. What is equality? Part 2: equality of resources. *Philosophy and Public Affairs* 1981, **10**: 283–345.

Frey RG. Medicine, animal experimentation, and the moral problem of unfortunate humans. *Social Philosophy and Policy* 1996, **13**: 181–211.

Günzberg WH and Salmons B. Xenotransplantation: is the risk of viral infection as great as we thought? *Molecular Medicine Today* 2000, **6**: 199–208.

Hughes J. Justice and third party risk: the ethics of xenotransplantation. *Journal of Applied Philosophy*, 2007, **24**: 151–168.

McCarthy D. Rights, explanation and risks. *Ethics* 1997, **107**: 205–225.

Mill JS. *On Nature*, Watts & Co. for the Rationalist Press, 1904: Also available http://www.lancsac.uk/users/philosophy/texts/mill_on.htm

Nuffield Council on Bioethics. *Animal-to-Human Transplants: the Ethics of Xenotransplantation*, London: Nuffield Council on Bioethics 1996.

Rawls J. *A Theory of Justice*, London: Oxford University Press 1971.

Regan T. *The Case for Animal Rights*, London and New York: Routledge 1988.

Shrader-Frechette KS. *Risk and Rationality*, Berkeley, CA: University of California Press, 1991.

Singer P. *Practical Ethics*, Cambridge: Cambridge University Press 1993.

UK Transplant. *Transplants Save Lives*, 2005. http://www.uktransplant.org.uk/ukt/newsroom/fact_sheets/transplants_save_lives.jsp.

Veatch RM. *Transplantation Ethics*, Washington, D.C: Georgetown University Press 2000.

Wolff J. Fairness, respect and the egalitarian ethos. *Philosophy and Public Affairs* 1998, **27**: 97–122.

Yang Y et al. Mouse retrovirus mediates porcine endogenous retrovirus transmission into human cells in long-term human-porcine chimeric mice. *Journal of Clinical Investigation* 2004, **114**: 695–700.

105

Pharmacogenomics

RUTH CHADWICK

PHARMACOGENETICS AND PHARMACOGENOMICS

Although the terms pharmacogenetics and pharmacogenomics are to some extent used interchangeably, it is possible to distinguish between them. The term 'pharmacogenetics' was coined in the 1950s to indicate the study of genetic differences between individuals that influence drug response and susceptibility to adverse effects. In the case of a given drug, we may know that it will help a certain proportion of people whereas others will suffer from adverse reactions. Pharmacogenetics enables the identification of who will likely be benefited and who will likely be harmed, so that prescribing the product to the latter group can be avoided. It affects, potentially, the whole of health care, not only that part which deals with genetic disorders or with genetic susceptibility to common disease; it has implications for both therapy and clinical trials. It raises the issue of genetic exceptionalism anew for several reasons: it has been argued that it will individualize medicine and challenge professional roles and that even as compared with other areas of genetics, the relevant ethical considerations and principles are different (Roses, 2000). There might even be a temptation to coin the term 'pharmacogenetic exceptionalism'.

In this chapter I shall outline the possible applications in research and treatment, with their associated ethical issues, identify some questions specific to patient groups, different products and prerequisites for implementation of pharmacogenomics in clinical practice, and close with a brief assessment of the extent to which pharmacogenomics *is* exceptional from an ethical point of view.

John Bell, writing in the *British Medical Journal*, predicted that pharmacogenetics might lead to a new understanding of disease (Bell, 1998). Whereas common diseases are currently defined by their clinical appearance, it will become possible to subdivide heterogeneous diseases into discrete conditions, in other words, change our perception of what the condition is for which the treatment is sought (Bell, 1998). As genetic variants are identified that are associated with drug response a move has been predicted towards widespread testing before prescribing – in fact, it may come to be considered unethical not to carry out such tests. The type of testing involved, however, is different from testing for single gene disorders: it will involve testing for single nucleotide polymorphisms (SNPs) or copy number variants (CNVs) and thus the transferability of guidelines developed for other kinds of testing cannot be assumed (Roses, 2000). CNVs relate to the number of copies of a sequence a person has, and thus the dose, or amount, of a genetic factor, rather than the presence of the genetic factor itself.

In the post-genome era, pharmacogenomics, as opposed to pharmacogenetics, uses the information arising out of the Human Genome Project to establish associations between genetic factors and drug response. It is concerned with the genome-wide study of the relationship between pharmaceuticals and gene expression. For the sake of simplicity, in the remainder of this chapter I shall use the term pharmacogenomics for both.

POSSIBILITIES

Although pharmacogenomics has been 'sold' on the basis of a promise of personalized medicine, as already hinted at above, the relationship between genetics and pharmaceuticals has several different aspects during the research and development process, and there are associated ethical issues at different stages. I shall distinguish between research issues and clinical practice issues.

Principles of Health Care Ethics, Second Edition   Edited by R.E. Ashcroft, A. Dawson, H. Draper and J.R. McMillan
© 2007 John Wiley & Sons, Ltd

RESEARCH

Although much of the popular discussion of pharmacogenomics has tended to focus on the promises of individualized medicine at the treatment stage, the role of pharmacogenomics in research is also important, both morally speaking and in policy terms (UK Pharmacogenetics Study Group, 2006). Genomic information is relevant, first, in identifying targets for drug development, but from an ethical point of view what is higher up the agenda is its influence on the design and conduct of clinical trials. If differences in response to a new molecule can be identified at an early stage in clinical trials, then later stages can be restricted to those with suitable genotypes, thus reducing the size and expense of those trials (Roses, 2004). This possibility offers potential benefits in a number of ways – to the pharmaceutical industry, clearly, from a financial point of view, but beyond that, it may reduce the number of molecules that are stopped from further development at that stage on the grounds that they show efficacy in only a certain proportion of the population. This would be to the benefit of those who could be helped by the drug, who might have been denied it without pharmacogenomics.

On the contrary, there are worries about a future in which drug development might be restricted to those with suitable genotypes (Breckenridge et al., 2004), and that new classes of orphan patients might arise not only with reference to one disease or drug but also in relation to large numbers of drugs for common diseases (Breckenridge et al., 2004). Some take the view that the longer-term effects of clinical trials organized according to genotype might actually be an increase in adverse reactions once a drug is on the market (Breckenridge et al., 2004).

As Allen Roses has pointed out, up to now, the fact that a molecule is only effective in, say, 30% of the population has not necessarily prevented its further development – in fact some *have* been licensed on the basis of only 30% efficacy (Roses, 2004). The severity of potential adverse responses also has to be taken into account.

Where safety as opposed to efficacy is concerned, the possibilities of pharmacogenomics has led to discussions of 'drug resuscitation' – bringing back drugs which have been taken off the market because of adverse effects, with proviso that in future they be prescribed only to that segment of the population identified as genetically suitable. Although Roses takes the view that this is one of the more popular 'myths' surrounding pharmacogenomics (Roses, 2004), which is unlikely to come to fruition because patents on such products are likely to be running out, Daar and Singer (2005) see it as a real opportunity, especially in developing countries, citing the example of Bidil, which has been resuscitated for African Americans, having not shown suitability for a mixed population. In such cases, however, there are clear dangers of 'off-label' prescribing which underline the need for public and professional acceptance of the new developments (see 'Prerequisites' below). Any drug marketed for a restricted population would have to be issued with a test, but Daar and Singer argue that this does not necessarily mean testing each individual.

TREATMENT

In the absence of everyone having their full genetic profile accessible to health care professionals, either on a chip or database, the implication of the implementation of pharmacogenomics in treatment is pre-prescription testing or screening. The possibility of individual *testing* has encouraged some of the literature on this topic to describe developments in pharmacogenomics as facilitating 'personal pills' (Persidis, 1998), the suggestion being that awareness of genetic variation between individuals will facilitate prescribing in accordance with the specific needs of the individual, thus arguably in accordance with a principle that heath care resources should be allocated according to need at the point of delivery. Pharmacogenetics has the potential to personalize prescribing by affecting a prescribing decision for a given patient in at least three different ways: (1) adjustment of dosage of drug A; (2) a choice between prescribing drug A or drug B; (3) drug A or nothing (where there is no alternative treatment available). Monitoring of appropriate dosage as compared with choice of medication needs to be considered. The situation where the choice is between drug A and *no* medication gives rise to the ethical problem of perceived or actual abandonment.

Ethical issues also arise in relation to someone not wanting to take the test, but still wanting access to the medicine. The reason why someone might not want to take a test may be because of some perception of genetics in general or because of worries about what the specific test may reveal. Clearly there are also resource implications in terms of access to testing in the first place, which are unlikely to be available in all locations, hence exacerbating the concerns about differences in access to what benefits pharmacogenomics has to offer.

If on the contrary population screening is what is envisaged, then some thought has to be given to the relation of pharmacogenomic screening to genetic screening in general. Criteria for the introduction of screening programmes include the nature of the condition sought and the scope for action in the event of a positive result (Danish Counsil of Ethics, 1993; Chadwick, 1999). Unlike screening for susceptibility to a disease, however, the 'condition sought' is susceptibility to adverse reactions. The scope for action, however, may be negative, that is 'stop taking the tablets'. In cases where there is no other treatment available, however, patients might still wish to take a risk, especially in the light of genetic test results being probabilistic, quite apart from any placebo effect.

PATIENT GROUPS

Testing and screening attempt to classify patients as 'genetically suitable' or not – although the fact that someone is genetically suitable does not necessarily equate to clinical suitability, as other factors may affect whether a patient is suited for a medication. Concerns have been expressed about such patient stratification on genetic lines, although against this it is argued that patient stratification has always been part of the traditional practice of medicine (Breckenridge et al., 2004).

The worry about patient stratification is that it could have discriminatory implications. One possibility is that genetic susceptibility might be correlated with some other characteristic such as ethnicity, leading in effect to a presumption of an effective treatment for that condition for that particular group although there might be considerable variation within the group. The Council on Ethical and Judicial Affairs of the American Medical Association, in an article on 'Multiplex genetic testing' in the *Hastings Center Report,* argued that

'ethnic heritage may contribute to particular concerns, it is clinically relevant and should be considered. Offering multiplex tests that are bundled according to race or ethnicity, however, serves to categorize patients rather than to address their distinct needs. The profession can ill afford the perception that science is being used to bring attention to the genetic flaws present in lines of inheritance' (Council on Ethical and Judicial Affairs, 1998).

Some see in pharmacogenomics, however, an opportunity to redress a balance here – certainly in relation to geographical ancestry. Daar and Singer, for example, argue that '[d]eeper understanding of genotypes of local populations may make it possible to predict drug responses without the need to treat each individual' (Daar and Singer, 2005), with potential benefits for developing countries.

The fact that drug testing has traditionally tended to be done on very limited segments of the population (e.g. excluding pregnant women and elderly persons) has long been considered to raise potential ethical problems in terms of prescribing them to others. It has been argued, for example, that evidence-based medicine may discriminate against women (Rogers, 2004). Segmentation of the market may go some way to addressing this. Children, however, remain problematic in relation to pharmacogenomics, not only because they are not included in clinical trials but also because they metabolize drugs differently and because insofar as they might have genetic predispositions which are likely to affect drug response, there are particular concerns about genetic testing in children unless the information gained can be used for their therapeutic benefit. While this may be the intention, additional concerns would arise if the testing detected information which related to long-term consequences, such as a predisposition to a late onset disorder for which there

was no effective treatment. This is part of a general worry about pharmacogenetic testing, the extent to which it is likely to reveal other information apart from that directly relevant to drug prescription.

PRODUCTS

There is a question as to whether issues in pharmacogenomics relate primarily to the development and use of *new* drugs or also to already licensed drugs. The answer is – potentially both. As already indicated in relation to the possibility of drug resuscitation, however, the fact that a drug is no longer patent protected, or nearing the end of its patent protection, militates against the possibility that pharmaceutical companies will have an interest in doing further research to assess its pharmacogenetic potential. A similar issue arises regarding the difference between brand name drugs and generics. It has been suggested that the manufacturers of generics are unlikely to have the requisite research and development funds to undertake pharmacogenetic research in relation to them (Nuffield Council on Bioethics, 2003).

New kinds of product will increasingly emerge – drugs licensed along with a test. It is not likely, however, that this will be the case with all new drugs. The most likely product areas in which this will happen are those where existing treatments have a narrow therapeutic index (Stix, 1998).

PREREQUISITES

For pharmacogenomics to be implemented routinely in health service delivery, there are certain prerequisites which have ethical dimensions. These include public and professional acceptability.

The effectiveness of any kind of pharmaceutical treatment depends on much more than genetic factors. Diet, age and interactions of different products all play a part – as does whether the patient accurately follows the prescribed regime (Stix, 1998). In relation to pharmacogenomics, the extent to which there is public acceptance and trust is another factor, particularly in relation to those who may be denied access to a drug for factors related to genetics such as their membership of particular groups. In the case of pre-prescription genetic testing, possible misperceptions of what is being tested for are an issue, although research conducted in the north west of the United Kingdom has elicited perceptions of potential benefits, including a reduction in the amount of time it takes to get the medicine with the highest efficacy (in place of trial and error) and more personalized side effect profiles (Fargher et al., 2006).

It is not just in relation to the public or publics that there may be an issue about acceptability. The introduction of pharmacogenomics also requires a shift in culture among health care professionals in relation to prescribing practice, including the perception that there is some added value to be had. In the case of many drugs, where safety is not a major concern and where the therapeutic index is wide, this may not occur, as indicated above. Health care professionals may be concerned also about the consequences of *withholding* a drug in certain circumstances on the basis of genetic information.

Questions for professional ethics arise when considering how pharmacogenomics will affect health care delivery. Different modes of delivery will raise different ethical questions, and countries may differ in how they integrate pharmacogenomics into health care. If genetic testing becomes a standard accompaniment of prescribing, there are questions about how this will be carried out. Doctor–patient interactions could be 'geneticized', with all the associated concerns about the potential use, misuse, understanding and misunderstanding of genetic information. There may be an expanding role here for pharmacists, however, if for example doctors *prescribe* generically and pharmacists *dispense* according to genotype. The last scenario may be more appropriate in certain applications of pharmacogenetics, for example when the choice is between drug A and drug B.

Changes in professional roles, if the situation develops in this way, suggest a need for education and training in the ethical implications. What form this training should take will depend on how the ethical issues should be addressed, and this is one respect in which the question of appropriateness of existing ethical frameworks becomes significant. As Allen Roses suggests 'It is . . . incumbent that medical guidelines for mendelian- or susceptibility-gene testing do not extend automatically to discussions of other types of genetically based profiles in pharmacogenetics. Clear language and differentiation of respective ethical, legal and societal issues are required . . .' (Roses, 2000).

In the case of both public and professionals, a major prerequisite is quality assurance. External quality assessment schemes (EQAs) of genetic tests in Europe have demonstrated a low but significant error rate in cystic fibrosis testing (Ibarreta et al., 2004), and the number of laboratory tests carried out annually as pharmacogenetic testing comes on stream is set to increase dramatically. Mistakes may arise not only through technical error but also out of clerical error or sample mix-up (Ibarreta et al., 2004). The possibility of errors in genetic testing, which may form part of the patient's record for considerable amounts of time, makes it imperative that there is some quality control of associations and of testing in this area, such as an independent body to assess clinical validity and utility (Breckenridge et al., 2004).

PRINCIPLES

What ethical frameworks are appropriate in thinking about pharmacogenomics? This is a field in which the ethical debate has to a large extent been led by the historical assessment of pharmaceuticals. As safety and efficacy have been the paramount considerations in relation to drugs, these have also driven the ethical debate about pharmacogenomics. This is in contrast to the food context, where food products are subject only to safety tests, though with the increasing popularity of functional foods and the possibilities of nutrigenomics, the boundary between the two contexts is growing fuzzier.

Autonomy, then, has less attention than it does in other fields, although there clearly are important considerations of autonomy to consider. In the research context it has been recognized that there are pharmacogenomics-related issues of informed consent (Chadwick, 2001). Participants in clinical trials that have a genetic dimension may have to address the issues not only of taking a new drug (or being in a control group) but also of giving a sample of DNA for analysis, possibly to be stored for considerable time. They may also have to consider issues of secondary use of that sample and the information it contains. The issues of pharmacogenomics are thus closely related to those concerning genetic databases and storage of samples.

Other autonomy-related issues concern control of an individual's information and the choice over whether to take a genetic test or not. A major feature of the debate about the introduction of population screening programmes has been the 'right not to know' question – it has been argued that there might be a right not to know information about, for example, one's future health status. It might appear that the same considerations would not apply in relation to susceptibility to drug toxicity – surely it could only be beneficial to have information enabling one to avoid the side effects of drugs (presuming the information is accurate). A right to know one's genetic status vis-à-vis such susceptibility might be supported by an autonomy-based argument where autonomy is interpreted in terms of self-determination – facilitating the choice of the individual in relation to treatment. On the contrary, the knowledge that one has a higher risk of toxicity might in itself increase that risk (e.g. where the issue is *how much* to take). Further, genetic susceptibility to toxicity might in some contexts have insurance implications in the way that genetic predisposition might have to health problems – people who are slow because of their genotype to clear drugs from their bodies, or to convert them into non-toxic form, might be identified as belonging to a higher insurance risk category.

SAFETY AND EFFICACY

Safety and efficacy have tended to dominate the debate so that in relation to the 'four principles' of biomedical ethics, the ones that have had priority are non-maleficence and beneficence. There have been explicit suggestions, however, of a need to move beyond the four principles in this context, as in other genetic health care contexts (Chadwick and Berg, 2001; Knoppers and Chadwick, 2005; Lunshof, 2006).

Where an argument for the moral urgency of pursuing the pharmacogenomic approach to health care is put forward, attention is typically drawn to the mortality and morbidity arising from adverse drug reactions (ADRs), or to the number of hospital beds occupied by ADRs at any given time. For example, a commonly quoted figure is that 100 000 people die from ADRs every year in the United States (Stix, 1998; Schmidt, 1998). This suggests that the paramount consideration is considered to be safety. Although this reflects the ethical importance of doing no harm, it is important to have regard to the commercial interests at stake in drug development and to the fact that pharmaceutical companies as well as patients and health care providers have a clear interest in the avoidance of ADRs.

In terms of the moral and commercial argument for pharmacogenomics, then, efficacy comes in second place. It might be argued that from a moral point of view it is more important to avoid doing harm than it is to promote benefit – a version of the 'negative/positive' distinction, and therefore, priority should indeed be given to avoiding ADRs than to improving the efficacy of pharmaceutical products.

The situation is not, however, one where there is a clear choice between safety and effectiveness. An improvement in safety might at the same time in certain circumstances facilitate an improvement in effectiveness. What this discussion may overlook, however, is that there are choices to be made about different ways of preventing harm and about which harms are prevented. One criticism of the hype surrounding pharmacogenomics is that it distracts attention from other ways of reducing adverse responses, such as better management of prescribing (Webster et al., 2004).

A long-standing ethical issue in the context of pharmaceuticals has been the existence of orphan diseases for which there is no treatment available. To fail to develop treatments for such diseases is to fail to prevent harm that is, in principle at least, avoidable. The question arises as to which is the greater harm, the failure to develop medicines for orphan diseases or to fail to prevent ADRs through pharmacogenomics.

EQUITY

The discussion of orphan diseases and avoidable harm is closely connected to discussions about equity. Pharmacogenomics has the potential either to increase or to decrease health inequalities and in fact some take the view that this is possibly the main concern (Breckenridge et al., 2004). Fears that it will increase them are associated with the idea that only in rich countries will the development of personalized medicine be affordable, and that new orphan populations

will be produced if there are commercial incentives to develop products designed only for good responders. The possibilities of increased patient stratification are potentially associated with new forms of health inequality.

PERSONALIZATION

In addressing the equity aspects of pharmacogenomics it is thus necessary to discuss the issues of personalization. A criticism of the four principles of biomedical ethics has been that they represent a largely individualistic model of ethics, as they are primarily concerned with protecting the interests of individuals in medical contexts. Individualism has been predominant in biomedical ethics since the second half of the twentieth century at least. The 'personalization' project fits in this very nicely. What personalization means, however, is not transparent, and as a result it is not clear whether personalization is desirable or not.

Personalization as a project has far wider implications than in the context of pharmacogenomics. As the Food Ethics Council has pointed out, personalization is both a political project and an economic project (Food Ethics Council, 2005). It is associated not only with the rhetoric of 'choice' (and autonomy), but also with facilitating more individual responsibility for health. As applied to pharmacogenomics, personalization means therapy 'tailored' (Department of Health, 2003) to the individual's genotype, and is justified, as indicated above, more by considerations of safety and efficacy than of autonomy.

This model of implementation of pharmacogenomics has been referred to as the 'boutique' model (Daar and Singer, 2005) and has been countered by the proposal of Daar and Singer that there are moral considerations in favour of, rather, looking at the differences between population groups (Daar and Singer, 2005) – although treating people as members of a group rather than as individuals has its own dangers as we have seen.

NEW ETHICS?

This seems to be the key issue in pharmacogenomics – the extent to which it will reinforce existing inequalities, promising personalized medicine for some which is not affordable for all, or be used to reduce the inequity of the status quo. This question raises the wider issue of directions in the development of ethical frameworks. There has been a considerable amount of attention paid to the question of the extent to which developments in genetics require new thinking in ethics. Pharmacogenomics represents an important example of how the applicability of traditional ethical frameworks themselves is coming under challenge (Lunshof, 2006). Justice, privacy, informed consent, and autonomy: all these are subject to reconstrual in the light of developments in genetics, and in particular it has been suggested that frameworks such as the 'four principles', although they should by no means be abandoned, are not best suited to addressing the questions raised by population-based genetic research, which is closely connected to pharmacogenomics (Chadwick and Berg, 2001; Knoppers and Chadwick, 2005; Lunshof, 2006). This area of biomedical ethics, in particular, suggests the need to be sensitive to the possible inappropriateness of a model which uncritically takes pre-existing theories and principles with a view to 'applying' them to (pharmaco)genomics. Unfortunately the 'personalization' agenda makes this more likely.

REFERENCES

Bell J. The new genetics in clinical practice. *Brit Med J* 1998; **316**: 618–620.

Breckenridge A, Lindpainter K, Lipton P, McLeod H, Rothstein M, Wallace H. Pharmacogenetics: ethical problems and solutions. *Nat Rev Genet* 2004; **5**: 676–680.

Chadwick R. Criteria for genetic screening: The impact of pharmaceutical research. *Monash Bioethics Rev* 1999; **18**(1): 22–26.

Chadwick R. Informed consent and genetic research. In: Doyal L, Tobias J, eds. *Informed Consent in Medical Research*. London: BMJ Books, 2001.

Chadwick R, Berg K. Solidarity and equity: New ethical principles for genetic databases. *Nat Rev Genet* 2001.

Chadwick R, ten Have H, Shickle D, eds. *The Ethics of Genetic Screening*. Dordrecht: Kluwer, 1999.

Council on Ethical and Judicial Affairs, American Medical Association. Multiplex genetic testing. *Hastings Center Report* 1998; **28**(4): 15–21.

Daar AS, Singer PA. Pharmacogenetics and geographical ancestry: Implications for drug development and global health. *Nat Rev Genet* 2005; **6**: 241–246.

Danish Council of Ethics. *Ethics and Mapping of the Human Genome*. Copenhagen: Danish Council of Ethics, 1993.

Department of Health, UK. *Our Inheritance, Our Future: Realising the Potential of Genetics in the NHS*, 2003.

Fargher FA, Fargher EA, Eddy C, Payne K, Tricker K, Elliott RA, Qasim F, Bruce I, Shaffer J, Griffiths C, Moriarty K, Pearson C, Newman W. Exploring patients and healthcare professionals' views of pharmacogenetic testing. Poster presentation. Symposium From Genes to Patients: New Perspectives on Personalised Medicines. Warwick University, 5 July 2006.

Food Ethics Council. *Getting Personal*. Food Ethics Council, 2005.

Ibarreta D, Elles R, Cassiman J-J, Rodriguez-Cerezo E, Dequeker E. Towards quality assurance and harmonization of genetic testing services in the European Union. *Nat Biotechnol* 2004; **22**: 1230–1235.

Knoppers B, Chadwick, R. Human genetic research: Emerging trends in ethics. *Nat Rev Genet* 2005; **6**: 75–79.

Lunshof J. Personalised medicine: New perspectives – new ethics? *Personal Med* 2006; **3**(2): 187–194.

Nuffield Council on Bioethics. *Pharmacogenomics: Ethical Issues*. London: Nuffield Council on Bioethics, 2003.

Persidis A. The business of pharmacogenomics. *Nat Biotechnol* 1998; **16**: 209–210.

Rogers W. Evidence-based medicine and women: do the principles and practice of EBM further women's health? *Bioethics* 2004; **18**(1): 50–71.

Roses AD. Pharmacogenetics and future drug development and delivery. *Lancet* 2000; **355**: 1358–1361.

Roses AD. Pharmacogenetics and the practice of medicine. *Nature* 2000; **15**: 857–865.

Roses AD. Pharmacogenetics and drug development: The path to safer and more effective drugs. *Nat Rev Genet* 2004; **5**: 645–656.

Schmidt K. Just for you. *New Sci* 1998; **160** (21660): 32–36.

Stix G. Personal pills. *Sci Am* 1998; **279**(4): 10–11.

UK Pharmacogenetics Study Group. *Policy Issues in Pharmacogenetics*, 2006.

Webster A, Martin P, Lewis G, Smart A. Integrating pharmacogenetics into society: In search of a model. *Nat Rev Genet* 2004; **5**: 663–669.

World Health Organization. *The Ethical, Legal and Socio-Cultural Implications of Pharmacogenomics in Developing Countries*. Geneva: World Health Organization, 2006.

106

Ethical Issues in Human Gene Transfer: A Historical Overview

ERIC T. JUENGST AND HANNAH GRANKVIST

One of the most striking features of the history of human gene transfer has been the extent to which science has been influenced by concerns over social values and the public's voice. From the beginning, human gene transfer research seems to have been recognized to involve social value commitments that require the approval of the democratic process. Forty years ago, R.D. Hotchkiss set the tone by concluding the essay in which he coined the phrase 'genetic engineering' by prescribing that

> The best preparation will be an informed and forewarned public, and a thoughtful body scientific. The teachers and the science writers can perform their historic duties by helping our public to recognize and evaluate these possibilities and avoid their abuses. For these things surely are on the way (Hotchkiss, 1965, p. 202).

In the early 1970s, prospective gene therapists such as W. French Anderson made this point the cornerstone of their arguments about how society should proceed, proposing that 'only the conscience of an informed society as a whole should make these decisions' (Anderson, 1972). This point of view found fertile ground in society's new interests in controlling the 'biological revolution', and, in the United States, the national public review process established through the Recombinant DNA Advisory Committee (RAC) was explicitly designed to help achieve that goal. In the years since, the ethos that has shaped the professional and public policy discussions of human gene transfer research has remained grounded in the remarkably populist view that 'the public review provided by the RAC assures both policymakers and the general public that they are well informed about developments in gene therapy and thus partners in the progress of this exciting new field' (Capron et al., 1993). With the development of analogous national review

processes in the United Kingdom and Europe (de Wachter, 1993), Institutional Biosafety Committees, and the RAC's *Points to Consider* for the design of human gene transfer research, first human gene transfer trials have had the distinction of being the most thoroughly reviewed experiments in the history of biomedical research.

This populist tradition is important to recall, because it is the backdrop against which new professional ethical and social policy issues in gene transfer research are and will be framed. There are four possible types of human gene transfer interventions that can be performed on individuals. Such interventions can be targeted either towards an individual's somatic cells or towards the germ-line cells, and the goal of the intervention can be either the cure of disease or the enhancement of human capabilities (Walters and Palmer, 1996). In this chapter, our goal is to review the ethical issues that arise with the first two of the four possible combinations of target cells and goals: somatic cell gene therapy, and germ-line gene therapy. In each case, our focus will be on the intersection of the ethos that guided the birth of gene therapy and the challenges that the field's future will bring, and on the implications of that intersection for professional practice and public policy.

ETHICAL ISSUES IN SOMATIC CELL GENE TRANSFER RESEARCH

The literature that captures the public discussion of the ethics of human gene therapy displays an interesting metamorphosis between the early 1970s and the 1980s. The first wave of writing was characterized both by an awe in the face of the 'New Biology' and by a sense of being ethically disoriented by its prospects. This period's response to these

Principles of Health Care Ethics, Second Edition   Edited by R.E. Ashcroft, A. Dawson, H. Draper and J.R. McMillan

challenges was a sweeping reach of reflections that quickly took investigators to questions of philosophy and theology in search of moral bearings (Ramsey, 1972). Much of this early work is still fresh and valuable at those deeper levels. But it was difficult to translate this work into practical policies for scientific research, and not much concrete policy development emerged from it.

In the early 1980s, galvanized by the prospect of clinical trials for somatic cell therapy at the US National Institutes of Health (NIH) (Anderson and Fletcher, 1980), the discussion of gene therapy became more focused. In the United States, this second wave of discussion is captured best in the reports on human gene therapy by the President's Commission for Ethical Issues in Medicine and Biomedical and Behavioural Research (1982) and the Congressional Office of Technology Assessment (US Congress, 1984). It culminated in the publication of the NIH's *Points to Consider* document in 1990 (Subcommittee, 1990). In these reports, the biomedical community seems to have gained a moral compass that could allow policy to be developed without having to triangulate against deep questions of individual belief. As a result, commentators could already write: 'From the present vantage point, it may be hard to remember that in 1980, when the Commission began its work, critics (including respected religious groups) argued that 'fundamental dangers' were posed by any alteration of human genes' (Capron, 1990).

This new sense of direction reflects the hybridization of two sets of ethical deliberations that occurred in United States over the course of the 1970s: the discussion of biomedical research with human subjects and the debate over the use of recombinant DNA technology (Areen, 1985). Neither of these discussions was conducted with human gene therapy in mind, but together they provided the investigators of the 1980s with a repertoire of widely recognized and well-grounded moral and policy considerations that was unavailable to the investigators of the first phase. With the formation of the RAC's Working Group on Human Gene Therapy in 1985, these two discussions came together. Collectively, through the RAC's *Points to Consider* document, their moral considerations still form the ethical framework against which protocols for human gene transfer research are evaluated and the substantive principles for the next phase of deliberations.

The first important accomplishment of this second wave of discussion was to clarify and integrate into public policy the basic conceptual distinctions between the four possible types of human gene transfer introduced above (President's Commission for the Study of Ethical Problems, 1982). This led to the recognition that somatic cell gene therapy, if it worked, would simply be an extension of traditional medical efforts to modulate the expression of genes (such as transplantation or gene product therapy) and did not raise the special problems created by the other possible forms of gene transfer. Because the science required for successful germ-line interventions in humans was also undeveloped, this allowed the public discussion simply to table the most problematic issues until further notice and concentrate on helping to launch the first form of gene transfer research in a responsible manner.

Framing somatic cell gene therapy as an extension of traditional medical approaches was progress because it allowed the public review process to assess gene transfer research protocols through the ethical questions that had already become normative within biomedical research with human subjects: questions that have to do with the anticipated benefits and risks of the intervention (including biosafety risks), the selection of research subjects and the protection of the rights of research subjects and their proxies to informed consent, free withdrawal and privacy. Ironically, however, framing somatic cell gene transfer research as simply another form of innovative medical therapy also sowed the seeds of views that challenged the need for any special societal oversight of investigators' ability to address these questions.

RISKS AND BENEFITS

Concerns about the relative risks and benefits of gene transfer interventions reflect a commitment to the basic principle of research ethics that 'risks to the subjects [must be] reasonable in relation to anticipated benefits, if any, to subjects, and the importance of the knowledge that may be reasonably expected to result' (45 CFR, Section 46.111a). Thus, the RAC says in the introduction to its *Points to Consider*:

> In their evaluation of proposals involving the transfer of recombinant DNA into human subjects, the RAC and its subcommittee will consider whether the design of such experiments offers adequate assurance that their consequences will not go beyond their purpose, which is the same as the traditional purpose of all clinical investigations, namely to protect the health and well-being of individual subjects being treated while at the same time gathering generalizable knowledge (Subcommittee on Human Genome Therapy, 1990, p. 96).

In practice, this concern means that human gene transfer researchers must have enough prior knowledge to believe that the probable benefits to the subject outweigh both the possible risks of the experiment and the known benefits of any alternative treatments available. Thus, it lies behind the RAC's questions about, and the community's discussion of, the safety and efficacy of somatic cell gene therapy techniques, the adequacy of preliminary animal studies and the relative value of emerging therapeutic alternatives (Brenner, 1995).

Moreover, one of the striking legacies of the recombinant DNA debate in the public discussion of gene therapy is the acceptance of the need to prepare for the unforeseen as well as predictable risks in designing gene transfer research. In the public review of gene transfer protocols, this concern has concentrated primarily on the 'biosafety' risks involved in gene transfer. Here, the community seems to agree with the molecular geneticist Howard Temin, when he wrote that

> There are often unexpected effects of new technologies. . . . The use of retrovirus vectors for somatic therapy of human genetic disease can be looked upon as either a novel improvement on present means of drug delivery or as the introduction of potentially dangerous technology. Although scientists and physicians may believe the first characterization is correct, I am convinced that we must act as if the second characterization is correct. We must design vector systems and protocols so that even quite unrealistic fears about safety are allayed (Temin, 1990).

As a result, the RAC and the scientific community have gone to unprecedented lengths to assess and minimize both the risks of 'insertional mutagenesis' involved in the delivery and integration of exogenous DNA into the subject's cells and the risks that vectors may infect germ-line cells as well as their targets, even when the risks seem quite remote. Over the first decade of human gene transfer research, questions were raised about this work from both directions: first by those who thought it erred too far on the side of caution and then by those who questioned its ability to safeguard this technology.

THE PROBLEM OF 'COMPASSIONATE USE'

One consequence of the public's preoccupation with the special risks of gene transfer research has been its relative inattention to the issues involved in defining the *benefits* of gene transfer research, and that is where issues emerged in the 1990s. Despite the fact that all initial gene transfer experiments are ostensibly only phase I investigations of the safety of a particular protocol, some patients and physicians seek to become involved in gene transfer research out of hope of clinical benefit. In situations in which no alternative treatment exists and death is imminent, the risks of gene transfer pale, and any possibility of benefit, no matter how remote, seems worth attempting. Because little generalizable

new knowledge can be expected from these situations, they raise a fundamental professional and public policy question: when should we move beyond gene transfer research, with its elaborate process of public review and approval, and to treat gene therapy as simply another innovative medical practice, performed at the discretion of clinicians and their patients in full acceptance of the risks?

The American experience with this issue to date is instructive. In 1992, the NIH was asked to grant an exemption to the regular review process for gene therapy protocols, on the basis of the clinical need of a particular patient. Borrowing the notion of 'compassionate use' from the US Food and Drug Administration (FDA), the investigator argued that a protocol involving the use of gene therapy for brain tumours that had not yet been approved by the RAC should be allowed to be performed on a terminally ill patient. After initially denying the request, the Director of the NIH, Dr Bernadine Healy, granted the exemption on compassionate grounds and instructed the RAC to develop guidelines for the expedited review of such requests in the future (Thompson, 1993).

In defending her decision to grant an exemption from public review for this intervention, Healy offered an interesting response. She suggested that far from relinquishing public review of gene transfer, the time had come to expand that review beyond the research setting and to establish a public review mechanism that could oversee even the emergency clinical use of gene transfer interventions (even if that meant bringing them to the public's attention of the fact) (Healy, 1993). The RAC took that invitation seriously and developed an oversight process for the compassionate use of gene transfer in 'single-patient protocols' that makes such uses the single hardest form of clinical care to perform Legitimately in modern medicine. By requiring Institutional Review Board and Institutional Biosafety Committee (IBC) approval, declaring all gene transfer interventions as 'experimental', and advocating the use of the *Points to Consider* as review standards, the RAC essentially argues that emergency clinical uses of gene transfer should meet the same tests as research studies (Recombinant, 1993). This is a conservative standard: more conservative than that imposed by the FDA for the compassionate use of investigational drugs (Flannery, 1985) and even more conservative than the standards used to implant the first artificial heart (Annas, 2000). Many felt that, in view of the fact that none of the special hypothetical risks of gene transfer research had materialized over the first five years of clinical research, the time had come to loosen the apron-strings of this technology, and in 1998 a new NIH Director decided that the RAC's review process should no longer serve a gatekeeping function in the regulation of this technology.

THE PROBLEM OF LATROGENIC RISKS

Unfortunately, the wisdom of the RAC's clinical conservatism was confirmed almost as soon as the committee ceded its regulatory power to the Food and Drug Administration.

In September 1999, 18-year-old Jesse Gelsinger became the first person to die as a direct result of participating in a gene transfer study. Gelsinger suffered from a rare disorder called partial ornithine transcarbamylase (OTC) deficiency, an X-linked defect of the urea cycle which affect the nitrogen metabolism, leading to a spectrum of neurological symptoms including mental retardation and seizures in severe infantile cases, and manageable, non-neurological problems in its milder form (Shreenivas, 2000). The purpose of this phase I study was to determine the maximum safe dosage level of a gene transfer vector that scientists at the University of Pennsylvania had developed to treat this disease. Of the 17 patients who preceded Gelsinger in the trial, no other patients in their cohort experienced any reaction to the vector or were unable to tolerate it. However, Gelsinger's case quickly turned into a tragedy as he, within hours of the injection, developed a high fever which caused an acute respiratory distress syndrome (ARDS), and he died four days later of multiple organ failure due to anoxia. It was later suggested that the vector used had caused systemic inflammatory response syndrome (SIRS), which is associated with ARDS (Hollon, 2000).

The death of Gelsinger revealed that the lead investigators in the clinical trial misrepresented clinical findings to the National Institute of Health (NIH) and the Food and Drug Administration (FDA) (Couzin and Kaiser, 2005). In fact, it seemed to be a widespread non-compliance with federal requirements for clinical research studies were NIH-supported investigators had violated federal mandates by deviating approved study design, taking risks involving human subjects, and not reported adverse events to appropriate authorities. As a response, the Food and Drug Administration (FDA) shut down human gene transfer research at several major medical centres and issued sanctions for non-compliance with human research regulations (Steinbrook, 2002).

Meanwhile, during this same period, a European group was facing exactly the kind of biosafety issues predicted by Temin a decade earlier, in their otherwise successful attempt to use gene therapy to treat severe combined immunodeficiency disease in children. In Britain, Italy and France, 17 out of 18 children born with the rare immune disorder X-linked severe combined immune deficiency, X-SCID, or adenosine deaminase-deficiency (ADA⁻/SCID) were successfully treated by genetically modified bone marrow stem cells, and heralded as a positive counterpoint to the Gelsinger case (Cavazzana et al., 2004). In late 2002, however two children in the French trial developed leukaemia after a vector inserted near an oncogene, that is a cancer-promoting gene, called LMO2 (Berns, 2004). One of the children died in October 2004. A third case of leukaemia has recently occurred in France which again halted the clinical trial (Couzin and Kaiser, 2005).

These episodes served to confirm that the early hypothetical concerns about the potential risks of human gene transfer cannot yet be put to rest. As a result, the drive to 'normalize' human gene transfer as a clinical practice has abated, to be replaced by a new concern over how the subjects for gene transfer research are selected and recruited.

SELECTION OF SUBJECTS

The development of national policies for research with human subjects in the 1970s was motivated in part by a concern that the burdens of participating in biomedical research were unfairly distributed among particularly vulnerable populations within society, including children and the seriously ill. Children have traditionally been viewed as vulnerable because of their inability to consent to research, and the seriously ill, like the parents of sick children, are capable of neglecting important risk considerations out of clinical desperation, to their own detriment. As a result, whenever it is possible, new biomedical interventions are usually first tested for their safety in healthy adult volunteers in phase I trials before being tested for efficacy in patient – subjects or children (Levine, 1986). Indeed, this was the primary rationale for recruiting adults like Jesse Gelsinger for the Penn OTC trial: while they did not face the severe disease burdens of infants (and thus had 'more to lose'), they could take on those risks voluntarily and serve as a buffer for those who could not. But both children and the seriously ill have been prominent among the initial subjects of human gene transfer phase I trials, and the decision to test the OTC vector on adults instead of infants was criticized as unethical in some quarters (Shreenivas, 2000).

Children have usually been involved in gene transfer trials when the diseases targeted are fatal in childhood, making their selection as initial subjects unavoidable. Seriously ill adult patients, however, have been typically selected as subjects against another rationale: like cancer patients in chemotherapy trials, they are recruited because they are the least likely to suffer the consequences of any unanticipated harms from gene transfer research, and they have the most to gain from any unanticipated benefits. This justification depends heavily on the assumption that, like chemotherapy, gene transfer involves serious potential 'toxicities' that would not be appropriate to impose on healthy subjects with nothing to gain. If it were only a matter of distributing potential benefits, the argument would fail: the expectation of benefit from a phase I study is by definition 'unreasonable', and can only become a factor against the backdrop of the risks involved (King, 1999).

RESPECTING THE RIGHTS OF SUBJECTS

The need for informed consent by patient-subjects is one of the central tenets of research ethics. Thus, it is no surprise that this issue would be considered in ethical discussions of gene transfer research, although the challenges in securing voluntary and informed participation do not differ in principle from other areas of biomedical research. Two complicating features of the gene transfer context are worth noting. First, the proposed interventions in gene transfer experiments are usually at the cutting edge of research and require that subjects or their proxies have at least a basic understanding of molecular biology. Effective techniques for conveying complex technical information to lay people do exist and should be employed in the consent process for these research protocols. Second, to the extent that subjects are also patients, those securing their participation should be especially sensitive to the fact that prospective subjects will often be in relatively desperate clinical circumstances, which can exert a powerful influence on the motivations of the subjects, their families and their physicians. One crucial precaution in this regard is to avoid fostering the 'therapeutic misconception' that can be created when terms suggesting clinical benefit are used to describe basic research interventions. Thus, for many protocols, it is preferable to use the phrase 'human gene transfer' rather than 'gene therapy' to emphasize the remoteness of therapeutic benefit (King, 1999).

The protection of privacy and confidentiality for the subjects in gene transfer research has also been important. In other cases involving innovative therapy – for example, in the early heart transplants – a virtual media circus has surrounded both the subjects and the research team. Thus, the RAC's *Points to Consider* asks researchers to provide plans for dealing with the public disclosure of their research in responsible ways. A proper approach to subjects will not isolate them from public view, but will attempt to strike a balance between disclosure to an interested public and respect for the subject's privacy.

In sum, the national public review process that has overseen the development of human gene transfer research has been the victim of its own success. With the widespread public acceptance of the idea of gene therapy and the successful review of over 200 pioneering protocols, the RAC and its process are often held up as a model of

other scientific policy-making challenges (Wolf, 1997). However, that very success has led to challenges on three fronts: (1) Some argue that the similarity between human gene transfer and other innovative medical therapies has become so strong that the prospects of clinical benefit from gene transfer interventions now justify decisions to apply gene transfer techniques to seriously ill patients in the clinical setting without prior public discussion and review; (2) others argue that the risks of gene transfer have now been reduced to the point that it is time to shift to a more traditional biomedical research and development paradigm and to test new interventions for safety on normal volunteers before recruiting seriously ill patients; and (3) still others argue that both the risks and benefits of somatic cell gene therapy are unremarkable enough to no longer need public discussion at the national level over and above the ordinary system of research review. As the field of human gene transfer research matures and proliferates, each of these arguments is likely to be pressed further. At the same time, the next phase of our national conversation about the ethics of human gene transfer remains to be addressed.

ETHICAL ISSUES IN HUMAN GERM-LINE GENE TRANSFER

One of the problems that would be created by a premature dismantling of the public review process for human gene transfer research is that the issues that were set aside during the development of criteria for assessing somatic cell gene therapy would be left unaddressed at the national level. This would be an important loss because these issues – the challenges raised by the prospect of germ-line gene transfer interventions and the uses of gene transfer for enhancement purposes – were the ones that provoked the development of this process in the first place. As the discussion to date already shows, both of these categories raise fundamental social policy issues that require widespread public reflection and debate (cf. Chapman and Frankel, 2003; Rasko et al., 2006).

The major difference between somatic cell gene therapy and clinical techniques aimed at germ-line genetic intervention is that the latter would produce clinical changes that could be transmitted to the offspring of the person receiving the intervention. This simple difference is often the only consideration cited in the many official statements that endorse somatic cell gene therapy while proscribing or postponing research aimed at developing human germ-line gene therapy (Bonnicksen, 2000). Behind these official statements, however, lies a longer argument, revolving around four sets of concerns: scientific uncertainties, the need to use resources efficiently, social risks and conflicting human rights concerns.

SCIENTIFIC UNCERTAINTIES

Even the proponents of germ-line gene therapy agree that human trials under our current state of knowledge would be unacceptable. For gene-therapy techniques to be effective, the genes must be stably integrated, expressed correctly and only in the appropriate tissues, and reliably targeted to the correct location on a chromosome. If the intervention cannot eliminate the parents' risks of transmitting the alleles they carry or can only do so by substituting other genetic risks, its promise remains weak. Critics maintain that, given the complexity of gene regulation and expression during human development, germ-line gene transfer experiments will always involve too many unpredictable long-term Iatrogenic risks to the transformed subjects and their offspring to be justifiable (Council for Responsible Genetics, 1993).

Proponents, however, respond that our current ignorance only justifies postponing human trials of germ-line therapy techniques until their promise can be improved. A more optimistic reading turns the argument around in that to the extent that the barriers to effective therapy can be overcome, its promise should encourage research to continue (Munson and Davis, 1992). Proponents add that by focusing on the obvious barriers to performing clinical trials today, critics of germ-line gene therapy ignore the fact that it will take future research to determine whether or not they are right. So the question remains as to whether current barriers should ultimately dissuade society from contemplating clinical trials in the future (cf. Resnik et al., 1999).

Moreover, advocates can point out that, whether unintentionally or not, we have already crossed the boundary between somatic and germ-line interventions in humans, or could easily do so, through a number of routes unrecognized by our current regulatory schemes. For example, attempts to avoid genetic mitochondrial diseases by transplanting mitochondria-rich cytoplasm from one egg into another have already effected inheritable genetic changes in human beings, by permanently importing new mitochondrial DNA (Parens and Juengst, 2003). Does it matter that, in these cases, the inheritability of the new mitochondrial genome is only an unintended byproduct of the attempt to prevent the embryo's eventual somatic cell deficiencies? If not, how should we classify scenarios for *in utero* somatic cell gene transfer experiments that pose similar risks of accidentally transducing germ-line cells? For that matter, some studies of somatic cell gene transfer have already shown the risk of inadvertent germ-line transmission: to what extent should the risks of such side effects be tolerated in exchange for an effective therapy (King, 2003)? It may well be that the moral challenge that provoked us to draw the somatic/germ cell distinction in the first place – the prospect of creating inheritable changes in our children – will actually appear at one of these scientific side-doors long before it arrives at the front door of 'germ-line gene transfer', where we have been waiting for it.

ALLOCATION OF RESOURCES

One common criticism of the argument from medical utility is that it betrays a reductionistic attitude towards illness that fails to appreciate approaches that could achieve the same ends more efficiently. Because it must become possible to identify pre-embryos in need of therapy before their transformation, the argument goes, it would be more efficient simply to use the same techniques to identify healthy pre-embryos for implantation (Davis, 1992). Many clinical geneticists argue that even our current methods of prenatal screening serve this function. Against these convenient, effective approaches, they conclude, germ-line gene therapy will never be cost-effective enough to merit high enough social priority to pursue.

One scientific rejoinder to this argument is that screening will not help with all cases. Presumably, for example, as more beneficiaries of somatic cell gene therapy survive to reproductive age, there will be more couples whose members are both afflicted with the same recessive disorders (Wivel and Walters, 1993). Gene therapy strategies that affect the germ-line may also be the only effective ways of addressing some genetic diseases with origins very early in development. Moreover, by preventing the transmission of disease genes, germ-line gene therapy could obviate the need for screening and somatic cell gene therapy in subsequent generations of a family.

SOCIAL RISKS

Proponents of germ-line gene therapy research also point out that screening prevents genetic disease only by preventing the birth of the patients who would suffer from it. This, they point out, is a confusion of therapeutic goals that runs the long-term risk of encouraging coercive eugenic practices and tacitly fostering discrimination against those with genetic disease. By attempting to prevent disease in individuals rather than selecting against individuals according to genotype, germ-line gene therapy would allow us to maintain our commitment to the value of moral equality in the fact of our acknowledged biological diversity (Juengst, 1995).

Critics reply to this that, to the contrary, it is germ-line therapy that has the more ominous social implications, by opening the door to genetic enhancement. One line of argument recalls the historical abuses of the eugenic movement to suggest that, to the extent that the line between gene therapy and enhancement would increasingly blur, germ-line interventions would be open to the same questions about the proper vision of human flourishing that eugenics faced. Even those who dispute the dangers of the 'slippery slope' in this context take pains to defend the moral significance of the distinction 'between uses that may relieve real suffering and those that alter characteristics that have little or nothing to do with disease' (Fletcher, 1985, p. 303). Proponents must then argue that appropriate distinctions among these different uses can be confidently drawn (Anderson, 1989) and point out that the same eugenic challenges already face those engaged in pre-implantation screening or prenatal diagnosis (Fowler et al., 1989).

HUMAN RIGHTS CONCERNS

Finally, however, some critics argue that the focus of germ-line gene therapy on the embryonic patient has other implications that foreclose its pursuit. If the primary goal of the intervention is to address the health problems of the pre-embryo itself, germ-line gene therapy becomes an extreme case of foetal therapy and the pre-embryo gains the status of a patient requiring protection. Germ-line gene therapy experiments would involve research with early human embryos that would have effects on their offspring, effectively placing multiple human generations in the role of unconsenting research subjects (Lappe, 1991). If pre-embryos are given the moral status of patients, it will be very hard to justify the risks of clinical research that would be necessary to develop the technique.

This objection to human germ-line gene therapy research is framed in several ways. For European commentators, it is often interpreted as the right to one's genetic patrimony (Mauron, 1991) in that germ-line gene therapy interventions would violate the rights of subsequent generations to inherit a genetic endowment that has not been intentionally modified. For advocates of people with disabilities, this concern is interpreted in terms of the dangers of society's willingness to accept their differences (Buchanan, 1996). Some feminists join this position as well, out of a concern for the impact on women of taking the pre-embryo too seriously as an object of medical care (Minden, 1987).

Proponents can offer several responses to these concerns. First of all, some of these appeals, such as the appeals to the rights of future generations to an unmodified 'genetic patrimony', can be criticized simply on scientific and conceptual grounds as incoherent (Juengst, 1998). Beyond that, proponents also argue that germ-line gene therapy is a reproductive health intervention aimed at the parents, not the embryo (Zimmerman, 1991). Its goal is to allow the parents to address their reproductive risks and have a healthy baby, in cases in which the parents' own views prohibit pre-

implantation screening and embryo selection. In taking this position, proponents acknowledge the moral uncertainty over the status of the pre-embryo and defend parental requests for germ-line therapy as falling within the scope of their reproductive rights. Their argument is that, as a professional policy, medicine should continue to accept and respond to a wide range of interpretations of reproductive health needs by prospective parents, including requests for germ-line interventions (Fowler et al., 1989).

Germ-line gene transfer has traditionally been perceived as scientifically remote. However, the development of techniques in reproductive medicine, like *in vitro* ovum nuclear transfer (Rubenstein et al., 1995), makes the prospect of applying somatic cell gene transfer techniques to pre-implantation embryos a good bit more realistic. Although the application of gene transfer techniques at that stage would still lack adequate background evidence of safety and efficacy, the relatively unregulated environment in which innovations in reproductive medicine are introduced increases the risks that such experimentation could occur. The danger of muting the public discussion of human gene transfer at the national level, of course, is the risk of creating a climate in which such experimentation could proceed without prior knowledge or review.

ACKNOWLEDGEMENTS

This chapter is an updated adaptation of an essay by E. Juengst and LeRoy Walters (1999). Dr Walters has entrusted his coauthorship role to Ms Grankvist for this revision, but much of what remains reflects his invaluable contributions to the original and we remain in his debt. The research conducted for this revision was supported in part by National Institutes of Health grant RO1 HG-1446-02.

REFERENCES

Anderson F.W. Genetic therapy. In: Hamilton M, ed. *The New Genetics and the Future of Man*. Grand Rapids, MI: W. B. Eerdmans, 1972, pp. 110–125.

Anderson FW. Human gene therapy: Why draw a line? *J Med Philos* 1989; **14**: 681–693.

Anderson FW, Fletcher J. Gene therapy in human beings: When is it ethical to begin? *N Engl J Med* 1980; **303**: 1293–1297.

Annas G. The Phoenix heart: What we have to lose. *The Hastings Center Report* 1985; **15**: 15–16.

Areen J. Regulating human gene therapy. *W Va Law Rev* 1985; **88**: 153.

Berns MA. Good news for gene therapy. *NEJM* 2004; **350**: 1679–1680.

Bonnicksen A. Gene therapy ethics: International perspectives. In: Murray T, Mehlman M, eds., *Encyclopedia of Ethical, Legal and Policy Issues in Biotechnology.* New York: John Wiley & Sons, Inc., 2000, pp. 275–285.

Brenner M. Human somatic gene therapy: Progress and problems. *J Intern Med* 1995; **237**: 229–239.

Buchanan A. Choosing who will be disabled: Genetic intervention and the morality of inclusion. *Soc Philos Policy* 1996; **13**: 18–47.

Capron A. The impact of the report, splicing life. *Hum. Gene Ther.* 1990; **1**: 69–73.

Capron A, Leventhal B, Post L, Walters L, Zallen D. Requests for compassionate use of gene therapy: Memorandum from the subcommittee to the RAC. *Hum Gene Ther* 1993; **4**: 199–200.

Cavazzana-Calvo M, Trasher A, Mavilio F. The future of gene therapy – Balancing the risks and benefits of clinical trials. *Nature* 2004; **427**: 779–781.

Chapman A, Frankel M, eds. *Designing Our Descendants: The Promises and Perils of Genetic Modifications.* Baltimore, MD: Johns Hopkins University Press, 2003.

Council for Responsible Genetics. Position paper on human germ line manipulation (Fall 1992). *Hum Gene Ther* 1993; **4**: 35–37.

Couzin J, Kaiser J. As Gelsinger case ends, gene therapy suffers another blow. *Science* 2005; **307**: 1028.

Davis B. Germ-line gene therapy: Evolutionary and moral considerations. *Hum Gene Ther* 1992; **3**: 361–365.

de Wachter M. Ethical aspects of germ-line gene therapy. *Bioethics* 1993; **7**: 166–178.

Flannery E. 1986. Should it be easier or harder to use unapproved devices? *The Hastings Center Report* 1986; **16**: 17–23.

Fletcher JC. Ethical issues in and beyond prospective clinical trials of human gene therapy. *J Med Philos* 1985; **10**: 293–309.

Fowler G, Juengst E, Zimmerman B. Germ-line gene therapy and the clinical ethos of medical genetics. *Theor Med* 1989; **10**: 151–165.

Healy B. Remarks for the RAC regarding compassionate use exemption. *Hum Gene Ther* 1993; **4**: 195–197.

Hollon T. Researchers and regulators reflect on first gene therapy death. *Nat Med* 2000; **6**: 6.

Hotchkiss R. Portents for a genetic engineering. *J Hered* 1965; **56**: 197–202.

Juengst E. 'Prevention' and the goals of genetic medicine. *Hum Gene Ther* 1995; **6**: 1595–1605.

Juengst E. Should we treat the human germ-line as a global human resource? In: Agius E, Busuttil S, eds. *Germ-Line Intervention and Our Responsibilities to Future Generations.* Dordrecht, The Netherlands: Kluwer, 1998, pp. 85–102.

Juengst E, Walters L. Ethical issues in human gene transfer research. In: Friedman T, ed. *The Development of Human Gene Therapy.* Cold Spring Harbor, NY: Cold Spring Harbor Press, 1999, pp. 691–713.

King N. Rewriting the 'Points to Consider': The ethical impact of guidance document language *Hum Gene Ther* 1999; **10**: 133–139.

King N. Accident and desire – Inadvertent germ-line effects in clinical research. *The Hastings Center Report* 2003; **33**(2): 23–30.

Lappe M. Ethical issues in manipulating the human germ-line. *J Med Philos* 1991; **16**: 621–639.

Levine RJ. *The Ethics and Regulation of Clinical Research*, 2nd edition. New Haven, CT: Yale University Press, 1986.

Mauron A, Thevoz J-M. Germ-line engineering: A few European voices. *J Med Philos* 1991; **16**: 649–666.

Minden S. Patriarchal designs: The genetic engineering of human embryos. In: Spallone P, Steinberg D, eds. *Made to Order: The Myth of Reproductive and Genetic Progress.* Oxford: Pergamon Press, 1987, pp. 102–109.

Munson R, Davis L. Germ-line gene therapy and the medical imperative. *Kennedy Inst Ethics J* 1992; **2**: 137–158.

Parens E, Juengst E. Inadvertently crossing the germ line. *Science* 2001; **292**: 397.

President's Commission for the Study of Ethical Problems in Medicine and Biomedical and Behavioral Research. *Splicing Life: A Report on the Social and Ethical Issues of Genetic Engineering with Human Beings.* Washington, D.C.: U.S. Government Printing Office, 1982.

Ramsey P. Genetic therapy: A theologian's response. In: Hamilton M, ed. *The New Genetics and the Future of Man.* Grand Rapids, MI: W. B. Eerdmans, 1972, pp. 1570–1579.

Rasko JE, O'Sullivan GM, Ankeny RA. *The Ethics of Inheritable Genetic Modification: A Dividing Line?* Cambridge: Cambridge University Press, 2006.

Recombinant DNA Advisory Committee. Procedures to be followed for expedited review of single patient protocols. *Hum Gene Ther* 1993; **4**: 307.

Resnik D, Steinkraus H, Langer P. *Human Germline Gene Therapy: Scientific, Moral and Political Issue.* Austin, TX: R.G. Landes, Co., 1999.

Rubenstein DS, Thomasma DC, Schon EA, Zinaman J. Germ-line gene therapy to cure mitochondrial disease: Protocol and ethics of in vitro ovum nuclear transplantation. *Camb Q Healthcare Ethics* 1995; **4**: 316–339.

Shreenivas S. Who killed Jesse Gelsinger? Ethical issues in human gene therapy. *Monsh Bioethics Rev* 2000; **19**: 35–43.

Steinbrook R. Protecting research subjects – the crisis at Johns Hopkins. *New Eng J Med* 2002; **346**: 716–720.

Subcommittee on Human Genome Therapy (Recombinant DNA Advisory Committee, National Institutes of Health). Points to consider in the design and submission of protocols for the transfer of recombinant DNA into the genome of human subjects. *Hum Gene Ther*

Temin HM. Safety considerations in somatic gene therapy of human disease. *Hum Gene Ther* 1990; **1**: 111–123.

Thompson L. Gene therapy: Healy approves an unproved treatment. *Science* 1993; **259**: 172.

US Congress (Office of Technology Assessment). *Human Gene Therapy.* Washington, D.C.: U.S. Government Printing Office, 1984.

Walters L. Palmer J. 1996. *The Ethics of Human Gene Therapy.* Oxford: Oxford University Press, 1996.

Wivel NA, Walters L. Germ-line gene modification and disease prevention: Some medical and ethical perspectives. *Science* 1993; **262**: 533–538.

Wolf SM. Ban cloning? Why NBAC is wrong. *The Hastings Center Report* 1997; **27**: 12–15.

Zimmerman BK. Human germ-line therapy: The case for its development and use. *J Med Philos* 1991; **16**: 593–612.

The Ethics of Ageing, Immortality and Genetics

DANIELA CUTAS AND JOHN HARRIS

The questions we address are the following: are we entitled to access life extension therapies? Must we draw the line at some point (say 120 years, the maximum life span so far, or maybe even earlier) and decide that that's that and now we must die? Are there considerations that might make either living or making it possible to live after a certain ages immoral? Does justice require forgoing life extension therapies, or does it require the development and application of these therapies (for a more exhaustive analysis of arguments for and against life extension, see Harris, 2002)?

In this chapter immortality covers all stages from modest life-extending therapies to indefinite survival and presupposes a delay or an arrest of the ageing process. We assume that a world of immortals would not be a world of frail, diseased people kept alive indefinitely; few, including the population of life-extended individuals, would want this. On the contrary, a world with substantially extended life expectancy would be a world where people would not suffer the deleterious effects of ageing or will suffer them later than they do nowadays. And even if ageing were indefinitely postponed, death would still occur because of accidents, diseases, wars and murders. Thus the only cause of death which would be eliminated, or delayed, would be the death-causing diseases of old age.

There are broadly three ways of achieving immortality: extending life by postponing old age-related death in people already alive (for instance, by alleviating or curing illnesses that affect people in old age – in this case, immortality would become a 'side effect' of prevention and treatment of diseases); extending life indefinitely by the abolition of ageing in people who are now alive; and engineering immortality into gametes or early embryos, who would thus be born immortals.

In the literature, the proponents of life extension are often referred to as prolongevitists, meliorists or life extensionists; among these are Caplan (1992; 2005), Harris (2002), de Grey (2003), Kirkwood (1999); and its opponents are referred to as apologists, quietists, thanatophiles, deathists for example, Callahan (1995), Fukuyama (2002), and Kass (2002). The two categories are not always clear cut, as there are authors who do not contest the good of 'quality life' extension and at the same time do not believe in the possibility of overcoming ageing (Olshansky and Carnes, 2001, for example).

OVERPOPULATION

The worry in terms of overpopulation is so pervasive that if unchallenged may come to seem convincing. Overpopulation is often pointed out as a source of misery in the developing world and is a considerable part of the most pessimistic picturing of the doomed future of mankind. Several confusions lie at the core of these dark expectations. First, it is unclear (at least) why in the context of overpopulation worries we should be suspicious of life extension, instead of fertility rates, overwhelmingly lower in states that would be more likely to benefit from life extension therapies than in states where life expectancy is lower and which are far less likely to benefit from life extension therapies in the near future. According to the website of the CIA[1], last updated in January 2006, the population growth rates in states such as the United Kingdom (0.28%, life expectancy 78.38, fertility rate per woman 1.36 children), the United States (0.92%, life expectancy 77.71, fertility rate 2.08), France (0.37%, life expectancy 79.6, fertility rate 1.85), Italy (0.07%, life

---

[1]CF. Central Intelligence Agency, www.odci.gov/cia/publications/factbook.

Principles of Health Care Ethics, Second Edition Edited by R.E. Ashcroft, A. Dawson, H. Draper and J.R. McMillan
© 2007 John Wiley & Sons, Ltd

expectancy 79.68, fertility rate 1.28), Spain (0.15%, life expectancy 79.52, fertility rate 1.28), Switzerland (0.49%, life expectancy 80.39, fertility rate 1.42) are far lower than in states where the death rate is much higher, such as Somalia (3.38%, life expectancy 48.09, fertility rate 6.84), Gabon (2.45%, life expectancy 55.02, fertility rate 4.77), Kenya (2.56%, life expectancy 47.99, fertility rate 4.96), Uganda (3.31%, life expectancy 51.59, fertility rate 6.74), the Democratic Republic of Congo (2.98%, life expectancy 51.1, fertility rate 6.54), and both lists continue. It is worth noting that population growth comprises the immigrants, usually numerous in many of the developed countries, and that as it is obvious from the figures, in the countries of the former lot, population growth is still remarkably inferior than in the latter lot, in spite of the higher mortality and reduced life expectancy that the former experience.

Second, it is not self-evident that if overpopulation occurs, the only proper response is to let older people die. There is no well-recognized obligation that physicians refuse to treat people with life-threatening conditions because their dying decreases the number of "mouths that must be fed". What makes it ethical to save the lives or postpone the deaths of one particular category of people rather than another, and why is it that not allowing the death rate to decrease is the optimal solution, rather than, for instance, slowing the fertility rates? (see More, 2001).

The readiness from some opponents of life extension to suggest that there is a point where there has been enough life and room needs to be made for others raises questions as to why it is that the old have to sacrifice themselves for others. Even if we accept the fact that life extension creates a wide array of difficulties (more overpopulation, heavier taxes, more burdens for their families and health care systems, higher unemployment, etc. the likeliness of all of which being yet to be established), it does not follow that the old have any kind of obligation to accept their deaths without a fight. Indeed, as Overall stresses,

> [t]he very fact that older people are expected, without need for further argument, to accept their deaths and not struggle to prolong their lives - an expectation that is not foisted on individuals belonging to other social groups – is indicative of the deep, naïve, and unquestioned ageism that lies at the heart of many of the claims on behalf of apologism. In general, I see no reason to decide on the basis of age that certain individuals must be prepared to die for the alleged greater benefit of the human species (Overall, 2003).

As Overall points out within the same argument, there are categories of people in our societies who create more of a burden on others than immortals would, such as people with illnesses and severe disabilities, people chronically poor and, we may add, people imprisoned for life. Yet those who oppose life extension because of immortals being burdens do not also advocate for the moral obligation of the above-mentioned groups

to die. It is important here to re-emphasize that life extension is not advocated as the prolongation of frail and disabled old age but as the delaying of the devastating effects of ageing. Thus the immortals would not be old and dependent people being kept alive to the detriment of the living standards and life opportunities of all, but active people able to function for longer than they do today. Which again creates a corresponding worry for the apologists: enjoying life actively (including by pursuing professional careers) might make it more difficult for younger people to do the same. Therefore, the only escape seems to be, some would say, that older people retire and die. One can wonder what the apologists would propose if, for instance, a population were to become immortal by accident or if a plant were discovered that would stop the ageing process in people who ingested it (or if any other version of the 'fountain of youth' myth were to become real). In the first example, would the accidentally immortal be given a deadline by which they should be killed? In the second example, would the use of the plant (or whatever source of eternal youth) become illegal? Would the plant have to be destroyed for the sake of the young?

As Max More insists (More, 2001) and as it is obvious from the data quoted above, population growth is much more closely related to fertility rates than to longevity. Thus, correlating life extension treatments with improving access to health care and education for contraception may well have better overall results than refusing to treat old age diseases for fear that people will live too long and crowd the planet.

THE RIGHT TO LIFE: A RIGHT WITH A DEADLINE?

The right to life is a very popular concept. A simple Google search for 'right to life' gives hundreds of thousands of results. However, surprisingly or not, the overwhelming majority of these results do not have anything to do with life-prolonging interventions in the sense that interests us in this chapter. Instead, the supposed right is generally correlated with the issue of abortion, embryonic stem cell research, embryo experimentation and euthanasia–in most cases, the right to life is invoked as an objection to all such practices. It is as if the most passionate proponents of the right to life only uphold it when it is of no meaning for its holder (the embryo) or when it is not wanted by its holder (the irreversibly comatose human being for which it may be indifferent, or who when still a self-conscious person objected to being kept alive should such a state occur, or the terminally ill person asking to be allowed to die).

Christine Overall addresses the matter of the right to life in the context of life extension, but does not think that there is a positive right to life, that is, an 'entitlement to all possible assistance to preserve, enhance, and extend life' (Overall, 2003, pp. 109, 193). Also, Overall writes that a positive right to life would 'devour resources' (Overall, 2003 p. 116). However, we do not see why the acknowledgement of a positive right to life would have to lead to such consequences. Indeed, positive rights need not be absolute rights, but rights that require more than non-interference (the obligation classically entailed by negative rights). Even if it was accepted that we do not have rights to be provided with the means to life extension, forbidding life extension altogether, in principle, can very well be described as a violation of a negative right to life, the right to not being prevented from continuing one's life. Thus, either as a negative or as a positive right, the right to life seems to support allowing (the negative version), if not providing when accomplishable (the positive version) access to life extension treatments.

The acceptance of a right to life does not allow discrimination on grounds of age, as long as morally justifiable reasons cannot be advanced for the distinction between older and younger people, of a nature to show that the former are less entitled to life. Surely it cannot be the quantity of life that one has had, as different people have different lives, which can be more intense for some, or more burdened, more satisfying or more frustrated. Deciding on how much life is enough is likely to result in more injustice for people who, although they have lived many years, have had fewer opportunities and fewer chances to flourish in their previous years (for an extensive argument in this sense, see Overall, 2003: examples focus especially on women, generally both the longer lived and the least advantaged gender). The value of persons' lives is not dependent upon the quantity of life at one end or the other, but on their respective capacities to value their own lives, whatever the content of that which they actually value (for a more detailed account of this position, see Harris, 1985).

An argument in terms of rights that is often advanced in opposition to immortality therapies is that allowing existing people to live longer violates either the right to reproduce or the rights of future generations, or both. Regarding the former, we do not deny that the interest that people may have to become parents is worthy of moral consideration; however, we cannot see how it would be so strong as to demand that existing people die to make room for offspring (in fact, people tend to think it cynical and disrespectful when such expectations are declared). We think it is rather obvious that the interest in continuing one's existence cannot be simply trumped by the interest in parenting. Among other reasons, this is because living is often a much stronger interest than parenting (maybe except for the cases of people who are willing to give up their own life for the sake of reproducing, but surely such can only be a personal decision and not a requirement for all others), and the loss of a life one does not wish to lose is usually considered more of a tragedy than not experiencing parenthood. Concluding otherwise demands that solid arguments be advanced for preferring to respect the interest in reproduction than to respect the interest in continuing existence.

Regarding future generations, we agree that there are many ways in which we can now harm them, but halting reproduction is not one of these, simply because if we do not reproduce there are no future generations to be harmed. Again, we cannot compare the right that people have not to lose their lives with an alleged right to be created.

Besides the ageist flavour, the arguments in terms of the right to reproduce and the rights of future generations assume that, first, life extension would be indefinite and immortals would be invulnerable and second, that killing people may be a optimum solution in the race for space. However, invulnerability does not appear to be even foreseen by scientists anywhere in the near future (if indeed it ever becomes possible), which means that 'some' reproduction is likely to remain not only possible but also necessary, and therefore a decision between not allowing people to live longer lives (and continuing to reproduce) and halting reproduction altogether (and living longer) is not a priority at the moment.

In another context, Joel Feinberg (1992) proposes what he calls 'the right to an open future', a right to be held 'in trust' for a child to exercise when he or she has the competence that makes the right relevant. According to Feinberg, children must be 'permitted to reach maturity with as many open options, opportunities, and advantages as possible' (Feinberg, 1992, p. 80). If, then, it were the case that the most successful and enduring life-enhancing modifications would have to be made on the embryo, the right to an open future might well require parents to give their children the option of immortality in order to ensure for their child that such an important option is available when he or she reaches maturity. So it seems, plus because immortality does not imply invulnerability, that once the children reach adulthood, if immortals decide that they do not want immortality, they can always choose to die. Feinberg had in mind a range of options that would present themselves 'simultaneously', so to speak, to individuals on reaching maturity, like a number of doors on different possible futures among which to choose. However, extended life span will principally present options sequentially in addition to simultaneously to future individuals. Even allowing for some discounting of future options they are nonetheless real options, and when (and if) the future become less problematic the discounting may seem less psychologically appealing and its illogicality will seem more obvious.

This raises the very interesting and vexed question of the extent and nature of parental duties to children. Whether parental obligations to children include trying to extend their life expectancy and how binding or enforceable such obligations might be is of great interest and complexity. Could the obligation to provide life-extending treatments to the embryo be greater or lesser than the obligation of mothers to take folic acid during pregnancy or to avoid smoking?

In the end, life saving is just death postponing with a positive spin. If it is right and good to postpone death for a short while, it is difficult to see how it would not be better and more moral to postpone death for longer – even indefinitely. If we accept an ethic of life saving we are committed to death postponement. So the obligation to extend life does not necessarily have to be a dimension of a right to life, but also part of an obligation that most people accept that they should save the lives of others if they can and certainly that they should not stop their fellows from saving others if they wish to do so. The rule of rescue is one form of expression of this truth (for debates on the duty to rescue, see Kleining, 1976; Weinrib, 1980; Harris, 1985; McIntyre, 1994; Barry, 1995).

WHAT JUSTICE REQUIRES AND WHAT IT DOES NOT REQUIRE

One of the frequently voiced worries regarding immortality is that the technologies that would bring it about are likely to be expensive, at least initially. The extremely rich might afford it, or maybe governments in rich countries would provide them to all their citizens. In either of these cases, the problem of access would increase the divide between high-income individuals or countries and low-income individuals or countries, with the latter practically denied access. However, if immortality or increased life expectancy is a good, it is unclear in what way its denial for everyone would assist the unfortunate who could not afford it. As long as the criteria for offering the treatment are not unjust in themselves, the mere fact that it cannot be provided to all is no reason to abandon it altogether; the fact that all lives cannot be saved is not a reason to refuse to save any lives. If access to life extension is only awarded to the rich, and if life extension is a good, and if this is considered problematic in terms of justice, then surely justice would rather be achieved by some sort of redistribution and not by universal prohibition. In addition, we cannot yet know who will and who will not afford immortality; some authors even argue that, once achievable, immortality may well rapidly become widely accessible, maybe in a way similar to the case of antibiotics (see de Grey, 2003; de Magalhaes, 2005).

If, instead, immortality is not a good, as some apologists would argue, then of course its possession by some is not unjust for the others who do not have it. Its effects, instead, are what may make it unjust: immortals, some argue, would lead to the overcrowding of the planet, aggravating resource exhaustion, would compete with the young for jobs and so on. In the previous section we have seen which are some of the problems inherent in this interpretation.

Prohibiting immortality would also entail deciding not to treat people for old age-related diseases, at least in some cases (maybe after a certain age, say 120), on the grounds that such treatments would abolish old age, and deciding to deny those suffering from treatable disease the chance of a cure. If, then, justice demands the limiting of life expectancy for some, so that it matches others, we will have to face up to the deliberate curtailing of lives that would otherwise continue, with all the additional problems that this would entail. This way of achieving justice, some may argue, is far from being fair (see the previous section).

The supposed toll on health care that immortality would cause, creating injustice and unaffordable care, is also related to the misunderstanding according to which immortals would be people kept old and disabled for longer. In fact, it is likely that immortality would be cost-effective because although people might live longer, they would be on average healthier throughout their lives and might have much shorter periods of health care dependency at the end of life. Thus, despite the greater span of consumption resources, the actual consumption might be reduced for immortals and therefore economic arguments for penalizing such individuals might well fail. Moreover, it can be argued that immortality would rather dramatically reduce health costs (the same conclusion of the cost-effectiveness of immortality is reached by de Grey, 2003; and de Magalhães, 2005). There may be an economic discounting argument for public funding of immortality interventions. Let us see how this might look (the example and the calculations have been suggested by Søren Holm in a personal communication):

1. For both mortals and immortals there is the same period of old age with increased health care costs (say 10 years, but the length does not matter for the argument) and the same costs of treatment during those years (let's say £10, 000 on average).
2. The mortals will reach this period in 70 years and the immortals in 1, 000 years.
3. There is a 1% per year rate of real economic growth.

Thus, the present-day discounted costs of treating a person in 70 years' time will be £4948 whereas the present-day cost of treating the same person in 1000 years' time will be 43 pence. Therefore, it does make economic good sense to invest now and postpone health care costs from 70 years into the future to 1000 years into the future, and as is evident from the figures, it makes sense even if immortals would have a much longer and more costly old age (because of the discounting even a tenfold increase in costs would not matter). Add to this the probability that a greater number of immortals would die as the result of accidents rather than long drawn-out illnesses, and the economic arguments grow stronger still (not to mention that their organs might be usable for transplants for much longer). However, even if the reverse were the case, it is still not clear that it would be justifiable to distinguish between older and younger citizens in terms of access of health care.

CONCLUSION

We have discussed some of the arguments for and against immortality. Far from suggesting that immortality does not raise problems, we have emphasized that often the difficulties and burdens associated with it are overstated, or the interest that people may have to desire immortality are understated. We strongly think that it is important to take seriously all proposals and implications of life extension therapies, and this is partly because failing to do so is likely to leave us unprepared to deal with the issue when the pace quickens. There is also a risk associated with fears and misrepresentations that threaten to overcome the public discourse in a way similar to the issues related to cloning, for instance. In this sense, it may be easier to approach life extension-related topics not as 'immortality' but as the 'conquest of disease, suffering, and infirmity', thus shifting the attention from any 'boundary crossing' to values that most of us embrace. This approach has been suggested by Steven Austad in a lecture given at a conference organized in Cambridge in 2003 by the International Association of Biogerontologists (IABG), and in its turn has its problems because detractors may claim that it involves an attempt to 'hide' the realities of what is being proposed.

We have thus discussed objections in terms of overpopulation and justice, which are occasioned by the thought of immortality, and showed that they show a number of weaknesses. We have also discussed the right to life and the obligation to save lives, not for the most part much emphasized in the literature. If there is a right to life, or if we accept that there is a duty to rescue (even a weak one), and if these do not have a deadline, then many of the objections to immortality appear less powerful.

REFERENCES

Barry B. *Justice as Impartiality.* Oxford: Clarendon Press, 1995.

Callahan D. *What Kind of Life: The Limits of Medical Progress.* Georgetown: Georgetown University Press, 1995.

Caplan A. *If I Were a Rich Man Could I Buy a Pancreas? And Other Essays on the Ethics of Health Care.* Bloomington, IN: Indiana Bloomington Press, 1992.

Caplan A. Death as an unnatural process. Why is it wrong to seek a cure for ageing? *EMBO Reports* 2005; 6: S72–75.

de Grey, A. Why we should do all we can to hasten the defeat of human aging. http://www.gem.cam.uk/sens, 2003.

de Magalhaes JP. *Should We Cure Aging?* http://www.senescence.info/myths.html, 2005.

Feinberg J. *Freedom and Fulfilment: Philosophical Essays.* Princeton, NJ: Princeton University Press, 1992.

Fukuyama F. *Our Posthuman Future: Consequences of the Biotechnology Revolution.* London: Profile, 2002.

Harris J. *The Value of Life: An Introduction to Medical Ethics.* London: Routledge, 1985.

Harris J. Intimations of immortality: the ethics and justice of life-extending therapies. In: Freeman MDA, ed. *Current Legal Problems.* Oxford: Oxford University Press, 2002; Vol. 55.

Kass L. *Life, Liberty and the Defense of Dignity.* San Francisco: Encounter Books, 2002.

Kirkwood T. *Time of our Lives: The Science of Human Ageing.* London: Weidenfield & Nicolson, 1999.

Kleining J. Good Samaritanism. *Philos Public Aff* 1976; **5**(4): 391–413.

McIntyre A. Guilty bystanders? On the legitimacy of duty to rescue statutes. *Philos Public Aff* 1994; **23**(2): 157–171.

More M. Life extension and overpopulation. www.maxmore.com/LifeExtensionandOverpopulation.htm, 2001.

Olshansky J, Carnes B. *The Quest for Immortality: Science at the Frontiers of Aging.* New York: W.W. Norton 2001.

Overall C. *Aging, Death, and Human Longevity.* Berkeley, CA: University of California Press, 2003.

Weinrib E. The case for a duty to rescue. *Yale Law J* 1980; **90**: 247–293.

108

Ethical Issues of Enhancement Technologies

RUUD H.J. TER MEULEN, LISBETH NIELSEN, LAURENS LANDEWEERD

Both in popular media and in academic publications, serious discussions take place about the prospects of the enhancement of human capacities by the application of new biotechnologies and other emergent technologies like nano-technologies. Biotechnologies may be applied to make people think better, to make them feel happier, to make them live longer or to improve their functioning in sports and athletics. These envisaged improvements or enhancements have their roots in the 'normal' application of such technologies, namely the healing of illness and the relief of suffering. The effectiveness and power of these technologies in the area of therapy have come to a second use in the efforts to elevate human feeling, improve cognition and intelligence and raise physical performance to higher levels. Although these new possibilities are for some authors a reason to envisage a new utopia, and see the new application as essentially 'good', there are also serious ethical concerns. These concerns have to do with the impact of the new technologies on fundamental values like the freedom and autonomy of the individual, the nature of humanity and justice in society and health care.

In this chapter we will present an overview of the ethical debate on the application of new technologies to enhance human capacities. We will start with a discussion about the moral value of enhancement, particularly in its distinction from therapy. The distinction between therapy and enhancement is often seen as an effort to separate the 'good' and 'the bad', with therapy as the good strategy and enhancement as the bad one. The background of this normative distinction must be found in the history of eugenics, in which primitive ideas about genetic inheritance were used to legitimize the sterilizing and even killing of people with 'undesirable' characteristics. But is therapy always good and enhancement always bad or at least dubious and thus unacceptable?

A second issue is the way the concept of human nature is used for the moral evaluation of enhancement technologies. A possible negative stance on enhancement is sometimes caused by the fear that, by improving human capacities, medicine and biotechnology are irreversibly changing human nature. However, is human nature a valuable and reliable anchor-point to evaluate the new technologies? Should this principle (including its reliance on certain ideas of natural preservation) be applied to the ethical and political assessment of the new technologies?

A third issue has to do with the relation between enhancement and health. Enhancement is sometimes seen as unhealthy, not because of its risks, but because it seems to interfere with 'normal functioning' of the body which, according to some philosophers, is central to the concept of health. Does the enhancement of human capacities contribute to the improvement of health and to the goals of medicine and health care?

The answer to this question is relevant for the access to the enhancement technologies and the problem of the just distribution of the benefits these technologies may bring to us. Society is said to have a moral obligation to help those persons who are in need of care and treatment because of handicaps or disease. However, enhancement is seen by many as a mere preference and not as a health need. According to some authors, then, society has no obligation to fund the access to enhancement technologies. Other authors are of the opinion that enhancement may improve the opportunities of individuals in society and that access to these technologies should be guided by concerns about justice.

Principles of Health Care Ethics, Second Edition   Edited by R.E. Ashcroft, A. Dawson, H. Draper and J.R. McMillan

The final issue in this chapter concerns authenticity. If we change our capacities in the field of intelligence, mood or physical performance, are we not changing our fundamental and authentic selves? Or, more fundamentally, are we not focusing too much on our individuality and neglecting our relation with others and with society in general?

THE MORAL VALUE OF ENHANCEMENT

In order to get a better understanding of the moral value of enhancement, its goals are often juxtaposed with those of therapy. Though therapy is in most cases the source of enhancement technologies, enhancement is often considered as something new, and often something negative. Although enhancement basically means improvement or adding of a new capacity, its application in the field of mood, intelligence and cognition as well as physical capacities seem to evoke negative sentiments by many. Enhancement then is an ambiguous concept which can mean better and more, but also something that many people may think to be less desirable and that should be avoided. For example, genetic doping in sports may be highly valued by some athletes, but may be judged negatively by many others because it may result in unfair competition. Extending the life span seems to go beyond the normal or 'natural' range of the human life cycle with many negative social and psychological consequences. But is enhancement always bad or at least dubious and thus unacceptable? Moreover, therapy and enhancement are to a certain extent overlapping; all successful therapies are a kind of enhancement, even if not all enhancements can be called therapeutic. The improving and regenerating of organs and tissues in the elderly may be seen as enhancement, but it can be considered to be a therapy as well.

The negative evaluation of enhancement is partly the result of the history of eugenics in the first decades of the twentieth century. Many handicapped persons and people with psychiatric and psychogeriatric disorders were sterilized and killed because they did not meet the ideals of race and humanity. People with physical and learning disabilities have the feeling that the application of enhancement technologies as a new kind of eugenics might result in a less favourable view of handicaps and disabilities, and even on their existence as members of society. One can argue that some kinds of enhancement can indeed be considered as eugenic. An example may be the genetic improvement and genetic selection through prenatal and pre-implantation genetic diagnosis (PGD and PIGD). However, the proponents of these new technologies argue that there is a big difference with the approach of the 'old' eugenics because of the emphasis in the 'new' eugenics on free choice and autonomy ('liberal eugenics'). Nonetheless, the basic idea is the same, namely the weeding out of undesirable physical and psychological traits, and one should be aware that a broad application of enhancement can indeed lead to discrimination of handicapped persons.

Though the discussion about enhancement versus therapy has taken its point of departure in ethical concerns about the new 'liberal' eugenics, the enhancement-therapy discussion goes way beyond the field of eugenics. Therapeutically aimed research of diseases such as Alzheimer's and disorders such as ADHD, OCD and depression also brings a potential for enhancement of both cognition and mood by pharmacological means. There is a long list of drugs developed with the purpose of treatment of illness, but with the potential for enhancement, if used on 'normal' (i.e. not diagnosed ill) persons: psychopharmacological drugs such as Modafinil (increases alertness) and antidepressants such as Prozac, Seroxat and Cipramil (SSRIs), synthetic growth hormones such as EPO may all be used for other purposes than medical treatment in the 'strict' sense. Likewise, the doping problem within sports is the result of the desire for enhancement of human capacities, in order to improve physical performance.

One of the major arguments in the debate on human enhancement is that it will lead to homogenization. This is of course to be seen in the light of the history of eugenics. However, although one might think that a broad application of new technologies beyond treatment purposes could lead to one ideal type, the future will not necessarily be populated by a homogeneous mass. According to the proponents of enhancement technologies, we will not share the same appearance, talents or traits, as what is considered to be ideal and what not will appear to be as diverse in practice as it is in contemporary society (Buchanan et al., 2001). The diversity of conceptions of the good life gives rise to a broad diversity of life-styles, subcultures and human potential in our society. So why would this be any different in a future scenario with a broad application of enhancement technologies? The enhancement of human capacities does not necessarily have to result in Huxley's *Brave New World* as one would be inclined to think.

The debate on enhancement technologies has suffered from a rather one-dimensional view on what an enhancement is supposed to be. Many theorists are tempted by the idea to rank selectable traits in a linear way, presupposing a criterion for what should count as obligatory forms of treatment and prevention, what should count as less obligatory and supererogatory forms of prevention, and what should count as non-obligatory forms of treatment and prevention. Very often the criterion is sought in the goals of medicine, that is belonging to the 'normal' applications of medical technology, or falling outside of it.

But things are not so easy. In his article 'Normal Functioning and the Treatment-Enhancement Distinction' Norman Daniels begs the question whether one can make a clear-cut distinction between treatment of a child with growth hormone deficiency that is the result of a brain tumour and an enhancement of one's child's height because of a normal hereditary shortness (Daniels, 2000). Both children have the same height, but it is a height that is seen as inferior according to our cultural standards. However, in the first case, the problem has a medical cause, namely the tumour. In the second case, the child's (future) shortness is part of a normal variance in human height. The big question is, do the two cases fall within the area of medical necessity and if yes, do they qualify for medical treatment or not? This is not only an issue of reimbursement by an insurance company but also a general issue whether we should allow for an intervention in such a case at all.

According to some authors, the distinction between disease or disability and health or normality is culturally defined. Engelhardt, for example, argues that concepts of health and disease are guided by value judgements and prejudices that may change over time (Engelhardt, 1996). Examples are masturbation which was for a long time considered a disease, and homosexuality which was only recently removed from the *Manual of Psychiatric Disorders* (DSM). Efforts to limit access to certain technologies because they fall outside the prevailing definitions of disease can be considered to be biased and an inconsistent application of our values. This could imply that the distinction between normal and enhanced is basically normative rather than objective or universally valid. One can also argue that the distinction between treatment and enhancement is based on a culturally defined definition of what counts as a disease and what not. If one follows that argument, the distinction between therapy and enhancement will become highly questionable and nothing will stand in the way of the application of biotechnologies outside the medical domain.

ENHANCEMENT AND HUMAN NATURE

Apart from the reminder of the eugenic movement, enhancement is considered morally problematic by some because it is seen as a violation of the integrity of the human body and mind. They argue that the enhancement of human capacities is challenging the concept of human nature: for them the distinction between enhancement and therapy is essential. Therapy is considered natural and enhancement as unnatural; therapy is seen as a way to assist the natural healing process, whereas enhancement is adding something – possibly detrimental – to the human being that is considered as unnatural (President's Council on Bioethics, 2003). However, proponents of enhancement justify their arguments on the basis of the concept of nature as well: they claim that the desire and pursue of enhancement by the development of new technologies is part of human nature and must be considered as morally good. Because of his nature, man is enabled and even morally obliged to enhance his capacities.

In order to understand why some authors state that enhancement of human capacities is a violation of human integrity and others see it as a moral obligation, it is necessary to look in detail at the perceptions of human nature that underlie the debate. According to the proponents of the moral distinction between enhancement and therapy, the ethically suspect element of 'enhancement' lies within the idea of changing human nature through the addition of non-native skills or qualities:

> When a physician intervenes therapeutically to correct some deficiency or deviation from a patient's natural wholeness, he acts as a servant to the goal of health and as an assistant to nature's own powers of self-healing, themselves wondrous products of evolutionary selection. But when a bioengineer intervenes for nontherapeutic ends, he stands not as nature's servant but as aspiring master, guided by nothing but his own will and serving ends of his own devising (President's Council on Bioethics, 2003).

In this view, nature is seen as a process (i.e. the reference to self-healing and evolutionary selection) that constitutes the human being as well as the world as a whole. This approach is reminiscent of the Aristotelian definition of nature as a self-moving process. In his lecture on Physics, Aristotle explains nature as an ongoing process mastered by an intrinsic causality. In this approach, the human being is part of and dependent on cosmic natural processes and can only to a limited extent master his own physical nature.

However, in a different perspective on enhancement, some authors make use of a distinction between nature and human nature. They argue that, as opposed to other living beings, only human beings possess the potential to master their physical and cognitive capacities to an extent that goes beyond the element of natural chance. The idea of the human being as capable of mastering nature dates back to the Enlightenment and the Cartesian philosophical tradition. The ability to act according to free will is what distinguishes the human being from other living beings. At the same time it is exactly this ability that constitutes the moral dilemma, as free will makes it possible for human beings to act against the laws or processes of nature. But is intervening in the natural process for non-therapeutic ends morally wrong because of an intrinsic value of the natural process itself? Or is it rather the element of 'aspiring master' that causes ethical concern?

Enhancement can be interpreted both as part of human nature and as a potential violation of human nature. Some would claim that nature and natural process are fragile, and that any interference in them must be approached with precaution. The unknown long-term effects of the new enhancement technologies make our own desire for enhancement of human capacities a potential danger for present and future generations. Others would claim that the desire for enhancement of human capacities is to be pursued:

> In the end, this search for ways to enhance ourselves is a natural part of being human. The urge to transform ourselves has been force in history as far back as we can see. It's been selected for by millions of years of evolutions. It's wired deep in our genes – a natural outgrowth of our human intelligence, curiosity and drive. To turn our backs on this power would be to turn our back on our true nature (Naam, 2005).

A radical elaboration of this approach is represented in the idea of trans-humanism or post-humanity. Proponents of this line of thought claim that enhancement of existing human capacities will make us overcome our current vulnerability, and will result in a post-human state that is no longer dependent on our natural surroundings (Bostom, 2005). The possibility, for example, of uploading our brains like computers and growing new organs by using of human stem cells will eventually make us able to deal with human vulnerability to disease and damage. However, such radical alterations will change the core nature of *Homo sapiens* and turn us into post-humans.

The concept of nature and of human nature is often referred to as a moral anchor to evaluate the enhancement technologies. However, the complexity of the concept makes it clear that, when used as a normative benchmark, the concept of nature will not help to create consensus on the moral status of enhancement. Nonetheless, the concept cannot be dismissed entirely as invalid for the ethical evaluation of enhancement technologies. As both proponents as adversaries of human enhancement by way of biotechnologies make use of the concept of 'nature', the analysis of the concept, and of its use, in the ethical debate may help to better understand the lack of consensus within this debate.

ENHANCEMENT AND JUSTICE

The debate about the distinction between enhancement and therapy is not merely an academic one. This distinction is particularly important for policymaking on the funding by society for the access to these technologies. It is a deep understanding that as a society we have an obligation to help those persons who are in need of medical treatment. This obligation is based on our solidarity with the weaker groups in society and particularly with those persons who cannot help themselves. In medical ethics, this obligation is theoretically analysed by the concept of distributive justice. This concept says that there should be a reasonable distribution of the benefits and the burdens of medical treatments between the individuals in our society. Within this perspective we will find it hard to accept that societal resources are spent on technologies that are only fulfilling individual preferences, for example to lead a happier life or to enhance physical performance in sport, instead of fulfilling a need for medical treatment because of serious illness or disease.

Justice in health care is narrowly linked with the perspective of the goals of medicine and health care. For treatments to be funded, most health care systems in the world have as a condition that they should fall within the medical domain. This is a necessary, but not a sufficient condition: there are medical treatments, like advanced cancer drugs or transplantations, which may very well be considered as medical treatments, but they may be so expensive that society cannot afford to pay for these treatments for those who are in need. It is generally recognized that the goals of medicine, which characterizes the medical domain, include the preservation and restoration of health by the fight against disease. However, it is less clear how to define health and disease. The following concepts can be distinguished.

First of all there is the individual-oriented or liberal concept of health. According to this concept, health can be considered as the equilibrium between the goals an individual wants to realize on the one hand and the capacities to reach these goals on the other hand (Whitbeck, 1981). The individual-oriented concept of health puts the autonomous decisions of individuals at the basis of health and of what society should provide individuals in the area of health care. Within this perspective the societal funding of access to enhancement technologies will be justified when these technologies enable individuals to reach their own goals. For example, when a person wants to be an Olympic gold medal winner in the Marathon, he or she could claim genetic therapeutic interventions to enable him or her to reach this goal.

The individual-oriented concept of health has been criticized because of the lack of criteria regarding the reasonableness of the goals individuals set for themselves. When individuals set unreasonable or unreal goals for themselves, for example, winning an Olympic gold medal, they will be considered ill when they are not able to reach them. The individual concept could in fact lead to a huge number of claims on the health care system, including access to enhancement technologies, as every claim has an equal value compared to other claims. It will not only be very difficult to make decisions between the access to various services and priority-setting, but also between what counts as therapy and what as enhancement on the basis of individual preferences and life-style. In other words, a distinction between individual needs and wants will be difficult to make.

Communitarian philosophers like Daniel Callahan have criticized this approach as individualistic and not in the interest of society as a community of individuals. According to Callahan, health should be understood as a common benefit, something we need for our life together, not just one by one (Callahan, 1990). Health and health care should be related to the functioning in society and to the well-being of society and of the individuals living in that society. The communitarian perspective advocates the society-oriented approach to health: health care should contribute to the functioning of individuals in society and to strengthen the bonds between individuals. Funding of health care services should be directed at enabling individuals to function again in society in case of disease or handicap. One could argue then that in a communitarian perspective, society would have an obligation to fund enhancement technologies if they contribute to an improved functioning of individuals in society.

The third approach is the biological one which tries to base heath and disease on the biological functioning of individuals. The best known example is the bio-statistical theory of Christopher Boorse (1977). According to Boorse health should be defined in terms of the biological functioning that is typical functions for individuals of a certain species. Typical functions are that contribute to the goals of the organism, and these goals can be conducted from the 'natural design' of that organism. On the basis of empirical investigation, Boorse argues that the main biological functions are survival and procreation. Health means 'normal functional ability', that is functioning according to the 'natural design' of the species. Disease is then any state that interferes with this normal functioning. This means that Boorse's account of the concepts of health and disease is heavily dependent on an objective image of 'nature', 'natural' or 'normal functioning'.

Boorse's biostatistical design has met with much criticism because it rules out many conditions, like mental or physical handicaps, that have nothing to do with 'normal species functioning'. Amongst others, Engelhardt criticizes this naturalist approach to the conceptualization of diseases. According to him, one cannot analyse concepts of health and disease solely on the basis of the biological nature of the organism and its functioning, as one also needs to take its context into account. In this normative approach, diseases are seen as contextual (Engelhardt, 1996). They are normative constructions with a specific socio-cultural background, rather than a natural given within a bio statistical framework.

In spite of these criticisms, the philosopher Norman Daniels took Boorse's concept of normal functioning as one of the basic elements for his approach to justice in health care (Daniels, 1985). According to Daniels, normal functioning is a condition to have access to the range of opportunities that are open to individuals in society according to their abilities. Disease hinders normal functioning; this is the reason why there is a moral obligation on society to restore individuals with disease to normal functioning. According to Daniels, protecting normal functioning contributes

to protecting normal opportunities. By keeping close to normal functioning, health care preserves people's ability to participate in political, social and economic life. On the basis of Daniels' concept of justice in health care (which is based on Rawls' *Theory of Justice*), Buchanan et al. argue that there is no moral obligation on society to fund enhancement technologies as they are not focused on the restoration of 'normal functioning'. In their view, the distinction between enhancement and therapy is relevant as the basis for decision-making about the kind of medical and biotechnical services that should be supplied by society (Buchanan et al., 2001).

This view is challenged by some authors who argue that in Daniels' view there will still exist differences among individuals in their possession of capabilities in society, which might hinder some of them from reaching good positions in society. For example, intelligence and a good memory might be essential for success in the competition for social positions. The application of enhancement technologies might result in a more even distribution of these capabilities among individuals which would be more just from an egalitarian point of view. There are two theories defending this position. The first is called 'resource egalitarianism' and is advocated by Amartya Sen. This theory says that if resources ought to be distributed equally and natural resources are resources, then we ought to intervene in the natural lottery whenever doing so would be the best way of equalizing resources (Sen, 1990). The second theory is called the 'brute luck theory' and is advocated by Thomas Scanlon. This theory holds that persons should not have fewer opportunities as a result of factors that are beyond their control. These circumstances do not only include the effects of the social lottery, like poverty or ethnic discrimination, but also the consequences of the natural lottery like genetic differences (Scanlon, 1989).

Both 'resource egalitarianism' and 'brute luck theory' are committed to the thesis that justice may require interventions to counteract natural inequalities by means of biotechnological interventions, whether they constitute diseases or not. In fact, they advocate that there is an obligation within our society to supply enhancement technologies, not just treatments, whenever a natural inequality can be prevented by enhancement. In this view, the distinction between enhancement and therapy is disappearing. Buchanan et al. argue that, certainly in a market-oriented society, it can be expected that genetic technologies and other biotechnologies will be used by the rich and powerful beyond the medical domain, in order to enhance their capacities and opportunities in social life. They recognize that from the viewpoint of justice regulations may well be in place in order to prevent a widening gap between the better-off and the worse-off in respect with social opportunities. However, that is no reason to equalize the differences in capacities by funding access to enhancement technologies for all members of our society. Such a policy would seriously affect the possibility of competition in our society and of the principle of liberty which is a major principle in Rawls' *Theory of Justice*:

> Just as we do not owe it to our friends or others in general to contribute our resources to make them feel happy when they are unhappy because they have developed extravagant tastes, we do not owe it to others to improve any and every capability that they judge to be disadvantageous to them, given their plans of life (Buchanan et al., 2001).

Although radical egalitarianism does not see a difference between enhancement and therapy, as they both affect the chances of individuals in society, the mitigated liberalism of Daniels and others sticks to this divide as it would seriously affect liberty in our society. However, they do advocate access to biotechnologies where they restore normal functioning. Access to technologies for the purpose of enhancement of capabilities falls outside the domain of health care and should be regulated within the broader social context.

ENHANCEMENT AND AUTHENTICITY

In his book *Better than Well* Carl Elliott tries to find an answer to why enhancement technologies have become so popular in contemporary society (Elliott, 2003). According to Elliott, the answer can be found in the ideal of authenticity which has become so dominant in our society. Elliott refers to the work of Charles Taylor, who tried to uncover the roots of this ideal in the history of western culture (Taylor, 1991). According to Taylor, this ideal meant that to reach an understanding of our moral directions and obligations we should have contact with our feelings. This ideal was first put forward by Romantic philosophy in the early eighteenth century. Particularly important is the work of the German philosopher Herder, who put forward the idea that every person has an original way of being human and that this difference has an important moral significance. Taylor summarizes this view as follows: 'There is a certain way of being human and that is my way. I am called to live my life in this way, and not in imitation of anyone else's. But this gives a new importance to being true to myself. If I am not, I miss the point of my life, I miss what is being human for me' (Taylor, 1991). Authenticity has become a powerful ideal in our culture; it means that we have to get in contact with ourselves, with our own inner nature, our inner voice, particularly when it is threatened to become lost because of the pressure of external conformity. It is strongly linked to the idea of originality; each voice has something of its own to say. External sources of moral conduct are not important: I can only find these directions within myself.

According to Elliott, it is the ideal of authenticity that drives the language of people using biotechnologies and other technologies to enhance their functioning. From Prozac to face-lifts, using these technologies or drugs make people feel more authentic, more 'being themselves' (Elliott, 2003). He gives the example of Jan Morris, who made herself transform from a man into a woman. She felt after the sex-reassignment surgery that she had found her true self and that her life became fulfilled by the procedure. She was very happy because of this, and 'fulfilment requires being true to that inner voice' (Elliott, 2003). Another example mentioned by Elliott is persons who had their limbs amputated at their own request: 'I have always felt I should be an amputee. It is a desire to see myself, be myself, as I "know", or "feel" myself to be' (Elliott, 2003).

A critique of the preoccupation with the self is voiced by communitarian philosophers who argue that the self can only realize itself in the community with others. In contemporary culture, the search for the self has resulted in narcissism and estrangement from others, a process that is reinforced by the use of enhancement technologies. In its discussion of the role of Prozac and other SSRIs in mood enhancing and mood elevation, the President's Commission states that by the availability of mood-enhancing drugs individuals become so preoccupied with their state of mind 'that they remove themselves increasingly from active participation in civic life, discarding those attachments without which they cannot achieve the happiness they seek and without which the community cannot survive and flourish' (President's Council on Bioethics, 2003). The first danger of a widespread use of mood enhancing drugs, according to the Commission, involves the 'solipsistic self worried only about the state of his feelings, who uses psychopharmacology to ensure a flat and shallow self regarding psychic pleasure'.

Taylor agrees that the ideal of authenticity in its modern variant has indeed transformed into an inward-looking, solipsistic kind of individuality. According to Taylor this decline into solipsism must be seen as a deviation from and as a wrong interpretation of the original idea of authenticity. Originally, the change to authenticity was considered a more subtle and personal way of connecting to a larger whole, be it society or nature or the cosmos. It was a new way or manner of relating to the social and (supra-) natural world. This meaning of authenticity has gradually been hidden and forgotten, in favour of an obsession with the manner itself (instead of the goal). Real authenticity is reached only by a relation to a world outside of us, or, in Taylor's words, a horizon of meaning that exists independent of us.

It is not said that enhancement technologies cannot enable individuals to reach such a richer way of relating to the outside world. The President's Council on Bioethics might be too pessimistic about the way enhancement reduces social and civic life. In his contribution to *Prozac as a Way of Life*, Tod Chambers gives examples of how spiritual lives have been changed by the impact of Prozac. After taking Prozac, one devout Christian felt 'like living again. And I began to experience God like I never had before' (Chambers, 2004). In his book *Listening to Prozac*, Peter Kramer gives examples of how patients by using Prozac felt more able to cope with ordinary life, overcoming shyness and social inhibition (Kramer, 1993).

Enhancement technologies do not necessarily create solipsistic, selfish individuals, searching for their own selves. If there is a tendency of individuals to use enhancement technologies for this purpose, it is not the technology that is to blame, but the social and cultural process that is driving individuals into this sort of behaviour. Enhancement can very well be applied to 'open up' individuals to play an active life in the community and to search for meaning by relating to moral and spiritual sources.

CONCLUSION

Biotechnologies and other technologies are increasingly invading our life as tools to enhance our capacities in mood, cognition and physical performance. Although the use of enhancement technologies is often seen as matter of free choice and personal life-style, there are important ethical questions that go beyond this individual perspective. In this chapter, some of these issues are dealt with like the access to the enhancement technologies, their impact on the position of the handicapped individuals, their influence on our conceptions of human nature as well as the impact they might have on our way of life and our self-image as modern individuals. For this reason, the introduction of enhancement should not be left to the free forces of our society but should be guided by ethical debate. An important issue in this debate should be the distinction between enhancement and therapy and the possible role this distinction should play in public policymaking on the acceptance and accessibility of the enhancement technologies.

REFERENCES

Boorse C Health as a theoretical concept. *Philos Sci* 1977; **44**; 542–573.

Bostrom N. A history of transhumanist thought. *J Evol Technol* 2005; **14**(1); 1–27.

Buchanan A, Brock D, Daniels N, Wikler D. *From Chance to Choice. Genetics and Justice*. 4th edition. Cambridge: Cambridge University Press, 2001.

Callahan D. *What Kind of Life. The Limits of Medical Progress*, New York: Simon and Schuster, 1990.

Chambers T. Prozac for the sick soul. In: Elliott C, Chambers T. eds. *Prozac as a Way of Life*. Chapel Hill, NC: University of North Carolina Press, 2004; p. 199.

Daniels N. *Just Health Care*. Cambridge: Cambridge University Press, 1985.

Daniels N. Normal functioning and the treatment-enhancement distinction. *Camb Health Ethics Q* 2000; **9**; 309–322.

Elliott C. *Better than Well. American Medicine Meets the American Dream*. New York: W.W. Norton, 2003.

Engelhardt HT. *The Foundations of Bioethics*. 2nd edition. Oxford: Oxford University Press, 1996.

Kramer P. *Listening to Prozac*. New York: Viking, 1993.

Naam R. *More Than Human – Embracing the Promise of Biological Enhancement*, Broadway Books, 2005.

President's Council on Bioethics. *Beyond Therapy – Biotechnology and the Pursuit of Happiness, a Report of the President's Council on Bioethics*, Washington, DC: US Government Office, 2003 www.bioethics.gov.

Scanlon T. A good start: reply to Roemer. *Boston Rev* 1989; **20**(2); 8–9.

Sen A. Justice: means versus freedoms. *Philos Publ Aff* 1990; **19**; 111–121.

Taylor C. *The Ethics of Authenticity*. Cambridge MA: Harvard University Press, 1991.

Whitbeck CA. Theory of health. In: Caplan AL, Engelhardt HT, McCartney JJ eds. *Concepts of Health and Disease. Interdisciplinary Perspectives*. London: Addison-Wesley Publishing Company, 1981; pp. 57–81.

Psychosurgery and Neuroimplantation: Changing What is Deep Within a Person

GRANT GILLETT

Psychosurgery and neuroimplantation are two overlapping sets of procedures both aimed at 'the source of our pleasure, merriment, laughter and amusement, as of our grief, pain, anxiety and tears' (Hippocrates, 1978). Some of the techniques involved have demonstrable and relatively objective results but some do not; some have well-established indications and measures of success but others are controversial; all share the excitement of the new and appeal to both theorists and therapists. Such is the current interest in the interconnections between neuroscience and ethics that the term 'neuroethics' has been coined to cover the innovative academic (and not-so-academic) writing in this area (Journal of Medical Ethics).

The ethical aspects of interventions in the stuff of mind are best considered against a philosophical understanding of the mind or soul in relation to the brain. I will explore an Aristotelian understanding of that relation (1986) because it renders the mind/brain relation comprehensible and accessible to detailed discussion. It therefore allows a perceptive purview of the implications of mind/brain for psychosurgery, neural repair and neural enhancement with cybernetic technology in relation to issues of both well-being and identity.

ARISTOTLE ON THE SOUL

The Aristotelian soul is part of a holistic conception of human beings in which both matter and subjectivity are important (as it is for thinkers from St Thomas Aquinas to present day naturalistic philosophers). A helpful analogy is the form of a statue – say a statue of Diana – that exists as such in virtue of a particular configuration of a piece of bronze. The same bronze, recast into a statue of Apollo, becomes a different thing with a distinctive nature, properties and significance. The form of a living human being is, however, not just an inanimate shape but also a holistic, subjective and embodied reality underpinning all our thinking in biomedical ethics (Gillett, 2004, pp. 6–7).

Aristotle's view conceives of human beings as social animals who exhibit reason and reflection (Aristotle, 1925; Barnes, 1982): 'if the eye was an animal, then sight would be its soul' (Aristotle, 1986 p. 158). The human soul 'is defined by ... the nutritive, perceptive, and intellective faculties and movement' (Aristotle, 1986 p. 160) of an integrated being. Our human reason and social function (or relatedness) result in an identity which evolves over time, a stream of conscious experience, and a moral standing as a socially situated agent whose life-story is lived among other human beings. A formative part of this life-story relates to caregivers in the context of intense interpersonal activity in which we are loved by and learn to love other people. The human soul, we might say, comprises an emergent set of functions reflecting the interrelatedness of reason, emotion and action in human life. Thus (after Wittgenstein, Bruner, Harre and others) an exclusive focus on 'intellective' functions in human nature overlooks the complexity of our function as members of a collective group bound to each other in familial and cultural ways.

Our brains, as the Hippocratics noted, relate us to a natural and human environment and also to formative cultural symbols and myths so that the tools of cognitive adaptation are holistically informed by the interaction with the world and others. For this reason the relatively rich term 'soul' is preferable to the term 'mind' in discussing the human psyche as it engages with psychiatry and human dysfunction (Gillett, 1999).

Principles of Health Care Ethics, Second Edition   Edited by R.E. Ashcroft, A. Dawson, H. Draper and J.R. McMillan
© 2007 John Wiley & Sons, Ltd

Two conclusions follow:

(1) We are beings-in-relation-to-others; and
(2) We are beings who are constantly remoulding ourselves.

Over time a human being develops life skills through training in a highly articulated relational milieu that is discursively productive.

Our discursive system structures both our cognitive skills and our moral framework. The resulting 'mental map' is, in an important way, *holistic* so that our knowledge is suffused by knowledge of the significance or worth of things for critters like me. Wittgenstein, after he had crystallized semantics into an austere philosophical form in the *Tractatus Logico-Philosophicus*, discarded the mathematically perfect picture of the mind, the world and the relation between them in that work and turned his attention to our shared activity and the language that informs it as the *fons et origo* of our understanding of the world and ourselves (Wittgenstein, 1953). These thoughts are crucial in understanding the special ethical challenges of psychosurgery and neuro-modification.

The present view is that the soul arises during an individual's life as a subjective body among others and is not a composite of an inner ghostly substance called a mind and an outer physical substance called a body or brain. It can be summarized as follows:

1. The soul is the expression of patterns of activity laid down in the brain.
2. The brain records significant patterns of information arising in human life.
3. These patterns reflect both the regularities of nature and social and cultural reality.
4. A study of human discourse replete with the relationships in which it occurs is needed to understand the human soul which is a holistic configuration of cognitive, conative, relational and cultural functions unique to a given person and crucially dependent on brain function for their integrity.

When we bend our minds onto psychosurgery and neuroimplantation, we take from this framework the thought that ethical thinking concerns the needs, vulnerabilities and interests of holistic creatures like us so that they become proper subjects of 'reactive attitudes' (Strawson, 1974).

PSYCHOSURGERY

Psychosurgery uses neurosurgical techniques to try to alleviate psychiatric disorders (Manshour, 2005). It has a controversial history, punctuated by the debates to the fore

in works such as *One Flew over the Cuckoo's Nest* and *Fire and Rain*.

In 1848, Phineas Gage, a railroad gang foreman described as 'the most efficient and capable' man, was supervising the blasting of some rock, when a tamping iron sparked off the blasting powder he was using and blasted into his brain, damaging the prefrontal areas of both hemispheres. He was so radically transformed that a medical commentator described him as

> fitful, irreverent, indulging at times in the grossest profanity which was not previously his custom, manifesting but little deference for his fellows, impatient of restraint or advice when it conflicts with his desires, at times pertinaciously obstinate, yet capricious and vacillating, devising many plans of future operation, which are no sooner arranged than they are abandoned (Damasio, 1994, p. 28).

Gage remained a medical curiosity, graphically illustrating the serious effects of damage to the so-called 'silent' areas of the brain – now associated with executive intelligence and the integration of social and personality function.

The frontal lobes were considered 'silent' because bedside neurological examination and cognitive capacities measured by standard psychological tests did not adequately probe the complex and integrated activity required in everyday intelligent function. Gage's injury 'compromised his ability to plan for the future, to conduct himself according to the social rules he previously had learned and to decide on the course of action that would be most advantageous to his survival' (Damasio, 1994, p. 33); he was, in a word, 'not the same Gage' (a severe blow for a railway foreman).

Phineas Gage should have sounded warning bells for Egas Moniz and Almeida Lima (in Lisbon) who, following nineteenth-century work by Burkhardt, began operating to divide frontal lobe connections in psychiatric patients. Initial reports of success in patients regarded as hopeless led to the widespread adoption of their technique. Between 1936 and 1978, in the United States alone, some 35,000 patients had frontal leucotomy. Moniz received a Nobel Prize (partly for his work on cerebral angiography) but, even as scientific accolades resounded in the medical world, ethical concerns were raised.

First, there are problems about the rationale, indications and efficacy of the surgery. In fact, the very idea that a destructive brain lesion would unravel a significant 'Gordian knot' in the psyche seems naive. Janet Frame's (1961) critique is eloquent.

> After her operation Louise became more docile, less inclined to fly into a rage if people refused to hear her 'story'; she wet her pants and giggled delightedly, and yet began to take a pride in her appearance, but one is not sure how far that was the result of the operation or of the changed attitude towards her. She was given every attention and plied with curious morbid

questions by the nurses who shuddered when they looked at her and at the others with their bald heads and said, amongst themselves, 'I'm glad it's not me. It gives you the creeps'.

Louise improved. The doctor came to see her twice in 1 week! And then, as she stayed day after day in Lawn Lodge, and the novelty of the operation wore off, and the doctor had no more time to see her twice a week, although still docile, she grew more careless about her appearance, she did not mind wetting her pants, and the nurses, feeling cheated, as people do when change refuses to adopt the dramatic forms expected of it, at the sight of the 'old' Louise still settled comfortably under the 'new', gave up trying to reeducate her, and very soon she was again just one of the hopping, screaming people in the dayroom (Frame, 1961, p. 111).

Frame noticed multiply interactive influences on Louise's psychology demanding balanced assessment rather than acceptance of the therapeutic intervention as a success. In many cases it was impossible to say what a lobotomy achieved and the procedure has undergone continuous changes in indication, method and even site of operation since its beginnings explaining the 'collective uncertainty which should not be eliminated from judgments of psychosurgical efficacy' (Kleinig, 1985, p. 110).

A further problem concerns the 'old unacceptable personalities' (Frame, 1961, p. 111), and is seen in Phineas Gage. Gage survived his horrendous accident but *as whom* did he survive? Is the personality of the patient modified or destroyed? The popular image is that lobotomy makes people into 'zombies' exhibiting 'Inertia, unresponsiveness, decreased attention span, blunted or inappropriate affect and disinhibition' (Mashour et al., 2005, p. 412). These cognitive and psychic injuries and the alteration of self by lobotomy have led to continuing attempts to refine or limit the procedure but we should question whether we should allow this to happen at all.

During the lobotomy years, psychologists and neurologists were trying to understand the limbic system, its connections and its role in behaviour and personality, work which led to the development of a series of more targeted procedures such as anterior cingulotomy (for obsessive compulsive disorder—OCD) (Bear, 1995); subcaudate tractotomy' for depression and OCD (Hodgkiss, 1995); limbic leucotomy and stereotactic lesions including amygdalotomy (Korzenev, 1995). Recent refinements include stereotactic radiosurgical procedures such as cingulotomy and amygdalotomy to minimize the side effects of the procedures while preserving their beneficial effects, in so far as these can be measured in refractory psychiatric conditions (Kim, 2002).

The overall ethical justification for continuing use of psychosurgery is that we may lack any other effective therapy in some serious psychiatric conditions and yet recognize the therapeutic imperative to do something, and there is some evidence of efficacy for such procedures. Given that the indications are agreed by suitable health care professionals and those properly consulted over the decision (patient, family, counsellors and so on), it seems that psychosurgery might still represent a beacon of hope for some patients with debilitating problems (such as severe OCD).

Despite its refinements and the mitigation of its worst features, psychosurgery remains somewhat experimental in terms of its theoretical underpinning and actual results so that '[w]here the existing evaluative data is deficient, it is important that patients be made aware of the experimental character of the therapy which is being ... recommended to them' (Kleinig, 1985, p. 111). Many surgical treatments have experimental aspects, but in the case of psychosurgery there is great potential to damage the 'substrate of the soul'. What is more, the indications for surgery may be based on the way the person interacts with others and therefore be partly for the sake of others as in the case of intractable aggression by cognitively impaired patients, overactive or self-damaging children and violent offenders (Merskey, 1999, p. 285). Psychosurgery therefore raises serious questions about the criteria for benefit, the risks of therapy, and the adequacy with which we can obtain consent for what is planned. Those problems have made it almost impossible to have major psychosurgery performed in many countries.

Even if psychosurgery offers relief from a debilitating psychiatric condition, the deeper worry is that we are not curing a disorder but rather transforming a person into someone who is more acceptable to the rest of us (Pressman, 1998, p. 10). Gosta Rylander, a Swedish psychiatrist, commented in 1947 that some of his lobotomy patient's families had said things like 'she is my daughter but yet a different person'; 'She is with me in body but her soul is in some way lost'; or 'his soul appears to be destroyed' (Pressman, 1998, p. 328). The issue of 'old unacceptable personalities' and questions of identity, spirit, relationship, integrity and human flourishing not only bedevil the ethics of destructive psychosurgery but also arise in patients surviving moderately severe head injuries causing profound changes in character, temperament and cognitive ability, and can be deeply disturbing for those who care about them.

I have prefaced my remarks with a holistic view of the human soul because psychosurgery affects the substrate of the person's soul. The issue of consent to such a procedure is made vivid if we compare the choice to that of spinal patients asked about life-saving measures after their life-changing injury. The patients might make a powerful plea that even if they will survive and learn to make the best of their life as a survivor, they do not want to be that kind of person. The analogy is close because the person may seem so different after psychosurgery that we do think in terms of a discontinuity of identity and we are potentially altering the mind or soul in a way that may be irreversible. The problematic nature of this decision explains the demanding ethical requirements for these interventions, (Veatch 1995; 1996) in terms of both 'objective good' and the subjective wishes of the patient such that the procedure can go ahead only when the two seem clearly to be aligned.

I have noted, however, that the relevant assessment is affected by the evaluative and observer-dependent nature of the judgements involved. The 'Stepford husbands' believed their wives were happier after their treatment and their wives seemed to agree but, as the story unfolds, that judgement is radically problematized. It is not as if these questions are unique to psychosurgery, in fact they can be raised about ECT, psychotropic medication in general (particularly with cognitively marginal patients in institutional settings) and even behavioural management (think of *The Clockwork Orange*). In each case we wonder about our entitlement to alter a person so as to make them more 'normal' according to well-developed cultural stereotypes. I will return to these issues of identity in the context of cybernetic enhancement.

It is true that far more circumscribed and directed interventions constitute the modern face of psychosurgery and that it is carefully monitored and surrounded by patient safeguards, but it is important to note that we are still embroiled in the intense debates between biological and social-humanistic schools in psychiatry that polarized the profession and its research and treatment paradigms in the 1950s and 1960s (Gillett, 1999).

Having explored the destructive 'surgeries of the soul', we can now turn to the equally but distinctively problematic reparative interventions.

NEUROIMPLANTATION

Neuroimplantation makes use either of cellular grafting techniques (which may use stem cells) and/or of increasingly sophisticated artificial technology to compensate for defects such as blindness, strokes and degenerative diseases.

There is ongoing experimental work on the use of foetal tissue grafts in patients who have a variety of neural disorders such as Parkinson's disease, Alzheimer's disease and spinal injury (Macklin, 1999). The ethics of foetal tissue transplants is, however, confounded by debates about the status of the human embryo or foetus (Jones, 1991).

The embryo or foetus has the potential to become a fully functioning human being, and some ethicists argue that destroying an embryo is equivalent to killing a human being (Holland, 1990). If foetal tissue transplants are inseparable, ethically, from the foetal sacrifice providing the brain tissue then this stance seems justified, but the link between the two is arguable. If, for instance, one were offered kidneys from a murder victim or a young woman killed by a drunken driver, we would not argue that the transplant doctor colluded with either death. Therefore, only if the foetal tissue transplant and the abortion are morally inseparable as, for instance, if a couple were to conceive a child merely to provide tissue for transplantation into the brain of their favourite uncle, could the one be ethically linked to the other. In such a case one may want to say that there has been a cynical creation and sacrifice of a young human life to allow the cannibalization of the brain for spare parts. That observation would not close the issue but at least would usher that debate onto the stage. Creation for sacrifice is not the case in most centres where such work is done so that the link cannot be made.

Some would argue that (*de facto*) a clear separation between an abortion decision and the transplant decision it makes possible does not excuse us from entering the debates about the moral status of the embryo. Even if we would not have to create embryos especially to do stem cell research so that debates about the creation of human beings merely for the purposes of medical science (cf. the couple with their to-be-aborted foetus) are not to the point, the stem cells used in a procedure may, in fact, be obtained from embryos (perhaps 'spare' embryos from centres providing Assisted Human Reproduction programmes) rather than from adults or children. Some ethicists would go further, arguing that because the cells being used, even if not from embryos, may be indistinguishable from human organisms at certain stages of embryonic development, they are equivalent to embryos. We can, however, resist this view.

Our diverse moral intuitions about embryos are best understood if we adopt the view that an embryo should be seen in the context of human growth and development (Copland, 2003). In general, the way we think of a thing depends on our general knowledge about the world. Now, imagine that I have a ticket to the Boxing Day cricket test and my wife uses it to start the fire. Fleeing for her life, she remarks, 'But what are you so upset about, it was only a bit of paper?' In one sense, she is right – my ticket is just a piece of paper – but it has a value 'not dreamed of in her philosophy'. Similar points are relevant in the case of the embryo.

The human embryo develops from a scrap of tissue into a living, loving and loved child. Thus, like a painting, it takes shape gradually, its value increasing as it develops. But if a painting is destroyed after only a few brushstrokes on the canvas, it is a lesser thing than destroying it when it is complete. Analogously we might opt for the gradualist position whereby a human organism accrues value as it forms so that the embryo is precious but not in the same way as a child or adult who is truly one of us.

This line of ethical reasoning is compatible with the idea that embryos do not change into human beings but are human beings from their conception. We recognize increasingly, especially in an age of assisted reproductive technologies, that a given embryo or pre-embryo may not follow that path. Therefore, we should ensure that in our treatment of embryos and foetuses we neither lose sight of the inherent value attached to a human life from its beginning nor overinflate it. Arguably it is as respectful to use embryos to provide tissue for healing as it is to dispose of them when it is clear that they will not be implanted and develop into human beings among us.

The argument that we should accept technologies involving stem cells is strengthened when the process begins with adult human tissue, even if it does involve something like an embryo, because that entity is specifically created as part of the stem cell repair process and, therefore, does not have a normal developmental trajectory. There is not, we could say, any embryo being killed that would otherwise live to become a child, so the embryo debate is irrelevant. But the other ethical issues remain pressing.

NEURAL REPAIR AND CLINICAL ETHICS

Stem cells offer hope that we can not only repair but also regenerate damaged and impaired bodily tissues to restore adequate function. This idea is especially exciting for clinicians dealing with diseases where the lost tissues and their functions seem irreplaceable and the resulting disabilities are major (as in neural implantation). But a number of other ethical problems must be solved by those interested in neural repair.

Stem cell technology is closely related to genetic engineering and, in fact, often contributes to genetic research. There are, however, distinct questions associated with genetic transfer which are not inherently part of the ethics of stem cell neural repair even though these debates are important, ongoing and concern ethical problems such as the enhancement of human beings and the creation of a society in which genetic determinism influences our attitudes to human beings. I will not discuss those issues.

Some ethicists argue that experimental procedures aimed at repair and restoration of function should be done given that they may help the recipients. Others argue that these are major experimental operations on a vulnerable and often desperate group of patients with no proven results to support their use. Assessing this argument is difficult because of the well-known problems in the early evaluation of a new medical technique, (Jennett, 1986, p. 244) and a kind of 'scientific pragmatism' tends to win the day (Jones, 1991). But even if neural tissue grafting is going to help a large number of patients, the early results are likely to be mixed or even disappointing. Thus the arguments based on 'scientific pragmatism' are likely to be quite inconclusive in ways that affect stem cell repair and neuroimplantation in general.

A CLUSTER OF CLINICAL ETHICAL PROBLEMS IN NEURAL REPAIR

THE SELECTION OF PATIENTS

This is doubly problematic: first any intervention carries a risk of making the patient worse; and second, those with complete loss of function probably have the least chance of success. Unfortunately the more intact the patient is, the more they have to lose if neuroimplantation causes damage, but if we work solely with patients who have profound lesions then we may not realize that we have made small but important steps toward the techniques and combinations of interventions that offer the maximal chance of viable repair by seeing marginal improvements of function.

THE PLACEBO EFFECT

The placebo effect is greatest when the gains from treatment are subjective as is the case with some of the gains in function expected from foetal tissue transplantation (increased facility of movement or proprioception). Therefore, the ethical issue of subjecting patients to sham neuroimplantation has to be faced. The justification of sham surgery depends on safety, the need to distinguish between genuine and placebo outcomes, and the openness of disclosure to patients (they should know that randomization to the control arm dictates that they may have a sham procedure).

THERAPEUTIC PRESSURE

Clinicians are constantly being pressured, both by patients and by commercial ventures interested in medical innovation, to do new procedures as soon as they look promising. Many desperate patients volunteer for high-risk, low-benefit surgery in the hope of improvement and there are rich pickings available from patents and devices spawned by new techniques. On the face of these pressures, it is hard for clinicians doing this work to maintain their standards of clinical judgment and ethical practice.

LONG-TERM COMPLICATIONS

Animal studies increasingly show that neural repair is 'a long haul' and that we may need to wait months or years before an intervention produces clear benefits to the patient. However, waiting so as to carefully assess the results of interventions is difficult, and some of the potential complications (e.g. from neural tumours) are delayed in their manifestation. Thus the first tentative steps with a new technology such as stem cell repair are taken under a cloud of risks and uncertainties. These clinical ethical concerns tend to support a cautious policy with neuroimplantation using stem cells even when the sourcing issues have been resolved.

We must now consider the neural interventions which radically affect our conception of human identity and the moral community of which we are a part.

CYBORGS

Neuroscience and intelligent technology now, as never before, pose the problem of cyborgs – part-human and part-machine complexes functioning as integrated wholes. In fact the insertion of a shunt for hydrocephalus is an example of the creation of such a hybrid. But developments integrating intelligent components into human neural function raise the debate to a new level, posing questions about what is a person and how we should regard beings who are part artefacts in ways that possibly affect the nature and functioning of their soul or psyche.

Supplementing our cognitive abilities by using artificial devices such as diaries, cell phones, tape recorders and so on is a common feature of human life. However, when we extend this technology inwards we quickly encounter neuro-ethical versions of the paradox of the heap. Such paradoxes (Sorites paradoxes) focus on a category based on a quantifiable attribute – such as baldness. We notice that a bald man does not become hirsute (or not bald) if he has *only one* hair on his head. But what goes for *one* can go for *one plus one* and so on, until we have a man with, say, 10,000 hairs (or whatever it takes so that he is no longer bald). We then realize that it looks as if at some point a bald man becomes not bald by merely adding one more hair to his head. We must therefore ask, 'When does a human being become a robot or vice versa by adding just one more artificial (neuro-cognitive) function?'

This type of problem affects all our thinking about complex objects; for instance, I might have had my grandfather's axe for 30 years, having fitted it with five new handles and three new heads. You may ask, 'So why is this not a new axe?' The problem is 'What change in an object results in a metaphysical difference so we now have a different object (or kind of object) from the one with which we started?' I am the person whom people regard as me when I use my diary or computer, I am myself when I take my antidepressant medication, but what if I incorporate cybernetic technology to enhance my thought and personality and how much techno-replacement is too much? Would I still be myself

if my thinking resulted in part from a device simulating a young male adult psyche perhaps upgradable like a games system as fashion changes?

Our intuitions here resonate with the initial remarks on the soul; they reflect an informal evaluation of the myriad cues manifest in our forms of life. These cues and clues arise in our dealings with each other as members of human society (even though we can be fooled). Our moral reactions to cyborgs are, therefore, not a product of disengaged metaphysical speculations but of engaged and holistic discourse in which our ways of knowing the moral sphere and its inhabitants are themselves moral (or ethical). For this reason we extend the benefits of existing relationships to each other even where we are changed (as in psychosurgery or severe brain damage) and even though the changes may create nasty strains on those relationships. In near-human cases, we hope we will not slip too easily into judgement mode but rather explore the path of acceptance and a charitable deployment of our reactive attitudes. In a cybernetic age, we may find that we are living at a frontier where all things are matters of degree; but the human mind constantly negotiates that kind of moral terrain, a feat requiring both humanity and phronesis.

THE SCHISM – BIOLOGY AND THE PSYCHE

The technologies of the psyche are deeply problematic in that they straddle a deep-seated ideological divide. I have argued that the human psyche is not comprehensible in the language of physical objects, causality and objective consequences and is unavoidable because it is at the heart of ethics. Worries about what we are doing to the human psyche occur in both psychosurgery and neuroimplantation, and in both we flirt with reductive attitudes to human beings. Wittgenstein remarks, 'The way in which some reality corresponds – or conflicts – with a physical theory has no counterpart here' (Wittgenstein, 1965, p. 24) and warns us against expecting too much precision in our deliberations: 'It is a great temptation to try and make the spirit explicit' (Wittgenstein, 1980, p. 8). I have espoused a neo-Aristotelian position whereby the individual elaborates a psyche in the complex relationships and encounters of ordinary human life. On that basis we extend to those altered by brain injury or psychiatric disorder or who are complexes, part-human and part-artefact, a morally informed set of attitudes embodying reason and sympathetic reflection. The Hippocratic imperative to learn about human illness and develop our healing techniques means we cannot turn our back on the challenges and opportunities of these new technologies, but addressing them requires philosophical work on ourselves and our way of seeing things, (Wittgenstein, 1980, p. 16) and also on our profession and our relationships with patients, industry and each other. We would do well, given the nature of the soul and its vulnerability to the contingencies of embodiment, to heed the warning: 'Don't play with what lies deep in another person!' (Wittgenstein, 1980, p. 23).

REFERENCES

Aristotle, *Nicomachean Ethics* (Translated by Ross D). Oxford: Oxford University Press, 1925; 1097b, 9–11; 1098a, 1–15.

Aristotle. *De Anima* (Translated by Hugh Lawson-Tancred). London: Penguin Books, 1986.

Baer L, Rauch SL, Ballantine HT, Martuza R, Cosgrove R, Cassem E Girinius I, Manzo PA, Dimino C, Jenike MA. Cingulotomy for intractable obsessive-compulsive disorder: prospective long term follow up of 18 patients. *Arch Gen Psychiatry* 1995; **52**: 384–392.

Barnes J. *Aristotle*. Oxford: Oxford University Press, 1982.

Copland P, Gillett G. The bioethical structure of a human being. *J Appl Philosophy* 2003; **20**:123–132.

Damasio A. *Descartes' Error*. New York: G.P. Putnam, 1994.

Frame J. *Faces in the Water*. London: The Women's Press, 1961.

Gillett G. *Bioethics in the clinic*. Baltimore, MD: Johns Hopkins University Press, 2004.

Gillett G. *The Mind and its Discontents*. Oxford: University Press, 1999.

Hippocrates, *Hippocratic Writings*. ed. Lloyd CEM. London: Penguin Books, 1978.

Hodgkiss AD, Malizia AL, Bartlett JR, Bridges PK. Outcomes after the psychosurgical operation of stereotactic subcaudate tractotomy. *J Neuropsychiatry Clin Neurosci* 1995; **7**: 230–234.

Holland A. A fortnight of my life is missing: a discussion of the human 'pre-embryo'. *J Appl Philosophy* 1990; **7**: 25–37.

Jennett B. *High Technology Medicine*. Oxford: Oxford University Press, 1986.

Jones G. Fetal neural transplantation: placing the ethical debate within the context of society's use of human material. *Bioethics* 1991; **5**: 23–43.

Journal of Medical Ethics, 32.2.

Kim M-C, Lee T-K, Choi C-R. Review of long-term results of stereotactic psychosurgery. *Neurologia Medico-Chirurgica* 2002; **42**: 365–371.

Kleinig J. *Ethical Issues in Psychosurgery*. London: Allen and Unwin, 1985.

Korzenev AV, Shoustin VA, Anichkov AD, Polonskiy JZ, Nizkovolos VB, Oblyapin AV. Differential approach to psychosurgery of obsessive disorders. *Stereotact Funct Neurosurg* 1997; **68**: 226–230.

Macklin, R. The ethical problems with sham surgery in clinical research. *N Engl J Med* 1999; **341**: 992–995.

Mashour GA, Walker EE, and Martuza RL. Psychosurgery: past, present and future. *Brain Res Rev* 2005; **48**: 409–419.

Merskey H. Ethical aspects of the physical manipulation of the brain. In: Bloch S, Chodoff, P, Green S. eds. *Psychiatric Ethics*. Oxford: Oxford University Press, 1999; pp. 275–300.

Pressman J. *The Last Resort: Psychosurgery and the Limits of Medicine*. Cambridge: Cambridge University Press, 1998.

Strawson P. *Freedom and Resentment and Other Essays*. London: Methuen, 1974.

Veatch R. Abandoning informed consent. *Hastings Cent Rep* 1995; **25**(2): 5–12.

Veatch R. Letter in reply: abandoning informed consent. *Hastings Cent Rep* 1996; **26**(1) 2–4.

Wittgenstein L. *Philosophical Investigations* (Translated by Anscombe GEM). Oxford: Blackwell, 1953.

Wittgenstein L. Lecture on ethics. *Philos Rev* 1965; **74**: 3–26.

Wittgenstein L. *Culture and Value* (Translated by Winch P). Oxford: Blackwell, 1980.

Resisting Addiction:
Novel Application of Vaccines

ANDREAS HASMAN

Vaccination against infectious diseases is a contentious issue in biomedical ethics, and the literature on ethical implications of vaccines against, for example, polio, malaria and influenza is well established (Paul and Dawson, 2005; Kilama, 2005; Kitalik, 2005). A new breed of vaccines is now seeing the light of day, however, which gives rise to a rather different and arguably much broader set of ethical problems. What these new vaccines have in common is their capacity to reduce or eliminate the neurological effects of substances that are known to be addictive. They are, in effect, interventions against drug dependence and addiction[1] and I shall refer to them as drug vaccines. This chapter discusses this novel application of vaccination technology, but rather than give a full overview of the technical aspects of the innovation, it focuses on the main moral pitfalls that emerge as the development of this technology continues.

Even though the drug vaccination technology is still in its infancy, it is clear that vaccines have the potential to become a potent public health measure one day to combat drug addition, and a means to address problems of antisocial and criminal behaviour, which sometimes result from substance use and abuse. However, drug vaccination also gives rise to ethical concerns not normally associated with immunotherapy. Although these new technologies are vaccines in the sense that they generate specific immune resistance, unlike traditional vaccines, they have modification of individual behaviour and life-style as a major component of their effectiveness. They are medical interventions, which impact profoundly on individual choice and personal identity and if used without consent, they may eventually do more harm

than good. They may even be an infringement of fundamental individual rights.

The discussion in this chapter will centre on the most probable future potential of drug vaccines. Although fully effective and irreversible vaccination is not currently a therapeutic option for drug dependence, the implicit assumption in what follows is that permanent vaccines will one day become the state of play, and that the possibility of life-long immunity to a wide range of illegal and legal substances will eventually be achieved. However, as the direction of scientific progress is sometimes unpredictable (Nye, 2006), this may prove to be too much of an assumption. After all, political priorities might change, cutting funding for research, or irresolvable technical problems may be encountered in later stages of development of this particular technology. Nevertheless, the aim of the chapter is to explore the ethical consequences if (or indeed when) the most likely prospects materialize.

Recent advances in drug vaccination technology have centred on the development and testing of vaccines against nicotine and cocaine dependency (Carrera, 2004; Henningfield, et al., 2005). Initial steps have also been taken in the development of a similar vaccine for methamphetamine (Haney and Kosten, 2004). This is perhaps not a coincidence. Tobacco smoking is understood to be one of the major causes of preventable disease in the developed world, and cocaine has in recent years become the most commonly used illicit drug after cannabis (UNODC, 2005). Use of methamphetamine is also on the up, especially among younger people in rural America (BBC,

---

[1]The World Health Organization and some commentators prefer the term 'substance dependence' to 'drug addiction'. I will use both terms interchangeably.

Principles of Health Care Ethics, Second Edition   Edited by R.E. Ashcroft, A. Dawson, H. Draper and J.R. McMillan
© 2007 John Wiley & Sons, Ltd

News online, 2005; Colfax and Shoptaw, 2005). The discussion here will centre on these emerging technologies, but because it is by no means inconceivable that initial success for vaccines against cocaine, nicotine and methamphetamine will lead to development of vaccines for other substances such as heroin, marihuana, alcohol and caffeine, I will focus on generic issues that would supposedly apply to all drug vaccines. In addition to such generic issues, however, each individual vaccine will probably give rise to a host of unique practical and ethical problems. If an anti-heroin vaccine one day becomes available, for example, it could be a practical and ethical problem that those vaccinated no longer would be susceptible to the most commonly used anaesthetics. Although such drug-specific questions are likely to be instrumental in determining the future success of drug vaccination programmes, I will not be able to pursue them in the space available here.

The chapter first sets out the current and future potential of vaccines against substance use and misuse, and second, outlines and discusses the main ethical problems that these vaccines will give rise to if or when they are in routine use.

DRUG VACCINATION

Drug vaccines are different from other vaccines in that, rather than targeting viral and bacterial infections, they generate specific immune responses to substances which are known to be both addictive and systematically abused. There are other differences as well. Unlike vaccines against infectious diseases, herd immunity is not an issue with regard to drug vaccines because drug addiction is not a communicable disease. The implication is that compulsory immunization, which is sometimes justified in the context of public health protection to effectively prevent the spread of disease, will not be justified in the case of a drug vaccine (Hasman and Holm, 2004).

Stimulants such as nicotine, cocaine and methamphetamine are widely believed to trigger dependence by elevating certain brain chemicals. They are powerful central nervous system stimulants that either directly or indirectly promote the release, or block the reuptake, of neurotransmitters like dopamine, norepinephrine and serotonin, each of which controls the brain's messaging system for reward and pleasure, sleep, appetite and mood. Their immediate effect is a sense of euphoria and increased energy, and they suppress appetite. Adverse effects related to the frequent use of the drugs are both short term and chronic, including (to a varying degree for each type of drug) respiratory failure, stroke, cardiac problems (Weber et al., 2003), depression and psychosis (Gawin, 1988; Platt, 1997; Hunt, Kuck and Truitt, 2005). Unlike cocaine

and methamphetamine, nicotine is not an illicit drug, and it is its mode of administration (i.e. tobacco smoking), rather than the drug itself, which has the most serious adverse effects on health (Henningfield et al., 2005). Diseases which have been linked to smoking include cancer, cardiovascular disease and lung disease (Mannino, 2006). Varied and limited success of existing treatment options for substance abuse has led to a search for more effective alternatives, in order to increase treatment retention and reduce relapse (Nutt and Lingford-Hughes, 2004; Catalano et al., 1990–91). Immunotherapy holds particular promise in this respect because vaccinations have the potential to specifically target the physiological aspects of addiction.

Vaccines against nicotine, cocaine and methamphetamine are conjugate vaccines, and they consist of a virus-like particle protein carrier that incorporates a derivative of the active substance (i.e. nicotine, cocaine or methamphetamine). Whilst in the blood, the protein induces the production of a specific antibody, which binds the active substance and prevents it from crossing the blood-brain barrier. The active substance is therefore retained in the bloodstream (eventually it is secreted through the kidneys) and never reaches the neural receptors in the brain to produce neurological effects. The vaccine effectively removes the addicted user's ability to satisfy cravings by taking the substance and, in the case of the not yet dependent user, makes it difficult to experiment with the drug for recreational purposes.

Phase I and II trials have shown nicotine and cocaine conjugate vaccines to be safe and well tolerated in humans, and creating specific immune responses (Xenova, 2006). A limitation of current vaccines, however, is that the immune response they generate is only temporary and can be subverted by increasing the dose of the active substance. Immunity over prolonged periods of time therefore requires frequent 'booster jabs', but even then the user can still 'annul' the vaccine by increasing drug intake. For the individual patient this shortcoming of the technology introduces increased risk and discomfort relating to repeated injections, as well as inconvenience and uncertainty. Experience from other vaccination programmes shows that a need for repeat injections has severe negative effects on concordance and outcomes (Van Damme and Van der Wielen, 2001). Solutions to the problem of elapsing effect may soon be on the horizon, however, in the form of either mechanisms for slow release of vaccine in the body (Telegraph, 2006) or gene therapy (van Drunen and den Hurk, 2006). The argument put forward in this chapter is that although fully effective and permanent drug vaccination is probably some way off, current trends in science suggest that such vaccines will become a reality and that this needs to be taken into consideration in the ethical debate.

ETHICAL ISSUES

There are various ways in which one could address the ethical issues pertinent to conjugate vaccines against drug addiction. Readers of this volume will not be strangers to Beauchamp and Childress's conceptual framework for analysis of ethical issues in biomedical ethics, and because this approach seems to lend itself well to the issues that are relevant in this context, I will take a principles-based approach as a starting point for the discussion. In the following sections I will in turn discuss issues around beneficence and non-maleficence (risk and benefits), personal autonomy (informed consent) and justice.

RISKS AND BENEFITS

If we found that the benefits of drug vaccines overwhelmingly outweigh the risk of harm from vaccination, then there could be a case for compulsory treatment of those who are already addicted and potentially also those who are at risk of becoming addicted in the future. Even in the case where benefits are found to outweigh harms to some extent, we may still want to argue that vaccines should be made available, although it would be difficult to find moral justification for a programme of compulsory immunization, and we would have to consider aspects other than the potential for benefit when deciding who should be vaccinated. If, on the contrary, harms overwhelmingly outweigh benefits then a case could be made for barring therapeutic uses of conjugate vaccines in treatment of drug abuse or, in any event, to call a complete halt to any further development of the technology.

Some people would probably claim that a halt should be called on this type of research because it is mainly aimed at resolving what is arguably a 'non-medical' problem and because vaccine development requires testing on animals in order to assure the safety and efficacy of the treatment. In their view, drug addiction is not an illness and its treatment does therefore not provide sufficient justification for the sacrifice of animals. However, even without the assertion that addiction is a medical condition (a question which is outside the scope of this account), it is clear that drug vaccines have the potential to bring sizeable benefits to a great number of people which arguably outweigh at least a reasonable sacrifice of animal life.

A group of people who could have obvious benefits from vaccination are those who are addicted to a substance and want to end their misuse, but for whom alternative therapeutic options are inadequate or inappropriate. There may also be groups of prospective addicts who, for example, for social reasons, are particularly susceptible to substance abuse and who want the vaccine to save themselves the potential anguish of first addiction and then withdrawal. Benefits

would, moreover, not be restricted to those actually abusing substances. In the case of the nicotine vaccine, reduced nicotine addiction would inevitably lead to fewer people smoking and hence to less exposure to passive smoking for non-smokers. Also, if fewer people are addicted to illicit substances such as cocaine and methamphetamine, crime rates could possibly fall, resulting in fewer victims of crime among non-addicts. Finally, society at large would enjoy indirect benefits because reduced use of health hazardous substances could lead to increased productivity and savings on health care budgets. We could argue, therefore, that if therapies exist which make it easier for those abusing drugs to end their addiction, then it would be harmful and unethical to restrict access to such therapies.

It is, on the contrary, not all substance users who are ready to relinquish the physiological effects of drugs such as nicotine and cocaine. Some people may feel that they benefit from the stimulating effects of the drugs or find that they help them to control their weight effectively. Vaccinating against the effects of drugs will therefore necessarily lead to a loss of benefit, although this seems largely unproblematic as long as benefit gained outweighs benefit lost. In addition to the problem of loss of benefit, however, there is also a potential for direct harm from vaccination. Blocking the neurological effects of addictive substances once dependence has developed will cause temporary but potentially serious, physical withdrawal symptoms, including irritability, aggression, anxiety, cognitive disturbances and sleep disruption. More importantly perhaps, a permanent vaccine would be traceable in the blood for the rest of a person's life, bearing witness to previous drug abuse and potentially compromising confidentiality and privacy (Ashcroft, Campbell and Capps, 2005). Other potential sources of harm from the vaccines are perhaps less obvious. For example, although direct therapeutic effects of nicotine, cocaine or methamphetamine are either very limited or nonexistent, it may still be harmful to completely destroy the possible future use of these drugs in a clinical context. In what has come to be known as *therapeutic switching*, drug manufacturers are now systematically searching for new indications for known compounds and substances. Substances deemed harmful at one point in time may later turn out to be beneficial in a different context. The case of the drug thalidomide is possibly the most famous example of this actually happening. In 1960, thalidomide was found to be teratogenic in foetal development after having been originally approved and marketed as a treatment of morning sickness in pregnant women. Around 15 000 foetuses were damaged by the drug world-wide, and of those about 12 000 babies were born with significant birth defects. Despite the enormity of this medical scandal, however, thalidomide was again approved as a medicine in 1998, this time as a treatment of erythema nodosum leprosum associated with leprosy and has later been found to be also effective in the treatment of multiple myeloma, prostate cancer, glioblastoma, lymphoma, Crohn's disease and Kaposi's sarcoma (Mary, 2006). This once highly dangerous drug is now a life-saver in areas of medicine which have lacked therapeutic options. It was, of course, never possible to vaccinate against the effects of thalidomide, but the radically changed application of this drug illustrates the problem of definitively forfeiting any physiological effects of known substances. What is deemed harmful today could be found to be beneficial tomorrow, and the next few decades may see new therapeutic uses for nicotine, cocaine and amphetamine, or some of those other drugs it may be possible to vaccinate against in the future. Those who have been vaccinated would potentially be harmed as they would no longer be able to benefit from treatment.

The balance between benefits and harms of drug vaccination will inevitably depend on how advanced the technology is. With the current level of technology, that is with no option of permanent irreversible vaccination, the argument could be seen to be weighted slightly towards compulsory vaccination (or at least heavily incentivized uptake) because potential future harms, such as the forfeiting of future therapeutic effects of known substances and loss of privacy, can still be avoided. Although the need for repeat injections poses some risk of harm to the individual (i.e. infection and damage to veins), this is probably outweighed by the benefits of treatment. This position may change, however, as the technology advances. When immune resistance is permanent the potential for harm to the individual may be much greater. Although individual and societal benefits arguably would still outweigh potential harms to some extent, this would no longer be overwhelmingly so. The previous section argued that because it is likely that the development of this technology will lead to irreversible, permanent vaccines, the ethical discussion should be had on the basis, and it is my contention, therefore, that the balancing of harms and benefits will not on its own give sufficient indication as to what is the proper use of immunotherapy in this area. To get a more complete answer to the question, we will need to draw on other moral considerations. Those considerations relate to respect for individual autonomy and justice.

INFORMED CONSENT

Requirements for informed consent are now an integral part of standards governing clinical medicine, public health and research involving human subjects. On one conception, informed consent is defined as an autonomous decision by which the individual authorizes a health care professional or scientist to perform a procedure, intervention or course of treatment. In order to qualify as an informed consent, the decision must be made intentionally, with understanding,

and without controlling influences from others (i.e. coercion, persuasion and manipulation (Faden and Beauchamp, 1986).

Informed consent to treatment for substance misuse and addiction is a traditionally contentious issue, and this is especially the case where illicit substances are concerned. In most countries drug treatment under legal coercion is an established judicial arrangement in which treatment is offered as an option to persons who have been convicted of an offence to which their drug dependence is thought to have contributed. The option is typically provided as an alternative to imprisonment and under the threat of subsequent imprisonment if the person refuses or fails to comply with the requirements of treatment (Hall and Carter, 2004). Such a threat is clearly a controlling influence (it is intended as such), and the offender will not give an informed consent. The main justification for legal coercion is that the offender's risk of reoffending will be reduced if their drug misuse is treated (Hall, 1997). What makes this justification seems somewhat problematic, however, is that what is deemed unacceptable substance misuse often depends as much on cultural values as on crime statistics. For example, alcohol is probably the most abused substance in the western world, with excessive drinking causing widespread social problems and violent crime, yet alcohol is banned nowhere outside the Islamic world. It should also be a concern that, unlike some current treatment options, drug vaccines would affect only the neurobiological effect of drug addiction and leave untouched any underlying behavioural pathology and dependence that are often seen as the actual cause of criminal behaviour (Telegraph, 2006; Cohen).

According to a World Health Organization consensus panel it is, nevertheless, justified to disregard the need for informed consent and impose compulsory drug treatment provided that the rights of individuals are protected by 'due process', and that effective and humane treatment is provided (Porter, Curran and Arif, 1986). However, considering that a future drug vaccine could be irreversible and thus would have more serious long-term implications than any current treatment for drug addiction, this rationale should probably be revisited. Bearing in mind the increased risk of harm to those vaccinated in the form of severe withdrawal syndrome, loss of privacy and loss of future treatment options, it might be discriminatory and unjustified, and thus essentially inhumane, to treat a group of criminal drug abusers without their consent.

Even in the absence of direct coercion, informed consent to permanent drug vaccination is ethically problematic, with more subtle controlling influences originating from other sources. Once effective drug vaccines have become available, various parties will have an interest in these technologies becoming widely used. The drug companies that have developed the vaccines are likely to enjoy substantial financial rewards if they can tap into the enormous markets of current drug users. If the vaccines are perceived to be the most effective intervention against substance abuse, governments may want to further incentivize the uptake in order to improve public health and reduce drug-related crime. Employers may require key staff (such as famous footballers or designers) to be vaccinated to minimize the risk of them harming the business by developing a drug addiction. There may also be a potential efficiency gain from vaccination because reduced drug use in the workforce could lead to staff needing fewer and shorter breaks (in the case of the anti-nicotine vaccine), less absence due to sickness and less drug-related crime in the workplace. Parents may also be interested in reducing their children's susceptibility to addictive drugs in order to improve educational outcomes or future career prospects, and the large majority who do not smoke or use cocaine will want to see less use of these substances because that would potentially reduce their own exposure to second-hand smoke, crime and antisocial behaviour. It is probably inevitable therefore that in some cases drug users will be influenced by this unidirectional social pressure to the extent where they accept treatment they would not otherwise have accepted. They may be persuaded to consent to vaccination, even when their preference is for another treatment option or indeed for no treatment altogether, and social pressure could be seen to render any informed consent to irreversible vaccination invalid.

A final problem relating to informed consent is that at least some drug users' ability to consent to treatment will be impaired because drug addiction impacts on judgement and reduces the individual's ability to act intentionally and with understanding of consequences. Again, it is probably necessary to make a distinction among the drugs that are being abused. Whereas most people would agree that a majority of smokers can make an informed decision to treat their dependence effectively (thereby balancing the personal benefits and disbenefits of vaccination), they will probably see long-term crack cocaine addicts to have that ability to a lesser extent – or not at all. Obtaining informed consent to vaccination is in any event problematic, and a judgement would have to be made on a case-to-case basis. Some drug users would not be able to consent meaningfully, and unfortunately they are likely to be the users with the most serious problems of addiction and abuse. A possible response to these concerns is that the problem of coercion through social pressure by no means applies exclusively to vaccines. Most people who have experienced addiction of some sort can probably testify to pressure to stop from family, friends, work colleagues and the health service to seek treatment for their dependence. However, although it is probably true that consent to any form of drug treatment and rehabilitation involves some degree of social pressure, it is also true that these vaccines have the potential to have more far-reaching consequences for the individual than any of these other options.

JUSTICE

Three broad issues of justice are pertinent to irreversible vaccination for drug dependence. First, we will need to ask if it is just to make the vaccines a priority for research and health care funding if this means that other patient groups, as a consequence, are deprived treatment options. Second, it is relevant to ask whether the distribution of the vaccines will be just, that is, will the benefits and potential harms of the treatment be distributed justly among drug users and addicts. Third, there are particular issues relating to parents' rights to make long-term treatment choices for their children.

Under resource scarcity, scientific progress in one area may come at the cost of lost opportunity in other areas. In theory, designating research resources to the development of an effective vaccine for drug dependence means that other areas of vaccine development, such as vaccines for tropical diseases or cancer, could lose out. It could be argued that this is unjust either because drug addiction is not an illness in the usual sense, because there is an aspect of individual responsibility to drug abuse, or because other patient groups are generally more deserving.

Most people would probably intuitively make a distinction between diseases such as pneumonia or cancer and drug addiction. They would probably argue that patients with pneumonia or cancer should be of higher priority for research and treatment than those who are addicted to drugs. Arguably, this intuition has nothing to do with the severity of the condition because drug abuse can be as life-threatening as those other conditions in extreme circumstances, but relates instead to social perceptions of what it means to have a disease. Most smokers and drug users would probably share this intuition and strongly object to being branded as 'sick' or having an illness (FOREST). One possible explanation for this intuition is that addiction is sometimes seen to involve an element of personal responsibility and that psychological dependence is interpreted, to an extent at least, as the consequence of a personal choice. In other contexts, addiction is seen as the symptom of an actual disease (such as depression or obsessive compulsive disorder) or as the side-effect of some other treatment (for example, pain relief), rather than as a disease in its own right. If the position is that illness should be treated before symptoms of illness, or that drug dependence is a life-style choice, then naturally it will not be justified to make the treatment of drug dependence a high priority for funding. Even if it is accepted that drug addiction is a disease on a par with other life-threatening conditions, it may still be argued that it is unjust to make the drug vaccine a priority, essentially because other patients would be more deserving than those benefiting from effective treatment of drug abuse. Other patient populations could be seen to be more deserving if, for example, the disease they suffer is considered more severe than drug dependence, if it is under-researched, or if its occurrence is not linked to personal life-style choices. However, it is, of course, difficult to assess the precise implications an increased focus on development and provision drug vaccines have for other patients. Progress on a drug vaccine could plausibly advance effective treatments in other areas and the argument may not be so straightforward. It should be a concern, however, that other patients can be seen to lose out as effective vaccines against drug addiction are developed.

It will also be a concern that access to drug vaccination may turn out to be inequitable. In the previous section it was argued that it would probably not be possible to obtain a meaningful informed consent from drug users with the serious problems of dependence and that coercing this group into treatment with a permanent, irreversible vaccine would be discriminatory. The implication is, however, that if vaccination is only available to patients who can give informed consent, then provision will also be inequitable, and would potentially exclude the patients who would benefit the most.

Finally, the vaccines raise questions about the right of patients to make treatment decisions for their children that could have consequences for many years into future (Hasman and Holm, 2004). Parents may see advantages of a preventive use of vaccination as an opportunity to protect the child from self-inflicted harm later in life. Because drug dependence arguably is more damaging than most of the infectious diseases that children are already vaccinated against (Nutt and Lingford-Hughes, 2004), it seems an unproblematic proposition to add drug vaccines to current immunization programmes. There is, however, at least one important difference between drug vaccines and vaccines for diseases such as, measles or rubella. Using a substance for recreational purposes is not the same as having a disease, regardless of whether *addiction* to that substance is considered a disease, and although substance misuse may lead to an increased risk of addiction, there is no direct causal relationship between the two. Whereas current smokers and recreational drug users will have an opportunity to balance the benefits and risks of using substances such as nicotine and methamphetamine and to make an informed choice whether or not to relinquish the ability to have an effect from these, children will be denied such a choice. Permanently vaccinating children against the physiological effects of known substances would not only mean a risk that they will be unable to benefit from potential future therapeutic uses of those substances, it would also unjustly deny them the right to an open future in which to assess the benefits and harms from substance use and to make that informed choice for themselves. In a related argument, virtue ethicists may point out, moreover, that parental (prophylactic or therapeutic) uses of drug vaccines would obstruct the opportunity of children to exercise virtue in resisting the temptation of drugs both now and later in life (Foot, 1997). The argument does not apply exclusively to children, of course (adults who are vaccinated would essentially also lose their opportunity to be virtuous), but it is particularly important in relation to children as vaccination would potentially impede their moral development and would be an injustice.

CONCLUSION

Substance abuse and dependence are a serious global problem and there are growing efforts to identify effective treatment options. Immunotherapy holds promise as a potent tool in future therapeutic regimens. However, the effectiveness of vaccines for nicotine, cocaine and methadone dependence, for example, will depend on whether limitations in the current technology can be successfully resolved. The next generations of drug vaccines will probably be fully effective, so that they cannot be subverted by increased doses of drugs, and irreversible, so that repeated 'booster jabs' are no longer necessary and relapse to drugs misuse cannot occur. Provided the technology can be improved along these lines, drug vaccines have the potential to improve the lives of a great many people. Those seeking treatment for drug addiction will benefit from more effective treatment and society at large will potentially see benefits from, for example, reduced crime, improved productivityand savings on health care.

However, it inevitably complicates matters that although the potential benefits of vaccination seem overwhelming, there is also a potential for harm to those who are vaccinated. Sudden withdrawal after prolonged periods of substance misuse causes quite serious, albeit temporary, symptoms. More importantly perhaps, permanent vaccines could compromise confidentiality and privacy, and potentially limit options for medical treatment in the future.

Other ethical issues will have to be taken into account alongside considerations for benefits and harms, and in this chapter I have discussed problems relating to the difficulties obtaining informed consent from the patients most severely affected by drug addiction, issues around distributive justice and limits of parental rights to make treatment decisions on behalf of their children. These issues are perhaps less urgent as long as the effectiveness of vaccination as a treatment for drugs misuse remains limited. Over time, however, the technology may well move on to make drug vaccination one of the most controversial topics in biomedical ethics.

REFERENCES

Ashcroft R, Campbell AV, Capps B. *Ethical Aspects of Developments in Neuroscience and Drug Addiction*. London: 2005.

BBC News online. *Rural US Gripped by Meth Epidemic*. Wednesday, 6 July 2005, http://news.bbc.co.uk/1/hi/world/asia-pacific/4654503.stm (accessed March 2006)

Carrera MR, Meijler MM, Janda KD. Cocaine pharmacology and current pharmacotherapies for its abuse. *Bioorg Med Chem* 1 October 2004; **12** (19): 5019–5030.

Catalano RF, Hawkins JD, Wells EA, Miller J, Brewer D. Evaluation of the effectiveness of adolescent drug abuse treatment, assessment of risks for relapse, and promising approaches for relapse prevention. *Int J Addict* August 1990-91; **25** (9A-10A): 1085–1140.

Cohen P. Immunisation for prevention and treatment of cocaine abuse: Legal and ethical implications. *Drug Alcohol Depen* 1997; **48**: 167–174.

Colfax G, Shoptaw S. The methamphetamine epidemic: Implications for HIV prevention and treatment. *Curr HIV/AIDS Rep* November 2005; **2** (4): 194–199.

Faden RR, Beauchamp TL, *A History and Theory of Informed Consent*. New York: Oxford University Press, 1986.

Foot P. Virtues and vices. In: Crisp R, Slote M, eds. *Virtue Ethics*. Oxford: Oxford University Press, 1997, pp. 163–177.

FOREST, *Smoking: addiction or habit?* Freedom Organisation for the Right to Enjoy Smoking Tobacco, http://www.forestonline.org/output/page134.asp

Gawin FH, Ellinwood EH. Cocaine and other stimulants: Action, abuse and treatment. *N Engl J Med* 1988; **318**: 1173–1182.

Hall W. The role of legal coercion in the treatment of offenders with alcohol and heroin problems. *Austral NZ J Criminol* 1997; **30**: 103–120.

Hall W, Carter L. Ethical issues in using a cocaine vaccine to treat and prevent cocaine abuse and dependence. *J Med Ethics* 2004; **30**: 337–340.

Haney M, Kosten TR. Therapeutic vaccines for substance dependence. *Expert Rev Vaccines* February 2004; **3** (1): 11–18.

Hasman A, Holm S. Nicotine conjugate vaccine: Is there a right to a smoking future? *J Med Ethics* August 2004; **30** (4): 344–345.

Henningfield JE, Fant RV, Buchhalter AR, Stitzer ML. Pharmacotherapy for nicotine dependence. *CA Cancer J Clin* 1 September 2005; **55** (5): 281–299.

Hunt D, Kuck S, Truitt L. *Methamphetamine Use: Lessons Learned*. Cambridge, MA: Abt Associates, 2005, www.cjpf.org/methuse_lessonslearned.pd (accessed December 2005)

Kilama WL. Ethical perspective on malaria research for Africa. *Acta Trop* September 2005; **95** (3): 276–284.

Kotalik J. Preparing for an influenza pandemic: Ethical issues. *Bioethics* August 2005; **19** (4): 422–431.

Mannino et al. The natural history of chronic obstructive pulmonary disease. *Eur Respir J* 2006; **27**: 627–643.

Mary K. The Return of Thalidomide, *About.com*, 2006, http://rarediseases.about.com/cs/autoimmune/a/042603.htm (accessed March 2006)

Nutt D, Lingford-Hughes A, Infecting the brain to stop addiction. *Proc Natl Acad Sci USA* 2004, **101** (31): 11193–4,http://www.pnas.org/cgi/content/full/101/31/11193 (accessed January 2006)

Nye D. *Technology Matters: Questions to Live With*. Cambridge, MA: MIT Press, 2006.

Paul Y, Dawson A. Some ethical issues arising from polio eradication programmes in India. *Bioethics* August 2005; **19**(4): 393–406.

Platt JJ. *Cocaine Addiction: Theory, Research and Treatment*. Cambridge MA: Harvard University Press, 1997.

Porter L, Curran WJ, Arif A. Comparative review of reporting and registration legislation for treatment of drug and alcohol dependent persons. *Int J Law Psychiatry* 1986; **8** (2): 217–227.

Telegraph. Lifelong vaccine will end booster jab ordeal. *The Daily Telegraph*. Saturday, 18 March 2006.

United Nations Office on Drugs and Crime (UNODC). *World Drug Report 2005*. Vienna, Austria: UNODC, June 2005.

Van Damme P, Van der Wielen M. Combining hepatitis A and B vaccination in children and adolescents. *Vaccine* 21 March 2001; **19** (17-19): 2407–2412.

van Drunen S, den Hurk LV. Novel methods for the non-invasive administration of DNA therapeutics and vaccines. *Curr Drug Deliv* January 2006; **3** (1): 3–15.

Weber JE, Shofer FS, Larkin GL, Kalaria AS, Hollander JE. Validation of a brief observation period for patients with cocaine-associated chest pain. *N Engl J Med* 6 February 2003; **348** (6): 510–517.

Xenova Group Limited. *Drug Candidates Overview*. 2006, http://www.xenova.co.uk/dc_overview.html (accessed January 2006).

Index

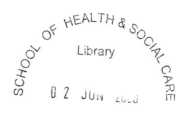

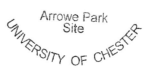

Principles of Health Care Ethics, Second Edition   Edited by R.E. Ashcroft, A. Dawson, H. Draper and J.R. McMillan
© 2007 John Wiley & Sons, Ltd